The New
**Lexicon**
Illustrated **Medical Encyclopedia**
and Guide to
**Family Health**

# The New
# LEXICON
# Illustrated
# Medical

the enlarged and revised **8**th edition

# Encyclopedia

## and Guide to

# Family Health

Edited by Robert E. Rothenberg, M.D., F.A.C.S.

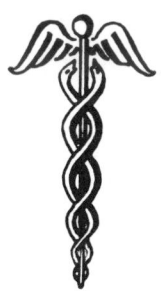

**LEXICON PUBLICATIONS, INC.**

95 Madison Avenue, New York, N.Y. 10016

In loving memory of Caroline, Simon, Alan, and Joel

# Acknowledgements

THE EDITOR wishes to express his sincere gratitude for the exceptional cooperation he has received from the contributors in revising and updating the 7th edition of the *Medical Encyclopedia.* The assignment to distill the essence from the huge amount of medical information each possesses was a task of immense proportions, yet each met the challenge successfully.

R.E.R.

Library of Congress Cataloging in Publication Data

Main entry under title:

The New illustrated medical encyclopedia for home use.

Includes index
1. Medicine, Popular. I. Rothenberg, Robert E.
II. Medbook Publications, inc.
RC81. A2N44 1982      616.02'4      81-7981
ISBN 0-8109-1441-7                  AACR2

**Enlarged and Revised 8th Edition,
Updated 1988**

**STAFF OF THE 8th EDITION**
The Editors of Lexicon Publications, Inc.
Editorial Director: Donald D. Wolf
Design and Layout: Margot L. Wolf

# CONTRIBUTORS
## AND EDITORIAL CONSULTANTS

**DAVID I. ATKINSON**
Diplomate, American Board of Anesthesiology; Fellow, American Academy of Anesthesiology; Director of Anesthesiology, Cabrini Medical Center, New York; Attending Anesthesiologist, St. Vincent's Hospital and Medical Center, New York.

**SELWYN J. BAPTIST**
Clinical Assistant Professor of Pathology, New York Medical College; Diplomate, American Board of Pathology; Associate Attending Pathologist, Cabrini Medical Center, New York.

**AARON J. BERMAN**
Diplomate, American Board of Neurosurgery; Fellow, American College of Surgeons; Attending Neurosurgeon, Mount Sinai Hospital, New York; Attending Neurosurgeon, Jewish Hospital and Medical Center of Brooklyn; Attending Neurosurgeon, Beth Israel Medical Center, New York; Chief Neurosurgeon, Bronx V.A. Medical Center.

**ARCANGELO M. CALOBRISI**
Clinical Professor of Psychiatry, New York University and Postgraduate School of Medicine; Diplomate, American Board of Psychiatry; Past Director of Psychiatry, Cabrini Medical Center, New York; Associate Attending Psychiatrist, University Hospital, New York; Chairman, Professional Advisory Board, New York Council on Alcoholism.

**MARTIN FINKEL**
Assistant Clinical Professor of Medicine, Mount Sinai Medical College, New York; Diplomate, American Board of Internal Medicine (Gastroenterology); Fellow, American College of Physicians; Associate Attending Physician, Mount Sinai Hospital, New York.

**A. JAMES GEWIRTZ**
Assistant Professor of Dermatology, New York University School of Medicine; Diplomate, American Board of Dermatology; Consultant Dermatologist, Jewish Hospital and Medical Center of Brooklyn and Kingsbrook Hospital, Brooklyn.

**RICHARD J. HIRSCHMAN**
Assistant Clinical Professor of Medicine, Mount Sinai Medical College, New York; Diplomate, American Board of Internal Medicine (Hematology); Diplomate, American Board of Internal Medicine (Oncology); Fellow, American College of Physicians; Attending Physician and Chief of Medical Oncology, Cabrini Medical Center, New York.

**JONATHAN A. KORN**
Professor of Orthopedics, New York College of Podiatric Medicine; Diplomate, American Board of Orthopedic Surgery; Fellow, American College of Surgeons; Associate Attending Orthopedist, Cabrini Medical Center, New York; Consultant Orthopedist, Gracie Square Hospital, New York.

**RAYMOND D. LaRAJA**
Associate Professor of Surgery, New York Medical College; Clinical Associate Professor of Surgery, New York University School of Medicine; Diplomate, American Board of Surgery; Fellow, American College of Surgeons; Director of Surgery, Cabrini Medical Center, New York; Attending Surgeon, Bellevue Hospital, New York.

**ALFRED E. MAMELOK**
Clinical Associate Professor of Ophthalmology, Cornell University Medical College, New York; Diplomate, American Board of Ophthalmology; Fellow, American College of Surgeons; Attending Ophthalmologist, New York and Manhattan Eye, Ear and Throat Hospitals.

**CHARLES P. MELONE, JR.**
Assistant Professor of Orthopedics, New York University School of Medicine; Diplomate, American Board of Orthopedics; Director of Hand Surgery, Cabrini Medical Center, New York; Fellow, American Academy of Orthopedics; Attending Surgeon, Bellevue Hospital, New York.

**DAVID MERKSAMER**
Diplomate, American Board of Allergy and Immunology; Diplomate, American Board of Pediatrics; Consultant Allergist, Jewish Hospital and Medical Center of Brooklyn; Past President, New York Allergy Society.

**PAUL S. METZGER**
Diplomate, American Board of Obstetrics and Gynecology; Fellow, American College of Surgeons; Fellow, American College of Obstetrics and Gynecology; Assistant Attending Obstetrician and Gynecologist, Mount Sinai Hospital, New York.

**NORMAN OSTROV**
Diplomate, American Board of Otolaryngology; Fellow, American College of Surgeons; Chairman, Department of Otolaryngology, St. Clare's Hospital, New York; Attending Otolaryngologist, St. Luke's Hospital, New York.

**LAWRENCE S. REED**
Assistant Professor of Surgery, New York Medical College; Diplomate, American Board of Plastic Surgery; Director, Plastic Surgery, Metropolitan Hospital, New York; Attending Plastic Surgeon, Cabrini Medical Center, New York, and New York Eye and Ear Infirmary.

**ALFRED ROSENBAUM**
Clinical Assistant Professor of Radiology, Mount Sinai Medical College, New York; Diplomate, American Board of Radiology; Member, American College of Radiology; Assistant Attending Radiologist, Mount Sinai Hospital, New York.

**ROBERT E. ROTHENBERG**
Clinical Professor of Surgery, New York Medical College; Diplomate, American Board of Surgery; Fellow, American College of Surgeons; Attending Surgeon, Jewish Hospital and Medical Center of Brooklyn, 1954-64; Attending Surgeon, French-Polyclinic Hospital and Medical School, New York, 1962-75; Attending Surgeon, Cabrini Medical Center, New York; Director, Surgical Research, Cabrini Medical Center, New York.

**HOWARD A. RUSK**
Professor and Chairman, Department of Rehabilitation, New York University School of Medicine; Diplomate, American Board of Physical Medicine and Rehabilitation; Diplomate, American Board of Internal Medicine; Director, Institute of Rehabilitation, New York University School of Medicine; President, World Rehabilitation Fund.

**GERALD M. SPIELMAN**
Clinical Assistant Professor of Pediatrics, Cornell University Medical College, New York; Diplomate, American Board of Pediatrics; Director, Developmental Disabilities Clinic, Cornell University Medical College and New York Hospital; Fellow, American Academy of Pediatrics.

**STANLEY J. WITTENBERG**
Diplomate, American Board of Internal Medicine; Fellow, American College of Physicians; Past Director of Medicine, Cabrini Medical Center, New York; Associate Physician, University Hospital, New York.

**ADRIAN W. ZORGNIOTTI**
Clinical Professor of Urology, New York University School of Medicine; Diplomate, American Board of Urology; Director of Urology, Cabrini Medical Center, New York; Attending Urologist, University Hospital, New York.

# CONTRIBUTIONS*

**DAVID I. ATKINSON** *Anesthesia.*

**SELWYN J. BAPTIST** *Laboratory (Pathology) Tests and Procedures.*

**AARON J. BERMAN** *Neurology; Neurosurgery; The Pituitary Gland.*

**ARCANGELO M. CALOBRISI** *Alcoholism; Mental Health and Disease; Sex and Human Sexuality.*

**MARTIN FINKEL** *Endoscopy; Parasites and Parasitic Diseases.*

**A. JAMES GEWIRTZ** *Dermatology (Skin and Subcutaneous Tissues).*

**RICHARD J. HIRSCHMAN** *Blood and Lymph Diseases; Cancer and Other Malignant Growths; The Spleen.*

**JONATHAN A. KORN** *Bones, Muscles, Tendons, and Joints.*

**RAYMOND D. LaRAJA** *The Intensive Care Unit (ICU); The Liver; The Pancreas; The Parathyroid Glands; The Thyroid Gland.*

**ALFRED E. MAMELOK** *The Eyes.*

**CHARLES P. MELONE, JR.** *The Hand; Replantation Surgery.*

**DAVID MERKSAMER** *Allergy.*

**PAUL S. METZGER** *Birth Control; The Female Organs; Pregnancy and Childbirth; Sterility, Fertility, and Male Potency.*

**NORMAN OSTROV** *The Ears; The Lips, Jaws, Mouth, Teeth, and Tongue; The Nose and Sinuses; The Salivary Glands; The Throat.*

**LAWRENCE S. REED** *Plastic Surgery.*

**ALFRED ROSENBAUM** *Sonography; X ray.*

**ROBERT E. ROTHENBERG** *Abscesses and Bacterial Infections; Appendicitis; Blood Vessel Surgery; The Breasts; Cancer and Other Malignant Growths; The Esophagus; First Aid in Emergencies; Gall Bladder and Bile Ducts; Hernia; Peritonitis; Pilonidal Cyst; Preoperative and Postoperative Routines; The Rectum and Anus; The Small and Large Intestines; The Spleen; The Stomach and Duodenum; Transplantation of Organs.*

**HOWARD A. RUSK** *Physical Therapy and Rehabilitation.*

**GERALD M. SPIELMAN** *Child Behavior; Contagious Diseases; Immunizations and Vaccinations; Infant and Childhood Diseases; Infant Feeding and Bowel Function; Inherited and Congenital Conditions; The Newborn Child.*

**STANLEY J. WITTENBERG** *Arthritis; Diabetes Mellitus; Diet; The Heart; Infectious and Virus Diseases; The Lungs; Medications and Drugs; Rheumatic Fever; Tuberculosis; Upper Respiratory Diseases; Vitamins.*

**ADRIAN W. ZORGNIOTTI** *The Kidneys and Ureters; The Male Organs; The Prostate Gland; Sterility, Fertility, and Male Potency; The Urinary Bladder and Urethra; Venereal Disease.*

*Revisions and contributions by Doctors Atkinson, Baptist, Berman, Calobrisi, Finkel, Gewirtz, Hirschman, Korn, LaRaja, Ostrov, Reed, Rosenbaum, Spielman, Wittenberg, and Zorgniotti are based in part upon earlier revisions and contributions by Doctors F.P. Ansbro, J. Bergida, A. Ellman, E.H. Feiring, H.R. Fisher, I.S. Freiman, M. Goodman, I.N. Holtzman, T.G. Holzsager, J.J. Kelter, O.C. Kestler, B. Kissin, M. Krinsky, P. Rosenblatt, B. Small, and A.K. Swersie.*

# AUTHOR'S PREFACE

IT IS UNFORTUNATE that physicians are so busy caring for the seriously ill that they frequently do not have time to answer all the questions patients or their families wish to ask. Furthermore, there is a general reluctance on the part of most people to make too many inquiries for fear that they will impose upon their doctor's valuable time. This situation is often aggravated by the desire of patients to obtain additional data about their illness long after they have left their physician's consulting room. As a consequence, much important medical information fails to be transmitted at times when it would be most helpful.

This book is predicated upon the conviction that people have the right to medical knowledge should they seek it, and that the widespread dissemination of accurate information about health and disease can lead only to a healthier population.

Included in this work are more than 7,500 questions and answers pertaining to the various branches of medicine and surgery. The chapters have been written by qualified specialists who have compiled those questions most often asked them by their patients. Nontechnical language has been used wherever possible, so that there will be no difficulty in understanding the text.

The statements of the contributors represent their own independent medical thinking. Somewhat different responses may be given in discussion of similar topics, but it should be remembered that Medicine has always embraced differences of opinion, and that its ultimate goal, attainment and maintenance of health, can be achieved by varied approaches.

The use of this book will be facilitated by reference to the Contents to help locate the topic in which the reader is interested. If a subject cannot be located readily in the Contents, we suggest that the Index be consulted.

Every effort has been made by the participating doctors to provide the soundest and most up-to-date information and advice. Events in the medical world are happening with great and sometimes surprising rapidity. Thus, new discoveries may take place even while the book is being printed. Each contributor has reviewed his material in the light of current developments at the very last moment, making this encyclopedia, in our belief, as complete as it is possible to make it.

R.E.R.

# CONTENTS

**Chapter 1**   GENERAL INSTRUCTIONS TO PATIENTS  1
Selecting a Doctor — Medical Fees — Hospitalization — Nursing Services — Periodic Health Examination — The Medical Record — Compensation and Liability Cases.

**Chapter 2**   ABSCESSES AND BACTERIAL INFECTIONS  5
Prevention of Infections — Blood Poisoning — Treatment for Abscesses and Infections.

**Chapter 3**   ADOLESCENCE  8
Onset — Menstruation and Adolescence — Breast Development — Skin Changes — Psychological Problems — Sexual Development — Hormones in Adolescence.

**Chapter 4**   THE ADRENAL GLANDS  11
Function of the Adrenals — Pheochromocytoma — Addison's Disease — Cushing's Disease — Surgery of the Adrenal Glands.

**Chapter 5**   AGING  14
Onset of Aging Process — Longevity — Inheritance and Aging — Potency and Aging — Alcohol and Aging — Diet and Aging — Work and Aging — Life Expectancy — Aging — Alzheimer's Disease.

**Chapter 6**   ALCOHOLISM  18
Causes of Alcoholism — Addiction to Alcohol — Inheritance — Physical Effects of Alcoholism — Delirium Tremens — Alcoholism and Insanity — Alcoholism and Childbearing — Alcoholics Anonymous — Treatment.

**Chapter 7**   ALLERGY  20
General Discussion of Allergy — Hay Fever — Bronchial Asthma — Food Allergy (Gastrointestinal Allergy) — Skin Allergies — Drug Allergy — Insect Allergy — Physical Allergy.

**Chapter 8**   ANESTHESIA  29
The Specialty of Anesthesiology — Preanesthetic Medication — Induction of Anesthesia — General Anesthesia — Spinal Anesthesia — Epidural and Caudal Anesthesia — Regional Anesthesia — Intravenous Anesthesia — Topical Anesthesia — Endotracheal Anesthesia — Anesthetic Reactions and Complications.

Chapter 9     APPENDICITIS  33
Diagnosis — Laxatives and Appendicitis — Diet and Appendicitis — Treatment — Rupture of the Appendix — Postoperative Routines.

Chapter 10    ARTHRITIS  37
Rheumatoid Arthritis — Osteoarthritis — Gouty Arthritis — Traumatic Arthritis — Bacterial Arthritis — Cortisone and Arthritis — Salicylates and Arthritis — Other Methods of Treatment in Arthritis.

Chapter 11    BIRTH CONTROL  41
Abstinence — The Rhythm Method — Withdrawal — Intercourse Without Orgasm — Condoms — Douches — Vaginal Diaphragms, Contraceptive Jellies, Foams, Creams, Suppositories — Intrauterine Devices (IUD's) — Birth Control Pills — Surgical Birth Control.

Chapter 12    BLOOD AND
LYMPH DISEASES  48
General Discussion — Anemias — Polycythemia Vera — Blood Poisoning — Hemophilia and Other Bleeding Tendencies — Infections of Lymph Glands — Leukemia — Lymphoma — Hodgkin's Disease — Non-Hodgkin's Lymphoma.

Chapter 13    BLOOD VESSELS AND BLOOD VESSEL
SURGERY  55
Arteriosclerosis (Hardening of the Arteries) — Raynaud's Disease — Buerger's Disease (Thromboangiitis Obliterans) — Thrombosis — Embolism — Aneurysm — Thrombophlebitis — Blood Vessel (Vascular) Surgery — Varicose Veins — Blood Vessel Tumors — Arteriovenous Fistulas.

Chapter 14    BONES, MUSCLES, TENDONS, AND
JOINTS  69
Birth Deformities of the Extremities — Amputations — Lower Back Pain — Slipped Disk — Scoliosis and Spondylolisthesis — Bursitis — Wry Neck (Torticollis) — Bunions and Corns — Plantar Warts — Flat Feet — Hammer Toe — Torn Cartilage of the Knee (The Deranged Knee) — Osteomyelitis (Bone Infections) — Neuromuscular Disorders — Bone Diseases: Paget's Disease (Osteitis Deformans) — Osteitis Fibrosa Cystica (Hyperparathyroidism) — Osteomalacia — Osteoporosis — Reconstructive Surgery upon the Bones, Joints, and Muscles — Arthroplasty and Joint Replacement — Fractures — Fracture Charts — Tumors of the Bone — Segmental Resection of Bone.

Chapter 15    THE BREASTS  93
Function — Self-Examination — Breast Infections — Breast Tumors and Cysts — The Male Breast — Surgery of Breasts — Results of Breast Surgery — Plastic Surgery of the Breasts — Cancer Prevention — Cancer Detection — Treatment — Cures of Cancer — Nonsurgical Anticancer Treatment.

Chapter 16    CANCER AND OTHER MALIGNANT GROWTHS  100
Prevalence — Susceptibility to Cancer — Inheritance Factors — Causes of Cancer — Cancer Prevention — Cancer Detection — Treatment — Cures of Cancer.

Chapter 17    CHILD BEHAVIOR  107
Crying — Thumbsucking and Similar Habits — Breath-Holding — Temper Tantrums — Tics — Masturbation — Night Terrors — Nightmares — Sleepwalking — Fears — Speech Defects — Bedwetting (Enuresis) — Sleep Problems — Learning Disability — Hyperactivity — Parenting.

Chapter 18    CONTAGIOUS DISEASES  116
Chickenpox — Diphtheria — German Measles (Rubella) — Measles — Mumps — Poliomyelitis (Infantile Paralysis) — Roseola (Exanthem Subitum) — Scarlet Fever — Whooping Cough (Pertussis) — Contagion Charts.

Chapter 19    DIABETES MELLITUS  131
Symptoms — Diagnosis — Prevention — Insulin and Diabetes — Infection and Diabetes — Complications of Diabetes — The Outlook for Diabetes.

Chapter 20    DIET  134
Obesity (Overweight) — Underweight — Reducing Diet — Low-Fat Diet — Low-Salt Diet — High-Residue Diet — Low-Residue Diet — Gout (Low Purine) Diet — High-Calorie Diet for Underweight — Ambulatory Ulcer Diet — Full Liquid Diet — Elimination (Allergic) Diet — Percentage of Carbohydrates — Low-Carbohydrate Diet — Caloric Value Chart.

Chapter 21    THE EARS  145
Hearing — Wax (Cerumen) in the Ears — Pain in the Ear Canal — Middle Ear — Middle Ear Infection (Otitis Media) — Mastoid Infection — Deafness — Otosclerosis — Treatment for Deafness — Surgery for Deafness — Equilibrium — Acoustic Nerve Tumors — Ménière's Syndrome — Plastic Surgery of the Ear — Congenital Disorders of the Ear.

**Chapter 22** ENDOSCOPY  154

Esophagoscopy — Gastroduodenoscopy — Proctoscopy — Sigmoidoscopy — Colonoscopy.

**Chapter 23** THE ESOPHAGUS  156

Function of the Esophagus — Birth Deformities — Inflammation of the Esophagus (Esophagitis) — Injuries of the Esophagus — Diverticulum of the Esophagus — Achalasia (Esophageal Spasm) — Varicose Veins of the Esophagus — Tumors of the Esophagus.

**Chapter 24** THE EYES  161

Eye Examinations — Nearsightedness (Myopia) — Farsightedness (Hyperopia) — Astigmatism — Conjunctivitis — Lacerations, Abrasions, Ulcerations, and Foreign Bodies of the Cornea — Styles and Cysts of Eyelids — Entropion and Ectropion — Dacryocystitis — Iritis — Glaucoma — Cataracts — Strabismus (Crossed Eyes) — Detached Retina and Retinal Tears — Diabetes Mellitus — Tumors of the Eye — Retinal Thrombosis — Sympathetic Ophthalmia — Trachoma.

**Chapter 25** THE FEMALE ORGANS  177

**The External Genitals:** Anatomy and Function — The Hymen — The Bartholin Glands — Leukoplakia — Cancer of the Vulva — The Vagina — Douching — Prolapse of the Uterus — Cystocele and Rectocele — Vaginal Repair Operations — Vaginitis — Gonorrhea.

**Menstruation:** Absent or Scant Menstruation — Excessive Menstruation — Irregular Menstruation — Painful Menstruation — Premenstrual Tension.

**The Cervix:** Anatomy and Function — Inflammation of the Cervix — Cauterization of the Cervix — Cancer (Papanicolaou) Smears — Polyps — Cancer of the Cervix.

**The Uterus:** Anatomy and Function — Tipped Womb — Curettage — Endometritis — Polyps of the Uterus — Endometrial Hyperplasia — Cancer — Fibroids — Surgery of the Uterus — Hysterectomy — Endometriosis.

**Abortion:** Spontaneous Abortion — Induced Abortion — Threatened Abortion — Treatment for Abortion — Therapeutic Abortion.

**The Fallopian Tubes:** Anatomy and Function — Salpingitis (Inflammation of the Tubes) — Ectopic Pregnancy (Tubal Pregnancy) — Cancer of the Fallopian Tubes.

**The Ovaries:** Anatomy and Function — Infection of the Ovaries — Ovarian Dysfunction — Follicle Cysts — Corpus Luteum Cysts — Dermoid Cysts — Papillary Cysts — Tumors of the Ovary — Surgery of the Ovary.

**The Menopause:** Natural and Artificial "Change of Life" — Symptoms — Treatment of Menopause — Sex and Menopause.

Chapter 26    FIRST AID IN
EMERGENCIES  209

Animal or Human Bites — Insect Bites — Snake Bites — Burns and Frostbite — Choking — Convulsions — Drowning — Electric Shock — Fainting, Dizziness, and Vertigo — Foreign Bodies — Stab and Gunshot Wounds — Fractures, Dislocations, Sprains — Gas Poisoning — Heat Stroke and Heat Exhaustion — Hemorrhage — Lacerations, Abrasions, and Contusions — Poisons — Radiation Exposure — Shock — Suffocation or Strangulation — Cardiopulmonary Resuscitation (CPR) — Bandaging.

Chapter 27    GALL BLADDER AND BILE DUCTS  221

Anatomy and Function of the Gall Bladder — Gall Bladder Inflammation — Gallstones — Disgnosis of Gall Bladder Disease — X rays of Gall Bladder and Ducts — Treatment for Gall Bladder and Bile Duct Disease — Surgery of the Gall Bladder — Diet and Gall Bladder Disease.

Chapter 28    THE HAND  227

Injuries to the Hand: Fingertip Injuries, Nerve and Tendon Injuries, Baseball Finger (Mallet Finger), Dislocated Finger, Skier's Thumb, Fractures — The Wrist — de Quervain's Disease — Trigger Finger — Carpal Tunnel Syndrome — Pinched Nerves — Dupuytren's Contracture — Tumors in the Hand — Infections of the Hand — Birth Deformities of the Hand — Surgery of the Hand.

Chapter 29    THE HEART  231

Anatomy and Function of the Heart — Smoking and the Heart — Alcohol and the Heart — Impaired Heart Function and Heart Disease — Heart Failure — Blood Pressure — Congenital Heart Disease — Coronary Artery Disease (Angina Pectoris and Coronary Thrombosis) — Heart Irregularities (Cardiac Arrhythmia) — "Athlete's Heart" — Palpitation — Paroxysmal Arrhythmia — Heart Block — Fibrillation — Heart Murmers — Heart Valve Infection (Bacterial Endocarditis) — Heart Surgery — The Cardiac Care Unit (CCU).

Chapter 30    HERNIA  247

Causes of Hernia — Frequency of Hernia — Types of Hernia — Trusses and Hernia — Surgery for Hernia — Strangulated Hernia — Results of Surgery — Postoperative Care.

Chapter 31    IMMUNIZATIONS AND VACCINATIONS  252

Immunity, Active and Passive — Schick Test — Tuberculin Test — Smallpox Vaccination — Polio Vaccination — Measles Vaccination — German Measles Immunization — Mumps Immunization — Typhoid Fever Vaccination — Tuberculosis Vaccination — Rabies Vaccination — Other Disease Vaccinations — Travel to Foreign Countries — Immunization and Vaccination Chart — Immunization Chart for Infants and Children.

**Chapter 32** INFANT AND CHILDHOOD DISEASES 260

Croup — Celiac Disease — Cystic Fibrosis — Hirschsprung's Disease (Megacolon) — Nephrosis (see Chapter 37, on The Kidneys and Ureters) — Rheumatic Fever (see Chapter 62, on Rheumatic Fever) — Erythroblastosis — Amaurotic Family Idiocy (Tay-Sachs Disease) — Niemann-Pick Disease — Down's Syndrome (Mongolism) — Retrolental Fibroplasia — Hyaline Membrane Disease (Respiratory Distress Syndrome) — Atelectasis, of the Newborn — Hemorrhagic Disease of the Newborn — Tetany of the Newborn — Sepsis of the Newborn — Thrush — Omphalitis — Congenital Laryngeal Stridor.

**Chapter 33** INFANT FEEDING AND BOWEL FUNCTION 269

Breast Feeding — Bottle Feeding — Formulas — Vitamins — Solid Foods — Colic — Bowel Movements — Diarrhea.

**Chapter 34** INFECTIOUS AND VIRUS DISEASES 279

Causes of Infectious and Virus Diseases — Typhoid Fever — Virus Pneumonia (see Chapter 41, on The Lungs) — Malaria — Yellow Fever — Dengue Fever — Relapsing Fever (Recurrent Fever or Tick Fever) — Infectious or Epidemic Jaundice (Spirochetal Jaundice or Weil's Disease) — The Rickettsial Diseases — Tularemia (Rabbit Fever) — Brucellosis (Undulant Fever, Malta Fever, Mediterranean Fever, Gibraltar Fever — Plague (Black Plague, Bubonic Plague) — Leprosy — Infectious Mononucleosis (Glandular Fever) — Rabies (Hydrophobia) — Tetanus (Lockjaw) — Anthrax — ECHO Virus — Cholera — AIDS.

**Chapter 35** INHERITED AND CONGENITAL CONDITIONS 287

Definition of Inherited Characteristics — Definition of Congenital Conditions — Dominant vs. Recessive Characteristics — Marriage and Inherited Characteristics — Children and Congenital Characteristics — Cancer and Inheritance — Prevention of Inherited Abnormalities — Longevity and Inheritance — Mental and Physical Retardation — Genetic Medicine.

**Chapter 36** THE INTENSIVE CARE UNIT (ICU) 292

Definition and Function of the ICU — ICU vs. Routine Hospital Care — ICU Tests and Procedures — Special Equipment — Patients Eligible for the ICU.

Chapter 37   THE KIDNEYS AND URETERS  294
Anatomy and Function — Glomerulonephritis — Nephrosis — Uremia — Pyelonephritis (Kidney Infections) — Kidney and Ureter Stones — Kidney Tumors — Cysts of the Kidneys — Congenital Defects (Birth Abnormalities) of the Kidneys — Kidney Injuries — Tuberculosis of the Kidneys — "Dropped Kidney" or "Floating Kidney" (Nephroptosis) — Tumors of the Ureter — Ureterocele — Transplantation of Kidneys.

Chapter 38   LABORATORY (PATHOLOGY) TESTS AND PROCEDURES  305
Definition and Duties of a Pathologist — Hematological Blood Tests — Serological Tests — Bone Marrow Analysis — Blood Transfusions — Blood Banks — Blood Chemistry — Glucose Tolerance Test — Blood Cultures — Blood Bases and Acid-Base Status — Urine Analysis — Pregnancy Tests — Rh Test — Gastric Analysis — Papanicolaou Test — Biopsy — Sputum Analysis — Stool Analysis — Pus Cultures — Lung Taps (Thoracentesis) — Abdominal Taps (Paracentesis) — Spinal Taps — Guinea Pig Inoculations.

Chapter 39   THE LIPS, JAWS, MOUTH, TEETH, AND TONGUE  316
The Lips: Lip Infections, Lip Tumors, Harelip — Cleft Palate — The Jaws: Jaw Infections, Fractured Jaw, Cysts and Tumors of the Jaw — The Mouth: Bad Breath, Pyorrhea, Trench Mouth (Vincent's Angina) — Leukoplakia — The Teeth: Cavities of the Teeth, Abscess of the Teeth — The Tongue: Inflammation of the Tongue (Glossitis), Appearance of the Tongue in Health and Disease, Tumors of the Tongue.

Chapter 40   THE LIVER  323
Anatomy and Function of the Liver — Jaundice — Cirrhosis — Fatty Liver — Cancer of the Liver — Infectious Hepatitis — Serum Hepatitis (Homologous Serum Jaundice) — Toxic Hepatitis — Surgery of the Liver.

Chapter 41   THE LUNGS  330
Anatomy and Function of the Lungs — Smoking and the Lungs — Coughing Blood — Atelectasis — Emphysema — Spontaneous Pneumothorax — Pneumonia — Lung Abscess — Pulmonary Embolism and Infarction — Dust Diseases (Pneumoconioses) — Sarcoidosis — Mucoviscidosis — Surgery of the Lungs — Bronchiectasis — Empyema — Tuberculosis — Injuries to the Lungs or Chest Cavity — Cysts of the Lungs — Lung Tumors.

Chapter 42   THE MALE ORGANS  339
(The Penis, Scrotum, and Testicles)
Anatomy and Function of the Penis — Circumcision — Tumors of the Penis —
The Scrotum and Testicles — Injuries to the Testicle — Tumors of the Testicle
— Undescended Testicle — Hydrocele — Torsion (Twist) of the Testicle — Infection
of the Epididymis (Epididymitis) — Varicocele.

Chapter 43   MEDICATIONS AND DRUGS  345
General Information about Medications — Drug Addiction — Antibiotic Drugs
— Sulfa Drugs (Sulfonamides) — Pain-Relieving Drugs (Analgesics) —
Barbiturates — Tranquilizers — Narcotics — Laxatives (Purgatives) — Weight-
Reducing Drugs — Hormones — Stimulating Drugs — Psychedelic or Hallucina-
tory Drugs — Venereal Disease Drugs (see Chapter 77, on Venereal Disease)
— Vitamins (see Chapter 78, on Vitamins).

Chapter 44   MENTAL HEALTH AND DISEASE  354
General Discussion and Definition of Neurosis and Psychosis — Insomnia —
Hysteria — Psychosomatic Symptoms — Mental Institutions — Psychotherapy
— Psychotic Disorders: Depression (Melancholia), Shock Treatment, Manic-
Depressive Reactions, Schizophrenia, Paranoid Reactions — Mental Deficien-
cy: Idiots, Imbeciles, Morons — Aptitude Tests — Stress.

Chapter 45   NERVOUS DISEASES  362
(The Brain, Spinal Cord, and Nerves)
Anatomy and Function of the Nervous System — Neuritis — Herniated Disk
— Shingles (Herpes Zoster) — Trigeminal Neuralgia — Facial Paralysis (Bell's
Palsy) — Cerebral Palsy — Brain Tumors — Encephalitis — Meningitis — Syphi-
lis of the Nervous System — Cerebrovascular Accidents (Strokes) — Epilepsy
— Fainting — Coma — Headache — Vertigo — Ménière's Disease — Muscular
Dystrophy — Multiple Sclerosis (Disseminated Sclerosis) — Parkinsonism
(Shaking Palsy) — Lumbar Puncture (Spinal Tap) — Brain Tests: Cat Scan,
Pneumoencephalography, Electroencephalography.

Chapter 46   NEUROSURGERY  372
(Brain, Spinal Cord, and Nerve Surgery)
Surgical Approach to the Brain — Skull and Brain: Head Injuries (Lacerations,
Concussion, Fracture), Surgical Infections of the Skull and Brain, Tumors of
the Brain (CAT Scan, Angiogram), Intercranial Hemorrhage, Abnormalities
of Blood Vessels of the Brain — Miscellaneous: Trigeminal Neuralgia, Surgery
for Epilepsy, Surgery for Mental Disease, Surgery for Parkinsonism (Shaking Palsy), Hydrocephalus — Spinal Cord: Birth Deformities (Congenital Malformations, Developmental Anomalies), Tumors of the Spinal Cord, Ruptured
Intervertebral Disks (Herniated, Slipped Disks), Spinal Cord Injuries, Surgery
for Intractable Pain — Peripheral Nerves.

Chapter 47    THE NEWBORN CHILD  384
Shape of the Head — Soft Spot in the Skull — Care of the Scalp — Care of the Eyes, Ears, and Mouth — Jaundice in the Newborn — Blemishes and Marks on Body — Weight of the Newborn — Eye Focus — The Newborn's Breasts — Circumcision — Care of the Umbilical Cord — Bathing — Room Temperature — Going Out of Doors — Visitors — Premature Babies: Chances for Survival, Incubator Care, Feeding the Premature Baby, Prematurity and Mental Development.

Chapter 48    THE NOSE AND SINUSES  389
Anatomy and Function of the Nose and Sinuses — Fractured Nose — Deviated Septum — Nasal Polyps — Nasal Sinuses: Infections, Surgery for Sinus Infections — Tumors of the Nose and Sinuses — Nosebleeds — Plastic Surgery of the Nose (Rhinoplasty).

Chapter 49    THE PANCREAS  397
Anatomy and Function of the Pancreas — Pancreatitis (Inflammation of the Pancreas) — Abscess of the Pancreas — Diabetes (see Chapter 19, on Diabetes) — Hyperinsulinism (Hypoglycemia) — Cysts of the Pancreas — Benign Tumors of the Pancreas — Cancer of the Pancreas.

Chapter 50    PARASITES AND PARASITIC DISEASES  402
How Parasites Gain Entrance into the Body — Prevention of Parasitic Disease — Amebiasis — Amebic Dysentery — Trichomonas Vaginitis — Leishmaniasis — African Sleeping Sickness — Schistosomiasis — Chagas' Disease — Malaria — Worm Diseases: Roundworms, Whipworms, Hookworms, Pinworms, Ascaris, Filariasis, Flukes, Tapeworms, Echinococcus Cyst.

Chapter 51    THE PARATHYROID GLANDS  407
Anatomy and Function of the Parathyroid Glands — Overactivity of the Parathyroids (Hyperparathyroidism) — Osteitis Fibrosa Cystica — Surgery of the Parathyroid Glands — Underactivity of the Parathyroid Glands (Hypoparathyroidism) — Cause of Hypoparathyroidism — Medical Treatment for Underactivity of the Parathyroid Glands.

Chapter 52    PERITONITIS  410
Causes of Peritonitis — Symptoms of Peritonitis — Prevention of Peritonitis — Treatment of Peritonitis — Outlook for Recovery from Peritonitis.

Chapter 53   PHYSICAL THERAPY AND REHABILITATION 412

General Discussion — Heat Therapy — Ultraviolet (UV) Light Therapy — Hydrotherapy — Electrical Stimulation — Massage — Exercise — Rehabilitation — Physical Therapy and Rehabilitation for Older People.

Chapter 54   PILONIDAL CYST 416

Definition — Cause of Pilonidal Cyst — Surgical Treatment of Pilonidal Cyst — Aftertreatment — Recurrence Following Surgery.

Chapter 55   THE PITUITARY GLAND 418

Anatomy and Function of the Pituitary Gland — Giantism and Acromegaly — Cushing's Disease — Oversecretion and Undersecretion of Pituitary Hormones — Surgery of the Pituitary Gland — Diabetes Insipidus — Dwarfism.

Chapter 56   PLASTIC SURGERY 422

Plastic vs. Cosmetic Surgery — Indications for Plastic Surgery — Skin Grafts: Pinch Grafts, Split-Thickness Grafts, Full-Thickness Grafts, Pedicle Grafts, Mesh Grafts, Flaps, Free Flaps — Results of Skin Grafting.

Chapter 57   PREGNANCY AND CHILDBIRTH 426

**The Prenatal Period:** Symptoms of Pregnancy — Signs of Pregnancy — Examinations and Tests to Determine Pregnancy — Diet — Iron and Vitamins — Physical Activity — Care of the Breasts — Intercourse and Pregnancy — Visits to the Obstetrician — "Lightening" — Morning Sickness — Hemorrhoids — Varicose Veins — Vaginal Discharge — Backache — Heartburn — Dizzy Spells.

**Labor (Delivery and Confinement):** Positions of the Baby — Onset of Labor — The Stages of Labor — The Length of Labor — False Labor — Going to the Hospital — Induced Labor — Natural (Prepared) Childbirth — The Progress of Labor — Pain During Labor — Anesthesia and Labor — Checking the Baby During Labor — Episiotomy — The Afterbirth — The Umbilical Cord — Forceps Delivery — Breech Delivery — Prolapsed Cord — Multiple Births (Twins, Triplets, and Quadruplets) — Inertia Labor — Cesarean Section — Postpartum Hemorrhage (Hemorrhage Following Delivery).

**The Postpartum Period (After Delivery):** Getting out of Bed — Catheterization — Bowel Function — The Breasts — The Vagina and Anus — Length of Hospital Stay After Delivery — Returning to Normal Activity — The Return of Menstruation — Resuming Sexual Relations — Special Treatments and Exercises After Delivery — Having Another Baby.

**Complications of Pregnancy:** Heart Disease in Pregnancy — Pyelonephritis in Pregnancy — Diabetes in Pregnancy — Toxemia of Pregnancy: Preeclampsia — Eclampsia — Placenta Previa — Abruptio Placenta.

Chapter 58 PREOPERATIVE AND POSTOPERATIVE
ROUTINES 447
**Preoperative Measures:** Informed Consent — Advice re Smoking, Drinking,
Sleeping, Bowel Function, Food Intake, Sedatives, Narcotics — Preparation
of the Wound Area — Intravenous Fluids — Blood Transfusions — Stomach
Tubes — Catheterization.

**Postoperative Measures:** Recovery Rooms — Intensive Care Unit (ICU) —
Position in Bed — Airways — Ambulation — Stomach Tubes — Food and Fluid
Intake — Catheterization — Narcotics — Antibiotics — Blood Transfusions —
Enemas — Wound Dressings — Suture Removal — Blood Tests — Hospital
Discharge.

Chapter 59 THE PROSTATE GLAND 450
Anatomy and Function — Infections of the Prostate — Benign Enlargement of
the Prostate (Prostatism) — Removal of the Prostate (Prostatectomy) — Cystostomy — Cancer of the Prostate — Impotence and the Prostate Gland.

Chapter 60 THE RECTUM AND ANUS 455
Anatomy and Function — Bowel Function — Laxatives and Lubricants — Consti-
pation — Bowel Symptoms — Hemorrhoids ("Piles") — Sigmoidoscopy — Co-
lonoscopy — Fissure in Ano — Abscesses and Infections About the Anus
(Perirectal and Perianal Abscess) — Fistula in Ano — Pruritus Ani (Itching Anus)
— Prolapse of the Rectum — Polyps of the Rectum and Anus — Cancer of the
Rectum and Anus.

Chapter 61 REPLANTATION SURGERY 463
Definition and Function of Replantation — Procedures Prior to Replantation
(Saving the Amputated Part) — Advances in Replantation Surgery — Parts of
the Body Favorable to Replantation — Surgical Procedures — Recovery.

Chapter 62 RHEUMATIC FEVER 465
Definition of Rheumatic Fever — Cause — Relationship of Rheumatic Fever
and Heart Disease (Myocarditis, Endocarditis, Pericarditis) — Rheumatic Joints
— Recurrent Attacks of Rheumatic Fever — Chorea (St. Vitus' Dance) — Treatment of Rheumatic Fever — Rheumatic Fever and Other Infections.

Chapter 63 THE SALIVARY GLANDS 468
Definition of Salivary Glands — Infection of the Salivary Glands — Stone in the
Salivary Duct — Salivary Gland Tumors — Surgery of the Salivary Glands —
Removal of the Parotid Gland and Injury to the Facial Nerve.

Chapter 64    SEX AND HUMAN SEXUALITY  471
Determination of Sex — Amniocentesis — Hermaphrodites and Pseudoher-maphrodites — Children and Sex Information — Masturbation — Sexual Contact — Sexual Desire — Sexual Variations — Frigidity — Impotence — Premature Ejaculation — Homosexuality — Sexual Relations — Climax — Painful Intercourse — Sexual Normality vs. Abnormality — Causes for Lack of Sexual Fulfillment — Remedy for Common Sexual Malfunctions — Middle Age and Sexual Activity — Effect of Alcohol and Drugs on Sexual Activity.

Chapter 65    SKIN AND SUBCUTANEOUS TISSUES  476
Skin Care — Acne — Skin Planing (Dermabrasion) — Impetigo — Athlete's Foot — Eczema — Bathing and the Skin — Perspiration and Body Odors — "Cold Sores" (Herpes Simplex) — Shingles (Herpes Zoster) — Ringworm — The Hair: Baldness, Alopecia, Washing, Excessive Growth on Body, Electrolysis, Dyeing the Hair — Seborrheic Dermatitis and Dandruff — Chilblain — Keloid — Scabies — Lice — Psoriasis — Lupus — Pityriasis Rosea — Vitiligo — Poison Ivy.

**Surgical Conditions of the Skin and Subcutaneous Tissues:** General Discussion — Sebaceous Cysts (Wens) — Moles — Warts — Blood Vessel Tumors — Fibrous Tumors (Fibromas) — Fatty Tumors (Lipomas) — Ganglions — Skin Cancer.

Chapter 66    THE SMALL AND LARGE INTESTINES  486
Anatomy and Function — Chronic Constipation — Diarrhea — Gastroenteritis — Regional Ileitis — Meckel's Diverticulum — Intussusception — Volvulus — Diverticulitis and Diverticulosis — Colitis: Spastic or Mucous Colitis, Chronic Ulcerative Colitis, Colitis Due to Bacteria or Parasites — Intestinal Obstruc-tion — Hirschsprung's Disease (Megacolon) — Tumors of the Small and Large Intestine.

Chapter 67    SONOGRAPHY  500
Definition and Function of Sonography — Sonography vs. X rays — Sonogra-phy and Pregnancy — Diagnostic Applications of Sonography: Detection of Abnormalities in the Lung, Liver, Pancreas, Kidney, Aorta, Abdominal Cavi-ty, Female Organs; Gallstones; Enlarged Lymph Nodes.

Chapter 68    THE SPLEEN  502
Anatomy and Function — Congenital Hemolytic Anemia — Thrombocytopen-ic Purpura — Hypersplenism — Tumors of the Spleen — Sickle Cell Anemia — Gaucher's Disease — Cooley's Anemia — Rupture of the Spleen — Enlarge-ment of the Spleen and Its Significance — Surgery of the Spleen (Splenectomy).

Chapter 69    STERILITY, FERTILITY, AND MALE POTENCY 506

Definition of Sterility — Incidence of Sterility — Orgasm and Conception.

**Female Sterility:** Causes — Fertile and Barren Periods — Ovulation — Endometrial Biopsy — Blocked Fallopian Tubes — the Rubin Test — Hysterogram — Glandular Imbalance — Sperm Penetration of the Cervix — Fibroids and Sterility — Ovarian Cysts and Sterility — Emotional Factors in Sterility — Artificial Insemination — Sperm Donors.

**Male Sterility:** Definition of Sterility — Sperm Counts — Causes of Absent or Reduced Sperm — Treatment of Male Sterility

**Male Potency and Impotence:** Definition — Incidence of Impotence — Causes of Impotence — Premature Ejaculation — "Male Menopause" — Treatment of Impotence (Psychotherapy, Hormones, Surgery).

Chapter 70    THE STOMACH AND DUODENUM 513

Anatomy and Function — Indigestion (Dyspepsia) — Stomach Acidity — Acute Gastritis and Gastroenteritis — Chronic Gastritis — Inflammation of the Duodenum (Duodenitis) — Peptic Ulcer (Ulcers of the Stomach, Duodenum, or Esophagus) — Surgery for Peptic Ulcer — Pyloric Stenosis (Obstruction of the Outlet of the Stomach in the Newborn) — "Upside-Down" Stomach (see Chapter 30, on Hernia) — Cancer of the Stomach.

Chapter 71    THE THROAT 523

The Tonsils and Adenoids: Anatomy and Function, Tonsillectomy and Adenoidectomy, Allergy and Tonsillectomy, Poliomyelitis and Tonsillectomy, Tonsillitis, Quinsy Sore Throat, Hemorrhage and Tonsillectomy — Pharyngitis (Sore Throat) — The Larynx: Anatomy and Function, Laryngitis, Tumors of the Larynx — The Trachea (Windpipe): Tracheitis, Tracheotomy (Tracheostomy) — Branchial Cysts (Gill Slits).

Chapter 72    THE THYROID GLAND 531

Anatomy and Function — Basal Metabolism Test (BMR) — Colloid Goiter — Nodular Goiter — Hyperthyroidism (Overactivity of Thyroid) — Thyroiditis (Inflammation of the Thyroid) — Surgery of the Thyroid Gland.

Chapter 73    TRANSPLANTATION OF ORGANS 535

Grafting — Homotransplantation — Autotransplantation — Rejection Reaction — Organs Surgically Transplantable — Arteries and Blood Vessels — Synthetic Grafts — Extending Life Span Through Organ Transplantation.

Chapter 74    TUBERCULOSIS  538

Types of Tuberculosis — Methods of Getting Tuberculosis — Prevention —
Symptoms — Diagnosis — Tuberculin Test — Incidence of Tuberculosis — Prima-
ry Tuberculosis — Tuberculosis of the Lung — Active vs. Inactive Tuberculosis
— Treatment in Tuberculosis: Medical Treatment, Surgical Treatment (see
Chapter 41, on The Lungs) — Tuberculosis and Pregnancy.


ULTRASOUND

See Chapter 67, on Sonography.


Chapter 75    UPPER RESPIRATORY DISEASES  543

The Common Cold — Laryngitis — Bronchial Tubes: Acute and Chronic Bron-
chitis, Bronchoscopy, Bronchiectasis — Influenza (the Flu) — Asiatic and Hong
Kong Influenza — Pneumonia (see Chapter 41, on The Lungs) — "Swine"
Influenza.


Chapter 76    THE URINARY BLADDER AND URETHRA
594

Anatomy and Function — Bladder Infection (Cystitis) — Cystoscopy — Bladder Fistulas — Bladder Stones (Calculi) — Tumors of the Bladder — Surgery
of the Bladder — The Urethra: Strictures of the Urethra, Caruncles of the
Urethra, Diverticulum of the Urethra, Ininfections of the Urethra, Hypospadias and Epispadias.


VASCULAR SURGERY

See Chapter 13, on Blood Vessels and Blood Vessel Surgery.


Chapter 77    VENEREAL DISEASE  557

Definition — Modes of Contraction — Syphilis: The Chancre, Prevention of
Syphilis, Blood Tests, Treatment, Complications of Syphilis, Cure of Syphilis
— Gonorrhea: Symptoms, Diagnosis, Treatment, Complications — Herpes:
"Cold Sores"(Herpes Simplex), Shingles (Herpes Zoster), Genital Herpes.


Chapter 78    VITAMINS  561

Definition — The Need for Vitamins — Vitamin Deficiencies — Foods Rich in
Vitamins — Requirements of Vitamins — Supplementary Vitamins — The Value
of Taking Vitamins.

Chapter 79    X RAY  564

Definition of X rays — The Ownership of X-ray Films — Fluoroscopy — The Safety of X ray and Fluoroscopy — CAT Scan — The Value of X rays in Viewing Specific Organs — Radiation Therapy (X-ray Therapy) — The Value of X-ray Therapy in Treating Specific Organs and Diseases — Radon — Radioactive Isotopes — The Value of Radioactive Isotopes — Nuclear Scanning.

DEFINITIONS OF MEDICAL TERMS  571

INDEX  643

ACKNOWLEDGEMENTS TO SOURCES OF ILLUSTRATIONS  678

# CHAPTER 1

# GENERAL INSTRUCTIONS TO PATIENTS

*(See also Chapter 26 on First Aid in Emergencies; Chapter 79 on X ray)*

## SELECTING A DOCTOR

**What is the best way to select a doctor?**

If you do not know a doctor personally in your community, call your county medical society. It will give you the names of reputable physicians who practice in your vicinity.

**Is it wise to depend completely on the advice of friends in selecting a physician?**

No. Your friends, while well-meaning, may not be in a position to judge the professional competence of a doctor.

**How can a patient find out about the professional qualifications of a physician?**

Either by calling the hospital with which he is affiliated or by calling the county medical society.

**In these days of specialization, what value does a family physician have?**

He has great value. Many family physicians are now qualified specialists in the field of Family Practice and hold Board certification in that field. Such physicians are therefore excellently qualified to treat the great majority of ills.

**How can one tell whether he is sick enough to require a physician's service?**

Call your doctor on the phone. He will ask you for a description of your symptoms. Let him decide whether or not you must be seen.

**When is it safe for a patient to treat himself?**

This is a dangerous procedure. A telephone call to your physician will reveal whether expert medical care is necessary. If you are not sick enough to require a visit, your doctor will tell you.

## MEDICAL FEES

**How can a patient tell if he is able to afford a doctor's fees?**

People should hold frank discussions of costs *before* they embark upon a course of medical treatment.

**Is it ethical for people to discuss with their doctor, or their doctor's nurse, the cost of medical service?**

Yes.

**Will doctors adjust their fee schedule if the patient finds himself unable to pay the full fee?**

Yes. Physicians will modify their fees if they are convinced that there is a real inability to pay.

**Why do doctors have different fees for different patients?**

Because the nature of the services almost always varies from case to case. Also, some patients require more time, expert skill, and attention than others.

**What is the best way to budget for medical expenses?**

By procuring as comprehensive a health insurance policy as possible.

**What is the best type of health insurance to purchase?**

This depends upon the community in which you live. It is always advisable to read a health insurance policy thoroughly, to be sure what is included or excluded. A policy that covers your expenses for medical services rendered in the doctor's office and your home, as well as expenses incurred in the hospital, is the best type to buy. Remember that 90 percent of all illness is treated *outside* of hospitals. Of course those eligible for Medicare should take advantage of the medical insurance benefits. Those not eligible for Medicare who cannot afford private care should seek assistance from the Medicaid program.

## HOSPITALIZATION

**What is the best way to choose a hospital?**

As a rule, patients should go to the hospital where their physician has a staff appointment or courtesy privileges.

**Can your doctor take you to any hospital you may choose?**

No. In most areas in this country, hospitals have closed staffs. Only those physicians who are on the staff can admit patients. It is therefore necessary to go where your physician can treat you.

**What is the best way to budget for hospital expenses?**

By purchasing hospital insurance, preferably the nonprofit, Blue Cross type. This is a valuable insurance policy and will entitle you to semiprivate care for a period of three or more weeks.

**To what services do hospital insurance policies usually entitle the patient?**

a. Room and board.
b. Floor (not special) nursing care.
c. Ordinary drugs and medications.
d. Treatments such as injections and intravenous solutions, etc.

*(continued)*

e. The use of the operating room and the x-ray department.
f. The use of hospital laboratory facilities.

## What hospital services are usually not included under hospital insurance?

a. Rare or expensive medications or treatments.
b. Special nursing care.
c. Blood transfusions.
d. Anesthesia when given by a physician.
e. The physician's or surgeon's fee.

## What items should a patient take with him to the hospital?

a. A hospital insurance card, if any.
b. A checkbook.
c. Sufficient money to make payment for the hospital stay if there is no hospital insurance.
d. A small watch or clock.
e. A toilet kit.
f. Pajamas, slippers, and bathrobe.
g. Pen, pencil, stationery, and stamps.
h. A small suitcase.

## Do hospitals have adequate provisions for the safekeeping of valuables?

It is wisest not to bring jewelry or other valuable possessions to a hospital, for many do not have adequate provisions for storing them safely.

# NURSING SERVICES

## When are special-duty nurses necessary?

When the patient is seriously ill.

## How will the patient know if special nurses are advisable?

The doctor in attendance will notify the patient or his family.

## In acute illness, how many nurses may be required to give full twenty-four-hour coverage?

Three, as it is now customary for nurses to work on eight-hour shifts.

## For how long a period of time will special nurses be required?

Your physician will advise you when you can discontinue them.

## Why can't floor nurses give all the attention necessary?

The nursing shortage in the United States is so acute that floor nurses cannot give too much in the way of individual attention. They must act as floor supervisors and must help the special nurses in getting supplies and giving treatments.

## What purpose do practical nurses serve?

They have proved of great value during the present shortage of registered nurses, and will perform many of the same duties.

## When are home nurses required?

Your physician will always advise home-nursing service when necessary.

# PERIODIC HEALTH EXAMINATION

## How often should periodic health examinations be performed?

In people under forty-five years of age, once a year—after that, a checkup twice a year is advisable.

## Should one undergo a periodic health examination even when he feels perfectly fit?

Yes. This is the most improtant time to be examined. Many conditions of a serious nature can exist for a long time without producing symptoms.

## What are other advantages of a periodic health checkup when one feels well?

Disease can sometimes be spotted in its very early stages, when it is easiest to cure.

## What specific tests should a periodic health examination include?

Your physician will be able to determine this after a thorough physical examination. It will vary widely, depending upon his findings.

## Should one undergo a periodic cancer detection test?

If one has a thorough periodic general health examination it will reveal the need for any special cancer detection examinations, and your doctor will advise them for you. Don't forget that it is just as important to detect other diseases that are a good deal more common than cancer.

## Is a Total Body Scanner (CAT scan) test advisable for healthy people?

It may be valuable, but the test is so expensive that it should be reserved for those who are suspected of having a serious disease such as cancer.

## To whom should one go for his periodic health examination?

The family physician. He will send you to specialists if he thinks additional tests or examinations are required.

# THE MEDICAL RECORD

## Is it safe to confide intimate personal information to your physician?

Yes. Your medical record is a completely confidential document. Contents of this medical record will not be revealed, without your permission, to anyone, including your husband or wife.

## What is the significance of the medical record?

A thorough medical record with notations after each visit is extremely valuable in giving the physician a running picture of your health over the years. Your physician will repeatedly refer to the medical record to see if certain conditions were present years before.

## Can the patient himself obtain information about his own medical record?

Yes. Your physician will be most willing to inform you of your past or present health status and will, almost always, give you information about his findings.

## Will a physician forward to insurance companies or to other physicians data from his medical record?

Yes, but only with the patient's written permission.

## Who owns the patient's medical record?

The physician owns the record. He will often give you a copy of the material contained therein, although it is seldom that he will relinquish the original record itself.

## Who owns the x rays the physician takes?

The physician. This is part of his medical record. Patients do not buy their own x rays. They pay their fee for the interpretation of the x rays.

## COMPENSATION AND LIABILITY CASES

## What is a compensation case?

It is a case in which an injury or illness arises out of, and in the course of, employment.

## Does each state have its own compensation laws?

Yes, and they vary from state to state.

## What are the purposes of compensation laws?

a. They provide for the reimbursement, through insurance policies paid for by the employer, of injured or ill workers whose disabilities have arisen out of employment.
b. Compensation insurance policies enable employers to insure themselves against the costs of medical care and provide funds to pay sick or injured employees.
c. Compensation policies provide for the payment of medical and hospital bills, special nursing, needed appliances, convalescent and rehabilitation care. The extent of coverage differs in various states.

## Is compensation reimbursement dependent upon the amount of money a worker earns?

Yes. The greater the earning capacity, the more compensation will be paid.

## Are workers specially compensated for permanent injuries?

Yes. Specified sums of money are often awarded for loss of various parts of the body, such as an eye, a finger, or an entire limb.

## If a worker is permanently disabled, will compensation payments be made to him for the rest of his life?

In most states compensation will continue indefinitely.

## Are various kinds of permanent disability considered?

Yes. Most disabilities are divided into two main categories:
a. Total permanent disability.
b. Partial permanent disability.
Naturally, payments will be scaled according to the percentage of total disability that exists.

## Are compensation payments usually equal to the worker's earnings?

No. In most states they are three-quarters, or less, of the weekly earnings. Thus, there is an incentive for the patient to recover and to resume work.

## What is the definition of total disability?

It is a disability that prevents a worker from performing any type of work. This does not necessarily mean that the injured worker is so completely incapacitated that he must be confined continuously to bed. As an example, a machine operator can be declared totally disabled if but one finger is injured or infected.

## What is the definition of partial disability?

A worker is considered partially disabled when he can perform some part of his regular work or can be assigned to do some different kind of work that will not be influenced by the injury.

## Are there various degrees of partial disability?

Yes. Usually, the degree is calculated in percentage of total disability.

## Who determines whether a worker has a compensation illness or injury?

When a worker is injured or has a work-connected illness, he goes to see his own doctor or one recommended by his employer. After the worker gives his history, substantiating that his condition has arisen out of employment, the physican will fill out a compensation form and will send a copy to the employer and to the compensation insurance authorities in the state. The employer will also file a form and will notify his compensation insurance carrier that the worker is injured or sick. This procedure is all that is necessary for a doctor to treat his patient as a compensation case. However, if the compensation insurance carrier wants to make his own determination that the condition is work-connected, he has the privilege of having one of his own physicians conduct an independent examination of the patient.

**What happens if the worker claims his condition to be a compensation case, but the employer or the employer's insurance company disagrees with his claim?**

The issue is put before an impartial referee, who rules whether or not the injury or illness is compensable.

**What happens if the worker's physician differs with the employer's insurance carrier on the extent of the injury?**

The issue is usually decided by an impartial referee, who thoroughly studies and reviews the case.

**Do all doctors treat compensation cases?**

Not in all states. Some physicians, a minority, prefer not to treat compensation patients and therefore do not apply for compensation ratings.

**Can any doctor treat any kind of compensation case?**

Doctors are licensed by state agencies, and if the particular state authorizes him to treat any and all illnesses when he receives his medical degree, he would theoretically be permitted to administer to any type of illness. However, most states recognize that this is an era of specialization and have therefore es-

tablished special medical compensation boards, which authorize care only by those who are specialists in various categories. Thus, only a qualified neurosurgeon will be authorized to operate upon a worker who has sustained a brain or spinal cord injury; only an ophthalmologist will be authorized to treat a serious eye injury.

**Is the injured worker entitled to legal services to help him collect his claim?**

Anyone can retain an attorney to assist him in collecting a claim. This is often unnecessary, as disagreement may not develop. On the other hand, if there is dissatisfaction on the part of the claimant, he should most certainly obtain legal help.

**What is meant by the term "liability case"?**

It refers to a personal injury or accident for which another individual or individuals are liable. Under this category come cases in which negligence is involved.

**Who determines responsibility in liability cases?**

The ultimate authority rests with the courts in the various states. Often, liability cases are settled without resorting to court action, merely upon agreement between the involved parties.

**Can an individual protect himself against liability damages?**

Yes. It is wise for everyone to take out liability insurance policies so that if an injury occurs in his home or on his property, or is caused by his automo-

bile, his insurance company will assume payment for damages.

**Is liability insurance compulsory?**

There are several states that insist that all automobile owners take out liability insurance; in other states it is voluntary.

**What are some of the things that determine the amount of damages in an accident case?**

a. The severity of the injury and its degree of permanence.
b. The presence or absence of disfigurement.
c. The extent of medical and hospital expenses.
d. The amount of wages or earnings lost because of the injury.
e. The degree of pain and suffering that has been incurred.

**What is meant by the term "third-party action"?**

It is the right of an individual injured while at work to collect damages from the individual or party who caused the injury. He may receive compensation payments and at the same time, in most states, take legal action against a third party.

**Can someone collect both compensation monies and damages from a third party?**

Yes, but monies paid out by the compensation insurance company are returned to it after the claimant has received a settlement as a result of his third-party action. In such cases, the compensation insurance company obtains a lien against possible third-party recovery.

CHAPTER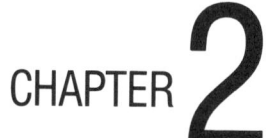

# ABSCESSES AND BACTERIAL INFECTIONS

*(See also Chapter 8 on Anesthesia; Chapter 19 on Diabetes Mellitus; Chapter 34 on Infectious and Virus Diseases; Chapter 38 on Laboratory Tests and Procedures; Chapter 43 on Medications and Drugs)*

**What causes abscesses, pimples, boils, carbuncles, or other infections associated with pus formations?**

Various bacteria. There are literally dozens of different types of bacteria capable of producing infections.

**Is there any difference between an abscess and a boil?**

They are the same thing.

**What is the difference between an abscess and a carbuncle?**

A carbuncle is a more extensive infection, usually coming to a head in several areas rather than in one area.

**Are there special times when people are particularly susceptible to abscesses or infections?**

Yes, when they are anemic, undernourished, overtired, or when they are suffering from diabetes or some other debilitating disease. Women who have just recently given birth are also particularly susceptible to infection.

**Do infections or abscesses tend to run in crops?**

Yes, because the patient has built up no resistance against the particular germ that has entered the body.

**Does a series of boils or abscesses indicate that there is something wrong with the patient's blood?**

Usually not. However, the blood should be examined to be certain the patient is normal.

**What is the best way to avoid a serious infection?**

a. Report to your physician for periodic health examinations to make sure that you have no underlying disease.

b. Clean all scratches or cuts thoroughly with plain soap and water and then cover them with a clean bandage.

c. Never squeeze or pick or open even the smallest pimple or boil.

d. Avoid using substances on the skin to which you may be sensitive. Some people are sensitive to deodorants or cosmetics.

e. A spreading infection should be treated by bed rest and antibiotic medications.

f. Apply warm compresses to any inflamed area.

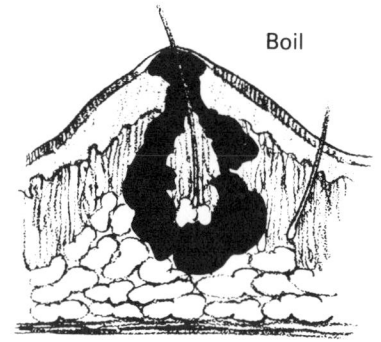

Boil

g. Consult your doctor on the telephone. He will tell you if any special medication, such as an antibiotic, is indicated.

**Are there any regions of the body in which abscesses or infections are particularly dangerous?**

Yes, the region of the upper lip, the nose, and the face. This is because there is a direct connection through the system of veins between these areas of the skin and the veins within the skull.

**What is septicemia?**

This is commonly called blood poisoning, a disease in which bacteria are living, growing, and circulating in the bloodstream.

**Is blood poisoning curable?**

Yes. With the use of antibiotic drugs, most patients with septicemia can now be rescued. However, certain infections cannot be overcome even with the use of antibiotics.

**Should patients medicate themselves with antibiotics?**

No. This is a dangerous procedure.

**What is done when a patient develops an allergy or sensitivity to an antibiotic drug?**

There are now so many excellent antibiotic drugs on the market that your physician will undoubtedly find one to which you are not allergic or sensitive.

*The Difference between a Boil and a Carbuncle. A boil, as shown at left, has one opening or "head." A carbuncle, as shown below, has several openings.*

Carbuncle

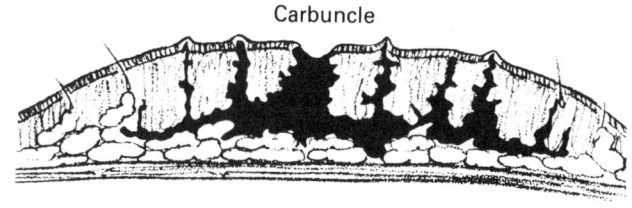

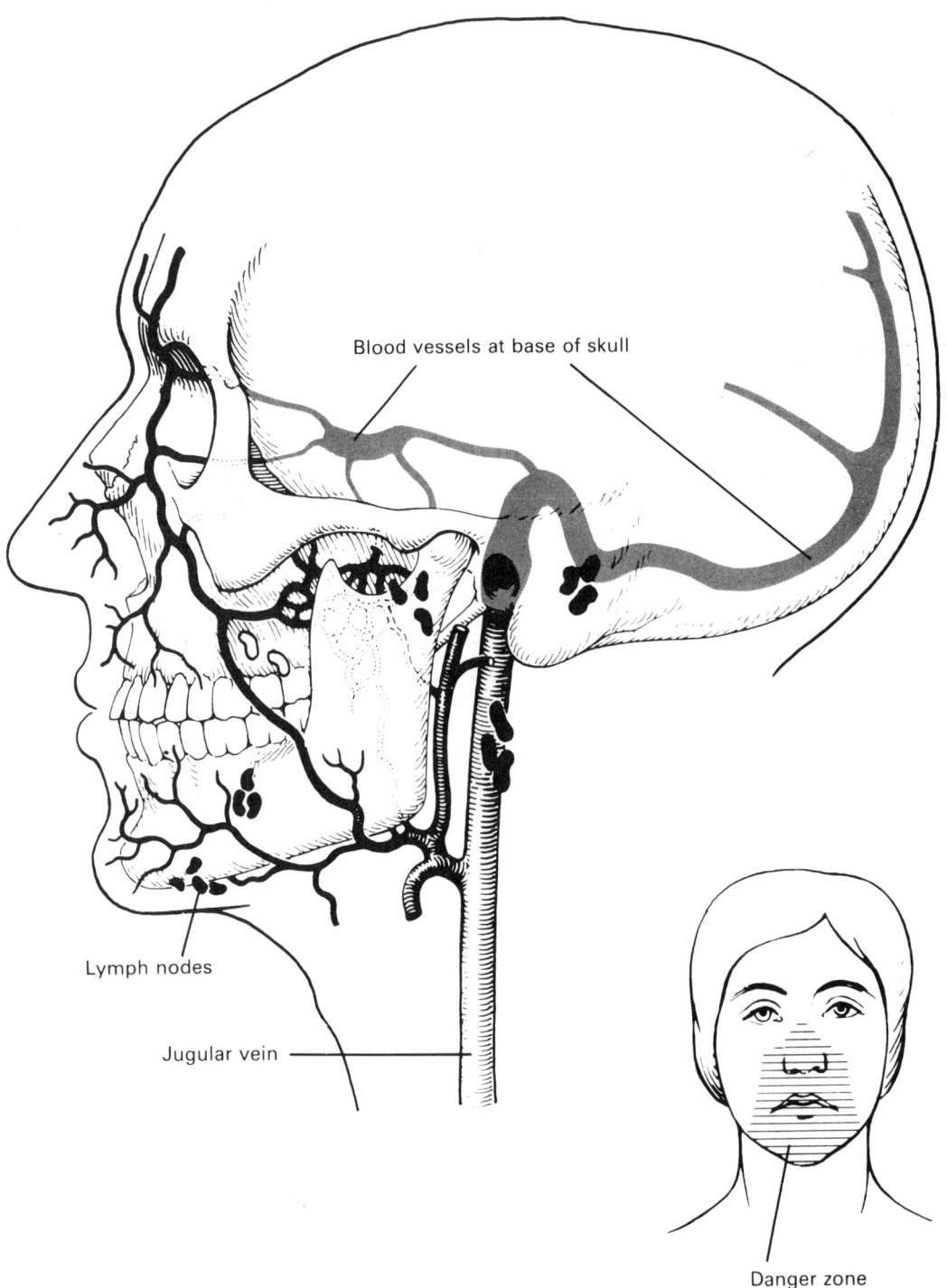

Blood vessels at base of skull

Lymph nodes

Jugular vein

Danger zone

**Dangerous Areas of Infection on Face.** *It is dangerous to prick or squeeze a pimple about the upper lip, nose, or cheeks, as the blood and lymph channels from these areas drain directly into the skull at the base of the brain. Because of this anatomical structure, serious brain infections may sometimes result. Young people especially should be warned never to squeeze pimples or boils in these areas.*

# ANATOMY
# OF THE
# HUMAN BODY

### A SERIES OF VIEWS
### SHOWING THE PRINCIPAL PARTS OF
### THE MALE AND FEMALE BODY

SUPPLEMENT TO
THE NEW ILLUSTRATED
MEDICAL ENCYCLOPEDIA FOR HOME USE

Enlarged and Revised
8th Edition
EDITED BY ROBERT E. ROTHENBERG, M.D., F.A.C.S.

Harry N. Abrams, Inc.,
Publishers, New York

# INDEX TO PLATES

In the list below, the names of the principal parts of the human anatomy are given in English (insofar as this is possible). The number immediately following the name of that part is the identification number that locates the part on the drawing; the letter or letters following it indicate the View or Views in which it is shown. See page 10 for numerical Latin listing.

Abdominal muscle, rectus, 98: **A, B**
Abdominal muscle, transverse, 109: **A, B**
Adductor brevis muscle, 67: **G**
Adductor longus muscle, 68: **F, G, L**
Adrenal gland, 44: **E, F, L**
Aorta, 3: **E, F, J, K, L**
Aponeurosis, external oblique, 4: **A**
Appendix, 5: **D, M**
Arcuate line, 58: **B**
Atrium, left, 19: **K**
Axillary artery, 6: **E, F, L**
Axillary vein, 178: **C, J, K**

Biceps brachialis muscle, 69: **E, F, J, K**
Bile duct, common, 35: **D, E, J, K, M**
Brachial artery, 7: **E, F, L**
Brachial artery and vein, 179: **C, H, J, K**
Brachial muscle, 70: **L**
Brachial plexus, 140: **E, F, G, L**
Brachiocephalic arterial trunk, 164: **E, L**
Brachiocephalic vein, 180: **C, D, J, K**
Brachioradialis muscle, 71: **L, M**
Bronchus, main, 20: **E, L**
Buccinator muscle, 72: **A**

Carotid artery, common, 8: **E, L**
Celiac arterial trunk, 165: **E, J, L**
Cephalic vein, 183: **C, D, H, I, K, L, M**
Cerebellum, 22: **K, L**
Cerebrum, 23: **K, L**
Clavicle, 24: **A, B, G, H, I, L**
Colon, ascending, 25: **C, D, M**
Colon, descending, 26: **C, D, M**
Colon, sigmoid, 27: **C, D, M**
Colon, transverse, 28: **C, D, K**
Coracobrachialis muscle, 73: **E, L**
Corpus callosum, 32: **K, L**
Cranium, 33: **B**

Deltoid muscle, 74: **E, F, H, I, L**
Depressor muscle, 75: **A, J**
Diaphragm, 34: **B, C, D, E, F, I, J, K, L**
Digastric muscle, 76: **C**
Duodenum, 37: **E, M**

Epigastric vessels, inferior, 169: **E, H, I**
Esophagus, 122: **E, F, L, M**
Extensor carpi radialis longus muscle, 77: **L**

Falciform ligament, 53: **C, I**
Falx of the cerebrum, 38: **M**
Femoral artery, 9: **E, F, L**
Femoral nerve, 114: **G, L**
Femoral vein, 184: **E, F, L**
Femur, 39: **G**
Flexor carpi radialis muscle, 78: **L**
Fossa ovalis, 40: **H**
Frontal bone, 126: **C, G**
Frontal sinus, 153: **B, C, D, E, F, G, K, L, M**
Fundiform ligament, 54: **A**

Gall bladder, 200: **C, D, J, K**
Gastric vessels, 170: **K**
Gastroepiploic vessels, 171: **J**
Glans penis, 46: **A**
Gluteus medius muscle, 79: **A, E, F, G, L**
Gluteus minimus muscle, 80: **G**
Gracilis muscle, 81: **F, G, L**

Humerus, 48: **G**

Ileum, 49: **L**
Iliac artery, common, 10: **E, F, L**
Iliac artery, external, 11: **E, F, L**
Iliac artery, internal, 12: **E, F, L**
Iliac muscle, 82: **G, L**

Iliac spine, anterior superior, 159: **A, B, G, H, L**
Iliac vein, common, 185: **E, F, L**
Iliac vein, external, 186: **E, F, L**
Iliac vein, internal, 187: **E, F, L**
Iliohypogastric nerve, 115: **G**
Ilioinguinal nerve, 116: **G**
Inguinal ligament, 55: **A, B, C, E, F, H, M, L**
Inguinal ring, deep, 1: **A, B**
Inguinal ring, superficial, 2: **A**
Intercostal muscle, external, 83: **A**
Intercostal muscle, internal, 84: **B, I**
Ischium, 127: **G**

Jugular vein, internal, 188: **C, D, E, J**

Kidney, 149: **E, F, L**

Lacrimal gland, 41: **B**
Larynx, 51: **D, G, K, L**
Ligamentum teres, 56: **B, I**
Linea alba, 57: **A, B, H**
Liver, 47: **C, D, I, J, K**
Lumbosacral plexus, 141: **G**
Lung, 146: **C, D, E, F, J, K, L**

Mandible (lower jaw), 61: **A, B, C, D, E, F, G, K, L**
Masseter muscle, 85: **A**
Maxilla (upper jaw), 62: **B, C, D, E, F, G, K, L, M**
Maxillary sinus, 154: **B, C**
Median nerve, 117: **E, F, L**
Medulla oblongata, 63: **K, L**
Mesenteric artery, inferior, 14: **E, F, L**
Mesenteric artery, superior, 15: **L**
Mesenteric vein, inferior, 189: **M**
Mesenteric vein, superior, 190: **E**
Mesenteric vessels, inferior, 173: **M**
Mesenteric vessels, superior, 174: **E, M**
Mesocolon, transverse, 66: **K**
Mylohyoid muscle, 86: **B, C**

Nasal septum, 152: **E, F, M**
Nasal turbinate, inferior, 29: **D, G, K, L**
Nasal turbinate, middle, 30: **D, G, K, L**
Nasal turbinate, superior, 31: **D, G, K, L**

Oblique muscle, external, 87: **A, H**
Oblique muscle, internal, 88: **A**
Obturator nerve, 118: **G**
Occipital bones, 128: **D, E, G**
Omentum, great, 123: **J**
Omentum, lesser, 124: **C, D, I, J, K**
Omohyoid muscle, 89: **A, B, I**
Orbicularis oris muscle, 90: **A**
Ovarian vessels, 175: **L**
Ovary, 135: **L**

Pancreas, 136: **E, M**
Parietal bone, 129: **C, G**
Parotid gland, 42: **A, B**
Pectoral muscle, major, 91: **A, B, E, H, I, L**
Pectoral muscle, minor, 92: **B, E, I, J, K**
Penis, 137: **B, C, E**
Pericardium, 138: **J**
Phrenic nerve, 119: **J**
Platysma muscle, 139: **H, I**
Pons, 144: **K, L**
Portal vein, 191: **E, K, M**
Pronator teres muscle, 93: **L**
Prostate gland, 145: **F**
Psoas major muscle, 94: **G, L**
Pterygoid muscle, medial, 95: **B**
Pubic bone, 130: **C, F, G, L, M**

Pulmonary artery, 16: **E, J, K, L**
Pulmonary vein, 192: **K, L**
Pylorus, 147: **M**

Quadratus lumborum muscle, 96: **L**
Quadriceps femoris muscle, 97: **C, D, E, F, L**

Rectum, 148: **G, L**
Renal artery, 17: **F, L**
Renal vein, 193: **F, L**
Rib, 125: **A, B, G, I**
Root of mesentery, 65: **D, K**

Sacrum, 131: **G**
Sagittal sinus, inferior, 156: **M**
Sagittal sinus, superior, 157: **M**
Saphenous vein, great, 194: **H, I**
Sartorius muscle, 99: **A, B, I**
Scalene muscle, anterior, 100: **L**
Scapula, 150: **G**
Scrotum, 151: **A, B, E**
Semilunar line, 59: **A, B, H, I**
Seminal vesicle, 202: **F**
Serratus muscle, anterior, 101: **A**
Small intestine, 50: **C, D, J, K**
Sphenoid bone, 132: **G**
Sphenoid sinus, 158: **D, E, F, G, K, L, M**
Spinal medulla, 64: **G, L**
Spleen, 52: **E, M**
Splenic artery, 13: **E**
Splenic vessels, 172: **M**
Sternocleidomastoid muscle, 102: **A, B, H, I, J**
Sternohyoid muscle, 103: **A, B, I**
Sternothyroid muscle, 104: **B, I**
Sternum, 160: **A, B, H, I**
Stomach, 196: **C, D, J, K**
Styloglossal muscle, 105: **C**
Subclavian artery, 18: **E, F, L**
Subclavian vein, 195: **C, D, J, K**
Submaxillary gland, 43: **A, B**

Temporal bone, 133: **C, G**
Temporal muscle, 106: **A**
Tensor fascia lata muscle, 107: **A, E, F, L**
Tentorial sinus, 155: **M**
Tentorium cerebellum, 161: **K, L**
Testicle, 162: **E**
Testicular vessels, 176: **E, F**
Thoracic muscle, transverse, 110: **B, I**
Thoracic vessels, internal, 177: **I, J**
Thyrohyoid muscle, 108: **B**
Thyroid cartilage, 21: **C**
Thyroid gland, 45: **C, D, J, K**
Tongue, 60: **C, D, E, F, G, K, L**
Trachea, 163: **E, F, L**
Trapezius muscle, 111: **E, F, J, L**
Triceps muscle, 112: **E, F, L**

Ulnar nerve, 120: **E, F, L**
Umbilical fold, medial, 142: **I**
Umbilical fold, median, 143: **I**
Ureter, 166: **E, F, M, L**
Urinary bladder, 201: **C, D, E, F, M**
Uterus, 167: **L**

Vagina, 168: **L**
Vagus nerve, 121: **L**
Vas deferens, 36: **E, F**
Vena cava, inferior, 181: **E, F, K, L**
Vena cava, superior, 182: **D, E, J, K**
Ventricle, left, 198: **C, D, J, K**
Ventricle, right, 197: **E, J, K**
Vertebra, 199: **F, G, K, L**

Zygoma, 134: **A**
Zygomatic muscle, major, 113: **A, J**

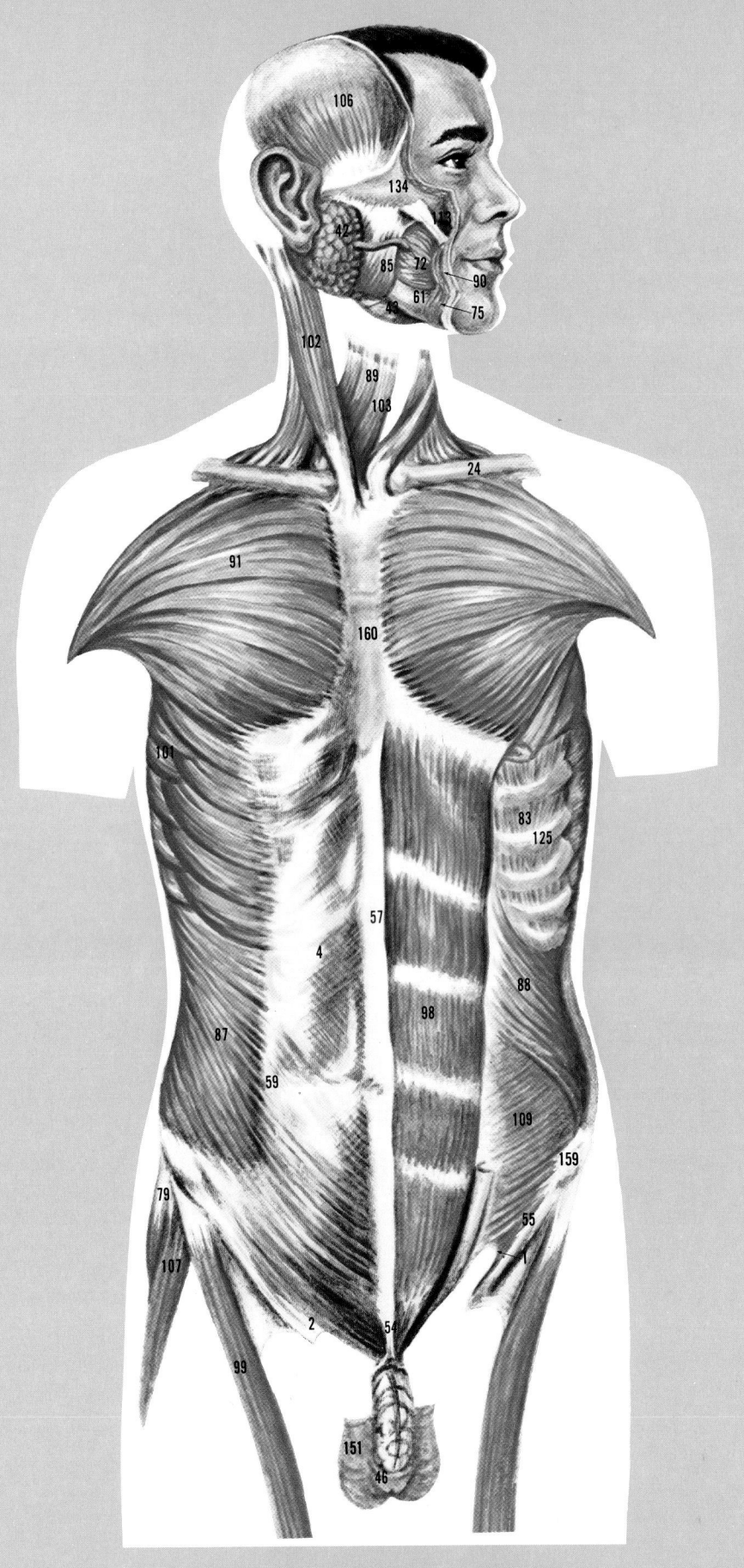

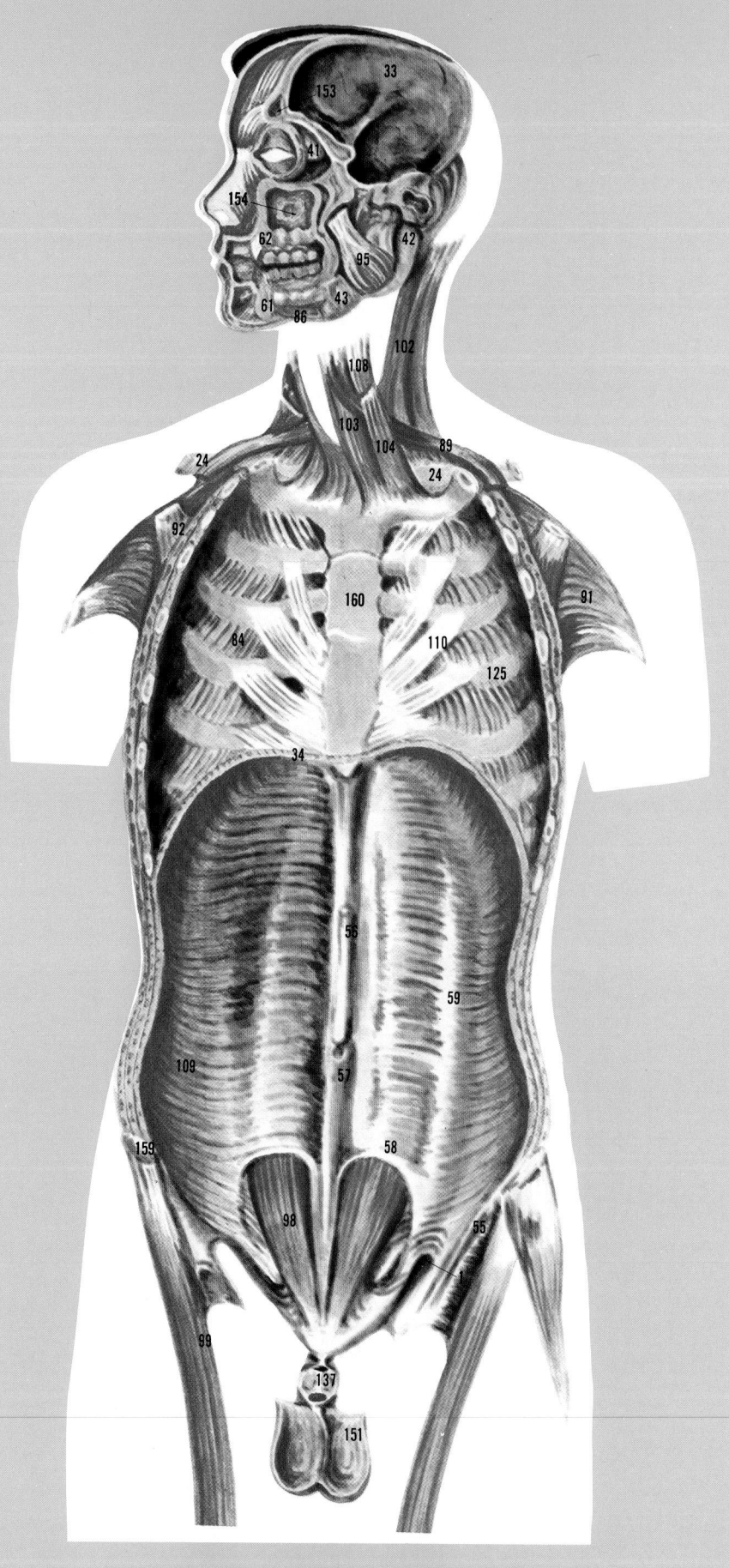

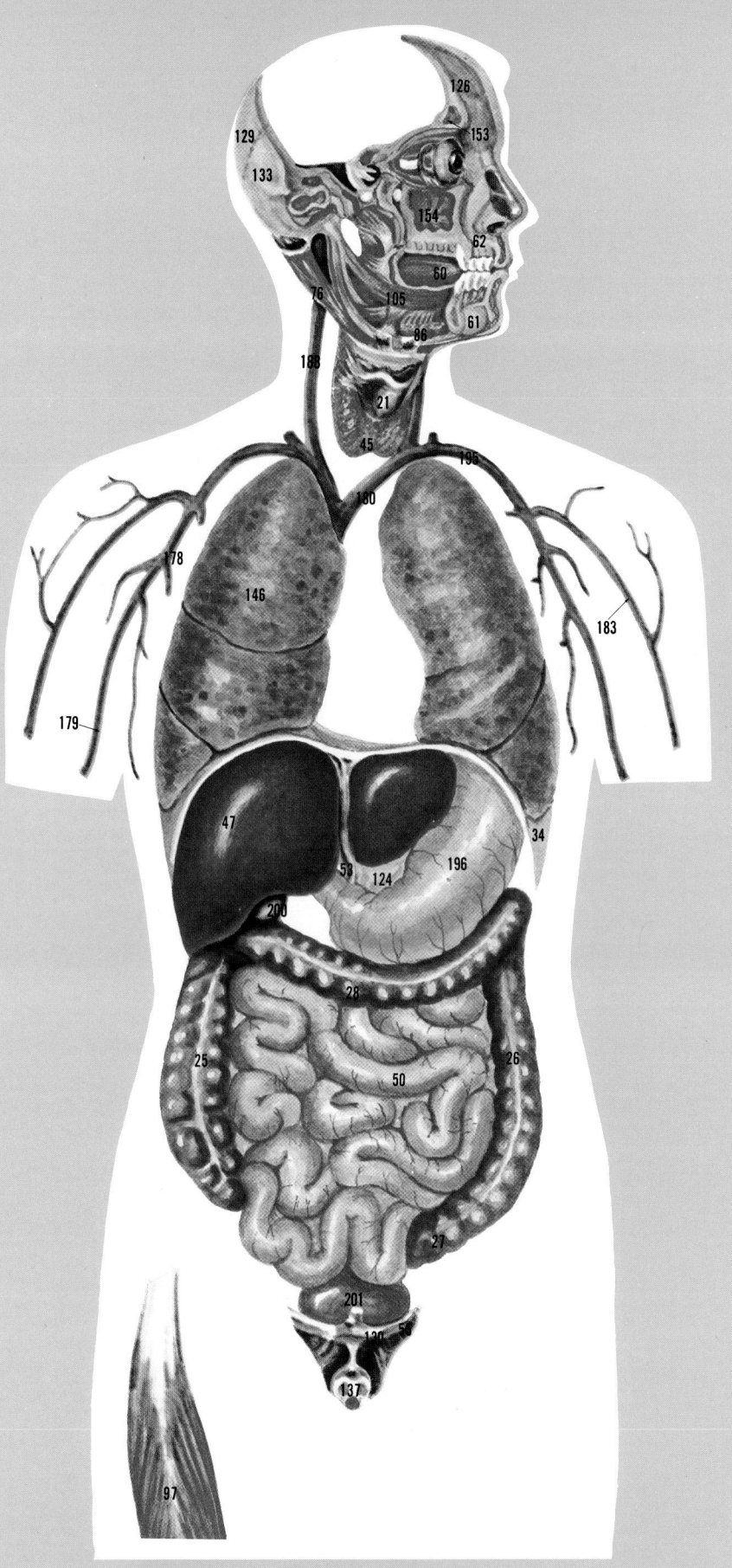

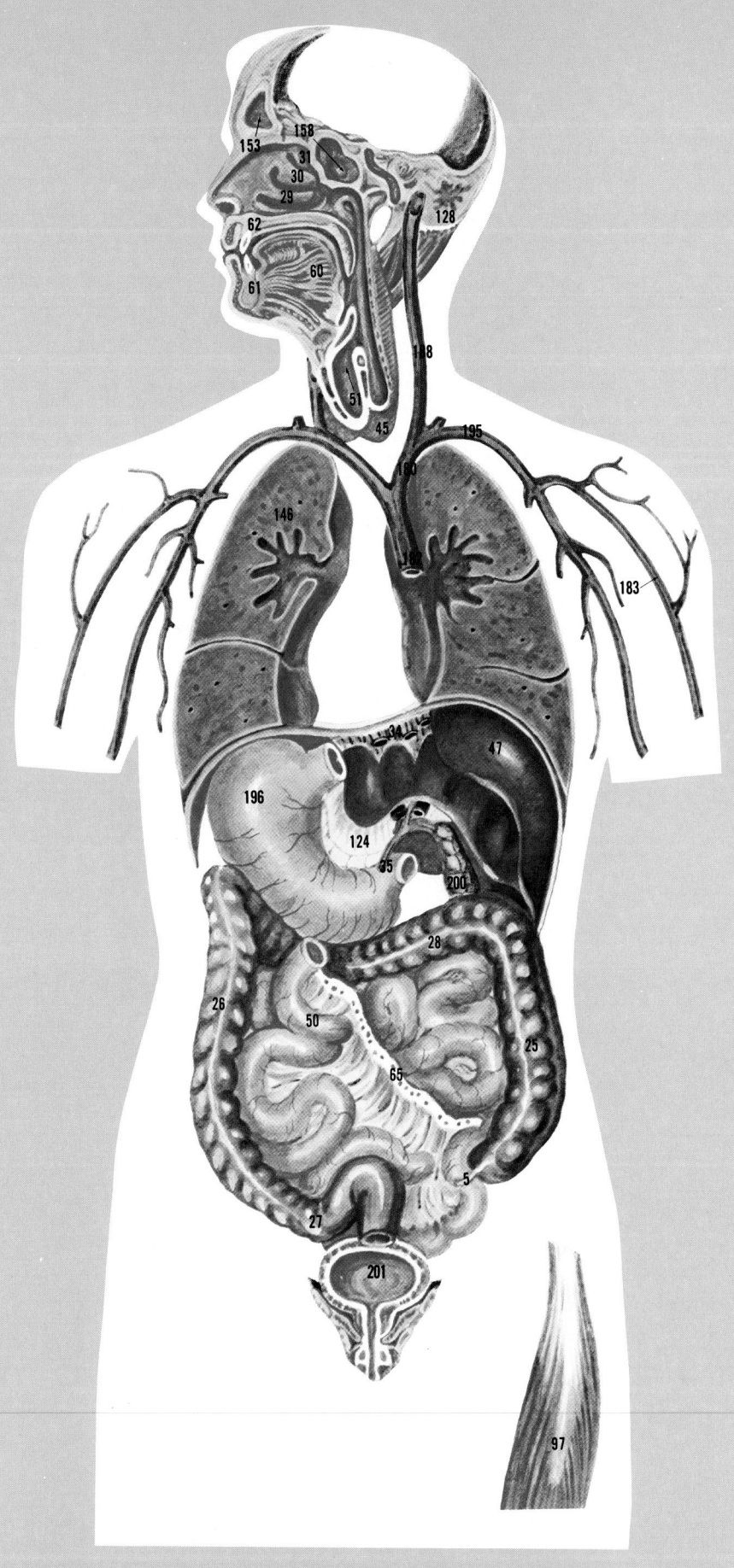

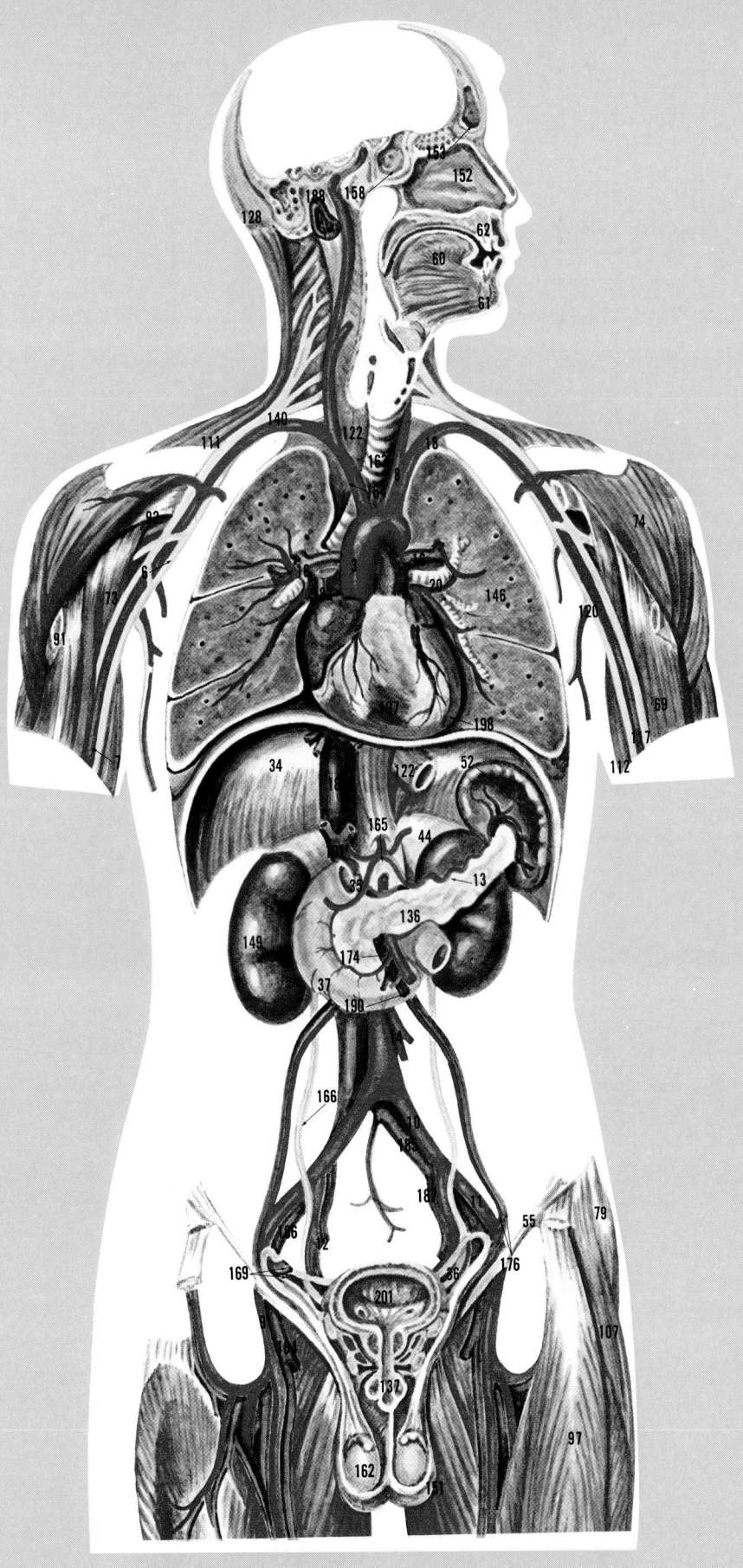

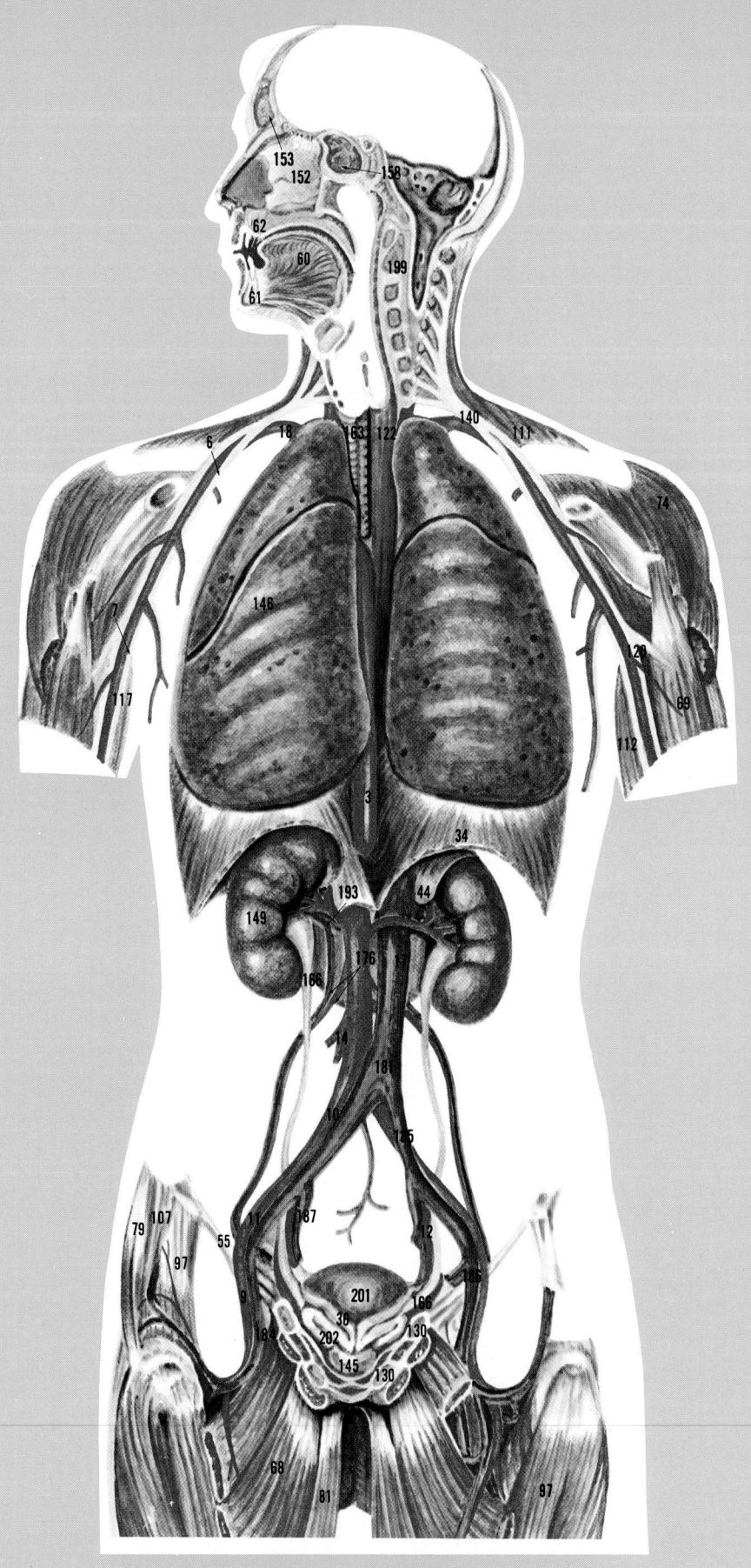

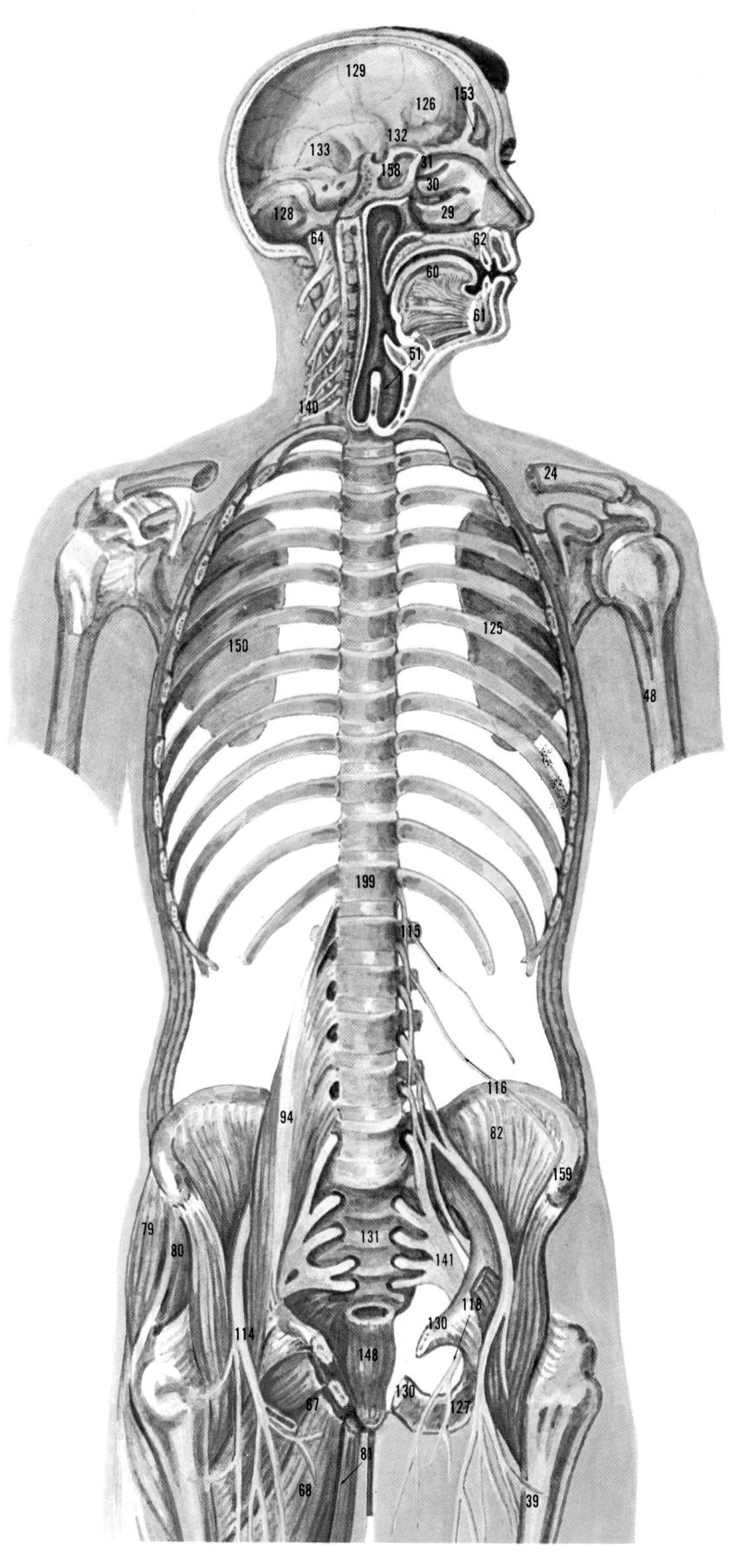

# KEY TO NUMBERING
## PLATES A–M

In Views A–M each part of the body has an identification number. This identification number appears at the left in the list below. The letter or letters following the part name indicate the View or Views in which this part of the body is shown. See page 2 for alphabetical English listing.

Abbreviations: A. (Arteria); L. (Ligamentum); M. (Musculus); N. (Nervus); and V. (Vena).

1. Anulus inguinalis profundus, **A, B**
2. Anulus inguinalis superficialis, **A**
3. Aorta, **E, F, J, K, L**
4. Aponeurosis m. obliquus externus abdominis, **A**
5. Appendix vermiformis, **D, M**
6. A. axillaris, **E, F, L**
7. A. brachialis, **E, F, L**
8. A. carotis communis, **E, L**
9. A. femoralis, **E, F, L**
10. A. iliaca communis, **E, F, L**
11. A. iliaca externa, **E, F, L**
12. A. iliaca interna, **E, F, L**
13. A. lienalis, **E**
14. A. mesenterica inferior, **E, F, L**
15. A. mesenterica superior, **L**
16. A. pulmonalis, **E, J, K, L**
17. A. renalis, **F, L**
18. A. subclavia, **E, F, L**
19. Atrium sinistrum, **K**
20. Bronchus principalis, **E, L**
21. Cartilago thyreoidea, **C**
22. Cerebellum, **K, L**
23. Cerebrum, **K, L**
24. Clavicula, **A, B, G, H, I, L**
25. Colon ascendens, **C, D, M**
26. Colon descendens, **C, D, M**
27. Colon sigmoideum, **C, D, M**
28. Colon transversum, **C, D, K**
29. Concha nasalis inferior, **D, G, K, L**
30. Concha nasalis media, **D, G, K, L**
31. Concha nasalis superior, **D, G, K, L**
32. Corpus callosum, **K, L**
33. Cranium, **B**
34. Diaphragma, **B, C, D, E, F, I, J, K, L**
35. Ductus choledochus, **D, E, J, K, M**
36. Ductus deferens, **E, F**
37. Duodenum, **E, M**
38. Falx cerebri, **M**
39. Femur, **G**
40. Fossa ovalis, **H**
41. Glandula lacrimalis, **B**
42. Glandula parotis, **A, B**
43. Glandula submandibularis, **A, B**
44. Glandula suprarenalis, **E, F, L**
45. Glandula thyreoidea, **C, D, J, K**
46. Glans penis, **A**
47. Hepar (liver), **C, D, I, J, K**
48. Humerus, **G**
49. Ileum, **L**
50. Intestinum tenue, **C, D, J, K**
51. Larynx, **D, G, K, L**
52. Lien (spleen), **E, M**
53. L. falciforme hepatis, **C, I**
54. L. fundiforme penis, **A**
55. L. inguinale, **A, B, C, E, F, H, M, L**
56. L. teres hepatis, **B, I**
57. Linea alba, **A, B, H**
58. Linea arcuata, **B**
59. Linea semilunaris, **A, B, H, I**
60. Lingua (tongue), **C, D, E, F, G, K, L**
61. Mandibula, **A, B, C, D, E, F, G, K, L**
62. Maxilla, **B, C, D, E, F, G, K, L, M**
63. Medulla oblongata, **K, L**
64. Medulla spinalis, **G, L**
65. Mesenterium, **D, K**
66. Mesocolon transversum, **K**
67. M. adductor brevis, **G**

68. M. adductor longus, **F, G, L**
69. M. biceps brachii, **E, F, J, K**
70. M. brachialis, **L**
71. M. brachioradialis, **L, M**
72. M. buccinator, **A**
73. M. coracobrachialis, **E, L**
74. M. deltoideus, **E, F, H, I, L**
75. M. depressor anguli oris, **A, J**
76. M. digastricus, **C**
77. M. extensor carpi radialis longus, **L**
78. M. flexor carpi radialis, **L**
79. M. gluteus medius, **A, E, F, G, L**
80. M. gluteus minimus, **G**
81. M. gracilis, **F, G, L**
82. M. iliacus, **G, L**
83. M. intercostalis externus, **A**
84. M. intercostalis internus, **B, I**
85. M. masseter, **A**
86. M. mylohyoideus, **B, C**
87. M. obliquus externus abdominis, **A, H**
88. M. obliquus internus abdominis, **A**
89. M. omohyoideus, **A, B, I**
90. M. orbicularis oris, **A**
91. M. pectoralis major, **A, B, E, H, I, L**
92. M. pectoralis minor, **B, E, I, J, K**
93. M. pronator teres, **L**
94. M. psoas major, **G, L**
95. M. pterygoideus medialis, **B**
96. M. quadratus lumborum, **L**
97. M. quadriceps femoris, **C, D, E, F, L**
98. M. rectus abdominis, **A, B**
99. M. sartorius, **A, B, I**
100. M. scalenus anterior, **L**
101. M. serratus anterior, **B**
102. M. sternocleidomastoideus, **A, B, H, I, J**
103. M. sternohyoideus, **A, B, I**
104. M. sternothyreoideus, **B, I**
105. M. styloglossus, **C**
106. M. temporalis, **A**
107. M. tensor fasciae latae, **A, E, F, L**
108. M. thyrohyoideus, **B**
109. M. transversus abdominis, **A, B**
110. M. transversus thoracis, **B, I**
111. M. trapezius, **E, F, J, L**
112. M. triceps brachii, **E, F, L**
113. M. zygomaticus major, **A, J**
114. N. femoralis, **G, L**
115. N. iliohypogastricus, **G**
116. N. ilioinguinalis, **G**
117. N. medianus, **E, F, L**
118. N. obturatorius, **G**
119. N. phrenicus, **J**
120. N. ulnaris, **E, F, L**
121. N. vagus, **L**
122. Oesophagus (esophagus), **E, F, L, M**
123. Omentum majus, **J**
124. Omentum minus, **C, D, I, J, K**
125. Os costale, **A, B, G, I**
126. Os frontale, **C, G**
127. Os ischii, **G**
128. Os occipitale, **D, E, G**
129. Os parietale, **C, G**
130. Os pubis, **C, F, G, L, M**
131. Os sacrum, **G**
132. Os sphenoidale, **G**
133. Os temporale, **C, G**
134. Os zygomaticum, **A**
135. Ovarium (ovary), **L**

136. Pancreas, **E, M**
137. Penis, **B, C, E**
138. Pericardium, **J**
139. Platysma, **H, I**
140. Plexus brachialis, **E, F, G, L**
141. Plexus lumbosacralis, **G**
142. Plica umbilicalis medialis, **I**
143. Plica umbilicalis mediana, **I**
144. Pons, **K, L**
145. Prostata, **F**
146. Pulmo (lung), **C, D, E, F, J, K, L**
147. Pylorus, **M**
148. Rectum, **G, L**
149. Ren (kidney), **E, F, L**
150. Scapula, **G**
151. Scrotum, **A, B, E**
152. Septum nasi, **E, F, M**
153. Sinus frontalis, **B, C, D, E, F, G, K, L, M**
154. Sinus maxillaris, **B, C**
155. Sinus rectus, **M**
156. Sinus sagittalis inferior, **M**
157. Sinus sagittalis superior, **M**
158. Sinus sphenoidalis, **D, E, F, G, K, L, M**
159. Spina iliaca anterior superior, **A, B, G, H, L**
160. Sternum, **A, B, H, I**
161. Tentorium cerebelli, **K, L**
162. Testis, **E**
163. Trachea, **E, F, L**
164. Truncus brachiocephalicus, **E, L**
165. Truncus celiacus, **E, J, L**
166. Ureter, **E, F, M, L**
167. Uterus, **L**
168. Vagina, **L**
169. Vasa epigastrica inferior, **E, H, I**
170. Vasa gastrica, **K**
171. Vasa gastroepiploica, **J**
172. Vasa lienalis, **M**
173. Vasa mesenterica inferior, **M**
174. Vasa mesenterica superior, **E, M**
175. Vasa ovarica, **L**
176. Vasa testicularis, **E, F**
177. Vasa thoracicae internae, **I, J**
178. V. axillaris, **C, J, K**
179. V. comitans a. brachialis, **C, H, J, K**
180. V. brachiocephalica, **C, D, J, K**
181. V. cava inferior, **E, F, K, L**
182. V. cava superior, **D, E, J, K**
183. V. cephalica, **C, D, H, I, K, L, M**
184. V. femoralis, **E, F, L**
185. V. iliaca communis, **E, F, L**
186. V. iliaca externa, **E, F, L**
187. V. iliaca interna, **E, F, L**
188. V. jugularis interna, **C, D, E, J**
189. V. mesenterica inferior, **M**
190. V. mesenterica superior, **E**
191. V. portae, **E, K, M**
192. V. pulmonalis, **K, L**
193. V. renalis, **F, L**
194. V. saphena magna, **H, I**
195. V. subclavia, **C, D, J, K**
196. Ventriculus (stomach), **C, D, J, K**
197. Ventriculus dexter, **E, J, K**
198. Ventriculus sinister, **E, J, K**
199. Vertebra, **F, G, K, L**
200. Vesica fellea (gall bladder), **C, D, J, K**
201. Vesica urinaria, **C, D, E, F, M**
202. Vesicula seminalis, **F**

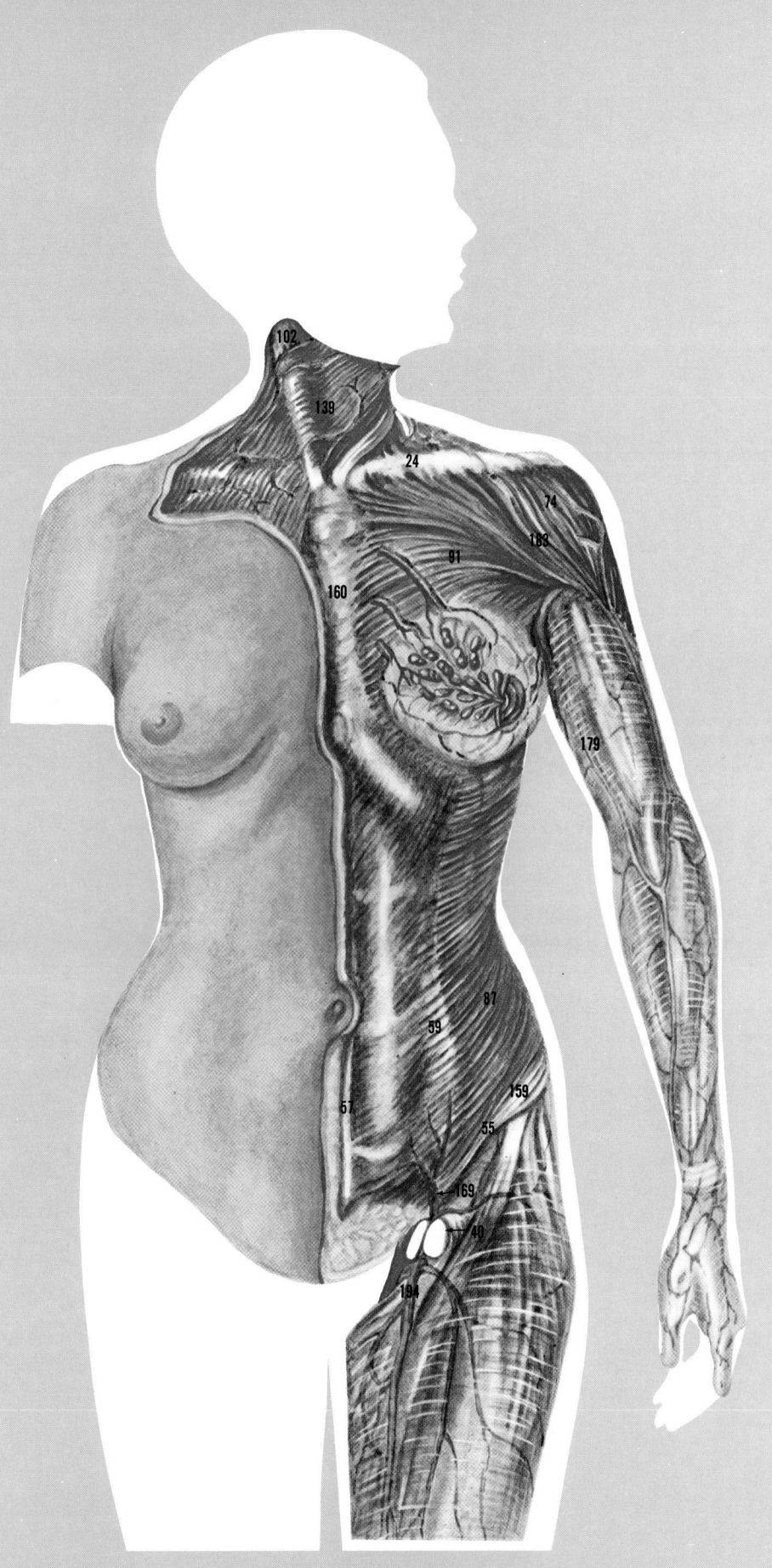

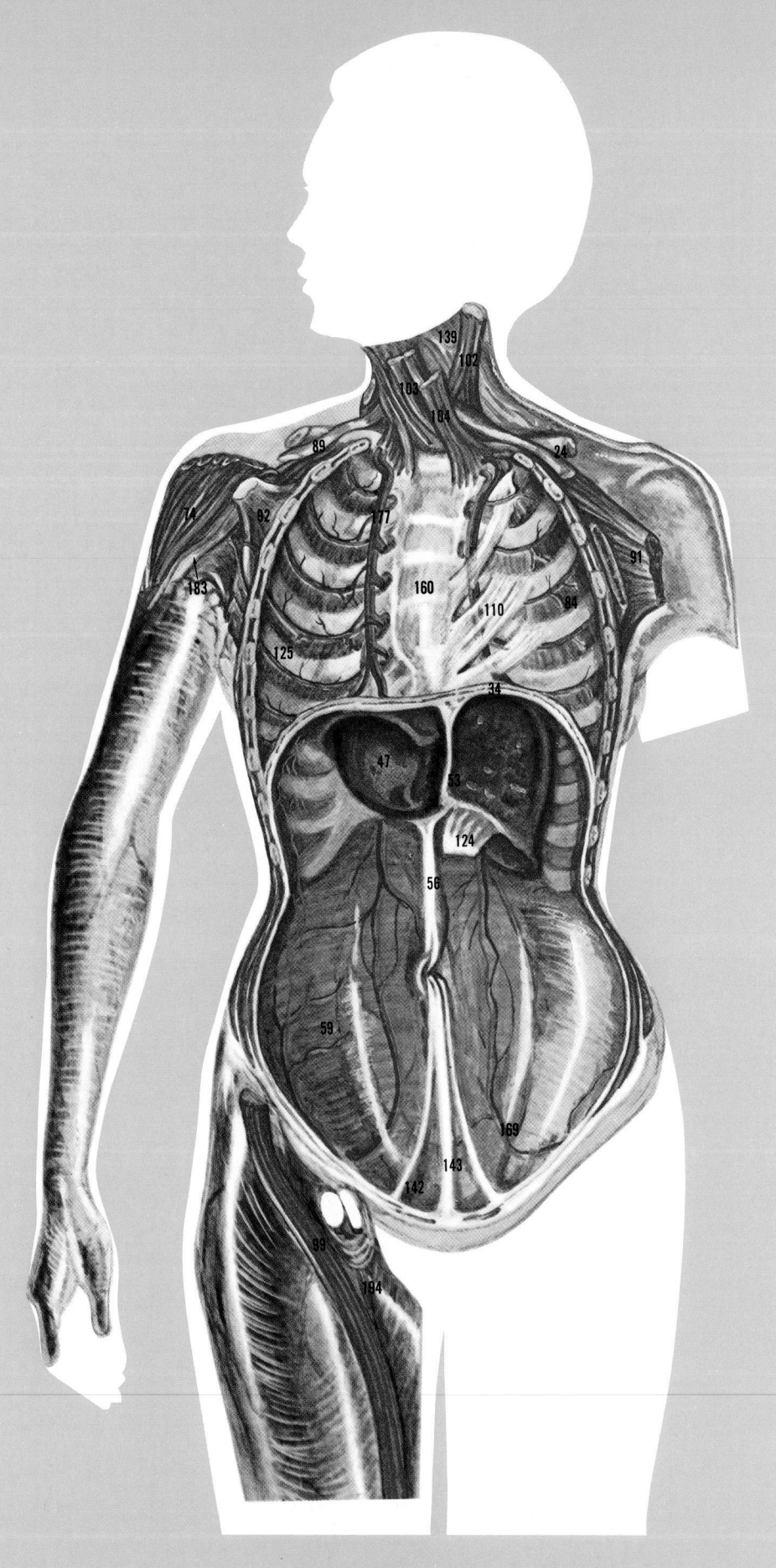

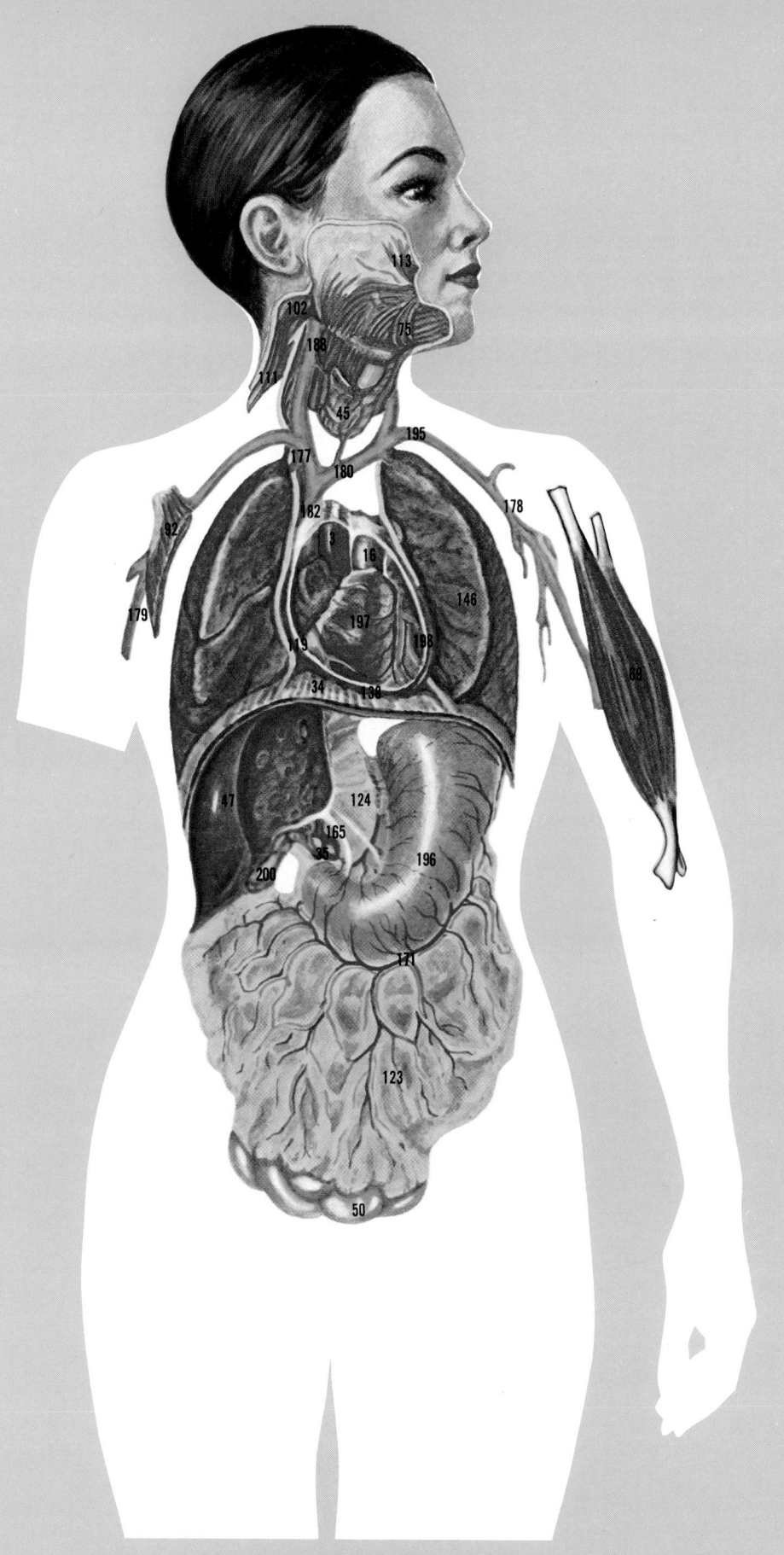

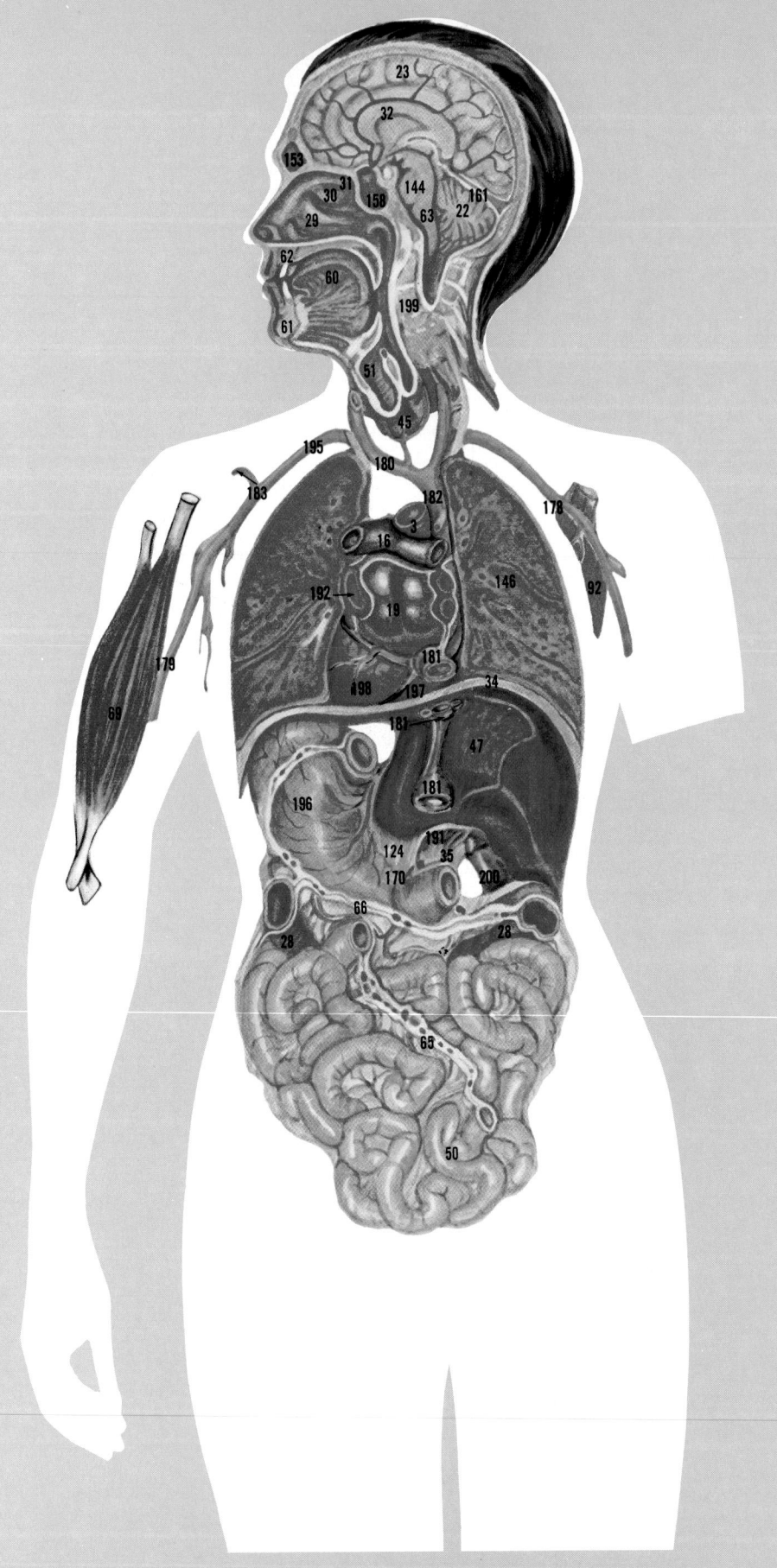

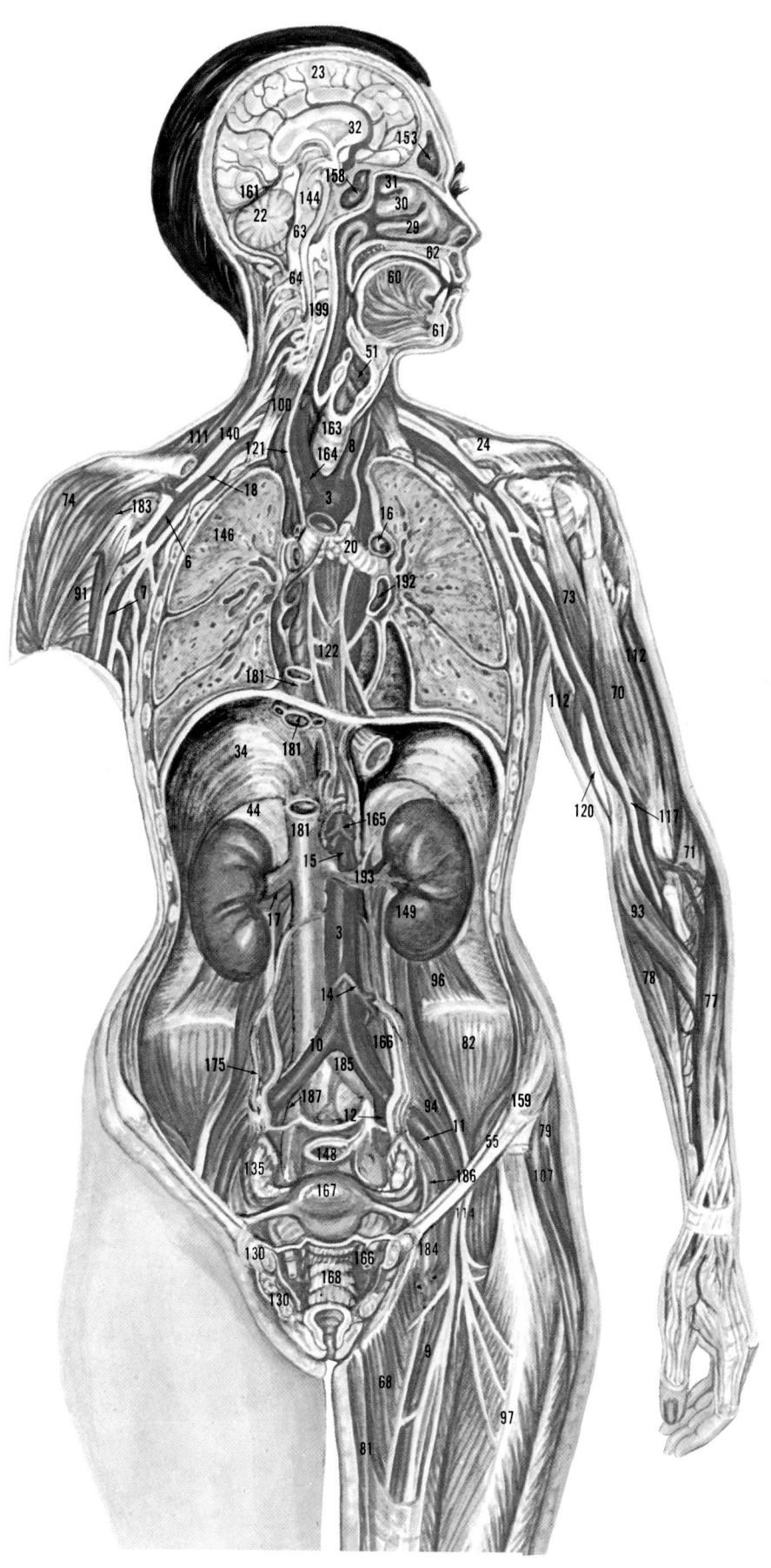

## VIEW M Posterior

See pages 2 and 10 for key to numbers

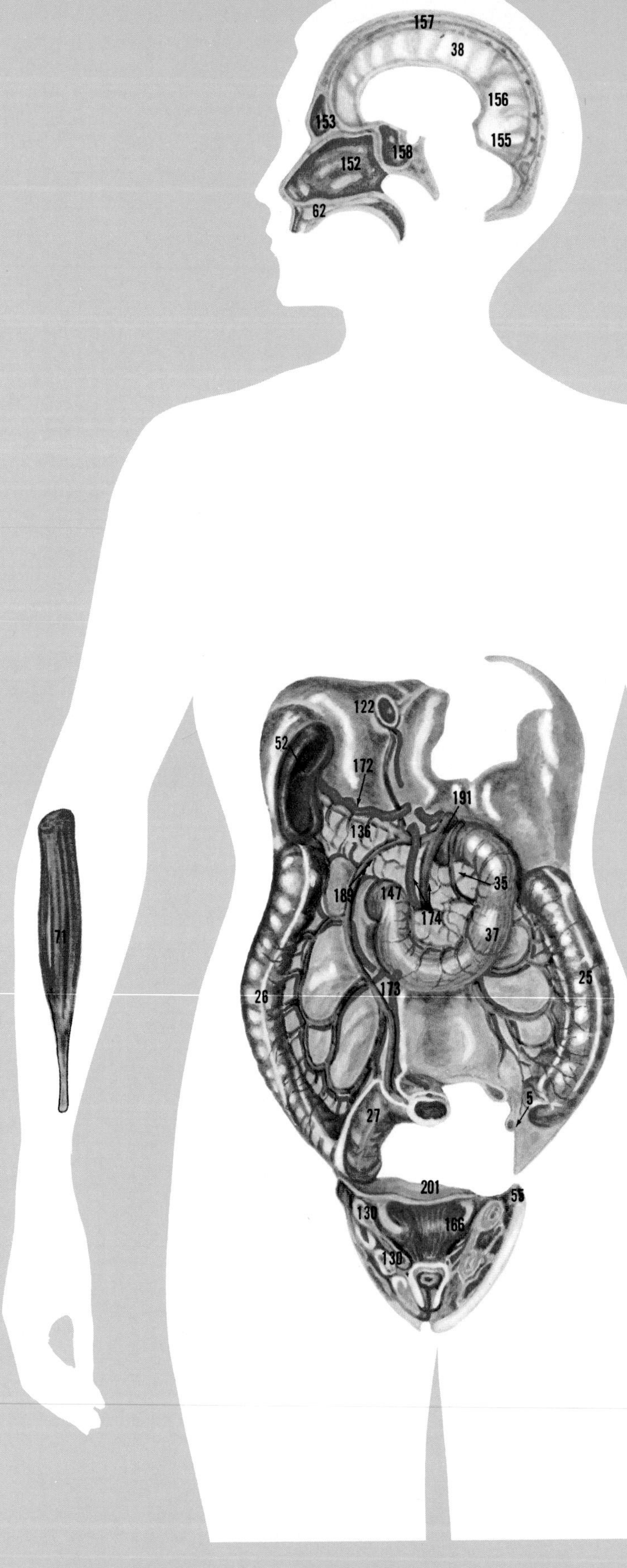

**Should the patient always tell his doctor which antibiotic he is allergic or sensitive to?**

Yes. This information is essential for the doctor to have before he prescribes for you.

**Does picking or squeezing an abscess cause more of them to develop?**

In all probability, it does.

**How does one bring an abscess to a head?**

By using warm compresses, which your doctor will prescribe for you.

**Are ointments valuable in bringing an abscess or infection to a head?**

No.

**What is the treatment when an infection or abscess has come to a head?**

The abscess or infection should be opened surgically by your doctor.

**Do abscesses and infections often subside by themselves?**

Yes. With the proper use of warm compresses and antibiotics, many infections will not have to be opened by your surgeon.

**When is an abscess or infection drained?**

When the surgeon feels that pus will exude from the region for several days, he will often place a drain to guide the pus out of the abscess or infected region.

**Should one go to work with an abscess or infection?**

Not if his temperature is elevated or if he has to use the part of the body that is involved in an abscess or infection.

**Is is often necessary to amputate a limb because of a severe infection?**

This is becoming less and less necessary all the time. There is one notable exception, namely, when the patient has gangrene of the part, as in diabetic gangrene, or when a limb has an infection secondary to the loss of its blood supply.

**What interferes with the cure of an infection of an extremity involved in diabetic gangrene?**

Diabetic gangrene is often impossible to cure because in this type of case the circulation to the extremity is so poor.

**Are vaccines helpful in preventing recurrence of infections?**

Only occasionally.

**What is the best way to prevent recurrence of infections?**

By receiving a thorough physical examination and removing any underlying cause for them.

**Do viruses or fungi often cause abscesses?**

Usually not, although both may cause severe infections. Viral pneumonia, viral hepatitis (inflammation of the liver), viral meningitis (inflammation of the membranes surrounding the brain and spinal cord), are examples of serious viral infections, but they are not accompanied by abscess formation. (See Chapter 34, on Infectious and Virus Diseases.)

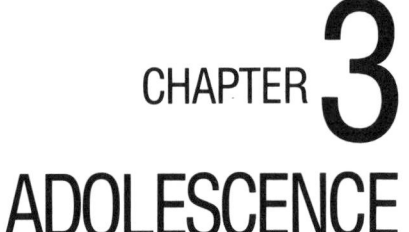

# CHAPTER 3
# ADOLESCENCE

*(See also Chapter 15 on Breasts; Chapter 17 on Child Behavior; Chapter 25 on Female Organs; Chapter 32 on Infant and Childhood Diseases; Chapter 44 on Mental Health and Disease; Chapter 64 on Sex; Chapter 65 on Skin).*

**What is considered to be the adolescent period of development?**

The teenage period, between the ages of twelve and twenty years.

**What is meant by puberty?**

This is the period when sex functions mature, roughly between twelve and fifteen years of age in girls, and thirteen and sixteen years of age in boys.

**Why is the adolescent period of life so important?**

Because it is the time when there is the most rapid growth and the most sudden changes in physical, psychological, and physiological development.

**What are the major evidences of puberty in young girls?**

a. Breast development.
b. The appearance of pubic and axillary hair.
c. The assumption of the female type of figure.
d. The onset of menstruation.

**What are the major evidences of puberty in a boy?**

a. Increase in size of the external genitals.
b. The appearance of pubic and axillary hair.
c. The appearance of hair on the face and upper lip.
d. Voice changes, with deepening in tone.
e. The development of muscles and the masculine figure.

**Does puberty tend to take place at the same age in boys and girls?**

No. Girls tend to mature one to two years earlier than boys.

**Do all girls tend to mature at the same age?**

No. There is a great latitude in the age at which these changes take place.

**Does the age at which puberty takes place tend to be the same for all the females in a family?**

Yes. It is common to find that all the girls will develop early in one family or will develop late in another family. Usually, at the onset of menstruation, a girl will be the same age her mother was when she began to menstruate.

**Is there a tendency for the age at which menstruation begins to vary in different races and in different climates?**

Yes. In warmer climates, the girls tend to mature and to menstruate at an earlier age.

**When menstruation starts, is it usually irregular for the first few months or year or two?**

Yes. It may occur every two to three weeks or may occur only once in every two to three months. Also, the amount of flow varies widely.

**How long does it usually take before a regular menstrual cycle establishes itself?**

Anywhere from one to three years.

**Is early menstrual irregularity an abnormal finding?**

No. The irregularity will usually correct itself and requires no treatment.

**Is there any relationship between the onset of menstruation and the rate of growth in a girl?**

Yes. Growth is usually completed when the menstrual cycle has become regular.

**If a young girl is irregular in her periods for a year or two, is it wise to have her examined?**

Yes. A rectal examination will give the necessary information as to the state of the uterus and ovaries. It is not necessary to do a vaginal examination on these young girls.

**At what age to the breasts usually begin to develop?**

About one year before the onset of menstruation.

**Is it common for one breast or one nipple to develop before the other?**

Yes. This happens in a fair number of children and is perfectly normal.

**Does the unequal development of the breasts mean that one breast will always remain larger than the other?**

No. The other breast will eventually catch up in its development, and both breasts will be approximately the same size.

**Is it normal for there to be pain and tenderness in the developing breasts?**

Yes. This requires no treatment, unless it is very severe.

**Should a young girl be told about menstruation before it appears?**

Yes. At about ten to twelve years of age all girls should be told about menstruation so that they are prepared for its onset. At the first signs of breast development, explanations concerning the nature of menstruation should be given.

**Who should instruct girls about adolescence, puberty, and sexual changes?**

Preferably, the child's mother. If the

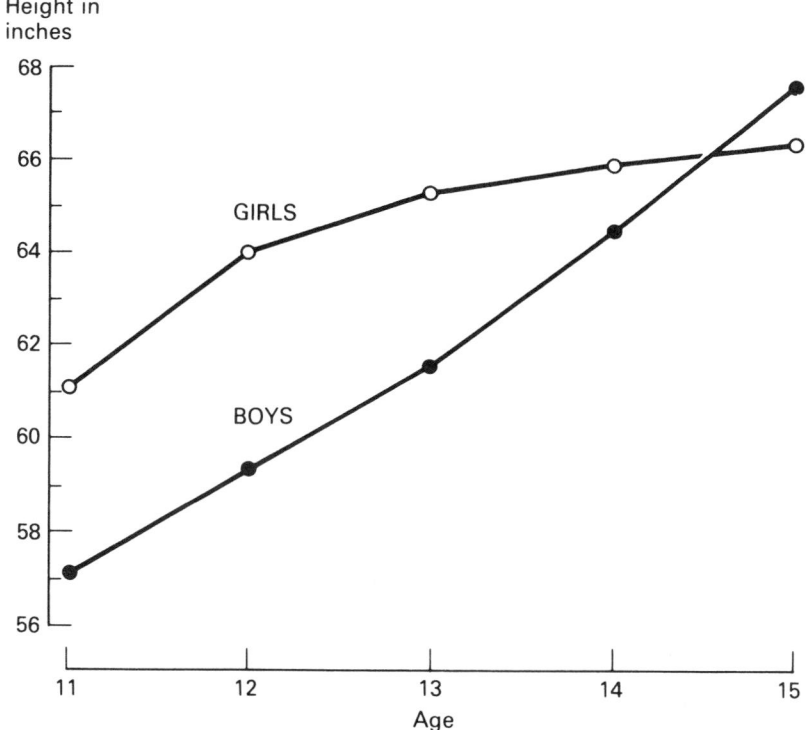

Height in inches

*Growth Chart. At the age of 11, girls are normally taller than boys. From this age on, boys grow faster, and, by the time they are 15, they are normally taller than girls.*

mother is not able to do it, then someone who is educated in the field, such as a schoolteacher or physician, should inform the child. It is best that she get the information factually from an older person rather than from her friends, who may be misinformed.

### What organs are responsible for the onset of adolescence?

The pituitary gland, the ovaries, and the testicles begin to secrete larger quantities of the sex hormones and thus bring on the changes seen in adolescents.

### Is breast enlargement ever seen in a boy during puberty?

Yes. There may be a nodule formed beneath the nipple at some time or other in boys between the ages of eleven and fifteen years.

### Does this enlargement of the

breast remain as a permanent change?

No. It usually disappears spontaneously within a few months and requires no treatment.

### Is it natural for the skin to undergo changes during the adolescent period?

Yes. Both boys and girls tend to develop pimples and blackheads during this period. This condition is called acne.

### What should be done in the way of treating acne?

There are certain specific measures, including special diet, special methods of keeping the face clean, and medications, that prove helpful.

### What are some of the more important psychological changes that take place in the adolescent boy and girl?

This is a period when a child is striv-

ing to break away from parental dependence. Such children wish to assert themselves and prepare for adult life. It is therefore a period of great conflict between parents and children. This period is characterized by a good deal of aggressiveness, restlessness, disobedience, disrespect, and awkwardness. However, during this period, a mature, warm affection develops between children and parents, provided the parents handle adolescents in a sympathetic and intelligent manner.

### How should a parent handle the psychological problems of adolescence?

First of all, the parents must recognize that this is a trying period for the child, during which he or she is undergoing many conflicts. This is a time when a child needs assurance and encouragement, warmth, love, and proper guidance.

### Why does the adolescent feel such a strong urge to be with a group of other children?

Because they are all going through the same difficult period together, and they derive comfort from associating with others with similar problems. This herding together of adolescents gives them strength to combat parental domination and to assert their individuality through group activity.

### Is it common for the adolescent child to have wide swings in his or her emotions?

Yes. During adolescence such rapid changes take place that the child is often childlike in certain respects and extremely grown-up in others.

### Is it common for children to overeat during adolescence or, in certain instances, to starve themselves?

Yes. There are all sorts of extremes of conduct and behavior during adolescence. The main effort by the parents should be directed toward sympathetic understanding of the problems their children face.

### Does major intellectual growth accompany physical growth during the period of adolescence?

Yes. Adolescents usually show tremendous intellectual strides and demonstrate widened interest in the world about them.

### What attitude should the parents adopt concerning the increased sexual urges of their children during adolescence?

This is a natural phenomenon and need not be discouraged. It is normal for boys and girls to want to get to know one another and to want to get along with each other. Sexual curiosity is part of that desire to learn more about the opposite sex and does not necessarily lead to complete sexual relations or to promiscuity. During this period, sexual curiosity should be controlled gently, and children should be directed so that their curiosity does not result in harmful pursuits.

### At what age should sex education begin?

A child should be educated gradually from his or her earliest years when he or she first evinces interest in sex. By the time adolescence is reached, children should know a great deal about sex so that they are better able to manage their sexual urges. Ignorance about sexual matters often results in unwanted pregnancies or venereal infections among young people.

### Is it natural for boys and girls to masturbate during the adolescent period?

Yes. It is important not to make them feel guilty about this practice.

### Should the adolescent be permitted to get married during the teen years?

This is usually unwise, since emotional maturity is rarely complete in teenagers. If there is a true love, it will survive the adolescent period, and there will be ample time for its full expression when both of the young people have reached maturity.

### Does late adolescence or delayed adolescence require medical treatment?

In the great majority of cases, in both boys and girls, late or delayed adolescence requires no treatment. Eventually, all children reach physical maturity without the need for medical treatment.

### Can the giving of hormones to bring about an earlier adolescence be harmful?

Yes. In certain cases the giving of hormones is not only unnecessary but may actually have a harmful effect. This is due to the fact that there is a tendency toward a slowing up of glandular function when the hormones have been discontinued.

### When should treatment be started if a girl is late in starting to menstruate?

If her physical development has otherwise been normal, it is safe to wait until she is sixteen or seventeen years of age before consulting a gynecologist. Girls who go beyond the age of seventeen or eighteen without menstruating will probably require some treatment.

### Is any treatment necessary for boys who fail to grow or develop other evidences of approaching maturity?

In the great majority of cases, unless there is an obvious defect in the function of their pituitary or thyroid gland, they will require no treatment. Eventually, they will reach maturity without treatment.

### Should precocious adolescence require the treatment of a physician?

There are unusual cases of girls who begin to mature and to menstruate at the age of seven, eight, or nine years. Also there are boys who may develop voice changes, genital enlargement, and a beard at a similar age.

These cases usually signify that there is an abnormality in the development of one of the glands. These children should have a thorough investigation by a physician. Certain cases of tumor of the pineal gland in the base of the brain will lead to such precocious development.

# CHAPTER 4

# THE ADRENAL GLANDS

*(See also Chapter 44 on Mental Health and Disease; Chapter 55 on Pituitary Gland; Chapter 72 on Thyroid Gland)*

## Where are the adrenal glands located, and what do they look like?

There are two adrenal glands, one on each side of the body, located just above the kidneys. They are somewhat triangular in shape and measure approximately two by one inches in diameter.

## What are the components of the adrenal glands?

They are each composed of two separate parts: a cortex and a medulla.

## Do these two parts of the adrenal gland have similar functions?

No. In reality they constitute two separate organs.

## What is the function of the adrenal medulla?

This portion of the gland secretes the chemical substances known as adrenalin and noradrenalin. These are hormones that are secreted into the bloodstream.

## What are the effects of adrenalin and noradrenalin?

a. They stimulate the heart by increasing the force of contraction.
b. They increase the concentration of sugar in the blood, thereby making the sugar more available to the tissues.
c. They increase the rate of coagulation of the blood.
d. They decrease muscular fatigue, thereby allowing more vigorous and more sustained physical exertion.
e. They cause blood vessels to contract, thereby channeling blood from one part of the body to another, where it may be needed more urgently.

## What is the overall effect of the secretion of adrenalin?

It prepares the body for action in response to danger or stress. It is the secretion that prepares the body for "fight or flight."

## Is the medulla of the adrenal gland ever involved in disease processes?

Yes. A tumor known as pheochromocytoma sometimes occurs within the medulla of the adrenal gland.

## What effect does a tumor of the adrenal medulla have upon the body?

This tumor will cause elevated blood pressure, attacks of anxiety, palpitation, overactive metabolism, and increased blood sugar.

## Is there any treatment for pheochromocytoma?

Yes. The tumor can often be cured by surgical removal through an incision made in the flank or through the abdomen.

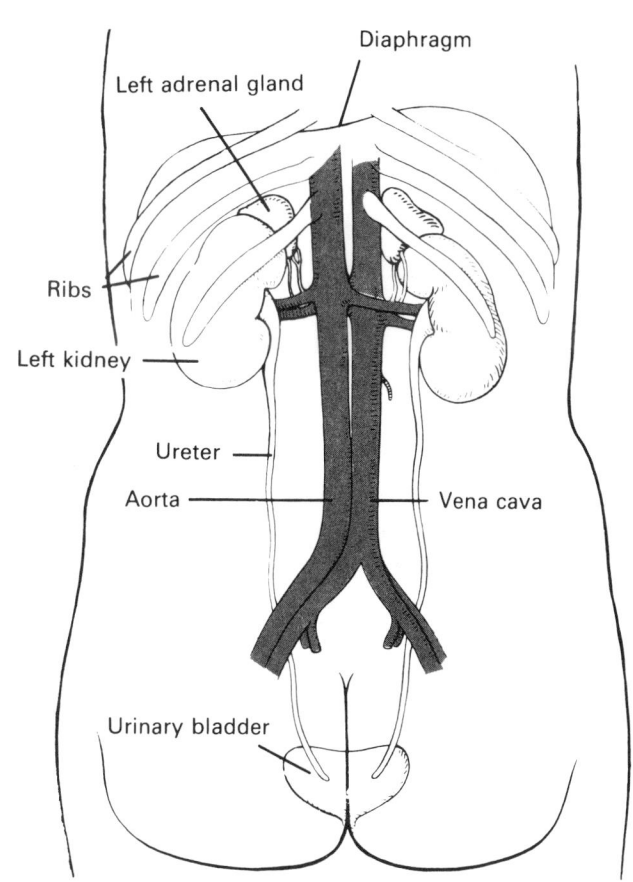

*Anatomy of the Adrenal Glands. The adrenal glands measure approximately two by one inches in diameter and are located just above the kidneys in the upper posterior part of the abdomen. They are very important organs because of the hormones and chemicals they manufacture and secrete into the bloodstream. The diagram to the left shows the view from the back, looking anteriorly.*

**Does recovery from this type of tumor usually take place after surgery?**

Yes.

**What is the function of the cortex of the adrenal gland?**

This is a very important structure, as it manufactures hormones that influence the following body functions:

a. The utilization, storage, and maintenance of body sugars, proteins, and fats.

b. The balance of water and minerals in the body.

c. The secretion of certain male and female sex hormones.

d. The manufacture of chemicals concerned with the body's response to stress, strain, and injury.

**What happens if the adrenal glands are removed or fail to function?**

The presence of the adrenal glands is important to the continuation of life. Their total removal will lead to loss of weight, debility, and eventually to death unless cortisone is given continually to maintain chemical balance by controlling salt and water quantities in the blood.

**Are there any diseases in which the cortex of the adrenals fails to function properly?**

Yes. Addison's disease is a condition in which there is a chronic deficiency of the adrenal cortex. It is a rare disease, occurring in one in a hundred thousand people.

**What are the symptoms of Addison's disease?**

There is a gradual increase of fatigability, weakness, weight loss, loss of appetite, nausea, vomiting, and emotional instability. There is also a peculiar discoloration and pigmentation of the skin and mucous membranes.

**What is the outcome of untreated Addison's disease?**

Eventually it is fatal.

**What is the present treatment of Addison's disease?**

It can be successfully treated by the use of cortisone-like hormones, which correct adrenal deficiency.

**Are there other diseases of the adrenal cortex?**

Yes, Cushing's disease. This condition is caused by an excessive production of the hormone of the adrenal cortex.

**What are the characteristics of Cushing's disease?**

a. Redistribution of fat to the upper torso, neck, and shoulders, giving the patient a "buffalo" appearance.

b. A fattened and rounded "moon" face.

c. Peculiar purplish streaks in the skin of the abdomen, thighs, and arms.

d. The development of male body characteristics in a female.

e. Elevated blood pressure.

f. Elevated blood sugar content.

**Is Cushing's disease a common disease?**

No.

**What causes Cushing's disease?**

In certain cases, a tumor of the adrenal cortex is the cause. In other cases, overactivity of normal adrenal cortex function.

**Can Cushing's disease be treated sucessfully?**

Yes.

**What is the treatment for Cushing's disease?**

a. X-ray treatment of the pituitary gland in the skull. This will cut down its stimulation of the adrenal gland, resulting in lessened adrenal secretion.

b. Surgical removal of part of the adrenal glands, or removal of any tumor that may be found to be present within the gland substance.

**What will happen if Cushing's disease goes untreated?**

The patient will succumb to it eventually, usually after a period of several years.

**Can the adrenal gland be studied through x rays?**

Yes, in certain cases, by the use of specialized techniques.

**What is Conn's syndrome?**

Recently a newly discovered entity has been described, known as Conn's syndrome. It is allegedly caused by tiny tumors of the adrenal glands, which manufacture a specialized hormone concerned with the normal maintenance of body minerals and body fluids. Patients with Conn's syndrome may display a variety of symptoms. One of the most common is high blood pressure. It has been said by authorities in this field that these tumors may be more common than hitherto believed and may be present in about 10 percent of all people who, at the present time, are grouped under essential hypertension or ordinary high blood pressure. In addition to high blood pressure, these patients may or may not display generalized weakness, periodic paralysis, excessive thirst, excessive urination, and headaches. These patients may also show a diabetic tendency. The diagnosis of this condition is quite complex and specialized. Its presence may be suspected from the aforementioned signs and symptoms, but the exact diagnosis can be made only at a few specialized research institutions. In the future, it is anticipated that such a diagnosis will be more routine and that surgery for the removal of these tumors may become a significant factor in the cure of people with high blood pressure.

**Can a patient lead a normal life with only one adrenal gland?**

Yes, if the remaining gland is normal.

**Are the adrenal glands ever removed surgically to slow down the spread of a cancer?**

Yes. It has been found in occasional cases of cancer of the breast that removal of both adrenal glands will inhibit the spread of the cancer. This form of treatment is extremely drastic and usually advocated only in those cases where cancer has already been widely disseminated throughout the body. The operative procedure is known as adrenalectomy. However, with the use of chemotherapy, adrenalectomy is used much less frequently.

**How effective is removal of the adrenal glands in cases of disseminated cancer?**

It may result in prolongation of life for a few months, or, at best, a year or two.

**Are portions of the adrenal glands ever transplanted from their normal anatomical position to another position in the body in an attempt to slow the growth of cancer?**

Yes. If both adrenal glands have been removed in an attempt to slow down the growth and spread of a breast or other cancer, it is essential that cortisone be given indefinitely. Recently, however, it has been discovered that if a portion of one gland is transplanted to a new location in the inner, upper aspect of the thigh, sufficient cortisone may reach the bloodstream to maintain life without disturbing the beneficial effects of adrenalectomy. Unfortunately, only a small percentage of these transplants survives.

**Is there any way to prevent disease of the adrenal glands?**

No way is known at present.

# CHAPTER 5

# AGING

*(See also Chapter 10 on Arthritis; Chapter 13 on Blood Vessels and Blood Vessel Surgery; Chapter 29 on Heart; Chapter 44 on Mental Health and Disease; Chapter 56 on Plastic Surgery; Chapter 59 on Prostate Gland; Chapter 73 on Transplantation of Organs)*

## Are aging processes fully understood?

No. This entire subject is now undergoing widespread investigation, and many of our present thoughts will eventually be modified or changed.

## When do people start to grow old?

There is no set age at which people show signs of growing old. Some people demonstrate aging in their twenties, while others are young in their sixties or seventies.

## Are there evidences of aging in childhood?

Yes. Certain anatomic changes indicate that the aging process begins at birth. Thus, our span depends to a great extent on how slow or how rapid the process may be.

## Do various organs in the body age at different rates of speed?

Yes. Someone in his seventies may have certain organs that show practically no evidence of degeneration, while other structures show extreme evidences of deterioration. In a woman, for example, the ovaries age at the change of life, long before there may be overt evidence of aging elsewhere in the body.

## Do mental aging (senility) and physical aging tend to go together?

Not necessarily. Many people become mentally senile at a time when their bodies are in good condition, whereas others retain alert, young minds long after their physical structures have become old. The latter situation occurs more often than the former.

## What determines longevity?

There are so many important and qualifying factors that it is impossible to list them specifically. The type of organs and the type of body structure one has inherited are important factors, but so are the many illnesses, stresses, and the degree of wear and tear to which the body is subject throughout a lifetime. A frail body that has not been afflicted by ravaging illness, organ damage, or other stresses may outlive a strong body that has experienced serious and repeated assaults of disease and injury.

## Is longevity inherited?

The type of anatomical structures one possesses as well as their susceptibility to stress and illness is, to a great extent, inherited. However, longevity will depend on what happens to these organs in the course of a lifetime. For instance, good blood vessels will afford no protection against the development of a fatal infection or malignant tumor. Therefore, it can be said that we inherit only a *tendency* toward longevity.

## Does an early adolescence have any bearing on the age at which one will show signs of growing old?

No.

## What bearing does a late adolescence have on the aging process?

None.

## Do all members of one family have the same tendencies as far as aging is concerned?

No. Each member of a family has his own combination of inherited genes. *Tendencies* toward longevity may be present in some members of a family and absent in others.

## Do strenuous physical exercise and athletics in youth influence the rate at which one ages?

No, unless one has seriously damaged an organ or structure in youth. This happens only rarely. It is *not* true that athletes have a tendency to die young.

## Does sexual activity influence the rate at which one ages?

No.

## What effect does illness in earlier life have upon aging?

If there has been serious chronic or recurrent disease in earlier life, it can damage important organs and lead to premature aging.

## Will well-regulated physical exercise during early and middle age tend to lengthen life?

Insofar as it aids someone in keeping his body fit, intelligent exercise will aid longevity. It has been demonstrated statistically and it is the common belief of most heart specialists that moderate exercise, such as walking, swimming, golfing, cycling, etc., has a beneficial effect upon heart muscle and heart blood vessels, and that the incidence of heart attacks appears to be less in those so engaged.

## Is there any way in which a physician can predict at what age a young person will begin to show signs of growing old?

Only if there are obvious signs of disease in major organs.

## Are there any laboratory or clinical tests that can give an accurate indication of early aging before it is noticed on physical examination?

No, but certain tests may show diminished function of the vital organs. In this way, one may learn of the possibilities for continued good health.

**Does one inherit a tendency toward the premature aging of certain organs? For example, if one's parents showed early loss of sight or early loss of hearing, will the children have the same tendency?**

One may inherit a tendency, but it is not always confined to specific organs.

**What determines the age at which a man loses potency?**

This will vary markedly, as loss of potency is more likely to be a psychological rather than a physical phenomenon. Many men may retain their potency well into the eighth decade of life.

**Are there any medications or hormones that can be taken to forestall the onset of aging?**

Not at present, but there are certain substances that may, at some time in the future, be beneficial in this regard.

**Are there any rejuvenation operations that are valuable or successful?**

Not at the present time.

**Does excessive drinking of alcoholic beverages result in premature aging?**

It may, if continued over a period of many years. Large quantities of alcohol may interfere with a well-regulated diet and may lead to liver disease, or disease of other vital organs.

**What part does adequate sleep play in the aging process?**

Inadequate sleep is definitely detrimental and may be a factor in premature aging. Loss of sleep cannot be made up.

**Does smoking tend to make one grow old prematurely?**

The weight of accumulating evidence would indicate that smoking, especially one or more packages of cigarettes a day, predisposes the body to cancer of the lung, cancer of the bladder, coronary artery disease, heart attacks, chronic bronchitis, and pulmonary emphysema. It has also been shown statistically that relatively heavy smokers of cigarettes have a reduced longevity due both to the causes just mentioned and to others not quite understood at the present time.

**What role does diet play in the rate at which one grows old?**

Diet plays an extremely important role in longevity. An inadequate or suboptimum diet often leads to defective body metabolism. On the other hand, a high cholesterol diet may lead to premature arteriosclerosis. Also, obesity due to overeating can place an inordinate strain upon the heart and blood vessels.

**Can an emotionally disturbed life lead to premature aging?**

Yes.

**Will the bearing of many children cause a woman to age prematurely?**

No.

**Is it true that people who work particularly hard at physical labors tend to grow old earlier?**

No. Other things being equal, sedentary people are more prone to earlier aging.

**What diseases lead to premature aging?**

Any serious, chronic, or recurrent disease.

**Will medical science ever prolong the span of life beyond the proverbial "three score and ten"?**

Yes.

**How does the span of life today compare to that of fifty years ago?**

It is much longer today.

**What is the average life expectancy for healthy young adults today?**

For men, about seventy years. For women, about seventy-four years.

**Is it true that people tend to live longer in warm, equable climates?**

Not necessarily, but it is true that extremes of temperature are difficult for some individuals to tolerate and may play a role in shortening their lives by causing them to take ill more frequently.

**Do people who have undergone frequent surgery tend to have shorter lives?**

Not necessarily, if recovery was complete and the conditions for which they underwent surgery were of a curable type.

**Do married people tend to live longer?**

Yes, probably because they monitor one another's health and thus seek medical help earlier than single people.

**Can a physician tell if a patient is aging prematurely?**

Yes, by performing a thorough physical examination.

**Do lapses in memory, occurring in middle life, indicate that one is growing old prematurely?**

No. These are most often emotional in origin.

**Should physical exercise be abandoned when one reaches middle age?**

Not if one has been accustomed to regular exercise during younger life.

**Does vitamin intake have any effect upon the length of life?**

If there is a chronic vitamin deficiency from an inadequate diet, life may be shortened. The life span is not lengthened when a healthy person takes excess vitamins.

**Does an early menopause indicate that a woman is aging prematurely?**

No. It indicates merely that the female organs are aging prematurely. This may or may not be associated with premature aging of other structures.

**At the time of the menopause is there any advantage in artificially stimulating periodic menstrual cycles by taking female hormones?**

During the past few years, a new school has arisen composed of endocrinologists and gynecologists who feel that the aging processes seen after the menopause, such as skin changes, bone changes, coronary artery changes, and other signs of aging, can be delayed by supplying hormones either by mouth or by injection on a cyclical basis. However, at the present time, there is insufficient data to substantiate these dramatic claims, and it is possible that there are dangers in pursuing such a program, such as an increased incidence of cancer of the uterus.

**Is it true that people tend to have their best ideas when they are young or in middle life, and that people are not as creative when they reach their sixties and seventies?**

This as a general rule, is true. However, there are innumerable exceptions.

**Is it possible to live into the seventies and eighties even if one has hardening of the arteries, high blood pressure, or heart trouble?**

Yes.

**Do people who look old tend to live shorter lives?**

No. The appearance of the skin is but one small diagnostic finding and does not necessarily indicate the state of health of the vital organs.

**Is premature graying of the hair an indication that one is aging prematurely?**

No.

**Do people with well-developed muscles and good physiques tend to live longer than people with poor muscular development?**

Not necessarily, but it is true that a routine of sensible physical exercise is conducive to maintaining good health.

**Do thin people tend to live longer than fat people?**

Yes.

**Does the early loss of teeth indicate premature aging?**

Not necessarily. Premature loss of teeth may be the result of neglect.

**Is there any way to slow up the aging process once it has begun?**

Yes, by eating a sensible diet, avoiding overweight, avoiding excesses of all types, attempting to reduce the stresses and strains of daily living, and receiving prompt treatment for any prevailing illness.

**What is Alzheimer's Disease (AD)?**

Alzheimer's Disease is a progressive disorder of the brain causing loss of memory or serious mental deterioration. Little is known about the cause of this disorder, but research shows that nerve endings in the cortex of the brain degenerate and disrupt the passage of electrochemical signals between the cells. The areas of degeneration have a characteristic appearance under the microscope and are called "plaques." In addition, the nerve cells, themselves, develop abnormal fibers called neurofibrillary tangles. The larger the number of these two abnormalities—plaques and tangles—the greater the disturbance in intellectual function and memory.

The condition is not caused by

hardening of the arteries, nor is it contagious. It is estimated that the disease affects from 500,000 to 1.5 million middle-aged and older Americans, or about 2-3 percent of the general population over 60 years of age. AD does not usually affect more than one member of the family.

**What are the symptoms?**

There are many patterns in the type, severity, and sequence of mental changes in A.D. Usually, the symptoms are progressive but vary greatly in the rate of change from person to person. In a few cases, there may be rapid mental deterioration, but often, there are long periods in which little change is noted. However, the progressive deterioration which occurs is a source of deep concern and frustration for both the victim and the family.

As the disease progresses, the changes in the nerve cells produce simple forgetfulness and increasingly more noticable memory loss. Changes in thought, language, personality, and behavior can eventually render the person incapable of taking care of himself or communicating his needs to others.

**How is the Diagnosis Made?**

The diagnosis of Alzheimer's Disease is made after other illnesses (affecting memory loss) area ruled out; such as brain tumors, strokes, infections, and spinal-cord abnormalities. Diagnostic techniques are needed to differentiate the various causes of dementia. These techniques include computer tomography (CT scan), studies of the spinal fluid system and electroencephalography (EEG). Comprehensive blood studies and metabolic tests are also conducted.

A thorough physical, neurological, and psychiatric examination is necessary to rule out several other conditions which mimic the symptoms of AD. Some of these related disorders are Creutzfeld-Jakob disease, Pick's disease, or cerebral vascular disease. A diagnosis of AD can be made on the basis of history, mental status and course of the disease.

### What is the Treatment?

Medical care can *relieve many of the symptoms* of AD but prevention or cure of the disease is not known. Counseling can help the victim and his family in coping with the illness. A neurologist, psychiatrist, or family physician should closely monitor treatment and have the time and interest to answer the variety of questions that arise. Medication can be prescribed to improve sleeping patterns. Proper nutrition, exercise and physical therapy can aid difficulties that arise in physical functioning. Social contacts should be encouraged. A list of daily tasks, written reminders, and safety measures can assist the individual in day-to-day living. It is best to maintain an ordered environment so that the afflicted person does not have to continuously learn new things.

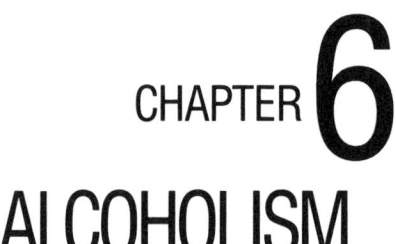

# CHAPTER 6

# ALCOHOLISM

*(See also Chapter 40 on Liver; Chapter 43 on Medications and Drugs)*

## What is alcoholism?

Alcoholism is a chronic ailment associated with prolonged heavy alcohol abuse. It is manifested by an inability to control drinking and by the consequences of repeated inebriation. Alcoholism usually results in impairment of family relationships and working activities. Eventually, alcoholism leads to damage to one's physical and mental health.

## Are there various stages in alcohol addiction?

Yes. It may begin with just occasional episodes of drunkenness, with brief periods of incapacitation. These episodes are repeated more often until heavy drinking on a regular basis ensues. Finally, the individual loses control over his drinking and shows marked emotional, psychological, social, and physical impairment.

## How does one distinguish between a heavy drinker and a true alcoholic?

A true alcoholic loses control over his drinking and shows signs of physical and psychological impairment. The heavy social drinker does not proceed to the above state, but maintains a workable control over his alcohol intake.

## Does alcoholism tend to be hereditary?

The *tendency* is now thought by a great many investigators to have hereditary aspects. Recent studies of identical twins indicate this tendency. An interesting hereditary pattern relates to the fact that depressive male parents frequently have alcoholic daughters.

## What is a blackout?

This condition, also known as alcoholic amnesia, is a period of memory loss associated with heavy drinking. A person experiencing a blackout may engage in complicated social or working functions, awaken after the episode is over, and have no recollection of the previous period of activity.

## What are some of the causes of alcoholism?

The exact cause is not known. However, some of the predisposing causes are:

a. A family history of alcoholism.

b. Anxiety states, which lead an individual to reduce his anxiety through drinking.

c. A state of depression, which leads a person to seek relief through alcohol.

d. Social pressures within a family where heavy drinking is an accepted activity.

e. A combination of the above situations may lead to alcoholism, particularly in a predisposed individual.

## Can alcoholism be prevented?

Yes, if efforts are aimed at therapy of the children of alcoholics during their formative years. Also, people who have a family history of alcoholism should be urged never to drink at all.

## Is it possible to foretell by physical examination whether one is predisposed to becoming an alcoholic?

No. (At one time it was thought that people with chronically low blood pressure or glandular deficiencies were more prone to becoming alcoholics. This has not proven to be true.)

## Are the breathing tests and blood tests accurate in determining whether a person is under the influence of alcohol?

Yes. Alcohol intoxication can be diagnosed by either method.

## What organs are most affected by alcoholism?

a. The nervous system. Both brain cells and nerves in the arms and legs can be permanently damaged by alcohol addiction.

b. The esophagus (foodpipe), stomach, and duodenum may become involved in severe chronic inflammation or ulcer-formation as a result of chronic alcoholism.

c. Cirrhosis of the liver with death of liver cells is a common complication of chronic alcohol abuse.

d. The heart. The muscles of the heart may become markedly weakened and the process of arteriosclerosis may be hastened.

## Does chronic alcoholism often shorten the life span?

Definitely, yes. First of all, fatal accidents occur with much greater frequency among alcoholics. Secondly, damage to the brain, the nervous system, the liver, the heart, and the gastrointestinal tract often results in premature death.

## What are the most common alcohol-related damages to the nervous system?

a. Loss of brain power and intelligence if the alcoholism persists over a long period of time.

b. Acute episodes of irrational behavior with loss of contact with reality, as in delirium tremens (D.T.'s) or Korsakoff's psychosis.

c. Permanent loss of balance due to damage to nerves.

d. Pain and loss of sensation in the arms and legs.

## What are the symptoms of delirium tremens (D.T.'s)?

A state of psychosis (insanity) in an

alcoholic, who, following a heavy bout of drinking, abruptly interrupts his alcohol intake. The condition is manifested by exhaustion, marked agitation, visual hallucinations, tremors, and severe perspiration. Sometimes, high fever, metabolic imbalance, and death can ensue if treatment is not begun promptly.

### Can chronic alcohol abuse in a pregnant woman affect her unborn child?

Yes. It has been noted that children born to alcoholic mothers have a tendency to be smaller than normal and underweight at birth. They learn to talk much later than normal children, and they tend to have low I.Q.'s (intelligence quotients). Also, as they develop, they tend to have difficulty getting along with other children.

### What is the "fetal alcohol syndrome"?

It is associated with the deficiencies listed above, taking place in the children of alcoholic mothers.

### During what period of pregnancy is it most dangerous for women to drink?

During the first three months, when the child is developing so rapidly.

### Can an alcoholic woman avoid damage to a subsequent pregnancy by stopping all drinking before and during the pregnancy?

Yes.

### Are intoxicated people dangerous?

Yes. Statistics show that 60 percent of fatal automobile accidents, suicides, and murders are alcohol connected.

### Is alcoholism limited to one period of life?

No. It can affect children, adolescents, young adults, middle-aged people, and the elderly.

### Is alcoholism more common among males?

It was formerly, but now alcoholism is approximately as prevalent among both sexes. However, women more often hide their affliction.

### What is the modern approach toward the treatment of alcoholism?

It will consist of medical, psychiatric, social, and self-help therapy. Most effective treatment will include the use of group therapy, the administration of a medication known as Antabuse, and participation in an organization called Alcoholics Anonymous.

### What is Antabuse?

The drug Antabuse, also known as disulfiram, when taken with alcohol, will form a toxic substance, which makes the patient extremely sick. Knowing that he will become very sick, the person taking Antabuse often refrains from drinking.

### Should alcoholics take tranquilizers regularly?

No. The prolonged use of tranquilizers merely attempts to substitute one dependency for another. However, in certain acute phases of alcoholism such as delirium tremens or in situations where an alcoholic becomes violent, tranquilizers may be beneficial.

### What are the indications for intensive psychiatric treatment in alcoholism?

Psychiatric therapy is indicated in the alcoholic who also has an emotional or mental disability. Good results are obtained when psychiatric care is aimed at the control of the underlying depression, which may have been an important factor in the development of alcoholism.

### Is it true that alcoholics can revert to controlled drinking?

Although some studies have indicated the possibility of reduced drinking as a means of cure among alcoholics, this is generally regarded as the exception, not the rule. Alcoholism is considered to be a progressive process of lifelong duration that can only be controlled by a state of sobriety. In the light of present knowledge, the aphorism of A.A., "Once an alcoholic, always an alcoholic," appears to be true.

### What is the treatment for D.T.'s?

Patients with delirium tremens are best treated in a hospital where they can receive sedation in the form of tranquilizer drugs, intravenous medications, and vitamins. Usually the illness subsides within three to five days.

### What is a comprehensive treatment program for alcoholics?

A comprehensive treatment program includes a biomedical approach, with psychotherapy when indicated, and efforts directed toward long-range vocational rehabilitation. These goals are best achieved in Centers in which all supportive facilities are available. Specifically, comprehensive treatment should include the following:

a. A short period of hospitalization, including detoxification.
b. Partial hospitalization to foster sobriety. This phase is accomplished in facilities known as "halfway" or "quarter-way" houses.
c. The continued use of Antabuse.
d. For some patients, the drug lithium carbonate may be prescribed on an ongoing basis.
e. Membership in Alcoholics Anonymous and full participation in its activities.
f. Frequent attendance at group therapy sessions.
g. Psychotherapy when indicated.

### Can true chronic alcoholism ever be cured?

Yes. Contrary to common belief, success is often obtained, especially among those who follow the program outlined above.

# CHAPTER 7

# ALLERGY

*(See also Chapter 24 on Eyes; Chapter 43 on Medications and Drugs; Chapter 48 on Nose and Sinuses; Chapter 65 on Skin and Subcutaneous Tissues; Chapter 75 on Upper Respiratory Diseases)*

### What is an allergy?

Allergy is a state of abnormal sensitivity to a substance or substances that ordinarily cause little or no irritation to people without this sensitivity.

### What kinds of things may produce allergy?

Almost anything that we touch, swallow, or inhale may cause an allergic response. Substances that produce allergies are called allergens. There are literally hundreds of allergens.

### What are some of the most common allergens?

The pollen of trees, grasses, and weeds; mold spores, house dust, animal hairs; certain foods, drugs, dyes, cosmetics, chemicals, etc.

### How can one tell if he has an allergy?

The most common symptoms are sneezing paroxysms and nasal stuffiness, wheezing and shortness of breath, itching of the skin, large swellings, and hives. Also, it is known that allergies can manifest themselves in vomiting, diarrhea, abdominal cramps, headaches, severe rashes, and other symptoms.

### Can allergies be dangerous?

Yes. Untreated hay fever may develop into asthma and sinusitis. Asthma, when not brought under control, can cause chronic disability and make a person susceptible to other serious respiratory conditions.

### Is it important to make an early diagnosis of an allergic condition?

Yes. By treating certain allergies in their early stages, more serious complications, such as asthma or permanent lung conditions, can be avoided. This is particularly important with children, who may become markedly retarded if their allergies are not brought under control at an early age.

### What are some of the most common allergic diseases?

a. Hay fever.
b. Perennial allergic rhinitis or vasomotor rhinitis.
c. Bronchial asthma.
d. Eczema (atopic dermatitis).
e. Hives (urticaria) or giant hives (angioedema).
f. Contact dermatitis, such as poison ivy.
g. Migraine (sick headache).

### Are allergies curable?

In a great many instances, the removal of the cause of the allergy (the allergen), such as a dog or a cat, may cure the patient permanently. In other instances, a course of hyposensitization injections may relieve the patient completely.

### Must allergy patients be treated indefinitely?

Not always. A degree of hyposensitization can sometimes be obtained so that no further treatment is necessary. However, a great many people have to be treated as long as the allergen continues to cause symptom.

### Can allergies be prevented?

In a general way, yes. People who know they are allergic can avoid the substances that are the cause of their allergy. Thus, they should avoid drives into the country during the pollen season; keep away from house dust as much as possible; try not to breathe fumes from paint; and they should attempt to avoid fatigue and excess emotional strain.

### What are the common causes for allergies in small infants and young children?

The foods they eat and the substances that are used to care for their bodies.

### Can allergies be prevented in children who, by inheritance, will have unusual allergic tendencies?

Yes. Boiled milk and evaporated milk should be used, as they are less likely to cause allergy than raw milk. All new foods should be added to such an infant's diet one by one, so that the mother can tell when an allergic response occurs. Solid foods such as egg and fish should be added to the diet at a later age. The bedroom and playroom should be as dust free as possible, and animals such as dogs, cats, and birds, and even stuffed animal toys, should be kept away from these children. It is very important to inform the attending pediatrician of the infant's family history of allergy.

### Are allergies inherited?

Most allergists believe that the tendency to develop the disease, rather than the disease itself, is inherited. This means that a child whose father or mother is allergic is much more likely to develop an allergy than one whose parents are not allergic.

### Do children tend to develop the same allergy as their parents?

Not necessarily. A child whose parent has hay fever may develop asthma, eczema, or another allergic condition.

### Do children of two allergic parents develop allergies more readily than those with one allergic parent?

Yes. They develop their allergies earlier and in a more serious form.

**If both parents are allergic, what are the chances of the children being allergic?**

Fifty percent of them will be allergic. When one parent is allergic, the possibility is approximately 25 percent.

**Do allergies ever subside and go away by themselves?**

Yes, but not very often.

**Do allergies tend to recur after they have been cured or arrested?**

Occasionally, yes. Or, more commonly, the patient may develop a new sensitivity.

**Are allergies ever fatal?**

They are only rarely fatal. Occasionally, a marked sensitivitiy to a drug may prove fatal. Also, once in a great while, death may result from the stings of bees, yellow jackets, hornets, or wasps if the individual is extremely sensitive.

**Do allergies tend to be seasonal?**

Some are, some are not. People sensitive to tree pollens will have symptoms in April and May; those sensitive to atmospheric molds will have symptoms during hot, humid weather; and those allergic to grasses will have their hay fever in May and June. Most hay fever occurs in August and September, when the weeds, especially ragweed, pollinate.

**What are pollens?**

They are fine, powdery, yellowish grains, microscopic in size, which are the fertilizing elements of flowering plants, trees, grasses, and ragweed.

**Are allergies ever contagious, like colds?**

No. Allergies are not transmitted from person to person by contact.

**Are any age groups particularly prone to allergy?**

No. Allergy may develop at any age.

The most common time to develop allergies, however, is in childhood.

**Why is it that someone who is well for many years can suddenly develop an allergy?**

It is a well-known fact that prolonged contact with certain substances is necessary in some cases before allergy will develop. Also, emotional disturbances, excessive fatigue, and infection are among the potent causes for the abrupt development of allergic symptoms in a person who has previously had no symptoms. Changes that occur in an individual at puberty, menopause, or during pregnancy are also great influences that may upset an allergic balance and cause symptoms of an allergy to appear.

**Is it true that for a person to become allergic he must have had allergic tendencies all his life?**

Yes. He will develop an allergy when, because of some disturbance, he is thrown out of allergic balance.

**Are allergies psychosomatic?**

No. It is true that emotions such as anxiety, fear, anger, and strong excitement may precipitate or intensify an allergic attack. It is also true that certain allergies will tend to disappear when the patient is receiving psychiatric help. However, this does not deny the physical basis of allergy, for the presence of an allergic tendency exists despite one's state of mind. Parents of allergic children should try to maintain an attitude of reassurance and calm, for in such an atmosphere the child will react less violently to his allergies.

**Does nervousness ever cause allergy?**

No. However, there is a definite relationship between the two.

**How common is allergy in the United States?**

At least 30 percent of the population

of this country has some kind of allergy. Allergic disorders are third in the U.S. Public Health Service list of chronic diseases. Only arthritic and cardiovascular disorders are more frequent.

**Are allergic people usually sensitive to more than one substance (allergen)?**

Yes.

**What are the most common causes of allergy?**

Pollen, mold spores, dust, strong fumes, animal hairs, feathers, and various foods. Also, drugs, serums, antitoxins, dyes, perfumes, plastics, and numerous other chemicals used in the home and in industry, as well as the bites or stings of insects.

**How can a patient learn whether or not he is allergic and what substance is causing it?**

His physician will take a thorough history and make a study of his environment at home and at work, his living habits, and his recreations. From this study he will determine the extent of these factors and will resort to certain laboratory tests. Using extracts of many of the more common allergens, he will perform various skin tests for evidence of hypersensitivity. It is real detective work, requiring skill and patience.

**Are skin tests always reliable?**

Unfortunately, no. An individual may show certain positive reactions without being really sensitive to those agents causing the reaction, or he may show negative reactions and still be sensitive. The interpretation of the skin test depends upon the physician's knowledge and experience in the field of allergy. Skin tests with inhalants are much more reliable than those with foods.

**Are skin tests painful?**

Not when properly performed. There may be a slight sting when the tests are made, but this should not cause much discomfort.

## What is the indirect method of performing allergy tests?

In this method, serum obtained from the blood of the allergic patient is injected into several sites in the skin of a nonallergic individual. After a certain length of time has elapsed, the allergy tests are then done on these sites. This method is used when the patient himself has a poor or diseased skin, which is not suitable for the allergy tests.

## Should allergic patients be particularly careful about taking medications or injections for conditions other than allergic conditions?

Yes! It is wise for an allergic patient to inform his physician about the allergy before taking any new medication or injection.

## How are allergies treated?

The first and most important step is diagnosis. The allergist will attempt to determine, by taking a detailed history, just what is causing the trouble. He may insist that the patient keep a diary of his activities and everything he eats. He may place him on trial diets. Extensive skin tests may be necessary. When the causes are found, and there may be several, avoidance of these causes is prescribed. If there is no practical way to avoid the responsible allergen, the allergist will prescribe drugs that tend to suppress allergic symptoms. He may give the patient gradually increased injections of the substance involved, such as pollen, molds, or dust. These injections help to increase the patient's tolerance to the allergen and consequently will effect a subsidence or arrest of the symptoms.

## If it is found that an animal is the cause of an allergy, should the individual give up the pet?

Yes. It is almost impossible to fully desensitize an allergic patient to a house pet.

## If the patient discovers that the allergen is in a food, can he always avoid eating that food?

This is very difficult, as some of these ingredients are not obvious in certain foods. But the patient must learn to avoid those foods containing substances to which he is allergic.

## How effective are the antihistaminic drugs?

The antihistaminic drugs, and there are many of them on the market, are very helpful in reducing the symptoms of hay fever and hives, but are not very effective in reducing the discomfort of asthma. In fact, they should not be given to adults with asthma. Occasionally, asthma in young children is helped by the administering of antihistaminic drugs.

## How effective are ACTH, cortisone, and other steroid hormones in the treatment of allergic conditions?

They are very effective in depressing the symptoms of all allergic conditions, including asthma. However, the conditions reappear as soon as the drugs are discontinued, unless the allergic cause has been otherwise removed. Since these drugs are too potent and have too many undesirable side effects to be prescribed continuously, they are best used only in an emergency or for the most stubborn type of case.

## Are there advantages to the patient in going to an allergist who specializes in the field, or can any physician serve as well?

Wherever possible, the patient should be directed to a specialist in the field. Allergy has become such a complex specialty that only those who have devoted years of study, thought, investigation, and experience to the field are properly equipped to treat allergies successfully.

## Will taking vitamins help to eliminate allergy?

No.

## Are sinus infections caused by allergy?

No. Sinus infection is not caused by allergy, but allergic people are particularly susceptible to the development of such infections. Conversely, many conditions labeled sinus infection are really nothing more than nasal allergies.

## Is acne or psoriasis caused by an allergy?

No.

## What is a mold?

Mold is a fungus, which grows on vegetable matter. Housewives know it as something that spoils bread or mildews clothes. Molds grow on wheat, corn, oats, grasses, leaves, and soil and thrive during the warm months of the year. The spores of molds are even smaller than pollen and are found in the air in large numbers. Next to pollen, mold spores are the most important cause of seasonal allergy of the respiratory organs. The season of mold allergy is long. Mold spores may be present in the air at all times of the year except when there is snow on the ground.

## Where does house dust come from?

The sources of house dust are woolen carpets and rugs, feather pillows, hair- and cotton-filled mattresses, quilts, comforters, heavy draperies, and upholstered furniture. House dust is present in large quantities in rooms in which these materials are found, regardless of the fact that thorough housecleaning has been done.

# HAY FEVER

## What is hay fever?

A respiratory allergy caused by sensitivity to pollens or molds, or both. The spring and summer types are due mainly to the pollen of trees and grasses and to mold spores. The autumn type, which begins about the middle of August and lasts until the end of September or until early frost, is usually caused by ragweed pollen and mold spores.

## What are the symptoms of hay fever?

Inflamed, itchy, and weepy eyes, a stuffed-up, clogged, or running nose, burning and itching of the nose, the eyes, the palate, and the throat. There are paroxysms of sneezing, which come on suddenly and continue for a few minutes to a few hours. Infections of the sinuses are commonly associated with hay fever. In some cases, asthma may develop during the hay fever season.

## How does hay fever get into the body?

The pollen is inhaled. In certain people, the inhaled pollens or molds (allergens), after repeated exposure, produce antibodies within the body. It may take months or years before these antibodies are formed. Until such time, no symptoms occur. However, when sufficient numbers of these sensitizing antibodies have been produced, repeated contact of the pollen, mold, or dust with the tissues will produce hay fever.

## Is rose fever the same as hay fever?

Rose fever is a name that has more or less fallen into disuse but is used to describe a form of hay fever. It is not caused by roses but by the pollen of grasses.

## Is hay fever caused by goldenrod?

No. It is caused by the pollen of ragweed in most cases.

## Is hay fever contagious?

No.

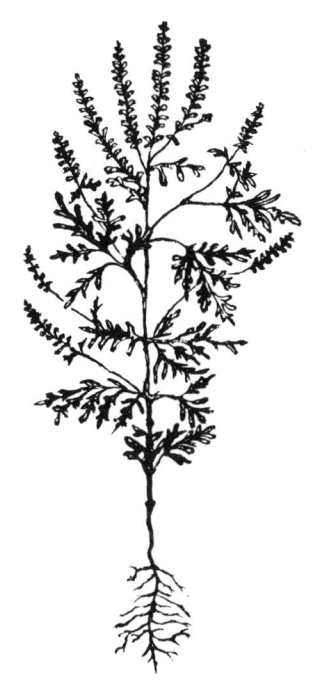

*Ragweed Plants Whose Pollen Causes Hay Fever.* The ragweed plant is one of the greatest causes of hay fever in this country. A tremendous amount of pollen is released by a single ragweed cluster (right) during the course of one day. This pollen is wind-borne and may travel for hundreds of miles before it settles.

## Is hay fever inherited?

The tendency is definitely inherited.

## What is year-round hay fever?

This condition is also called allergic rhinitis and frequently is confused with inflammation of the sinuses. In year-round hay fever, the itchy, watery eyes, sneezing, and running nose continue all year. However, it is caused by nonseasonal allergens, such as house dust, feathers, animal hairs, or even foods. In some cases, bacterial infection may be the cause.

## What is the influence of weather on hay fever?

The severity of hay fever depends upon the amount of pollen in the air and the degree of sensitivity of the patient. On a cool, cloudy, windless, or rainy day, the average patient may have practically no symptoms. When the weather is hot, dry, sunny, or windy, the patient will have increased symptoms. If patients are susceptible to wet or dampness, their symptoms become worse on cool or rainy days. Most pollen is released from the plants between 6:00 A.M. and 1:00 P.M. Therefore, this is the worst time of day for hay fever patients.

## How common is hay fever?

Approximately 4 percent of the population of the United States is affected by hay fever.

## How is hay fever diagnosed?

By a study of the history of the patient, and by skin tests with pollens and molds.

## Can substances other than the pollen aggravate hay fever?

Yes. During the pollinating season, such things as tobacco smoke, fresh paint, strong perfumes, spray insecticides, and house dust may be responsible for aggravating the symptoms of hay fever. Also, the eating of chocolate, corn, melons, especially cantaloupe and honeydew, and other seasonal fruits, such as cherries and peaches, may aggravate the symptoms.

## Does hay fever ever clear up without treatment?

Yes, but very infrequently.

## What can happen if hay fever is not treated?

In the East, approximately 25 to 30 percent of untreated hay fever patients eventually will develop asthma; in the Midwest, approximately 50 to 60 percent of untreated patients will develop asthma.

## What is the treatment for hay fever?

There are three main methods:
a. Coseasonal method. In this method the patient is treated during the period when the plants are

pollinating. Treatment must be given daily, or every other day, to control the symptoms.

b. Preseasonal method. Here, treatment is begun about three months before the pollinating season starts, and the injections are given at five- to seven-day intervals to build up a tolerance that will be maximal before the season begins.

c. Perennial method. In this method, after the injections have been gradually built up to a maximum, at weekly intervals, the injections are continued at three- or four-week intervals throughout the year, with the idea of maintaining maximum tolerance.

These methods are modified by the allergist according to his own experience and preferences.

## Is it necessary for the patient to cooperate in order to get good results?

Yes. He must have patience if the symptoms are not relieved quickly, and he must not tempt fate by deliberately exposing himself to the offending agents in order to see if the shots are doing any good. If dietary restrictions are imposed, he must follow them carefully.

## How early in life can hay fever treatment be started?

A child is never too young for treatment to be started. The earlier the treatment is started, the better the results.

## Are hay fever injections dangerous?

There is virtually no danger in taking injections from an experienced physician.

## What about the "one shot" treatment of hay fever?

The "one shot," or repository, method of treatment has not been accepted by all allergists. In fact, it has been disapproved of by the Food and Drug Administration.

## Can people with other serious diseases, such as heart trouble, take hay fever injections?

Yes. Such injections will do them no harm.

## Are hay fever injections painful?

They cause only slight pain.

## Are there any aftereffects from the injection treatment of hay fever?

Occasionally there may be a swollen arm, or the patient may have some general symptoms, such a generalized itch or an increase in the severity of an allergic attack, etc. These symptoms usually occur within a few seconds to a half hour after the injection is given. It is therefore wise for a patient to remain in an allergist's office for this length of time after an injection.

## What can be done to alleviate the reactions to a hay fever injection?

The allergist has medications that he gives to bring about prompt relief from any of these reactions.

## Are the antihistaminic drugs effective in treating hay fever?

They can help considerably in relieving the symptoms of hay fever, but most of these drugs produce undesirable side effects, such as drowsiness and dizziness. They should not be used as a substitute for the injection treatment. Furthermore, they do not prevent bronchial asthma from coming on as a complication of hay fever.

## Is hay fever effectively treated with the steroid drugs, such as cortisone, etc?

They are helpful in relieving symptoms, but they should not be used in place of the standard treatment.

## Are air conditioners and home

filters in rooms helpful in treating hay fever?

Yes. The amount of relief will depend upon how much of the day is spent in such an atmosphere.

## Are air conditioners ever harmful in hay fever?

Occasionally there are patients whose symptoms are made worse by air conditioning. Before investing in an air conditioner, a patient should determine for himself its effect on his symptoms.

## Does hay fever recur if it has once subsided and been cured?

Yes. A patient may have no symptoms for several years and then suddenly have a severe recurrence.

## Must a hay fever patient take treatment all his life?

Not necessarily. There is no way of predicting in advance how long a patient will require injections, but in many cases the treatment can be discontinued within three to five years.

## When will an allergist discharge a patient from further hay fever treatment?

After the patient has had two successive years with no symptoms while under treatment.

## Do the emotions have any effect on hay fever?

Yes. Emotional upsets of any kind are apt to make symptoms worse.

## Should hay fever patients restrict their physical activity?

Yes. Excessive physical exertion resulting in fatigue seems to increase the symptoms of hay fever.

## Should surgery be carried out during the hay fever season?

Hay fever sufferers should have only emergency surgery performed during the season. A patient who sneezes violently is not a good surgical risk. Anesthetics may act as irritants to the nose of the hay fever patient. Asthma is more likely to occur in a hay fever patient operated upon during the season.

**When should children with hay fever have their tonsils removed?**

After the hay fever season is over, in the late fall or early winter. Tonsillectomy should not be performed just before the onset of the season.

**Should the pregnant hay fever patient be treated?**

Yes. Many hay fever patients have an aggravation of their condition during pregnancy.

**Does diet have anything to do with hay fever?**

Yes. Certain foods may aggravate the symptoms.

**What is the effect of alcoholic beverages on hay fever?**

It makes the symptoms worse during the hay fever season.

**Does hay fever occur more often in one sex than in the other?**

No. It occurs just as often in males as in females.

**Is it wise for a hay fever patient to change his residence?**

There are certain places in this country that have a particularly low pollen count. Great relief can be obtained by going to these places during the height of the hay fever season.

**What are some of the places that have low ragweed pollen counts?**

In the New York area, there are the eastern Long Island area, the Pine Hill area in the Catskills, and the Raquette Lake area in the Adirondacks. Also, there are certain areas in the Northwest, Bermuda, the Virgin Islands, Nassau, Miami Beach, Nova Scotia, and several places in Maine,

New Hampshire, and northern Michigan. Of course, an ocean voyage is always safe. There is virtually no ragweed in the British Isles or on the European continent.

**Should the hay fever patient have animal pets?**

It is better not to have such pets. Allergic patients tend to develop allergy to animal hairs. Also, animals that run out in the open may bring pollen into the house.

**Why can't ragweed be eliminated entirely?**

Because such a plan of eradication would have to be statewide or nationwide. It is of little value to eradicate pollen in one town or in one city, since the pollen is carried in the air for long distances.

## BRONCHIAL ASTHMA

**What is bronchial asthma?**

This condition, associated with an obstruction of the bronchial tubes, is characterized by a hard cough and difficult breathing. It is a chronic disease, which usually begins in childhood or early adult life.

**What causes bronchial asthma?**

Any common allergen, such as pollen, mold spores, house dust, animal hair, foods, or drugs.

**When is the most common time for asthmatic attacks to occur?**

In the early morning hours.

**What are the most common symptoms of asthma?**

Wheezing, a sense of suffocation, a hard, dry cough, and an inability to expel air easily from the lungs.

**What precipitates asthmatic attacks?**

Acute respiratory infection or exposure to an extremely strong dose

of one of the allergens. Also, emotional disturbances, exertion, or sudden changes in temperature.

**Do asthmatic attacks tend to come on suddenly?**

Yes.

**What takes place in the body during an asthmatic attack?**

There is swelling in the mucous membranes of the bronchial tubes and in the smaller bronchioles within the lungs. This causes narrowing of the passageway for air. The mucus glands within the bronchial tubes secrete an increased amount of mucous, thus further obstructing the passage of air.

**How common is asthma?**

It is estimated that 3 to 4 percent of the entire population of the United States has asthma.

**Is asthma ever outgrown?**

No. It is a popular misconception that children will outgrow their asthma.

**Does asthma usually clear up without treatment?**

No. On the contrary, it tends to become worse when not properly treated.

**What is the treatment for asthma?**

a. Finding an allergen that has caused the asthma and then instituting hyposensitization injections.
b. Giving steroid (cortisone) medications.
c. To relieve acute attacks, injections of adrenalin or epinephrine are given.
d. The inhalation of special medications to relieve bronchial spasm often relieves acute attacks.

**Is hospitalization ever required for an asthmatic?**

Yes. In an acute asthmatic attack,

which is very severe, hospitalization is often necessary to prevent suffocation.

### Does asthma ever cause tuberculosis or cancer of the lungs?

No.

### Can even the most severe asthmatic attack be brought under control temporarily?

Yes. There are drugs that can effectively relieve the acute severe attack.

### Does asthma ever lead to heart disease?

In certain cases of chronic asthma, heart disease may be caused by the increased strain of the repeated attacks. This takes a long time, however, and is not a very common occurrence.

### What diseases of the chest can asthma produce?

Emphysema, bronchiectasis, and other lung diseases can be caused by asthma.

### Will a change of climate help asthma?

It may be valuable if the allergic causes of asthma are not present in the new location.

## FOOD ALLERGY
### (Digestive or Gastrointestinal Allergy)

### What are digestive allergies?

Disorders of the stomach and intestines caused by foods to which the individual is sensitive.

### What are some of the symptoms of digestive allergies?

Belching, nausea, vomiting, abdominal pain, constipation, diarrhea, and even canker sores in and about the mouth.

### How can one tell what food is causing the digestive allergy?

By eliminating all foods for a day or two and then slowly adding one substance at a time to the diet. When the culprit is discovered, it is eliminated from the future diet of the patient.

### What is the treatment for food allergies?

a. The elimination of the offending substance.
b. The giving of antihistaminic or other drugs to relieve the acute attack.

### How soon after eating a food can an allergic reaction take place?

The allergic reaction may occur immediately, or within a few minutes, or be delayed from a few hours to approximately thirty-six hours after a food has been eaten.

### If a food has once caused an allergic reaction, will it always produce such a reaction?

Not necessarily. The patient may build up a tolerance for such a food.

### Should a patient test himself by taking a food that he is known to be sensitive to?

This is not always a wise procedure if the allergic reaction has been violent. However, if the patient does test himself, a very small amount of the food should be taken.

### How common is food allergy?

Many people have some type of food allergy, but most of them are unaware of it.

### Are food allergies ever fatal?

No.

### Do food allergies ever cause abdominal symptoms that suggest a surgical condition?

Yes. Occasionally a diagnosis of appendicitis or gall bladder disease is made when, in reality, the patient is suffering from a food allergy.

## SKIN ALLERGIES

### What are some of the common skin allergies?

a. A contact dermatitis, which is caused by the irritation of substances to which one is sensitive.
b. Poison Ivy.
   (This is really a form of contact dermatitis.)
c. Atopic dermatitis—or eczema.
d. Urticaria (hives).

### What is contact dermatitis?

This is one of the most common of all allergic diseases. It is caused by exposing the skin to a substance to which the patient is hypersensitive. One example of it is poison ivy. The symptoms of contact dermatitis are itching and redness of the skin, with swelling, blisters, oozing, crusting, and scaling. It may occur in one spot, or it may cover the entire body surface.

### What are some of the common substances that may cause contact dermatitis?

Chemicals, plant oils, cosmetics, deodorants, mouthwashes, medicines, clothing, plastics, dyes, etc. Sensitivity to such substances varies widely.

### What is the treatment for contact dermatitis?

The giving of the antihistaminic drugs to relieve the acute symptoms and the application of medication to relieve the skin irritation. Also, the discovery of its cause and avoidance of the offending irritant. Frequently, it is necessary to resort to the use of a steroid, such as cortisone.

### What is atopic dermatitis?

It is a skin eczema, often occuring in infants, and is usually caused by a food sensitivity. There is almost always a family history of allergy in these patients.

### What is urticaria (hives)?

This is a skin allergy characterized by wheals of various sizes and number on the skin surface. These wheals are swellings, which may be very large and which cause an intense amount of itching. They sometimes occur on the lips, face, tongue, throat, eyelids, ears, or any other part of the body.

### What causes urticaria or hives?

Hives are usually caused by an allergy to a food or a drug.

### What are the symptoms of urticaria?

Itching is the most distressing symptom.

### What are the usual allergens causing urticaria?

Fish, seafood, highly seasoned foods, and aspirin are the most frequent causes.

### How are hives treated?

By the elimination of the offending irritant and by the giving of antiallergent medications. The acute attacks are often relieved by giving adrenalin and like substances.

### Does urticaria tend to recur once it has been cured?

Yes, if the same offending irritant is eaten again.

### Do children tend to outgrow skin allergies?

Yes.

### Do children with skin allergies tend to develop other allergies as they grow older?

Yes, as the skin allergy is just one manifestation of an allergic tendency.

## DRUG ALLERGY

### What drugs can cause an allergic reaction?

Practically any drug, if the patient is sensitive to it.

### Can one tell in advance if he is allergic to a drug?

No.

### How is the diagnosis of drug allergy made?

From the patient's history.

### What are the symptoms of drug allergy?

It may cause running nose, hives, asthmatic attacks, or a skin eruption.

### Are drug allergies ever dangerous?

Yes. A patient who is sensitive to a drug such as aspirin may die after taking even one aspirin tablet.

### Is drug allergy inherited?

No. It is an acquired form of sensitivity.

### Can skin tests be done to determine drug sensitivity?

No.

### What is the treatment for drug allergies?

The antihistaminics and the steroids are most helpful in the treatment of drug allergies.

## INSECT ALLERGY

### Can patients allergic to the bites of bees, hornets, wasps, and yellow jackets do anything to avoid being stung?

Yes. The likelihood of stings can be lessened by taking certain simple precautions:

a. Any sort of food will attract these insects. Outdoor cooking or eating, feeding pets out-of-doors, garbage cans left uncovered, the dribble from a child's Popsicle or candy—all will attract insects. Keeping food covered until the moment of disposal, meticulous cleaning about the garbage area, and repeated spraying of outdoor recreational areas and garbage cans with insecticides will tend to keep insects away.

b. Gardening should be done cautiously; electric hedge clippers, tractors, and power mowers should not be used.

c. Since perfumes, hair sprays, hair tonic, suntan lotion, and many other cosmetics attract insects, these substances should not be used. Flowing garments in which insects might become caught, bright colors, flowery prints, and black should be avoided. Light colors, such as white, green, tan, and khaki, are thought neither to attract nor to antagonize bees.

d. Shoes should be worn at all times when outdoors except on a hard, sandy beach.

e. Plain common sense will prevent many a sting. Calm, quiet behavior without sudden movements or flailing of arms, avoidance of situations known to attract insects, and keeping a sharp lookout usually will prevent trouble.

### What other precautions can insect-sensitive patients take?

These people, when outdoors, should always keep with them a kit containing epinephrine for injection, antihistamine tablets, and a tourniquet. On being stung, these drugs should be used immediately, and a physician should be seen.

### Can patients sensitive to insect stings be treated prophylactically?

Yes. They can be tested with extracts of the insects and then hyposensitized with the appropriate extract. Recently, venom extracts have been used instead of extracts of the insect's whole body.

## PHYSICAL ALLERGY

### What is physical allergy?
An abnormal reaction caused by some physical agent, such as heat, cold, light, or mechanical irritation.

### What are the symptoms of physical allergy?
There are two types of reactions: the contact reactions and the reflex reactions. The contact reactions occur at the site of contact with the physical agent—for example, hives, which develop on portions of the body exposed to cold. Reflex-like reactions may be generalized or developed in remote tissues of the body, as, for example, an asthmatic attack or hives, which can result from exposure to heat or cold. Reflex-like reactions following exposure to an irritant may be so severe that they might cause fainting or loss of consciousness and may even explain certain deaths from drowning.

### What is the treatment for physical allergies?
Treatment may consist of exposing the patient to a small degree of heat or cold or other irritant in short, daily exposures over a long period of time. The patient may then develop a tolerance for the specific physical agent. For instance, daily baths, which are gradually made colder or warmer, as the case may be, may sometimes desensitize a patient to heat or cold. Occasionally, the antihistaminic drugs will bring about desensitization.

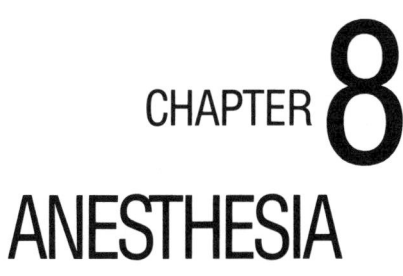

# CHAPTER 8

# ANESTHESIA

*(See also Chapter 58 on Preoperative and Postoperative Routines)*

## Is the physician-anesthesiologist a specialist like the surgeon?

Yes. Both are graduated from approved medical schools, and both have had internships and resident training in their specialties.

## Should anesthesiologists be physicians?

It is best to have a physician specializing in anesthesia administer the anesthetic. In addition to knowledge and skill in the area of anesthesia, a physician is better able to diagnose and treat medical problems that would otherwise divert the surgeon's attention from the operation.

## What is an anesthesiologist's training?

After internship he spends approximately two years as a resident in an approved hospital, where a regular course of study is pursued in the administration of anesthesia. Following these two years, he must spend three more years in practice and then take a rigorous series of examinations to qualify as a Diplomate of the American Board of Anesthesiology.

## Are nonmedical anesthetists still in practice?

Yes, in certain parts of the country there are not enough trained medical doctors to fill the demand. Certified Registered Nurse Anesthetists (C.R.N.A.'s) are the best category of nonphysician anesthetists and have taken training and passed an examination in the administration of anesthesia.

## Why do I pay a separate fee to the anesthesiologist?

The anesthesiologist, like the surgeon, is in private practice and is not employed or paid by the hospital. He will submit a bill for his services.

## Are the services of an anesthesiologist advisable for delivery of a baby?

Yes. The anesthesiologist has cut down on maternal and fetal complications remarkably. And if difficulty is anticipated with the newborn, it may be advisable to have a neonatologist* or second anesthesiologist present.

## What is meant by the term "preanesthetic evaluation and premedication"?

The anesthesiologist will study the patient's medical record and past history before he determines which type of anesthesia to give. If an anesthesiologist is not satisfied that the patient will come safely through the surgery and anesthesia, he will recommend the postponement or cancellation of the operation. Medications such as narcotics and sedatives are usually given before anesthesia, in the patient's room. This puts the patient in a drowsy, comfortable frame of mind so that the onset of anesthesia is smooth and easy.

## Is a great deal of pain necessary during childbirth?

No. In modern methods of anesthesia, only the beginnings of labor pains must be endured by the mother. Most severe pain can be abolished and the delivery of the baby effected without harm to it or to the mother.

## If the baby is to be born through Cesarean section, will an anesthesiologist be used?

Yes. Anesthesia for a Cesarean section is a complex procedure involving the care of *two* patients.

## What is meant by "the induction of anesthesia"?

These are the initial stages of anesthesia. Today, induction is accomplished without excitement or fear. Preliminary medications, or the induction of sleep by an intravenous injection, make the anesthesia relatively painless and pleasant.

## What are the most common types of anesthesia?

a. General inhalation anesthesia is being used today more than any other type. However, most anesthesiologists utilize what is known as *balanced anesthesia.* This means that several agents are administered during the course of any one anesthesia. To put the patient to sleep, an intravenous drug such as Pentothal or some similar medication is given. Then, nitrous oxide and oxygen are administered to overcome pain sensations. Finally, when muscle relaxation is required so that the surgeon can carry out his technical maneuvers, one of the muscle-relaxant drugs is given intravenously. As the operation progresses, additional doses of the above agents are applied as the need arises.

The tremendous increase in the use of various kinds of electrical equipment in the operating room, combined with the development of nonflammable anesthetic agents, has led to the virtual abandonment of explosive anesthetic agents such as ether and cyclopropane.

---

*A neonatologist is a pediatrician with special training in the care of the newborn.

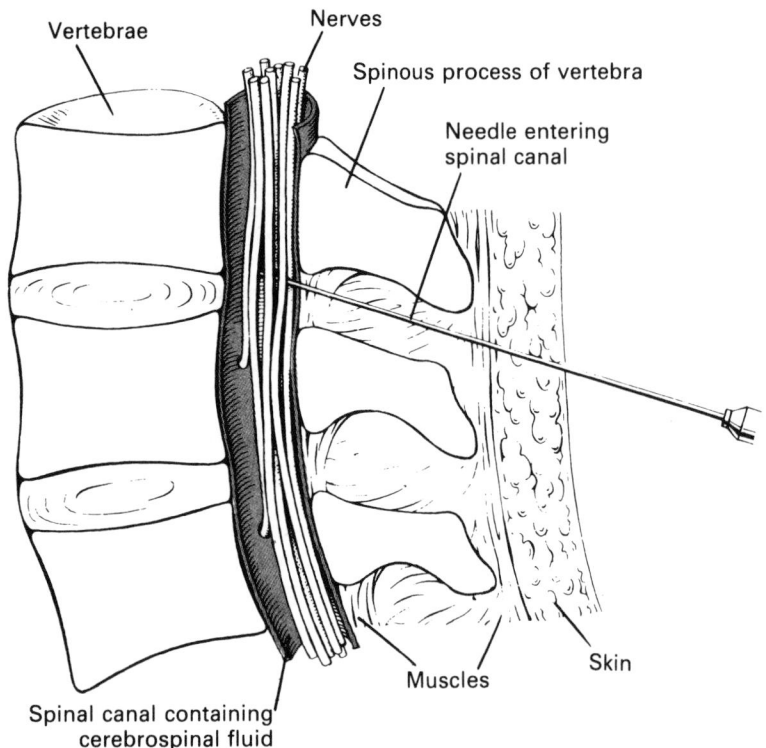

Vertebrae

Nerves

Spinous process of vertebra

Needle entering spinal canal

Skin

Muscles

Spinal canal containing cerebrospinal fluid

*Spinal Anesthesia Showing Needle in Spinal Canal. This diagram shows the needle in place within the spinal canal. The anesthesiologist will withdraw some of the spinal fluid and mix it with an anesthetic agent such as procaine (Novocain). He will then inject it into the spinal canal, and in a few minutes anesthesia of the lower part of the body (from the chest down) will result. The spinal puncture is practically painless, as the skin is anesthetized before the needle is inserted into the spinal canal.*

Fluothane (halothane) is a non-flammable and nonexplosive vapor, which has been widely used until recent years. It is unfortunate that rare instances of liver damage have led to a decline in the use of this valuable agent. In fact, studies suggest that halothane is one of the safest anesthetics so far discovered.

Ethrane (enflurane) is a potent, nonflammable, short-action agent for inhalation anesthesia. It has the advantages over halothane of providing considerable muscle relaxation and having less association with possible liver problems.

b. Spinal anesthesia. This type is usually used for an operation from the waist down. It is carried out by injecting Novocain or some like substance into the spinal canal.

This form of anesthesia makes numb that part of the body to be operated upon and allows the patient to remain awake. Today, spinal anesthesia is given most frequently in conjunction with intravenous agents that permit the patient to doze during the operation.

c. Epidural and caudal anesthesia. These types are similar to spinal in that they block the spinal nerves, thus anesthetizing various regions of the body. They differ from spinal anesthesia only in that the anesthetic agent is injected outside the spinal fluid rather than into the spinal fluid.

d. Local or regional anesthesia. Procaine is the most widely used agent for local anesthesia and is used by injection into the nerves that supply certain parts of the body. Unfortunately, its effect is of rather short duration, and to overcome this characteristic, other agents have been developed in an attempt to obtain a longer period of pain obliteration. Some of these agents are Xylocaine, Carbocaine, and Lidocaine. Although these latter agents will result in longer periods of anesthesia, they are somewhat more toxic, and greater caution must be taken in their use. It is frequently possible to prolong local or regional anesthesia by adding a small amount of adrenalin to the anesthetic mixture before injecting it. Adrenalin causes a contraction of blood vessels in the area and thus diminishes the amount of anesthetic agent that is absorbed into the bloodstream and carried away from the surgical site.

e. Intravenous anesthesia. There are several drugs that, when administered intravenously, produce unconsciousness. The most commonly used intravenous drugs are Pentothal, Innovar, and Valium. These agents cannot be used as the sole drug for anesthesia because their main function is to produce sleep (narcosis) rather than to obliterate pain sensations. For this reason, they are given essentially to assist the anesthetic agent, and once the patient has gone to sleep, he is maintained in an anesthetic state by the administration of nitrous oxide and analgesics such as Demerol. In performing anesthesia in this manner, the anesthesiologist is always careful not to give too large a quantity of intravenous medications because they may have a tendency to depress vital functions such as respiration.

f. Topical anesthesia. This consists of applying an anesthetic solution directly to a mucous membrane, such as the mouth, the nose, the eye, etc. Some anesthetic solutions may be applied with a cotton applicator or spray; others can be dropped onto a mucous membrane with an eye dropper. The chemicals most widely used for topical anesthesia are cocaine and Xylocaine.

## What gases and vapors are used in administering anesthesia?
Nitrous oxide, halothane, and enflurane.

## Are these gases unpleasant to smell?
No.

## Will the patient positively be asleep before the operation is begun?
Yes. Surgery is never begun before anesthesia has taken complete effect.

## Is it wise for a patient to select his own anesthesia?
No. The surgeon and the anesthetist are in a much better position to know the best anesthesia to give a patient for a particular operation.

## Do patients ever give away important secrets while talking as they go under anesthesia?
No. This is a very common misconception.

## Does the anesthesia ever wear off before the operation is over?
No. An anesthesiologist knows when additional anesthesia is necessary and will administer it during the course of the operation.

## How long does it take for anesthesia to wear off after the operation is completed?
This varies widely according to the amount of anesthesia administered and the type of anesthetic. Spinal anesthesias usually wear off within one to three hours after an operation is over. General anesthesias may wear off within a few minutes after the operation is over or may last for several hours.

## What is the safest type of anesthesia?
Today all anesthetics are safe when administered by well-qualified anesthesiologists. Serious anesthetic accidents are so rare that they consti-

tute a very minor problem in surgery today.

## Is one type of anesthesia safer than another?
There is no absolute rule about this. It depends on the type of operation, the surgeon, the patient, etc. It is best to accept the advice of your anesthesiologist regarding the choice of anesthesia.

## What is the best method of preventing complications from anesthesia?
Seeing to it that the patient has a sufficient supply of oxygen intake troughout the entire operative procedure, and also making sure that there is a proper airway from the outside into the patient's lungs. Both of these measures are always provided during competently administered anesthesia.

## How long is it safe to continue an anesthesia?
It is safe to continue an anesthesia many hours—provided the patient receives good care. With the new

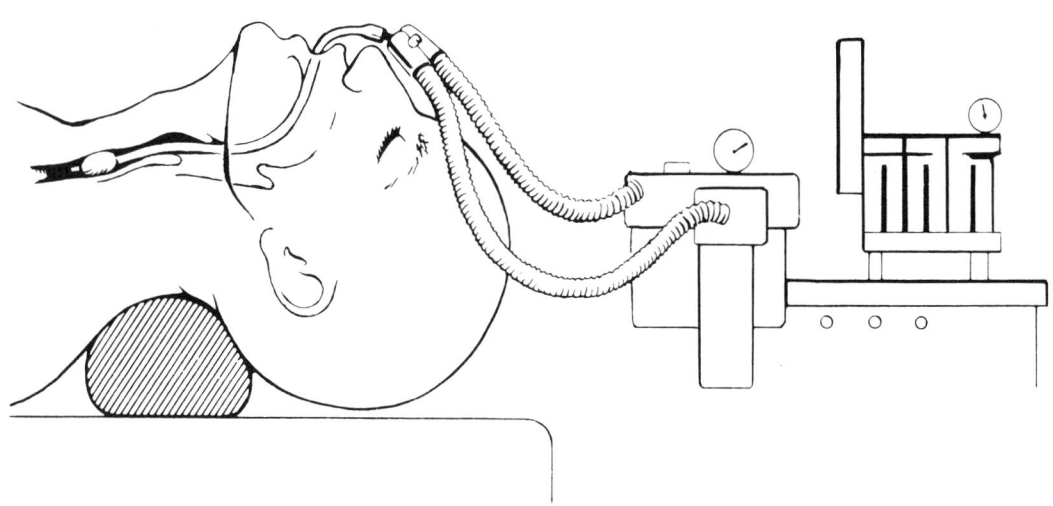

***Endotracheal Anesthesia.*** *The anesthesia machine is connected to the patient by means of a tube inserted into the trachea. The strength and quantity of the mixture of oxygen and gases can be adjusted and controlled by the anesthesiologist.*

types of operations being performed in all fields of surgery today, it is not at all uncommon for a patient to be kept continually under anesthesia for many hours.

## What is meant by endotracheal anesthesia?

This is a method of administering an inhalation anesthesia by the placing of a tube through the mouth or nose directly into the trachea. It is the safest way to give an inhalation anesthesia, because breathing can be controlled most efficiently through this method.

## Are headaches after spinal anesthesia very common?

About one in twenty people develop postspinal headaches. These can now be prevented or treated successfully.

## How long do postspinal headaches last?

On the average, about two to three days.

## What is the treatment for postspinal headache?

a. Drink large quantities of water, eight to ten glasses daily.

b. Analgesics such as aspirin.
c. Certain injections to increase the water content of the spinal canal.

## Do children and infants take anesthesia as well as adults do?

Yes. Infants and young children tolerate general anesthesia extremely well.

## Is the anesthesiologist responsible for the general condition of the patient during the operation?

Yes. He watches not only the breathing of the patient but also the pulse, heart action, and blood pressure. The anesthesiologist frequently advises the surgeon and gives him periodic reports on the condition of his patient while under anesthesia.

## If a patient has once had a bad anesthetic reaction at a previous operation, does it mean that he will again react poorly?

No. Advances in anesthesia have been so great that patients who had adverse reactions years ago do not necessarily have the same reactions today.

## Should the patient tell the anesthesiologist about a previous bad anesthetic reaction?

Yes. It is always wise to let the anesthesiologist know of past difficulty that you or a member of your family may have suffered.

## Should the patient tell the anesthesiologist if he has eaten prior to surgery?

Yes. It is most important that a patient come to anesthesia with an empty stomach. If a patient has taken food or drink before surgery is to be performed, it is essential that he or she so inform the anesthesiologist.

# TYPES OF ANESTHESIA
## USUALLY GIVEN FOR THE FOLLOWING OPERATIONS

| OPERATION | ANESTHESIA |
|---|---|
| **Brain:** | General or, occasionally, local, with or without intravenous agents. |
| **Eye:** | General, topical, or regional nerve-block anesthesia. |
| **Bone:** | General, spinal, or regional nerve-block anesthesia. |
| **Mouth:** | Local or regional nerve block. |
| **Tonsils:** | In children: general. In adults: local or general. |
| **Thyroid:** | General, often through an endotracheal tube. Regional or local, only occasionally. |
| **Breast:** | General anesthesia. In exceptional cases, local anesthesia may be employed. |
| **Heart and lungs:** | General anesthesia. |
| **Abdominal organs:** | General or spinal anesthesia, according to the particular case. When spinal anesthesia is used, intravenous agents are often added to put the patient to sleep. |
| **Kidneys, bladder, and prostate:** | General or spinal anesthesia. |
| **Rectum, anus, and genitalia:** | General, spinal, caudal, or local anesthesia, often with intravenous agents to produce sleep. |
| **Upper extremity:** | General, local, or regional nerve-block anesthesia. |
| **Lower extremity:** | General, spinal, local, or regional anesthesia. |

# CHAPTER 9

# APPENDICITIS

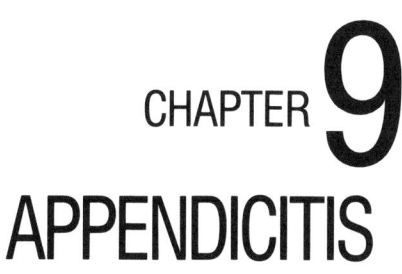

*(See also Chapter 8 on Anesthesia; Chapter 52 on Peritonitis)*

## What is the appendix and where is it located?

The appendix is a wormlike extension of the cecum (large bowel), measuring three to five inches in length, located in the lower right portion of the abdomen at the very beginning of the large intestine. Normally, it is about the thickness of a lead pencil.

## What is its function?

It serves no function in humans and is thought to be a remnant of our primitive past.

## What is appendicitis?

Appendicitis is an inflammation of the lining of the appendix that spreads to its other portions, thus involving the entire structure. When involved in an acute inflammation, the appendix may become filled with pus. When the infection spreads through the wall of the appendix, it may become gangrenous and may rupture.

## What causes appendicitis?

Appendicitis may be caused either by bacterial inflammation or by obstruction of the blood supply to the appendix by a hardened particle of feces that blocks its passageway and presses upon the blood vessels in the region.

## How common a condition is appendicitis?

Before the era of antibiotics, appendicitis was one of the most common of all surgical conditions within the abdomen, but today it occurs much less frequently. It is seen most often in young adults in their twenties, thirties, or forties, although it can occur in infants or old people. Rarely does it occur in children under three years of age.

## Is the incidence of appendicitis decreasing?

Yes. For some unexplained reason, appendicitis occurs less often today than twenty to thirty years ago.

## How can one tell if he has appendicitis?

By noting the symptoms of generalized abdominal cramps, nausea or vomiting, and localization of pain to the lower right side of the abdomen. These symptoms persist over a period of several hours and tend to become more severe. There is also a slight temperature rise and an increase in pulse rate. Lack of appetite and constipation are also frequent findings in appendicitis.

## Can appendicitis develop from swallowing foreign bodies, such as pits of fruits, chewing gum, etc.?

No.

## Does appendicitis tend to run in families or be inherited?

No.

## What types of appendicitis exist?

a. Acute appendicitis, which usually begins with abdominal cramps, nausea, vomiting, and subsequent localization of pain to the lower right side of the abdomen. This sequence of events takes place within a few hours' time.

b. Recurrent appendicitis, characterized by repeated attacks of mild appendicitis, which subside spontaneously, only to return at intervals of several months or years.

## When should a laxative be given for abdominal pain?

Never! The most dangerous thing to do is to give a laxative. This may cause an inflamed appendix to burst.

## Should an enema be given for abdominal pain?

No! Unless a physician has examined the patient and has specifically ordered it.

## Should appendicitis be operated upon once it has been diagnosed?

Yes, as the acute variety rarely subsides spontaneously, and in many cases the inflammatory process may lead to rupture and peritonitis.

## Is there any method of preventing appendicitis?

No.

## Is appendicitis caused by dietary indiscretion?

No.

## What laboratory test is performed to help establish the diagnosis of appendicitis?

A blood count is taken. The white blood cell count is usually elevated above normal in cases of acute appendicitis.

## How soon after the diagnosis is definitely made should an operation be performed?

Within several hours.

## What occurs if the appendix bursts?

Pus from the appendix spreads into the abdominal cavity and causes peritonitis. This is a very serious condition. (See Chapter 52, on Peritonitis.)

## Can one cure an attack of acute appendicitis by the use of ice bags?

No, but a certain number of mild cases will subside spontaneously without any treatment.

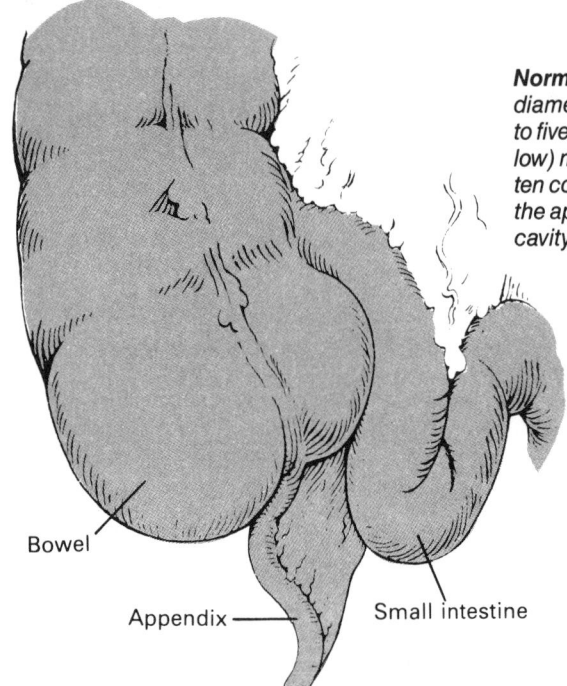

**Normal and Inflamed Appendix.** *The normal appendix (left) is about the diameter of an ordinary lead pencil, is pinkish gray in color, about three to five inches long, and has a glistening coat. The inflamed appendix (below) may be several times the normal thickness, altered in color, and often contains pus. Should the inflammatory process continue for too long, the appendix may burst, allowing the pus to seep out into the abdominal cavity.*

Bowel

Appendix —

Small intestine

— Acutely inflamed appendix

**If a mild attack does subside by itself, is there a tendency for another attack to take place at a later date?**

Yes, and a subsequent attack may be much more serious than the initial attack.

**Can appendicitis be cured medically, without surgery?**

In a small number of cases, appendicitis can be successfully treated with large doses of the antibiotic drugs. However, this is not good treatment, as it carries with it greater risks than surgery.

**What is the best treatment for appendicitis?**

Surgical removal of the appendix.

**How serious an operation is appendectomy?**

When performed for an early case of appendicitis, the procedure is not at all serious. When performed upon a patient whose appendix has ruptured and who has developed peritonitis, it is a serious operation.

**How long does it take to perform an appendectomy?**

Anywhere from a few minutes in an uncomplicated case, to an hour or two in a complicated, long-standing case.

**What are the chances for recovery after an appendectomy?**

In these days of improved surgery and the antibiotic drugs, recovery takes place in almost all cases.

**What are some of the complications of appendicitis?**

The greatest complication is rupture, with the development of peritonitis. In a small number of untreated cases, pus from the appendix may spread to the liver, causing liver abscesses.

**What anesthesia is used in operating upon the appendix?**

Inhalation anesthesia, utilizing nitrous oxide and the muscle-relaxant drugs, or in some hospitals, spinal or epidural anesthesia.

**How long a period of hospitalization is necessary?**

In the uncomplicated case, approximately five days to a week. If rupture has occurred, the patient may be in the hospital for several weeks.

**Where is the incision made in performing an appendectomy?**

In the lower right portion of the abdomen. Incisions are made either in an oblique direction or longitudinally. They usually extend two to four inches in length.

**Is the length of the incision important?**

Absolutely not. Some surgeons prefer to work through larger incisions than others. It should be known that all incisions heal from side to side, so that a long incision will heal just as quickly as a small one.

### Are special preoperative treatments necessary?

Not in the uncomplicated case. In the complicated case it may be necessary to give intravenous fluids and large doses of antibiotics before surgery is performed. Also, a tube may have to be passed through the nose down into the intestinal tract in order to empty the tract of fluid and gases that might interfere with the surgery.

### Are special private nurses necessary after surgery?

Not for the usual case of appendicitis.

### Is the postoperative period particularly painful?

No.

### What special postoperative treatments are carried out?

There are no extraordinary postoperative procedures in the ordinary, uncomplicated case. However, follow-ing surgery for a ruptured appendix, it may be necessary to withhold fluids by mouth and to give fluids by injection into the veins. Also, to keep the intestinal tract empty and to combat distention, a tube may be inserted through the nose into the stomach. Where rupture has taken place, large doses of antibiotics are given to combat peritonitis.

### How soon after appendectomy can a patient get out of bed?

In the uncomplicated case the patient can get out of bed the day after surgery. When peritonitis is present, the patient may be forced to remain in bed for several days or even weeks.

### How long does it take the wound to heal?

In the simple, uncomplicated case the wound will heal within a few days to a week. Where a drain has been inserted, as in a ruptured appendix, it may take several weeks for an appendectomy wound to heal.

### Is it common for an appendectomy wound to become infected?

Yes, since an infected organ (the appendix) has been removed through the wound and may have caused some contamination of the abdominal wall while being removed.

### Is serum frequently found in wounds following appendectomy?

Yes. A light pinkish fluid frequently collects in the wound several days after operation. The surgeon drains this off by inserting a clamp. Very little discomfort is occasioned by this procedure.

### Is special convalescent care required after appendectomy?

Not in the uncomplicated case.

### Are there any permanent after-effects of appendectomy?

No.

### Is the scar disfiguring?

Not in the uncomplicated case. How-

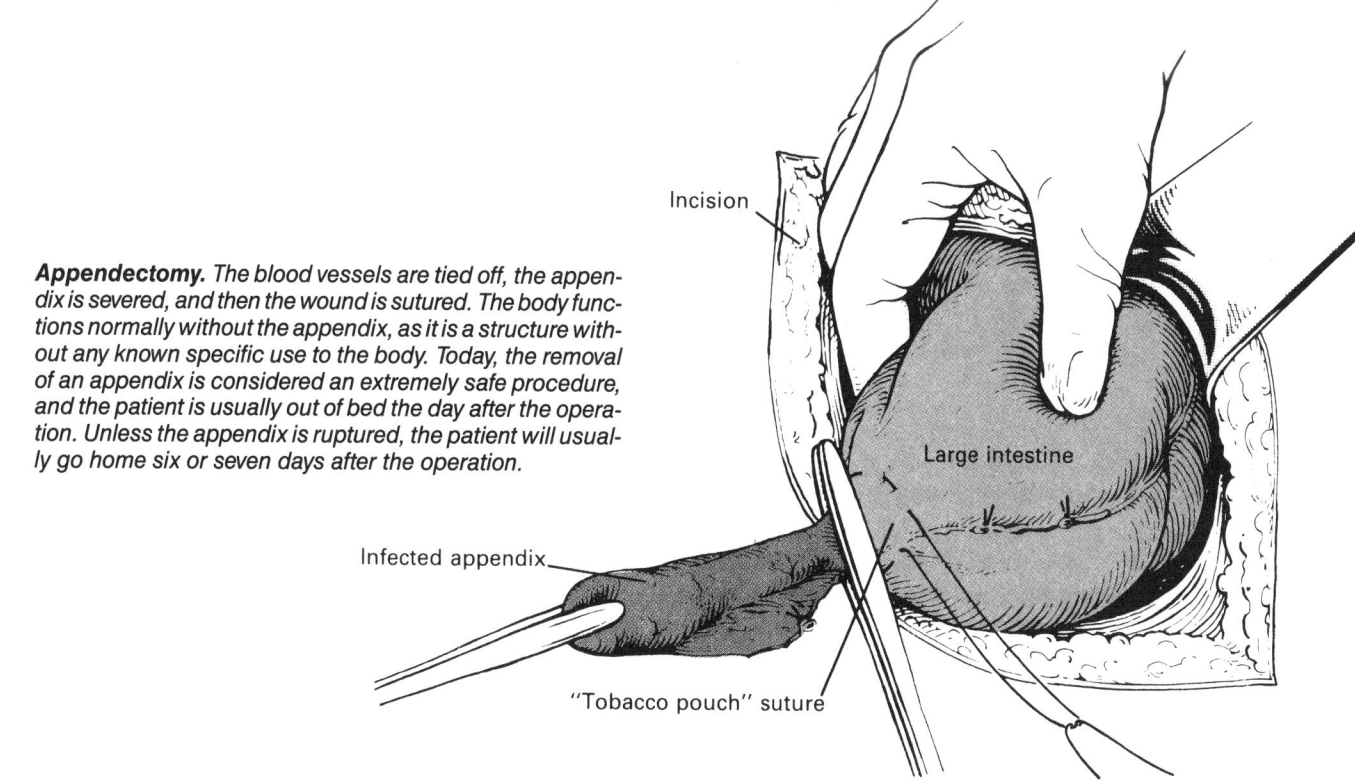

*Appendectomy. The blood vessels are tied off, the appendix is severed, and then the wound is sutured. The body functions normally without the appendix, as it is a structure without any known specific use to the body. Today, the removal of an appendix is considered an extremely safe procedure, and the patient is usually out of bed the day after the operation. Unless the appendix is ruptured, the patient will usually go home six or seven days after the operation.*

Incision

Large intestine

Infected appendix

"Tobacco pouch" suture

ever, if a drain has been inserted and infection of the wound has set in, a rather disfiguring scar may be seen in the lower right side of the abdomen.

**Does the intestinal tract return to normal function after removal of the appendix?**

Yes.

**Does appendicitis ever recur after it has been operated upon?**

Not if the appendix has been removed. In a very small percentage of cases, where a ruptured appendix has been encountered or where the appendix is in an inaccessible position, the surgeon may elect merely to drain the abdominal cavity and to leave the appendix in place for removal at a later date.

**Why is the appendix sometimes left in place during an appendix operation?**

Because pus can easily spread farther in the abdominal cavity in attempting to remove certain appendices, especially those in which a localized abscess has formed. Simple drainage of the appendiceal abscess is carried out in these cases and will result in recovery. It is important to insist that the patient return for subsequent appendectomy, as recurrent attacks are a constant threat whenever the appendix has been left in.

**Can a woman permit herself to become pregnant after an appendix operation?**

Yes.

**Are special diets necessary after appendectomy?**

No.

**Is it usual to have pain in the wound area after appendectomy?**

Yes. For several weeks thereafter, slight pain may be noted.

**How soon after uncomplicated appendectomy can one do the following?**

Bathe:
    Whenever the wound has healed.
Walk out in the street:
    Seven days.
Walk up and down stairs:
    Seven days.
Perform household duties:
    Three weeks.
Drive a car:
    Three to four weeks.
Resume sexual relations:
    Three to four weeks.
Return to work:
    Three to four weeks.
Resume all physical activity:
    Six weeks.

# CHAPTER 10
# ARTHRITIS

*(See also Chapter 5 on Aging; Chapter 14 on Bones, Muscles, Tendons, and Joints; Chapter 53 on Physical Therapy and Rehabilitation)*

## What is arthritis?

Any inflammatory or degenerative condition of a joint or joints.

## What is rheumatism?

It is a term commonly used to describe a large, diversified, and often vague variety of aches and pains of the the muscles, joints, tendons, bursae, and other parts of the musculoskeletal system.

## What are the most common types of arthritis?

a. Rheumatoid arthritis.
b. Osteoarthritis.
c. Gouty arthritis.
d. Traumatic arthritis.
e. Bacterial arthritis.
f. Arthritis caused by chemical or hormone upset.

## What is the place of cortisone in the treatment of arthritic conditions?

Cortisone is far from being the panacea that many consider it. The main use of cortisone today resides in its ability to counteract inflammatory reaction and thus relieve the pain, swelling, and disability associated in the many forms of arthritis. At the present time, cortisone is used only when all other less dangerous therapies afford the patient inadequate relief.

## Can cortisone cure an arthritic condition?

No. It only gives relief while it is be-

ing used. It does not halt the basic underlying process.

## Does cortisone prevent joint damage?

Recent studies seem to indicate that it does not. On the other hand, there are a number of competent experts in this field who claim otherwise.

## Is cortisone safe?

Yes, but only under strict medical supervision.

## What is the place of aspirin in the treatment of arthritis?

It is one of the better drugs for relief of symptoms.

## Can aspirin be taken safely over prolonged periods of time without medical supervision?

No. There are many reactions to the use of aspirin, and it should be taken under medical supervision.

## What are salicylates?

A general category of drugs, of which aspirin is one, helpful in relieving the symptoms of arthritis.

## What are some of the other drugs that are helpful in the treatment of arthritis?

Indocin, Motrin, Butazolidin, Naprosyn, and Clinoril are drugs that often bring relief of symptoms for sufferers of arthritis.

## Do special diets help the arthritic patient?

As a rule, diets are ineffectual. The only exception is that in gout a special low-purine diet may decrease the frequency of attacks.

## Does local heat or diathermy help arthritis?

Only insofar as it may give some temporary relief.

## Does extraction of teeth alleviate arthritis?

Usually not. Removal of teeth should

be performed purely on the basis of whether it is indicated dentally. The removal of sound teeth is to be condemned.

## Does removal of tonsils alleviate arthritis?

The answer is the same as for the preceding question.

## Does change of climate help an arthritic?

Some arthritics feel more comfortable in a warm, dry climate.

## How effective are spas in the treatment of arthritis?

They are not curative, but benefits felt by patients visiting spas are due to an accumulation of factors such as rest, relaxation, physiotherapy, and a change of environment. There is no scientific evidence that the mineral content of spa water is of specific value for arthritics, either by bathing or by drinking.

## Does constipation affect arthritis?

No.

## Is periodic purging with laxatives of any value?

No.

## Do colonic irrigations help the arthritic?

No.

## Have any specific vaccines been discovered that will help the arthritic?

Not as yet.

## Will the antibiotic drugs help arthritis?

Only when the arthritis has been caused by a bacterial agent such as gonorrhea or a streptococcal infection, etc.

## Can surgery help those afflicted by arthritis?

Yes. Reconstructive and corrective surgical procedures have been devised recently, and they have proved most beneficial to those suffering from chronic joint deformities.

## RHEUMATOID ARTHRITIS

### What is rheumatoid arthritis?

A specific type, which has its onset in young adults and occurs approximately three times as frequently in females as in males. It is characterized by varying degrees of inflammation, pain, swelling, and destruction of joint tissues. The course of the disease is chronic, and there may be periods of quiescence and periods of flare-up. If the disease is untreated and progressive, severe disabling and deforming joint destruction may occur.

### What joints are most commonly affected in rheumatoid arthritis?

Joints in the fingers, wrists, knees, ankles, and spine.

### Are there other symptoms in rheumatoid arthritis besides joint symptoms?

Yes. Fever, weakness, weight loss, and anemia may accompany the joint symptoms.

### What is the cause of rheumatoid arthritis?

The cause is not actually known.

### What is the outlook for patients suffering from rheumatoid arthritis?

If untreated, approximately 10 to 15 percent recover from the initial attack spontaneously and remain perfectly well thereafter. Thirty-five percent show improvement, with only mild "leftovers." About 50 percent develop persistent, progressive, and disabling involvement of the joints. Twenty percent eventually become severely crippled.

### What is the treatment for rheumatoid arthritis?

a. General measures include adequate rest, the elimination of as much emotional stress as possible, and the maintenance of a well-balanced diet.
b. Local physiotherapy, such as baths and diathermy to affected joints.
c. Drugs such as:
1. Salicylates (sodium salicylate and aspirin) often give great relief from pain, although they are not curative.
2. Cortisone, ACTH, and related chemicals will frequently bring about subsidence of symptoms, but symptoms recur when these drugs are discontinued. Often cortisonelike drugs are injected into particularly severely affected joints when all other modalities of therapy are ineffective.
3. Gold salts, which are taken by injection, help some people with rheumatoid arthritis, but the injections must be administered cautiously because of potentially severe toxic reactions.
4. Certain antimalarial drugs have been found of value in the treatment of rheumatoid arthritis in some patients.
5. New medications such as Indocin, Motrin, Naprosyn, and Clinoril have been found to be helpful in the treatment of rheumatoid arthritis.
d. Reconstructive surgery can help remedy some deformities that result from chronic arthritis.

### How effective are treatments for rheumatoid arthritis?

It must be admitted that there is presently no known *cure* for rheumatoid arthritis. The treatments outlined above serve mainly to relieve symptoms and to carry the patient through an acute phase in the course of his disease. By causing abatement of an acute episode, treatment may lessen permanent joint damage, but it cannot bring about a reversal of damage already in existence.

### What is Still's disease?

A form of rheumatoid arthritis occurring in children.

### What is spondylitis?

A specific form of arthritis that attacks the vertebrae and connecting bony and ligamental structures. It occurs most frequently in young adult males.

## OSTEOARTHRITIS

### What is osteoarthritis?

A disease of the joints, which occurs predominantly in middle-aged and elderly people. It is generally thought to be caused by years of wear and tear with inadequate or faulty repair of the joint tissue and certain metabolic changes.

### What joints are most commonly involved in osteoarthritis?

The weight-bearing joints such as the knees, hips, and spine, plus the joints near the tips of the fingers.

### What are the usual symptoms of osteoarthritis?

A gradually increasing stiffness, discomfort, or pain in the affected joint. This is especially noted when the joint is used after a period of rest, and may occur in the morning or after sitting or standing in one place for some time. After such a period of inactivity, it takes the patient a little while to "limber up" or "oil up" the joint while in motion to get the "kinks" out. The joint may become mildly swollen, and a sense of grating may be felt if the palm of the hand is held over the joint while it is flexed and extended.

In the great majority of cases the

disease does not lead to real crippling or deformity but rather to varying degrees of stiffness and pain—forcing the individual to slow down and to engage in more limited physical activities.

## What is the outlook for osteoarthritis?

Most people with this condition need not worry about becoming bedridden, severely restricted, or crippled.

## Can osteoarthritis be prevented?

Not really. But maintenance of correct posture, correction of flat feet and other orthopedic defects, the avoidance of obesity, exercise, proper diet and living habits, and good general care will contribute greatly to joint endurance and will lessen the chances of developing this condition.

## Can osteoarthritis be helped or cured?

It can be helped by physiotherapy, weight loss, medications to relieve joint inflammation, and advice concerning avoidance of strain upon involved joints. Also, reconstructive joint surgery may help to overcome some of the deformities that result from the arthritic process.

## What is the significance of the bulbous knobs seen so often at the last joint of the fingers?

These are osteoarthritic nodes, which sometimes cause stiffness and pain but will not result in serious crippling of the fingers.

# GOUTY ARTHRITIS

## What is gout?

A disorder in body chemistry, that results in the excessive manufacture of urates. Abnormal amounts of these urates are then deposited in the cartilages, bones, kidneys, skin, bursae, and other tissues.

## Do these deposits lead to impairment of function and damage to the organs in which they occur?

Yes.

## Can gout ever result in the loss of a limb?

No.

## What is gouty arthritis?

An inflammation of one or more joints associated with deposits of uric acid. At times, this type of arthritis is accompanied by excruciating pain.

## Can gouty arthritis be treated effectively?

Yes. There are several medications that will prevent most attacks of gout. The one most widely used is allopurinol (Zyloprim). Medications that can relieve acute attacks include colchicine, Butazolidin, Benemid, and other noncortisone, antiarthritic drugs. Combinations of these drugs, if taken regularly, usually prevent most attacks of gout.

## Can early treatment of gout or gouty arthritis prevent permanent damage to the joints and also prevent recurrent attacks?

Yes.

## Does gout tend to run in families?

Yes.

## Is gout more common in men than in women?

Yes, by twenty to one.

## What factors are apt to bring on an attack of acute gout?

Attacks commonly occur following surgery, dietary excesses, excessive alcoholic indulgence, emotional upsets, and excessive chilling. Certain drugs, especially oral diuretics, appear to elevate the blood uric acid and precipitate acute attacks of gout. However, none of the aforementioned factors need be present prior to an acute attack.

## Is gout really a "rich man's disease"?

This is not true. It can, and does, occur in all economic strata.

## What are the physical manifestations of localized gout?

Pain, tenderness, and swelling in the region of a joint.

## What is the course of untreated gout?

An acute joint attack may last two to fourteen days. These attacks may recur at intervals of several months to a year or longer. In the intervening period the patient is usually completely devoid of any joint pain or symptoms. If untreated, after a number of years these attacks occur more frequently, last longer, and leave more profound joint damage. Finally, the joints, especially those of the hands and feet, may become severely warped and irreparably damaged, causing considerable crippling.

Extremely important is the fact that untreated gout can lead to the formation of kidney stones and serious kidney disease.

## How can one corroborate the clinical diagnosis of gouty arthritis?

By finding a high content of uric acid in the blood.

# TRAUMATIC ARTHRITIS

## What is traumatic arthritis?

Any inflammation of a joint caused by an injury, such as a severe blow or strain, which may affect a joint.

## What is the treatment for traumatic arthritis?

Immobilization of the joint in a snug bandage or cast until the inflammation subsides completely.

## What is meant by "water on the knee"?

This is a form of traumatic arthritis of

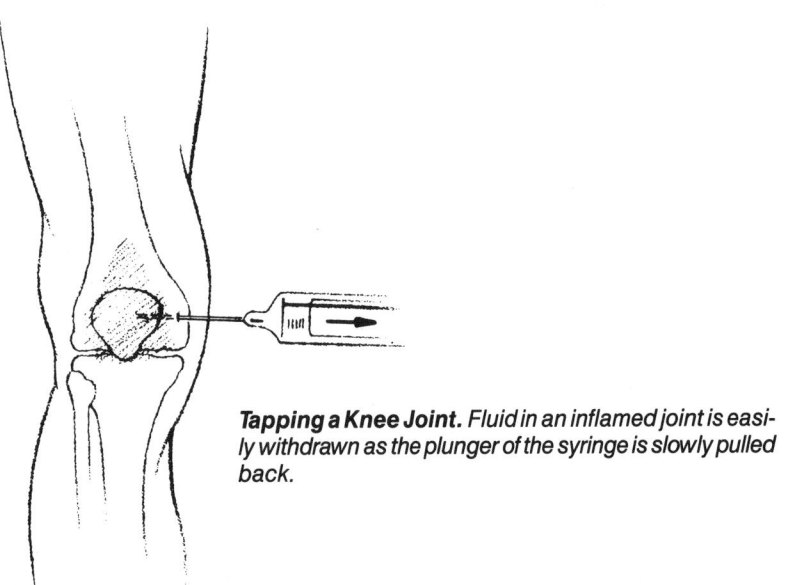

*Tapping a Knee Joint. Fluid in an inflamed joint is easily withdrawn as the plunger of the syringe is slowly pulled back.*

the knee joint, usually caused by a sprain or direct injury.

**What is meant by "tapping" a joint?**
When a joint is injured it often collects fluid within it. Relief of pain and marked improvement usually follow withdrawal of the fluid by "tapping" the joint with a needle.

**Does full recovery usually follow traumatic arthritis?**
Yes. Most injuries of this kind will heal completely within a few weeks.

## BACTERIAL ARTHRITIS

**What is bacterial arthritis?**
It is an infection of a joint space, caused by bacteria such as streptococci, staphylococci, gonococci, etc.

**What is the treatment for bacterial arthritis?**
If the infection is severe, it may become necessary to drain the joint surgically to permit exit of the pus. The antibiotic drugs are very helpful in controlling such infections.

**Is permanent damage to the joint possible following bacterial arthritis?**
Yes. In some cases the lining membrane of the joint is destroyed by the infection and a stiff joint results.

**Is bacterial arthritis very common today?**
No. Early treatment of infections elsewhere in the body usually prevents the bacteria from invading the joints. The advent of the antibiotics has done much to decrease the incidence of arthritis due to gonorrhea and staphylococcic and streptococcic infections, etc.

# CHAPTER 11

# BIRTH CONTROL

*(See also Chapter 25 on Female Organs; Chapter 42 on Male Organs; Chapter 57 on Pregnancy and Childbirth; Chapter 64 on Sex; Chapter 69 on Sterility, Fertility, and Male Potency)*

### What is birth control?

Birth control, also known as contraception, refers to the prevention of fertilization, the union of the sperm and the egg. Birth control is sometimes called Family Planning.

### What circumstances affect whether or not contraception is employed?

a. Religious beliefs. Many devout Catholics and some orthodox Jews feel very strongly that the practice of birth control is sinful. If one partner in a marriage holds this view while the other doesn't, it is good practice to talk out the matter with a leader of their faith. Recent statistical surveys reveal that the majority of women of childbearing age in the United States use some form of birth control, *no matter what religion they espouse.* Despite this revelation, one should not abandon a firmly held religious belief merely because others have done so. Such a course of action may lead to a deep sense of guilt resulting in major emotional disturbances.

b. Age. Couples in their early twenties are much more likely to want to use birth control for a period of years than are older couples, who may want to have a child soon after they marry. There are many reasons why older couples, especially women in their thirties, want to have a child soon after they get married. Statistics show that there are more birth defects in children born to women over thirty years of age. Also, an older man may want to have children soon after he marries so that he will be able to enjoy his child's growing years.

c. Mental and physical health. If a woman is in poor health, she may decide to practice birth control until she is better able to go through with a pregnancy. Similarly, a man with a serious illness may not want to risk having a child for fear of leaving the child fatherless at an early age. If either the man or the woman is mentally ill, it is wise not to permit pregnancy to take place until full recovery from the illness. An emotionally disturbed or mentally ill individual will make an extremely poor parent for a newborn child.

d. Family Planning. If a couple has all the children that they want, it is natural for them to wish to practice birth control. Some parents may have a desire for more children but would like to space them out. These people often practice periodic birth control. Finally, economic factors often play a significant role.

e. Previous Cesarean sections. As a general rule, a woman who has had two to three Cesarean section deliveries will either practice birth control or will give permission to her obstetrician to have her tubes tied off at the time of her last operation.

f. Inherited deformities and diseases. There are a considerable number of conditions that are transmitted from generation to generation through the chromosomes and genes. (Hemophilia is one of the best known of these diseases.) It has been discovered that families in which there are known cases of inherited deformities are much more likely to have other children born with these defects. Families who have no history of inherited diseases or deformities have a much greater chance to have normal offspring. If a physician informs a couple that they have a greater than average chance of having a defective child, they might decide to practice birth control. It must be appreciated, however, that even in the families where inherited conditions do appear, the chances are that a normal child will follow the birth of a deformed one. Fortunately, both inherited diseases and abnormalities are recessive traits and therefore show up only occasionally.

### Is there a need for birth control in the world today?

Most emphatically, yes! Philosophers, sociologists, ethnologists, scientists, and many of the world's spiritual advisers agree that the population explosion is far outstripping our ability to adequately feed, clothe, shelter, and supply sufficient economic income to all the inhabitants of this earth.

### Why is the need for birth control so critical?

Because it is the poor and underprivileged peoples of the world who are reproducing in such large numbers. The problem would be of much less significance if the population explosion affected mainly those countries that required an increase in their people and had the means to support them.

### How large a segment of the world's population is in need of advice regarding planned parenthood and birth control?

It is estimated that two-thirds of the world's four-and-a-quarter billion people are ill-clad, ill-housed, ill-fed, and unable to earn a decent wage. Surely, they need information relating to birth control.

**If the population continues to grow at its present rate, will world food supplies be adequate?**

Authorities estimate that within a few short generations there may not be sufficient food to feed the globe's inhabitants unless vast new sources of supply are tapped. The farming of the sea and the development of synthetic foods may be possible future sulutions to this grave problem.

**How can one teach the uneducated and primitive peoples birth control?**

This is exceedingly difficult. At present, it appears that large-scale utilization of intrauterine devices will be the best approach to this problem. Also, surgical sterilization programs may be a solution.

**Do the financially secure peoples tend to over-reproduce too?**

No. One of the great problems facing the world today is the fact that those most able to support large families are having relatively small ones. Statistics show that the more educated and well-off people are, the more they limit family size.

**Are there organizations that give out information and teach people about birth control?**

Yes. Birth control clinics are set up in many areas of the country. In addition, there are local chapters of an organization known as Planned Parenthood throughout the United States. Also, the United Nations will make birth control data available to anyone who asks for it.

**What are the various methods of birth control?**

There are approximately a dozen methods of contraception; some are effective in only about 85 percent of cases, others are almost 100 percent effective. The methods most widely used are:
a. Abstinence.
b. Rhythm.
c. Coitus interruptus (withdrawal).
d. Condoms.
e. Douching.
f. Vaginal diaphragm and contraceptive jellies, foams, creams, and suppositories.
g. Intrauterine devices.
h. Oral contraceptives (birth control pills).
i. Surgical sterilization.

**Is abstinence advisable as a method of contraception?**

No. Prior to the advent of effective methods of contraception, physicians used to say that the only truly safe method of birth control was abstinence. Of course, we now know that there are extremely effective methods that approximate 100 percent, if used properly. Moreover, even abstinence is not 100 percent effective, as there are cases on record, admittedly very few in number, where a woman has become pregnant without having had actual intercourse. In these cases, it has been shown that semen that is ejaculated near the entrance to the vagina may come into contact with a virginal hymen (maidenhead), and the sperm may travel through the small opening in the virginal hymen and gain access to the vagina. It is well known, through tests, that sperm have the ability to leave the ejaculated semen and to swim alone along the walls of the vagina until they reach the entrance to the uterus. Few marriages could survive among young people if abstinence were the sole method of birth control.

## RHYTHM METHOD

**What is the rhythm method?**

It is a partial form of abstinence, using the supposition that there is a certain time in each month when the woman is least likely to become pregnant.

**How does the rhythm method work?**

A normal female of childbearing age sheds an egg from her ovary each month. This is known as *ovulation.* The average woman with a regular twenty-eight-day interval between menstrual periods ovulates at some time in the middle of this interval. She would be most likely then to ovulate about fourteen days after the onset of her menstruation. However, even if she is usually very regular, she might ovulate on the twelfth, thirteenth, fifteenth, or sixteenth days rather than the fourteenth day. Furthermore, even a woman who is habitually regular is subject to conditions that might throw her period temporarily off its usual timing. Should this happen, and if she should perchance have a twenty-four-day interval instead of her usual twenty-eight-day interval, she might ovulate as early as ten days after the onset of her previous period. By the same token, if she happens to be late one month and has a thirty-two-day interval, she might ovulate as late as the twentieth day after her previous menstrual period.

It is thought that sperm can live for at least two days within the Fallopian tubes, the site at which fertilization takes place. Therefore, a woman who unexpectedly has a twenty-four-day interval between periods may have an egg reach her Fallopian tube on the tenth day after the beginning of her last period. Sperm from intercourse that took place two days previously may be waiting in the Fallopian tubes when the egg arrives. *In such a case, fertilization with pregnancy may occur only eight days after the beginning of her menstrual period.* If this woman happened to have a menstrual period in that particular month that lasted for six days, then she actually becomes pregnant from intercourse that takes place only two days after her last period ended.

Similarly, if a woman who habitually has a twenty-eight-day interval unexpectedly has a thirty-two-day interval between periods, her egg may reach the Fallopian tube on the twentieth day after the beginning of her last period. It is thought that an egg spends two days passing down the Fallopian tube toward the uterus and that it is capable of being fertilized during both of these two days. Thus, such a woman can become pregnant from intercourse that takes place as late as twenty-two days after the onset of her last period.

From the foregoing, it is obvious that the rhythm method is not always accurate, and if couples had intercourse a hundred times or more during the course of one year, the chances are considerable that pregnancy would follow a menstrual irregularity.

### Do most physicians recommend the rhythm method?

No, because it is thought to be effective only in about 85 to 90 percent of cases. Statistically, therefore, a woman who has intercourse a hundred times during a year is exposed to the possibility of pregnancy on about ten to fifteen of those occasions.

### How can a woman know when she ovulates?

There is a technique for finding out the approximate time each month when a woman sheds an egg from her ovary. She takes her rectal temperature at the same time each morning before getting out of bed. The temperature record is kept for a period of several months. It will be noted that there is one morning each month when the temperature is a half degree or more above that of the other mornings. This record is kept along with an accurate record of the onset of each menstrual period. Ovulation is thought to occur the day that the temperature is elevated, and

by noting similarities in the temperature chart of each month, one can discover the time each month that the woman is most likely to ovulate. Of course, these determinations can be made only on a woman whose menstrual periods are regular.

### Can one rely completely on ovulation predictions?

No, because even the most regular individual may unexpectedly have an earlier or later ovulation. If she is following her usual period of abstinence during that month and her ovulation is off by several days, she may be exposed to pregnancy.

## COITUS INTERRUPTUS

### Is coitus interruptus a satisfactory technique for birth control?

For millions of people throughout the world, this, the oldest method of birth control, is still quite acceptable. If the male has proper control and the couple has no objection to the method, there are no medical contraindications to its use.

### Can any harm ensue from the practice of withdrawal?

No.

### Does withdrawal frequently interfere with a female orgasm?

Yes, because some women reach a climax only when their partner ejaculates within them.

### Is withdrawal a completely safe method of contraception?

No. From time to time a man may think that he is fully withdrawn before he ejaculates, but, in reality, some of the semen has been deposited in the vagina.

### When is coitus interruptus most dangerous to practice?

When the man has poor control over

ejaculation or when he suffers from premature ejaculation.

### What is meant by the term "intercourse without orgasm"?

Some men, in order to gratify their partners, and at the same time relieve any existing fear of pregnancy, will indulge in intercourse but will withhold their orgasm. As a regular practice, this should be condemned as a method of birth control. A man has a great need for completing the sexual act once he has started. Also, if utilized repeatedly, it will undoubtedly build up tensions and resentments.

## CONDOMS

### What are condoms?

They are thin latex sheaths that are placed on the male organ as a means of containing the semen following ejaculation.

### Are condoms used very widely today?

Their use has decreased markedly within the United States in recent years since the advent of the diaphragm and jellies and the birth control pills. However, they were the most frequently employed method of contraception until some thirty to forty years ago.

### Is it good practice for a condom to be used as a birth control measure?

Yes, if for some reason or another the woman has not been fitted for a diaphragm, has not purchased contraceptive jellies or creams, and has not been instructed in the taking of birth control pills.

### Are condoms safe to use?

Yes, providing they do not break and providing they are discarded after each ejaculation.

## Do condoms alter the sensations during intercourse?

Yes, most men object to the exclusive use of condoms as they state that it decreases sensations during intercourse. Some women, too, complain that they enjoy intercourse much less when their partner uses a condom.

## What are the main objections to the use of a condom as the sole method of contraception?

a. Decreases sensation during intercourse.
b. The fact that one must interrupt lovemaking in order to get the condom and put it on.
c. If the condom is not properly used, it may break during intercourse.
d. Some condoms are defective and have tiny holes in them, thus allowing some of the semen to leak out.
e. Condoms sometimes slip off after orgasm before the male has withdrawn his organ from the vagina.

## What is the proper way to use a condom?

Most condoms are packaged in a rolled state. They can be unrolled, inflated with air blown from the mouth, and tested to see if they have a hole in them. If found to be intact, the condom is again rolled and then is unrolled onto the male organ. It is necessary that at least one inch of the condom remains loose at the tip of the penis. By so doing, it permits space for the ejaculation and will also reduce friction on the latex. When rolling on a condom, one should twist the loose end so that no air remains in the tip. Failure to do this may cause the condom to burst during intercourse. When unrolling a condom, it should be unrolled completely so that the shaft of the male organ is sheathed. Before commencing intercourse, a lubricating jelly or contraceptive jelly should be applied liberally to the condom. This will reduce any possible pain from friction and will reduce the chances that the condom will rupture during the sexual act. After completion of intercourse, the man should withdraw before the penis has become entirely flaccid. If this is not done, there is a possibility of spillage of semen from around the condom. When withdrawing, the base of the condom should be held with the fingers, in order to make sure that it does not slip off and remain in the vagina. Naturally, the condom should never be used again if intercourse is resumed after a period of rest. Semen may leak to the outside during the rest interval. Prior to second intercourse, the condom should be discarded; the man should urinate and thoroughly wash his genitals and hands. He may then apply another condom.

## What should a woman do if a condom does break and ejaculation has taken place?

The woman should immediately place one or two contraceptive suppositories, or a liberal supply of contraceptive jelly or foam, deep into her vaginal canal. She should *not* douche.

# DOUCHES

## What is a douche?

It is a cleansing of the vaginal canal by use of a syringe and stream of water.

## Is the method of a douche after intercourse an effective method of contraception?

No. It is one of the poorest methods because it is difficult to wash out all the semen that has infiltrated all the crevices and folds of the vagina. In addition, within three minutes after ejaculation, millions of active sperm will have penetrated into the cervix, and douching will not flush them out.

# DIAPHRAGMS, CONTRACEPTIVE JELLIES, FOAMS, AND CREAMS

## What is a vaginal diaphragm?

It is a circular rubber device that fits tightly in the vagina and completely covers the cervix. It is one of the most frequently used methods in the United States at this time.

## Should a woman consult a physician before purchasing a diaphragm?

Yes, because a physician must first determine what size diaphragm is required and then give instruction to the woman on how it should be inserted.

## What position should a woman assume when inserting a diaphragm?

Whatever position is easiest. Some women prefer to insert a diaphragm while lying flat on their backs with knees bent up onto the abdomen; others prefer to insert it while standing with one foot resting on a chair or toilet seat; and still others find it easiest to sit on the toilet while inserting the diaphragm.

## What is most essential in the placement of a diaphragm?

It must be slid across the *back* wall of the vagina as far as it will go. The front end of the diaphragm will then be tucked in back of the pubic bone.

## Is it necessary to use an applicator in inserting a diaphragm?

There are specially designed applicators for this purpose, but many women prefer to insert the diaphragm without them.

## How can a woman be sure that the diaphragm has been inserted correctly?

By inserting a finger into the vagina, a woman should feel the cervix with the rubber over it.

## Should a woman feel the presence of a diaphragm inside her?

When a snug-fitting diaphragm is properly placed, it cannot be felt when a woman walks around, nor can it be felt during intercourse. If a diaphragm causes pain before or during intercourse, it has been inserted incorrectly and should be reinserted properly.

## Is a diaphragm, of itself, an effective contraceptive device?

The diaphragm affords some mechanical protection against sperm impregnation when it fits tightly in the vagina over the cervix. However, it is *not* recommended that it be used without the addition of a contraceptive jelly, foam, or cream. Sperm are so tiny that some can swim between the wall of the vagina and the most tightly fitting diaphragm.

## How effective is the diaphragm-jelly technique of birth control?

When used properly, it is approximately 99 percent effective.

## What are contraceptive jellies, foams, creams, tablets, and suppositories?

They are commercial products that are highly effective in destroying sperm within the vagina. When these substances are inserted properly in sufficient quantities within an hour prior to intercourse, they are a satisfactory method of contraception.

## How should contraceptive jellies, foams, or creams be used with a diaphragm?

Before the diaphragm is inserted, about one inch of jelly, foam, or cream should be placed on its concave surface. An equal amount should be spread around its rim. Most tubes of contraceptive jellies, foams, or creams bear explicit instructions on how to use them.

## When is a diaphragm removed after intercourse?

The next morning or about five hours after termination of relations.

## How is a vaginal diaphragm removed?

The index finger is placed under the diaphragm's rim and pressure is exerted in a downward direction. This maneuver permits the diaphragm to be grasped between the thumb and the index finger, thus making it easy to remove.

## What should be done for cleansing after the use of contraceptive jellies, foams, or creams?

Although it is not essential, a douche can be taken a few hours after intercourse.

# INTRAUTERINE DEVICES (IUD's)

## What is an intrauterine device (IUD)?

It is a plastic, or plastic-metal, object that the gynecologist inserts into the uterine cavity. IUD's come in varying sizes, manufactured to fit various-sized uterine cavities.

## How effective are IUD's?

They are approximately 98 percent effective.

## How is an IUD inserted?

The cervix is dilated, usually during a menstrual period, and the device is pushed into the uterine cavity.

## Is it painful to have an IUD inserted?

There is only mild discomfort. The procedure is performed in the gynecologist's office, without anesthesia.

## How do IUD's prevent pregnancy?

The exact mechanism is not known. Some investigators feel that the device blocks the entrance of the sperm into the Fallopian tube, where fertilization normally takes place.

Other investigators feel that the device causes a chemical or antibody reaction to be set up that interferes with the normal implantation of the fertilized egg into the wall of the uterus.

## How long should an IUD be permitted to remain in place?

It should be changed approximately every three years.

## Can all women use this method of birth control?

Women who tend to have heavy menstrual periods or those who have fibroid tumors or extremely painful menstruation are probably best not to have IUD's inserted.

## What are some of the disadvantages of the IUD?

a. Lower abdominal cramps in some women.
b. Excessive bleeding during menstruation, or bleeding in between periods, is occasionally encountered.
c. In a small number of cases, infection may ensue.

## What is done if the IUD causes any of the above complications?

The device is easily and promptly removed, and the cramps and excessive bleeding will subside spontaneously. Any infection can be treated effectively with antibioitics.

## Who are the best candidates for the use of the IUD?

Women who have already had children. While women who have not borne any children may safely use the device, most authorities feel that because of the possibility of an infection and its possible effect upon future fertility, they are best advised to try other methods of birth control.

## Can a tumor of the uterus result from prolonged use of an IUD?

In rare instances, some investigators believe that an IUD has stimulated a growth. However, this complication is so rare that it does not constitute a real threat to the average woman.

### How can a woman tell if an IUD has been expelled by the uterus?

The devices have a string attached to them, which protrudes from the cervix into the vagina. Patients are instructed to feel the string periodically with a fingertip. If the device is partially or wholly in the vagina, it will be apparent. Also, patients with IUD's are instructed to undergo periodic gynecological examinations.

### What if pregnancy occurs even though one has used an IUD?

The device should be removed promptly within a few days after the woman knows she is pregnant. In such cases, no harm will come to the pregnancy.

## BIRTH CONTROL PILLS
### (Oral Contraceptives)

### How do birth control pills work?

These pills, which are taken orally, are *anovulatory*. This means that they inhibit ovulation or egg formation. Without ovulation, pregnancy is impossible regardless of how many sperm enter the vagina and reach the Fallopian tubes.

### What is the composition of the birth control pill?

Each tablet contains two female hormones, one an *estrogen,* the other a *progesterone.*

### How effective are these pills?

They are 100 percent effective when taken as prescribed.

### What is the prescribed schedule for taking the pills?

They are taken once a day, at approximately the same time, for three weeks (twenty-one days). Then they are stopped for seven days, following which they are resumed for another twenty-one days. Some of the pills are packaged with seven blank tablets in a different color for those individuals who do not wish to be bothered stopping for a week each cycle. These packages are known as "Twenty-eights."

### Should a woman consult a physician before taking the Pill?

Absolutely! It should be prescribed only after she has been given a complete physical examination. In addition, there are several excellent pills on the market, and the physician may decide that one kind will be best suited to a particular patient.

### What are the advantages of the Pill over other forms of contraception?

Most users find this by far the best method of birth control. It permits intercourse without any immediate preparation or halt in foreplay. It requires no after-chores, such as removing a diaphragm or douching. The contact situations are completely natural and unaffected by the feel of a diaphragm and sticky jellies or cream or a condom. It permits falling off to sleep without having to get out of bed to cleanse away excess jelly or cream. It also eliminates any disagreeable contraceptive odor.

### What is indicated when a woman stains or bleeds during the time she is taking the Pill?

This "breakthrough bleeding" usually indicates that a larger dose of the medication is required. It does not affect the efficiency of the birth control.

### Are there any complications from taking birth control pills?

Yes, but they do not affect the majority of women. Some of these complications are headache, nausea, a bloated feeling with some weight gain due to fluid retention. In rare instances, a heart attack or an embolus is attributed to the prolonged use of the Pill, the latter condition affecting women with marked varicose veins or phlebitis. Also, some women may develop high blood pressure while on the Pill.

### Do some women develop swelling and tenderness in the breasts as a result of taking birth control pills?

Yes, but these symptoms tend to lessen, and often disappear, within a few months.

### Does the Pill cause phlebitis?

The Surgeon General of the United States Public Health Service has stated that birth control pills do *not* cause plebitis (inflammation of the veins in the legs) in a normal woman. However, if a woman has marked varicose veins, or gives a history of once having had phlebitis, it is best that she not use the pills.

### Who should not use oral contraceptives?

a. Markedly obese women.
b. Women who have marked varicose veins or evidence of phlebitis.
c. Women with chronically high blood pressure.
d. Those with a known liver disorder.
e. Heavy smokers, especially older women who smoke heavily.
f. Women with fibroids of the uterus.
g. Women who have had a breast tumor or who have cystic disease of the breasts and a family history of breast disorders or tumors.

### Are the pills conducive to cancer?

No.

### Does the taking of birth control pills interfere with pregnancy after a woman stops taking the pills?

Some gynecologists advocate stopping the pills for three months before attempting to become pregnant.

### Is there a birth control pill that men can take?

Not yet, but several drugs are being

researched that seem to interfere with the production of sperm.

## SURGICAL BIRTH CONTROL

### What surgical techniques are used for birth control in the female?

a. An incision is made in the lower abdomen, the tubes are grasped with a forceps and tied in their midportion, or tied and cut in their midportion, or are cauterized with an electric cautery.

b. A *laparoscope* is inserted through a tiny incision in the navel. The laparoscope is a hollow, lighted metal instrument through which the gynecologist looks into the abdomen. An electric cautery passes through the laparoscope and, under direct vision, the gynecologist applies the cautery to the midportions of the Fallopian tubes.

### How effective is interruption of the Fallopian tubes in preventing pregnancy?

If done properly, it is almost 100 percent effective.

### Does this operation affect a woman in any way?

No. The patient continues to ovulate and menstruate as before, and there is no effect upon sexual function or desire.

### How long is the recovery period after surgical sterilization?

a. A female remains in the hospital for about five to six days if her abdomen has been opened surgically.

b. If the tubes have been cauterized through a laparoscope, the patient will remain in the hospital overnight.

c. Male patients can readily undergo vasectomy in a doctor's office or can be hospitalized for a day or two.

### How soon after a woman has undergone surgical sterilization can she resume sexual relations?

In approximately three weeks.

### What is vasectomy?

It is the technical name for cutting the vas deferens, thereby making the male infertile.

### Should a man who has undergone vasectomy have his semen checked before resuming sexual relations?

Yes. It is important that the semen show no sperm. Some sperm that have already passed up the vas deferens prior to vasectomy may still be alive and may be stored in the seminal vesicles.

### When is tubal ligation performed?

When a woman has had several children and feels positive that she wants no more and does not care to be involved in the continuing use of other forms of contraception. Most often, it is advised for women with an incurable physical or mental illness, who would be unable to care for a child. The operation is also performed upon women who wish to avoid transmitting a serious inherited disease. A woman who is to be ligated, and her husband, must give written consent to the procedure.

### How does cutting the vas deferens in the male prevent conception?

The severing of the vas deferens prevents sperm from being ejaculated during orgasm.

### When is it performed?

When a couple has had many children and the husband wishes to spare the wife the discomfort of surgery. Cutting the vas deferens in no way interferes with a man's potency or ability to have or enjoy intercourse.

### Will reoperation restore the ability to have children in females and males who have undergone these surgical procedures?

Surgical repair and restoration of the structures that have been cauterized, ligated, or cut is only successful in a minority of cases. Restoration of the male vas deferens, using microsurgical techniques, is more successful than restoration of the Fallopian tubes in the female.

# CHAPTER 12

# BLOOD AND LYMPH DISEASES

*(See also Chapter 13 on Blood Vessels and Blood Vessel Surgery; Chapter 34 on Infectious and Virus Diseases; Chapter 38 on Laboratory (Pathology) Tests and Procedures; Chapter 50 on Parasites and Parasitic Diseases; Chapter 68 on Spleen)*

**What is blood?**

Blood is the fluid circulating through blood vessels. It contains red blood cells, white blood cells, platelets, and a pale, yellowish liquid known as plasma.

**What are the major functions of plasma?**

a. It acts as a fluid medium for the suspension of blood cells.
b. It transports dissolved nutriments to the tissues.
c. It carries waste products from the tissues to the organs of excretion, such as the lungs and the kidneys.
d. It contains substances necessary for blood clotting.

**What are the major functions of red blood cells?**

Red blood cells contain hemoglobin, the oxygen-transporting red pigment of the blood. Oxygen is thus carried to all the tissues of the body.

**What is the main function of the white blood cells (leukocytes)?**

White blood cells are part of the body's defense against infection. Some combat invading bacteria and viruses by engulfing and destroying them, while others produce infection-fighting proteins called antibodies.

**What is the function of blood platelets?**

Platelets are small, circulating cells that prevent and stop bleeding by plugging up holes in blood vessels and by promoting the clotting of blood.

**Where are the elements of blood manufactured?**

The red cells, white cells, and platelets are produced in the marrow of the bones of the body (bone marrow). During the development of the embryo, blood is also formed by other organs, such as the spleen.

## ANEMIA

**What is anemia?**

A condition in which the blood has too few red cells.

**What is the main harmful effect of anemia?**

It results in a lessened ability of the blood to supply oxygen to the tissues. This results in weakness, lassitude, and pallor.

**Are there there different types of anemia?**

Yes. They are usually classified according to the cause of anemia.

**How can one tell if he or she has anemia?**

By having a complete blood count performed by a competent laboratory.

**Is it normal to develop a certain amount of anemia in the winter months when there is less sunshine?**

No. A person may, however, look paler during this time of year.

**Can one tell by the color of the skin whether anemia is present?**

No. Unless the anemia is marked, it is not possible to tell by observing skin color. Many people who seem to be pale have normal red blood cells and are not anemic at all.

**Is it common for females who are in the age groups that menstruate to be anemic?**

Yes. The loss of blood during menstruation must be replaced by new blood produced in the bone marrow. This requires that the female have sufficient iron in her diet. If the iron is insufficient, anemia will result.

**What is sickle-cell anemia?**

It is a type of anemia occurring most frequently in members of the black race. It is characterized by a chemical abnormality of the hemoglobin, which results in the sickle-cell shape of the cells. These cells do not survive and circulate normally, and as a consequence, the patient develops anemia.

**Can one be tested for sickle-cell anemia?**

Yes. Accurate tests will tell whether an individual has inherited a sickle-cell trait (the carrier state) or whether he has inherited the disease.

**What are the chances of passing sickle-cell disease from parent to child?**

If only one parent has the sickle-cell trait, the offspring will not have the disease, but 50 percent will inherit the trait. If *both* parents have the sickle-cell trait, there is a 25 percent chance that an offspring will develop sickle-cell disease.

**What are the symptoms and signs of sickle-cell anemia?**

A severe anemia is usually present, and many children with this condition are moderately jaundiced. Older children may have long, thin arms and legs, short torsos, and protruding abdomens. Pain in the abdomen and legs occurs periodically. It is thought to be caused by sludging of the sickle cells and by failure of blood to circulate satisfactorily within the affected parts of the body.

### What is the treatment for a sickle-cell anemia?

Blood transfusions are given to restore red cells when the anemia is severe, and antibiotics are given to protect the child against infection. Treatment also involves relieving the pain that occurs during crises. Good nutrition, plenty of fluids and vitamins, especially folic acid, are recommended and may prove helpful.

### Should two people with sickle-cell traits marry?

It is perfectly all right for them to marry, but they should receive expert genetic counseling before they decide to have children.

### Why is it that some physicians recommend taking pills for anemia whereas others give injections?

It depends upon the cause of the anemia. If the anemia resulted from iron deficiency, iron pills are sufficient. However, if the anemia is associated with Vitamin $B_{12}$ deficiency, the vitamin must be administered by injection.

### Is it safe to buy patented medicines and medicate oneself for anemia?

No. If true anemia exists, the cause should be determined, and medical treatment should be carried out by a physician.

### How often should one have a blood count taken?

This should be performed about once a year as part of a general physical checkup.

### Will anemia cause increased susceptibility to infections?

Yes.

### Can a person be stout and anemic?

Definitely, yes.

### What effect does diet have on anemia?

Inadequate diet is one of the most common causes of anemia.

### What effect does a lack of vitamins have on anemia?

Vitamin B and C deficiencies, as seen in beriberi and scurvy, can cause severe anemias. Minor deficiencies may be a contributing factor to anemia.

### Can minor blood loss over a long period of time, such as bleeding from hemorrhoids, produce anemia?

Yes.

### What is a deficiency anemia?

It is an anemia caused by lack of a substance necessary for the *formation* of blood.

### What are some of the deficiency anemias, and what is lacking in the blood in these conditions?

a. Simple nutritional anemias are generally due to the lack of sufficient iron or vitamins in the diet. They are often encountered in infants who are on a milk diet or in adults whose dietary habits are poor.
b. Pernicious anemia results from a deficiency of Vitamin $B_{12}$ in people who are unable to absorb it from their intestines.
c. Iron-deficiency anemia can also be caused by acute or chronic loss of blood. This type of anemia can be treated by blood replacement or by giving iron pills, which promote the formation of new red blood cells.

### Is pernicious anemia a serious disease?

Yes. In former years it was frequently fatal. However, since the discovery of Vitamin $B_{12}$, this disease can now be controlled, and people having the disease can look forward to a normal lifespan.

### Must people with pernicious anemia take Vitamin $B_{12}$ throughout life?

Yes.

### How can one make a definite diagnosis of pernicious anemia?

a. By the characteristic findings on examination of the blood and bone marrow as seen under the microscope.
b. By finding no hydrochloric acid in the stomach on gastric analysis.
c. By determining the level of Vitamin $B_{12}$ in the blood.

### What are congenital anemias?

These anemias occur in individuals who are born with innate defects in the blood. The blood cells are generally more fragile than normal and more readily destroyed in the body. These anemias tend to be familial and are often racially distributed.

### What are some of the congenital anemias?

a. Cooley's anemia, or Mediterranean anemia. This occurs most frequently in people of Italian or Greek origin.
b. Sickle-cell anemia. This type is seen mainly in members of the black race.
c. Hemolytic anemia. These diseases, in which blood cells are destroyed more rapidly than normal, run in families and are of variable degrees of severity.

### Can anemia be caused by injury to the bone marrow where blood is formed?

Yes.

### What can cause injury to the bone marrow and thus produce an anemia?

Toxic agents such as x rays, benzene, lead, certain drugs, and other agents that are as yet unknown.

### Are toxic anemias serious?

Yes. Prompt removal of the toxic agent is necessary before the patient can get well.

### Do toxic anemias result in death?

On occasion this can happen. Overdose of radiation or toxic drugs can sometimes cause a fatal anemia.

### What are the hemolytic anemias?

Those anemias resulting from the abnormal and excessive destruction of blood cells. The destruction may be due to inherited defects in the blood itself, such as in congenital hemolytic anemia, or they may be acquired as the result of infections, specific poisons, toxins, or other diseases.

### Can the existence of a serious disease elsewhere in the body produce anemia?

Yes. This is one of the most common causes of anemia. Such a disease may interfere with blood formation by depressing the bone marrow or by actually destroying the red blood cells. People with extensive cancers often fall into this category.

### What are some common signs and symptoms of anemia?

The patient may feel weak, look pale, have palpitation of the heart, shortness of breath, and headache.

### How is anemia best treated?

This will depend entirely on the cause for the particular anemia. In deficiency anemias, the substance that is lacking must be replaced. In toxic anemias, the specific poison must be eliminated from the diet or environment. If the anemia is severe,

blood transfusions must be given as a temporary replacement measure.

### Are blood transfusions curative in the treatment of most anemias?

No. It is necessary to find the underlying cause and to eliminate it. Blood transfusions are usually of temporary benefit only, except when they are used to replace sudden loss of blood.

## POLYCYTHEMIA VERA

### What is polycythemia vera?

A condition in which the body produces too many red blood cells.

### What is the significance of polycythemia?

The blood is thickened, tends to clot too readily, and may result in clotting within the blood vessels.

### Is polycythemia a serious condition?

It can be, because it may cause thrombosis (clotting) in blood vessels.

### What is the treatment for polycythemia?

It is treated by frequent bleedings (phlebotomy) of the patient or by the administration of certain drugs, which reduce the number of red blood cells.

### Can people with polycythemia lead normal lives?

Yes, but they must be kept under constant medical observation and control.

### What is the cause of polycythemia vera?

The cause is unknown.

### How can one tell if a patient has polycythemia?

The patient may complain of weakness, headache, and other vague

symptoms. There may be hemorrhages in the skin and mucous membranes. A common feature is a dusky, blue-red flush to the skin. Examination may reveal that the spleen is enlarged, and a blood count will show an excess of red blood cells.

### How is the diagnosis established positively in polycythemia?

By a combination of findings, including a high red blood count and an enlarged spleen.

### Is polycythemia inherited?

No.

## BLOOD POISONING

### What is blood poisoning?

A condition in which bacteria are found in the blood. If the bacteria cause fever and intoxication, the condition is known as septicemia. When the bacteria are merely present for a short period of time, the condition is called bacteremia.

### How does blood poisoning occur?

By germs extending from some infected area in the body into the bloodstream. This is most usually a complication of a neglected or badly treated abscess or other infection.

### Is septicemia fatal?

Sometimes. In former years, those who developed septicemia usually died. Today, however, by identifying the offending bacteria by blood culture and by treating the patient with the appropriate antibiotic drug, most patients with septicemia will get well.

### How does one decide what medication to give in a case of blood poisoning?

A blood culture is taken from the vein of the patient, and the bacteria are grown in a culture medium in the laboratory. The germ's sensitivity to various antibiotic drugs is determined, and the specific antibiotic to which the bacteria is most sensitive is given.

### How can one tell if he is recovering from septicemia?

By taking repeated cultures of the blood. When the blood is sterile on several cultures and when the temperature has maintained a normal level, the patient can be considered to have recovered.

### What are some of the complications of septicemia?

Since germs are circulating throughout the blood, they may lodge and form abscesses or secondary infections anywhere in the body—in the tissues under the skin, the lungs, the liver, the brain, etc.

### Is surgery ever indicated in septicemia?

Not for removing the bacteria from the bloodstream. However, surgery is sometimes necessary for the complications of septicemia, as in the surgical drainage of abscesses that may have formed as a result of bacteria lodging in certain areas of the body.

## HEMOPHILIA AND OTHER BLEEDING TENDENCIES

### What is hemophilia?

A hereditary disease characterized by delayed clotting of the blood and a consequent abnormal tendency to bleed or hemorrhage.

### Is hemophilia hereditary?

Definitely, yes.

### How is hemophilia transmitted?

It is inherited by males through the mother.

### What causes hemophilia?

A deficiency within the plasma of a clotting factor, which is present in normal individuals.

### Do females ever get true hemophilia?

It is almost exclusively a male disease.

### How common is hemophilia?

It is a rare condition.

### Can a hemophiliac marry?

Yes. If he has children, his sons will be normal, but his daughters will be carriers of the disease.

### Should a female member of a hemophiliac family marry?

Marriage is is in no way contraindicated. However, such a female may be a carrier of the hemophiliac factor.

### What will happen to the children of a woman from a hemophiliac family?

Half of her sons will have hemophilia, and half of her daughters will be carriers.

### How is the diagnosis of hemophilia made?

A history of abnormal bleeding would lead a physician to order thorough blood examinations, including the testing of the blood-clotting mechanisms. Such tests would reveal the missing factor responsible for hemophilia.

### Are other blood findings normal in patients with hemophilia?

Yes. The only abnormality is the absence of a specific clot-promoting factor.

### What are some of the signs and symptoms of hemophilia?

Continued and prolonged bleeding after a minor injury. Bleeding into the muscles or joints is also characteristic of the condition. The disease is frequently discovered early in infancy when circumcision is performed.

### Does bleeding ever take place in

the hemophilia patient without an actual cut or laceration?

Yes. Bleeding under the skin with large black-and-blue-areas, or bleeding into one of the joints, may take place merely from a contusion or fall.

### What is the local treatment when a hemophilia patient sustains a laceration?

Application of firm pressure over the injured area.

### What treatment is given the hemophilia patient who continues to bleed?

He is promptly given an intravenous injection of concentrated plasma containing large amounts of the antihemophilic factor. This substance is commonly known as AHF.

### What is the outlook for the individual who has hemophilia?

With the availability of concentrated AHF, the outlook has improved dramatically. Many hospitals throughout the country have special provisions for handling hemophilia patients so that it is rare today for such a patient to die from bleeding. Actually, many hemophilia patients have learned to treat themselves at home.

### Can a patient with hemophilia live a normal span of life?

Yes, providing he is treated promptly when bleeding occurs.

### What is the future outlook in the treatment of hemophilia?

More efficient and cheaper ways of producing and giving AHF are being developed. Also, in some areas, hemophilia patients are receiving prophylactic treatment for their condition.

### What is meant by bleeding tendencies?

There are people with bleeding tendencies who do not have true hemophilia. Such conditions often affect females as readily, if not more so, as males. They are due to some deficiency within the blood, which either prolongs the bleeding time or retards the clotting mechanism.

### What are some diseases associated with bleeding tendencies?

a. Thrombocytopenic purpura. This condition is associated with an abnormally low blood platelet level. (See Chapter 68, on The Spleen.)

b. Diseases due to lack of vitamins, such as scurvy. (See Chapter 78, on Vitamins.)

c. Cirrhosis of the liver. (See Chapter 40, on The Liver.)

## INFECTIONS OF LYMPH GLANDS

### What are lymph nodes (glands)?

These are small, oval-shaped structures, which drain the lymph channels. They exist everywhere in the body and can be felt under the skin in the neck, under the armpits, in the groin, etc. They vary in size from one-eighth to one-half inch in length.

### What are the functions of the lymph glands?

The lymph glands ward off and block the spread of infection or disease.

### What happens when bacteria or toxins reach these lymph glands?

The result is an inflammation of the glands known as lymphadenitis.

### What is lymphangitis?

An inflammation of the lymphatic channels leading to the lymph glands.

### How can one tell if there is an infection of the lymph channels (lymphangitis)?

There are red streaks seen in the skin along the course of the lymph channel. These can be seen along a leg or arm extending from an infection of a foot or hand.

### What is the treatment for lymphangitis?

Surgical incision and drainage of the infection at its primary site. Also, antibiotics will control infection within a lymph channel.

### What happens when infection has involved the lymph glands?

a. The gland becomes enlarged and tender.

b. If the infection can be successfully combated by the cells within the glands over a period of time, the infection will subside and the swelling of the glands will go down.

c. The infection may be stopped at the lymph glands, but the lymph gland itself may be severely damaged. In this event, an abscess of the lymph gland will develop.

d. If the infection is overpowering, it may pass straight through the lymph gland into the lymphatic channels, which lie beyond the lymph glands, and then on into the bloodstream. In this event, blood poisoning (septicemia) may result.

### What must be done when lymph glands are involved in abscess formation?

Surgical incision and drainage of the abscess must be performed.

### Can inflammation of the lymph glands be successfully treated with medications?

Usually, antibiotic drugs will control infection of the lymph glands. However, once pus has formed, it must be drained surgically.

### Where does one commonly see infected lymph glands?

a. When the scalp is infected, there will be enlarged lymph glands in the back of the neck. When the ear is infected, there may be enlarged glands in front of and behind the ear. When the face or nose and throat are infected, the glands in the neck may be enlarged and tender.

b. An infection of the toes or feet will show enlarged glands in the groin.

c. An infection of the finger or hand may show enlarged glands under the arms.

### Do the lymph glands ever become enlarged because of conditions other than infection?

Yes. One of the most common modes of spread of cancer is through the lymph channels. Thus, cancer often spreads to the lymph nodes, causing them to enlarge.

### What glands are most commonly affected by the spread of cancer?

The lymph glands under the arms are frequently involved in cancer that has spread from the breast. The glands in the neck may be involved in cancer that has spread from the nose and throat or from the thyroid gland. The glands in the groin may be affected because of the spread of cancer from the lower extremities. All internal organs have adjacent lymph glands, and these are frequently involved in the spread of cancer.

### Are the lymph glands ever involved in tuberculosis?

Yes. Tuberculosis of the lymph glands in the neck used to be a common complication of tuberculosis of the tonsils. This is not seen very often today, since pasteurization has eliminated infected milk.

## LEUKEMIA

### What is leukemia?

Leukemia is a malignant disease of the bloodforming tissues, wherein abnormal white blood cells are found in the bloodstream in unusual numbers.

### Are there various kinds of leukemia?

Yes. They are classified not only according to the cell type, but also according to the clinical course. The course may be rapid (acute), or slowly progressive (chronic).

**Is leukemia a form of cancer?**
Yes.

**How can one diagnose the different forms of leukemia?**
By noting the particular type of white blood cell that is involved in the cancerous process.

**What is the cause of leukemia?**
The cause is unknown. However, it seems to occur more frequently in people exposed to radiation and certain chemicals.

**How common is leukemia?**
It is not an uncommon disease. About twenty thousand new cases occur in the United States each year.

**What are the different types of leukemia?**
There are two forms of the acute, or rapidly progressing, type, and two forms of the chronic, or slowly progressing, type of the disease. The various types are determined by microscopic examination of the blood cells and cells taken from the bone marrow.

**Where does leukemia usually begin?**
Probably in the bone marrow, where the white blood cell elements are formed. It may first become clinically apparent by enlargement of the lymph nodes (glands), the spleen, or the liver.

**What are the symptoms of leukemia?**
Pallor, loss of weight and appetite, excessive weakness, and fatigue. The patient may be anemic, may run a slight fever, and may bleed excessively after a minor injury.

**What is the average length of sur-**

vival for the chronic forms of leukemia?
Approximately three to five years from the onset of the disease. However, sometimes leukemia can be controlled for an indefinite period of time.

**Does the height of the white blood cell count in the blood directly influence the disease?**
In chronic leukemia, very high white counts can be tolerated for long periods of time.

**What is the general aim of treatment of leukemia?**
The goal is to cure the patient of his disease. Unfortunately, this is only possible in a minority of cases. In the others, the goal is to induce and maintain a remission for as long as possible.

**Can remissions be obtained in most cases of leukemia?**
Yes, and the remissions may last for several years.

**Do the various treatments now available prolong the life of the average leukemia patient?**
Definitely, yes.

**What is the future outlook for leukemia?**
A great deal of productive research is going on in this field. Some patients can now be cured; others can live much longer than they would have some ten years ago.

## LYMPHOMA

**What is meant by the term lymphoma?**
A lymphoma is a malignant tumor of lymphoid tissue. Lymphomas are subdivided into Hodgkin's disease and the Non-Hodgkin's lymphomas.

**How is the diagnosis of lymphoma suspected?**
By noting enlargement of lymph nodes, often in the neck, under the arms, or in the groin. Enlargement of the spleen or liver may be the first evidence of the presence of a lymphoma. It should be emphasized, however, that simple enlargement of the lymphoid tissues is usually due to causes other than malignancy.

**How can a positive diagnosis be made?**
By removing one of the glands surgically and submitting it to microscopic examination by a pathologist.

## HODGKIN'S DISEASE

**What is Hodgkin's disease?**
A malignant lymph gland disease, which falls into the category of the lymphoma group.

**Is Hodgkin's disease common?**
It is a relatively uncommon disease.

**Who is most likely to get Hodgkin's disease?**
It can occur at any age but is found most often in the third and fourth decades of life. It is more common among males than females.

**Is Hodgkin's disease inherited, or does it tend to run in families?**
No.

**What is the cause of Hodgkin's disease?**
The cause in unknown.

**What are the symptoms of Hodgkin's disease?**
At the outset there is usually none, and the only evidence of the disease may be the painless swelling of lymph glands. Later on there may be abdominal discomfort due to an enlarged spleen, bouts of fever, and weight loss. Eventually, the patient

may become anemic and suffer all of the associated symptoms of anemia.

### What organs are involved in Hodgkin's disease?

The lymph glands, liver, spleen, and bone marrow are most commonly involved. Other organs, too, may be involved in the process.

### How is the diagnosis of Hodgkin's disease made?

By the surgical removal of one of the glands and by noting characteristic findings on microscopic examination.

### What is the usual course of Hodgkin's disease?

Most patients with Hodgkin's disease can now be cured with radiation therapy and/or chemotherapy, providing they are diagnosed and treated during the earlier stages of the disease.

### Is Hodgkin's disease a form of cancer?

Although opinion is somewhat divided, most physicians believe that the condition is a type of malignancy.

### What is the treatment for Hodgkin's disease?

Many cases are treated primarily with radiation (x ray, cobalt, etc.) therapy; others are treated with chemotherapy. A combination of both methods often brings about the best results. Dramatic improvement in the cure rate and quality of survival has been achieved through modern treatment.

## NON-HODGKIN'S LYMPHOMA

### What is Non-Hodgkin's lymphoma?

It is a form of lymphoma that differs from Hodgkin's disease in its microscopic characteristics and in its pattern of spread.

### Is Non-Hodgkin's lymphoma ever localized to one area of the body?

This does occur occasionally, but most cases show early spread of the disease.

### What is the treatment for Non-Hodgkin's lymphoma?

The localized form of the disease is treated by radiation therapy. When the disease is widespread, it is treated by chemotherapy.

### Can people with Non-Hodgkin's lymphoma live for prolonged periods of time?

Yes. Patients generally survive many years, and some are cured.

CHAPTER **13**

# BLOOD VESSELS AND BLOOD VESSEL SURGERY
## (Vascular Surgery)

*(See also Chapter 5 on Aging; Chapter 19 on Diabetes Mellitus; Chapter 29 on Heart; Chapter 73 on Transplantation of Organs)*

## ARTERIOSCLEROSIS
### (Hardening of the Arteries)

**What is arteriosclerosis, or hardening of the arteries?**

The normal wall of an artery is strong, supple, and elastic so that it can expand and contract in adjustment to the changes in the blood pressure, which take place with every heart contraction. When an artery becomes hardened or arteriosclerotic, its walls are rigid and pipelike instead of elastic. This is caused by abnormal deposits within the walls of the artery that cause gradual narrowing and may eventually seal the vessel completely so that no blood can pass through it.

**What causes arteriosclerosis?**

The exact cause is unknown, but great advancements have been made within recent years in investigations as to the cause. Current thinking tends to favor the theory that wear and tear upon the blood vessels and faulty metabolism of fatty substances (such as cholesterol) produce arteriosclerosis.

**Why does hardening of the arteries take place at an earlier age in some people than in others?**

It is thought that there is an inborn factor that predisposes some people toward earlier hardening of their arteries. The body chemistry of each individual and his dietary habits seem to influence the development of arteriosclerosis.

**What types of people are more prone to develop early arteriosclerosis?**

a. People with diabetes.
b. Overweight people.
c. People with high blood pressure.
d. Those who have a particularly high fat content within their blood.

**Does early arteriosclerosis tend to run in the family or to be inherited?**

It is not inherited, but a tendency toward early arteriosclerosis does exist in families. On the other hand, certain families seem to develop very little hardening of the arteries until extremely advanced ages. It is highly probable that environmental factors and diet are of greater significance than heredity.

**What are the symptoms of arteriosclerosis?**

This will depend entirely upon the location and the degree of the condition. Basically, the symptoms are those caused by decreased blood flow through the artery. For example, if the coronary arteries of the heart are involved, the individual may experience angina pectoris upon exertion. If the arteries of the legs are involved, the patient may experience intermittent claudication (severe cramps and pain in the muscles of the legs on walking).

**How is the diagnosis of arteriosclerosis usually arrived at?**

There are many ways in which this can be done. For instance, an examination of the eye grounds through an ophthalmoscope will often reveal hardening of the arteries in the retina. Hardening of the arteries of the arms and legs can often be determined simply upon feeling the vessels with the examining fingers. X-ray examination of various structures often will reveal the characteristic picture of hardened blood vessels. Special x-ray examinations called arteriograms will show narrowing of the passageways of blood vessels, thus indicating the presence of arteriosclerosis.

**Is there any sure method of preventing hardening of the arteries?**

No. However, if one is overweight, he should reduce. If one is accustomed to eating foods rich in cholesterol, he should eliminate these from his diet. If high blood pressure is present, this should be brought under control. These measures may tend to slow down the arteriosclerotic process.

**Does hardening of the arteries always produce symptoms?**

No. A minimal amount of arteriosclerosis may cause no symptoms whatever. Also, it is not unusual for some of the smaller blood vessels to be uninvolved in a sclerotic process. These vessels may take over the work that was formerly done by the larger arteriosclerotic vessels. Thus, a leg with marked hardening of the main arteries may function normally as a result of this "collateral circulation."

**Are there any satisfactory treatments for arteriosclerosis?**

Yes. Certain people can be helped greatly. There are drugs that will relieve the spasm that accompanies hardened blood vessels, thus permitting them to carry more blood. Certain physiotherapy procedures will also relax spasm and thereby increase the blood supply in the area. In addition, there are a number of

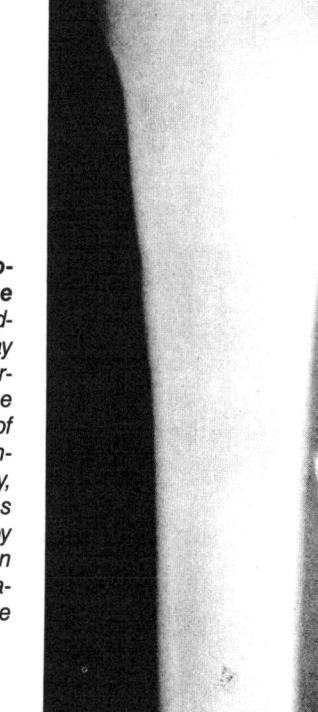

*X ray Showing Arteriosclerosis of the Main Artery in the Leg.* Should such hardening advance to any great extent, it may cause pain on walking or exercising (claudication). In extreme conditions of arteriosclerosis of the main vessels in a limb, gangrene may set in. Fortunately, the very small arteries have less of a tendency to be affected by arteriosclerosis, and they often take over the function of the major vessels, thus preserving the circulation within the limb.

surgical procedures that have been developed in treating arteriosclerosis. (See the section on Blood Vessel Surgery in this chapter.)

**Is bed rest helpful in cases of arteriosclerosis?**

Yes, when an acute complication, such as an infection or an ulcer, has set in. Also, if the blood flow to an organ is diminished, it will require more rest in order to perform its work.

**Should a patient with marked arteriosclerosis limit his physical activity?**

Yes. He must learn to function within the bounds of his restricted circulation.

**Does the excess drinking of alcohol over a prolonged period of time produce early hardening of the arteries?**

In all probability, this is not a major factor. On the other hand, there is a school of thought that believes that alcohol tends to *decrease* hardening of the arteries. However, there is no concrete evidence that this is true.

**Does smoking lead to early arteriosclerosis?**

There are recent statistical studies of considerable value that tend to indict smoking as a serious predisposing cause toward early arteriosclerosis.

**Does obesity encourage the early development of arteriosclerosis?**

Yes, because it places an additional load of work on the blood vessels.

**Does arteriosclerosis ever get well by itself?**

No, but there are many instances wherein the condition is relatively static, thus permitting the patient a completely normal span of life.

**Once arteriosclerosis has devel-**

oped, will special diet and proper rest cause the process to subside or disappear?

No. Once hardening has set in, there is no way to reverse the process.

**Is there a significant correlation between high blood cholesterol and arteriosclerosis?**

The fact has not been proved conclusively. However, it is known that high blood cholesterol and arteriosclerosis seem to coexist in a large proportion of cases.

**What are the greatest dangers of arteriosclerosis?**

Premature arteriosclerosis means early aging, with decreased vitality and decreased organ efficiency. If the heart is involved, coronary thrombosis may occur. If the brain is affected, senility, cerebral hemorrhage, or cerebral thrombosis may take place. If the extremities are involved, muscle cramps, impairment of blood supply, or even gangrene may ensue.

**How can a physician determine the rate at which arteriosclerosis is progressing?**

By periodic physical examination of the patient, with comparison of various findings.

## RAYNAUD'S DISEASE

**What is Raynaud's disease?**

It is a specific disease characterized by attacks of severe spasm of the blood vessels of the fingers or toes. Attacks of spasm are often brought on by emotional disturbances or by exposure to extreme cold or dampness. Occasionally, the ears, the tip of the nose, the chin, or the cheeks may be involved.

**What causes Raynaud's disease?**

The cause is unknown, but the disease tends to affect those who are thin, underweight, and exceptionally emotional.

**Are women more susceptible to Raynaud's disease?**

Yes.

**What are the symptoms of Raynaud's disease?**

During emotional excitement or on exposure to excessive cold, one or more fingers may turn white and then blue. The finger becomes numb, tingles, and aches with pain. This will last for a few minutes and then subside with return to normal circulation.

**What is the medical management for Raynaud's disease?**

a. Avoidance of dampness and extremes of cold.
b. The wearing of warm gloves and stockings.
c. The minimization of emotional stress.
d. The avoidance of tobacco in any form.
e. The administration of certain medications to cause dilation of blood vessels.
f. The administration of the drug Aldomet.

**What is the surgical treatment for Raynaud's disease?**

In severe cases, a sympathectomy is performed. This means cutting certain nerves (ganglia) that control the contraction and dilation of blood vessels in the extremities.

**Is the surgery for Raynaud's disease dangerous?**

No. It will consist of a sympathectomy in the region of the lower neck and upper chest. An incision is made on either side of the lower neck, and the nerves controlling contraction of the blood vessels in the arms are severed.

**Are the results of a sympathectomy for Raynaud's disease successful?**

Yes. This operation usually results in a cure of the condition and produces no unfavorable aftereffects.

**Does ulceration or gangrene of the fingers or toes ever take place in Raynaud's disease?**

Yes, in rare instances.

**How effective is the treatment of Raynaud's disease?**

One of the above forms of treatment usually brings about relief from the symptoms of this disease.

# BUERGER'S DISEASE
## (Thromboangiitis Obliterans)

**What is Buerger's disease?**

It is a chronic inflammatory disease of certain arteries and veins, principally of the extremities, usually terminating in clotting of the vessels. It occurs most often among men in their twenties, thirties, or forties.

**What causes Buerger's disease?**

The exact cause is unknown, but it is interesting to note that most of these patients are heavy tobacco smokers. In a certain small percentage of cases, it is thought that the eating of large quantities of rye bread may be associated with the onset of this condition.

**What are the symptoms of Buerger's disease?**

The symptoms are caused by inflammation of the blood vessels, which will eventually lead to occlusion. At first, the patient may experience coldness or an aching pain in one of his limbs. Next, he may have severe pain along the course of the blood vessels. Eventually there may be the consequences of the inadequate blood supply, with ulceration or areas of gangrene in the skin of the involved extremity. Finally, a toe or even an entire extremity may become gangrenous.

**Is this disease more common among Jewish people?**

It was once thought that this disease was predominant among Jewish people, but recent statistics have proved that its distribution is widespread and not limited to any one group.

**Does Buerger's disease ever affect the blood vessels of the heart, brain, kidneys, or intestines?**

Yes, but it is extremely difficult to confirm such a diagnosis.

**What is the medical treatment for Buerger's disease?**

a. *Smoking is absolutely forbidden.* Many patients will show immediate and remarkable improvement within a few weeks after they stop smoking.
b. Physiotherapy may be carried out to improve the blood supply to the extremities.
c. Medications to relax blood vessel spasm often prove helpful.
d. Nerve blocks (involving the blocking with Novocain of those nerves that cause blood vessels to contract) have proved to be helpful in certain cases.

**Is surgery ever beneficial in the treatment of Buerger's disease?**

Yes. In certain isolated cases, a lumbar sympathectomy in the lower back has helped by severing those nerves that stimulate blood vessel contraction.

**Is lumbar sympathectomy a dangerous operative procedure?**

No. Recovery will occur in practically all cases.

**How is lumbar sympathectomy performed?**

Through incisions made in the loins.

**What is the outlook for a patient with Buerger's disease?**

This disease tends to be chronic and lasts many years. If it has not progressed too far, and if the patient gives up smoking and carries out other measures listed above, he may avoid the most serious complication, gangrene of an extremity.

## THROMBOSIS

**What is a blood vessel thrombosis?**
The formation of a blood clot within the vessel, in either an artery or a vein.

**What causes thrombosis?**
There are many causes, some of which are not yet well understood. However, some of the more common causes are associated with conditions in which the blood vessel is diseased or injured, or a clot has broken away from a primary site and clogs a distant vessel. (See the section on Embolism in this chapter.) Also, disturbance in the blood-clotting mechanism may predispose toward a thrombosis. Thrombosis may also be caused by stagnation of blood within a vessel after an operation, or may be found in people who are debilitated and do no physical exercise.

**What can be the results of a thrombus?**
a. Interruption of the blood flow through the vessel, with consequent degeneration or gangrene of the organ ordinarily supplied with blood.
b. A piece of a thrombus in a vein may break off and travel to another part of the body (embolization), causing grave injury or death.

**When a thrombus breaks off and travels elsewhere, what is this called?**
This phenomenon is called an embolism.

**Does a thrombosis of a blood vessel ever get well by itself?**
Yes. Many vessels involved in thrombus formation will return to near-normal. The acute phase usually subsides with rest and the use of anticoagulant medications. The thrombus is eventually absorbed, and the aperture of the vessel is reestablished by the formation of new channels within its walls.

**What happens to an organ when it is supplied by a vessel that has undergone thrombosis?**
a. The organ may degenerate or become gangrenous.
b. Function may be severely damaged, but eventual recovery may take place by the absorption of the clot and reestablishment of the blood flow.
c. Minor blood vessels in the vicinity may dilate and transmit an adequate supply of blood to keep the organ alive and functioning.

## EMBOLISM

**What is an embolus?**
A piece of blood clot that has broken off from a thrombus in a vein or from the wall of the heart. An embolus travels through the bloodstream from one part of the body to another.

**What causes an embolus?**
It is felt that activity or strain by a patient who has a newly formed thrombus in a vein may cause a piece to break off. Clots of blood from the wall of the heart, or from heart valves, are usually fragile and break away readily. A poorly functioning heart, or a heart with an infection on a valve, is particularly prone to developing blood clots with subsequent emboli.

**What are the symptoms of embolism?**
There is often sudden and dramatic onset of shock. If the embolus has traveled to the brain, a stroke may take place. If the embolus has traveled to the lungs, there may be the sudden onset of shock, chest pain, spitting of blood, and difficulty in breathing. If the embolus has traveled to one of the limbs, the limb becomes cold and bluish, and pulsations are lost.

**Does embolism ever cause sudden death?**
It is one of the most common causes of sudden death!

**Does recovery ever take place after embolism?**
Yes, in a large percentage of cases, unless the embolus has traveled to the brain or the lungs and has interfered too extensively with the blood supply to these organs. In many instances where the brain or the lungs are involved, survival takes place.

**Is it ever possible to successfully remove an embolus and restore normal circulation?**
See the section on Blood Vessel Surgery in this chapter.

## ANEURYSM

**What is an aneurysm?**
It is a weakness in the wall of an artery resulting in a local dilatation or outpouching. It is analogous to a blister on a tire.

**What are some of the causes of aneurysm?**
a. An inherent weakness in the muscular coat of the vessel wall.
b. Injury to a blood vessel.
c. Disease of a blood vessel, such as arteriosclerosis, syphilis, or some other infection.

**At what sites are aneurysms most frequently found?**
They can occur anywhere within the body but have a tendency to occur in major arteries, such as the aorta, or in the groin, or behind the knee—or within the brain.

## What is the danger of an aneurysm?

The walls of an aneurysm are thin and lack a strong, inner elastic lining. Therefore they are apt to rupture and lead to a fatal hemorrhage.

## What aneurysms are most likely to rupture?

Those in the aorta, especially ones in the abdominal aorta.

## Can a patient ever be saved if an aneurysm ruptures?

Yes, if the diagnosis is made promptly, before too great a hemorrhage has occurred. (See the section on Blood Vessel Surgery in this chapter.)

## What is an arteriovenous aneurysm?

It is a connection between an artery and a vein, frequently the result of a severe injury.

## What harm is an arteriovenous (AV) aneurysm?

The connection between the artery and vein short-circuits blood away from the tissues ordinarily supplied by the artery. If the aneurysm joins a large artery and vein, it will place a great strain upon the heart.

## Is an arteriovenous (AV) aneurysm ever created purposely?

Yes, in patients with severe kidney disease who will require prolonged treatment with the artificial kidney (hemodialysis). In these patients, an artery and vein in the forearm are stitched to each other so that an aneurysm results. The aneurysm enlarges the vessels and makes it easy to stick a needle into them so as to connect the patient's circulation to the artificial kidney machine.

## What is the treatment for an aneurysm?

See the section on Blood Vessel Surgery in this chapter.

# THROMBOPHLEBITIS

## What is thrombophlebitis?

It is an inflammation of the wall of a vein associated with blood-clot formation and the stoppage of blood flow through the vessel.

## What are some of the factors predisposing toward the development of thrombophlebitis?

a. Stagnation of blood within a vein due to prolonged inactivity, prolonged standing in one position, and pressure upon a vein that cuts off its blood flow (tight garters may cause this).
b. A blood clot within a vein due to an injury, infection, or irritation of its wall.
c. Varicosities of the veins, with incompetent valves causing the blood to stagnate.
d. An increased tendency for the blood to clot due to some blood disease.

## Is there a difference between the type of phlebitis caused by an inflammation and the type usually seen after an operation?

Yes. The phlebitis sometimes encountered after surgery is called phlebothrombosis rather than thrombophlebitis. It signifies that the phlebitis has arisen as a result of inactivity and stagnation imposed by the operation. The inflammatory factor is much less evident in this form of phlebitis.

## Is it important for people to keep active and moving after major surgery in order to prevent phlebitis?

Yes. This is the underlying reason for getting people out of bed as soon as possible after a major surgical operation (early ambulation).

## Is thrombophlebitis a common condition?

Yes, it is an extremely common condition, particularly in today's society wherein people are less active physically and tend to stand in one position for long periods of time. In former years, when people were more active, varicose veins and phlebitis were less prevalent.

## Is phlebitis a common complication of pregnancy?

Yes. It is thought to result from the pressure of the fetus upon the great veins within the pelvis. This interferes with a free and easy flow of blood through the major veins toward the heart. When the blood stagnates, it has a greater tendency to clot.

## What kinds of people are more likely to develop thrombophlebitis?

Those in whom there is poor heart function, or those who are affected by some chronic disease. It is also more apt to occur in areas adjacent to an infection or injury.

## Does phlebitis tend to run in families or to be inherited?

It is not an inherited condition, but the type of blood vessels one possesses is inherited. Thus, people with fragile veins or varicose veins have a greater tendency toward the development of phlebitis. (Varicosities tend to run in families.)

## What actually takes place when a patient has thrombophlebitis?

There is an inflammation of the inner wall of the vessel, which causes blood in contact with the inflamed area to adhere and clot. The vessel may eventually become clogged to such an extent that blood must travel through other channels.

## What measures can be taken to prevent phlebitis?

a. Do not wear tight, circular garters.
b. Regular exercise, such as walking, is necessary for people who stand in one position for several hours at a time (barbers, machine operators, ushers, etc.).

*(continued)*

c. If one is a heavy smoker, it is perhaps best to discontinue the practice, since smokers have a greater tendency toward the development of phlebitis.

## What are the symptoms of thrombophlebitis?

a. There may be no symptoms at all or there may be a markedly swollen, red, hot, and tender leg.
b. There may be a tender cord felt along the course of an inflamed vein.
c. There may be a low-grade fever.

## What is the paramount danger in not following medical advice in thrombophlebitis?

The danger is that a piece of the thrombus (clot) may break off and travel to another part of the body, such as the lung.

## What is the treatment for thrombophlebitis?

a. Bed rest.
b. The giving of anticoagulant medications to prevent the spread of the clot.
c. Medications to relieve pain.
d. The giving of antibiotics to control infection, which may be present.
e. The wearing of bandages to give support to painful veins.
f. In certain cases, where the clot shows evidence of spreading despite adequate medical treatment, surgery may be necessary. This will consist of tying off the vein higher up so as to prevent further spread of the clot.
g. In some cases, the involved vein is exposed surgically and opened, the clotted blood is removed, and the opening in the vessel is sutured.

## Does thrombophlebitis tend to get well by itself?

Yes, but medical supervision is essential.

## What is the general course of thrombophlebitis?

The average case lasts from three to six weeks before it subsides completely.

## What are the permanent aftereffects of phlebitis?

If a large number of veins has been damaged by the process, blood may be slowed in its return course from the extremity to the heart. In such cases, there may be permanent swelling of the limb.

## Is hospitalization necessary for phlebitis?

If the patient has an acute phlebitis with elevated temperature, it is perhaps best that he be treated in the hospital, where antibiotics and anticoagulant medications can be given under supervision.

## Is there a tendency for thrombophlebitis to recur after it has once been arrested?

Yes. People who have had one attack must guard against a subsequent one.

## How can one prevent a recurrent attack of thrombophlebitis?

a. Improve the general health and treat any existing infection.
b. Obtain medical advice on the proper exercises for the extremities.
c. Avoid wearing tight, constricting garters around the legs.
d. Certain people should be placed on anticoagulant therapy for an indefinite period.
e. Stop smoking.

## Will the wearing of elastic stockings or elastic bandages help people who have a tendency toward thrombophlebitis?

Yes, as it will aid the return flow of blood from the extremity.

## Should elastic stockings be given to every patient with phlebitis?

No, only to those people who feel better when they wear the stockings. Those who have phlebitis of both deep and superficial veins may feel worse when wearing elastic supports.

## What surgical measures can be carried out to prevent subsequent attacks of phlebitis?

The ligation and/or ligation and stripping of incompetent varicose veins.

# BLOOD VESSEL SURGERY

## In what conditions is blood vessel surgery most helpful?

1. Lacerations (cuts) of major arteries or veins.
2. Arterioscleriosis.
3. Thrombosis of an artery or vein.
4. Thrombophlebitis (inflammation) of veins.
5. Embolism.
6. Aneurysm.
7. Cirrhosis of the liver.
8. Varicose veins.
9. Blood vessel tumors.
10. Fistulas between arteries and veins (arteriovenous fistulas).

## 1. Lacerations

## Can one bleed to death from a lacerated artery or vein?

Yes, but fatal hemorrhages occur mostly when a major vessel is severed, such as the jugular vein in the neck or the major arteries in the limbs. Bleeding from smaller vessels can be controlled usually by direct pressure over the bleeding point or by the temporary application of a tourniquet. (See Chapter 26, on First Aid in Emergencies.)

## Should lacerated blood vessels be tied off or repaired?

When a major artery, such as the

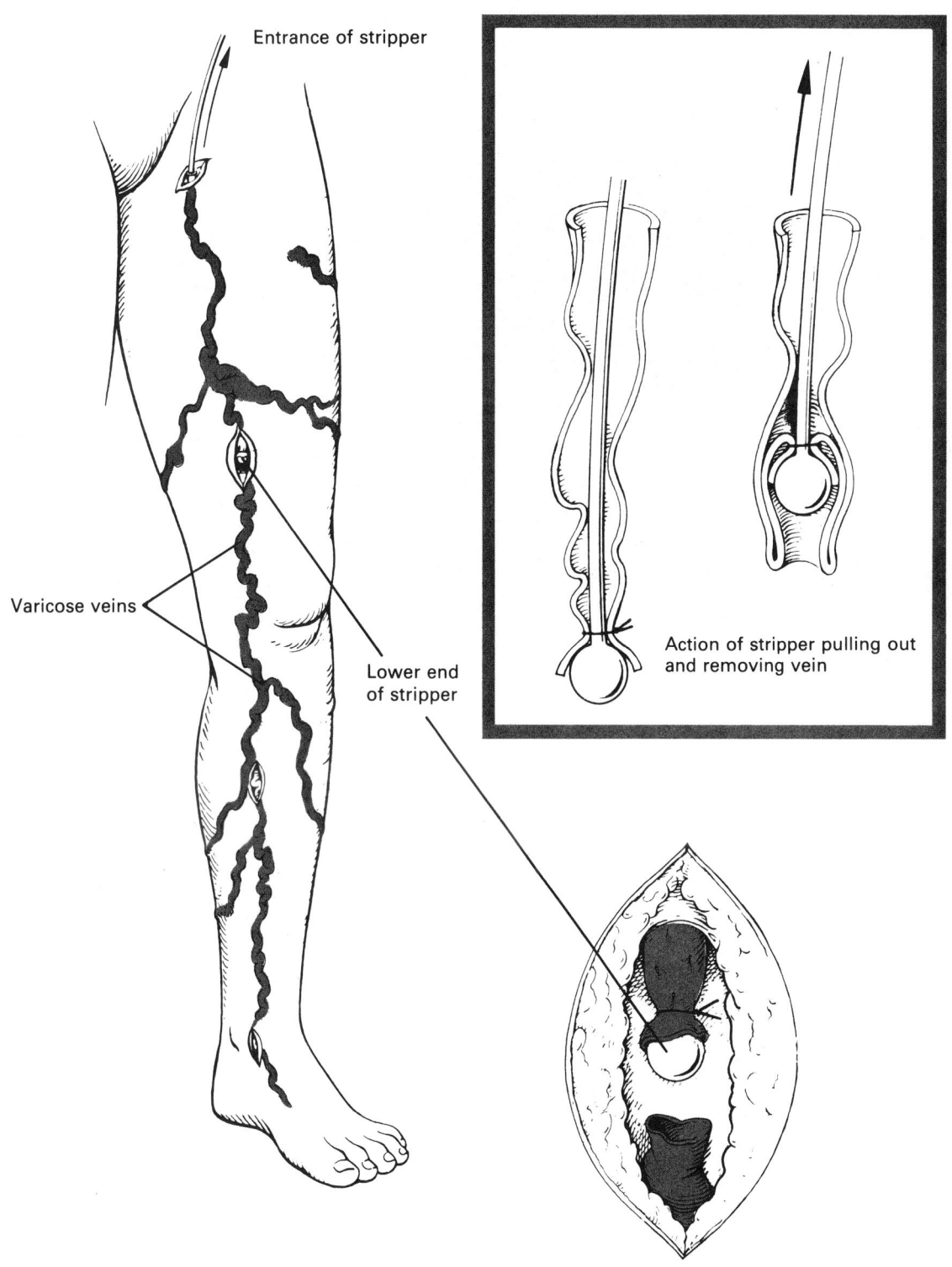

Entrance of stripper

Varicose veins

Lower end
of stripper

Action of stripper pulling out
and removing vein

*Varicose Vein Operation.* *Incisions are made over the largest varicosities, and a "stripper" is fed into each. The veins are then severed and the stripper is tied in. Withdrawing the stripper removes the diseased vein. Operations upon varicose veins are usually successful, although it is sometimes not possible to eradicate all of the varicosities. People with marked varicosities should seek medical advice early, before phlebitis or ulceration of the skin sets in.*

brachial artery in the upper arm or the femoral artery in the thigh, is injured, it should be repaired surgically. Many veins can be tied off, as other veins will take over the job of carrying blood back toward the heart.

### How soon after an injury to a major blood vessel should surgical treatment be started?

As soon as possible, especially if a major artery is involved. Loss of blood supply cannot be tolerated by tissues for more than thirty minutes to an hour. Moreover, continued bleeding from a major artery can lead to a fatality if the hemorrhage is uncontrolled.

### Can severed arteries and veins be repaired successfully?

Yes, careful suturing (stitching) of lacerated vessels, especially arteries, is possible in a great number of cases.

### What is done to prevent the blood from clotting within the passageway of an injured vessel?

Clots are removed, and heparin is injected. The heparin will help prevent further clots from forming.

## 2. Arteriosclerosis

### Is surgery helpful in the treatment of arteriosclerosis?

Yes, in special cases in which the arteriosclerosis involves a particular organ or region of the body.

### What are some of the arteriosclerotic conditions for which blood vessel surgery is beneficial?

a. Carotid surgery, in which there is arteriosclerosis of the major artery in the neck, which supplies the brain.
b. Coronary bypass and internal mammary artery implant operations in which arteriosclerosis involves the coronary arteries of the heart. (See also Chapter 29, on Heart Surgery.)
c. Loss of blood supply in a limb as the result of arteriosclerosis.
d. Arteriosclerosis of the renal artery supplying the kidney.
e. Removal of aneurysms. (See the section on Aneurysms in this chapter.)

### What are some of the surgical procedures recommended in arteriosclerosis?

a. Bypassing of obstructed arteries by use of segments of the patient's own veins or by use of plastic grafts.
b. Endarterectomy.
c. Patch grafts following endarterectomy.
d. Grafts, either substituting for, or bypassing, arteriosclerotic arteries.
e. Sympathectomy.

### What is sympathectomy, and when is it advocated?

It is an operation performed for the purpose of cutting sympathetic nerves, which cause contraction and constriction of blood vessels. These nerves lie along the spinal column and are approached surgically through incisions in the back or flank. Sympathectomy is advised in those cases of arteriosclerosis of the lower limbs in which it is felt that release of arterial spasm will permit greater blood flow. The operation is also advocated in certain cases of Buerger's disease and Raynaud's syndrome.

### What is endarterectomy, and when is it used?

It has been found that arteriosclerosis involves mainly the inner coats of an artery and that the outer coats remain relatively normal. Reaming out or coring out the sclerotic inner coat causes many of these vessels to regrow normal inner linings.

### In what conditions can endarterectomy be beneficial?

a. In patients who are showing signs of an impending stroke or in some who have had a stroke due to arteriosclerosis of the carotid artery in the neck. In some of the cases, coring out the inner lining of the artery and applying a plastic patch to widen the artery's passageway will bring about great improvement.
b. In certain cases in which the major artery to the leg—the femoral artery—has become markedly arteriosclerotic, endarterectomy followed by use of a patch graft will result in greatly improved circulation.
c. In occasional cases of marked arteriosclerosis of the abdominal aorta.
d. For coronary artery thrombosis. The reaming out of the coronary artery in the heart is a procedure purely in the experimental stage and is not recommended frequently. The coronary bypass operation has supplanted this procedure in most clinics throughout the country.

### Are patch grafts always used after performing an endarterectomy?

No. It is done only when it is thought that the graft will substantially widen the passageway of the artery.

### When are arterial grafts used in treating arteriosclerosis?

In patients who have impairment of circulation secondary to arteriosclerosis in major vessels such as the abdominal aorta and arteries leading to or in the lower extremities. The grafts, frequently made of Dacron, are used either to replace the sclerotic artery or are inserted alongside the diseased vessel.

When the lower end of the abdominal aorta and the iliac arteries in the pelvis are markedly sclerotic, replacement grafts are usually used. The healthy end of the aorta is stitched to the upper end of the graft, and the healthy lower ends of the iliac arteries are stitched to the lower end of the graft. (See diagram.)

When the main femoral artery in the upper thigh is diseased, a bypass graft is inserted alongside the iliac arteries in the pelvis and is inserted into the healthy portion of the femoral arteries in the lower thigh. This is known as an *iliofemoral* bypass operation.

When the lower end of a femoral artery is diseased in the lower thigh, a *femoropopliteal* graft is inserted beginning at the upper healthy portion of the femoral artery and extending to a healthy artery in the knee region.

When the lower aorta, the iliac arteries, and the upper ends of the femoral arteries are so involved in arteriosclerosis that the above grafts are not feasible, then a graft may be placed from the axillary artery in the armpit down through the tissues beneath the skin of the chest, abdomen, and pelvis to a healthy portion of the femoral arteries in the thigh. This procedure is known as an *axillofemoral* bypass.

### Can arterial grafts always be used in cases of arteriosclerosis?

No. It is essential that there is a relatively healthy portion of artery above *and* below the diseased portion of the vessel. If a vessel is uniformly arteriosclerotic throughout its course, a graft witll not work.

### Is it possible that arterial replacement with grafts will one day greatly affect longevity?

Yes. As we know, arteriosclerosis is the greatest cause of aging of an organ or limb. To slow down its process will prolong the life span.

### Can the coronary bypass operation help those with coronary artery disease?

Yes. It is estimated that at least a hundred thousand bypass operations are being performed in the United States each year.

### What maneuvers are carried out in doing a coronary bypass operation?

The long, superficial saphenous vein extending from the groin to the ankle is removed in one piece. The vein is then cut into appropriate-sized segments to be used as grafts to bypass obstructed areas of the coronary arteries.

While one member of the surgical team is preparing the vein for use as a graft, the other surgeon opens the chest and isolates the area or areas of the coronary artery that are obstructed and must be bypassed.

The vein graft is then attached to the aorta above the heart and to that portion of the coronary artery that is beyond the area of obstruction.

### Is only one graft usually placed in performing a bypass procedure?

No. It has been found that several areas of coronary obstruction often exist. Therefore two, three, four, or even five grafts are utilized.

### What are the results of the coronary bypass operation?

If the patient's main reason for surgery was heart pain—angina—the surgery relieves the condition in the great majority of cases. It has not yet, however, been proved conclusively that people with coronary arteriosclerosis have a prolongation of their life span because of the operation.

### How dangerous is a coronary bypass operation?

The risks, when the procedure is carried out by a surgical team with broad experience, are very low. The mortality rate is a good deal lower than one in twenty.

### Can anyone with coronary artery disease undergo a coronary bypass operation?

No. Intensive preoperative investigation and testing must be done before a patient is judged to be a good candidate for the operation. Elderly people, those who have had previous attacks of coronary thrombosis with extensive damage to the heart muscle, and those with unrelated but serious chronic diseases, may not be good candidates for bypass surgery.

### What is an internal mammary artery implant operation?

This procedure, performed to improve circulation to the heart muscle in coronary disease, dissects out the internal mammary artery beneath the breast bone and implants it into the wall of the heart.

### What is the purpose of the internal mammary artery operation?

The same as the coronary bypass procedure. Both operations have the goal of increasing circulation to the heart muscle.

### How effective is the internal mammary artery operation?

Those who perform large numbers of these operations claim that their results are as good as those obtained from the bypass operation. However, the procedure is not being employed very widely since the bypass operation has come into vogue.

### What harm results from arteriosclerosis of the renal artery to the kidney?

If circulation to the kidney is seriously impaired, high blood pressure will result. And if both renal vessels are arteriosclerotic, kidney function may fail, and the patient may become uremic.

### How is a diagnosis of renal artery obstruction established?

By arteriograms. These are x rays of the blood vessels supplying the kidneys, which are taken after the injection of radiopaque dyes into the circulation.

**What surgery is performed to help a patient with obstruction within a renal artery?**

The abdomen is opened, and the artery to the kidney is exposed. It is then incised, and its arteriosclerotic inner lining is cored out (endarterectomy). A bypass operation or plastic patch graft is then stitched to the artery, thus widening its passageway.

**Are operations on the renal arteries successful?**

Yes, in the great majority of cases. Kidney function and blood pressure levels often return to normal after this procedure. Moreover, the operation itself carries with it a low risk when performed by experienced surgeons.

## 3. Thrombosis

**Can thrombosis happen both in arteries and veins?**

Yes. A thrombosis is a clot, and it may cause clogging of either type of blood vessel.

**What surgery is helpful to a patient who has suffered a clot of a large vein in his leg or thigh?**

An incision is made, the vein is isolated and opened, and the clot is removed. Frequently, a clot that is several or many inches long can be extracted in one piece, thus permitting the vein to again carry blood.

**Can a thrombus in a vein in the brain be removed?**

This can take place in rare instances, but usually it is not a feasible operation.

**Can a thrombus in a main vessel in the lungs ever be removed successfully?**

Yes, in an occasional case. A pulmonary embolus—a clot propelled from some distant vein into the lungs—is a frequent occurrence, often accompanied by sudden death. However, it is possible in some instances to operate immediately and remove the thrombus (clot).

**Can surgery help a patient who has recently suffered an acute coronary thrombosis?**

No. Few people, if any, could survive such surgery immediately after a heart attack of this nature. Subsequent surgery may be beneficial.

**Must a thrombosed vessel be operated upon soon after the clot has formed?**

Yes, because clots tend to adhere very quickly to blood vessel walls, and unless they are removed within hours, or at the latest twenty-four hours after having formed, they cannot be removed.

## 4. Thrombophlebitis

**Can surgery often help those with thrombophlebitis?**

Since this condition is associated with an inflammation of the lining of a vein, surgery is not often beneficial. However, when pieces of blood clot break away from the main clot in the vein, surgery may be lifesaving. An embolus from a leg vein or vein in the pelvic region may travel to the lungs. In such cases, consideration must be given to tying off the vein high above the thrombophlebitis so as to prevent subsequent clots from reaching a vital organ.

**What operations are indicated to prevent serious consequences from thrombophlebitis?**

If the thrombophlebitis is in a superficial vein in the leg, the saphenous vein may be tied off in the groin to prevent clots from spreading. If the thrombophlebitis is in the thigh or pelvic region, tying off the vena cava in the abdomen, or inserting a sieve in the vena cava to stop clots from passing through, may be carried out.

## 5. Embolism

**Is it ever possible to successfully remove an embolus and restore normal circulation?**

Yes, in some instances.

**In what types of embolism can surgery overcome the condition?**

a. In patients who have an embolus blocking an artery in the arm or leg.

b. In some patients who have an embolus blocking an accessible blood vessel in the lung.

c. In rare cases in which the embolus has lodged in a blood vessel in the brain.

**Must surgery be carried out quickly after embolism has occurred?**

Yes, it requires emergency surgery. If the delay between embolism and surgery is more than several hours, little help can be afforded.

**Why must embolism surgery be performed so quickly?**

Because the tissues normally supplied by the blocked artery will die unless circulation is restored promptly.

## 6. Aneurysm

**Can surgery overcome an aneurysm?**

Yes, in a great many cases. The operative procedure consists of opening the aneurysm and replacing the damaged section of the artery with an arterial graft. The plastic arterial graft is stitched to the normal segments of the artery above and below the aneurysm.

**Is it necessary to remove the aneurysm portion of the artery after inserting the arterial graft?**

No. The tissues left behind can be wrapped around the graft, thus tending to eliminate adhesions to surrounding structures.

**At what sites can aneurysm surgery be performed?**

a. The abdominal aorta.

b. Certain cases of aneurysm of the aorta in the chest.

c. Some cases of aneurysm of arteries in the brain.

d. Aneurysms of vessels in the arms or legs.

**Are most operations for aneurysm successful?**

Yes, well over 95 percent are successful, provided they have been performed *before* the aneurysm has ruptured.

**Should a person with an abdominal aortic aneurysm have it operated upon even when he has few or minimal symptoms?**

Yes, because one day it might rupture and cause rapid death. Small aneurysms, less than two inches in size, may be observed to note whether they are getting larger. If they are, surgery should be carried out.

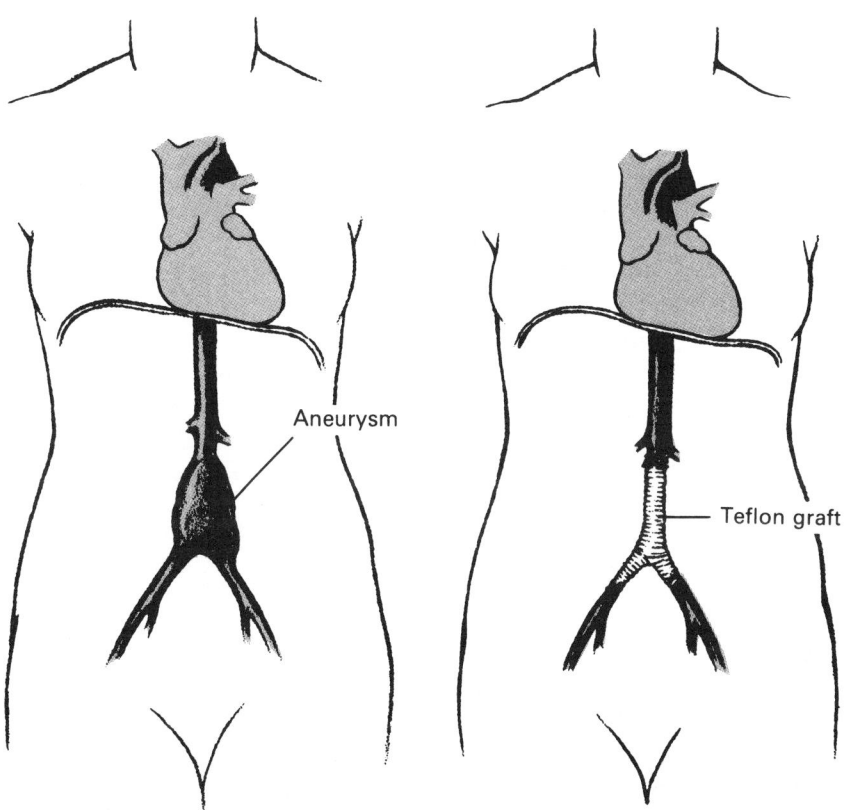

***Replacement of Aortic Aneurysm.*** *The diagram at left, shows a typical aneurysm of the aorta. At right, the aneurysm has been replaced by a Teflon graft.*

## 7. Cirrhosis of the Liver
*(See also Chapter 40 on Liver)*

**Can blood vessel surgery aid those who suffer from cirrhosis?**

Yes. The great danger of cirrhosis is hemorrhage from veins in the lower esophagus. In order to prevent this, various operations have been devised to shunt blood from the intestines away from the liver. In other words, blood is redirected so that it passes from the intestines into the vena cava rather than into the liver.

**What operations are performed to bypass the liver?**

a. A mesocaval shunt.

b. A portacaval shunt.

c. A lienorenal shunt.

**Are these procedures successful in curing cirrhosis?**

No, but they are beneficial in that

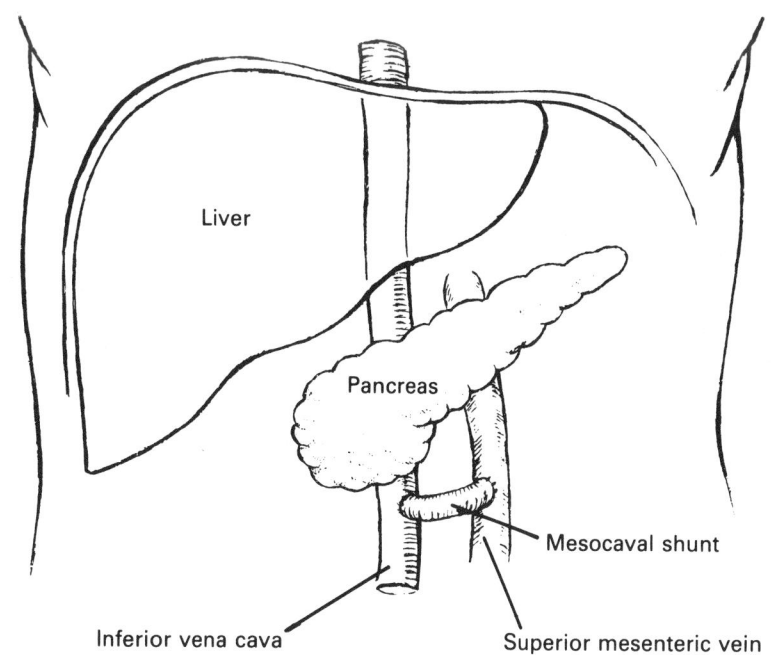

***Mesocaval Shunt.*** *A Teflon or Dacron graft is used to connect the superior mesenteric vein to the inferior vena cava. This operation is done frequently instead of the portacaval shunt to relieve the portal vein obstruction caused by cirrhosis of the liver.*

they cut down greatly on the incidence of fatal hemorrhage from rupture of varicose veins of the esophagus.

## What is a mesocaval shunt?

It is an operation in which a plastic graft is used to connect the superior mesenteric vein (carrying most of the blood toward the liver from the intestines) with the vena cava (the main vein carrying blood from the lower part of the body to the heart).

## Are mesocaval shunts often successful?

Yes. As a matter of fact, this procedure has replaced the portacaval shunt and the lienorenal shunt in many hospitals throughout the country.

## What is a portacaval shunt?

It is a procedure wherein the portal vein, carrying most of the blood to the liver from the intestines, is stitched directly to the vena cava. (See diagram in Chapter 40, on The Liver.)

## Are portacaval shunts successful in shunting blood away from the liver?

Yes.

## What is a lienorenal shunt?

This procedure involves suturing the main vein of the spleen to the renal vein of the left kidney. It is not done as frequently as the other two operations because these shunts carry less blood and have a greater tendency to close after passage of time.

## 8. VARICOSE VEINS

## What are varicose veins?

Enlarged, incompetent veins in which blood tends to stagnate.

## What causes veins to become varicosed?

Continued obstruction to venous blood flow often causes the valves within the veins to break down, resulting in stagnation and dilatation of the vessels.

## Who is most likely to develop varicose veins in the lower extremities?

People who have jobs requiring standing in one position for long periods of time.

## What is the incidence of varicose veins?

It it estimated that one out of every four men and one out of every two women over forty years of age have varicose veins.

## What symptoms are produced by varicose veins in the legs?

Small varicosities cause no symptoms. When they are large and numerous, they may cause a heavy, dragging sensation and tiredness in the legs.

## Is there a hereditary factor in the formation of varicose veins?

Yes. People tend to inherit the same type of blood vessels as their parents.

## What parts of the body are most prone to develop varicosities?

a. Veins in the legs and thighs.
b. Veins about the anus and rectum (hemorrhoids).
c. Veins in the scrotum (varicocele).

## What is the best way to prevent varicose veins from enlarging?

a. Avoid standing in one position for long periods of time.
b. Do not use constricting garters.
c. Exercise regularly.
d. Use elastic supports for the legs when forced to remain in a standing position for long periods.

## What is the best form of treatment for varicose veins?

Ligation and cutting of the main varicose vein (the saphenous vein) and its branches, and removing the veins through a procedure called "stripping."

## Is hospitalization necessary for this operation?

Yes, for two to three days.

## Is surgery the only form of treatment for varicose veins?

No. Injection of the veins with substances that cause clotting (sclerosing treatment) is often all the treatment necessary to obliterate the smaller varicosities.

## Is there a tendency for varicosities to recur or for new ones to develop after the injection treatment?

Yes.

## How effective is the injection treatment as compared to surgery?

Surgery is much more effective; the injection treatment is reserved for the treatment of mild cases of varicose veins and for the postoperative treatment of those varicosities that persist despite surgery.

## Do all varicose veins have to be operated upon or undergo injection treatments?

No. Small ones that cause no symptoms can be ignored.

## Do varicose veins tend to get well by themselves?

No. However, many varicosities that appear large during pregnancy tend to become smaller after childbirth.

## What is the best time for women to have varicose veins operated upon?

After the childbearing period.

## What happens to the blood flow after ligating or removing varicose veins?

The blood returns to the heart via the deep, nonvaricosed veins.

**Is circulation improved by cutting or removing varicose veins?**

Yes, since it does away with pooling and stagnation of blood, which had existed in the varicosities.

**Will wearing elastic stockings cure varicose veins?**

No. They merely relieve symptoms.

**What may happen if large varicose veins are left untreated?**

a. Ulcers of the skin of the legs may form (varicose ulcers).
b. Eczema of the skin of the legs may develop.
c. Phlebitis may develop within the veins.
d. The general health of the patient may eventually be impaired.

**Will varicose ulcers of the skin and eczema tend to heal after operating upon varicose veins?**

Yes.

**Do varicose veins, if untreated, ever hemorrhage through the skin?**

Yes. Severe bleeding can take place from an ulcerated, superficial varicose vein of the leg.

**What are the indications for surgery upon varicose veins?**

a. Pain in the legs and a generally fatigued feeling after a day's work.
b. Swelling in the legs as a result of the varicosities.
c. Unsightliness due to the large varicosities.
d. Hemorrhage.
e. A nonhealing varicose ulcer or chronic eczema.
f. When the general circulation of the body is impaired by the pooling of blood in the lower extremities.

**What precautions must a surgeon take before operating upon a patient with varicose veins?**

He must ascertain that the circulation through the deep veins is com-

petent. This is determined by various simple office tests. Proof that the deep venous circulation is adequate can be obtained by having the patient wear snug elastic bandages. If he obtains relief, it means the blood is traveling satisfactorily through the deeper channels. If it is painful to wear elastic bandages, the deeper circulation may be impaired, and it is perhaps wisest not to perform surgery.

**Can the little, bluish varicose veins be benefited by injections or surgical treatment?**

Usually not. In addition, no treatment is necessary for these veins, since they rarely cause symptoms.

**What are the results of the various forms of treating varicose veins?**

a. About 25 percent of people are helped permanently by the injection treatment.
b. About 80 percent obtain excellent permanent results from surgery.

**Are operations for varicose veins painful?**

There is moderate discomfort in the wound areas for four or five days after surgery.

**Are any special preoperative cautions necessary?**

No.

**Are operations upon varicose veins dangerous?**

No. They are simple operations.

**What type of anesthesia is used for these operations?**

Spinal anesthesia, epidural anesthesia, local procaine injections, or general anesthesia.

**Are the incisions for varicose veins unsightly?**

They are visible but are much less unsightly than the varicose veins themselves.

**Are there special postoperative measures after varicose vein surgery?**

Yes. The patient is advised to get up and walk as soon as the anesthesia wears off.

**Is it natural for blood clots to form in the vessels after surgery for varicose veins?**

Yes, particularly when ligation and cutting of the veins has been carried out. Such clots will seal off incompetent varicosities.

**Do varicose veins tend to recur even after surgery?**

Yes, in a small percentage of cases.

**Is there an improvement in the appearance of the leg after varicose vein surgery?**

Yes, although the appearance does not return to absolute normal.

**Are there any permanent limitations upon one's activities following varicose vein surgery?**

No.

**How often should one return for a checkup after varicose vein surgery?**

Approximately once a year.

## 9. Blood Vessel Tumors

**What is the most common tumor of blood vessels?**

The hemangioma. This may appear as a tiny red spot on the skin in some instances; in other cases it may form a large red blotch in the skin, or it may appear as a soft, bluish swelling beneath the skin.

**Do hemangiomas often turn into cancer?**

No, but if they are unsightly or disfiguring they may require removal. An electric needle or carbon dioxide snow is sufficient to destroy the small, superficial ones. Large hemangiomas may require more extensive excision and skin grafts.

### Do hemangiomas ever appear other than on the skin?

Yes, they may appear beneath the skin, in organs such as the liver, in the lining of the intestinal tract, or elsewhere.

### What symptoms are likely to occur with blood vessel tumors?

They usually produce no symptoms but some show a tendency to hemorrhage. Should this occur, surgery will be necessary.

### Are blood vessel tumors ever malignant?

The great majority of them are benign, but occasionally, a malignant blood vessel tumor will appear in an internal organ of the body.

### What is the treatment for blood vessel tumors?

The great majority of them, if they are surgically accessible, should be removed. Some of them, such as those that occur in the liver, may be left alone unless they show a tendency to grow rapidly or to hemorrhage.

### Is there any treatment except surgery for blood vessel tumors?

Yes. Certain of these tumors can be eradicated with x-ray therapy or by the application of radium. Others can be destroyed by applying carbon dioxide snow or with cryosurgery (intense cold applications to destroy the growth).

## 10. Arteriovenous Fistulas

### What is an arteriovenous fistula?

It is a connetion between an artery and a vein, resulting in the shunting of arterial blood into the venous circulation.

### What are the common types of arteriovenous fistulas?

There are three main types:
a. Congenital fistulas, which are false connections between an artery and vein present at birth.
b. Traumatic fistulas, resulting from injuries such as gunshot or stab wounds.
c. Surgically created fistulas, such as those created artificially in the forearm as an aid to dialysis (the use of the artificial kidney).

### What harm results from congenital or traumatic fistulas?

a. The heart must work extra hard to pump arterial blood to those parts of the body that lie beyond the fistula.
b. Both the artery and the vein in the area of the fistula become markedly distended, thus creating the danger of rupture.
c. The limb beyond the fistula may become greatly swollen and its function impaired.

### What is the benefit of an artificially created arteriovenous fistula?

The vessels in the region of the fistula become sufficiently distended so that it is a simple matter to insert a needle into them. This is important in continued dialysis, as the patient must have a needle inserted at repeated intervals in order to connect him to the artificial kidney. Patients themselves can learn to insert the needle at the fistula site.

### What is the treatment for congenital and traumatic arteriovenous fistulas?

The connection between the artery and the vein is removed surgically, following which the vessels are repaired.

### Are operations to remove arteriovenous fistulas successful?

Yes.

# CHAPTER 14

# BONES, MUSCLES, TENDONS, AND JOINTS

*(See also Chapter 10 on Arthritis; Chapter 26 on First Aid in Emergencies; Chapter 35 on Inherited and Congenital Conditions; Chapter 46 on Neurosurgery; Chapter 53 on Physical Therapy and Rehabilitation; Chapter 62 on Rheumatic Fever)*

## BIRTH DEFORMITIES OF THE EXTREMITIES

**What are some of the common birth deformities of the extremities?**

a. Clubfoot.
b. Congenital dislocation of the hip.
c. Absent limb, or absent part of a limb (phocomelia).

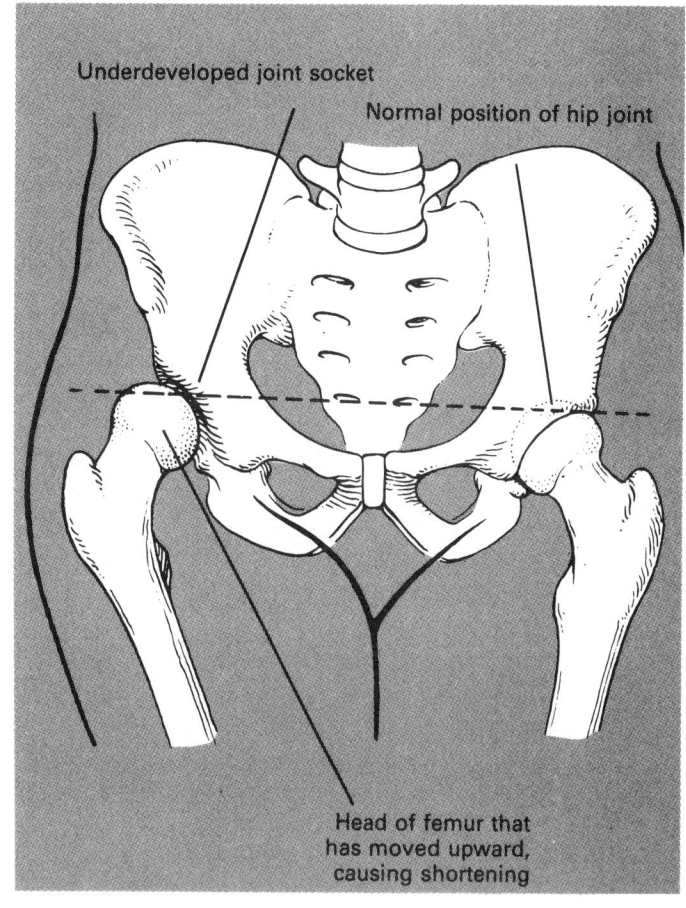

***Congenital Hip Dislocation.*** *A small number of children, particularly females, are born with the head of the thigh bone (femur) not within its proper socket at the hip joint. In some cases, this deformity can be corrected by manipulation, but in other cases, it is necessary to operate and construct a new hip socket for the head of the thigh bone. Operations of this type are usually successful.*

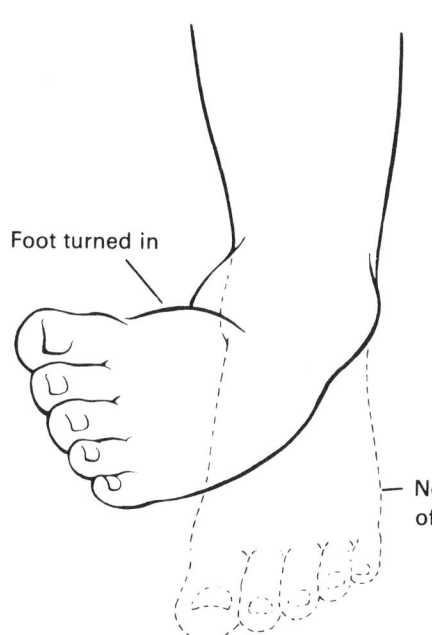

***Clubfoot.*** *Clubfoot is a not unusual birth deformity. Present methods of orthopedic surgery can bring about a cure in most cases, provided that the treatment is continued for one to two years. With proper treatment, it is no longer necessary for children to be permanently crippled by clubfoot.*

d. Extra digit (supernumerary digit or polydactylism).
e. Extra limb, or extra part of a limb.
f. Drug-induced deformities.

**What drugs can cause birth deformities in bones?**

There are many. The best advice to a pregnant woman is to avoid *all* drugs during pregnancy unless they are specifically prescribed by a physician.

**What is clubfoot?**

A birth deformity in which the foot is foreshortened, is flexed on the ankle, and turned inward.

## What is the treatment for clubfoot?

a. Medical management, with manipulation and placement of the foot and leg in a cast in an overcorrected position. The foot and leg will remain in a cast for several months.

b. Surgical treatment, which often involves cutting and stripping some of the fibrous tissues beneath the skin of the foot. In addition, procedures are carried out to lengthen some of the tendons to the foot.

## What causes clubfoot?

It is an inherited tendency and occurs only rarely in families that have no known history of birth deformities. In families with a history of birth abnormalities, it is seen more frequently.

## Can clubfoot be treated successfully?

Yes, results are excellent when proper medical or surgical treatment is carried out over a prolonged period of time. Cooperation of the parents is essential to a permanent good result.

## What is a congenital dislocation of the hip?

A birth malformation in which the head of the thigh bone fails to stay in its proper socket. As a result, the hip slides up high onto the bones of the pelvis. This condition affects females much more often than males.

## How is the diagnosis of congenital dislocation of the hip made?

If deformity is limited to one hip, a limp is noted when the child attempts to walk. The limp is caused by the fact that the limb on the involved side is shortened. There is a waddle when walking if both hips are involved.

## What is the treatment for congenital hip dislocation?

a. The conservative, nonoperative treatment will cure the majority of these children.

b. Surgical treatment is confined to those children who fail to respond to medical management. The best time for surgical treatment is early in life.

## What is the surgical treatment for congenital hip dislocation?

An incision is made on the front of the thigh over the pelvic bone. The underlying muscles are separated, and the head of the thigh bone (femur) is placed into its proper position in the hip joint. Either muscle or bone is altered to maintain position.

## Is surgery usually successful in curing congenital hip dislocation?

Yes. The results are most satisfactory in the great majority of cases.

## What causes a child to be born with an absent limb or an absent part of a limb?

A malformation in the development of the embryo within the uterus.

## Is this a frequent finding in newborns?

No, it is exceedingly rare.

## Who is more likely to have a child with an absent limb or an absent part of a limb?

This deformity occurs much more often in families that have a history of other birth abnormalities. Also, it is seen occasionally in women who have taken certain drugs, without the advice of their physicians, during the first few weeks of pregnancy.

## Who is more likely to have a child with extra digits (fingers or toes)?

This, too, is a rare birth deformity occuring in those families where there is a known history of similar or other deformities.

## What is the treatment for extra digits (polydactylism)?

It is a simple matter to remove a sixth finger or sixth toe. This can be accomplished without leaving a disfiguring scar.

## Are extra limbs seen frequently?

No. This is one of the rarest of all birth deformities.

## What is the treatment for an extra limb?

Almost all of these structures are deformed and underdeveloped. They should be removed surgically soon after the birth of the child, preferably before the child is taken home from the hospital.

# AMPUTATIONS

## What are the most common conditions requiring amputation of a limb?

a. Severe infections that destroy the blood supply to the extremity and which threaten life.

b. Gangrene secondary to arteriosclerosis or diabetes.

c. Malignant tumors of the bones or other structures of the extremities.

d. An accident or injury that has caused irreparable damage.

e. A crippling deformity that prevents the use of an artificial appliance or that interferes with the function of the extremity.

## What surgical principle guides the decision of whether or not to amputate a limb?

a. The most pressing consideration is whether or not the patient's life is endangered. Whenever a disease or condition in a limb has progressed so far as to endanger life, the surgeon will recommend amputation.

b. The ability of the patient to function better with an artificial limb.

## How is the level of amputation determined?

a. An attempt is made to preserve as much of the extremity as can safely be left in place.

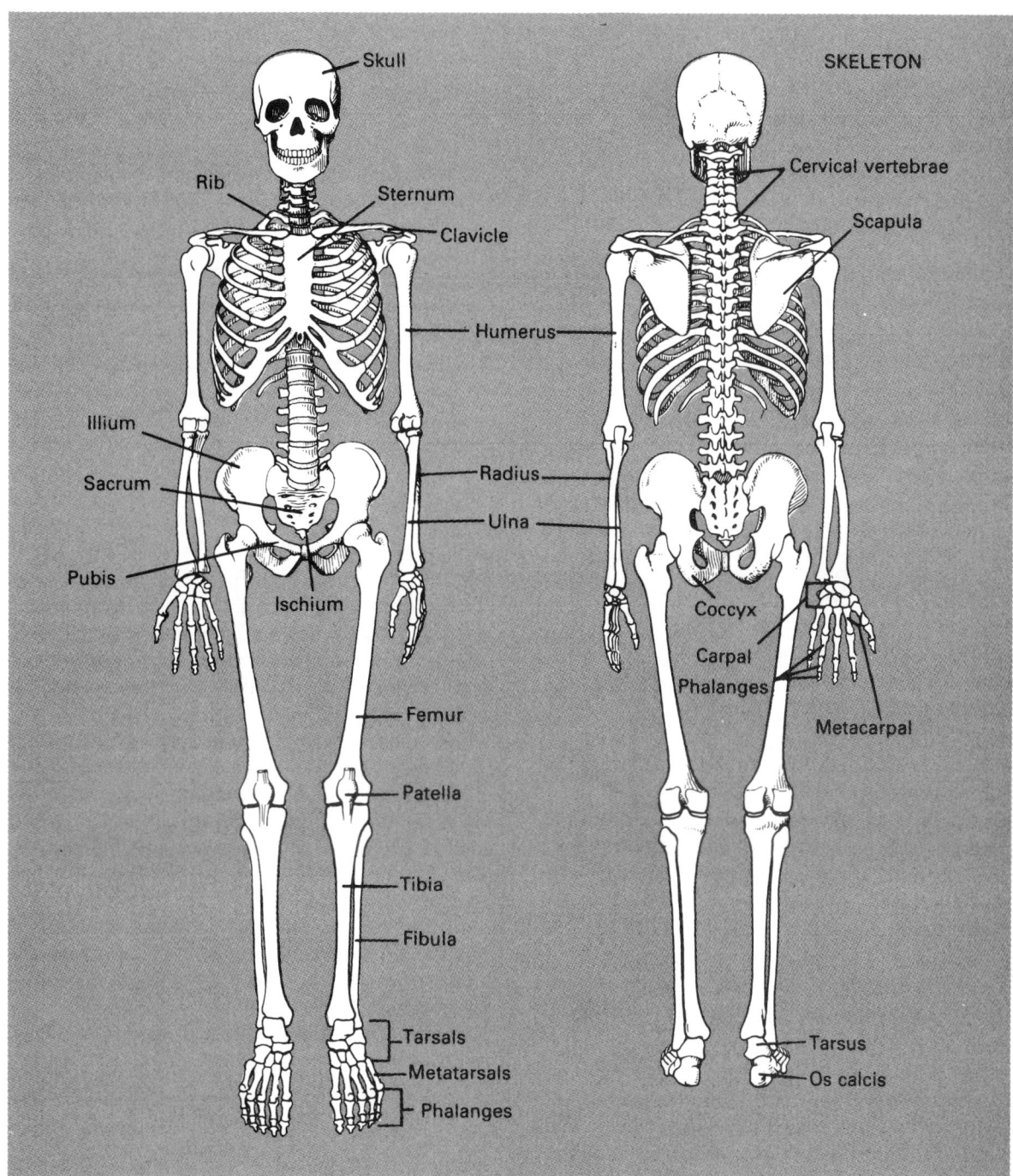

**The Bony Skeleton (anterior view).** *There are more than two hundred bones in the human body. Although bones tend to grow old as people age, it is remarkable that the skeletal structure of the body is so infrequently the seat of primary diseases (left).*

**The Bony Skeleton (posterior view).** *As the body ages, the cartilages that are attached to the ends of bones tend to shrink, so that people actually do get shorter as they grow older. This process is particularly noticeable in the vertebral column (right).*

b. Circulation must be adequate at the amputation site. The poorer the circulation, the higher the level of amputation.

c. A site is chosen that will permit the best usage of an artificial limb. (This important principle sometimes means amputation at a site higher than is required by the disease process.)

### Is amputation of a limb a dangerous operative procedure?

No, but there may be severe complications, because many patients who require amputation are sick people who are advanced in age and have accompanying infection, arteriosclerosis, and heart disease.

### Can the majority of people learn how to use an artificial limb satisfactorily?

Yes. Today there are excellent artificial appliances that can be used most effectively. Many amputees use their limbs so successfully that people are unaware that the amputee is wearing an appliance.

### How soon after an amputation can an artificial appliance be fitted?

This varies markedly, depending upon the level at which the limb has been amputated, the healing of the amputation stump, and the general health of the patient. If healing takes place at a normal rate, an artificial limb may be fitted six to eight weeks after amputation. Frequently, a temporary artificial limb is fitted in the operating room immediately following amputation.

### Can a person learn to walk if he has had both legs amputated?

Yes, but with greater difficulty than when only one limb has been removed.

### Does an artificial hand look and function like a real hand?

The most effective artificial hands are constructed of metal, and little attempt is made to imitate normal appearance. However, for purely cosmetic reasons, nonfunctioning or limited-functioning hands can be made to resemble the normal human hand.

### What is meant by the term "phantom limb"?

It is a sensation that an amputee experiences when he feels pain or sensation in the amputated extremity. It is thought to be caused by irritation of nerves that have been cut in the amputation stump.

### Is it ever necessary to reamputate a limb?

Yes. Certain amputations are done as emergency lifesaving measures without consideration for the future usefulness of the stump. In such cases, reamputation is necessary so that satisfactory artificial limbs may be fitted.

### If an amputation stump becomes useless because of poor circulation or ulceration, can a corrective operation be performed?

Yes, amputation at a higher level will often solve such a problem.

### Is there ever any regrowth of an amputated structure?

Never. However, occasionally an amputated limb can be successfully reattached. (See Chapter 61, on Replantation Surgery.)


## LOWER BACK PAIN

### What are some of the common causes of lower back pain?

a. Injury, from lifting heavy objects, for example, or from a fall with twisting of the back.

b. Arthritis of the spine.

c. Hernia of an intervertebral disk (slipped disk), or degeneration of the disks.

### What takes place when a slipped disk occurs?

Some of the cartilage that normally forms a cushion between the various vertebral bodies is dislocated and slips from its normal position into one in which it is subject to pressure each time a person moves. This creates great pain.

### Are there certain types of people who are more prone to lower back pain?

Yes, those who are born with weakness or abnormalities in the structure of the vertebrae in the lumbar or sacral regions or who have poorly developed back musculature.

### How can one tell beforehand whether his back is susceptible to sprain or to a slipped disk?

Usually this is not possible to forecast. In some instances, x rays will demonstrate malformations that should warn an individual against strenuous physical labors.

### If a patient has once had an attack of lower back pain, does this predispose him toward a chronic or recurring condition?

Yes.

### What is the difference between a sacroiliac sprain, the low back syndrome, and sciatica (sciatic neuritis)?

Sciatic neuritis is associated with pain along the course of the nerve, that is, pain starting in the lower back and descending to the buttock, back of the thigh, calf, and on to the foot. The low back syndrome usually relates to pain in the lower back that does not radiate down the legs.

### Will wearing a back brace—a strongly constructed corset—or other orthopedic appliance prevent one from developing pain in the lower back?

Only if one is susceptible to recurrent lower back pain.

## What is the usual medical treatment for chronic lower back pain?

a. Sleeping on a firm mattress with a board between the mattress and the bedspring and a pillow under the knees.
b. Taking pain-relieving medications and/or muscle relaxants.
c. Application of superficial and deep heat treatments.
d. Prescribed exercises to relieve spasm and strengthen the back musculature.
e. Avoidance of sudden movements and excess physical strain.

## Is there any satisfactory surgical treatment for chronic lower back pain?

If the pain is due to a birth deformity of the spine, a spinal-fusion operation will often eliminate the pain by stiffening and thus limiting painful movements of the vertebrae. If the pain is caused by a slipped disk, surgical removal of the dislocated disk will often bring about a cure.

## Do fat people have a greater tendency than thin people to develop chronic conditions of the lower back?

Yes.

## Can emotional imbalance cause chronic lower back pain?

Yes, but before it is decided that the symptoms are emotional in origin, it is essential to rule out all organic causes.

## Should people with chronic lower back pain perform heavy physical duties?

No.

## What motions are most likely to produce recurrences of lower back pain or sprain?

a. Sudden forward bending with the knees straight.
b. Sudden rotation of the trunk.
c. Unbraced lifting of heavy objects.

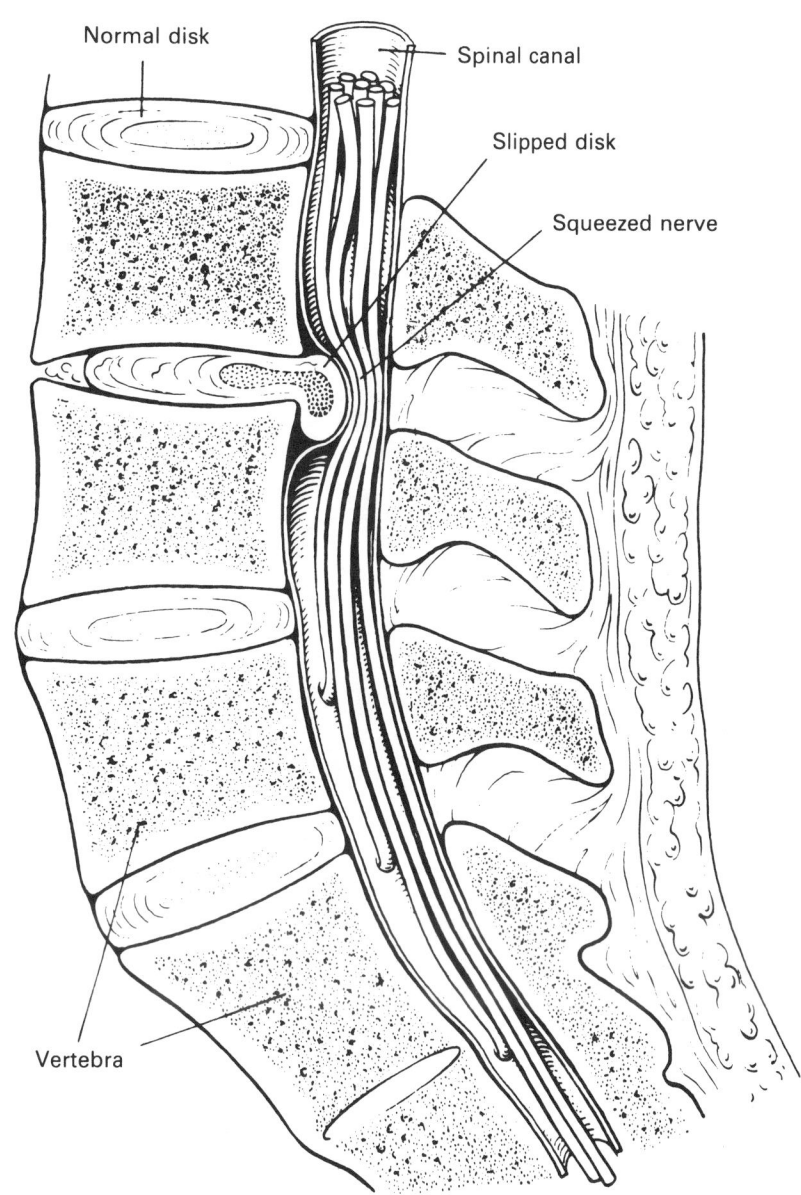

**Slipped Disk.** *This condition, also known as herniated disk or ruptured nucleus pulposus, is responsible for much of the back pain that occurs so commonly among people who do strenuous work. Most slipped disks can be relieved by traction, or by bed rest, and the application of braces to immobilize the back. A small number of cases must be operated upon to remove the herniated disk. The operation brings relief in the majority of cases.*

## How effective are physiotherapy treatments, such as diathermy, whirlpool baths, or muscle exercises, in relieving or treating chronic conditions of the lower back?

If used judiciously, these treatments are very helpful in relieving painful conditions of the lower back.

## Do infections, such as infected teeth, tonsils, or sinuses, play an important role in the causation of chronic conditions involving the lower back?

No. This was held to be true years ago, but today it is generally accepted that there is little correlation between infections and conditions

*X ray Showing Scoliosis (Curvature) of the Spine.* Scoliosis occurs most often in adolescent girls. Treatment of this condition is extremely difficult and must be carried out over a period of years.

*X ray of Normal Spine.* This x ray shows the various vertebrae in perfect alignment.

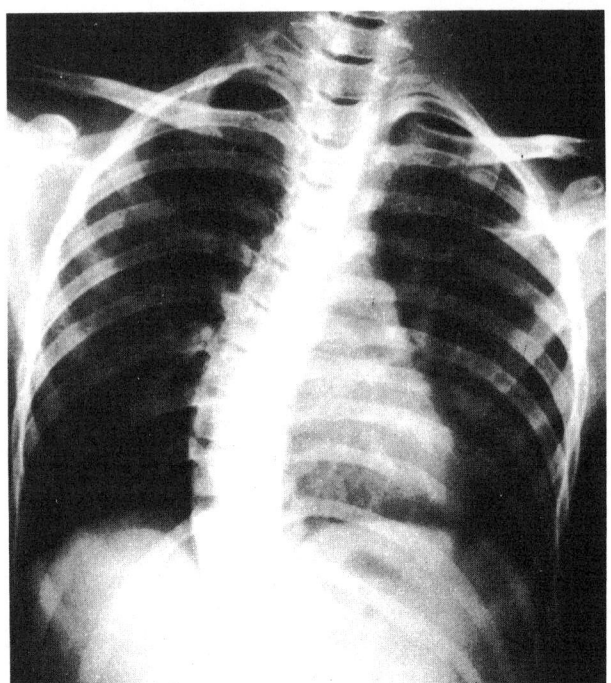

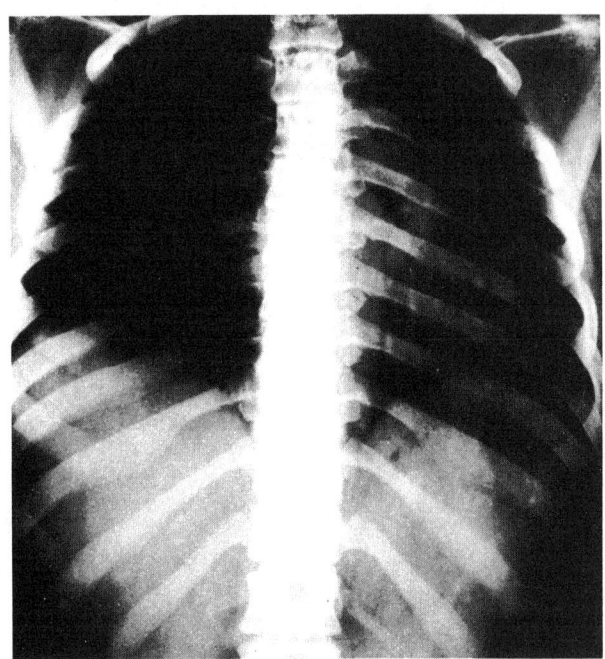

involving the muscles and bones of the lower back.

**How can one tell when to discard back supports or other orthopedic appliances?**

If pain and discomfort have ceased, gradual discontinuance of such appliances is permissible. At first, they should be discarded for short periods of time until finally, after several weeks of freedom from symptoms, they can be abandoned completely.

**Do x rays always reveal the presence or absence of conditions of the lower back?**

No. It is necessary, under certain circumstances, to perform highly specialized x-ray studies to uncover evidence of lower back disease. And

even when special studies are conducted, the x rays may not reveal the nature of the particular ailment.

## SCOLIOSIS AND SPONDYLOLISTHESIS

**What is scoliosis?**

A side-to-side curvature of the spine.

**How common is curvature of the spine?**

It is rather uncommon.

**Is scoliosis more common in girls than in boys?**

Yes, and it is seen most often during the rapid growth period of early adolescence.

**What causes scoliosis?**

The cause is unknown, except in those cases that follow neurological (nerve) diseases.

**Will bad posture habits cause curvature of the spine?**

No.

**Will physical exercises cure curvature of the spine?**

No.

**Is curvature of the spine (scoliosis) very painful?**

No.

**Does scoliosis ever correct itself without treatment?**

No, but in the majority of cases it is mild and reaches a stationary state beyond which it does not progress.

**Is surgery ever required to treat scoliosis?**

Yes, where the curvature of the spine is exceedingly marked and where it may interfere with normal heart action or normal development of the chest cavity.

### What operative procedures are carried out for scoliosis?

a. Spinal-fusion operations.
b. The insertion of metal devices such as Harrington rods.

### Are operations for scoliosis serious?

Yes, and the patient must often undergo treatment for many months or years following surgery.

### How much of the spine is fused when these operations are performed?

As much as one-third of the entire spinal column may be fused in order to establish stability.

### What is the operation employing the Harrington rods?

Long metal rods are inserted deep in the muscle tissues alongside the spine. By a system of pressures and counterpressures, these rods force the vertebrae into a straightened position.

### Are results encouraging following use of the Harrington metal rods?

Yes. They are very effective in the treatment of scoliosis.

### Are operations for scoliosis usually successful in preventing the extension of the spinal curvature?

Yes.

### Is it necessary to remove the metal rods at some future time?

Most of the rods will require eventual removal. However, the operation to execute their removal is not dangerous.

### How long a hospital stay may be necessary in cases of scoliosis?

Anywhere from three to six weeks.

### What is the course of scoliosis, if untreated?

In the great majority of cases the curvature of the spine will cease when maturity is reached. However, this may leave the patient with a markedly deformed spine and may interfere with normal heart and lung function.

### Are operations for fusion of the spine dangerous?

This is a major operative procedure, but one that seldom endangers life.

### For what other conditions are fusion operations of the spine advocated?

For spondylolisthesis.

### What is spondylolisthesis?

A slipping forward of one vertebra onto another because of a structural defect in the spine. This occurs most frequently when the fifth lumbar vertebra slides forward onto the first sacral vertebra.

### Is spondylolisthesis ever a cause of lower back pain?

Yes, but not often.

### What causes spondylolisthesis?

A deformity of the spine present since birth.

### How is the diagnosis of spondylolisthesis made?

By x-ray examination.

### Do all people with spondylolisthesis require treatment?

Only if they experience difficulty or pain.

### What treatment is carried out for painful spondylolisthesis?

A spinal-fusion operation in the lower back.

### Is treatment for spondylolisthesis successful?

Yes, in the great majority of cases.

## BURSITIS

### What is a bursa?

It is a saclike structure lying between muscles and joints, or between ligaments and bone. There are many throughout the body, and they serve to permit ligaments, muscles, and other structures to move freely and with a minimum of friction. The bursal sacs are lined with cells that secrete a small amount of fluid.

### Where are these bursae found?

Bursae are found over the bony prominences, as in the elbow region; between muscles and tendons and bone, as in the shoulder region, etc.

*X ray Showing Calcified Subdeltoid Bursitis. The arrow points to a deposit of calcium within the bursa around the shoulder joint. This is one of the most painful conditions affecting the joint areas.*

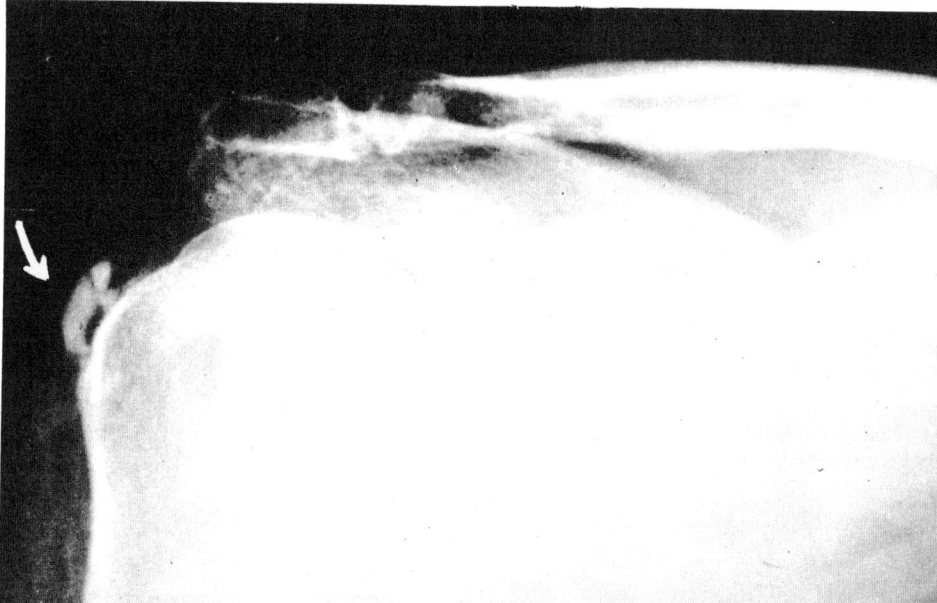

## What is bursitis?

It is an inflammation in which the fluid in the bursa is increased, or it is an inflammation of the lining of the bursa. In many cases, liquid calcium is present in the bursal fluid. Few conditions cause more excruciating pain than acute bursitis.

## Where are the most common sites for bursitis?

a. The shoulder region, as in subdeltoid and subacromial bursitis.
b. The elbow region.
c. The hip region.
d. The knee region.
e. The region near the big toe (bunions are actually inflammations of the bursae).

## What are the symptoms of acute bursitis?

a. Severe pain, worse when movement is attempted and worse at night.
b. Limitation of movement of the involved part.
c. Swelling, tenderness, and heat in the area of the acute inflammation.

## What is the treatment for bursitis?

a. Immobilization of the involved area.
b. Cold applications in the acute stages of the condition.
c. Aspiration of the inflamed bursa by inserting a needle into the bursa and withdrawing the fluid content and liquid calcium, and injection of hydrocortisone and Novocain.
d. Physiotherapy for the chronically inflamed bursa to relieve stiffness of the joints and muscles.
e. Surgical removal of the bursa, if the above measures fail.

## How effective is the treatment for bursitis?

In over 90 percent of cases, the aspiration of the bursa and the injection of hydrocortisone will bring about relief of the acute phase of the disease.

## If medical or injection treatment of bursitis fails, will surgery cure bursitis?

Yes, in most cases.

## How serious is the operation for removal of a bursa?

It is considered to be a minor operative procedure with minimum risks.

## How long can bursitis last?

If the acute phase subsides but calcium deposits and stiffness within the area persist, bursitis can become chronic and may last for months or years.

## Is there a tendency for bursitis to recur?

Yes, particularly among people in occupations in which trauma (injury) to the region tends to recur, as among orchestra conductors, painters, housemaids, etc.

## What can be done to prevent recurrent bursitis?

The avoidance of the activities that have caused it.

## Can an extremity or joint function normally after removal of a bursa?

Yes. Even though bursae are helpful in expediting the movements of muscles and tendons over bony prominences, they are not essential to normal function.

# WRY NECK (Torticollis)

## What is wry neck?

It is a deformity of the neck due to either muscle spasm or to a shortening of the muscles of the neck since birth. This deformity causes the head to rotate to one side and results in an inability to move the head freely in all directions.

## What causes wry neck?

a. A birth deformity with a shortening of the muscles of the neck.
b. Injury or infection of the neck muscles or soft tissues, with resultant muscle spasm.
c. A disease process within the spinal column in the neck region.

## What are the symptoms of wry neck?

If there is spasm, there may be great pain on any attempt to move the head. This may come on suddenly or may be gradual in onset. The pain is usually localized on one side of the neck, and marked tenderness is present when pressure is applied over certain muscles.

## What is the treatment for wry neck?

a. Medical treatment. This consists of giving medications to relieve muscle spasm, and physiotherapy, including various heat treatments. Also, repeated injections of Novocain, or like substances, to relieve muscle spasms.
b. Surgery may be indicated if the condition has been present since birth. This will consist of severing the shortened neck muscles and thus relieving the spasm and the rotation of the head upon the neck.
c. Traction (stretching).

## Is there a tendency for attacks of torticollis to recur?

Yes.

## Do infections or drafts predispose toward recurrent episodes of wry neck?

Yes.

## Will muscle strain or sleeping in awkward positions predispose toward development of an attack?

Yes.

# BUNIONS AND CORNS

## What is a bunion?

An inflammation of the bursa in the region of the base of the big toe, associated with an enlargement of the head of the first metatarsal bone.

## What causes bunions?

a. A malformation of the bony structure in the bone leading to the base of the big toe (metatarsal).
b. The wearing of too narrow a shoe and too high a heel.

## What is the treatment for bunions?

a. Wearing wider shoes and lower heels.
b. Surgical correction of the bony deformity with removal of portions of the metatarsal head and bone at the base of the big toe.

## How successful is the treatment for bunions?

Surgery is successful in curing bunions in almost all cases.

## Do bunions tend to recur once they have been satisfactorily treated?

Not if adequate surgery has been carried out and if the person stops wearing poorly fitting shoes.

## What causes corns?

a. Birth deformities of the toes, such as overlapping toes.
b. Deformity of the metatarsal arch of the foot.
c. Wearing too narrow shoes.
d. Improper gait.

## What is the treatment for corns?

a. Corrective shoes for fallen metatarsal arch and, in rare instances, surgical correction for the metatarsal arch.
b. Wearing corrective shoes.
c. Improving the gait.
d. Surgical correction of deformed toes.

## How effective are the corn remedies so widely advertised?

Since they do not attack the underlying cause, they can only serve as temporary relief.

## Can the wearing of improper shoes cause corns?

Yes, since they can cause pressure over an area exposed to undue friction.

## Should one go to a podiatrist for the treatment of corns, or should one see an orthopedic doctor?

A competent member of either profession can treat corns.

## PLANTAR WARTS

## What is a plantar wart?

A painful, calloused area on the sole of the foot. .-

## What causes plantar warts?

Warts are thought to be caused by a virus.

## What is the treatment for plantar warts?

Removal by one or more of the following means:
a. Surgical excision.
b. Electric cauterization.
c. Burning with caustic medications.

## FLAT FEET (Pes Planus)

## What is flat foot?

Flatness or depression of the longitudinal arch, sometimes associated with the turning outward of the heel of the foot.

## What causes flat feet?

a. Faulty development of bony structures.
b. Hereditary weakness of certain ligamentous structures.
c. Failure during babyhood and childhood to have proper orthopedic correction of foot weaknesses.

## How common are flat feet?

They are one of the most common structural defects in modern man.

## Will the wearing of improper shoes by children cause the development of flat feet?

It may not actually cause flat feet, but it will aggravate the tendency.

## How can flat feet be helped?

By regular visits to the orthopedist, who will recommend remedial measures such as exercises, the wearing of proper shoes, etc.

## Do flat feet always cause pain or other symptoms?

No.

## What are some of the symptoms of flat feet?

a. Tiredness in the legs.
b. Pain along the longitudinal arch.
c. Pain in the heels.

## What is the treatment for flat feet?

None is necessary if the patient is free of symptoms. Foot exercises and the wearing of arch supports often eliminate painful symptoms.

## Can flat feet be cured by wearing proper shoes?

No, but symptoms can usually be relieved.

## Should flat-footed people without symptoms wear arch supports or corrective shoes?

It is not necessary in such cases.

## What are the advantages of wearing arch supports?

In small children, it is possible that prolonged wearing of arch supports may influence the subsequent development of the longitudinal arch. In adults, arch supports serve only to relieve symptoms.

## Will exercises cure flat feet?

No.

## Can someone with flat feet indulge in physical activities?

Yes, providing corrective measures are undertaken to relieve symptoms.

## HAMMER TOE

### What is hammer toe?

A deformity in which the toe is bent upon itself and is mallet shaped.

### What causes hammer toe?

a. Birth deformity.
b. The wearing of improper shoes.

### What is the treatment for hammer toe?

Surgical correction of the deformed hammer toe, as well as the adjacent toes, which may also be somewhat deformed.

### Is surgery effective in curing hammer toe?

Yes.

## TORN CARTILAGE OF THE KNEE
### (The Deranged Knee)

### What happens when one of the knee cartilages is torn?

The cartilage is ripped from its attachment to the tibia (the main leg bone) and interferes with normal function of the knee joint.

### What is the most common cause of a torn cartilage in the knee?

A sudden, unexpected twisting motion of the knee as it is being bent. This is an injury occurring frequently among athletes.

### What are the symptoms of a torn knee cartilage?

a. Severe pain in the knee region.
b. In approximately half the cases a "locked joint" takes place, with inability to straighten the leg.
c. Tenderness when pressure is applied over the region of the torn cartilage.
d. Marked swelling of the joint, sometimes accompanied by fluid within the joint.

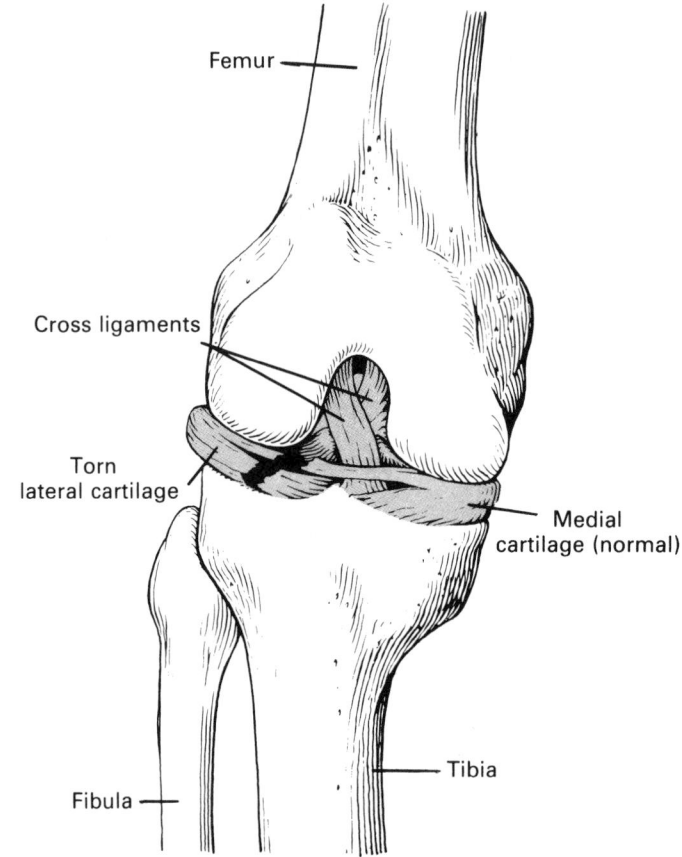

*Diagram of a Torn Cartilage of the Knee.* *A torn knee cartilage, or deranged knee, is one of the most common injuries of athletes and people who do strenuous work. It is likely to happen when the knee is twisted or subjected to extreme pressure while in a partially flexed position. A knee with a torn cartilage often locks and cannot be straightened. When locking occurs repeatedly, surgery is necessary to remove the torn cartilage. Results of such operations are excellent.*

e. Inability to stand or walk on the limb.
f. Buckling of the knee.

### Will a torn cartilage heal by itself?

No. Usually it remains a source of continuing difficulty until appropriately treated.

### How is a torn cartilage diagnosed?

a. By careful orthopedic examination.
b. By *arthroscopy* (looking into the knee joint with a special instrument).
c. By *arthrography* (a special x ray of the knee joint).

### What is the treatment for a torn knee cartilage?

For initial injuries, there is a trial period of medical management with immobilization of the leg in a splint or cast. If symptoms persist, or there is recurrent injury, the treatment is surgical.

### What operations are performed for a torn knee cartilage?

a. Through an incision in the knee region, the joint is opened and the torn portion of the cartilage is cut away from the bone and removed.
b. By removing the torn piece of cartilage through arthroscopy.

**Is an operation for a torn knee cartilage serious?**

No. It is a simple orthopedic procedure.

**Are there satisfactory results from operative treatment for a torn knee cartilage?**

Yes. A cure is obtained in most cases.

**Will the operation result in a stiff knee?**

No. Motion is begun very soon after the operation, and within several weeks the patient recovers.

**Can a patient who has recovered from a torn cartilage operation again indulge in physical exercise and athletics?**

Yes.

**Should the patient who has had a knee cartilage operation wear a support or brace?**

Yes, in some instances.

**Are special exercises advocated for these patients?**

Yes, bending and straightening the knee, usually against resistance, will lead more quickly to strengthening of the knee muscles.

**Do all torn cartilages have to be operated upon?**

No. Some will subside with rest.

**Which patients should be operated upon?**

Operation is advocated if the patient has had no relief from the pain and swelling or if locking of the knee recurs. Also, it is advocated for the patient who is subject to repeated injuries or whose injured knee buckles during the performance of his work.

**Is there a tendency for knee problems to recur in a joint that has been successfully operated upon?**

No, but it must be remembered that there are two of these cartilages in each knee joint. It is, therefore, possible to remove one cartilage and then discover at a later date that injury to the other cartilage has taken place.

## OSTEOMYELITIS
### (Bone Infections)

**What is osteomyelitis?**

An infection of the bone.

**What are the most common causes of osteomyelitis?**

An infection caused by a germ (bacteria) such as staphylococcus, streptococcus, etc.

**How common is osteomyelitis?**

Before the days of the antibiotic drugs, osteomyelitis of the bone due to bacteria was seen quite frequently following tonsillitis or other acute infections elsewhere in the body. Today it is a relatively uncommon condition, seen only occasionally in young children or after a severe injury.

**What are the symptoms of osteomyelitis?**

In the acute stages there is high fever and pain in the region of the bone infection. If the bone is near the skin surface, localized swelling, tenderness, heat, and redness may be noted. Superficial or deep abscesses may form in the bone or overlying the bone structure.

**Will osteomyelitis of the bone be visible on x-ray examination?**

Yes, but it may not be discernible until two or three weeks after the acute onset of the disease.

**What is the treatment for osteomyelitis caused by disease organisms such as the streptococci and staphylococci?**

a. Surgery, with scraping out of all infected bone.

b. Giving the specific antibiotic drug to which the bacteria are sensitive.

c. Complete bed rest for several weeks or months until complete bone healing has taken place.

d. Frequent x-ray examination to check the status of bone healing.

**How successful is treatment for osteomyelitis?**

a. Present-day treatment for tuberculous osteomyelitis is very successful providing other important organs are not too extensively involved.

b. Osteomyelitis caused by streptococci or staphylococci can be cured in almost all instances if proper treatment, as outlined above, is carried out.

## NEUROMUSCULAR DISORDERS

**What is meant by a neuromuscular disorder?**

This term applies to a group of diseases in which both the nerves and the muscles are affected.

**What are the results of disorders of the neuromuscular apparatus?**

a. Muscles may become paralyzed or may be tight and spastic.

b. The muscles may atrophy or waste.

c. The muscles may become extremely weak without any recognizable changes in the nerve structure.

d. The muscles may degenerate.

**What are some of the common diseases in which the neuromuscular apparatus is affected?**

a. Poliomyelitis (infantile paralysis). (See Chapter 18, on Contagious Diseases.)

b. Cerebral palsy. (See Chapter 45, on Nervous Diseases.)

c. Myasthenia gravis.

*(continued)*

d. Progressive muscular atrophy.
e. Muscular dystrophy.

## What is myasthenia gravis?

It is a rare disease characterized by great muscular weakness and rapid onset of fatigue.

## What causes myasthenia gravis?

A disturbance in the normal chemistry of transmission of nerve impulses to the muscle.

## What are the symptoms of myasthenia gravis?

There is progressive weakness of the muscles that move the arm, the facial muscles, and those muscles concerned with chewing and swallowing.

## Is there any effective treatment for myasthenia gravis?

Considerable benefit can be obtained by the administration of a drug called Prostigmin.

## Is myasthenia gravis an acute condition?

No. It tends to last over a period of many years and is characterized by very slow wasting of the muscles.

## What is progressive muscular atrophy?

It is a disease of the spinal cord characterized by a slow degeneration of some of the nerve cells within the cord. This degeneration of the nerves produces muscular wasting among certain muscle groups.

## What age group is mostly affected by progressive muscular atrophy?

People between the ages of twenty-five and forty-five.

## Is progressive muscular atrophy an inherited disease?

No.

## Is there any effective treatment for this disease?

No. The only beneficial effects, and these are minor, are obtained from massage and exercises and braces.

## What are the symptoms of progressive muscular atrophy?

Weakness of the muscles in the hands, arms, and shoulders.

## What is muscular dystrophy?

It is a primary disease of the muscles, which usually has its onset in early childhood.

## Who is most frequently affected by muscular dystrophy?

It is seen more often in boys than in girls and usually begins at the ages of five or six.

## How common is muscular dystrophy?

It is estimated that there are approximately a hundred thousand cases in the United States today.

## What are the symptoms of muscular dystrophy?

Weakness in the legs and excessive fatigue. There is a characteristic peculiar waddling gait in walking, and difficulty in climbing stairs. Children with muscular dystrophy have frequent falls on slight provocation.

## What is the cause of muscular dystrophy?

The cause is unknown, but there seems to be a hereditary factor.

## Do patients with muscular dystrophy ever get well?

There may be temporary periods of improvement, but they do not get well.

## Is there any effective treatment for muscular dystrophy?

No, but help can be obtained by systematic muscle training. Also, certain surgical operations that lengthen contracted tendons are helpful. Supportive braces also tend to aid the patient in walking.

## Are there any drugs that are helpful in treating muscular dystrophy?

Yes. Pilocarpine and similar drugs have given some benefit in certain cases.

## Is it possible that a cure for this condition will be found at some time in the future?

Yes.

## What is the eventual outcome of a case of muscular dystrophy?

Frequently the patient develops some other infection as a result of his lowered resistance.

# PAGET'S DISEASE
## (Osteitis Deformans)

## What is Paget's disease?

It is a chronic disease of the skeleton, which begins insidiously and manifests itself in progressive deformities in the long bones and in the skull.

## At what age is Paget's disease most likely to occur?

In middle and later life.

## What causes Paget's disease of the bones?

The cause is unknown.

## Does Paget's disease always affect all of the bones of the body or does it affect a single bone?

Paget's disease may be limited to one bone, but more often it affects many bones.

## What are the fundamental skeletal changes in Paget's disease?

There is a gradual thickening and bowing of the long bones, particularly those of the thigh and the shin. There is also thickening of the bones of the skull.

## What is the usual course of Paget's disease?

It does not seem to greatly affect the

length of life. However, spontaneous fractures may occur in the diseased bones, and deformity is usually progressive in nature.

**Is there any cure for Paget's disease?**

No, but treatment with a new medication is sometimes helpful.

## OSTEITIS FIBROSA CYSTICA *(Hyperparathyroidism)*

**What is generalized osteitis fibrosa cystica?**

It is a generalized disease of the bones characterized by the formation of cysts. These cysts occur particularly in the long bones of the body, in the skull, and in the spinal column.

**What are the symptoms of this disease?**

Deep-seated pain in the skeleton, with local swelling of the bones, and spontaneous fractures in the region of the cystic changes.

**What is the cause of osteitis fibrosa cystica?**

It has been definitely established that this disease is caused by a tumor within one of the four parathyroid glands, which are located in the neck.

**What is the treatment for this condition?**

Surgical removal of the diseased, tumorous parathyroid gland.

**Are all of the parathyroid glands removed in treating osteitis fibrosa cystica?**

No, only the ones involved in tumor formation. One gland should always be left in place to maintain vital parathyroid function.

**Can osteitis fibrosa cystica be cured by removal of the diseased parathyroid gland?**

Yes.

**Is osteitis fibrosa cystica a common condition?**

No. It is a relatively rare disease.

## OSTEOMALACIA

**What is osteomalacia?**

A generalized disease affecting and softening the skeleton as a result of the decalcification of the bones.

**What are the symptoms of osteomalacia?**

The bones become soft and bend and break and tend to form marked deformities.

**Does this disease tend to affect one sex more than the other?**

Yes, it affects mostly women, but children and elderly men are occasionally subject to this disease.

**What are the causes of osteomalacia?**

Although the exact causes are unknown, kidney disease or nutritional imbalance are thought to be the most frequent causes of the condition.

**What is the treatment for osteomalacia?**

Underlying kidney disease must be treated. Also, it is important that diet and nutrition be maintained at a good level and that orthopedic measures be instituted to forestall too many deformities of the softened bones.

## OSTEOPOROSIS

**What is osteoporosis?**

It is a disease occurring in the later years of life, affecting both sexes, characterized by decalcification of the bones.

**What causes osteoporosis?**

The slowing down of the normal process of bone-cell replacement by an aging body mechanism.

**Who is most likely to develop osteoporosis?**

People in the sixth, seventh, and eighth decades of life.

**What harm results from senile osteoporosis?**

When it affects the spine, as commonly happens, it is very painful. Furthermore, it may lead to a fracture of the involved bone because of its loss of strength due to decalcification.

**What is the best way to handle osteoporosis?**

a. Pain should be relieved by the giving of various hormone preparations, especially estrogen to women.

b. The patient is urged to be physically active.

## RECONSTRUCTIVE SURGERY UPON THE BONES, JOINTS, AND MUSCLES

**For what conditions can reconstructive surgery upon the bones, joints, and muscles be carried out?**

a. When fractured bones have healed in poor position, reconstructive surgery can be carried out to correct the defects.

b. Joints that are diseased and that are painful, or in which there is little or no motion, can be made useful again by reconstructive surgical measures.

c. Partially or totally paralyzed muscles can be substituted for by the transplantation of good muscles or good tendons from other parts of the extremity.

MUSCLES, POSTERIOR VIEW          MUSCLES, ANTERIOR VIEW

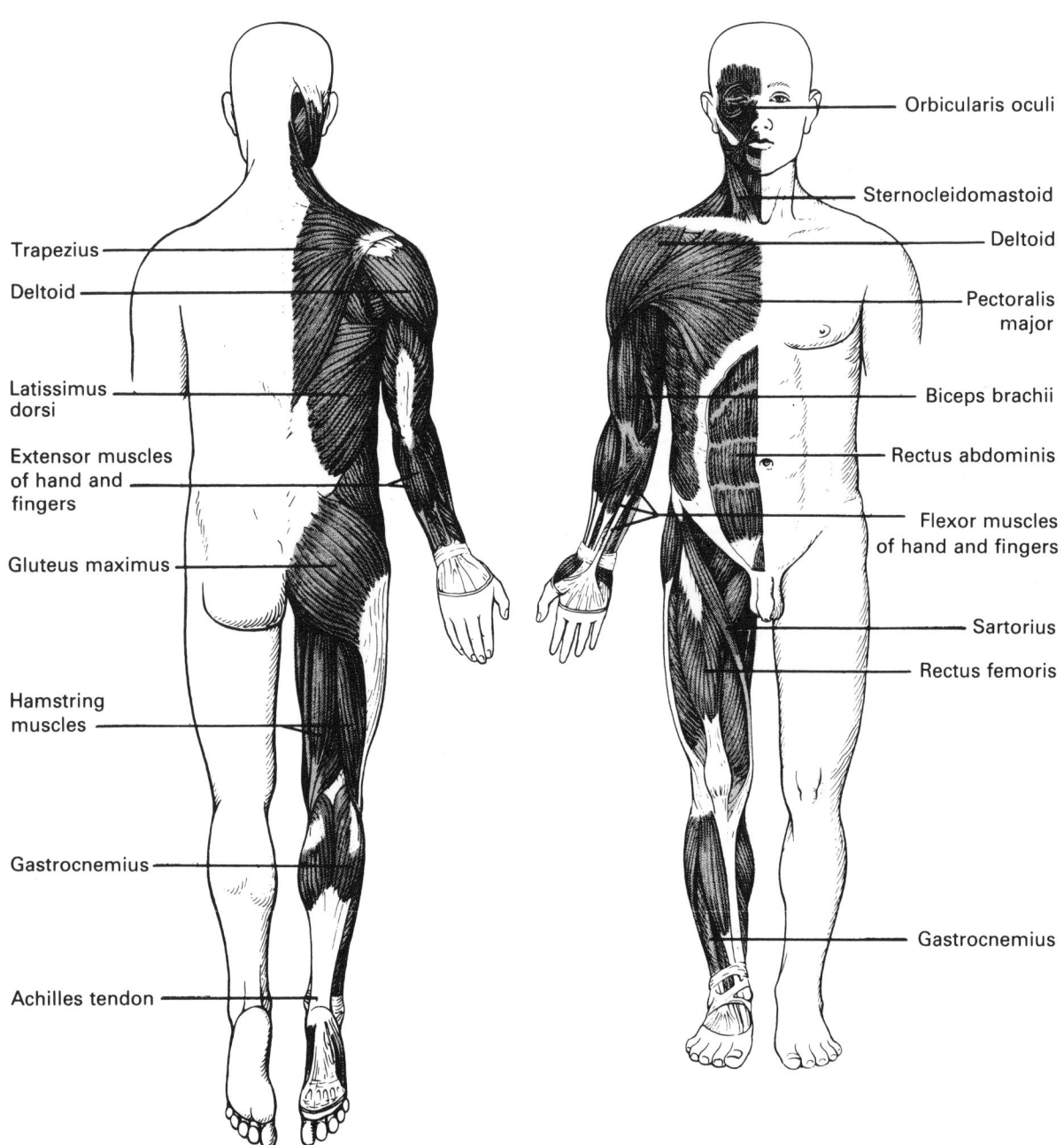

**Diagram of the Muscular System.** *Muscles are located beneath the skin and fatty tissues and are the means by which all movements of the body are made. There are many hundreds of muscles within the body, each having a function to flex, extend, or rotate movable parts in our body. Once a muscle cell or a whole muscle has been subject to serious disease and has died, it never regrows. Fortunately, the muscular system of the body maintains itself in remarkably good health throughout life.*

**How effective is reconstructive orthopedic surgery?**

This will depend upon how extensive the disability is and in what region it is located. In many conditions, reconstructive surgery is very beneficial.

**Can reconstructive surgery bring a paralyzed muscle back to life?**

No.

**Can people with severely arthritic joints be helped by reconstructive surgery?**

Yes, in a great many cases.

**Is it possible for the surgeon to determine which patient will be most benefited by reconstructive surgery?**

Yes. By careful analysis of the exact nature of the condition, it can usually be determined which patient can be helped by muscle or joint reconstruction.

**What types of reconstructive operations are performed?**

a. Joint replacements, including hip, shoulder, elbow, ankle, knee, wrist, and finger joints.
b. Arthroplasty, a surgical procedure to reshape a joint.
c. Operations for arthritis to decrease the amount of pain.
d. Osteotomy, an operation to realign a deformed or misaligned bone.
e. Fusion of a joint to stabilize a limb.

**When is it advisable to carry out a fusion operation?**

When joint replacement will not be beneficial or is too dangerous because of infection.

**Is reconstructive orthopedic surgery dangerous?**

No.

**Will transplanted muscles or tendons or fused joints continue to function as a child grows taller?**

Yes.

**Is it necessary to reeducate a transplanted muscle or tendon so that the patient can use it properly?**

This is very important. Actually, reeducation of the transplanted muscle or tendon is as important as the operation itself.

## ARTHROPLASTY AND JOINT REPLACEMENT

**What are arthroplasty and joint replacement?**

They are the terms used to describe the plastic reconstruction or surgical replacement of a joint.

*Hand, Before and After Surgery for Arthritis. Surgery for arthritis of the hand can do much to overcome the crippling effects of the disease. The photos show the same hand before (left) and (below) after corrective surgery.*

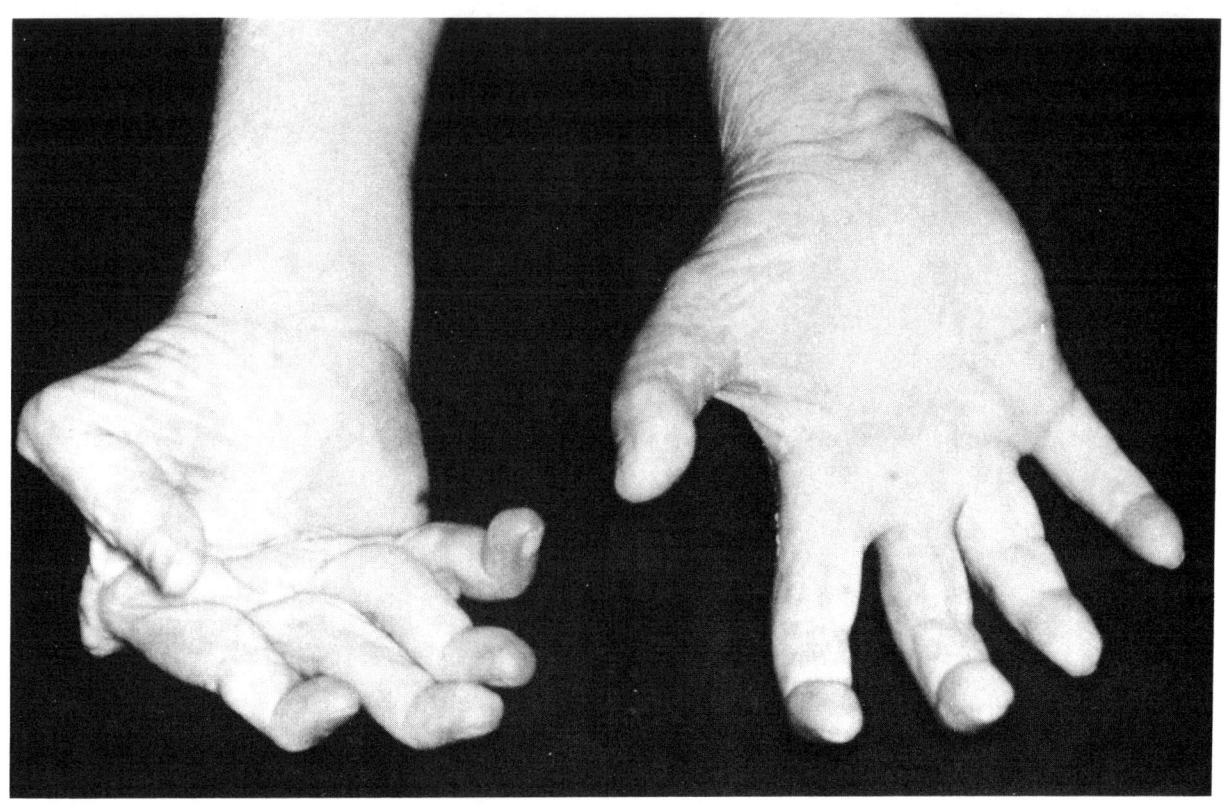

**For what conditions are these operations most frequently performed?**

a. In any condition accompanied by permanent, painful, restriction of joint motion.
b. When a joint has been irrevocably destroyed by a severe fracture with failure of normal healing processes.
c. When the bones making up a joint have been hopelessly destroyed by chronic arthritis or some other degenerative disease process.
d. When it is necessary to remove a joint, or part of a joint, because of a bone tumor.

**What are some of the joints that can be replaced?**

a. The hip joint.
b. The elbow joint.
c. The knee joint.
d. The ankle joint.
e. The wrist joint.
f. The shoulder joint.
g. Finger joints.

**What metals are used to replace the bones?**

One of several noncorroding metals.

**How successful are arthroplasty and joint replacement?**

Arthroplasty and joint replacement have made great strides in the last few years so that patients can expect great relief from pain and marked improvement in motion following surgery. Of course these are major operative procedures and must be performed only by specialists who have had wide experience in the field.

**How successful is hip replacement?**

Well over 90 percent of cases can be classified as successful.

**What is the most frequent cause of failure of an arthroplasty or joint replacement?**

Postoperative infection.

**If one procedure fails, is it possible to reoperate at a later date?**

Yes.

## FRACTURES

**What is a fracture?**

Any break in the continuity of a bone is called a fracture.

*X ray Showing Fracture of the Ankle (Fibula).* These x rays show what an actual fracture looks like. Note the break in the smooth contour of the bone about the ankle. When this fracture is set, the fragments of bone will come together and healing will take place between them. Although the process is slow, when a fractured bone has finally healed it is usually just as strong as it was before it was broken.

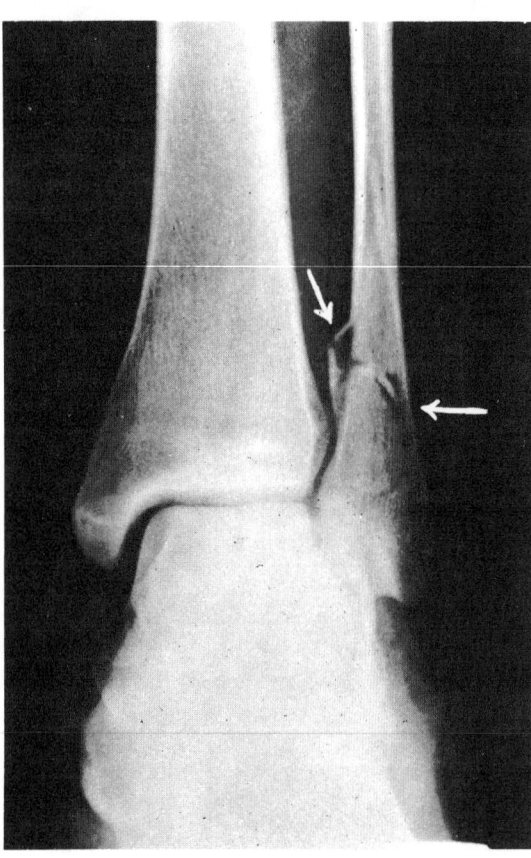
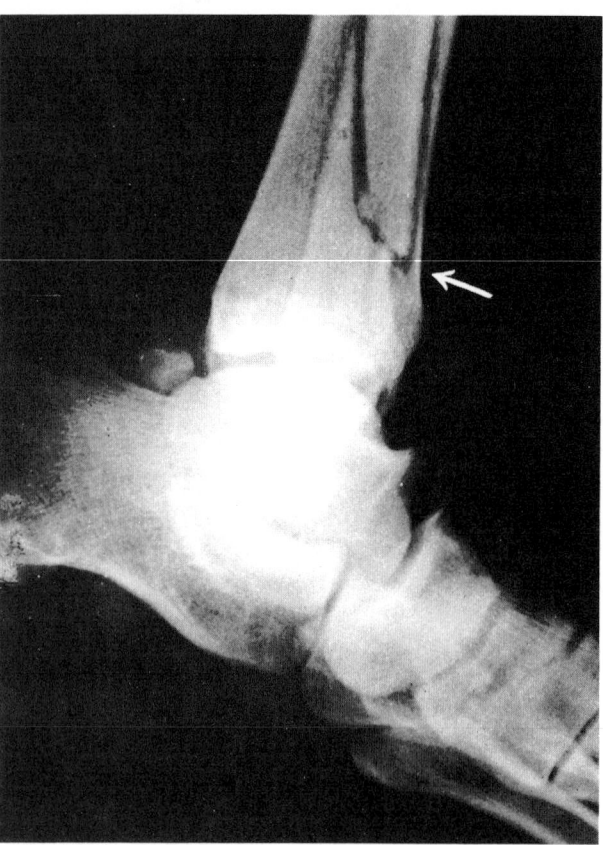

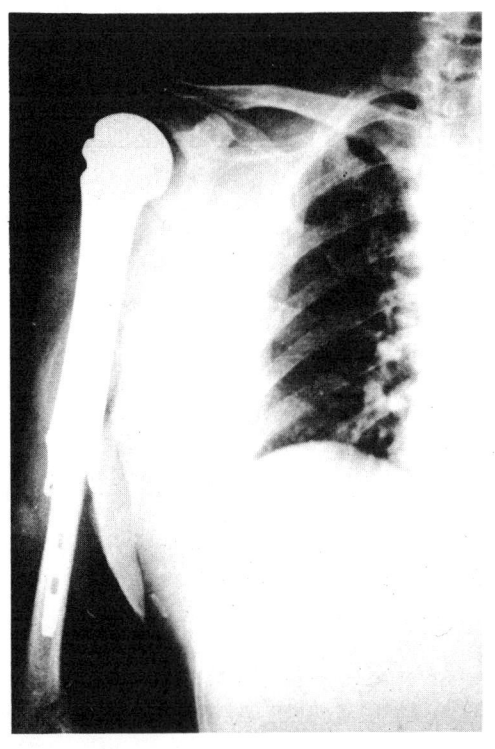

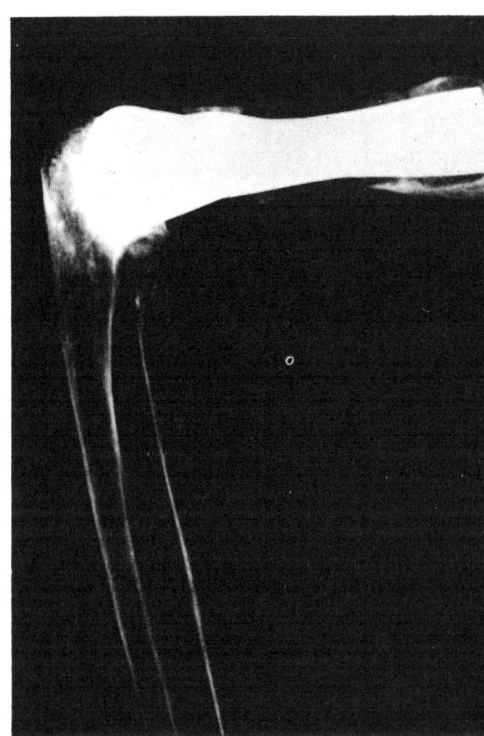

*Far left:*
***X ray of Shoulder Arthroplasty.*** *In this case the upper part of the humerus, connecting to the shoulder, has a metal replacement.*

*Left:*
***X ray of Elbow Arthroplasty.*** *This x ray shows a metal replacement of the crushed lower part of a humerus, the upper bone in the elbow.*

**Is there any difference between the terms "fracture" and "broken bone"?**

No.

**What types of fracture are there?**

a. Simple fracture; there is no connection between the skin surface and the broken bone.

b. Compound fracture; there is a skin wound and a connection between the fracture site and the skin surface.

**Why is it important to distinguish between these two types of fractures?**

Because the possibility of infection and poor healing is so much greater when there is a compound fracture.

**What other classifications of fractures are there?**

a. Transverse fracture; the fracture extends straight across a bone.

b. Spiral fracture; there is a spiral or twisting type of fracture along a bone.

c. Oblique fracture; one in which the break occurs at an angle through the bone.

d. Incomplete (greenstick) fracture; a fracture that does not extend all the way through a bone.

e. Comminuted fracture; the bone is broken into more than two fragments.

**How can one tell if he has a broken bone?**

The surest method is to have an x-ray examination performed.

**Can a physician often tell if a bone is broken without an x ray?**

Yes, in the great majority of cases. However, this should always be supported by an x-ray examination so that the exact nature of the break can be determined.

**Does one always hear a crack when a bone breaks?**

No.

**What are the basic underlying principles in treating all fractures?**

a. First, it is important to see that the general condition of the patient is taken care of. In other words, if a patient is in shock or has other serious injuries in addition to the fracture, he must be treated before attention is concentrated upon the broken bone.

b. To line up the broken parts of the bone so that they will heal in their normal position. This is called setting a fracture or reduction of a fracture.

c. To make sure that the fragments of the bone stay in good position until solid healing has taken place. This is called immobilization of the bone.

**Where should fractures be set?**

Minor fractures may be set in the surgeon's office; major fractures of the longer bones must be set in the hospital, where facilities are usually more adequate.

**What are some of the methods generally used in setting fractures?**

a. Closed reduction; the bones are brought into proper position by ex-

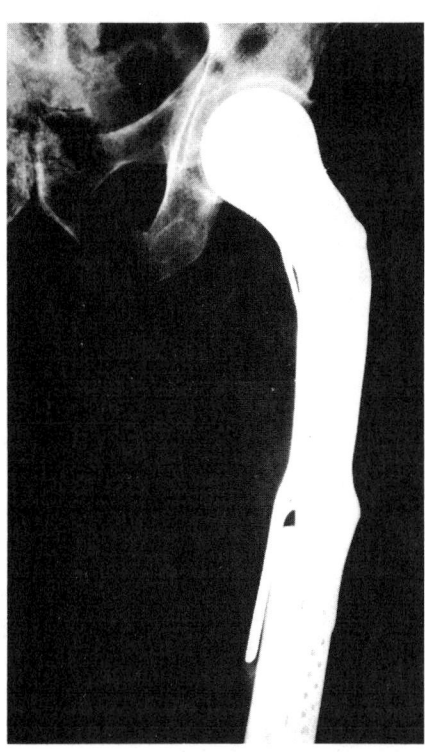

ternal manipulation of the fragments, without resorting to surgery.

b. Open reduction; surgery is performed, and the site of the fracture is exposed. The surgeon then gets the bones back into normal position by manually straightening them and bringing the ends together.

c. Maintaining the bones in proper position. This is carried out in one of several ways, as outlined below.

**What are some of the ways in which the fragments of fractured bones are maintained in proper position?**

a. By the application of a plaster cast, which will keep them in proper alignment.

b. By traction. This employs a system of weights and pulleys that are attached to the injured limb so as to line up the bones and to overcome muscle pulls, which might cause the fragments to slip out of alignment.

c. By the application of metal screws. Such screws are placed through the fragments of bone in order to keep them in alignment.

d. By wiring the bones, that is, by placing wire around the fragments to keep them in position.

e. By plating the bones, that is, by attaching a metal plate to the side of the bone and keeping the fragments in position by placing screws through the plate and bone.

f. By using metal nails or pins, which are hammered through the two fragments.

g. By medullary nailing, which involves the placement of a long steel or metal nail through the hollow portion of both fragments of the fractured bone.

h. By bone graft, which involves taking a piece of bone from some other part of the body and placing it alongside, or between, the bony fragments and then anchoring it in place.

**Are more fractures being treated today by operative intervention?**

Yes. Since surgery has become so much safer, it has been decided that a great deal of time can be saved by operative surgery.

**What is meant by "union of bones"?**

This means the healing of the bony fragments.

**What are the most common causes of nonunion or delayed union of fractures?**

a. Failure to immobilize the bony fragments.

b. Interference with the blood supply to the bony fragments.

c. Loss of bone substance, so that the broken ends do not come together.

d. Extensive injury to the soft parts,

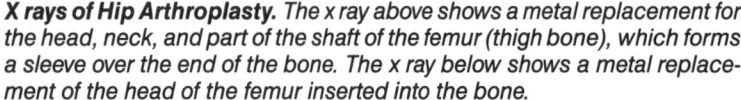

*X rays of Hip Arthroplasty. The x ray above shows a metal replacement for the head, neck, and part of the shaft of the femur (thigh bone), which forms a sleeve over the end of the bone. The x ray below shows a metal replacement of the head of the femur inserted into the bone.*

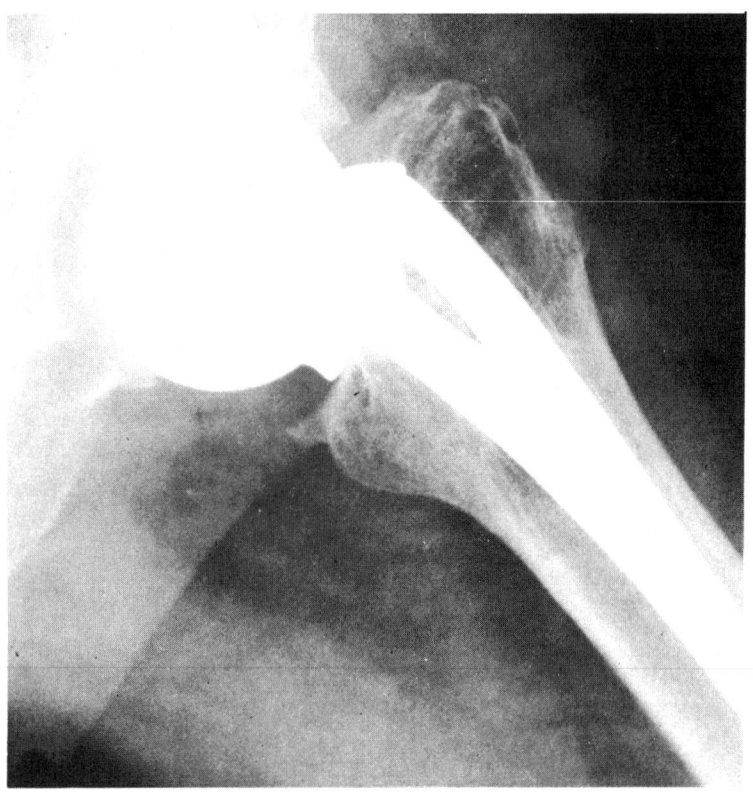

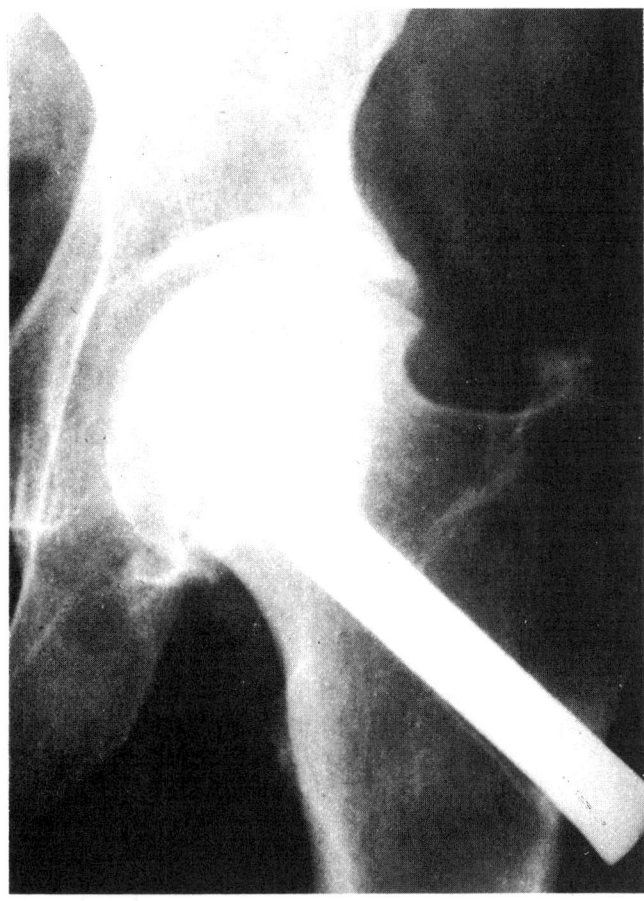

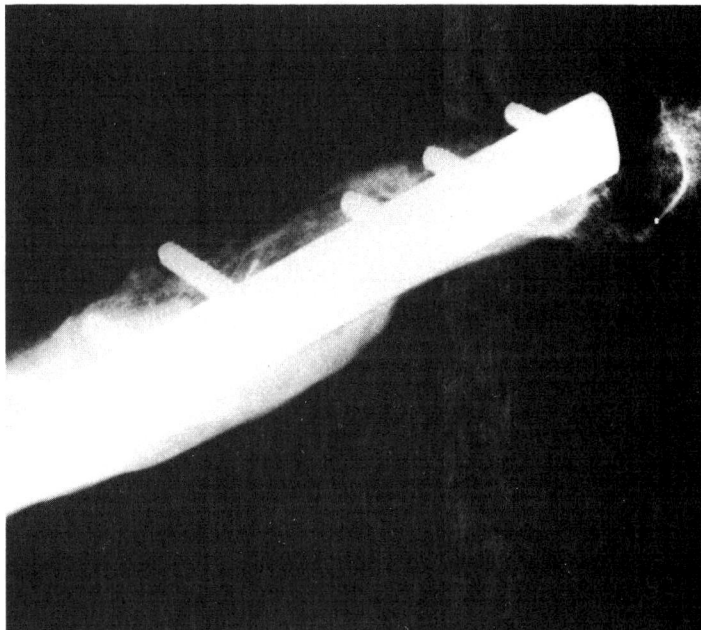

**Setting Fractured Bones.** *The x ray left shows a metal pin inserted into the head of the femur to set the fractured bone. The x ray below shows a fracture that has been set by screwing a metal plate into the bone.*

such as muscles or ligaments, surrounding the fracture.

e. Infection at the site of the fracture.

f. Excessive traction upon the fragments of the bone.

g. Muscle or fibrous tissues that intrude between the broken ends of the bones and prevent them from knitting.

h. Poor general health of the patient.

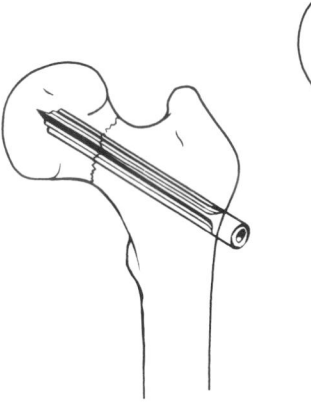
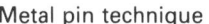
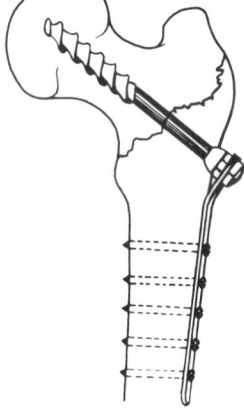

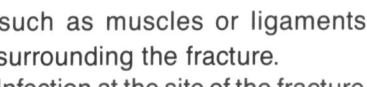
Metal pin technique      Plate and screw technique

**Can nonunion, or delayed union, be treated successfully by the orthopedist?**

Yes, either by surgery or by newly developed methods of electric current stimulation.

**Does the state of the general health of the patient often influence the rate at which fractures heal?**

Yes. The patient in poor general health may not heal his bony fracture.

**What is the first-aid treatment for a patient who has suffered a bone fracture?**

See Chapter 26, on First Aid in Emergencies.

**What is the basic principle underlying the first-aid treatment for all fractures?**

It is to splint the bony fragments so

that there is as little movement of the fractured bone as possible. *Anything* can be used as a temporary splint as long as it prevents the fractured parts from moving about.

**By what standards do orthopedists judge the results of the treatment of a fracture?**

a. Anatomical result.

b. Functional result.

## FRACTURES OF THE SHOULDER REGION AND ARM

| Bone Fractured | Usual Type of Treatment | Period of Immobilization | Usual Interval Until Full Recovery |
|---|---|---|---|
| **Shoulder Blade (scapula)** | a. Sling | 2-4 weeks | 4-6 weeks |
| **Collarbone (clavicle)** | a. Figure-of-eight bandage | 4-6 weeks | 6-8 weeks |
| | b. Closed reduction | 4-6 weeks | 6-8 weeks |
| | c. Open reduction with pin fixation | 3-4 weeks | 4-6 weeks |
| **Arm Bone (humerus)** | | | |
| **a. Neck of humerus** | a. Sling | 3-4 weeks | 8-12 weeks |
| | b. Velpeau's bandage (body and arm) | 3-4 weeks | 8-12 weeks |
| | c. Traction and cast | 4-6 weeks | 10-12 weeks |
| | d. Closed reduction (spica body cast) | 4-6 weeks | 10-12 weeks |
| | e. Open reduction by operation | 4-6 weeks | 10-12 weeks |
| **b. Shaft of humerus** | a. Hanging cast | 4-6 weeks | 10-12 weeks |
| | b. Closed reduction and spica cast (body and arm) | 6-8 weeks | 10-12 weeks |
| | c. Traction and cast | 6-8 weeks | 10-12 weeks |
| | d. Open reduction by operation | 6-10 weeks | 10-14 weeks |
| **c. Elbow region** | a. Plaster cast | 4-6 weeks | 10-12 weeks |
| | b. Traction and cast | 4-6 weeks | 10-12 weeks |
| | c. Closed reduction | | |
| | d. Open reduction by operation | 4-8 weeks | 12-16 weeks |
| **d. Epiphysial separation (at the growth line)** | a. Cast | 3-4 weeks | 8-10 weeks |
| | b. Closed reduction and cast | | |
| | c. Open reduction by operation | 3-6 weeks | 10-12 weeks |
| **Forearm Bones** | | | |
| **a. Radius** | | | |
| 1. Head of radius | a. Sling | 10 days | 10-12 weeks |
| | b. Plaster splint | 10 days | 10-12 weeks |
| | c. Closed reduction and plaster | | |
| | d. Open reduction by operation | 10 days | 10-12 weeks |
| 2. Shaft of radius | a. Cast | 6-10 weeks | 12-16 weeks |
| | b. Closed reduction | | |
| | c. Open reduction by operation | 6-8 weeks | 12-16 weeks |
| 3. Distal end (near wrist) | a. Cast | 4-6 weeks | 10-12 weeks |
| | b. Closed reduction plus cast | | |
| | c. Open reduction by operation | 6-8 weeks | 10-12 weeks |
| **b. Ulna** | | | |
| 1. Olecranon (elbow) | a. Cast | 4-6 weeks | 10-12 weeks |
| | b. Closed reduction and cast | | |
| | c. Open reduction by operation | 3-5 weeks | 10-12 weeks |
| 2. Shaft of ulna | a. Cast | 6-10 weeks | 12-16 weeks |
| | b. Closed reduction and cast | | |
| | c. Open reduction by operation | 8-10 weeks | 12-18 weeks |
| 3. Distal end (near wrist) | a. Cast | 4-6 weeks | 8-10 weeks |
| | b. Closed reduction and cast | | |
| | c. Open reduction by operation | 10 days | 4-6 weeks |
| **c. Radius and ulna combined** | a. Cast | 6-10 weeks | 12-16 weeks |
| | b. Closed reduction and cast | | |
| | c. Open reduction by operation | 6-10 weeks | 12-18 weeks |
| **d. Radius and ulna at distal end (wrist)** | a. Cast | 4-6 weeks | 10-12 weeks |
| | b. Closed reduction and cast | | |
| | c. Open reduction by operation | 4-8 weeks | 10-14 weeks |

| Bone Fractured | Usual Type of Treatment | Period of Immobilization | Usual Interval Until Full Recovery |
|---|---|---|---|
| **Wrist Bones** | | | |
| **a. Scaphoid** | a. Cast | 10-14 weeks | 14-20 weeks |
| **b. Other wrist bones** | a. Cast | 4-6 weeks | 6-10 weeks |
| **Hand** | | | |
| **a. Metacarpals** | a. Cast | 2-3 weeks | 4-6 weeks |
| | b. Closed reduction and cast | 2-3 weeks | 5-7 weeks |
| | c. Open reduction by operation | 2-3 weeks | 5-7 weeks |
| **b. Phalanges (fingers)** | a. Cast | 2-3 weeks | 4-6 weeks |
| | b. Closed reduction and cast | 2-3 weeks | 6-8 weeks |
| | c. Open reduction by operation | 2-3 weeks | 6-8 weeks |

## FRACTURES OF THE PELVIC REGION AND LEG

| Bone Fractured | Usual Type of Treatment | Period of Immobilization | Usual Interval Until Full Recovery |
|---|---|---|---|
| **Pelvis** | a. Bed rest | 4-8 weeks | 10-12 weeks |
| | b. Open reduction and wire fixation | 4-8 weeks | 10-12 weeks |
| **Thigh Bone (femur)** | | | |
| **a. Neck (near hip)** | a. Open reduction with nail fixation | 3-6 months | 12 or more months |
| **b. Intertrochanteric area (near hip)** | a. Traction | 3-6 months | 6-9 months |
| | b. Closed reduction and cast | 3-6 months | 6-12 months |
| | c. Open reduction and nail plate fixation | 3-6 months | 6-9 months |
| **c. Shaft of thigh bone** | a. Cast and brace | 3-6 months | 10-12 months |
| | b. Traction and cast or brace | 6-9 months | 10-12 months |
| | c. Closed reduction | | |
| | d. Open reduction with cast | 6-9 months | 12 months |
| | e. Open reduction without cast | 4-6 weeks | 12 months |
| **d. Supracondylar area (near knee)** | a. Cast | 3-4 months | 6-10 months |
| | b. Traction and cast or brace | 4-6 months | 8-10 months |
| | c. Open reduction without cast | 3-4 months | 6-8 months |
| **Kneecap (patella)** | a. Cast | 4-6 weeks | 10-16 weeks |
| | b. Open reduction plus cast | 2-5 weeks | 10-16 weeks |
| **Leg** | | | |
| **a. Shin bone (tibia)** | | | |
| 1. Condyle (upper end) | a. Cast | 10-12 weeks | 6-9 months |
| | b. Closed reduction and cast | | |
| | c. Open reduction and cast | 10-12 weeks | 6-9 months |
| 2. Midshaft | a. Cast | 3-5 months | 6-9 months |
| | b. Traction and cast or brace | 3-5 months | 6-9 months |
| | c. Closed reduction and cast | | |
| | d. Open reduction and cast | 3-5 months | 6-9 months |
| 3. Distal third (lower third) | a. Cast | 3-9 months | 9-20 months |
| | b. Closed reduction and cast | | |
| | c. Open reduction and cast | 3-9 months | 9-20 months |
| | d. Traction and cast or brace | 3-9 months | 9-20 months |
| **b. Fibula** | a. Bandage | 2-4 weeks | 6 weeks |
| | b. Cast | 2-4 weeks | 6 weeks |
| | c. Closed reduction and cast | | |
| | d. Open reduction and cast | | |

| Bone Fractured | Usual Type of Treatment | Period of Immobilization | Usual Interval Until Full Recovery |
|---|---|---|---|
| **Ankle** | | | |
| a. Medial malleolus (tibia) | a. Cast | 6-8 weeks | 9-12 weeks |
| | b. Closed reduction and cast | | |
| | c. Open reduction and cast | 3-6 weeks | 10-16 weeks |
| b. Lateral malleolus (fibula) | a. Cast | 6-8 weeks | 9-12 weeks |
| c. Bi- or tri-malleolar (tibia and fibula) | a. Cast | 6-12 weeks | 12-16 weeks |
| | b. Open reduction and cast | 6-12 weeks | 12-16 weeks |
| **Foot** | | | |
| a. Tarsals | | | |
|   1. Os calcis (heel bone) | a. Cast | 12-16 weeks | 5-6 months |
| | b. Open reduction and cast | 12-16 weeks | 5-6 months |
|   2. Others (foot bones) | a. Cast | 5-8 weeks | 8-12 weeks |
| b. Metatarsals | a. Cast | 5-6 weeks | 8-10 weeks |
| | b. Closed reduction and cast | | |
| | c. Open reduction and cast | 5-6 weeks | 8-10 weeks |
| | d. Bandage and crutches | | |
| c. Phalanges (toes) | a. Bandage or cast | 2-3 weeks | 4-6 weeks |

Hospital stay may be required for several types of fractures. Generally, closed reduction requires less time in the hospital than open reduction. Treatment by traction requires the longest stay in a hospital. Compound fractures are usually complicated fractures frequently requiring more than one procedure, and therefore longer hospitalization.

**What is the difference between the anatomical and functional result?**

The bones may be set in perfect alignment, and this will thereby constitute a fine anatomical result. Yet, in a certain number of these cases, the function of the extremity may be poor. Conversely, the bones may not be in strict anatomical alignment, but the extremity may be restored to completely normal function. This, then, will be a good functional result even though it is a poor anatomical result.

**Which is more important, a good functional result or a good anatomical result?**

Obviously, a good functional result is more important.

**What are the most common fractures, and what is the treatment for them?**

See the Fracture Chart in this chapter.

**What is a pathological fracture?**

One that takes place without injury or with a minimal injury. This happens most often when a bone is involved in a disease process, such as a cyst or a tumor.

**Should all fractures be set immediately after they occur?**

No. There are many fractures that have caused such injury and damage to the soft parts that it may be wise to wait a few days for these tissues to heal before attempting reduction of the broken bones.

**Is the treatment for compound fractures different from the treatment for simple fractures?**

Yes.

a. In compound fractures, the wound must be thoroughly cleansed, and if any dead tissue or foreign bodies are present, they must be removed from the fracture site.

b. Tetanus antitoxin and gas gangrene antitoxin may have to be given if the wound is dirty.

c. Large doses of the antibiotics are given to prevent infection in compound fractures. This measure is usually not necessary with simple fractures.

d. Surgery is indicated much more often in treating compound fractures.

**Do fractures with many fragments (comminuted) heal with more difficulty than simple fractures?**

Yes.

**Is an anesthetic usually used for the setting of a fracture?**

Yes. In simple and small fractures, local anesthesia may be used; in larger fractures, general anesthesia is usually employed.

**Does it hurt when a plaster cast is applied?**

No.

**Is it painful to have a plaster cast removed?**

No.

**Are casts applied only to the immediate area of fracture?**

No. They must be placed so that they

extend at least one joint above and one joint below the site of the fracture.

**Will pain continue for a day or two even after a cast has been applied?**
Yes. Within two to three days, however, the pain disappears.

**How long do casts have to be worn?**
See the Fracture Chart in this chapter.

**Is it ever possible to walk while wearing a cast on the leg?**
Yes, in certain simple fractures of the leg, walking upon the cast is permissible. This is accomplished by incorporating a special device into the structure of the cast.

**Are bones ever as strong after a fracture as they were before?**
Yes. A well-healed bone returns to normal strength.

**Is it necessary to exercise the muscles and tendons while the patient is in a cast?**
Yes, the orthopedist will prescribe the necessary exercises.

**Can a patient allow a cast to get wet?**
Yes, if it is made of special, water-resistant material.

**Is it often necessary to change or reapply a cast?**
Yes. This is done frequently as treatment of the fracture progresses over a period of weeks or months.

**How often is it necessary to x-ray a fracture?**
a. Immediately *before* it is set.
b. Immediately *after* it is set.
c. Approximately seven to ten days after it is set.
d. Approximately every few weeks if it is a slow-healing fracture.
e. After the cast has been removed.

**How do fractures heal?**
By the formation of new bone, called *callus,* in between the bony fragments.

**How long do fractures take to heal?**
See the Fracture Chart in this chapter.

**Are special diets necessary to help fractures heal more quickly?**
No.

**Is function of the limb normal immediately after removal of a cast?**
No. It is frequently necessary to take physiotherapy for several weeks or months in order to regain normal function.

**Is a bone, once fractured, more likely to become fractured again?**
No.

**Is it true that for months after a fracture has healed some people feel pain at the fracture site when there are changes in weather?**
Yes, but the reason for this sensation is not known.

**Is it common for an extremity to be somewhat shriveled after it has been in a cast for a long time?**
Yes. There is a certain amount of thinning of the muscles, but they will return to normal after resumption of activity.

**Is an arm or leg ever shorter after a fracture has healed?**
Yes, but it is usually only a slight shortening, which should not interfere with function unless a large portion of bone has degenerated or was lost when the fracture took place.

## TUMORS OF THE BONE

**What types of bone tumors exist?**
a. Benign tumors of the cartilage, such as chondromas, or benign tumors of bone known as osteomas, giant cell tumors, etc.
b. Malignant tumors of the bone, such as osteogenic sarcomas.

**How can one tell if he has a bone tumor?**
a. There is swelling in the vicinity of the tumor.
b. X-ray examination will show abnormal bone structure.

**How can one tell whether a bone tumor is benign or malignant?**
The history of onset, the physical examination of the region by a competent orthopedist, and characteristic x-ray findings will usually distinguish between a benign and a malignant bone tumor.

**How is a positive distinction made between a benign and a malignant bone tumor?**
Only by surgical removal of the tumor, or piece of the tumor, and examination under the microscope.

**What is the treatment for chondromas, osteomas, or other benign bone tumors?**
An incision is made over the region of the tumor, and the diseased bone is removed with hammer and chisel. If there is a resultant defect in the bone, a bone graft is inserted.

**Are operations for the removal of benign tumors serious?**
No. Recovery takes place without incident in almost all cases.

**What is the treatment for malignant tumors of the bone?**
After the diagnosis has been established positively by microscopic examination of the bone, it is often necessary to amputate the limb in order to save life. Amputation is followed in most cases by radiation therapy and treatment with anticancer chemicals and radioactive substances.

**Are there any forms of treatment, other than amputation, for malignant tumors of the bone?**

Yes, certain bone tumors respond well to radiation therapy; others can be destroyed by using cryosurgery (intense cold); still others can be destroyed by use of the laser beam (intense heat); and finally, some bone growths can be inhibited by use of radioactive medications and chemotherapy.

**Are malignant tumors of the bone always fatal?**

No. More and more people so afflicted are being saved all the time.

**When are malignant tumors of the bone most likely to occur?**

For some unknown reason, malignant bone tumors are much more common in children and young adults than they are in later life.

## SEGMENTAL RESECTION OF BONE

**What is segmental bone resection?**

It is the surgical removal of a portion of a bone, leaving the other tissues, such as muscles, nerves, and blood vessels, in place.

**What is used to replace the bone that has been removed?**

a. A piece of bone taken from some other part of the body.
b. A metal device shaped like the bone that has been excised.

**What are some common indications for segmental bone resection?**

a. Nonmalignant bone tumors or cysts that have caused extensive bone destruction.
b. Malignant bone tumors, particularly those that tend to be limited and will not recur when once removed.

**How successful is segmental bone resection with reconstruction by a bone graft or insertion of a replacement device?**

Results are constantly improving, and, in many instances, the patient can regain near-normal use of his limb. Of course, results are best when the bone resection has been carried out for a noncancerous condition.

# CHAPTER 15
# THE BREASTS

*(See also Chapter 3 on Adolescence; Chapter 16 on Cancer; Chapter 25 on Female Organs; Chapter 33 on Infant Feeding; Chapter 56 on Plastic Surgery; Chapter 57 on Pregnancy and Childbirth)*

**Are the two breasts always the same size?**

No. In many women one breast is slightly larger than the other.

**Is there a tendency for girls to develop the same kind of breasts as their mothers?**

Yes, the size and shape of the breasts tend to follow a familial pattern.

**Can small breasts be made larger?**

In most adolescents, underdeveloped breasts may be associated with slow development of the rest of the body and low production of female sex hormones. If this is the case, the breasts will enlarge spontaneously as the child matures. Within recent years, good results have been obtained by inserting a Silastic bag containing either saline or silicone gel beneath the breast to give it the appearance of being larger. This operative procedure is most successful when performed by plastic surgeons who have wide experience in the field of breast surgery.

**Are there any exercises that will prevent the breasts from sagging?**

No. This is a body characteristic not affected by exercise.

**What can be done to maintain the youthful contour of breasts?**

Wearing a good uplift brassiere is the best safeguard. Also, avoid marked fluctuations in weight, which tend to weaken the ligaments supporting the breasts.

**Does pregnancy alter the shape of one's breasts?**

Yes, but it does not necessarily lead to disfigurement. Many women discover that their breasts are improved by pregnancy and nursing.

**Should medications be given to ensure the ability of the breasts to produce milk after childbirth?**

This is actually not necessary, as only a small percentage of women will be unable to produce sufficient milk.

**Can the breasts be dried up when a mother wishes to stop nursing?**

Yes. There are several efficient drugs that will cause the breasts to stop secreting.

**Can breast contour be preserved as one enters the forties and fifties?**

Much can be done to maintain a youthful figure. Avoidance of overweight and the wearing of a proper breast support will help greatly.

**Are metal supports in brassieres harmful to the breasts?**

Not really, unless they press too strongly on one portion of the breast.

**Does nursing play a part in the subsequent development of breast tumors or breast cancer?**

There is no conclusive proof that nursing or failure to nurse plays a role in the subsequent development of breast tumors or cancer.

**What are inverted nipples?**

Nipples that are folded in upon themselves instead of protruding out from the surface of the body.

**Can inverted nipples be cured?**

If they are treated from earliest

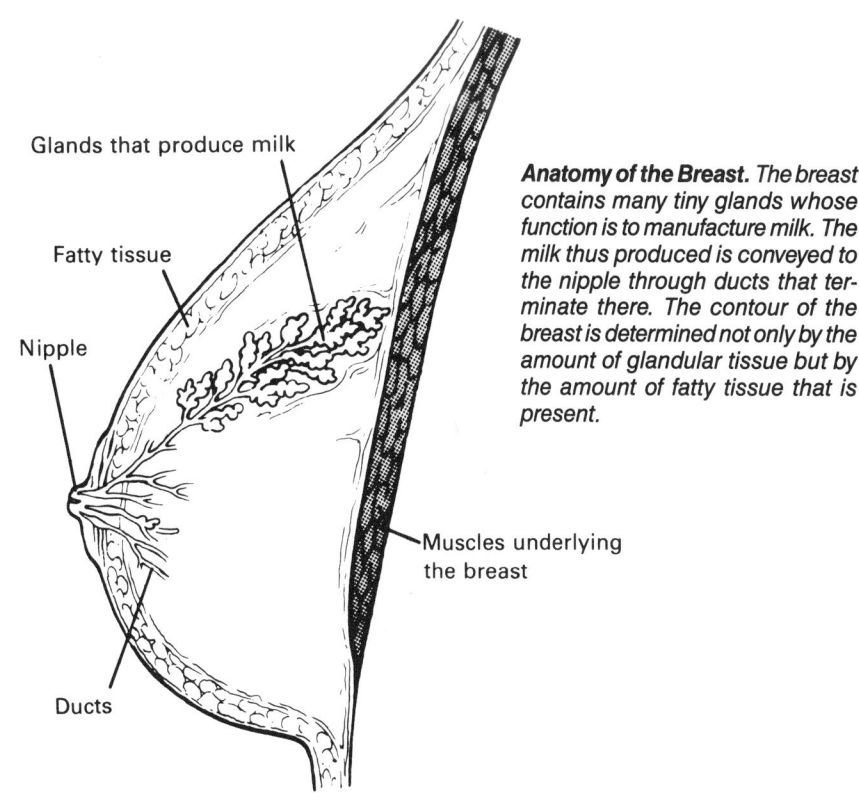

Glands that produce milk

Fatty tissue

Nipple

Ducts

Muscles underlying the breast

*Anatomy of the Breast. The breast contains many tiny glands whose function is to manufacture milk. The milk thus produced is conveyed to the nipple through ducts that terminate there. The contour of the breast is determined not only by the amount of glandular tissue but by the amount of fatty tissue that is present.*

youth, it is possible to prevent a certain amount of inversion. This involves daily treatment by everting and massaging them. It is important to do this during pregnancy if nursing is to be attempted.

### Can an injury to the breast produce a cancer?

No! This is a common misconception.

### Does breast size have anything to do with the development of breast tumors?

No. Tumors are just as common in large breasts as they are in small.

### Is it normal for breasts to become somewhat enlarged and tender just prior to a menstrual period?

Yes, in many women tenderness and engorgement of the breasts take place for a few days before a period and subside on the first or second day of the period.

### Can anything be given to decrease the sensitivity and engorgement of the breasts just prior to menstruation?

In the small number of patients in whom the sensitivity and tenderness is extreme, this condition can be relieved somewhat by restricting salt and fluid intake for the few days before menstruation and by giving large doses of Vitamin B complex. In the rare case, hormone therapy may be indicated.

### What is the significance of breast sensitivity and enlargement before a menstrual period?

This is a normal cyclic phenomenon related to hormone secretions.

### Is it safe to have hair removed from the breasts and nipples by electrolysis?

Yes. Electrolysis will often remove hair efficiently and with no ill effects.

### Is it common for the breasts to be injured by manipulation?

No.

### How often should a woman have her breasts examined?

Every woman should have her breasts examined at least once a year, or if she should feel something unusual or develop pain in a breast, she should seek medical attention at that time.

### Is self-examination of the breasts satisfactory?

Yes, but it should not be done as a substitute for periodic examination by a physician.

## SELF-EXAMINATION

### How is self-examination of the breasts carried out?

1. Lie flat in bed face up. Place a small pillow or large telephone directory under the right shoulder and back of your chest. This prevents the breast from sagging to the side of the body, thus permitting a more satisfactory examination.
2. Place your right arm on top of your head.
3. Place the fingers of your left hand together in a straight position and gently draw the flat portion of the fingers, not the tips, over the inner half of the breast, starting at the top and working down toward the bottom of the breast. It is easier to feel a lump if fingers are moistened with a little mineral or baby oil, or soap. This allows the fingers to glide smoothly over the breast.
4. Lower your right arm and place it at your side.
5. Again, take the flat portion of the fingers of your left hand and glide them over the outer half of the breast toward the nipple. Start this at the top of the breast and work down toward the bottom of the breast.
6. Repeat the above maneuvers, in

reverse, for examination of the left breast.
7. Milk each nipple gently but firmly to note any discharge. Normally there is no discharge.
8. After completing the above, stand in front of a mirror in a good light and inspect your breasts. Look particularly for the following abnormalities:
a. A sore or ulceration of the nipple.
b. A change in the size of a breast.
c. A change in the level of one of the nipples.
d. A change in the appearance of the skin overlying the breast, especially a dimpling or indentation in its contours.
e. The presence of a lump or a protrusion of any part of the breast.

## BREAST INFECTIONS

### Are breast infections common?

Yes, particularly in nursing mothers or women who have recently gone through pregnancy.

### Should nursing be discontinued from a breast that is inflamed or might be developing an abscess?

In some cases, yes; in other cases, nursing can continue without harming the child or mother.

### What is the treatment for breast abscess?

a. Apply warm compresses to the inflamed area.
b. See your physician, who will probably prescribe large doses of an antibiotic medication.
c. Incision and drainage of the breast if and when the abscess localizes.
d. Discontinue nursing if it becomes too painful to the mother or if the breast requires surgery.

### Is it necessary to go to the hospital to have a breast abscess drained?

Not for small abscesses. Large ones

must be opened under general anesthesia in the hospital.

**How long a hospital stay is usually necessary for a breast abscess?**

From two to three days.

**Can nursing be resumed after drainage of a breast abscess?**

It can continue in the opposite breast, but it is usually necessary to discontinue nursing in the infected breast.

**Are the breasts ever involved in infections not related to nursing or pregnancy?**

Yes. Occasionally, breast abscesses will form spontaneously in women who have not been pregnant. Such infections are treated in the manner outlined above. Rarely, a breast becomes involved in an infection caused by tuberculosis or syphilis. Such conditions are almost always secondary to tuberculosis or syphilis elsewhere in the body, and treatment is not limited to the local breast involvement.

## BREAST TUMORS AND CYSTS

**What are the most common growths found within the breasts?**

a. Cysts. These occur most often in women between the ages of thirty-five and forty-five. They appear as single small, rounded masses no larger than a pea, or they may grow to the size of a lemon or orange. Cysts tend to be multiple.

b. Adenomas, fibroadenomas, or cystadenomas. These are seen frequently as nontender, nonpainful lumps in young women between the ages of eighteen and thirty-five. They too can be as small as a pea or grow to the size of an orange.

c. Milk cysts (galactocele). These cysts are caused by blockage of a milk duct in women who have had children.

d. Intraductal papillomas. These tumors are warty growths within a breast duct and are first recognized because of a yellowish, greenish, or bloody discharge from the nipple. They may be so small that they cannot be felt by the examining physician. They tend to occur most frequently in women in their thirties or forties.

e. Fat necrosis and hematoma. These conditions are the result of an injury to the breast, such as a direct blow. They lead either to destruction of some fat tissue within the breast or to the collection of a blood clot as the result of hemorrhage from a blood vessel within the breast. The lump caused by fat necrosis can occasionally resemble the lump produced by breast cancer.

f. Cancer. These lesions first evidence themselves as small, painless, hard lumps, which can occur anywhere in the breast substance. Women in their forties and fifties are most prone to develop breast cancer, although the disease is also seen in young women in their twenties and thirties and in older women in their sixties and seventies.

## THE MALE BREAST

**Does the male breast ever become involved in disease?**

Yes, but not as frequently as the female breast.

**What are the commonest conditions found in the male breast?**

a. Adolescent nodule. This takes the form of a firm, round, tender swelling under the nipple of boys between the ages of eleven and seventeen. It requires no treatment and disappears spontaneously within a few months.

b. Gynecomastia. This is a peculiar condition wherein the breasts enlarge and take on the characteristics of a female breast. Studies of such men rarely reveal any other glandular abnormality. It requires no treatment unless the patient is psychologically disturbed by the condition. In such an event, the breast tissue is removed surgically. Gynecomastia is seen quite frequently in older men who are on medication for high blood pressure or heart disease.

c. Adenomatous disease. In men in their fifties, sixties, or older, the breasts sometimes undergo diffuse enlargement. It is best to remove such breast tissue to make certain it is not malignant.

d. Cancer. Cancer of the male breast is rare, but it does occur. It is treated in the same manner as cancer in the female breast.

## SURGERY OF THE BREASTS

**Should all localized lumps within the breast be operated upon?**

Yes, the safest procedure is to remove every localized lump from every breast. In this way many early malignancies will be discovered at the earliest possible time. In some cases in which a solitary cyst is present, needling of the cyst may be done instead of surgery.

**Is there an exception to the above rule?**

Yes. In cases of chronic cystic mastitis, where one has "lumpy" breasts containing innumerable areas of lumpy masses, surgery is not always advocated. However, this condition must be followed carefully, with frequent examinations of the patient.

**Can a surgeon tell before operation whether a lump is cancerous?**

In the great majority of cases he will

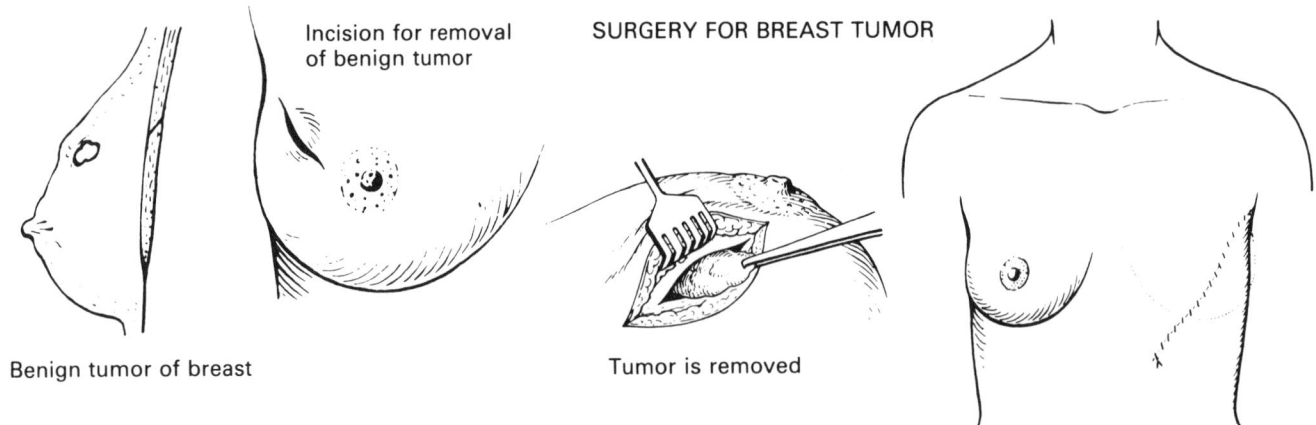

Incision for removal of benign tumor

SURGERY FOR BREAST TUMOR

Benign tumor of breast

Tumor is removed

Appearance of incision after breast removal for malignant tumor

*Breast Tumors. The accompanying diagrams show a benign tumor of the breast; the type of incision made for removal of a benign tumor; and the appearance of the scar after a breast has been removed for a malignant tumor. The breast is rarely removed for a benign tumor. The incision for breast removal is made in such a manner that the scar is not visible even when the patient wears a bathing suit or evening gown.*

be able to do so. However, because there is always a margin of error, surgical removal of the tumor is advocated so that microscopic diagnosis can be made.

**Can the presence of a breast tumor ever be detected before a lump appears?**

Yes; in some cases the presence of a lump can be diagnosed by x raying the breast. This procedure is known as mammography.

**If a breast x ray fails to show a tumor, is this a guarantee that none exists?**

No. A mammogram is only of value when it does show a tumor. A negative mammogram is *not* proof that the breast is free from tumor. Ten percent of breast cancers will not show on mammography.

**Are mammograms safe?**

Yes, but they should be taken only under specified circumstances, as when a woman has a family history of breast cancer, when she herself has had a previous breast tumor or cancer, etc. Modern techniques have reduced the amount of radiation greatly.

**Should mammograms be taken routinely every year?**

No. However, even if a woman did undergo a yearly mammogram for ten consecutive years, it would only increase her chances of getting a breast cancer from 8 to 9 percent.

**How soon after a lump has been discovered should surgery be performed?**

Within a period of two to three weeks, no longer.

**What is the usual type of surgery for a lump in the breast?**

An incision between one and two inches long is made over the lump, and the entire lump is removed. The lump is then submitted to microscopic examination to determine whether or not removal of the entire breast is necessary.

**What is meant by a biopsy?**

The removal of the isolated lump.

**What is meant by a frozen section examination?**

The lump is submitted to immediate microscopic examination while the patient is still under anesthesia. This is carried out by a special technique of preparing the tissue by freezing it before cutting and staining it.

**How accurate is microscopic examination in determining whether or not a lump is cancerous?**

It will give positive information in almost 100 percent of cases.

**Are operations upon the breast disfiguring?**

Not if a small incision is made to remove the localized tumor. If an entire breast is removed, there is a long scar across the chest, and the natural contour is altered. Incisions are made, however, so that a patient can wear an evening gown or bathing suit without any of the scar showing.

**What kind of anesthesia is used in performing breast operations?**

General inhalation anesthesia, often induced by intravenous Pentothal or a related drug.

**Are breast operations painful?**

Not particularly, although there is considerable discomfort for a few days following breast removal.

**Is there any way to avoid getting a breast tumor?**

No. However, early detection of

breast tumors by periodic examination will often prevent a breast tumor from reaching an incurable stage.

### What is the recognized treatment for a cancer of the breast?

Removal of the breast with or without its underlying muscles and the lymph glands that drain it. Some surgeons advocate a lesser procedure in which only the breast is removed, leaving the glands intact.

### What is a mastectomy?

The removal of a breast.

### Are special private nurses required after a mastectomy?

They are not absolutely necessary, but their presence for a few days can give great comfort.

### Is it common for there to be swelling of the arm after mastectomy?

Yes. This may be a permanent complication but is usually not disabling.

### Does the patient have full use of her arm after radical mastectomy?

Yes. Despite swelling, a full range of use is present.

### Is it common for the wound to drain following mastectomy?

Yes, the wound will drain for several days, or longer, after mastectomy.

### Is there any satisfactory treatment to reduce the swelling of the arm after mastectomy?

Elevating or bandaging the arm may reduce swelling temporarily.

### Are blood transfusions given during the performance of breast operations?

Not for the minor procedures, such as the removal of the lump. But when the breast is removed, blood transfusions are sometimes given.

### Can a woman hide the fact that her breast has been removed?

Yes. There are brassieres made to-day that can simulate accurately the appearance of the woman's breast.

### If a cancer of the breast has been found, will the surgeon tell the patient?

Most surgeons tell the patient the truth.

### Are x-ray or cobalt treatments advised after the removal of a breast?

If the tumor was found to involve the lymph glands in the armpit, x ray or cobalt treatments are often advised. If these glands are not cancerous, x ray and cobalt are not given. Some surgeons recommend chemotherapy for their patients who have undergone breast removal for cancer.

### What are the chances for a complete cure if a cancer of the breast has been found?

Approximately four out of five women with cancer of the breast can be saved if the operation is done before the cancer has spread to the glands under the arm.

### Are operations for removal of a breast dangerous?

No. Operative recovery takes place in almost all instances.

### How soon after breast operations can the patient get out of bed?

Usually the very next day.

### Do benign (noncancerous) lumps, if not removed, turn into cancer?

Most do not. Noncancerous lumps should be removed because it is not always possible to tell positively before surgery whether the lump is actually benign or malignant.

### Should a woman allow herself to become pregnant after the removal of a lump in the breast?

If the lump was a benign one, it is perfectly all right for her to become pregnant. If it was a cancer, it is advisable for her not to become pregnant again.

### Can people who have had breasts removed return to normal living?

Yes. This operation should in no way alter their activities.

### Is chemotherapy helpful in reducing the incidence of recurrence after surgery for breast cancer?

Yes, recurrence rates have been reduced markedly by its use.

### How long must chemotherapy be continued after breast removal?

Anywhere from one to three years.

### How often should patients return for follow-up examination after breast surgery?

Twice a year.

### Do tumors of the breast or cancer of the breast tend to be inherited or run in families?

There is no proof that tumors of the breast are inherited. Certain families, however, do have a tendency toward greater tumor formation.

### Is it permissible to have a breast operation during a menstrual period?

Yes.

## PLASTIC SURGERY OF THE BREASTS

### What are the indications for plastic surgery upon the breasts?

a. Marked enlargement or under-development.
b. Marked sagging (pendulous breasts).
c. Marked psychological disturbances caused by the feeling that one's breasts are ugly and that they interfere with one's happiness.
d. Breast reconstruction following mastectomy.

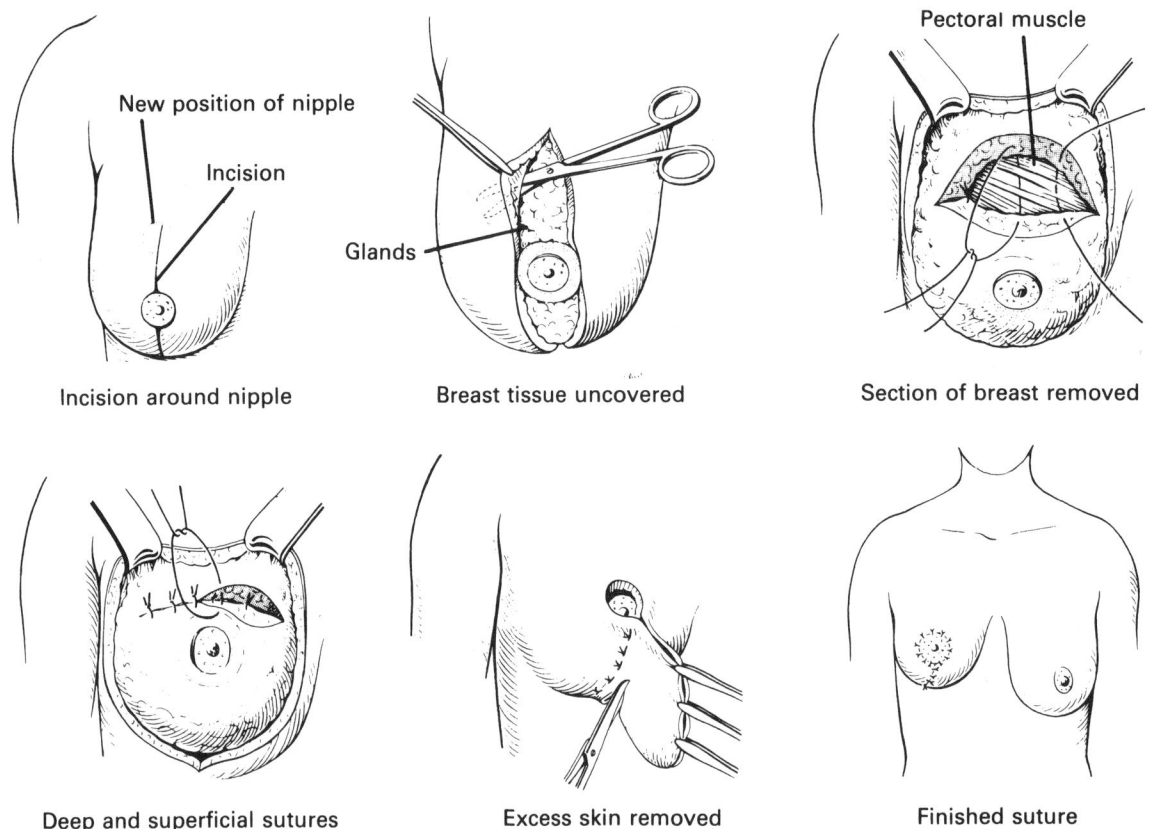

Incision around nipple

Breast tissue uncovered

Section of breast removed

Deep and superficial sutures

Excess skin removed

Finished suture

**Plastic Surgery for Pendulous Breast.** *This diagram shows an operation for making the breast smaller and reshaping it so that the nipple is in normal position. Such operations, while extensive and serious, can be carried out successfully when done by specially trained surgeons.*

**Can plastic operations be performed to make the breasts appear larger?**

Yes. A sac composed of a plastic material can be placed beneath the tissues of the breast. This sac is then filled either with a salt solution or a silicone gel. The sac may be inserted either through an incision made below the breast or around the nipple.

**Can a breast be reconstructed after mastectomy for cancer?**

Yes, in certain cases. A lapse of a year or more should usually exist between mastectomy and breast reconstruction.

**Do plastic operations interfere with breast sensation?**

No, but a breast reconstructed after mastectomy will not experience erotic sensations.

**Can a woman become pregnant after she has had a plastic operation upon her breasts?**

Yes.

**Is it possible to nurse a child successfully after breast plastic operations?**

Not usually.

**Are breast plastic operations successful?**

Yes, plastic surgery today can do much to beautify breast contour.

**Are plastic operations upon the breast serious?**

Yes. These operations should not be embarked upon lightly; they are major surgical procedures, to be performed only by experts in the field.

**When is the best time to undergo plastic surgery upon the breasts?**

The ideal time would be after a woman has finished childbearing. However, many young women wish to have breast plastic surgery performed. This is feasible as soon as maturity has been reached.

**What kind of anesthesia is used for these operations?**

General anesthesia.

**How long does it take to perform breastplasty operations?**

Anywhere from two to four hours.

**How long a hospital stay is necessary?**

From five to eight days.

**How can breasts, once removed, be reconstructed?**

a. If the major pectoral muscle has been left in place during a mastectomy operation, an implant is placed beneath it. This will produce a mound on the chest wall giving it the appearance of a breast.

b. If the pectoral muscle has been removed along with the breast, a flap of skin and muscle from the back of the chest or from the flank is brought onto the chest wall. This is done in a series of procedures using the principle of a pedicle graft. (See Chapter 56, on Plastic Surgery.)

**Can a new nipple ever be reconstructed?**

Yes, in some cases a rim of tissue around the opposite nipple is removed and is used as a free graft on the newly reconstructed breast. (See Chapter 56, on Plastic Surgery.)

**Do reconstructed breasts look normal?**

No, but they can give the outward appearance of a real breast.

**Are breast plastic operations always successful?**

Not always. A certain amount of asymmetry may result.

**Will breasts, once submitted to plastic surgery, retain their shape?**

Yes. Results usually are permanent.

**Are the scars following breast plastic surgery ugly or disfiguring?**

No. Most scars are placed beneath the breasts and appear only as thin white lines.

**Is it necessary to wear a special type of brassiere after plastic surgery upon the breasts?**

No.

**Can bathing suits or evening gowns be worn after breastplasty operations?**

Yes. No scars will be visible.

**How soon after surgery upon the breast can one do the following?**

Bathe:
Ten days.

Walk out in the street:
As soon as one leaves the hospital.

Walk up and down stairs:
As soon as one leaves the hospital.

Perform household duties:
Three to four weeks.

Drive a car:
Four weeks.

Resume sexual relations:
Four weeks.

Return to work:
Four to six weeks.

CHAPTER 16

# CANCER AND OTHER MALIGNANT GROWTHS

*(See also chapters dealing with specific organs)*

## What is cancer?

It is a disorderly wild growth of tissue cells. If the process continues unchecked, the normal structure and function of an organ are destroyed. Cancer cells may be likened to weeds in a well-kept garden, which get out of control and outgrow and kill the flowers. Eventually, if the weeds are not eradicated, the entire garden will be destroyed.

## Are there any organs that are exempt from cancer?

No. Any organ may be affected by cancer or a cancerlike growth.

## How prevalent is cancer today?

It is estimated that *one in four people* will at some time in their lives develop a cancer, and that *one in seven people* will lose his or her life as a result of cancer.

## Is cancer contagious?

No, but some investigators think that certain cancers are associated with virus invasion and therefore might conceivably be transmissible.

## Is there a tendency for cancer to occur more often in men than in women?

No. The incidence is approximately the same. However, certain types of cancer show up more often in one sex. For instance, lung cancer is more prevalent among men; breast cancer among women.

## How often does a noncancerous (benign) tumor turn into a cancer?

It is not possible to cite the precise number of cases, but this phenomenon takes place often enough to convince physicians that early treatment for all tumors is essential. Many lives are saved by the removal of benign tumors, which, if left alone, might have turned into cancer.

## Is cancer on the increase?

In all probability, cancer *is* on the increase. However, a good part of this increase can be explained by the fact that people live longer these days. Thus they live into the later decades when cancer is much more prevalent. Also, increased pollution of air and water and greater contacts with dangerous carcinogens may explain the increased incidence of cancer.

## Are there any age groups that are more prone to develop cancer?

Yes. Cancer occurs more frequently in the latter half of the life span.

## Are there any age groups that are less likely to develop cancer?

Young children, adolescents, and young adults, though they possess no immunity, develop cancer less often than older people.

## Is there a special type of person who is most likely to develop cancer?

No, but some investigators feel that stout people are somewhat more susceptible than thin people.

## Is there a type of person who has less chance of developing cancer?

No. However, the person who submits to thorough health examinations at regular intervals is better protected, since the presence of cancer may be detected at an earlier and more curable stage of its development.

## Does cancer tend to run in families or to be inherited?

Cancer is *not* inherited, but many physicians feel that a *tendency* toward cancer may be inherited.

## Should the history of cancer in a family cause one to hesitate to marry into that family?

No. There are practically no families in which some history of cancer cannot be found.

## Are certain races more likely or less likely to develop cancer?

No race is known to have any special immunity toward all forms of cancer.

## Are there certain ethnic groups that are more likely or less likely to develop cancer?

No, but certain peoples have habits peculiar to their own way of life that may predispose them to the more frequent development of certain types of cancer. Thus, in cultures where people smoke heavily, there may be a greater incidence of lung cancer than exists among peoples who use no tobacco.

## Does climate or the place in which one lives influence the incidence of cancer?

Cancer exists throughout the world. However, cancer is influenced by environmental factors. People who live in areas of least pollution may have a lower overall incidence of certain types of cancer.

## What causes cancer?

Cancer is not one but many diseases. The cause of certain cancers, such as cancer of the skin of the hands, found among those who work unprotected with petroleum products, is well known. Other cancers are thought to arise from other chronic irritants, such as tobacco. Some cancers are attributed to nests of primitive cells present since birth, which, suddenly in later life, undergo stimulation and grow wild. Now many investigators believe viruses are associated with the cause of many types of cancer.

**Does smoking have anything to do with the incidence of lung cancer?**

Yes. Lung cancer is much more common among smokers than among those who have never used tobacco.

**Does moderate drinking of alcoholic beverages have anything to do with cancer development?**

Not usually. However, alcoholics are more prone to develop certain types of cancer, especially cancer of the liver.

**How many different types of cancer are there?**

More than a hundred.

**Is there much variation in the virulence of cancer?**

Yes. Some cancers are extremely slow growing and will never destroy the host; others (like certain of the blood conditions, such as acute leukemia) may destroy the host within a few weeks.

**Is cancer caused by a blow or other physical injury?**

Practically never. This is a very common misconception.

**What actually takes place when an organ undergoes cancerous degeneration?**

The cancer cells outgrow the normal cells within the organ. They often use up most of the available nourish-

## 1988 ESTIMATED CANCER INCIDENCE BY SITE AND SEX†

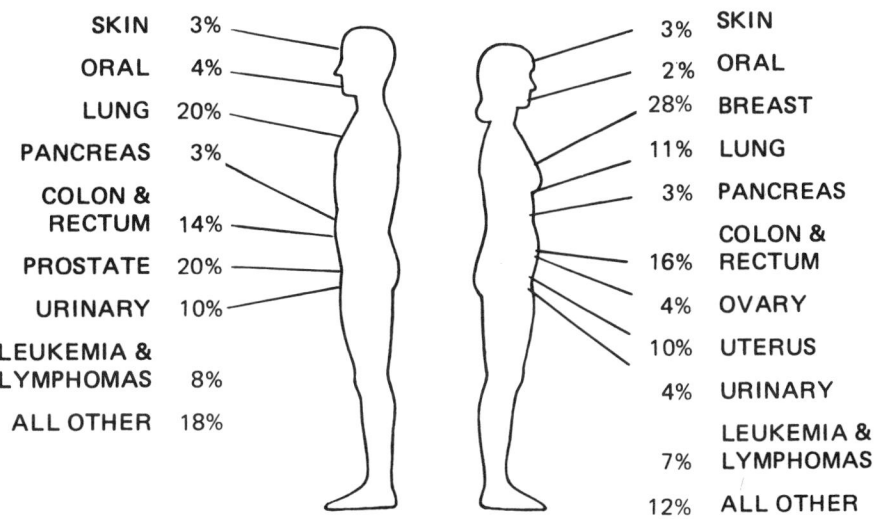

†Excluding nonmelanoma skin cancer and carcinoma in situ.

## 1988 ESTIMATED CANCER DEATHS BY SITE AND SEX

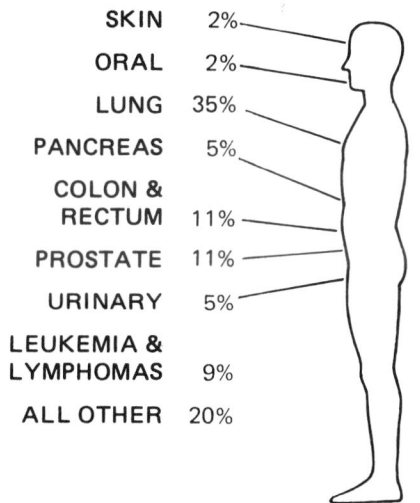
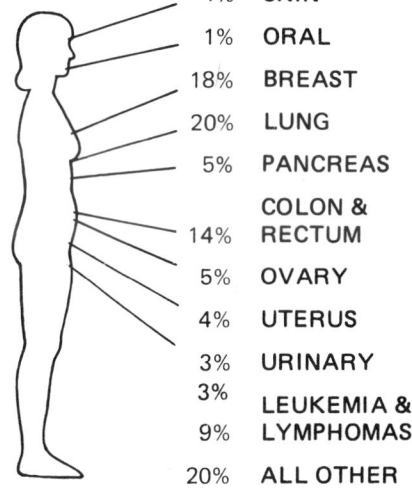

ment and oxygen meant for the normal tissues, thus causing the normal tissues to starve and die.

**How does cancer spread?**

There are three main routes:

a. By direct growth and extension to surrounding structures.
b. By spread through the lymph channels to distant organs.
c. By spread through the bloodstream to distant organs.

*Cancer Statistics, 1988. The estimates of the incidence of cancer are based on data from the National Cancer Institute's Surveillance, Epidemiology and End Results (SEER) program (1982–1984). Nonmelanoma skin cancer and carcinoma in situ have not been included in the statistics. The incidence of nonmelanoma skin cancer is estimated to be more than 500,000. Prepared by Edwin Silverberg, Supervisor, Statistical Information Services, and John A. Lubera, Statistical Information Technician, Department of Epidemiology and Statistics, American Cancer Society, New York, New York.*

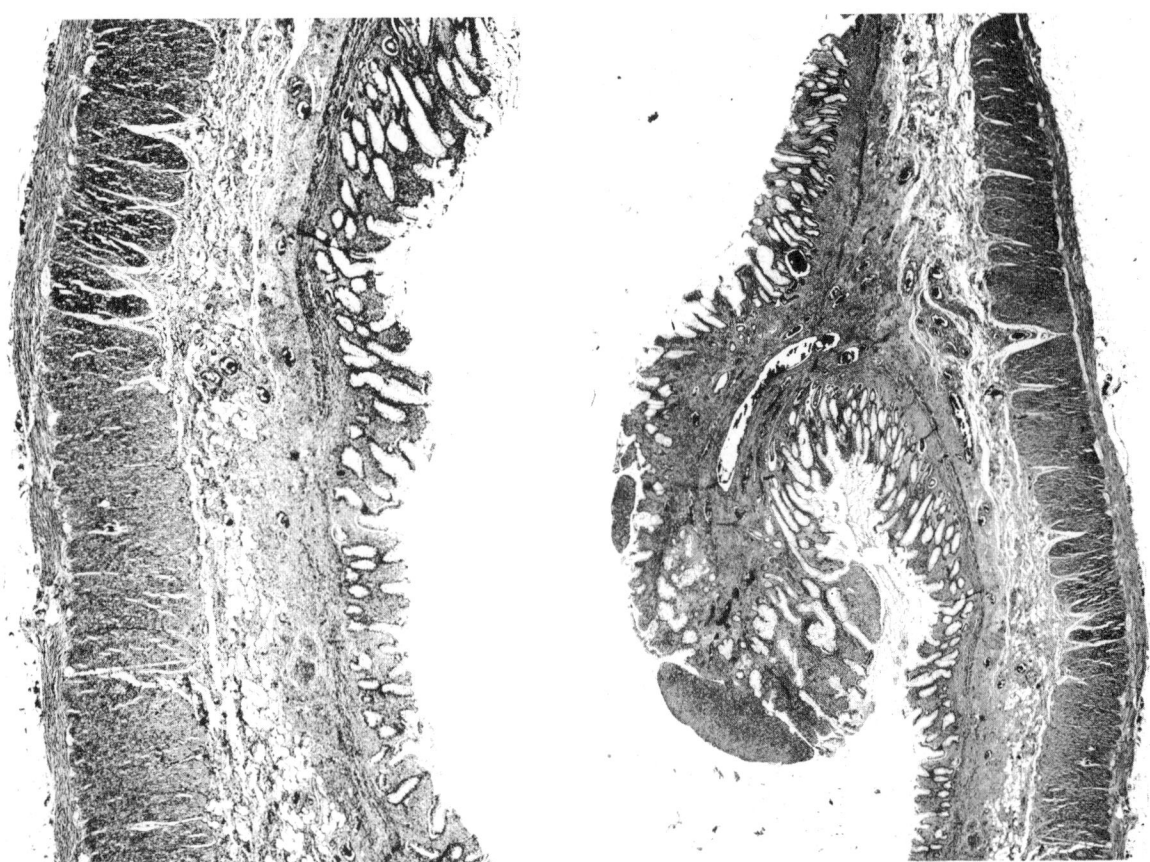

*Left:*
**Photomicrograph of a Section of Normal Bowel Wall.** *It should be noted that the mucous membrane is smooth, and that beneath it there is a normal construction of muscle and other tissues.*

*Right:*
**Photomicrographic Section Showing a Benign Polyp Protruding from the Bowel Wall.** *Here the mucous membrane is not smooth and straight, but it is protruding in one area, thus forming a polyp (a wartlike growth).*

*Below:*
**Photomicrograph Showing Early Cancerous Changes within a Polyp in a Bowel Wall.** *The few dark spots and the irregularly shaped cells within the polyp are evidence of early cancer.*

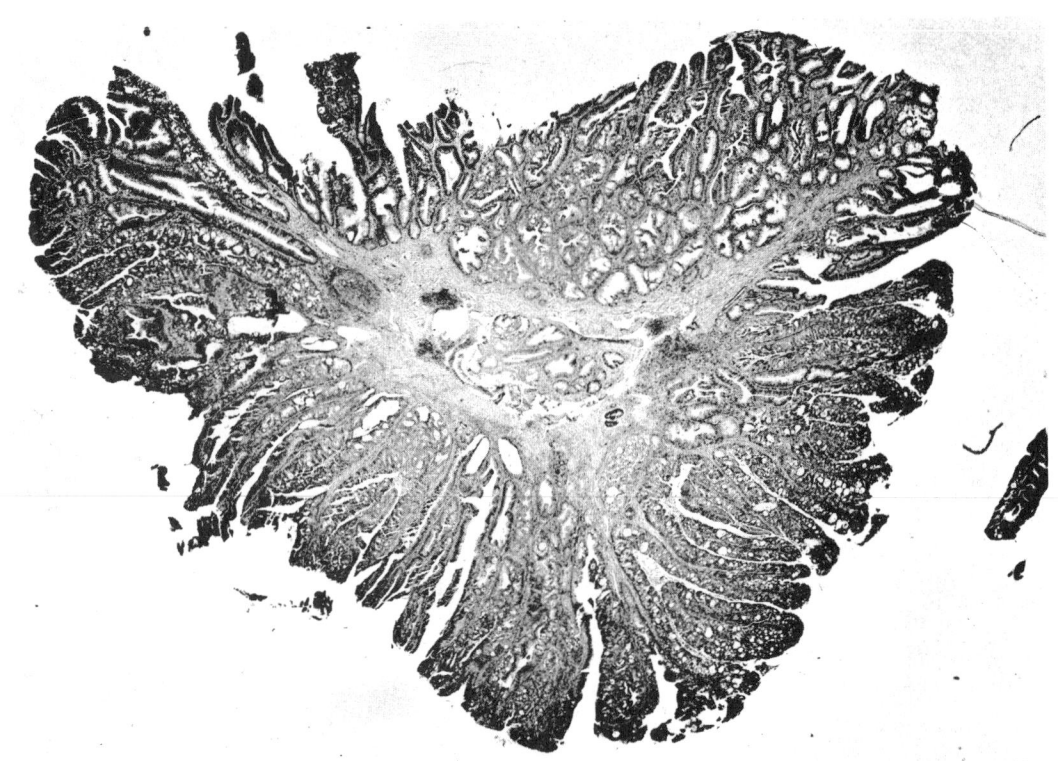

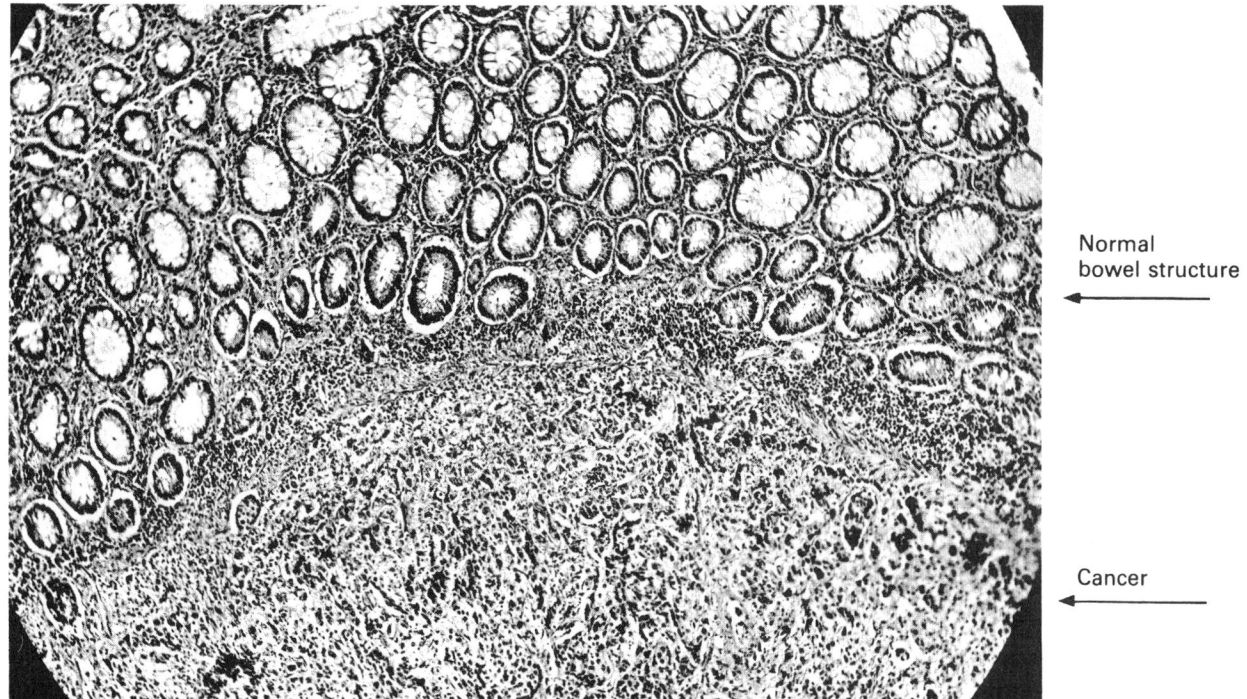

Normal
bowel structure ←———

Cancer ←———

*Photomicrograph Showing an Advanced Cancer of the Bowel Wall. The cancer has invaded the muscle structure and other layers of the bowel wall; note the difference between the appearance of these cells shown in the photomicrograph of the normal bowel wall.*

### What causes cancer to spread from one part of the body to another?

Cancer cells break loose from their site of origin and get into the lymph channels or blood vessels.

### Is there any way to prevent the spread of cancer from one part of the body to another?

Yes. By removal of the primary tumor when it is in an early stage of development.

### How can one tell if a cancer has already spread from its organ of origin?

A wide surgical removal of the primary tumor with surrounding normal tissue will often reveal, under microscopic examination, whether the cancer has already spread; that is, microscopic examination may spot cancer cells that have broken loose and become lodged in adjacent tissues. X rays such as bone scans and CAT scans (Computerized Axial Tomography) may show the cancer has spread.

### Is there any way to prevent cancer?

The best method is to have a complete physical examination once or twice a year. Also, report any unusual symptoms to your doctor at any time between regular examinations. The finding of a lump anywhere in the body or the occurrence of unexpected bleeding from any orifice in the body, while not necessarily indicative of cancer, should nevertheless stimulate a visit to your doctor.

### Is cancer on the increase among children?

No, but improved methods of cancer diagnoses may make it appear so.

### Are cancer detection examinations worthwhile?

Yes, but they should not be used as a substitute for a good general health examination.

### How can one tell if he has a hidden cancer?

Cancer does not often cause symp-

toms until it has existed for quite some time. This is another reason an annual or semiannual checkup is advisable.

### Are there any satisfactory blood tests to determine if one has cancer?

Not at present, but indications are that such tests will soon be a reality.

### Will cancer always show on x-ray examination?

No.

### Can a surgeon always tell whether a tumor is cancerous when he removes it?

No. It is frequently necessary to await the pathological, microscopic report.

**What tests are made to establish a positive diagnosis of cancer?**

The suspected tissue is taken and is subjected to microscopic examination. This procedure is known as a biopsy.

**How long may it take to get the microscopic report?**

Anywhere from fifteen to twenty minutes, in a frozen section examination, to one week for a more detailed report.

**Does an immediate frozen section microscopic examination in the operating room always give a conclusive diagnosis?**

No. It is often necessary to carry out further studies, which may take a few days.

**What is a biopsy?**

The microscopic examination of a tumor or piece of tumor tissue.

**Is the microscopic report accurate and reliable?**

Yes, in all but rare instances.

**Can cancer be diagnosed early by use of the CAT scan?**

Yes, this new x-ray technique, popularly called a CAT scan, of scanning the body can often pick up cancers deep within the body when they are in very early stages.

**Will cancer always end fatally if not treated?**

No. There are cases, by far the minority, where the cancer grows so slowly that the patient lives out his normal life span and dies of an unrelated condition. This is particularly true among old people.

**What are the chances for recovery in a patient with cancer?**

Certain types of cancer, such as skin cancers, are almost 100 percent curable. Other forms vary according to location and the stage at which they are first discovered and treated.

With early diagnosis, more than half the people with cancer can be saved.

**Must all cancer be treated surgically?**

No. There are several forms of this disease that are best treated with various medications or by x-ray therapy.

**Why is it that surgery is advocated for some patients with cancer while chemotherapy and x-ray treatment are advocated for other patients with cancer?**

Surgery, chemical therapy, and x ray are valuable forms of treatment, but certain cancers respond better to one type than to the other. A combination of the three often gives the best chance for recovery.

**How can one tell if he or she is cured of a cancer after its removal?**

The passage of time is the best evidence. Relatively few cancers recur after a ten-year lapse.

**Do cancer patients recuperate as easily as those who have had surgery performed for other conditions?**

No, but with modern surgical methods, the differences have been so minimized that cancer patients do almost as well after surgery.

**Can people recover from cancer if it has already spread beyond the point of origin?**

Yes, although the chances for recovery are markedly lessened. X-ray or cobalt treatments, radioactive isotopes, chemicals, or hormones may destroy those cells that have gotten beyond the original cancer site.

**Do cancer patients show weight loss early in the course of their disease?**

Not usually, but there are some types of the disease that do cause marked weight loss rather early.

**Do cancer patients usually show anemia early in the course of their disease?**

No, unless marked bleeding has been associated with the tumor.

**Do cancer patients often show loss of appetite early in the course of their disease?**

No, unless the tumor is in the stomach or esophagus.

**Does the size of a cancer have much to do with its degree of malignancy?**

Not necessarily. Many large cancers may have a low degree of malignancy, and many small cancers spread early, widely, and rapidly.

**Is it likely that a time will come when there will be *one* cure for all cancer?**

This is doubtful, since cancer is so many different diseases. Even now we have cures for some forms of cancer!

**Should a patient be told if he has a cancer?**

People have a right to know what is wrong with them *when they want to know*. If the patient would rather not know, then he should *not* be informed.

**What prevents the surgeon from removing a cancer completely?**

Surgeons always strive for complete removal, but sometimes the tumor has extended into vital organs that cannot be removed. Other times, the cancer has spread so extensively that it has gone beyond the help of surgery.

**Can a surgeon always tell if he has removed a cancer completely?**

No; a surgeon cannot operate microscopically, and a few cells may have spread beyond the reach of his scalpel. He will not, unfortunately, always be able to know this.

**Is there a tendency for cancer to recur after it has been removed?**

Yes, but periodic examinations may spot such a recurrence at a stage when it can be controlled or eradicated.

**How does one minimize the chances of recurrence of cancer?**

a. Wide, primary removal of the tumor.
b. Postoperative treatment with appropriate methods such as x ray, radioactive substances, chemotherapy, or hormones.

**Does diet have anything to do with the recurrence of cancer?**

No.

**If a patient has recovered from a cancer, can he return to a normal life?**

This depends upon the location of the cancer and the form of treatment that was administered. The great majority of those who have recovered from cancer *do* return to normal, or near-normal, activity.

**Is there a tendency for a patient who has had one cancer to develop another elsewhere in the body?**

Yes, but this situation can be handled satisfactorily by frequent, thorough medical surveys.

**Can pregnancy have a harmful effect upon a woman who has recovered from a cancer?**

Yes. It may sometimes reactivate the growth of tumors in certain organs that are influenced by the hormones of the body.

**After the successful treatment of a cancer, how often should one return to his doctor for follow-up examinations?**

This will vary according to the type of cancer. However, a semiannual visit is advisable and more frequent visits are preferable.

**What advances in the treatment of cancer can be foreseen at this time?**

Most physicians believe that the future treatment of cancer will revolve around vaccination and immunization, and around treatment with curative chemicals.

## NONSURGICAL ANTICANCER TREATMENT

**What is oncology?**

That branch of medical science dealing with tumors and malignant growths. An oncologist is a physician who specializes in the treatment of cancer and allied growths.

**What measures are used to treat cancer without surgery?**

a. Radiation therapy and the administration of radioactive substances such as iodine, phosphorus, gold, etc.
b. The use of hormone injections and tablets. It has been found, for example, that cancer of the breast is sometimes inhibited by male or female hormones; the growth of a cancer of the prostate is often inhibited by the administration of female hormones.
c. The administration of drugs (chemotherapy) that kill cancer cells.

**Has much progress been made in the application of x ray and radioactive substances in treating cancer?**

Yes. New techniques and new equipment have improved results remarkably.

**What is chemotherapy?**

A method of treating cancer and allied growths with chemicals.

**What is a chemotherapist?**

A physician who specializes in treating cancer and allied growths with various chemicals. Usually he is a physician trained in internal medicine, and often in hematology. (Hematology deals with disorders of the blood and blood-forming organs.)

**Is it likely that an ultimate cure for cancer will originate through the use of hormones?**

Most investigators agree that this approach to the treatment of cancer will not lead to a final cure as most cancers are uninfluenced by the administration of hormones.

**What appears to be the future of chemotherapy?**

New drugs are constantly being discovered that have greater and greater limiting effects upon the spread and growth of cancer. Some of these drugs are so effective that they can cause a cancer to disappear entirely. It is expected that new and better drugs will continue to be found and that the outlook for patients with cancer will continue to improve.

**Can cancer ever be *cured* by the use of x rays, radioactive substances, hormones, or chemicals?**

Yes. With the great new advances taking place in the nonsurgical anticancer methods, it is anticipated that the list of "curable" cancers will grow rapidly.

**What is immunotherapy?**

It is the prevention or treatment of disease through the production of immunity.

**Is it anticipated that immunotherapy will one day play an important role in the prevention and treatment of cancer?**

Yes. A tremendous amount of research is presently taking place throughout the world in this field. Since cancer is thought to be associated with virus invasion, it is hoped that a vaccine against such viruses will be discovered. Thus, the role of viruses as cancer-producing agents will be eliminated.

## What are some of the statistics regarding the benefits derived from the use of drugs and hormones in the treatment of cancer?

a. More than 90 percent of children with acute leukemia can be benefited through chemotherapy. Some can even be cured of their disease.

b. Seventy percent of children with kidney tumors (Wilms's tumors) can be benefited from chemotherapy.

c. Seventy percent of men with cancer of the prostate are benefited through the administration of hormones.

d. Sixty percent of women with cancer of the breast have years added to their lives through the administration of drugs and hormones.

e. Eighty percent of patients with chronic leukemia can be helped through chemotherapy.

f. Ninety percent of people with Hodgkin's disease will undergo remissions with courses of chemotherapy.

g. Eighty percent of men with cancer of the testicle will benefit from chemotherapy.

h. More than 40 percent of women with cancer of the ovary can be helped.

## Are the nonsurgical methods of cancer treatment often combined with surgical treatment?

Yes. It has been found that if the bulk of cancer cells in the body can be reduced through surgery, then the nonsurgical methods, including radiotherapy, chemotherapy, and hormone therapy, are more effective. Of course, there are certain conditions, such as leukemia and lymphoma, that do not lend themselves to the eradication of the bulk of tumor tissue in the body.

## Can cancer ever be helped by chemotherapy when the disease has spread throughout the body?

Startling as it may seem, there is a growing number of patients with widespread cancer who can be helped, and in some instances even cured, by the judicious use of chemical agents (drugs).

## Are the benefits from radiation, hormone, and chemotherapy of a temporary nature?

Yes, although life spans can frequently be extended, and the patient can live more comfortably after these treatments have been concluded. Furthermore, there is an ever-increasing number of patients who receive these forms of therapy who can be classified as cured.

# CHAPTER 17

# CHILD BEHAVIOR

*(See also Chapter 3 on Adolescence; Chapter 44 on Mental Health and Disease; Chapter 64 on Sex)*

## CRYING

**Why do infants cry?**

a. Because they are hungry.
b. Because they are wet or soiled.
c. Because they crave close contact with the mother's body.
d. Because they are sick or in pain. (Sickness and pain are the least common causes of crying.)
e. Because of colic in newborns.

**How can one discover which of the above reasons is causing a child to cry?**

If the crying is due to hunger, the child will stop crying when he is fed; if it is caused by discomfort, he will stop crying when his diaper is changed; if it is caused by a craving for affection or attention, he will stop crying when he is picked up; if he continues to cry, he may be ill.

**Is the crying of a sick child the same type as that heard in healthy infants?**

Usually not. Evidences of elevated temperature, a rash, vomiting, diarrhea, etc., will alert the parents so that they will be able to differentiate between the two types of crying. Furthermore, in illness, the mere demonstration of affection—or making the baby more comfortable—will not satisfy the child.

**Is it normal for a baby two to three months old to wish to be held constantly by a parent or nurse?**

Yes. Young infants will not be "spoiled" by frequent picking up. Later, if the behavior becomes manipulative, parents can gradually reduce holding and can engage the infant in play activities.

**Is a parent neglecting a child if he or she does not pick him up whenever he cries, or are they spoiling him if they pick him up too often?**

A compromise, after the age of six months, should be worked out. Intelligent parents will learn soon enough to distinguish when the child is in real need and when he merely desires to be pampered.

**Do babies tend to cry more at night?**

Yes, because they get less attention during the night. Also, some babies are aware of the "aloneness" of nighttime and wish to overcome it by calling people to them. Infants normally develop "separation anxiety" at about twelve to eighteen months of age.

**Is it permissible for a parent to "walk the floor" with a baby who cries or fusses at night?**

Yes, but it should not be overdone. Pick up the child for a little while and show affection. If he stops crying, put him down. If he cries again, it is perhaps wiser to let him alone. Just make him aware that you are nearby and can reach him if he is in real need.

**Does excessive crying ever cause a hernia (rupture) to develop?**

No.

## THUMBSUCKING AND SIMILAR HABITS

**Is thumbsucking considered a normal habit?**

Yes, in many young infants.

**Why do babies suck their thumbs?**

Psychological studies have shown that some infants have a sucking need greater than that met by feeding on either breast or bottle.

**Is it normal instinct for an infant to put things into his mouth?**

Yes. Touching things with his lips and tongue is a way of learning about them.

**Can thumbsucking be prevented by giving more time to the baby's feedings?**

It will help some children, but not others.

**When does thumbsucking usually stop?**

This is variable and may last only a few months in certain children. Others continue the habit until two to three years of age.

**When is thumbsucking harmful?**

Only when it continues too long, that is, when the child is four, five, or six years of age.

**Will thumbsucking affect the baby's teeth or the shape of its mouth?**

No, unless the habit lasts beyond six to seven years of age. It was formerly thought that deformity of the teeth was caused by thumbsucking, but most investigators now deny this.

**Do most children give up thumbsucking by themselves without treatment?**

Yes.

**What should be done if the baby falls asleep while thumbsucking?**

Nothing.

**Should restraints be used to stop thumbsucking?**

No. Thumb guards, elbow splints, bitter medicines, etc., usually do no good and are not considered advisable. In general, these methods tend to prolong the habit.

### Should a parent be concerned about thumbsucking?

Not in the young infant or young child. In fact, it is best to develop a calm, assured attitude toward the habit, knowing that it will pass without leaving any harmful effects.

### Is thumbsucking an indication that the child is tense or high-strung?

Not necessarily. Many calm babies also suck their thumbs.

### Can harmful psychological difficulties be created if there is too great an attempt on the part of the parent to stop the thumbsucking?

If the parent becomes tense and nags the child about the habit, it can do some harm. "Treatment" for thumbsucking includes planned ignoring.

### Is thumbsucking in an older child an indication of insecurity or a desire for greater love?

In an older child it may be part of a personality difficulty, but it may represent merely one manifestation of underlying tension or anxiety, or may indicate that he is unhappy.

### What should be done if thumbsucking seems to be associated with some psychological problem?

Consult your pediatrician or a psychiatrist.

### Are there any other habits that are similar to thumbsucking and that fall into the same category?

Yes. These are:
a. Hair-twirling.
b. Ear-twisting.
c. Sucking on toys, clothing, or blankets.

### Can a teething ring or pacifier prevent thumbsucking?

Yes, in many cases.

### Is the use of a pacifier harmful?

No. It is again thought to be a soothing device that does no psychological harm and may do good for tense babies.

### Can disease or infection be brought into the mouth by thumbsucking or by use of a pacifier?

Only in very rare instances. Pacifiers should be kept clean and washed often.

### Does thumbsucking ever produce finger calluses?

Yes, but they will disappear when the sucking stops. Calluses require no special attention.

### Is nailbiting related to thumbsucking?

Yes, but it usually occurs in older children.

### What is the treatment for nailbiting?

Interest the child in other pursuits. Too much attention to the problem may prolong the activity. Discussion with a pediatrician about underlying stresses on the child may prove helpful.

### What is the medical significance of teeth-grinding in sleep?

It has no medical significance.

### What significance does head-banging have?

It usually has no significance and disappears spontaneously within a short time.

## BREATH-HOLDING

### What are breath-holding spells?

The child will cry, hold his breath, turn blue, and seem to faint or become unconscious.

### How long do breath-holding spells tend to last?

No more than a few seconds, but they are very frightening to the parent.

### At what ages do these spells occur most frequently?

From about six months to four or five years of age.

### What brings on breath-holding spells?

Rage, fear, injury, plus intense crying.

### What can happen if a breath-holding spell lasts longer than a few seconds?

The baby may become limp and lose consciousness momentarily. In extreme cases a convulsion may take place.

### Are breath-holding attacks serious?

No. Although they may appear to be serious, they are not actually of great medical significance.

### Do breath-holding spells cause permanent damage to the child?

No.

### Does a baby ever die in a breath-holding spell?

No!!!

### How can breath-holding spells be stopped?

Once they have started, nothing can be done except to comfort the child. All of these spells end by themselves without requiring treatment.

### Should a child in a breath-holding spell be doused with cold water?

No.

### How can breath-holding spells be prevented?

By reducing the episodes of rage, fear, or injury that precipitate the attacks.

**Do breath-holding spells mean that the child is abnormally nervous?**

No.

**Will the attacks themselves affect the nerves?**

No.

**Will children outgrow breath-holding spells?**

Yes, they usually disappear by the time the child is two to three years of age.

## TEMPER TANTRUMS

**What are temper tantrums?**

Sudden outbursts of rage in young children.

**What brings on temper tantrums?**

Anger, displeasure, or failure of the child to get his own way.

**What forms do these attacks take?**

The child may throw himself on the floor, scream, kick about, bang the floor, strike his hands, feet, or head on the floor or against the wall, or he may claw at objects nearby. He may even tear and bite whatever is within reach.

**What should the parents' attitude be toward temper tantrums?**

Be calm, but firm. Do not give in to the child, for he will use these tantrums as a device to get his own way. If he sees that the tantrums are not effective and that they do not disturb you, he will soon abandon them.

**Is it necessary to use medicines or tranquilizing drugs for children who have frequent temper tantrums?**

No.

## TICS

**What are tics?**

They are jerky movements of the face or body that seem to have no purpose.

**At what age are tics most frequently encountered?**

Between seven and ten years.

**What are some of the common tics?**

Eye-blinking, head-jerking, face-twitching, shoulder-shaking, hawking or coughing sounds, mouth-twitching, etc.

**What causes tics?**

They may start because of an irritation or illness. For instance, a coughing tic may begin with a real cold, or a blinking tic may start as the result of an eye irritation or infection.

**What causes tics to continue?**

Even after the original irritating cause has disappeared, the movements may continue. This often begins as a voluntary movement, but later on the child may not even be aware that he is making the movements.

**Are tics an indication of nervousness?**

Yes, in most children they are the result of an emotional problem, probably related to the home or school or to the child's adjustment to his playmates.

**Do tics tend to recur often during the day?**

Yes, anywhere from every few minutes to every few seconds.

**Is it common for one tic to replace another tic as a habit?**

Yes.

**Can the child stop a tic voluntarily?**

In the beginning, yes; later on, no.

**Should a child be punished or warned about a tic?**

No. Nagging may intensify or aggravate the condition.

**At what age do most tics stop by themselves?**

Between ten and twelve years.

**What is the usual psychiatric treatment for a tic?**

When a tic is found to be due to a personality problem or some maladjustment, psychiatric treatment is directed at the child's underlying difficulty—not toward the treatment of the tic itself.

**Do tics ever continue on into adulthood?**

Occasionally they do. When this occurs, the patient is unaware that he is making these movements.

**What is the treatment for tics?**

At first, before the habit is well established, it might be best to disregard it. A great majority of tics, over 90 percent of them, will stop by themselves. However, if the tic continues, medical and psychiatric advice should be sought.

## MASTURBATION

*(See also Chapter 64 on Sex)*

**Is it common for young boys and girls to masturbate?**

Yes.

**What usually starts masturbation?**

It may begin because of an irritation or rash in the genital area that causes the child to explore the area. Often the child continues to masturbate after the original irritant has been eliminated.

**Can this type of masturbation be prevented?**

It can often be prevented by removing all possible irritants and by eliminating tight or wet clothing.

**Is masturbation harmful?**

No.

## Should masturbation be discussed with the child?

In general, it is wisest to disregard the practice. The child should not be given a sense of guilt about masturbation, nor should the parent be alarmed by the practice.

## Do older children masturbate?

Yes.

## Will masturbation result in any permanent harm to the sex organs?

No.

## Will masturbation result in any harm to the nervous system?

No.

## Does masturbation ever lead to insanity or mental deficiency?

Definitely not!

## Should children who masturbate be punished?

No.

## Will punishment aggravate masturbation?

It may, out of resentment to the parental authority.

## What should be done to diminish the habit of masturbation?

Arrange for the child to be kept busy most of the day and to have plenty of outdoor activity. There should be avoidance of long periods in which the child is left by himself.

## Does masturbation affect the ability to have normal sex relations in adult life?

No. However, if the parent makes a big issue of it and threatens the child because of it, it may produce emotional conflict that can have its manifestations in adult life.

## What is the best treatment for masturbation?

Judicious disregard of it by the parents.

# SLEEPWALKING

## Is sleepwalking very common in children?

No, it is rather rare.

## What can be done to prevent sleepwalking?

It is important to avoid any injury to the child during such episodes. A sedative is sometimes given to prevent episodes of sleepwalking.

# NIGHT TERRORS

## What are night terrors?

These are episodes, usually occurring in children between three and six years of age, in which the child awakens suddenly, about an hour or two after going to bed, and screams and cries out hysterically. He does not appear to know where he is and may tremble with fear.

## What is the cause of night terrors?

Although the exact cause is not known, it is thought that they may be caused by excessive excitement before retiring. In other instances, there may be psychological problems in the home environment that bring on the episodes.

## What is the treatment for night terrors?

It is important that the parent remain with the child to give comfort during these episodes.

## Do children remember night terrors the next morning?

Usually not.

## How can night terrors be prevented?

Simple measures—such as avoiding excitement and heavy meals before retiring—should be tried at first. If they fail, a mild sedative may be tried. In severe cases, it may be necessary to obtain expert psychiatric help.

## Do night terrors bear any relation to epilepsy?

No.

## Will most night terrors disappear in time?

Yes. Almost all cases will subside within a year or two.

# NIGHTMARES

## Are nightmares the same as night terrors?

No. In nightmares, the child usually remembers a specific dream, either during the night or when he awakens the next morning. The dreams are usually horrifying and frightening to the child.

## What should be done for nightmares?

At the time of awakening, reassurance and comfort must be given the child. The child may want to talk about and recount the dream, as this will convince him more certainly that it was unreal.

## How are nightmares prevented?

The same procedure should be carried out as for night terrors, that is, a light meal before bedtime and avoidance of excessive excitement before retiring. Children should not be allowed to watch horrifying television shows before going to sleep.

## Do children tend to have the same nightmares or other dreams over and over again?

This occurs in some cases. In such an event, psychiatric assistance should be considered.

# FEARS

## Is it normal for a child to experience fear?

Yes. Mild fear is normal and acts as a protective mechanism.

**When do fears become abnormal in children?**

When they are unwarranted and excessive and when they no longer serve the useful purpose of protecting the child.

**What causes abnormal fears in children?**

A very suggestible child will be frightened by a parent who urges him to stay away from possible sources of danger, such as fire, automobiles, animals, etc. Thereafter, the child's fears are enhanced and exaggerated.

**What is the best treatment for fear in young children?**

Constant reassurance from the parent; "talking out" the occurrences of fear will also help. It is often wise to attempt to associate the feared object with some pleasant experience that will serve to "recondition" the child's attitude.

**How should the fear of doctors or the fear of operations be treated in a child?**

By explaining honestly to the child what he may expect to find and what is going to be done to him. Preparation for the experience he is about to undergo is the best way to avoid inordinate fear. All questions should be answered honestly and as completely as the child's curiosity demands.

**Is it helpful to the child if the parent is available before and after he undergoes a surgical operation?**

Yes. Whenever it is possible, the parent should be available.

## SPEECH DEFECTS

**Why do children stutter?**

Although some investigators believe that stuttering is caused by a delay in the maturing of speech centers within the brain, most investigators believe that it is caused by anxiety and tension.

**Do girls stutter as frequently as boys?**

No. Boys are affected about four times more frequently.

**Is it common for all young children to stutter just a little bit while learning to speak?**

Yes. This is common in children from one to three years of age.

**Does the child who stutters occasionally usually become a permanent stutterer?**

No, but if stuttering persists for several years, it will probably require treatment.

**Is it good practice to correct the young child who stutters?**

No. This early hesitancy in speech will disappear spontaneously if there is not constant correction and attention directed to it.

**Will anxiety or tension in the child or parent make the child's stuttering worse?**

Yes. Home conflicts or conflicts with brothers or sisters or parents will aggravate the tendency.

**In what percentage of children does early stuttering continue into later childhood?**

In about 10 percent.

**What percentage of children continue to stutter into adult life?**

Only about 1 percent.

**When should stuttering be treated?**

As soon as it is realized that the condition is a real problem and not temporary. Usually, at about four to six years of age.

**Who should treat the child for stuttering?**

A competent speech therapist or a speech clinic associated with a school or hospital. Untrained personnel may only aggravate the condition.

**Do left-handed children stutter more than right-handed children?**

No.

**Is it advisable to change from left- to right-handedness?**

No.

**Is lisping always caused by a defect of the tongue?**

No. In most cases it is not caused by any anatomical defect but is associated with excessive use of baby talk in the home.

**Is it necessary to cut the little strand (frenum) under the tongue to prevent lisping?**

No. This is rarely done today. This structure will stretch with use, and needs to be cut only when it is very tight or very short.

**Is delayed speech in infancy a sign of mental retardation?**

Not always. Some children may not speak until they are two or three years old and yet be perfectly normal in all other respects. If delayed speech is associated with delays in development of other abilities—such as sitting up, standing, walking, comprehending—then it is a sign of mental retardation.

**What is the association of hearing to delayed speech?**

It is important to test hearing when there is delay in speech beyond two years of age. If there is a hearing defect, the child usually cannot learn to speak.

**Can a child be taught to speak if he does not hear?**

Yes, to a certain extent. There are several special hearing/speech centers throughout the country where even totally deaf children can be taught to speak if they are otherwise normal.

## BEDWETTING (Enuresis)

### What is bedwetting?
It is involuntary urination at night, usually occuring in children after the age of three or four years.

### Does bedwetting occur with the same frequency among boys and girls?
No. boys outnumber girls in this respect by about two to one.

### Is it normal for children to wet their beds up to the age of three to four years?
Yes.

### At what age do children gain daytime control of the bladder?
Usually at about two-and-a-half to three years of age.

### Do bedwetters often wet their beds more than once a night?
Yes.

### What causes bedwetting?
There are many causes. It is usually considered a developmental delay. Children who were dry and then begin to wet should be evaluated for an emotional problem.

### Does bedwetting tend to run in families?
Yes. It is sometimes found that the parent of a bedwetting child was also a bedwetter.

### Can bedwetting be corrected?
Yes. It requires a great deal of patience and cooperation among the parent, child, and physician.

### What are the most common physical causes of bedwetting?
An infection of the bladder or kidney, or a defect in the anatomical development of the urinary system.

### What are the emotional causes of bedwetting?
a. Too early an attempt at bladder training.
b. Excessive emphasis on bladder training.
c. Emotional immaturity or infantile behavior patterns.
d. Marked shyness.
e. Conflict between the parents.
f. Conflict between the child and his parent.
g. Rivalry among brothers and sisters.
h. Insufficient attention from the parent.
i. Excessive attention and oversolicitude.
j. Insecurity.
k. Problems of school adjustment.

### Do other behavior problems usually appear along with bedwetting?
Yes. These children often have nightmares, temper tantrums, excessive fears, and are thumbsuckers or nailbiters.

### Should the parent seek medical advice if the child continues to be a bedwetter?
Yes.

### What can be done to treat a mild case of bedwetting?
Restrict the fluid intake after dinner and wake the child at frequent intervals during the night to take him to the bathroom.

### Should a child who is a bedwetter be given fluids during the night even if he is thirsty?
No.

### Is it better to give a bedwetter a "dry" supper?
Yes.

### Should a salty diet be given at dinnertime to a bedwetter?
No. It will not improve the situation.

### How can the parent help the child who wets his bed?
The parent should find out at approximately what time bedwetting occurs and should wake the child about a half hour before that time in order to take him to the bathroom. Of course, all children should urinate before going to bed.

### Is it permissible to carry the child to the bathroom to urinate?
No. The child must be fully awake and go to the bathroom alone. Many parents make the mistake of carrying the sleeping or half-sleeping child to the bathroom to urinate. This only encourages his nighttime urination in his sleep.

### Does the child who bedwets have a smaller bladder capacity than normal?
Usually not.

### Does a bedwetting child produce more urine at night than during the daytime?
No.

### Should the bedwetting child be scolded?
No. This will usually aggravate the condition.

### Should the bedwetting child be rewarded for not wetting his bed?
Yes. A system of rewards for dry nights will often serve as an added incentive and is sometimes effective in stopping the habit.

### If a child is in the habit of wetting his bed more than once a night, should he be awakened more than once a night to be taken to the toilet?
Yes.

### Should bedwetters be made to sleep on rubber sheets?
No. Although it may help to keep the mattress dry, it is uncomfortable for most children to sleep on a rubber

sheet and may even aggravate the condition.

**How long does it usually take for the successful treatment of bedwetting?**

Several months to a year.

**Are there ever recurrences of bedwetting once it has been controlled?**

Yes. If the child is upset emotionally, or a new baby comes into the family, or the child develops an illness, there may be a relapse.

**What form of treatment should be carried out if there is a relapse?**

Return to the previous successful methods of treatment.

**Are the mechanical devices on the market to prevent bedwetting helpful?**

Usually not.

**Is there an electrical device that is helpful in the treatment of bedwetting?**

Yes. A new device has recently been devised whereby the first few drops of urine that touch an electric circuit in the bed pad will cause an alarm to ring, thus awakening the child so that he may go to the bathroom to complete his bladder emptying. This technique requires the child's cooperation.

**Are these electrical devices dangerous or harmful?**

No.

**If these electrical devices are to be effective, how long to they take to do their work?**

Several weeks.

**When should bedwetting be treated by a psychiatrist?**

When it is accompanied by other manifestations of emotional instability or when it is found in conjunction with other behavior problems.

**Do most children outgrow bedwetting?**

Yes.

**Are medications of much value in treating bedwetting?**

Yes, in more than half the cases, medications may be of temporary help.

**Are there psychological complications in adult life due to bedwetting in childhood?**

Usually not.

**What should the attitude of parents be toward a child who wets his bed?**

It is important for the parent not to be excessively concerned, because this may aggravate the child's anxiety and thus make the condition worse.

**What is the best method to prevent bedwetting?**

Avoidance of tension and anxiety in the home and an atmosphere of love and security for the child.

# SLEEP PROBLEMS

**How many hours of sleep does a baby require?**

This will vary with the age of the child. A newborn baby may sleep twenty hours a day; a six-month-old infant sleeps sixteen to eighteen hours a day; a one-year-old child requires fourteen to sixteen hours a day; and at two years the child requires about twelve to fourteen hours of sleep.

**How many hours do older children require?**

Three years old—about twelve hours.
Five years old—about ten to twelve hours.
Ten years old—about nine to ten hours.

**Until what age should the infant have two naps a day?**

Until twelve to fifteen months of age.

**When should a child have one nap a day?**

From three to five years of age.

**When does a baby begin sleeping throughout the entire night without awakening?**

This varies markedly. Some babies will sleep through the night right away; others not until eight months of age.

**Are sleep patterns definite?**

No. There is a great deal of variation according to the individual child.

**Should the parent be concerned if the child does not fit into any particular sleep pattern?**

No. Parents often become unduly concerned about the number of hours their baby sleeps. This anxiety is bad for the parent-child relationship.

**Is it normal to find a child in about the ninth or tenth month of life begin awakening during the night when he formerly slept through the night?**

Yes. These children are awakening because they are aware of being thirsty, uncomfortable, or wet. Changing the position, changing the diaper, or giving water will satisfy the child, and he will fall asleep again rapidly.

**Why do some babies between the ages of one and two years refuse to go asleep?**

Mainly because they have a fear that sleep means separation from their parents.

**Do older babies, between one and one-and-a-half years, often awaken during the night?**

Yes. This may be due to some of the above causes or to pain resulting from teething. It may also be caused by noises in the house or by too much light, poor ventilation, or improper covering.

**What should be done for the older child who refuses to go to sleep?**

It is important for the child to feel secure in the knowledge that his parent is nearby. It may be necessary to stay with the child for a time until he falls asleep. Sometimes a small light in the child's bedroom will help to dispel fear.

**Do children vary in their sleeping patterns from time to time?**

Yes. Parents should not become unduly alarmed by wide variations in sleeping patterns as children grow older. The important thing is to give the child affection, love, and a feeling of security.

**Is it permissible to rock a baby to sleep?**

Many physicians believe this will do no harm. If it is effective, it is permissible to do so until regular sleep habits have been established.

**What should be done about the older child of three to five years who gets out of bed during the night?**

In many instances, children do this because they have a feeling of being hemmed in by the crib. Such children will often do better if they are put into a youth bed or a regular bed without sides. They will then feel freer and will be less likely to get up during the night.

**What prevents children from falling asleep?**

Usually, excessive excitement, a heavy meal, or excessive play with parents or siblings just before bedtime.

**Will the loss of sleep do great harm to an infant?**

Not if it occurs occasionally.

**Is it wise for a child to sleep in a room by himself?**

Yes, whenever this is feasible.

**Is it unwise for a child to sleep in the same room as his parents?**

This should be avoided whenever possible.

**Is it permissible to leave a light in the baby's room during the night?**

Yes.

**Do most children require pillows?**

No.

**Should a child be placed in a special position in bed before going to sleep?**

No. The child can sleep in any position he finds most comfortable.

**Will children smother if they lie on their abdomen?**

No. A normal, healthy baby can turn his head to the side and will get adequate air intake.

**At what time should an older child be made to go to sleep?**

There seems to be a constant conflict between all parents and children as to the proper time to go to sleep. Parents want children in bed earlier; children want to stay up later. No set pattern can be presented. It will vary with the age and needs of the child, the activity in the household, the atmosphere of quiet or excitement in the household, the number of children, and the varying bedtimes of brothers and sisters. It may even depend upon the television programs that the child wants to see. Each parent must set the pattern, but the important consideration is that rules must be adhered to without wavering and indecision.

## LEARNING DISABILITY

**What is a learning disability?**

It is a condition in which the child

with normal intelligence finds it difficult to properly organize things seen and heard. Usually it presents a difficulty in reading (dyslexia), writing (dysgraphia), or calculating (dyscalculia).

**Is a learning disability a sign of brain damage?**

No. Some children with damage to the central nervous system may be learning disabled, but most children with learning disability have no history or evidence of such damage.

**Is learning disability the major reason for a child's school failure?**

No, it is only one of several possibilities, which may include poor preparation for learning, mental retardation, emotional or family problems. Children who are underachieving should have a complete psychological investigation to search for all possible causes.

**Are all learning-disabled children "hyperactive"?**

No!

**What is the treatment for learning disabilities?**

Learning disability is not really a medical problem. Special education techniques, started as early as possible, are utilized either in a regular school or in special education classes. The best approach is individualized and avoids frequent failure, which leads to poor motivation.

All learning-disabled children are entitled to special education under federal law.

## HYPERACTIVITY

**What is "hyperactivity"?**

Hyperactivity is a descriptive term that includes behavior such as short attention span, distractibility, impulsiveness, and excess movement.

Some or all of these behaviors can be seen in a "hyperactive" child.

### Is hyperactivity caused by brain damage?

Some children with known trauma to the brain exhibit these symptoms. Emotional problems can cause hyperactivity as well. Most often, no neurological abnormality is detected.

### Is hyperactivity associated with learning problems?

Often the two do coexist, but not necessarily.

### What can be done about hyperactivity?

First, a complete evaluation, including a history, review of family problems, medical examination, and psychological examination, should be performed. Once all factors are evaluated, treatment can be prescribed.

### What treatments are prescribed for hyperactivity?

a. In all cases, parents should be made aware of the problems their child is facing. Then, they should be counseled in ways to deal with their child's behavior and their own feelings about it. They can learn ways to modify their own behavior and reactions as well as their child's behavior.

b. Medications may be used in appropriate cases, but they do not cure the problem.

c. Special diets have sometimes been prescribed for hyperactivity, but results are not yet conclusive.

d. When necessary, special schooling in smaller, more structured classrooms than average may be needed.

## PARENTING

### How can parents know if they are doing the right things?

Parenting is hard work. No one approach is the right one. Children need warmth, love, and security. Their happiness and successful development are the clues to effective parenting.

### Are there ways to learn more about parenting?

Yes. One's pediatrician or family doctor can be a source of information about effective parenting. There are many books on the subject, as well as courses offered in effective parenting. In the absence of family support, frequent frank discussions about child behavior and development with the pediatrician should be a major part of child care.

CHAPTER **18**

# CONTAGIOUS DISEASES

*(See also Chapter 31 on Immunizations and Vaccinations; Chapter 32 on Infant and Childhood Diseases; Chapter 34 on Infectious and Virus Diseases; Chapter 75 on Upper Respiratory Diseases; Chapter 77 on Venereal Disease)*

## CHICKENPOX

**What is chickenpox?**

A contagious disease of childhood appearing anywhere from the third month of life through adolescence.

**What is the cause of chickenpox?**

Chickenpox is caused by a virus.

**How is chickenpox transmitted from one child to another?**

It is usually transmitted by direct contact.

**When is chickenpox infectious?**

It can be transmitted starting from the day before the appearance of the rash throughout the period of blisters, which extends for approximately seven days.

**Can it be transmitted later in the course of the disease?**

No.

**Does a child have fever with chickenpox?**

Yes. There is usually a slight elevation of temperature to 101°–102°F. In severe cases, there may be elevation of temperature up to 103°–104°F.

**Is treatment necessary for the fever in chickenpox?**

Appropriate aspirin, or similar medication, is often given.

**Can adolescents or adults contract chickenpox?**

Few children escape this disease. If it does not occur during childhood, it may develop during adulthood. It is usually more severe in adults.

**What does the chickenpox rash look like?**

At first there are many tiny spots spread over the body, largely on the chest and abdomen and on the upper part of the extremities. The spots start as small, reddish, pinpoint areas that become larger within a few hours and finally form blisters. For a day or two the blister will have clear fluid in it that changes to cloudy fluid a day or two later, and finally, after four to five days, each little blister will dry up and form a crust.

**On what parts of the body do the pox occur?**

They may appear anywhere on the body, including the hair, the scalp, the mouth, the palate, the eyelids, or in the genital area.

**Do all the spots appear at the same time?**

No. New crops will appear for the first three or four days of the disease. Eventually the entire series of blisters will dry up and form crusts or scabs.

**Can the fluid within the blisters transmit the disease?**

Yes.

**Will the scabs or crusts transmit the disease?**

Usually not.

**Do the spots itch?**

Yes, mildly.

**What can be done to relieve the itching?**

A soothing lotion such as calamine may be applied, or a paste made of bicarbonate of soda and water may be applied to each of the spots. This will relieve most of the itching.

**Is there any medication that can be taken internally to relieve the itching?**

Yes, there are several compounds that can be prescribed by a physician to give some relief from the itching.

**How many pox usually appear?**

There may be any number, from a handful to several hundred. The more severe cases tend to have more spots.

**How can one prevent chickenpox?**

At present there is no serum or vaccine available that is effective in the prevention of this disease.

**Is gamma globulin of any help in preventing or modifying chickenpox?**

No.

**What are the possible complications of chickenpox?**

a. There may be secondary infection of the spots on the body.
b. In rare instances, cases of encephalitis or brain inflammation have been reported.
c. Occasionally, pneumonia may follow chickenpox.
d. Inflammation of the middle ear occurs in a small percentage of cases.
All of these are rare complications.

**Should the child be prevented from scratching the pox?**

Yes. Excessive scratching of the spots may break the blisters and may add to the chances of secondary infection. Usually no harm results from moderate scratching.

**How can a child be prevented from scratching?**

If it is a very young child, it may be necessary to put mittens or gloves on his hands. Older children should be urged to cooperate in preventing scratching.

**Does a child with chickenpox require isolation?**

It is not necessary to isolate him from other members of the family, because it is almost impossible to prevent the spread of this disease among brothers and sisters. Of course, he should be kept away from children outside of his immediate family.

**How long should the child be isolated?**

About ten days from the onset of the disease, or until all the crusts have formed and are quite dry. In some localities, the school does not permit the child to return until the crusts have all fallen off, but in most cities the child may return to school in about ten days.

**Does chickenpox leave permanent scars?**

There may be tiny scars which appear after the crusts have fallen off. These scars are of short duration, are not permanent, and will disappear usually within several months to a year. If, however, the child has scratched the spots and they have become secondarily infected, the scars resulting from such infection may be permanent.

**Are antibiotics useful in treating chickenpox?**

No. They have no effect on the disease and should be used only if secondary infection ensues.

**Does the child need to be kept in bed during his disease?**

No.

**Should the child be bathed during the acute phase of chickenpox?**

If the child is terribly uncomfortable, a lukewarm bath will do no harm.

**Can chickenpox be contracted a second time?**

No.

# DIPHTHERIA

**What is diphtheria?**

It is a contagious disease of childhood affecting the throat and occasionally the larynx.

**What is the cause of diphtheria?**

It is caused by a bacillus (Klebs-Loeffler).

**Is diphtheria a common disease?**

No. It used to occur in epidemics, but since almost all children now get protective injections, it has become almost a medical rarity.

**How is diphtheria spread?**

It is spread from one patient to another through coughing, sneezing, or droplet infection.

**What are the symptoms of diphtheria?**

Mild fever and sore throat with the formation of a characteristic-appearing membrane on the tonsils or on the throat. When diphtheria involves the larynx or the nose, it causes obstruction to breathing.

**How can diphtheria be distinguished from ordinary tonsillitis?**

A physician will note the special characteristics of the diphtheritic membrane and will be able to make the correct diagnosis.

**What ages are affected by diphtheria?**

Children under the age of six months are usually immune to the disease. It can occur in any age group over six months.

**Can diphtheria be spread in any way other than by direct contact?**

Yes. Cases have been reported in which the drinking of infected milk caused the disease to spread.

**Is diphtheria a serious disease?**

Yes. It is serious because it may cause death by obstruction of the larynx when it involves that structure; or it may cause nerve paralysis of the larynx, thus interfering with breathing; or it may cause serious involvement of heart muscle.

**Is there any specific conclusive test to determine whether a child has diphtheria?**

Yes. A culture of the material in the throat or nose is taken and is grown to see whether the diphtheria germ is present.

**What is the treatment for diphtheria?**

As soon as the disease is suspected, the child should be given adequate dosage of diphtheria antitoxin.

**Are antibiotics effective against diphtheria?**

Once the disease has been established, the child must get antitoxin. Antibiotics may be given in addition but should not be used exclusively to produce a cure. Penicillin in large doses is effective against diphtheria and may be given in addition to antitoxin.

**What can be done for the difficulty in breathing in laryngeal diphtheria?**

If there is any obstruction to the breathing, the doctor should be called immediately, and in many instances a tracheotomy will be necessary. This will mean the opening of the trachea (windpipe) through an incision in the neck to permit freedom of breathing.

**What routine care is indicated in the treatment of this disease?**

The child must stay in bed for at least a week after the illness is over. He may be given a soft diet containing any foods that can be swallowed easily. Also, plenty of liquids should be given.

**Is it necessary for a child with diphtheria to be treated in a hospital?**

No. This condition can be treated at home unless complications develop.

## What are some of the complications of diphtheria?

The two serious complications are nerve paralysis of the larynx and sometimes a paralysis of the nerves of the palate so that normal speech is impaired. Another complication is damage to the heart muscle.

## Does immunity develop after one attack of diphtheria?

Yes, there is usually a lifelong immunity.

## Is there any test for immunity to diphtheria?

Yes, the Schick test has been devised for determining the presence of immunity.

## Can a child be immunized against this disease?

Yes, all children should be immunized against diphtheria by a series of injections, which are almost 100 percent effective. (See Chapter 31, Immunization Chart.)

## At what age should a child be immunized against diphtheria?

It is preferable to start these immunizations at two to three months of age.

## Are booster injections necessary?

Yes. (See Chapter 31, Immunization Chart.)

## How soon after diphtheria is over can a child be bathed?

Usually about a week after the disease has subsided.

## Are there any permanent aftereffects of diphtheria?

In an uncomplicated case, there are no untoward aftereffects.

## How soon after the disease can the child be permitted normal activities?

It is preferable to wait two or three weeks to be sure that there has been no heart involvement.

## When may the child be permitted to return to school after recovery from diphtheria?

In about two weeks.

## Is there any quarantine for a child with diphtheria?

Yes, the board of health in most cities requires that a child with diphtheria be quarantined until throat cultures are negative.

## What should be done if there has been contact with a person who has diphtheria?

Every child and adult who has been in contact with a diphtheria patient should be given diphtheria antitoxin. The dose will be determined by your physician.

## Must the contacts of diphtheria be quarantined?

In general, most health departments do not require this quarantine. However, it is preferable to take cultures of the throats of all contacts, since some people are carriers of this disease.

## What is meant by the term "diphtheria carrier"?

A diphtheria carrier is an individual who does not have the disease himself because he is immune, but who carries the potent organisms in his throat and can therefore spread the disease to others. Because of the existence of "carriers," it is essential that people who have been in contact with a case of diphtheria be watched very carefully.

## Are there many cases of diphtheria seen today?

No, this disease has been virtually eliminated in this country because of immunizations and boosters. However, there has been a reappearance of the disease in some areas due to neglect. Constant vigilance is still necessary.

# GERMAN MEASLES
## (Rubella)

## Is rubella another name for German measles?

Yes.

## What causes German measles?

It is an infectious disease believed to be caused by a virus.

## How does German measles manifest itself?

There are mild symptoms suggestive of a common cold, with slight elevation of temperature and a rash that starts on the face and extends down over the body. This takes place within a period of one day. The rash is made up of many small, isolated reddish spots that do not run together. On the first day the rash often resembles measles; on the second day it may resemble scarlet fever; on the third day it may disappear entirely. In addition, large lymph glands are usually felt at the back of the neck and behind the ears.

## Is German measles communicable?

Yes, but it is not as infectious or contagious as measles or chickenpox.

## At what age do most people get German measles?

It occurs more often in older children or adolescents. German measles occurs fairly frequently in adults, more so than the other contagious diseases.

## Does German measles occur in epidemics?

Yes, about once every three to seven years there is an epidemic of German measles in areas where vaccinations have not been carried out.

## Does German measles occur often in areas where vaccinations have been widely carried out?

No.

**At what season of the year is German measles most apt to occur?**

Most of the cases occur in the late winter and spring months.

**Do patients with German measles tend to run high fever?**

No. Only 100°-101°F.

**Is the patient very uncomfortable during German measles?**

No, but when it affects adolescents or adults, it may be more severe in its manifestations.

**How is German measles spread?**

By direct contact from one patient to another.

**Is German measles frequently confused with other conditions?**

Yes. It is often confused with measles, scarlet fever, or roseola.

**Are the eyes involved as they are in measles?**

No. All of the symptoms are milder in German measles than they are in measles.

**How long does the enlargement of the lymph glands last?**

About a week.

**Are there any complications to German measles?**

Complications are extremely rare.

**Is it necessary to isolate a child with German measles?**

Yes, one does not want to risk exposing a susceptible, pregnant woman.

**Why is it important for children, especially girls, to have this disease?**

German measles, though very mild in childhood, may be severe in adult life. More importantly, German measles during the early months of pregnancy may lead to serious defects in development of the embryo.

**What sort of damage may occur to the unborn child if the mother develops German measles during early pregnancy?**

Cataracts of the eyes, deafness, mental retardation, or heart abnormalities. These may occur as a single congenital defect, or they may appear in combinations.

**In what part of pregnancy is this disease dangerous to the embryo?**

During the first three months of pregnancy. However, some defects may occur if exposure takes place later in the pregnancy.

**In what proportion of cases do abnormalities develop in the baby when the mother has had German measles?**

From 15 to 50 percent of the cases. There is no agreement on the exact percentage.

**When can German measles do the least harm if contracted during pregnancy?**

During the last three months, when all the fetus's organs are formed.

**What can be done to prevent German measles?**

The German measles vaccine should be given to all children. It should also be administered to female adults of childbearing age who have not had the disease and who are not pregnant. They must be warned to avoid becoming pregnant in the two months following vaccination. Special care should be exercised in giving the vaccine to people who are allergic to eggs and to neomycin. Reports seem to indicate that immunity from the vaccine is of long duration and that booster shots may not be required.

**What can be done if a pregnant woman develops German measles?**

It would be best to consult her physician as to the proper course of action. It would vary, depending upon the age of the woman and whether she has other children.

**Can the physician tell before birth whether the embryo has been damaged by the mother having had German measles during pregnancy?**

No.

**What is the treatment for German measles?**

Bed rest, a light nutritious diet, and general cleanliness are all that are necessary.

**Are antibiotics effective against this disease?**

No. They should not be given unless some complication, such as an ear infection or a lung inflammation, sets in.

**How long is a child infectious with German measles?**

Usually for a day preceding the appearance of the disease and for three to four days thereafter.

**Are there any aftereffects of German measles?**

Usually none at all; complete recovery takes place in practically every instance.

**Can someone have German measles more than once?**

No.

## MEASLES (Rubeola)

**What causes measles?**

A virus.

**What is the difference between regular measles and German measles?**

They are two separate and distinct diseases, each caused by a different virus.

**Do young infants contract measles?**

Under six months of age, the child will be immune from measles if the mother has had it at some time in the past.

**Is measles seen very often?**

Not in areas where vaccination has been carried out extensively.

**Can measles be contracted twice?**

No. Once a child has had measles, he is immune for life.

**Is there any way to prevent getting measles?**

Yes, an extremely effective vaccine is available. It should be given to all children except those who have a current infection or a serious underlying disease. It should not be given to pregnant women.

**Is it worthwhile to give gamma globulin to produce a mild, modified case of measles in a child who has been exposed to measles?**

Until recently this was the procedure used in case a child was exposed to measles. Now it is better to give the measles vaccine even after exposure if the child has not had it previously. In this way, the disease will be modified in severity or prevented entirely.

**Does an attack of modified or very mild measles, such as that which follows the giving of gamma globulin, give permanent immunity?**

Yes.

**Is it possible to tell if a child has measles before the rash has appeared?**

Yes. A few days before the appearance of the measles rash there are certain characteristic spots (Koplik's spots) within the mouth, which will establish the diagnosis.

**Where does the rash usually appear first?**

On the face, behind the ears, on the forehead, and at the hairline. It then spreads down over the rest of the body.

**How close a contact is necessary for the transmission of measles?**

This is a very infectious disease and can be transmitted easily through sneezing, coughing, or close physical contact. In school, about 20 to 40 percent will contract the disease if one of the children in the class develops measles.

**Is there less likelihood of contracting measles if an exposure has taken place out of doors?**

Yes.

**How soon in the course of a disease can a child transmit measles to another child?**

As soon as he shows any of the early manifestations of the illness, such as fever, sneezing, coughing, or bleariness of the eyes. These signs appear about three days before the rash breaks out.

**When is a child no longer infectious and able to transmit measles?**

When the temperature has come down to normal, usually about four to five days after the rash has come out.

**Can a child who has had measles act as a carrier and transmit the disease from one of his brothers or sisters to some other children?**

No. Other children in the family may be permitted to attend school though they have a brother or sister who has active measles.

**How is it we hear so often that people have had two or three attacks of measles?**

This usually means that the diagnosis was not correct when originally made. What was diagnosed as measles may have been German measles, roseola, or a drug eruption. Such conditions are commonly misdiagnosed as measles.

**Is it necessary to keep a child out of school while he is incubating measles?**

No. He cannot transmit the disease to other children while he is in the incubation stage.

**How long does the incubation period last?**

About ten days after the original exposure. However, at the first sign of illness, such as fever or symptoms of a cold, the child should be withdrawn from school and should be isolated at home.

**Is it necessary to completely darken the room of a child with measles?**

No. This is an old-fashioned method of treatment, which was carried out to "protect the child's eyes." This has been shown to be unnecessary.

**How long should the child with measles be kept in bed?**

Until the temperature has been down to normal for three or four days and until the rash shows signs of fading.

**Should the room be at all darkened in cases of measles?**

No. The child's eyes should merely be protected from bright sunlight or from bright electric lights.

**Will reading or looking at television injure the child's eyes?**

No, unless the eyes are markedly inflamed and the child is extremely uncomfortable while looking at bright lights.

**What is the standard form of treatment for the ordinary case of measles?**

Bed rest, light diet, plenty of fluids, fresh air, cooling sponge baths, aspirin for the fever, and a cough medicine to reduce the cough.

**Are antibiotic drugs given in the treatment of measles?**

No.

**Is any special diet required by the measles patient?**

No. The ordinary light diet for any sick child with high fever is given.

**Is it necessary to keep the child with high fever well covered in bed?**

No. The old idea that a child with high temperature should be covered with many blankets is not sensible.

**What are the possible complications of measles?**

Today complications are quite rare. Formerly, the following complications were seen from time to time:
a. Inflammation of the ears.
b. Enlargement of the glands in the neck.
c. Pneumonia.
d. Inflammation of the brain (encephalitis).

**How frequent is encephalitis as a complication of measles?**

Although this is quite a serious complication, it occurs very rarely. Estimates are that it occurs only once in a thousand cases.

**Will antibiotics prevent or cure the encephalitis that sometimes occurs as a complication of measles?**

No. They act neither as a preventive nor as an effective treatment.

**Should children with measles ever be hospitalized?**

Yes. If the home facilities are not adequate to care for the child, or if the child has a complication like pneumonia or encephalitis.

**What are the possible dangers of not carrying out a doctor's orders in treating a patient with measles?**

The likelihood of complications is greater if there is improper care.

**Is measles ever a fatal condition?**

Measles itself is never fatal, but the complications of pneumonia or encephalitis may be fatal.

**Is it common for measles to affect the child's organs, such as the heart, kidneys, liver, etc.?**

No.

**How soon after an attack of measles can a child return to all physical activity?**

About ten to fourteen days, if there have been no complications.

**Is there very much danger if measles is contracted by a pregnant woman?**

No.

## MUMPS

**At what age do most people get mumps?**

Children under six months do not get mumps, and it is rare in adults, especially those over forty years of age. Many adults have had an unrecognized mild form of the disease in childhood.

**Should children who have not had mumps be purposely exposed to it?**

No. Formerly, before the advent of mumps vaccine, it was thought that children between the ages of five to twelve years should be exposed to mumps so that they would not get it after puberty, when complications could be serious. However, since the new mumps vaccine is so effective, this advice is no longer given. Over 95 percent of all children are completely immunized by mumps vaccine.

**Should all children be vaccinated with mumps vaccine?**

No. Those few children who are allergic to eggs should not be vaccinated because the vaccine is grown in chicken embryos, and serious allergic reactions might follow its use. It is best for these children to be exposed to mumps before they reach adolescence.

**Is mumps more serious in adulthood than in childhood?**

Yes. It is essentially a mild disease in childhood.

**Does the swelling in mumps always appear on the side of the face or cheek?**

No. The usual site of swelling is in the region of the parotid gland, which extends in front of, under, and behind the ear. In some cases, the salivary glands under the jaw and chin may be involved in addition to the parotid glands—or, sometimes, the salivary glands are involved and the parotid glands are not. Occasionally the swelling is so slight that it goes unrecognized. This condition exists in about 30-60 percent of the cases. Many people who think they have never had mumps have had this mild, unrecognized form.

**Is there any treatment for the pain and swelling of mumps?**

It is usually not necessary to treat the swollen area. When discomfort is marked, it is permissible to apply a hot-water bottle or electric pad, though some children may obtain more relief from cold applications. Aspirin may be given to relieve the discomfort.

**Are serums or antibiotics used in treating mumps?**

No.

**Is special mouth care necessary in mumps?**

Not ordinarily. It is advisable to avoid sour juices or foods that may be irritating; also, foods that require much chewing.

**Is there any special diet for the patient with mumps?**

Yes. A soft, bland diet containing large quantities of liquids.

**When may the child get out of bed and return to school?**

Mumps usually lasts seven to ten days. As soon as the fever and gland swellings have disappeared, the child may be allowed out of bed and may be permitted to return to school a day or two thereafter.

**If a child has mumps, can it be prevented in other members of the family?**

Prompt vaccination with live, attenuated (weakened) mumps virus may protect exposed persons from getting the disease.

**If mumps has developed on one side only, will the other side be affected at some later date?**

Mumps may involve one side first and then affect the other side two or three days later. In about half the cases, the disease remains limited to one side. Permanent immunity will develop whether one or both sides become involved!

**When is it best to get mumps?**

Before puberty.

**Do girls get inflammation of the ovary from mumps?**

This is extremely rare and occurs only after puberty.

**Will mumps cause sterility in a child?**

No. The fear of sterility produced by mumps is largely unwarranted. The complication of inflammation of the testicle occurs only in the mature testicle or in the child after puberty, not in the younger child.

**Will involvement of one testicle produce sterility?**

No.

**Will sterility result if both testicles are involved?**

Not necessarily; full recovery occurs in the majority of cases.

**How often is there involvement of a testicle in an adult?**

In about 20-25 percent of the cases.

**Are virility and the ability to have normal relations affected by testicular involvement?**

No. Virility is not affected by involvement of the testicle. Adults are more

frightened by mumps than they need be.

**Is it possible to prevent the testicle complication in a case of mumps?**

Various drugs and hormones have been given, but they have not been effective. Hyperimmune mumps serum and gamma globulin have also proved ineffective in preventing this type of complication.

**What are other possible complications of mumps?**

Occasionally a child develops headache, high fever, vomiting, and stiff neck several days after the onset of mumps. These symptoms are caused by an inflammation of the brain and its covering, known as meningoencephalitis. Such complications require careful medical supervision. Most complications clear up without serious aftereffects.

## POLIOMYELITIS
### (Infantile Paralysis)

**What is poliomyelitis (infantile paralysis)?**

An acute infection of the spinal cord and brain, caused by a virus.

**Is there only one virus causing the disease?**

No. There are many strains of the polio virus. These have been grouped into three types, known as Types I, II, III.

**What is the incidence of polio?**

There have been only a handful of cases of polio in the United States, in Europe, and in developed areas of the Orient in the past decade. However, it must be kept in mind that there are vast underdeveloped regions in Africa, Asia, India, the South Pacific, and Central and South America where children do not routinely receive polio vaccine. In these areas, polio is still potentially epi-

demic and is therefore just as dangerous a disease as it used to be in this country.

**When polio strikes, does it tend to run in families?**

In general, the paralytic form tends to limit itself to one member of the family, but there have been reports of several cases in a single family.

**Who is most likely to develop polio?**

Children from one to sixteen years of age, although it does occur among adults, particularly those under forty years of age.

**Does the disease tend to be more serious in older people?**

Yes. In general, the paralytic type of polio is more prevalent among adolescents and adults, and the severity of the disease is greater.

**Are boys more susceptible to polio than girls?**

Yes, slightly more susceptible; about 55 percent of the cases affect boys.

**Are pregnant women more susceptible to polio than nonpregnant women?**

Yes.

**Can polio occur in any part of the country?**

Yes. No areas are immune from polio if vaccination has not been widely carried out among the children.

**At what season of the year does polio occur most often?**

During the warm months, particularly summer and early fall.

**When is polio most prevalent?**

In August and September in temperate climates.

**How is polio spread?**

From person to person through direct contact, that is, by droplet infection or by coughing or sneezing.

**Can polio be spread by other means?**

Yes. It can also be spread by milk, drinking water contaminated by sewage, and possibly even by flies. These methods are not as important in the spread of the disease as direct contact.

**How does the polio virus get into the body?**

By inhalation of infected material. In some cases by drinking infected water or eating infected food.

**Will the use of chlorine in drinking water help to prevent the spread of polio?**

Yes, to a certain limited extent.

**How long does it take for polio to develop (incubation period)?**

Seven to fourteen days.

**When is polio communicable from one patient to another?**

Probably during the latter part of the incubation period and the first week of the acute illness, while fever is still present.

**Is the virus present in the nasal and throat discharges of a person with polio?**

Yes.

**Is the virus present in the stool (feces) of a polio patient?**

Yes, it may be present in the feces for as long as six to eight weeks after the onset of the disease, or it may persist for several months.

**Can healthy persons be carriers of the polio virus?**

They may be, although in some cases an apparently healthy person may really be suffering from a very mild form of the disease.

**Can very young infants develop polio?**

Most infants under the age of six months are immune because the mother has transmitted protective substances during her pregnancy, providing she is immune to the disease.

**What are the various forms of poliomyelitis?**

a. Abortive polio (very short-lasting disease with few symptoms).
b. Nonparalytic polio.
c. Paralytic spinal polio (involving the spinal cord).
d. Bulbar polio (involving the brain).
e. Polioencephalitis (involving the brain).

## POLIO VACCINATION

**Are there two types of polio vaccine?**

Yes, the Sabin vaccine, which is taken orally, and the Salk vaccine, which is given by injection.

**How are these vaccines given?**

The Salk vaccine is an inactivated (killed) vaccine and is given by injection in three doses about a month apart. The Sabin vaccine is an attenuated, but live, vaccine, which is administered orally on a sugar tablet or in a flavored syrup solution. It may be given at any time after the age of two to three months. Three doses are given about a month apart, followed by a booster a year later.

**Do these vaccines give permanent immunity?**

Yes, especially when booster doses are given a year or two later.

**Which is the preferred vaccine?**

The Salk vaccine, given by injection, is used very infrequently. It has been replaced almost everywhere in the world by the Sabin vaccine, taken orally, which appears to be somewhat more effective and is much easier to administer.

**Can vaccination eliminate polio?**

Yes. However, the sad fact is that not all children are able to receive the polio vaccine. In other words, it is a matter of distribution and administration, not a question of the effectiveness of vaccination.

**Is it permissible to give polio vaccination to children in an area where cases of polio have developed?**

Yes.

**Is it possible to get polio a second time?**

Yes, but it happens only very rarely.

**How is it that a second attack of polio can be contracted?**

The child may have developed immunity to only one type of polio virus and may be susceptible to other types of the virus.

**Should children who have already had polio be given polio vaccine?**

Yes, because they may be immune to only one type of polio virus.

**Should gamma globulin be given to members of a family in which there is a case of polio?**

No. It does not help.

**Since many adults are immune to polio, why should they be vaccinated against it?**

Only 80-85 percent of adults are immune, and since there is no practical way to determine who is and who is not immune, it is safer to advise *everyone* to take polio vaccine.

**Can polio vaccine do any harm?**

No. Reports of the U.S. Public Health Service state that no cases of polio have been caused by administration of vaccine.

**Should pregnant women be given polio vaccine?**

Definitely, yes! Pregnant women are more susceptible to polio and therefore need protection more than any-one else.

### Can polio vaccine harm the mother or unborn child?

No.

### When should polio vaccine be given to pregnant women?

As early as possible.

## ROSEOLA
### (Exanthem Subitum)

### What is roseola infantum?

It is a virus disease commonly affecting young children, characterized by a high temperature (104°-106°F.), which lasts for three days and then abruptly drops to normal on the fourth day. When temperature returns to normal, a rash appears over the entire body, which lasts one or two days.

### Are there any other symptoms of roseola?

Occasionally there may be convulsions at the onset of the disease. There may be a few respiratory signs and a slight sore throat. Roseola can be diagnosed before the rash appears by finding enlarged lymph glands at the back of the neck.

### At what age does this disease occur most often?

Somewhere between the ages of nine months and three years.

### What is the incidence of roseola?

About 50-75 percent of all children get this disease. It is often erroneously diagnosed as measles or German measles.

### Are there many complications to this disease?

Usually there are none.

### What does the rash look like?

It is made up of many fine, pinkish spots spread over the face, chest, abdomen, and extremities. When it disappears in about two days, it leaves no aftereffects.

### What is the treatment for roseola?

Aspirin is given for the high temperature. Sponging is also helpful during the period of high temperature. If there are convulsions, it may be necessary to give a sedative. Usually it is not possible to bring down the temperature to normal before the fourth day of the disease process.

### At what season is roseola seen most often?

In the winter and spring months, although it may occur at any season of the year.

### Is roseola highly contagious?

No.

### Does it occur in epidemics?

In some orphanages or institutions, epidemics take place, but it is not commonly encountered in epidemic form elsewhere.

### Is it necessary to isolate a child with roseola?

No.

## SCARLET FEVER
### (Scarlatina)

### What is scarlet fever?

It is a contagious disease of childhood usually caused by a streptococcus. It does not occur very frequently nowadays and seems to be getting progressively milder all the time.

### Who is most likely to develop scarlet fever?

Children of preschool and school age.

### Can babies develop scarlet fever?

Infants under six months usually do not get this disease, as they receive an immunity transmitted from the mother.

### How can one tell if the child has scarlet fever?

The disease usually starts with fever accompanied by sore throat, headache, vomiting, and, occasionally, abdominal pain. The glands in the neck may also be swollen. Within the next eighteen to forty-eight hours, a rash appears on the body.

### Does the rash in scarlet fever appear on all parts of the body?

No. It is usually not present on the face or the palms of the hands or the soles of the feet. It is most prominent in areas of pressure, in the folds of skin, as in the elbows or armpits, and in areas of excessive warmth.

### Does the child's face look flushed with scarlet fever?

Yes. The cheeks and chin are flushed, leaving the area around the mouth looking rather pale.

### Does the rash of scarlet fever usually itch?

No.

### Does the name scarlet fever denote the appearance of the rash?

Yes. The rash has an intensely reddish, scarlet appearance and is made up of tiny spots. These spots are slightly raised, so that when one rubs a hand over the skin it feels somewhat roughened, like sandpaper.

### What are the findings on examining the tongue and throat?

In scarlet fever, the child has a severe sore throat and a coating of the tongue, which are characteristics of the disease.

### Are there any tests to make a positive diagnosis of scarlet fever?

Yes. If one gets a culture of the throat, it will show the streptococcus.

**How long does the fever last?**

With modern treatment, the temperature usually drops to normal within two to three days. In an untreated case, it may last as long as five to seven days.

**Do any further changes take place in the skin of a patient with scarlet fever?**

Yes. About two to three weeks after the appearance of the rash, the child's skin will begin to peel. There will be a fine, flaky peeling of the skin of the abdomen, while the skin of the fingertips around the nails, the palms of the hands, and soles of the feet will peel almost like a glove.

**Do all cases necessarily have skin peeling?**

No. In some cases there is so little peeling that the disease is not recognized. Where peeling does occur, it proves definitely that the child had scarlet fever, even though it may have been a mild case.

**What is the treatment for scarlet fever?**

The child should be kept in bed and sponged if his temperature is very high. He should be put on a soft diet with moderate amounts of fluids. If he has pain he should be given aspirin, which may help alleviate the sore throat and reduce his temperature.

**Is hospitalization necessary in scarlet fever?**

No. Most cases can be treated satisfactorily at home. Only the very severe cases, or those with complications, need to be admitted to a hospital.

**How long a bed stay is necessary?**

In most cases, bed rest is not necessary.

**Are the antibiotics effective in scarlet fever?**

Yes. It is most important that the child be given penicillin. This antibiotic is very effective against scarlet fever and will promptly make the rash fade, the temperature come down, and all symptoms diminish or disappear.

**How should the penicillin be given?**

By injection for a few days, followed by medicine by mouth for ten days.

**Does the child with scarlet fever need to be quarantined?**

Yes, for about seven days. In some communities there is a longer period of quarantine, but this does not appear to be necessary with more modern methods of treatment.

**How long does the convalescent period last in scarlet fever?**

One to two weeks.

**Should the child be prevented from engaging in athletics during convalescence?**

Yes.

**Can the child return to school after the first week of the illness?**

Yes, the child may return to school, but he should be very careful to limit physical activity.

**How often do complications of scarlet fever occur?**

Very seldom.

**What are the complications of scarlet fever when they do occur?**

The most frequent complications are swelling of the glands of the neck, infection of the ears or sinuses, kidney infection or nephritis, and in some cases, rheumatic fever.

**If there are complications, when will they appear?**

The ear, sinus, and gland complications may appear during the height of the illness. Rheumatic fever or nephritis, if either ensues, may appear two to three weeks after the height of the illness.

**What treatment is carried out for the complications of scarlet fever?**

The ear, gland, or sinus infection is treated with antibiotics. Rheumatic fever or kidney complications should be treated by specific routines. (See Chapter 62, on Rheumatic Fever; and Chapter 37, on Kidney Disease.)

**Is it possible to prevent the development of complications?**

Yes. With adequate antibiotic therapy in scarlet fever, complications seldom occur.

**Is special diet necessary during scarlet fever?**

A mild, bland diet with plenty of liquids is indicated.

**Is a protein diet harmful, or will it lead to a kidney complication?**

No. It is not believed that the presence of meat or proteins in the diet will in any way affect the appearance of kidney complications.

**Is a child permanently immune after an attack of scarlet fever?**

Usually, yes. However, there have been instances of recurrence of this disease in a small percentage of cases.

**Will penicillin help to prevent scarlet fever from developing?**

Yes, and if it does develop, it will assume a mild form.

**Do the clothes and articles of the scarlet fever patient need to be sterilized?**

It is preferable that they be washed thoroughly with soap and water.

**Can scarlet fever be spread by contact with infected clothing?**

Yes.

**What should be done with contacts of a case of scarlet fever?**

All children who are exposed should be given penicillin, either orally or by injection, for several days. Throat cultures should be taken if they become ill.

## WHOOPING COUGH
### (Pertussis)

**What is whooping cough?**

It is a contagious disease of the respiratory system caused by a specific germ.

**How is whooping cough spread?**

By sneezing, coughing, or droplet infection from a child who has had the disease.

**Can young babies get whooping cough?**

Yes. There is no inherited immunity to this disease.

**What are the symptoms of whooping cough?**

It resembles an ordinary cold, for about a week. There is slight fever. In the second week, the child coughs a great deal and begins the characteristic whooping sound.

**Can the disease be recognized during the first week?**

Usually not.

**At what time of day does the child cough most?**

At night, or when indoors, or when eating.

**Is the characteristic cough easily recognized?**

Yes. The child looks "bleary-eyed" and has spasms of coughing associated with redness of the face and swelling of the eyes.

**What does the whoop sound like?**

After a series of coughs the child takes a deep, noisy breath that has a crowing sound.

**How long does the spasmodic coughing stage last?**

Anywhere from three to six weeks.

**Is there any vomiting after the cough?**

Yes. Vomiting is quite frequent after a series of coughing spasms.

**How long does it take until all of the coughing disappears?**

It may take six to twelve weeks before all coughing stops.

**Does a baby always cough and whoop?**

No. Some babies with whooping cough, particularly very young ones, may merely have a few coughing paroxysms and then seem to lose their breath.

**Does a child tend to cough more when lying down?**

Yes. The accumulation of mucus in the back of the throat tickles and causes more frequent paroxysms.

**How many paroxysms of coughing usually occur during a day?**

In mild cases, there may be only five to fifteen per day. In severe cases, there may be thirty, forty, or even more.

**Is there anything that can be done to help the child during a coughing spasm?**

Yes. Keep the child in an upright position during the paroxysm with the head bent somewhat forward.

**Are there any tests to make a more positive diagnosis of whooping cough?**

Yes. Cultures can be made from swabbings from the throat. Also, blood tests are sometimes helpful when the diagnosis is in doubt.

**Is it necessary to hospitalize a child with whooping cough?**

No. Only the severe cases, or very young children, need to be hospitalized.

**Does the child need to stay in bed?**

Yes, during the first week when there is an elevation of temperature.

**Can a child with whooping cough be allowed outdoors?**

Yes, after the first week when his temperature is normal.

**Should whooping cough cases be kept away from other children?**

Yes. The child should be quarantined if possible.

**For how long should the child be quarantined?**

In most communities, the quarantine period is from four to six weeks.

**Can the child transmit the disease during the entire coughing period?**

No. The disease is usually transmitted during the first four weeks, rarely thereafter.

**Can children attend school with this disease?**

No. They should not be in contact with other children.

**When may the child be permitted to return to school?**

Usually five weeks after the coughing has commenced.

**Are there ever recurrences of whooping cough?**

It is rare to have a recurrence, but there have been a few such cases on record.

**What are the aftereffects of whooping cough?**

For a year after an attack, it is not unusual for a child to develop paroxysms of coughing with each cold or upper respiratory infection.

**Are these recurrent paroxysms infectious?**

No.

**What is the treatment for whooping cough?**

The child should be kept at rest as much as possible during the first week of the disease.

**Is there any special diet in whooping cough?**

Yes. The diet should be light and bland.

**Will the nutrition suffer if there is repeated vomiting in a whooping cough case?**

Yes, it is one of the common complications. Young infants who vomit should be fed again within twenty to thirty minutes.

**Are drugs helpful in treating whooping cough?**

Yes. The antibiotics help considerably, although they do not cure the condition.

**Is there any serum that is useful in the treatment of this disease?**

Yes. Hyperimmune serum helps reduce the number of paroxysms.

**Can hyperimmune serum be used to prevent whooping cough?**

Yes. It helps prevent the disease when given to exposed contacts.

**What are the complications of whooping cough?**

Ear inflammations, pneumonia, or, in some severe cases, convulsions.

**How frequently do these complications occur?**

They are very infrequent at the present time.

**Can the complications be successfully treated?**

Yes. Pneumonia and ear inflammation are treated with the antibiotic drugs.

**Are the convulsions a serious manifestation of the disease?**

When convulsions occur, it is an indication of brain involvement and is usually a serious sign.

**Are there any other complications?**

Yes. Occasionally there is a small hemorrhage in the eye or small hemorrhages around the neck as a result of the coughing paroxysms. These are not serious complications and will disappear by themselves without treatment.

**Is there any way to immunize a child against whooping cough?**

Yes. Every child should be given whooping cough vaccine. (See Chapter 31, on Immunizations and Vaccinations.)

**Is there any harm from these injections?**

No. Millions of children have received them without harmful effects.

**Will whooping cough clear up by itself without treatment?**

Yes. It will last for six to twelve weeks and then disappear by itself.

**How soon can an infant with whooping cough be bathed?**

Sponge baths should be given until the fourth week of the disease; thereafter, a regular bath may be given.

**Will athletics or physical exertion induce paroxysms of coughing?**

Yes.

**Is it necessary to take x rays of the chest in the average case of whooping cough?**

No. But if there is anything suspicious about the cough or the diagnosis, it is best to have an x ray taken of the chest.

**What treatment should be given to contacts of a child with whooping cough?**

If the children have received inoculations previously, they should be given a booster injection when exposed to the disease.

**What should be done for exposed children who have never been inoculated against whooping cough?**

They should be given several doses of convalescent or hyperimmune serum.

**Should adults receive inoculations if they have been exposed to whooping cough?**

In most instances it is not necessary; most adults are immune to this disease.

**If an adult has not had whooping cough in childhood, can he contract the disease?**

Yes.

**Can a child get whooping cough even if he has been immunized?**

Yes. A milder form of the disease may be caused by a different strain of bacteria.

**Does the family have to be quarantined when there is a case of whooping cough?**

No. Unimmunized children should be kept away from others; but those who have been immunized, and the adult members of the family, can go about their normal activity.

**Is there any test to determine whether a child is immune after he has had the injections?**

Yes. There are tests, but these are usually not practical and are not used routinely.

**Does whooping cough occur more often during certain months of the year?**

Yes, it is most frequent in the winter and spring and least frequent in the summer and autumn.

*(continued)*

## CONTAGIOUS DISEASES

| Disease | Chickenpox | Diphtheria | German Measles |
|---|---|---|---|
| Other Names | Varicella | | Rubella |
| Cause | Chickenpox virus | Diphtheria bacillus | Rubella virus |
| How Transmitted | Direct contact, droplet infection | Contact with patient or carrier | Direct and droplet contact |
| Incubation Period | 14–21 days | 2–5 days | 14–21 days |
| When Communicable | One day before rash, 6 days after rash appears | From onset of disease until 2 weeks later | Two days before symptoms to 3 days after symptoms |
| Major Symptoms | Fever, rash, itching | Fever, sore throat, hoarseness, membrane in throat | Fever, slight respiratory signs, enlarged glands |
| Rash | Individual spots, blisters, scabs, crusts | None | Resembles measles first day. Resembles scarlet fever second day |
| Laboratory Tests | None practical | Culture of membrane, Schick test | None practical |
| Common Complications | Secondary infections, rare encephalitis | Myocarditis, neuritis, paralysis of palate, cervical adenitis | Encephalitis rarely, usually none |
| Treatment | Symptomatic for itching, fever, no antibiotics | Antitoxin, penicillin | General care, no antibiotics |
| Prevention | None | Immunization with diphtheria toxoid. See Immunization Chart, Chapter 31 | German measles vaccine |
| Quarantine | Not necessary | Yes, until 2 throat cultures are negative | None |
| Immunity | Permanent | Permanent, boosters for prevention | Permanent |

## CONTAGIOUS DISEASES

| Disease | Measles | Mumps | Poliomyelitis |
|---|---|---|---|
| **Other Names** | Rubeola | Epidemic parotitis | Infantile paralysis |
| **Cause** | Measles virus | Mumps virus | Polio virus: Types I, II, III |
| **How Transmitted** | Direct and droplet contact | Droplet and direct contact | Direct and droplet, possibly through infected water and food |
| **Incubation Period** | 10–14 days | 12–24 days | 7–14 days |
| **When Communicable** | One day before fever, to total appearance of rash | One day before swelling; as long as swelling lasts | Two days before onset until 3–6 weeks later |
| **Major Symptoms** | Fever, cough, conjunctivitis, Koplik's spots | Fever, swelling of face, swelling under jaws | Fever, nausea, vomiting, diarrhea, sore throat, headache, stiff neck, muscle pains, paralysis |
| **Rash** | From head downward: reddish-purple spots coalescing | None | None |
| **Laboratory Tests** | None practical | None practical | Spinal fluid examination |
| **Common Complications** | Ear infections, cervical adenitis, bronchopneumonia, encephalitis | Orchitis, pancreatitis, ovaritis, encephalitis | Various types; spinal, bulbar, respiratory |
| **Treatment** | Sponging, general care, no antibiotics | General care, no sour drinks, bed rest | Rest; symptomatic care; respirator if necessary; later, orthopedic care |
| **Prevention** | Measles vaccine. Also, gamma globulin for contacts | Mumps vaccine. Hyperimmune serum for adults | Polio vaccine |
| **Quarantine** | Until rash is fading | Duration of swelling | 10–30 days |
| **Immunity** | Permanent | Permanent | Permanent |

# CONTAGIOUS DISEASES

| Disease | Roseola | Scarlet Fever | Whooping Cough |
|---|---|---|---|
| **Other Names** | Exanthem subitum | Scarlatina | Pertussis |
| **Cause** | Virus | Streptococcus | Pertussis bacillus |
| **How Transmitted** | Not definitely known | Direct contact, occasionally by milk, maybe cooking | Direct contact and coughing |
| **Incubation Period** | 7–17 days | 2–7 days | 7–14 days |
| **When Communicable** | Not known | From onset of disease until 7 days later | During early states of cough, for about 3–4 weeks |
| **Major Symptoms** | Fever for 3 days, then rash appears; enlarged lymph glands | Fever, sore throat, headache, vomiting | Like cold at onset, later cough becomes paroxysmal; vomiting |
| **Rash** | Like many flea bites over body, may resemble mild measles | Pinpoint scarlet-colored rash on body, not on face | None |
| **Laboratory Tests** | None | Throat culture | Cough plate and blood count may help |
| **Common Complications** | Convulsions | Ear infections, adenitis, nephritis, rheumatic fever | Pneumonia, encephalitis |
| **Treatment** | General care | Penicillin for 10 days | Hyperimmune serum, antibiotics may help |
| **Prevention** | None | Penicillin for contacts | Vaccine injections in infancy, plus booster injections |
| **Quarantine** | None | 1 week | 3–4 weeks from school |
| **Immunity** | Permanent | Permanent | Permanent |

# CHAPTER 19

# DIABETES MELLITUS

*(See also Chapter 38 on Laboratory (Pathology) Tests and Procedures; Chapter 20 on Diet; Chapter 49 on Pancreas)*

### What is diabetes mellitus?

A chemical disorder of the body primarily involving an inability to utilize sugar and other chemical compounds properly. It is characterized by an elevation in the concentration of sugar in the blood and also by the appearance of sugar in the urine.

### What causes diabetes?

The inability of the pancreas to secrete sufficient amounts of insulin. However, there are many other complex chemical factors involving an imbalance between the various glands within the body. Recent research would indicate that many such patients have their insulin abnormally bound up with other proteins in the bloodstream so that it becomes ineffective.

### What are some of the predisposing factors in the development of diabetes?

Although the exact cause of this disease is unknown, it is known that the disease occurs much more frequently in people who have a family history of diabetes and who are overweight. Also, the disease will occur much more frequently in people who have abnormal function of the pancreas, liver, adrenal glands, pituitary gland, or other related structures.

### How common is diabetes?

It is estimated that 1.5–2 percent of the entire population has diabetes. Many of these people are unaware of its presence, because they have not been thoroughly examined for it.

### Does diabetes occur in children?

Yes, it can occur at any age.

### Does diabetes tend to run in families or to be inherited?

It is not directly inherited, but in about one out of four cases there is a family history of the condition.

### Does infection cause diabetes?

Not directly, but it is known that infection will aggravate or intensify a preexisting diabetes or make the condition more apparent. The only type of direct infection that will cause the disease is an abscess or infection that might destroy a large portion of the pancreatic gland. This is a rare occurrence.

### Will the eating of an excessive amount of sweets or carbohydrates cause diabetes?

No, but it may aggravate and bring to light an underlying tendency toward the disease.

### Will emotional strain cause diabetes?

Not directly, but it is known that diabetes may become worse or be brought to the fore by emotional crises.

### What are the symptoms of diabetes?

a. Mild cases may have no symptoms whatever. In this type of case, the disease may be discovered merely by the finding of sugar on routine urine analysis, or by blood sugar determinations.
b. In the more severe cases, symptoms include excessive thirst, excessive urination, weight loss, loss of strength and energy.

Occasionally, the first evidence of the disease may be the onset of coma (unconsciousness), because the disease has progressed to a profound stage without having been recognized.

### How can a positive diagnosis of diabetes be made?

a. By finding an elevated level of sugar on blood chemical analysis.
b. By finding sugar on urine analysis.
c. By finding a characteristic curve on performance of a glucose tolerance blood test.

### Does the presence of sugar in the urine always mean that the patient has diabetes?

No. There are a number of relatively uncommon conditions aside from diabetes that may cause the urine to show a positive test for sugar.

### Does the absence of sugar in the urine eliminate the possibility of diabetes?

No. Although there may be no sugar in the urine, there may be an elevated concentration of sugar in the blood.

### What is a glucose (sugar) tolerance test?

A patient is given a known quantity of sugar; blood samples are then withdrawn, and urine specimens are collected at intervals over a period of several hours. The concentration of sugar in both the urine and the blood is then calculated. Characteristic findings occur in those who have diabetes.

### Must all people who have diabetes take insulin?

No. This depends on the severity of the condition. Many patients can be controlled adequately by diet alone or by taking oral medication.

### Is there any way to avoid getting diabetes?

If one has only a mild tendency toward the disease, the eating of a balanced diet with a relatively low sugar intake and the keeping of the weight down to normal limits may forestall the onset of diabetes. Also, people should try to avoid infections that may aggravate or bring to the fore a tendency toward this disease.

### What is insulin?

A chemical substance normally secreted into the bloodstream by certain cells within the pancreas. Insulin is vitally important in the proper utilization and handling of sugar by the body. When it is secreted in insufficient amounts, diabetes may result.

### Can diabetes be controlled by giving insulin?

Yes.

### Can insulin be taken by mouth?

No. It must be injected under the skin.

### Who injects insulin?

Patients, even young children, can be taught to give themselves insulin by injection.

### Is it painful to inject oneself with insulin?

There is just a slight prick of the needle, which the diabetic becomes accustomed to within a very short period of time. Even children can be trained to give themselves these injections without minding the slight pain of the needle prick.

### How often is it necessary for diabetics to take insulin?

Usually once or twice a day, in varying amounts, as determined by repeated medical evaluation.

### Once a patient has had to take insulin for his diabetes, does it mean he will have to take it for the rest of his life?

Generally speaking, this is so, although there are a number of exceptions to this rule.

### Does the dosage requirement of insulin change from time to time?

Definitely, yes. It may increase or decrease at varying times.

### How does a patient know what his insulin requirements will be?

It is most important for all diabetics to test their urine themselves at regular intervals. It is also necessary for them to receive instructions from their physicians at regular intervals.

### Is it difficult to test one's urine for sugar?

No. This is a very simple test, which can be learned by anyone in a few minutes' time.

### Can medication taken by mouth control diabetes?

Yes, but it cannot be given to children and will not replace insulin in the more severe cases. Oral antidiabetic medications are most effective for those who contract diabetes later on in life, usually after the age of forty. However, there are certain disadvantages to prolonged use of oral antidiabetic drugs, and they should only be taken under a physician's strict supervision.

### How can a patient tell if his diabetes is being well controlled?

a. By examining his own urine.
b. By having a blood sugar test done at regular intervals.
c. By noting the presence or absence of diabetic symptoms such as excessive thirst, excessive hunger, weight loss, weakness, etc.

### What is meant by "insulin shock" (hypoglycemia)?

Occasionally, the dosage of insulin that the patient takes may cause the blood sugar to drop to an excessively low level. As a result, the patient may experience a variety of sensations, such as tremors, spots before the eyes, sweating, abrupt weakness, dizziness, confusion, and a hollow feeling in the pit of the stomach.

### What can be done to relieve insulin shock?

This can be accomplished readily and rapidly by the taking of orange juice, sugar, or any other substance containing sugar.

### What is meant by acidosis?

Acidosis is a condition denoting that the diabetes is out of control. It is evidenced by the presence of the chemical acetone in the urine. Patients must learn not only to test their urine for the presence of sugar, but also for the presence of acetone.

### Is acidosis harmful?

Yes, because it shows that the diabetes is not under control.

### What can cause acidosis in the diabetic patient?

a. Improper diet.
b. Improper dosage of insulin.
c. Any acute infection or illness that will upset the usual control of diabetes.

### Are diabetics particularly prone to infection?

Yes. In addition, their ability to combat infection is poorer than that of a nondiabetic patient. For this reason, a diabetic must be particularly careful in his personal hygiene and should consult his physician as soon as any minor infection takes place.

### What harm does diabetes do when it continues over many years?

The diabetic is more prone to develop hardening of the arteries (arteriosclerosis) than the nondiabetic. The diabetic has a tendency toward developing, earlier than most people, such illnesses as heart trouble, kidney trouble, eye trouble, nerve trouble, or difficulty with his lower extremities.

### Are these long-range complications of diabetes preventable?

Yes, some are preventable or can be minimized by meticulous care and cooperation between the diabetic patient and his physician. Other complications, unfortunately, are not preventable.

### Can a diabetic look forward to a long and healthy life?

Yes, provided he follows the path laid out for him by his physician. Many diabetics live longer than normal people because they see their physician more frequently and because they have a tendency to regulate their lives more strictly than the nondiabetic.

### What foods should be most carefully avoided by the diabetic?

Foods containing a large quantity of "free sugars," such as candy, pastries, ice cream, cake, and table sugar. Also, foods rich in starch, such as bread, potatoes, spaghetti, and rice, should be used in limited quantities.

### Should women with diabetes become pregnant?

Yes, but they will need special treatment by both their physician and their obstetrician during pregnancy, as complications are more prevalent among diabetics.

### Will diabetic women have normal children?

Yes. The great majority of diabetic women have completely normal children. (See Chapter 57, on Pregnancy and Childbirth.)

### What special care should the diabetic take to avoid infection?

The middle-aged diabetic who has signs of hardening of the arteries must exercise special care of his feet. Infections about the toes and toenails are extremely dangerous in the diabetic as they may lead to uncontrolled infection and gangrene.

### Should the diabetic consult his physician regularly about specific measures for the care and hygiene of the feet?

Definitely, yes.

### What can happen to the diabetic if he fails to take care of himself and to follow medical advice?

a. He may develop an uncontrollable infection leading to loss of a limb or even death.
b. If the diabetes is uncontrolled, acidosis, coma, and death may ensue.

### Does diabetes ever clear up by itself without treatment?

No, although it has been discovered that certain mild cases of diabetes that have been brought to light by an infection or by loss of dietary control will subside when the infection has disappeared or when proper diet has been resumed.

### Can diabetics be operated upon safely?

Yes. With modern methods of management, the diabetic patient can be operated upon with almost as much safety as the nondiabetic.

### Can the diabetic patient live a full, active life without restrictions upon physical activity?

Yes, but it must be remembered that physical activity burns sugar and may alter the requirements for insulin during such periods.

### Does diabetes shorten the span of life?

If a patient has been a diabetic for many years and has been under good control for many years, his life expectancy may approach that of the nondiabetic's. As stated previously, the diabetic's concern for his physical well-being, his care in avoiding infections and other diseases, will often lead to a longer-than-normal life span.

### Is it common for diabetic people to live into their seventies and eighties?

Nowadays this happens more often because of the better care that the diabetic takes of his body.

# CHAPTER 20

# DIET

*(See also Chapter 19 on Diabetes Mellitus; Chapter 29 on Heart; Chapter 40 on Liver; Chapter 70 on Stomach and Duodenum; Chapter 78 on Vitamins)*

## OVERWEIGHT

### What makes people overweight?

In the vast majority of cases, overeating is the sole cause for overweight. In other words, total caloric intake exceeds total caloric needs.

### Do the glands have any effect on one's weight?

There is very little evidence to prove that the glands have anything to do with overweight. Even people with underactive thyroid function can maintain normal weight if they limit their food intake.

### How often does a glandular disorder cause overweight?

Very rarely. The great majority of obese people are overweight because they eat more food than they need.

### Since the thyroid gland controls the metabolic rate, will the administration of thyroid extract cause an overweight individual to lose weight?

No. If an obese patient has normal thyroid function, the giving of thyroid extract will not usually change the metabolic rate. The patient's own thyroid will be less active when thyroid extract is given, and the sum total of thyroid will remain the same.

### Is there any harmful effect from taking too large a dose of thyroid extract in an attempt to reduce?

Definitely, yes. If excessive quantities of thyroid are taken, the metabolic rate may be increased beyond normal limits, and the patient may develop a condition similar to hyperthyroidism. This can, if continued for several months, lead to heart damage.

### Should injections be given for the purpose of weight reduction?

No. It had been the custom until recent years for some doctors to administer injections every few days to help patients lose weight. These medications usually consisted of diuretic drugs, and their results were only temporary because they caused water loss rather than loss of weight due to a decrease in fat tissue. The medical profession now frowns upon this form of treatment because it is convinced that no permanent weight loss results from its use.

### Is it dangerous to receive injections to lose weight?

Not if the medication contains only a diuretic drug. However, if continued for more than a few weeks' time, the medication may seriously alter chemical body reactions.

### Are there any effective medications that will make a patient lose weight?

No. There are some that will cut the appetite temporarily and thus enable the patient to take less food. However, these drugs do not actually create weight loss by altering body function, and their effect is seldom longlasting.

### What medicines are sometimes given to make people lose their appetites?

Most of the drugs belong to the amphetamine group (Benzedrine, Dexedrine, etc.). They often make people less hungry. There are also certain cellulose products that are bulk producers and are supposed to give the patient the sensation that his stomach is full. The amphetamines are habit-forming and should not be prescribed as weight-losing medications.

### Is it harmful to take these medications without a doctor's advice?

Yes. Both the amphetamines and the cellulose products can be very harmful.

### How effective is physical exercise in producing weight loss?

Exercise plays a definite and important role in weight loss. Short, irregular spurts of activity are ineffective, but regular supervised exercise will produce weight loss.

### What is the best way to lose weight?

To eat a properly balanced, medically approved, low-caloric diet. If the patient finds this difficult to do, artificial aids such as medications may be helpful for a short time.

### Should all obese people lose weight?

Yes. However, there are many people, such as those with ulcers or other intestinal upsets, who should lose weight at gradual rates of speed and only under close medical supervision.

### Is obesity hereditary?

No, but it is often influenced by environment. This means that a child who grows up in a family of big eaters will learn to become a big eater himself and therefore will tend to become obese.

### Why do certain individuals who eat huge quantities of food tend to remain thin?

These people may appear to eat tremendously, but in actuality they eat foods of low-caloric volume and often do not "snack." In addition, they are probably more active physically and burn up more calories in this manner. Then there are people who eat large quantities of foods, but who, because of illness such as diabetes and hyperthyroidism, lose weight.

## Why do some people fail to lose weight even when they diet strenuously?

Close study will usually reveal that these people do not diet as carefully or at sufficiently low level of caloric intake as they should to produce a significant weight loss. In control studies, it has been found that it is extremely rare for a patient to adhere to a prescribed diet and fail to lose weight.

## Will all overweight people who diet properly lose weight?

Yes, provided their caloric intake is less than their caloric need.

## Is it natural for women to put on weight at menopause?

Yes, but the menopause itself has relatively little to do with the problem. It is thought that there is a lessened caloric need in all people as they grow older, and many investigators feel that people need a hundred fewer calories a day for each ten years they advance in age beyond middle life. Thus, with the same caloric intake, every ten days an older woman may be receiving a thousand more calories than she needs. This can cause her to gain as much as a pound a month.

## Is there a relationship between the length of a life span and obesity?

Definitely, yes. Life insurance figures show that longevity is decreased in direct proportion to the degree of obesity.

## Of what value are the "miracle diets" one sees advertised so much in newspapers and magazines?

If they are low in caloric value they will cause weight loss. However, if they are unbalanced diets and are continued for any length of time, they may cause serious vitamin or protein deficiencies.

## What value are diets that claim that calories do not count?

All weight-reducing diets must take into consideration total calorie intake. If one eats a diet composed completely of fat, he can lose weight *provided the total calorie intake is below his body's needs.* On the other hand, if he eats a diet completely devoid of fat but containing a total caloric intake in excess of his basic requirements, he will gain weight!

## How does the emotional state of a person affect his weight?

People who are emotionally upset and under tension sometimes overeat and sometimes undereat.

## What is the relationship between overweight and coronary heart disease?

There is definite statistical evidence that coronary heart disease is greater among people who are obese and who eat a high-fat diet.

## What is cholesterol?

A fatty substance found in certain foods and also found on chemical analysis of blood. Cholesterol levels vary markedly in different people.

## Is there a tendency toward a greater incidence of coronary heart disease in people with elevated blood cholesterol?

Yes.

## How does excessive blood cholesterol tend toward coronary disease?

It is thought that high cholesterol levels lead toward premature arteriosclerosis of the coronary artery.

## Can one cut down on the blood cholesterol level by a low-fat, low-cholesterol diet?

This does not always take place, as the body produces its own cholesterol. Thus, strict limitation of cholesterol-rich foods is not always followed by a lowering of blood cholesterol levels.

## What types of fatty foods should be avoided?

Animal fats. Vegetable fats do not seem to cause very much harm or elevation in the blood cholesterol.

## Are massages, so-called slenderizing machines, various types of baths, etc., helpful in making one lose weight?

In actuality, they have no effect upon weight loss! However, they may influence people psychologically so that they tend to eat less. People who take special treatments and spend considerable sums of money do not want to fail or waste the money they are spending. Therefore they eat less.

## Should all people who are dieting strenuously take vitamin supplements?

Yes, if they are on an unbalanced, weight-reducing diet. However, a well-balanced, weight-reducing diet will not require the addition of vitamins.

## Do vitamins tend to increase one's normal appetite?

No.

## Should a patient who is dieting strenuously be checked frequently by his physician?

Yes.

## Is it true that there is a tendency to gain weight when one stops smoking?

Yes, because tobacco smoking has a tendency to cut one's appetite. Also, for want of something better to do, many people who stop smoking will reach for a sweet instead of a cigarette.

## Is it natural for some people to become constipated while they are on a weight-reducing diet?

This occasionally does occur because the total mass of food intake has been reduced. Under such circumstances, medical advice should be sought in order to aid bowel evacuation.

## Does strenuous dieting tend to make one nervous?

Only if the person feels frustrated by eating less than he wishes.

## What can one do to ease the hunger pangs that accompany a strenuous diet?

People who diet for a period of several weeks will become adjusted to the new low-calorie intake. If they can just muster the willpower to endure the first few weeks, they will discover that the hunger pangs will disappear.

## Should children, as well as adults, go on low-calorie diets to lose weight?

Actually, it is very important for children to maintain normal weight. If they develop poor eating habits and become obese in childhood, it will be much more difficult for them to stay thin when they mature.

## Is there such a thing as doing permanent harm to the body by losing too much weight too quickly?

Definitely, yes.

## Do obese people tend to get high blood pressure more often than thin people?

Yes.

## Do obese people tend to develop diabetes more often than thin people?

Yes.

## Do obese people have a tendency to develop tumors more frequently than thin people?

Statistics show that cancer is more common among the obese than among the thin.

## Should salt be restricted in weight-reducing diets?

Salt restriction permits a greater loss of fluid and therefore a greater weight loss. This, however, is a temporary loss.

## Will the drinking of alcoholic beverages tend to produce obesity?

Yes. An average drink contains about a hundred calories and also serves to stimulate appetite.

## Is it possible to carry out "spot" reducing?

No. All of the advertised means for losing weight in certain areas of the body, while not losing it in other areas, are fallacious. There is no efficient method of taking off weight in a particular area of the anatomy.

# UNDERWEIGHT

## What are the most common causes for underweight?

a. Chronic infections or diseases, such as tuberculosis, kidney ailments, chronic liver disorder, etc.
b. Glandular imbalance, such as excess activity of the thyroid gland or malfunction of the pituitary gland.
c. Neurotic manifestations with distaste for eating.
d. Poor eating habits, usually associated with an irregular life, excess physical activity, and too little sleep.

## Is the tendency toward being underweight inherited?

No, but there is a strong environmental factor. In other words, people who come from a family of poor eaters will tend to eat poorly themselves.

## Does emotion play a great part in underweight?

Yes. Some people who are under great emotional strain may eat less and thus lose weight.

## What is the best way to gain weight?

People who are underweight must eat more calories than they use so that there will be some left over to store as fat.

## Should a patient who is chronically underweight be subjected to a thorough examination?

By all means, yes. A thorough search must be carried out to make sure there is no infection or physical cause for underweight.

## Will excess smoking cause some people to be underweight?

Yes, if it interferes with their normal intake of food. The heavy smoker often lacks normal appetite.

## Why is it that some people eat tremendous quantities of food and still remain thin?

Because their tendency is to eat foods of low-caloric value. Such people should be placed upon foods containing higher caloric value, such as cream, eggs, carbohydrates, butter, etc. They may also burn up more energy with more-than-normal activity and less-than-normal amounts of sleep.

## Will vitamin pills help increase weight?

Not if the vitamin intake in the diet is normal. Vitamin pills are helpful only when there is definite vitamin deficiency.

## What is the best way to gain weight?

Eat several full meals a day consisting of foods containing high-caloric value. It may be necessary to develop new eating habits, with four or five meals a day instead of the usual three. Furthermore, if underweight has a psychological cause, it is necessary to get at the source of the emotional upset and attempt to eliminate it.

## How can children be made to gain weight?

By the establishment of regular habits and by training them to avoid excess physical activity and emotional strain. It is never helpful to threaten or punish children if they do not eat their food. This type of treatment may lead to rebellion and lessened food intake.

**Are there any medications that can aid one to eat more?**

There are stimulants that may increase the appetite, but their effectiveness is not great. It is important to discover, however, that no disease process is present that causes inadequate food intake.

## REDUCING DIET (1,000 calories)

|  | INCLUDE | AVOID |
|---|---|---|
| **Breads:** | 2 thin slices of whole wheat or enriched white bread | Hot bread, coffee cake, hot cakes, waffles, sweet rolls |
| **Cereals:** | None | All |
| **Soups:** | Clear broth, bouillon, vegetable soups made of skim milk and vegetables | Creamed or thickened soups |
| **Meat, fish, eggs or cheese:** | 5 ounces of lean beef, chicken, ham, lamb, veal, kidneys, liver, tongue, canned salmon, tuna, shellfish<br>1 egg<br>Dry cottage cheese | Fatty meats, such as goose, pork, sausage, fried meats, fish canned in oil<br>Cheese other than dry cottage cheese, pot cheese, or farmer cheese |
| **Vegetables:** | From 5 percent vegetable group, up to 12 grams of carbohydrates | Dried beans, dried peas |
| **Potato or substitute:** | None | All |
| **Fats:** | 2 teaspoons of butter<br>2 tablespoons of cream | Any other |
| **Fruits:** | Fresh, unsweetened, equivalent to 30 grams of carbohydrates | Sweetened, frozen, or canned fruit, avocado, dried fruit |
| **Desserts:** | Unsweetened custard of skim milk and egg allowance, unsweetened gelatin | Cakes, cookies, ice cream, pastries, puddings, other rich desserts |
| **Sweets:** | None, except saccharin | All |
| **Beverages:** | Coffee, tea, 1 pint of skim milk or fat-free buttermilk | Carbonated beverages, other sweetened drinks, whole milk |
| **Miscellaneous:** | Condiments, salts, and spices | Alcohol, catsup, chili, cream, sauce, gravy, nuts, pickles, relish |

## LOW-FAT (Low-Cholesterol) DIET

| | INCLUDE | AVOID |
|---|---|---|
| **Breads:** | Any made without eggs, butter, or milk | All made with butter, eggs, or milk |
| **Cereals:** | Any | None |
| **Soups:** | Vegetable soup without milk or meat stock | Cream soups, meat soups |
| **Meat, fish, eggs, or cheese:** | Lean beef, chicken, lean ham, lamb, veal, fish (not oily), egg white, dry cottage cheese, farmer cheese, pot cheese | Fatty meats, glandular meats (sweetbreads), fish canned in oil, egg yolk, all other cheese |
| **Vegetables:** | Any cooked without butter or fat | None |
| **Potato or subsitute:** | Potato, hominy, macaroni, rice, all cooked without fat or cream sauce | Noodles made with egg |
| **Fats:** | Vegetable cooking fats and oils (the oils are preferable) | Animal fats, butter, cream, lard, suet |
| **Fruits:** | Any | None |
| **Desserts:** | Angel food cake, gelatin, ices | Ice cream, pastry, Coca-Cola, pie |
| **Sweets:** | Jam, jelly, sugar, hard candy | Candy made with butter, cream, chocolate, cocoa |
| **Beverages:** | Buttermilk, skim milk, coffee, tea, carbonated beverages | Whole milk, cocoa, chocolate |
| **Miscellaneous:** | Popcorn, salt, spices, vinegar | Cream sauce, gravy, buttered popcorn |


## LOW-SALT (High Blood Pressure) DIET

| | INCLUDE | AVOID |
|---|---|---|
| **Breads:** | Salt-free bread and crackers | Any made with baking soda, salt, or baking powder |
| **Cereals:** | Salt-free cereal, puffed rice, puffed wheat, shredded wheat | Any other cereal |
| **Soups:** | Salt-free broth or cream soup with milk allowance | Soup made with salt |
| **Meat, fish, eggs, or cheese:** | Any meat, fowl, or freshwater fish prepared without salt; not more than 1 egg plus 1 egg yolk daily | Salted meats; smoked or canned meats or fish, saltwater fish, shellfish, glandular meat, except liver; all cheeses |
| **Vegetables:** | Any canned, cooked, or raw vegetables prepared without salt | Vegetables prepared with salt (Cardiac patients don't tolerate well: broccoli, brussels sprouts, cabbage, cauliflower, cucumbers, onions, dried peas, green peppers, radishes, turnips) |
| **Potato or substitute:** | Potato, hominy, macaroni, noodles, rice—all prepared without salt | Fried potatoes, potato chips |
| **Fats:** | Salt-free butter, 1/3 cup cream daily, lard, oil, salad dressing, vegetable fat | Salted butter, bacon fat, salted salad dressing |
| **Fruits:** | Any juice; canned, cooked, or raw fruit | Dried fruit with sodium benzoate |
| **Desserts:** | Salt-free desserts, custards, gelatin, ice cream made from milk allowance, unsalted fruit pie, puddings, rennet desserts | Desserts prepared with salt, baking powder, baking soda, or egg white |
| **Sweets:** | Candy, jam, jelly without sodium benzoate, sugar, syrup | Jam or jelly containing sodium benzoate |
| **Beverages:** | Carbonated beverages, coffee, milk (1 pint daily including that used in cooking) | Soft water |
| **Miscellaneous:** | Cocoa unsalted, cream sauce, herbs, spices and vinegar, unsalted nuts | Catsup, chili sauce, gravy, mustard, olives, peanut butter, pickles, popcorn, relishes, salt |

# HIGH-RESIDUE (High-Roughage) DIET

| | INCLUDE | AVOID |
|---|---|---|
| **Breads:** | Whole wheat, graham, dark rye bread | White, enriched, or fine rye bread, white crackers, toast |
| **Cereals:** | Whole-grain cereals | Refined cereals, corn, rice, wheat, dry cereals prepared from cooked oatmeal |
| **Soups:** | Cream soup, vegetable soup | Bouillon, broth |
| **Meat, fish, eggs, or cheese:** | Tough meat containing many fibers | Bacon, tender meat, fish, fowl, canned fish, eggs, cheese |
| **Vegetables:** | All, especially lettuce, celery, cabbage, endive, etc. | None |
| **Potato or substitute:** | Hominy, unrefined rice | Potatoes, macaroni, noodles, refined rice |
| **Fats:** | Any other | Butter, cream, margarine |
| **Fruits:** | All, including fruit skins | None |
| **Desserts:** | Desserts containing fruit or nuts | All plain cakes, cookies, custards, gelatin, ice cream, pies, puddings, rennet desserts without fruit or nuts |
| **Sweets:** | Candy containing fruit or nuts; jam | Hard candy, honey, jelly, sugar, syrup |
| **Beverages:** | Coffee, milk | Carbonated beverages (not iced), decaffeinated coffee |
| **Miscellaneous:** | Nuts, olives, pickles, popcorn, relish | Cream sauce, gravy, peanut butter, spices in moderation, vinegar |

# LOW-RESIDUE (Low-Roughage) DIET

| | INCLUDE | AVOID |
|---|---|---|
| **Breads:** | White, enriched, or fine rye bread, white crackers, toast | Whole wheat, graham, dark rye bread |
| **Cereals:** | Refined cereals, corn, rice, wheat, dry cereals prepared from cooked oatmeal | Whole-grain cereals |
| **Soups:** | Bouillon, broth | Cream soup, vegetable soup |
| **Meat, fish, eggs, or cheese:** | Bacon, tender meat, fish, fowl, canned fish, eggs, cheese | Tough meat containing many fibers |
| **Vegetables:** | None | All, especially lettuce, celery, cabbage, endive, etc. |
| **Potato or substitute:** | Potatoes, macaroni, noodles, refined rice | Hominy, unrefined rice |
| **Fats:** | Butter, cream, margarine | Any other |
| **Fruits:** | None | All, including fruit skins |
| **Desserts:** | All plain cakes, cookies, custards, gelatin, ice cream, pies, puddings, rennet desserts without fruit or nuts | Desserts containing fruit or nuts |
| **Sweets:** | Hard candy, honey, jelly, sugar, syrup | Candy containing fruit or nuts; jam |
| **Beverages:** | Carbonated beverages (not iced), decaffeinated coffee | Coffee, milk |
| **Miscellaneous:** | Cream sauce, gravy, peanut butter, spices in moderation, vinegar | Nuts, olives, pickles, popcorn, relish |

## GOUT (Low-Purine) DIET

| | INCLUDE | AVOID |
|---|---|---|
| **Breads:** | All | None |
| **Cereals:** | All | None |
| **Soups:** | Milk soups made with vegetables | Bouillon, broth, consommé |
| **Meat, eggs, fish, or cheese:** | Fish, fowl, shellfish, meats (except those excluded), eggs, cheese | Kidney, liver, meat extracts, sweetbreads, roe, sardines, anchovies, gravy, broth |
| **Potato or substitute:** | Potatoes, sweet potatoes, hominy, macaroni, rice | Fried potatoes, potato chips |
| **Fats:** | Butter or substitute in moderation | None |
| **Vegetables:** | All except those excluded | Asparagus, beans (lima, navy, or kidney), lentils, mushrooms, peas, spinach |
| **Desserts:** | Simple cakes, cookies, custards, gelatin desserts, puddings, rich desserts in moderation | Mince pie |
| **Sweets:** | All | None, except in cases of obesity |
| **Beverages:** | Carbonated beverages, coffee, milk or milk drinks, tea | None |
| **Miscellaneous:** | Condiments, cream sauce, nuts, salt, spices | Alcohol, gravy, yeast |

## FULL LIQUID DIET

| | INCLUDE | AVOID |
|---|---|---|
| **Breads:** | None | All |
| **Cereals:** | Strained farina, cornmeal or oatmeal gruel | Any other |
| **Soups:** | Broth, strained cream soups | Any other |
| **Meat, fish, eggs, or cheese:** | Raw eggs in beverages | Any other meat, fish, fowl, or cooked eggs |
| **Vegetables:** | Tomato juice and purees in soups, carrotjuice juice | All others |
| **Potato or substitute:** | None except puree in soup | All |
| **Fats:** | Butter, cream, margarine | Any other |
| **Fruits:** | Strained fruit juice | Any other |
| **Desserts:** | Thin custards, plain gelatin desserts, junket, ice cream, sherbet | Any other |
| **Sweets:** | Sugar, plain sugar candy | Any other |
| **Beverages:** | Carbonated beverages, coffee, milk, milk drinks, tea | None |
| **Miscellaneous:** | Spices, salt | Any other |

## AMBULATORY ULCER DIET

| | INCLUDE | AVOID |
|---|---|---|
| **Breads:** | White or fine rye dry toast, crackers, hard rolls | Hot bread, bread containing whole grain, flour, or bran |
| **Cereals:** | Refined corn, farina, rice, or wheat free from outer coating | Cereals containing whole-grain or bran |
| **Soups:** | Cream soup made with allowed vegetables | Meat broth or other cream soups |
| **Meat, fish, eggs, or cheese:** | Bacon, tender or scraped beef and chicken, lamb, liver, sweetbreads, fresh fish, canned tuna or salmon, eggs, cottage or cream cheese, cheddar cheese used in cooking | Any other meat, cheese, or fish |
| **Vegetables:** | Cooked asparagus, beets, carrots, peas, pumpkin, spinach, string beans, squash | Any other |
| **Potato or substitute:** | Potatoes, corn puree, lima bean puree, macaroni, noodles, refined rice | Any other |
| **Fats:** | Butter or substitute, cream | Any other |
| **Fruits:** | Ripe bananas or avocados, baked, canned, or stewed apples, apricots, cherries, peaches, or pears, puree of dried fruit—all without skin or seeds—orange juice diluted with an equal amount of water | Any other |
| **Desserts:** | Angel food or sponge cake, plain vanilla, arrowroot, or sugar cookies and custards, gelatin desserts, ice cream, rennet desserts, rice pudding, tapioca cream—all without fruit or nuts—apricots, prune whip | Any other |
| **Sweets:** | Jelly and sugar in moderation | Jam, marmalade |
| **Beverages:** | Milk, milk drinks, weak tea, decaffeinated coffee | Carbonated drinks, coffee, very hot or very cold drinks |
| **Miscellaneous:** | Cream sauce, salt | Alcohol, condiments, gravy, nuts, pickles, spices |

## HIGH CALORIE DIET FOR UNDERWEIGHT

| | |
|---|---|
| **Breads:** | Any, especially whole-grain or enriched bread |
| **Cereals:** | Any, especially whole-grain or enriched cereal |
| **Soups:** | Any |
| **Meat, fish, eggs, or cheese:** | At least 1 egg and two servings daily of meat or substitute, such as eggs or cheese |
| **Vegetables:** | Any vegetable canned, cooked, or raw |
| **Potato or substitute:** | Any |
| **Fats:** | Butter, cream, lard, margarine, oil, salad dressing |
| **Fruits:** | Any choice of fruit canned, cooked, dried, or fresh |
| **Desserts:** | Cakes, cookies, ice cream, pies, puddings, others |
| **Sweets:** | Candy, jelly, sugar, others |
| **Beverages:** | Any beverage, especially those high in calories |
| **Miscellaneous:** | Condiments, gravy, nuts, salt, spices, vinegar |

## ELIMINATION DIET FOR ALLERGIC PATIENTS

|  | INCLUDE | AVOID |
|---|---|---|
| **Breads:** | Quick bread, yeast bread, crackers—all made without eggs | Bread, quick bread, or rolls containing eggs or nuts |
| **Cereals:** | Any except chocolate-flavored | Chocolate-flavored cereals |
| **Soups:** | Any made from foods allowed | Unusual soups |
| **Meat, fish, eggs, or cheese:** | Any meat or fowl except fresh pork; cottage cheese | Fresh pork, fish, other seafood, cheese except cottage, eggs |
| **Vegetables:** | Common fresh vegetables in season year round, all canned or cooked vegetables | Seasonal vegetables such as corn, tomatoes |
| **Potato or substitute:** | Potatoes, hominy, macaroni, rice | Noodles containing eggs |
| **Fats:** | Butter, cream, French dressing without pepper, lard, margarine, oil | Salad dressings with pepper or eggs |
| **Fruits:** | Common fresh fruits in season all year round; all canned or cooked fruits | Fresh fruits in season only part of year, such as fresh berries or melon |
| **Desserts:** | All cakes, cookies, gelatin desserts, ice cream, puddings, rennet desserts—without chocolate, cocoa, eggs, or nuts | All baked custards—containing chocolate, cocoa, eggs, or nuts |
| **Sweets:** | Hard candy, honey, jam, jelly, sugar, syrup | Candy with chocolate, eggs, or nuts |
| **Beverages:** | Carbonated beverages, decaffeinated coffee, milk | Cocoa, coffee, tea |
| **Miscellaneous:** | Cream sauce, gravy, salt, most spices, vinegar | Chocolate, cocoa, nuts, pepper, any odd or unusual food or flavoring |

## LOW-CARBOHYDRATE DIET

|  | INCLUDE | AVOID |
|---|---|---|
| **Breads:** | 2 slices of plain bread | Any other type of bread |
| **Cereals:** | ½ cup of cooked cereal daily | Cereals with sugar added |
| **Soups:** | Bouillon, cream of vegetable | Thickened soups |
| **Meat, fish, eggs, or cheese:** | Any, plainly cooked in moderate amounts | Those cooked with excessive amounts of gravy |
| **Vegetables:** | Vegetables in the 5 or 10 percent grouping | Those in the 15 or 20 percent grouping |
| **Potato or substitute:** | None | Potatoes come in the 15 percent grouping and should be avoided |
| **Fats:** | Any in moderation | None |
| **Fruits:** | Any canned or cooked fruits without sugar, or fresh fruit in moderation | Ordinary canned fruit, dried or frozen fruit |
| **Desserts:** | Gelatin sweetened with saccharin | Cakes, pastries, pies, ice cream |
| **Sweets:** | Saccharin | All others |
| **Beverages:** | Coffee, tea, milk | Carbonated and other sweet beverages |
| **Miscellaneous:** | Condiments, dill pickles, spices, vinegar | Beer, catsup, cream sauce, gravy, sweet pickles, relishes, sweet wine |

## PERCENTAGE OF CARBOHYDRATES

| 5 percent<br>Vegetables | 10 percent<br>Vegetables and Fruits | | 15 percent<br>Vegetables and Fruits | 20 percent<br>Vegetables |
|---|---|---|---|---|
| asparagus | beets | lemons | artichokes | lima beans |
| string beans | pumpkin | grapefruit | potatoes | navy beans |
| watercress | turnips | cantaloupe | parsnip | fresh corn |
| beet greens | carrots | strawberries | baked beans | baked rice |
| celery | olives | pineapple | apples | |
| cucumbers | oranges | fresh string beans | bananas | |
| cabbage | | | huckleberries | |
| tomatoes | | | blueberries | |
| lettuce | | | pears | |
| eggplant | | | grapes | |
| dandelion greens | | | | |

## CALORIC VALUES

| Cereals & Breadstuffs | Calories |
|---|---|
| Bran muffin | 49 |
| Cornflakes, ½ cup | 50 |
| Cream of Wheat, ½ cup | 75 |
| Farina, ½ cup | 68 |
| Hominy (cooked) ⅔ cup | 88 |
| Melba toast, 1 slice | 25 |
| Oatmeal, ½ cup | 75 |
| Rice (boiled), ½ cup | 80 |
| Rye or white bread, 1 slice | 75 |
| Saltine cracker, 1 | 10 |
| Shredded Wheat, 1 biscuit | 105 |
| Uneeda Biscuit, 1 biscuit | 20 |

| Vegetables | Calories |
|---|---|
| Artichoke, 1 large | 64 |
| Asparagus, 8 tips | 20 |
| Beet soup, 1 cup | 90 |
| Beets, ¾ cup | 48 |
| Brussels sprouts, ⅔ cup | 20 |
| Cabbage (cooked), ¾ cup | 25 |
| Carrots, ¾ cup | 40 |
| Cauliflower, ¾ cup | 28 |
| Celery, 3 stalks | 15 |
| Cucumber, 10 slices | 15 |
| Eggplant, ½ cup | 25 |
| Endive, 10 medium stalks | 16 |
| Green peas (canned), ¾ cup | 56 |
| Green peas (fresh), ½ cup | 96 |
| Lettuce, ¼ small head | 15 |
| Lima beans (fresh), ¾ cup | 116 |
| Navy beans, ⅓ cup | 100 |
| Okra, ½ cup | 36 |

| | Calories |
|---|---|
| Onions, 4 small | 48 |
| Peppers, 2 small | 25 |
| Potatoes, ¼ cup mashed | 50 |
| Pumpkin, ½ cup | 24 |
| Radishes, 5 medium | 8 |
| Rhubarb, ¾ cup | 16 |
| Scallions, 3 small | 48 |
| Spinach (cooked), ½ cup | 30 |
| Spinach soup, 1 cup | 85 |
| Squash, ½ cup | 40 |
| String beans, ½ cup | 25 |
| Tomato (fresh), 1 medium | 20 |
| Turnips, ¾ cup | 35 |
| Vegetable soup, 1 cup | 75 |
| Watercress, 10 pieces | 8 |

| Beverages | Calories |
|---|---|
| Ale, 8 oz. | 130 |
| Beer, 8 oz. | 110 |
| Carbonated soda, 6 oz. | 80 |
| Chocolate malted milk, 10 oz. | 450 |
| Club soda, 8 oz. | 5 |
| Ginger ale, 6 oz. | 60 |
| Manhattan | 175 |
| Martini | 150 |
| Sherry, 2 oz. | 60 |
| Scotch, bourbon, or rye, 1 oz. | 80 |
| Tea or coffee, plain | 0 |
| Tea or coffee, with 2 tbsp.<br>cream and 2 tsp. sugar | 90 |
| Wine, 4 oz. | 80-120 |

| Meats & Fish | Calories |
|---|---|
| Bacon (crisp), 1 slice | 30 |
| Bass, 1 small piece | 45 |
| Brook trout, 1 small piece | 45 |
| Haddock, 1 small piece | 50 |
| Halibut, 1 small piece | 63 |
| Ham, 1 average slice | 100 |
| Hamburger steaks, 2 cakes | 85 |
| Lamb chop, 1 medium | 157 |
| Liver, broiled, 1 average slice | 100 |
| Oysters, 6 large | 50 |
| Pork chop (lean), 1 | 100 |
| Roast beef (lean), 1 slice | 85 |
| Roast lamb (lean), 1 slice | 95 |
| Round steak (lean), 1 slice | 85 |
| Salmon (canned), ½ cup | 100 |
| Tuna fish (canned), ½ cup | 100 |

| Dairy Products | Calories |
|---|---|
| American Cheese, 1 in. square | 87 |
| Butter, 1 tsp. | 50 |
| Buttermilk, 8 oz. | 75 |
| Cottage cheese, ¼ cup | 65 |
| Cream cheese, ⅜ cake | 87 |
| Cream (heavy), ½ tbsp. | 35 |
| Egg, 1 | 75 |
| Milk, 1 average glass | 125 |
| Skim milk, 6 oz. | 90 |
| Swiss cheese, 1 thin slice | 61 |

*(continued)*

| Fruits & Nuts | Calories |
|---|---|
| Apple, 1 small | 55 |
| Applesauce, ½ cup, no sugar | 84 |
| Apricots (fresh), 3 small | 56 |
| Banana, 1 small | 92 |
| Blueberries, ⅔ cup | 52 |
| Cherries, 12 medium | 68 |
| Cranberries, ⅔ cup | 44 |
| Grapefruit, ¼ small | 20 |
| Grapes (fresh), 24 | 89 |
| Lemon, 1 medium | 16 |
| Orange, ½ medium | 25 |
| Orange juice, ½ cup | 56 |
| Peach (fresh), 1 medium | 40 |
| Pineapple (fresh or canned) without sugar, 1 slice | 40 |
| Pear (fresh), 1 medium | 56 |
| Prunes, 3 cooked | 75 |
| Watermelon, ½ cup cut in cubes | 28 |
| Almonds, 10 | 130 |
| Cashews, 10 | 60 |
| Peanuts, 10 | 60 |
| Pecans, 10 halves | 150 |

| Desserts & Sweets | Calories |
|---|---|
| Chocolate bar | 190 |
| With nuts | 275 |
| Chocolate cream bonbon or fudge, 1 in. square | 90 |
| Custard pie, 1 average serving | 360 |
| Fruit pie, 1 average serving | 560 |
| Lemon meringue pie, 1 average serving | 470 |
| Pumpkin pie, 1 average serving | 460 |
| Fruit cake | 125 |
| Layer cake, iced | 340 |
| Ice cream, 1/6 qt. (vanilla) | 200 |
| Other flavors | 230 |
| Ice-cream soda, 10 oz. | 270 |
| Milk sherbet, 1/6 qt. | 250 |
| Sundae with nuts and whipped cream | 400 |

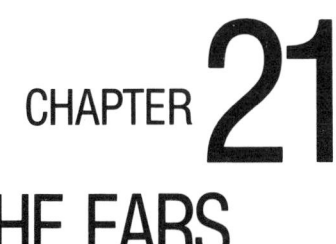

# CHAPTER 21
# THE EARS

*(See also Chapter 18 on Contagious Diseases; Chapter 48 on Nose and Sinuses; Chapter 56 on Plastic Surgery)*

**How does normal hearing take place?**

Sound waves enter the external ear canal and strike the eardrum, causing it to vibrate. On the inner aspect of the drum are three tiny bones—the malleus, incus, and stapes. Drum vibrations are transmitted to these bones, which, in turn, vibrate and transmit the impulses to the inner ear. The inner ear is filled with a fluid surrounded by a membrane. When the stapes vibrates, the impulses are conveyed through the fluid to special nerve endings. The impulses then travel up the nerve endings to the auditory nerve, which carries them to the brain, where they are recorded as hearing.

**Are there normal variations in sensitivity of hearing?**

Yes. Certain individuals have a more highly developed sense of hearing than others.

**How can one determine accurately how well he hears?**

Accurate measurements can be taken by use of an instrument called an audiometer. Such hearing tests will show accurately the range of hearing in each ear and thus determine sensitivity or loss.

**Is it true that if a person concentrates greatly on something, he may block out sounds that are taking place within earshot?**

Yes. Even though the sound waves are transmitted in the normal manner, the control of the brain is sufficiently strong so that it does not record in the conscious mind the sounds taking place.

**Can the ears be damaged by too loud a sound or by an explosion?**

Yes. Many men today have deficient hearing because of explosions that took place while they served in the armed forces. Also, exposure over a period of years to loud noises, as in factory work, may have a damaging effect upon hearing.

## WAX (CERUMEN) IN THE EARS

**Does wax occur normally in all ear canals?**

Yes. It is secreted normally in all people.

**What causes excessive wax in the ears?**

The exact cause is unknown, but for some reason the wax-secreting glands become overactive and may produce large quantities of the substance.

**What are the symptoms of excessive wax in the ears?**

Sudden loss of hearing. This may occur following a bath, shower, or a swim. The wax becomes softened by the water, and as it dries it forms in such a way that it closes and obstructs the ear canal.

**What is the treatment for wax in the ears?**

It should be removed by a physician. It must be done carefully to prevent damage to the eardrum. The physician may prescribe certain medications to be instilled in the ear canal for a day or two prior to syringing out the wax.

**Should an individual attempt to remove the wax by himself?**

Absolutely not. Great damage has been done to the ear and the eardrum by attempts to remove the wax by oneself.

**Does excessive wax cause permanent damage?**

No. If there is loss of hearing due to excessive wax, hearing will return immediately upon its removal.

**Should people with excessive wax formation receive periodic examinations?**

Yes. It is wise for them to have their physician examine their ear canals once a year, or whenever their ear canals appear to be obstructed.

## PAIN IN THE EAR CANAL

**What causes pain in the ear canal?**

It is usually inflammatory in origin and may be caused by a pimple, a boil, eczema, an injury, or a foreign body that has gotten into the canal.

**What is the treatment for an infection of the ear canal?**

a. Packing (medicated) inserted in the ear canal.
b. If an abscess has formed, it should be incised.
c. Medications to relieve the severe pain should be prescribed.
d. Antibiotics should be prescribed.

**Are fungus infections of the ear canal common?**

Yes. Some are chronic in nature and will require extensive treatment with antifungal drugs before subsiding.

## MIDDLE EAR

**Where is the middle ear and what is its function?**

It is on the inner side of the eardrum

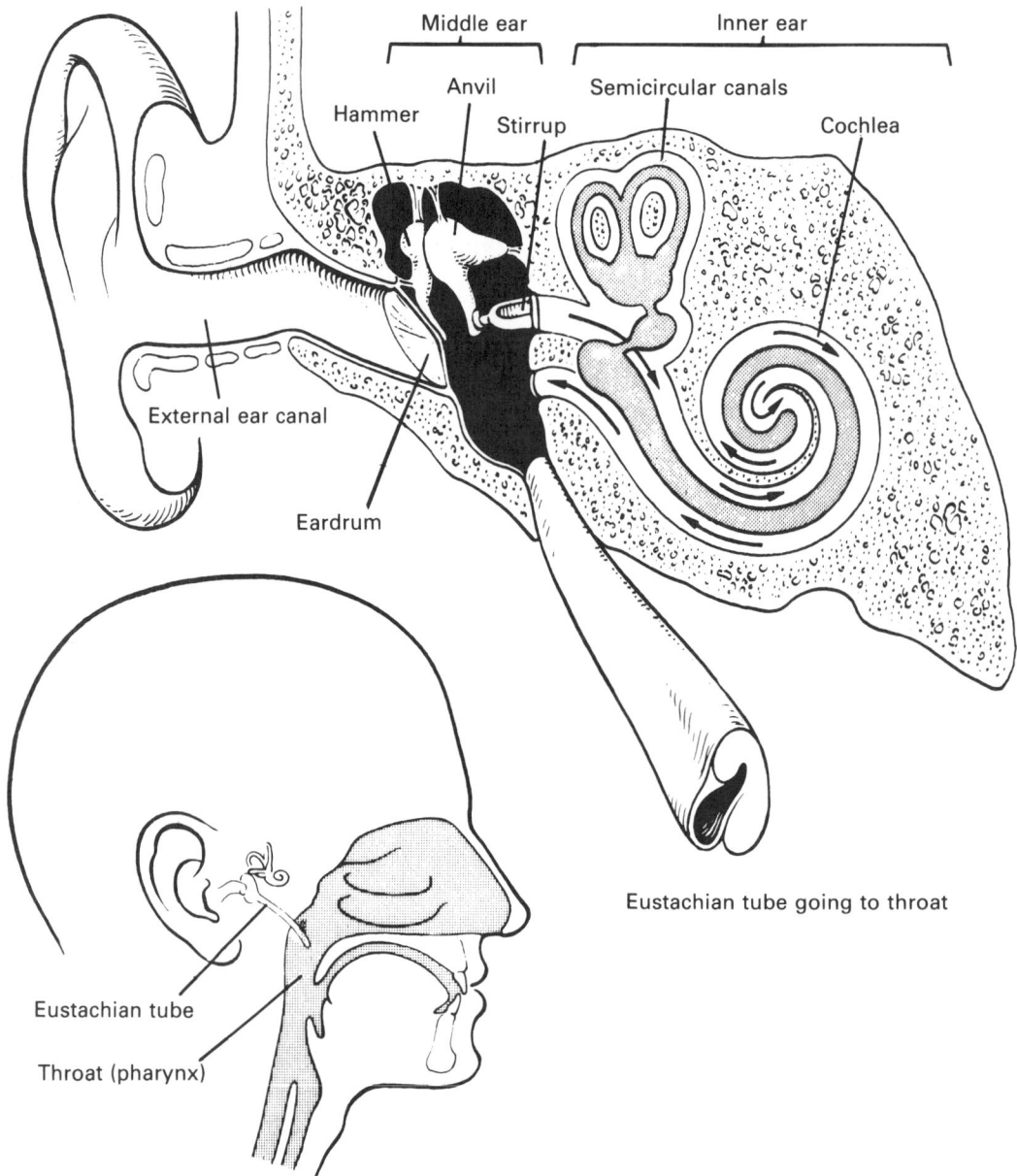

**Anatomy of the Ear.** *Sound waves are picked up and transmitted through the ear canal, eardrum, and the three small bones in the middle ear. The middle ear is connected to the throat by the Eustachian tube, which equalizes air pressure. From the stirrup, one of the three bones of the middle ear, the vibrations are passed through the oval window and into the fluid that fills the inner ear. The inner ear contains two sensory organs, one that controls hearing and one that controls balance (vestibular senses).*

and connects through a narrow passageway (the Eustachian tube) with the back of the throat. It also has a direct connection with the mastoid air cells lodged in the bone behind the ear. The middle ear houses the three little bones that form a link between the eardrum and the inner ear.

## What causes pain in the middle ear?

In most cases this is due to inflammation or infection. Such inflammation is usually secondary to infection of the nose and throat. In children, recurrent attacks of earaches can be indicative of enlarged adenoids. Oc-

casionally, ear pain is due to mucous collection and obstruction of the Eustachian tube.

## What other conditions give rise to ear pain?

Tonsillitis, abscessed teeth, inflammation of the pharynx, sinusitis, or a tumor growth in the middle ear region. There is frequently ear pain following removal of the tonsils.

## MIDDLE EAR INFECTION
*(Otitis Media)*

### What causes otitis media?

Infections of the middle ear are usually secondary to a spread, via the Eustachian tube, of an inflammation such as a cold, throat infection, or inflamed adenoids. The contagious diseases of children, since they are associated with throat inflammation, also lead to middle ear and mastoid infection.

### What are the symptoms of otitis media?

a. Pain in the ear.
b. Impairment of hearing.
c. Rise in temperature.
d. Red and swollen eardrum seen upon examination.
e. Pus discharge through the eardrum into the external ear canal if eardrum has ruptured.

### Are members of certain families more prone to develop otitis media than others?

Yes. Owing to the particular anatomy of the Eustachian tube, certain families inherit a straighter channel. It is easier for infection to travel along the straighter channel than it is when the Eustachian tube is curved and more likely to prevent the spread of infected material.

### What are the harmful results of middle ear infection?

a. Each attack results in slight thickening of the lining mucous membrane of the middle ear. Although one or even several attacks will not necessarily cause deafness, each additional inflammation leaves its mark, and the end result may be loss of hearing.
b. Middle ear infections may not subside and may extend into neighboring structures to cause mastoiditis, labyrinthitis, meningitis, or brain abscess. Repeated attacks of otitis media may result in a chronic middle ear infection, with a perforated eardrum and a persistent discharge of pus from the ear canal.

### What is the treatment for otitis media?

a. The best treatment is prophylactic. Children with diseased or markedly enlarged tonsils and adenoids should have them removed. People with colds should not go swimming or dive. Simple head colds should be treated and not neglected.
b. When infection of the middle ear has already taken place, adequate doses of antibiotics should be given. Nose spray or nose drops should be used to keep the nasal passages open.
c. Medications should be given to relieve the pain if it is very intense.
d. If there is a perforated drum and a discharge of pus from the ear, a specimen of the pus should be cultured and sensitivity tests performed to determine which antibiotic can be used most effectively.
e. In cases where medical measures have failed to overcome the infection, surgery is necessary.

### When is surgery necessary in middle ear infection?

If the eardrum is bulging because of fluid in the middle ear and the condition does not respond to the medical measures previously described, it is advisable to open the eardrums surgically. This procedure is called a myringotomy.

### How is myringotomy performed?

In adults it is done under local anesthesia in the patient's home or the physician's office. A specially devised knife is used, and a small incision is made in the drum to allow the fluid or pus to escape. Although there may be some pain, the entire procedure lasts but a moment or two. Children may require general anesthesia.

### How can one tell whether an infection of the middle ear has spread to involve the mastoid bone?

A mastoid infection should be suspected if:
a. There is an abrupt rise in temperature, with loss of appetite and swelling of the glands in the neck.

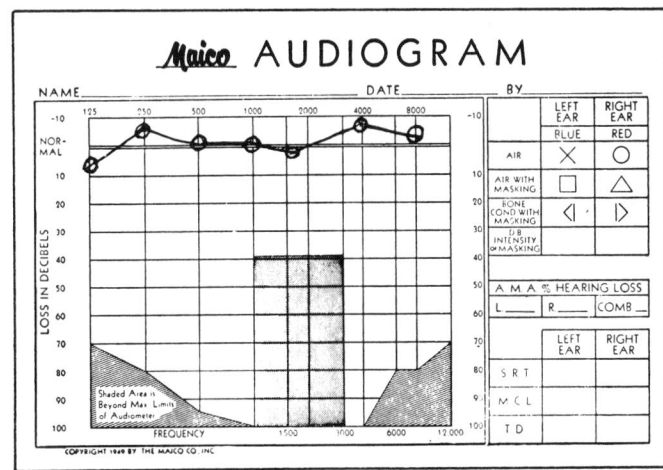

*Audiogram. The audiogram is a graphic summary of the measurements of hearing loss. The particular audiogram shown here demonstrates that the patient has normal hearing.*

b. There is pain behind the ear over the mastoid bone.

c. There is tenderness on direct finger pressure over the mastoid region.

d. There is a pouching forward of the back wall of the external ear canal.

e. There is an increase in the white blood cell count.

f. There are x-ray findings that indicate involvement of the mastoid bones.

g. There is impaired hearing.

h. There is swelling of the soft tissues behind the ear.

## Are mastoid infections very common today?

No. Because of the prompt and adequate treatment of middle ear infections with antibiotics, acute mastoiditis has become a rarity today. On the other hand, chronic mastoid infections are still encountered. Many of these cases are the result of inadequate treatment of a previous acute infection.

## What is the treatment for acute mastoiditis?

Before the advent of sulfa drugs and antibiotics, the wards of hospitals were filled with children suffering from mastoid infections. Today surgery is rarely necessary for this condition. However, when a neglected case of middle ear infection does involve the mastoid bones, intensive treatment with the appropriate antibiotics will frequently clear up the infection. If this does not take place, surgery, with removal of all the infected mastoid cells, is necessary.

## What may happen if a mastoid infection is permitted to go untreated?

a. Paralysis of the facial nerve may take place.

b. A bloodstream infection may take place.

c. Infection may extend into the skull and cause osteomyelitis, meningitis, or brain abscess.

d. A fatality may ultimately result if the condition goes untreated.

## How is a simple mastoidectomy performed?

It may be done through either the ear canal (endaural) or by the postauricular route. In the former, an incision is made within the ear canal extending from the drum outward. In the latter approach, an incision is made behind the ear. In both instances, the infected bone is chipped away until all of the cells are uncovered and found to be healthy. Recently, much more accurate determination of which cells are infected and which are healthy can be made by use of magnifying instruments, which are employed during the operative procedure.

## What type of anesthesia is used for a mastoidectomy?

General anesthesia with use of an endotracheal tube.

## Is mastoidectomy a dangerous operation?

No, but it is a serious one demanding expert skills.

## Is hearing affected by a mastoid operation?

a. Simple mastoidectomy does not impair hearing.

b. Radical mastoidectomy for a chronic ear infection will cause loss of hearing in that ear.

## What is the difference between simple and radical mastoidectomy?

A simple mastoidectomy involves removal of the mastoid air cells only. Radical mastoidectomy involves not only the removal of the mastoid cells but the removal of the eardrum and contents of the middle ear.

## How long does it take to perform a simple mastoidectomy?

Approximately one hour to one-and-a-half or two hours in the more extensive infections.

## Does the ear continue to drain pus even after a mastoidectomy?

Yes, for several days to several weeks.

## Are special preoperative or postoperative medications given with a mastoidectomy?

Yes. Large doses of antibiotics are utilized to control and prevent spread of infection.

## How long a hospital stay is needed for a mastoidectomy?

Seven to ten days.

## Will it be necessary to treat the patient for a long period of time after a mastoidectomy?

Yes, for several weeks.

## Is the scar of a mastoidectomy disfiguring?

No.

## Does mastoid infection often recur after surgery?

No.

## Does mastoidectomy carry with it a high mortality?

No. It is not a dangerous operation.

## Is there much pain after a mastoid operation?

Yes, especially when dressings are changed.

# DEAFNESS

## What causes deafness?

Impairment of hearing may be caused by any interference with the reception or transmission of sound waves along the canal through the middle ear to the inner ear and then along the auditory nerve to the brain.

**When there is deafness of one ear, will the other ear become involved too?**

Deafness may occasionally be limited to one ear when it is secondary to an infection, but this is not the general rule. In most cases, when one ear is involved, the other ear will show a loss of hearing sooner or later.

**Do both ears tend to go deaf at the same time?**

Not necessarily. There may be a wide interval, or there may be no impairment of hearing in the other ear if one ear is affected.

**What kinds of deafness are encountered?**

a. Congenital deafness.
b. Central deafness due to involvement of the brain.
c. Perceptive deafness due to involvement of the internal ear or auditory nerve.
d. Conductive deafness due to involvement of the middle ear or auditory canal.

**What is congenital deafness?**

This is a type with which one is born and is based upon the abnormal development, or lack of development, of the nerve of hearing (acoustic nerve).

**What causes congenital deafness?**

It is thought that many cases occurring in newborns are caused by diseases that the mother had during the first few weeks of the pregnancy. Toxins from certain diseases, such as German measles, are transmitted to the young embryo and cause maldevelopment of the hearing apparatus.

**What happens if a child is born deaf?**

The deaf child cannot hear; therefore, he cannot imitate and thus learn to talk. In other words, the deaf-mute *could* have talked if he had been able to hear and imitate the sounds of speech. There is nothing wrong with the speech mechanism of the deaf-mute.

**Do "deaf-mutes" prefer to be called "nonhearing" people?**

Yes. Many find the term "deaf-mute" objectionable.

**Can a person deaf since birth be taught to talk?**

Many of them can be taught through intensive teaching at schools for the deaf.

**What are some of the causes of inner ear deafness?**

a. Diseases such as mumps, influenza, scarlet fever, and malaria.
b. Drugs such as quinine and salicylates.
c. Occupations such as boilermaking, piloting an airplane, etc.
d. Fractures through the temporal bone of the skull that traverse the ear mechanism.
e. Allergic reactions involving the labyrinth, the inner portion of the ear.
f. Hemorrhage into the inner ear.
g. Tumors of the nerve of hearing.

**How can deafness caused by a defect in the inner ear be distinguished from deafness caused by trouble in the middle ear?**

Middle ear deafness does not involve disease of the transmission mechanism. Thus, if a vibrating tuning fork is held against the mastoid bone behind the ear, the vibrating sound is intensified as it can be transmitted through the undamaged inner ear. If the deafness is a result of disturbance in the inner ear or in the acoustic nerve, the tuning fork vibrations will not be heard.

**Can deafness be helped medically?**

a. If the deafness was caused by disease such as mumps, etc., nothing can be done to improve the hearing, except by the use of hearing aids.
b. If the deafness was caused by drugs and the use of the drug is stopped before permanent damage has occurred, hearing will improve by itself.
c. When deafness has been caused by exposure to loud noises or explosions, improvement may take place over a period of time if the patient is removed from such noises.
d. Deafness following fracture of the temporal bone or hemorrhage may recede as time passes, but little can be done medically to influence this change.
e. Deafness due to tumors of the acoustic nerve can be improved by surgical removal of the tumor.

**What causes middle ear (conductive) deafness?**

a. Impacted wax.
b. A foreign body in the external ear canal.
c. A discharge in the canal.
d. Narrowing of the canal due to inflammation of the skin of the canal.
e. Tumors of the external auditory canal.
f. Perforated eardrums.
g. Inflammation of the middle ear.
h. Tumor of the middle ear.
i. Lack of mobility of the stapes bone in the middle ear.
j. A blocked Eustachian tube.
k. A degenerative disease known as *otosclerosis.*

**What is the incidence of conductive deafness?**

It is estimated that about five out of every hundred people have deafness caused by disturbance in their conduction apparatus. Fortunately, only one of these five people has impairment to such a degree that it requires medical attention.

**Are hearing aids effective?**

Yes. There are wonderful new hearing aids being manufactured, and constant improvements are being made all the time. However, aids are not effective in all types of hearing loss.

## What are some of the medical measures used to improve conduction deafness?

If deafness has been due to wax in the external ear, to a foreign body in the canal, to an inflammation in the canal, to a middle ear infection, or to a blocked Eustachian tube, this can be helped readily by medical management by the nose and throat specialist. If, however, maximum benefit has been obtained from medical measures and marked impairment still exists, people with conductive deafness should use hearing aids.

## Is x-ray therapy or radium ever used for the treatment of deafness?

Formerly, x ray or radium was used to overcome blockage of the Eustachian tube by overgrowth of lymphoid tissue. It has been found, however, that this form of therapy may lead to cancer of the thyroid in later life, and it has therefore been abandoned.

## Is surgery helpful in the treatment of deafness?

Yes, in certain types of deafness. If the deafness is caused by the presence of fluid in the middle ear, an incision in the eardrum that permits the fluid to escape will often be followed by a complete return of hearing. In cases in which the deafness is secondary to rigidity of the stapes bone in the middle ear, surgery may bring about excellent relief.

## What is otosclerosis?

Otosclerosis is a disease of the inner ear.

## What are the harmful results of otosclerosis?

Otosclerosis is the most common cause of deafness, usually of the conductive type.

## Does otosclerosis always cause deafness?

No.

## What are the symptoms of otosclerosis?

Deafness is the outstanding symptom, but occasionally it causes noises in the ears. There are no abnormal ear findings on examination.

## What is the treatment for otosclerosis?

The operation performed most often now is *stapedectomy.* This operation is carried out under local anesthesia utilizing magnification instruments because of the small size of the parts being operated upon. A small incision is made adjacent to the eardrum and the drum is elevated, exposing the middle ear with its three small bones. The stapes (one of the three small bones) is then removed, thus uncovering an opening into the inner ear. This opening is covered with a small graft, usually a piece of vein or a plastic material. A small plastic tube or piece of stainless steel wire is attached to the graft and is then connected to the two remaining small bones of the ear (the incus and the malleus). When this portion of the operation has been completed, the eardrum is sutured back into its normal position.

## Is the fenestration operation performed frequently for deafness?

Not anymore. It has been found that the stapes operation results in a much higher percentage of cure, and, furthermore, recurrence of deafness is much less likely to take place after this procedure than following the fenestration operation.

## For what conditions is the stapes operation most effective?

Those cases of deafness caused by rigidity of the stapes bone of the middle ear and those caused by otosclerosis. For the stapes operation to be successful, the auditory nerve must function normally and the eardrum must be normal.

## Can the stapes operation be performed at any age?

Yes. This is not a major operation in the sense that it is dangerous or cannot be carried out at any age.

## Does hearing ever worsen after a stapes operation?

This occurs only in extremely rare instances.

## Is the stapes operation followed by very much pain?

No.

## Are there any scars visible following the stapes operation?

No, inasmuch as the incision is made within the ear canal.

## If the patient is deaf in both ears, is the stapes operation usually carried out simultaneously in both ears?

No, the usual practice is to perform them several weeks or months apart.

## How long following a deafness operation can the patient get out of bed?

In a day or two.

## Are there many complications following stapes surgery?

No. Those that do occur will usually disappear within a few weeks.

## What may be some of the complications following stapedectomy?

a. Failure to obtain improvement in hearing.
b. Noises in the ear.
c. Dizziness and headache.

## Are the benefits following surgery permanent?

Yes, in the great majority of cases.

**What percentage of patients who undergo deafness operations are benefited?**

With recent improvements in techniques, approximately 85 to 90 percent of patients will have improved hearing.

**If the initial operation for deafness has failed, is it possible to reoperate and obtain a better result?**

Yes. There have been many successes with secondary operations for deafness where the first operations have failed to obtain good results.

**How long after the surgery has been performed will the patient know whether hearing will return?**

If there is going to be a good result, it occurs almost immediately.

**How long a hospital stay is necessary after stapes surgery?**

Usually, no more than two to three days.

**When can a patient return to his usual work?**

Within approximately two weeks.

**Is the fenestration operation ever carried out following failure of a stapes operation?**

In isolated instances where the stapes operation has failed to obtain a good result, a satisfactory result may follow a fenestration procedure.

**How does the mobilization of the stapes operation differ from stapedectomy?**

In a mobilization operation, the stapes bone is not removed but is merely manipulated so as to free it from its adhesions or restrictions. It has been found that the adhesions may re-form after surgery; therefore removal of the stapes bone with a substitute graft has been found to be a more satisfactory operation.

**What is tympanoplasty?**

This is an operation performed to restore hearing by repairing the damage to, or by replacement of, the eardrum. The medical term for the eardrum is the tympanic membrane.

**How does the surgeon perform a tympanoplasty?**

He may merely mobilize the edges of the hole in the drum and stitch them together, or more commonly, if the drum is extensively damaged, he will replace it entirely with a vein graft. This type of surgery is usually performed using magnification because of the small size of the structures in the area.

**Is tympanoplasty a successful operative procedure?**

Yes, providing the underlying small bones of hearing and the inner ear are essentially normal. It will do little good to repair a damaged eardrum if the underlying bones are diseased or restricted by adhesions.

## EQUILIBRIUM

**What is equilibrium?**

It is both the inner consciousness and maintenance of the normal posture and balance of the individual in standing, walking, and carrying out normal physical activity.

**On what does equilibrium depend?**

It depends on three interrelated factors:
a. The eyes.
b. The skin and muscle-position sense.
c. The vestibular labyrinth mechanism of the inner ear and its connections to the brain.

**Must all three of these above factors be working perfectly in order to maintain equilibrium?**

No. Balance can be maintained if two of the above three factors function properly.

**What is meant by vertigo?**

Vertigo is a sensation of disturbed position, posture, or balance. In other words, it is an abnormality of the equilibrium. It is a symptom and not a disease.

## ACOUSTIC NERVE TUMORS

**Are acoustic nerve tumors common, and what is the treatment for them?**

Acoustic nerve tumors are rather common and must be treated by the neurosurgeon.

**What are the symptoms of an acoustic nerve tumor?**

a. Vertigo.
b. Buzzing, hissing, and ringing in the ear on the involved side.
c. Impairment of hearing.
d. Weakness or paralysis of the facial muscles.
e. Pain on the involved side of the face.
f. Headache.

## MÉNIÈRE'S SYNDROME

**What is Ménière's syndrome?**

It is a disease characterized by sudden attacks of vertigo, buzzing or ringing in the ears, impairment of hearing, with occasional episodes of headache and vomiting.

**What causes Ménière's syndrome?**

The cause is not known.

**What is the treatment for Ménière's syndrome?**

a. Medical treatment that consists of a low sodium (salt) diet and the use of nicotinic acid. In some cases this regime relieves the symptoms to a considerable extent.
b. Surgical treatment in severe cases. An operative procedure to decompress the endolymphatic

duct in the inner ear is sometimes performed. It has been found that by letting out some of this lymphatic fluid and thus reducing pressure, the dizziness (vertigo) of Ménière's syndrome may be relieved and hearing may be restored. If this operation fails, it may become necessary to cut part of the acoustic nerve (the nerve of hearing). Unfortunately, this surgical procedure may destroy hearing.

## PLASTIC SURGERY OF THE EAR

### For what conditions is plastic surgery of the ear recommended?
a. Protruding ears.
b. Folding or lop ears.
c. Deformities of the external ear.
d. Deformities of the external ear canal.

### What is the usual cause of these conditions?
They are deformities of the ear cartilage present since birth.

### Does the shape of the ear tend to run in families or be inherited?
Yes.

### Will an infant develop deformed ears because he lies upon them when they are in a folded position?
No. This is a common misconception.

### Are folded and lop ears seen on one side only?
Yes, but there are many cases in which both ears are misshapen.

### Is hearing disturbed by deformities of the external ear?
No.

### Will plastic surgery upon the external ear influence hearing?
No.

### Can large ears be made smaller?
Yes, through plastic surgery.

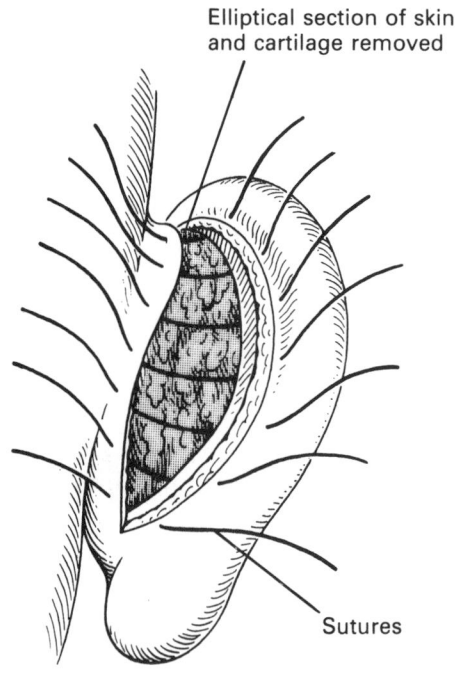

Elliptical section of skin and cartilage removed

Sutures

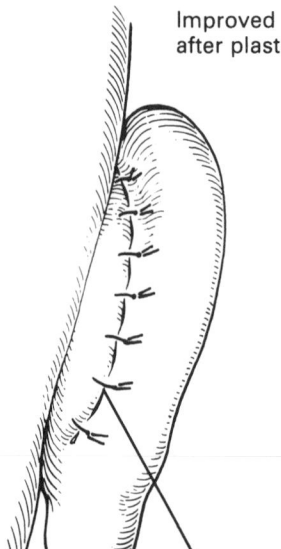

Improved position of ear after plastic surgery

Sutures

*Lop Ears.* The diagrams at left show how plastic repair of lop ears is carried out. It is a simple operation with excellent results. Children may become very self-conscious because of folded or lop ears, and it is unnecessary for them to go through life with such a deformity.

### Is plastic surgery upon the ears difficult?
No. The only difficult case is when the external ear is totally or partially lacking. In such an instance, very complicated skin grafting is required to create a new external ear.

### At what age should a child be operated upon for correction of deformed ears?
When the child is old enough to cooperate and not disturb his bandages. This means usually just before school age, between the ages of four and six. Some surgeons advocate not operating upon these children until they reach the age of thirteen or fourteen.

### What operative procedure is carried out for protruding or lop ears?
An elliptical skin incision is made behind the ear, and an elliptical section of skin and cartilage is removed. The skin edges are then sutured one to the other, which brings the ear back into normal position and appearance. A firm dressing is applied so that the ear will remain in its new position, the head is snugly bandaged, and the bandages are left in place for about ten days, until solid healing has taken place.

### Is there swelling of the ear following these operations?
Yes, but this will disappear within a few days to several weeks.

### Are the cosmetic results of these operations good?
Yes. In the great majority of cases they are excellent.

### What anesthesia is used for operations of this type?
For children, general anesthesia. For adults, local anesthesia.

### Are the scars of these operations visible?
No, as the incisions are behind the ears in the folds of the skin lines.

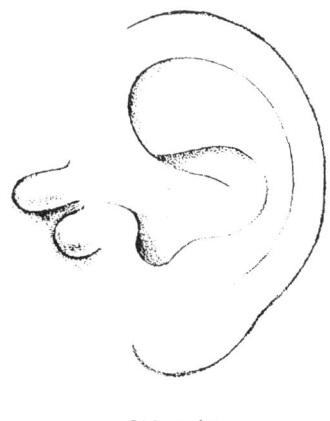

Skin tabs

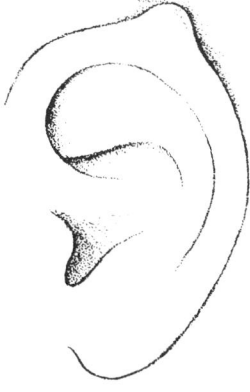

Darwinian tubercle

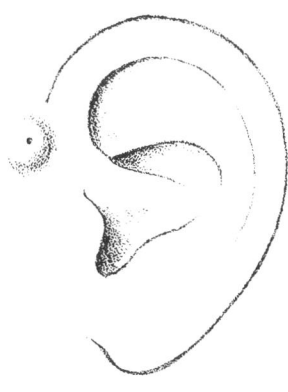

Opening of branchial cyst

*From Left to Right:*
**Congenital Deformities of the Ear.** *Extra skin tabs; a Darwinian tubercle; and the opening of a branchial cyst.*

**How long a period of hospitalization is necessary?**

From two to three days.

**If the results are not perfectly satisfactory, can these operations be done over again?**

Yes. Reoperation may correct residual deformities.

## CONGENITAL DEFORMITIES OF THE EAR

**What are the birth deformities of the ear?**

There are several forms:

a. Absence of the external ear canal. This is usually accompanied by maldevelopment of the middle ear, although the inner ear, which controls the sense of balance, is usually intact.

b. Absence of the external ear. In these cases, if there is a normally developed external ear canal, middle ear, and inner ear, hearing is not greatly interfered with.

c. Minor deformities of the external ear such as absent parts or extra tabs of tissue. These can usually be corrected without difficulty through plastic surgery.

d. A branchial cyst remnant in front of the ear. This represents failure of one of the gill slits to close during the life of the embryo. It will be diagnosed by a small opening usually in front of the ear. This may require surgery when the child has matured somewhat.

**How common are these congenital deformities of the ear?**

Absence of the external ear canal occurs in approximately one in two thousand cases of ear disease. Absence of the whole external ear is quite rare, but one does see partial deformities in the formation of the external ear. Both of these deformities are more likely to occur on one side than on both sides.

**Can surgery be helpful for congenital deformities of the ear?**

To construct an external ear canal in these cases is usually not of great value since hearing cannot be restored. This is due to the fact that the eardrum and the middle ear are usually underdeveloped. There are extensive plastic operations for the construction of a new external ear; these operations may be worthwhile psychologically, but the ultimate results are not too acceptable from a cosmetic point of view.

# CHAPTER 22
# ENDOSCOPY

## What is endoscopy?

Endoscopy is the study of internal organs with the use of optical instruments that permit direct viewing. The purpose of endoscopy is to aid in diagnosis and treatment.

Recent advances in fiber optical instruments have made endoscopy a safe and exceptionally useful procedure.

## What is esophagoscopy?

It is the study of the foodpipe (esophagus) with the use of an optical instrument. The lining of the esophagus can be seen and examined by peering through the esophagoscope, which transmits light.

## What is gastroscopy?

Gastroscopy is the study of the stomach with the use of an optical instrument. The instrument is passed through the mouth into the esophagus and down into the stomach. The source of light for all endoscopic instruments remains outside the body, and the light travels into the stomach by means of glass fibers.

## Are endoscopic instruments rigid or flexible?

The portion of the instrument within the body is flexible, unlike the old-fashioned gastroscope or the present-day proctoscopes and sigmoidoscopes.

## What is gastroduodenoscopy?

It is the combined study of both the stomach, and duodenum. (The duodenum is the first portion of the small intestine.)

## Is the same instrument used both for gastroscopy and gastroduodenoscopy?

Yes.

## What are the indications for doing an esophagoscopy, gastroscopy, or gastroduodenoscopy?

These procedures are helpful in making the following diagnoses:

a. The source of bleeding that may arise from a tumor or varicose vein in the esophagus, from a polyp, cancer, or ulcer of the stomach, or from an ulcer of the duodenum.

b. The presence or absence of an ulcer in the esophagus, stomach, or duodenum.

c. The presence of a tumor in the esophagus, stomach, or duodenum.

d. The presence of stones or a tumor in the common bile duct.

e. The presence of inflammation of the esophagus, stomach, or duodenum.

These procedures are also helpful in that biopsies, the snipping off of small pieces of tissue, can be taken from diseased areas of the esophagus or stomach, especially to determine if cancer is present.

## Is gastroduodenoscopy ever helpful in treating disease?

Occasionally, yes. Stones in the common bile duct can sometimes be removed with use of this instrument. The outlet of the common bile duct is stretched, thus permitting stones to pass into the duodenum. However, it must be noted that this procedure is not always successful.

## Is endoscopy of the esophagus, stomach, and duodenum painful?

No. Before the examination begins, the patient receives sedative and pain-relieving medications. Moreover, the instrument is made out of flexible, rather than rigid, material, such as metal.

## How accurate is endoscopy of the esophagus, stomach, and duodenum?

Approximately 90 percent of cases are diagnosed correctly. In many instances, the accuracy is checked by taking a biopsy.

## Does endoscopy of the esophagus, stomach, and duodenum make x-ray examinations unnecessary?

No. The procedures are complementary to x-ray studies and will not supplant them.

## What is proctoscopy?

Proctoscopy is the study of the rectum through direct viewing. Either a rigid metal or a flexible nonmetal instrument can be used for this examination. Through proctoscopy, diagnoses can be readily made by use of the proctoscope, biopsies easily taken, and certain lesions, such as polyps, can be burned or snared off. The average proctoscope is between five and six inches long.

## What is sigmoidoscopy?

Sigmoidoscopy is the study of the sigmoid colon—the portion of the colon that lies just above the rectum—with the use of optical instruments. It has the same diagnostic and therapeutic usages as the proctoscope but differs in that the instrument goes up ten to twelve inches, rather than five to six inches, from the anal opening.

## What is colonoscopy?

Colonoscopy is the study of the large intestine with the use of a flexible optical instrument. It is passed through the anus and is threaded through the entire extent of the colon, a distance of several feet.

## What conditions can be diagnosed through colonoscopy?

a. Inflammations of the colon, including the various types of colitis.
b. Diverticulosis or diverticulitis of the colon.
c. Polyps of the colon.
d. Cancer of the colon.
e. The sources of bleeding within the colon.

## Can biopsies be taken through a colonoscope?

Yes. This is one of its great values.

## Can polyps frequently be removed through a colonoscope?

Yes. This is a great asset since in many instances it does away with the need for an open surgical procedure.

## Is colonoscopy helpful in explaining puzzling findings on x-ray examination of the colon?

Yes. Frequently an x ray may point toward the presence of a tumor in the colon, but colonoscopy may prove no tumor to be present.

## Can colonoscopy ever reveal a tumor when x rays fail to show it?

Yes. This occurs on many occasions.

## Is colonoscopy painful?

Yes, at times it can be painful. For this reason sedatives and pain-relieving drugs are given prior to colonoscopy.

## How accurate are diagnoses made through colonoscopy?

There is a high degree of accuracy provided the examiner is well trained, the colon thoroughly cleansed prior to examination, and providing that bleeding has not obscured the site of disease.

## Can polyps and malignant tumors be removed through the colonoscope?

In many cases, polyps can be completely removed. However, if the base of the polyp is broad, it may not be possible to do so.

Malignant tumors of the colon must be removed surgically.

## What are examples of the rigid metal endoscopes?

a. The gastroscope. This is used infrequently now as it affords much less opportunity to view the entire lining of the stomach. However, it is a good instrument for removal of foreign bodies that have lodged in the esophagus or stomach.
b. The bronchoscope. This is still used, but to a lesser extent than the flexible instrument. However, the rigid metal bronchoscope affords a better way to remove foreign bodies.
c. The laparoscope. This is an instrument inserted through a small incision in the abdominal wall near the navel. Through it, one can view the abdominal organs. Recently it has been used widely to carry out sterilization in women. The Fallopian tubes are identified and are fulgurated (burned electrically) at their midpoint, thus blocking the passageway and preventing conception.
d. The culdoscope. Culdoscopy is a procedure whereby the instrument is inserted through the vagina into the abdominal cavity. Through its use the gynecologist can diagnose many abnormalities of the ovaries, Fallopian tubes, and the uterus. The doctor can also note the presence of blood in the abdominal cavity, often seen in tubal (ectopic) pregnancy.

e. The cystoscope. The instrument is passed through the urethra into the urinary bladder. (See Chapter 76, on The Urinary Bladder and Urethra.)

## Are there specialists in endoscopy?

Yes. Most gastroenterologists are trained in both upper and lower endoscopy. Gynecologists perform laparoscopy and culdoscopy whereas urologists perform cystoscopy. Most otolaryngologists and chest (thoracic) surgeons are trained in bronchoscopy.

## Is endoscopy painful?

The various procedures are uncomfortable, but pain is kept to a minimum by medications administered prior to endoscopy.

## Is anesthesia required for endoscopic procedures?

Anesthesia is not given for upper or lower endoscopy, but it may be given for laparoscopy, culdoscopy, and cystoscopy.

## Is endoscopy carried out in a physician's office or in a hospital?

Both places are utilized. To perform endoscopy in an office requires a special setup with special equipment to prepare the patient properly and highly trained personnel to assist the endoscopist.

## Are special courses given to train physicians in endoscopy?

Yes. The various procedures should be carried out only by those gastroenterologists or surgeons who have been specially trained.

# CHAPTER 23

# THE ESOPHAGUS

*(See also Chapter 70 on Stomach and Duodenum)*

### What is the esophagus?

It is a muscular tube that connects the pharynx, or back of the throat, to the stomach. Through it, swallowed food and fluid are conducted to the stomach. The esophagus has no digestive function, but acts merely as a conduit.

### Is the drinking of excessively hot liquids harmful to the esophagus?

Yes, as it may burn the lining membrane. Also, some investigators believe that the taking of extremely hot foods over a period of many years may stimulate cancer formation.

### Is the drinking of excessively cold liquids harmful to the esophagus?

No.

### Can one choke from swallowing too large a quantity of food at one time?

If food enters the esophagus and not the trachea (windpipe), choking does not take place. However, taking too much food in one swallow may cause it to become stuck somewhere along the course of the esophagus. This may require the passage of an esophagoscope to remove the excess food particles.

### What is the significance of inability to swallow?

It usually signifies an obstruction due either to a mechanical cause or to spasm.

### What does it mean if there is regurgitation of undigested food?

It signifies either an obstruction of the esophagus or the presence of an esophageal diverticulum (pouch).

### What is the significance of regurgitation of sour-tasting food or stomach contents?

This is caused in most instances by conditions within the stomach, duodenum, or gall bladder, and not by esophageal disease.

### What is the significance of tightness in the throat, especially in women in their forties?

This is a tightening of the muscles of the throat encountered in women during their menopausal years. It is not due to organic disease but is thought to be caused by the tenseness that many women exhibit during these years of their life.

### What are some of the common conditions affecting the esophagus?

a. Birth deformities.
b. Inflammatory conditions.
c. Injuries, including burns and foreign bodies.
d. Diverticulum of the esophagus.
e. Chronic spasm (achalasia).
f. Varicose veins.
g. Tumors.

## BIRTH DEFORMITIES

### What types of birth deformities of the esophagus are encountered?

The most common type of birth deformity is known as a tracheoesophageal fistula. This is an abnormal communication between the esophagus and the trachea (windpipe). As a result of such an abnormal opening, saliva, milk, or other swallowed materials get into the lungs and cause irritation, often resulting in pneumonia.

### Is tracheoesophageal fistula a serious condition?

Yes. If untreated, it always results in death.

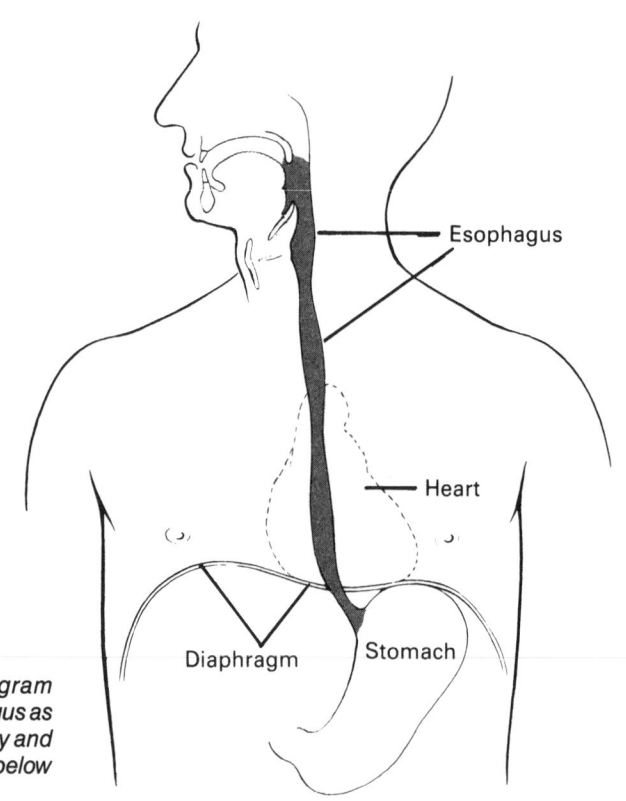

***Esophagus.*** *The diagram shows the normal esophagus as it traverses the chest cavity and empties into the stomach below the diaphragm.*

## What is the proper treatment for these fistulae?

Surgery must be performed promptly. This will involve severing the abnormal communication and stitching the openings left in the esophagus and trachea.

## What are the chances for recovery following this operation?

The mortality rate is approximately 25 percent. However, in the days before operation was feasible in this type of case, the mortality was 100 percent.

## Are there other birth deformities of the esophagus?

Yes. There may be an interruption in the continuity of the esophagus, with failure of the structure to reach the stomach. This is known as congenital atresia. Occasionally, a web, or diaphragm, is found coursing across the passageway. Such an abnormality may completely obstruct the channel of the esophagus.

## What is the treatment for an incompletely developed esophagus?

By an extremely extensive operation performed through the chest, the two normal ends of the esophagus are sutured together. If the lower half of the esophagus is not developed at all, it may be necessary to bring the stomach up into the chest and sew it to the lowermost portion of the normally developed section of the esophagus.

## Is there any urgency in the performance of this operation?

Yes. This operation must be performed as soon as the diagnosis of the congenital abnormality is made. If surgery is not instituted immediately, the condition will result in the death of the child.

## What procedure is carried out for a congenital web of the esophagus?

It must be removed surgically or dilated and stretched. This is not as serious an operation as for congenital atresia.

## INFLAMMATION OF THE ESOPHAGUS (Esophagitis)

## What conditions cause inflammation of the esophagus?

Inflammation of the esophagus (esophagitis) is either found in association with a hernia of the diaphragm (hiatus hernia) or with an ulcer in the stomach. In hiatus hernia, a portion of the stomach protrudes into the chest cavity through a widening of the opening in the diaphragm. This permits stomach contents and juices to go up into the esophagus, where they often cause irritation and set up a secondary inflammatory reaction. Patients with ulcers in the duodenum are also prone to regurgitate highly acid contents from the stomach into the lower portion of the esophagus. This may create an esophagitis.

## Is esophagitis a serious condition?

Yes. It is serious because it can result in an ulcer of the esophagus, bleeding, or stricture formation, with consequent interference with swallowing.

## What is the proper treatment for esophagitis?

The underlying cause must be removed. If a hiatus hernia is present, it should be corrected by surgery. If a duodenal ulcer is present, adequate medical treatment should be instituted. This should include a bland diet, drugs that prevent spasm, and medicines that counteract the excess acid secretions of the stomach.

## Is it ever necessary to surgically remove that portion of the esophagus affected by esophagitis?

If the esophagitis fails to respond to the usual medical measures, its removal, followed by reestablishment of the continuity of the esophagus, may be necessary to bring about a cure.

## Is removal of a portion of the esophagus a serious operation?

Yes, indeed; but approximately 90 percent of patients recover.

## INJURIES OF THE ESOPHAGUS

## What are some of the common injuries to the esophagus?

The most frequent injury to the esophagus is caused by the swallowing of corrosives such as lye. All too often this happens to small children because adults have carelessly failed to keep these dangerous substances out of a child's reach.

## What changes occur in the esophagus as a result of swallowing corrosive substances?

Severe esophagitis, complicated by stricture formation, may result.

## What is the treatment for this kind of injury?

The esophagitis is treated much the same as esophagitis from any other condition. If a stricture develops, it is treated by forceful, frequent dilatations over a period of several months. If dilatations do not produce a satisfactory increase in the diameter of the passageway, then removal of the constricted portion of esophagus may be required. If the involved area is extensive, it may be necessary to bring the stomach up into the chest and to suture it to that portion of esophagus that is normal and uninvolved in stricture formation.

## What other types of injury of the esophagus are encountered?

The esophagus is, on rare occasions, ruptured as a result of severe vomiting. It may also be perforated by the swallowing of a sharp foreign

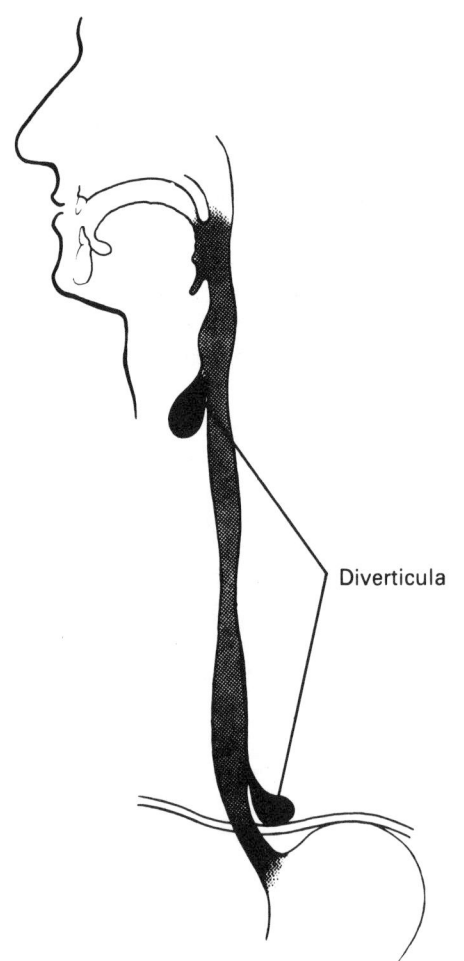

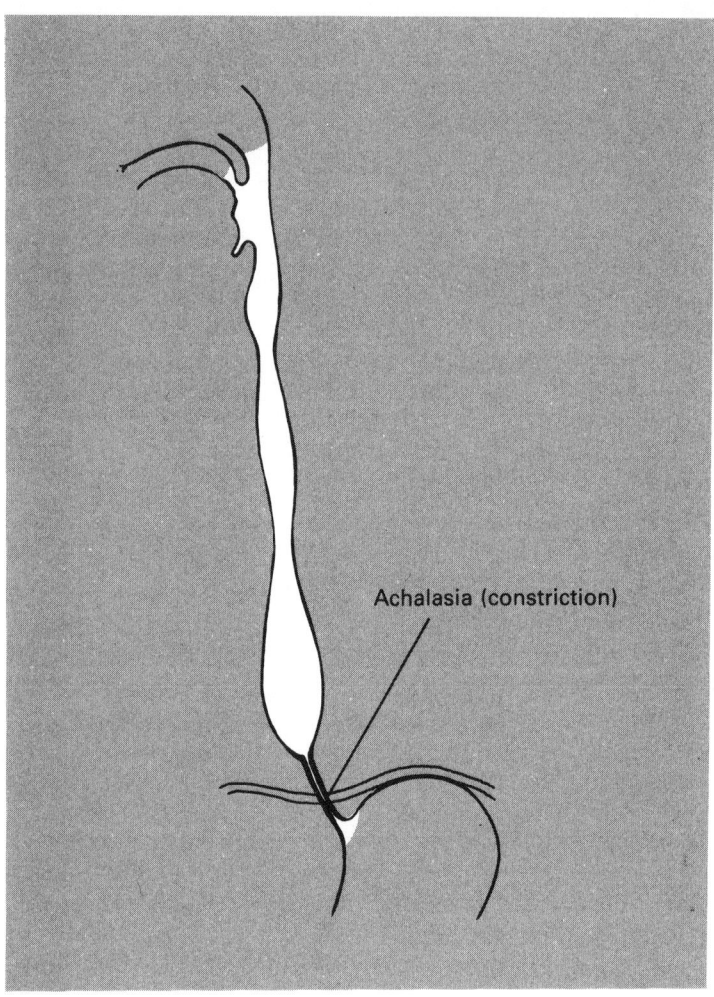

*Left:*
**Diverticula of the Esophagus:** *The diagram shows diverticula or outpouchings of the esophagus. Food tends to collect and stagnate within these pouches and to be regurgitated into the mouth from time to time, causing considerable discomfort. This condition can be cured by removing the diverticula surgically.*

*Right:*
**Achalasia.** *The diagram shows a condition affecting the esophagus known as achalasia or chronic constriction of the esophagus. Sufferers from achalasia are unable to hold down food thay have swallowed. If this condition continues for too long a time, it may cause fear of eating and even emaciation. Fortunately, this condition can now be relieved by a safe operative procedure.*

body such as a safety pin, a fishbone, or a denture.

### What is the management for a ruptured esophagus?

Rupture of the esophagus demands immediate surgery with closure of the opening and drainage of the chest cavity. On occasion, if the patient's condition is too poor to permit surgery, this condition may be treated conservatively by surgical drainage of the chest. In such cases, a permanent leak from the esophagus may develop, which will eventually require surgical correction.

## DIVERTICULUM OF THE ESOPHAGUS

### What is a diverticulum of the esophagus?

It is an outpouching, or hernia, of the mucous membrane through the muscle wall of the esophagus that produces a saclike protrusion in an otherwise smooth mucous membrane channel.

### Where are diverticula usually located?

The most common location is in that portion of the esophagus that traverses the neck. They may also be located within the chest, in the midportion of the esophagus, or in the lowermost portion, near the diaphragm.

## Do diverticula ordinarily produce symptoms?

Those in the neck usually cause symptoms because they tend to fill with fluid and grow larger, thus leading to obstruction of the esophagus. In addition, fluid or food that collects within the diverticulum may be ejected into the main passageway of the esophagus, thus causing regurgitation or vomiting. Occasionally, bleeding takes place from a diverticulum, and in rare instances, malignancy may develop within one of these sacs.

## Do all diverticula cause symptoms?

No. Only those that occur in the neck or in the lowermost portion of the esophagus are symptomatic. Those that occur within the midportion of the esophagus ordinarily do not cause symptoms.

## What treatment is recommended for diverticula of the esophagus?

Surgical removal of those diverticula that cause symptoms. If the diverticulum is located in the neck, the incision is made in the neck. If the diverticulum is located in the lowermost portion of the esophagus, the operation is performed through the chest cavity.

## ACHALASIA (Esophageal Spasm)

## What is achalasia, or spasm of the esophagus?

This is a condition in which certain nerves of the esophagus are absent, probably since birth. As a result of this deficiency, there is inability of the lower end of the esophagus to dilate and relax. As a consequence of this continued spasm, the esophagus above the area of spasm becomes tremendously widened and dilated.

## What causes achalasia?

It is thought to be associated with a birth deformity in which there is absence of certain nerve elements within the wall of the esophagus.

## What age groups are usually affected by this disease?

People in their twenties and thirties.

## What symptoms are associated with achalasia?

The most common complaint is inability to swallow normally. This symptom becomes progressive and severe. In addition, there is often a foul odor to the breath because of retained food particles within the esophagus. Sufferers from this condition are undernourished and show evidences of marked weight loss.

## What is the treatment for achalasia?

Seventy-five percent of patients with achalasia respond satisfactorily to repeated dilatations of the esophagus. However, about 25 percent require operation because they fail to obtain relief from repeated dilatations.

## What type of operation is performed for achalasia?

The thickened muscle fibers overlying the area of spasm are severed in a longitudinal direction. This permits outpouching of the mucous membrane of the esophagus at that site and creates an inability of the esophageal muscles to contract or become spastic.

## Is this a safe operative procedure?

Yes. It is carried out through an incision in the chest but is not associated with great surgical risk.

## What are the results of this operation?

The majority of patients are greatly improved, but an occasional patient may develop esophagitis as a complication.

## VARICOSE VEINS OF THE ESOPHAGUS

## What causes varicose veins of the esophagus?

Obstruction of the portal circulation, that is, the circulation of blood through the liver. This is seen in cirrhosis. (See Chapter 40, on The Liver.) Since the blood cannot get from the intestinal tract through the liver, it bypasses that organ and travels along the veins of the esophagus. This vastly increased blood volume causes the esophageal veins to dilate and become varicosed.

## What harm can result from esophageal varicosities?

Eventually, when the veins become too distended and dilated, they may rupture and cause a tremendous hemorrhage.

## How is the diagnosis of esophageal varicosities made?

a. By noting the evidences of cirrhosis of the liver.
b. By x-ray studies of the esophagus after taking a barium swallow.
c. By noting the bringing up of large quantities of blood through the mouth.

## What can be done to relieve esophageal varicosities?

a. Attempts should be made to relieve the portal circulatory obstruction. This is attempted by either suturing the large portal vein (in the abdomen) to the vena cava, by suturing the main vein of the spleen to the main vein of the left kidney, or by performing a mesocaval shunt. This operation entails placing a graft between the superior mesenteric vein (from the intestines) and the vena cava.
b. When life-threatening hemorrhage from esophageal varicosities is taking place, it may be necessary to open the chest, iso-

late and open the esophagus, and tie off the bleeding veins.

## TUMORS OF THE ESOPHAGUS

**What are the different types of tumors of the esophagus?**
a. Benign tumors.
b. Malignant tumors.

**What is the relative frequency of tumors of the esophagus?**
It is said that approximately 1 percent of all deaths from cancer are due to cancer of the esophagus. Benign tumors occur much less frequently.

**Is there any variation in the incidence of this disease in either sex?**
Yes. Males are much more commonly affected than females.

**What are the usual age ranges for cancer of the esophagus?**
Fifty to seventy years.

**What symptoms are associated with malignancies of the esophagus?**
a. Difficulty in swallowing.
b. Loss of desire to eat.
c. Weakness and weight loss.

**What is the treatment for cancer of the esophagus?**
Either surgery or x-ray therapy, or a combination of both.

**How effective are these forms of treatment in the cure of the disease?**
Radiation treatment rarely results in a cure for a cancer of the esophagus.

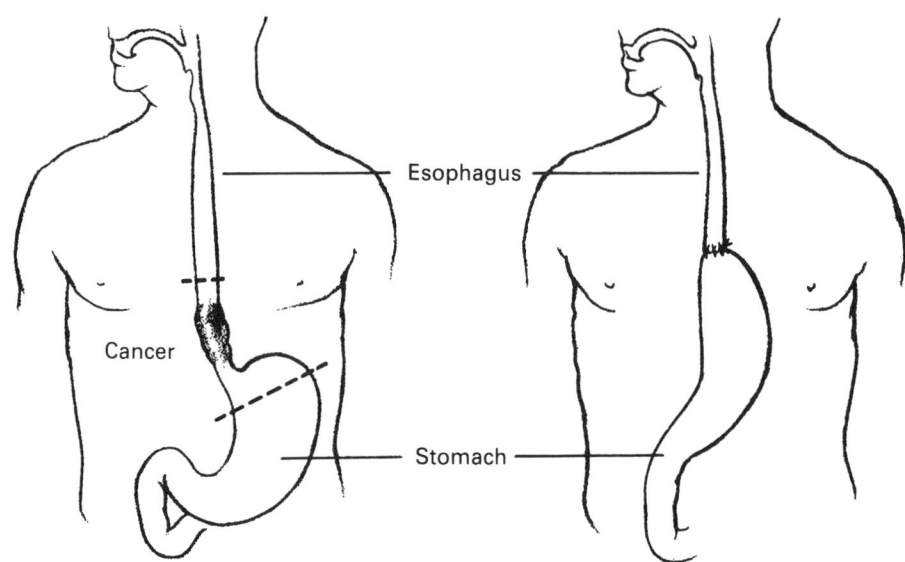

*Surgery in Esophageal Cancer.* In the diagram at the left, the affected part of the esophagus and a portion of the stomach to be removed with it are shown between the dotted lines. At the right, the stump of the stomach has been sutured to the cut end of the esophagus.

Surgery can effect a cure in approximately 20 percent of all patients with cancer involving the lowermost portion of the esophagus.

**Are benign tumors of the esophagus curable?**
Yes. Practically all patients with this condition can be cured by surgical excision of the tumor.

**What type of operation is performed for malignant esophageal tumors?**
Those that can be attacked most successfully are usually located in the middle or lower third of the esophagus. In these cases, through a chest incision, it is possible to remove that part of the esophagus involved in tumor formation and a generous portion of normal esophagus surrounding it. Through an opening made in the diaphragm, the stomach is drawn up into the chest and is sutured to the remaining stump of esophagus.

**What other forms of operation are available for cancer of the esophagus?**
In another, less commonly used operation, the tumor and adjacent esophagus are widely removed and replaced by a plastic tube. This has a disadvantage, however, of being followed in many cases by leakage.

**Are operations for removal of esophageal malignancy serious?**
Yes. They are among the most formidable of all operations and should be performed only by a specially trained surgeon.

# CHAPTER 24
# THE EYES

*(See also Chapter 7 on Allergy; Chapter 18 on Contagious Diseases; Chapter 26 on First Aid; Chapter 47 on Newborn Child)*

**Is it necessary for an eye specialist to perform an eye examination, or is an optometrist capable of performing the entire examination?**

When an optometrist works in association with an ophthalmologist, it is often sufficient to have him examine the eyes if it is solely for the purpose of obtaining eyeglasses. However, an examination by an ophthalmologist (eye specialist) is always advisable when the patient feels something is wrong with his eyes or when the optometrist notes some abnormality. Also, people over forty years of age should have a yearly examination by an ophthalmologist.

**How often should one have a routine checkup of the eyes?**

The average person should have his eyes checked at least every one to two years.

The nearsighted person should be checked once every six months to one year.

The farsighted patient under the age of forty should be examined at least every one to two years.

All people over the age of forty should be checked every one to two years.

All people over the age of sixty-five should be checked once a year.

**What are the common causes of eyestrain?**

a. The need for eyeglasses.
b. Reading under a poor light.
c. Reading in any position other than sitting up.
d. Reading for excessively long periods of time without resting the eyes.

**What are the symptoms of eyestrain?**

Blurring of vision, smarting and burning of the eyes, slight tearing, and headaches.

**Can eyestrain be caused by reading too much?**

Yes.

**What is the treatment for eyestrain?**

a. Wearing corrective glasses.
b. Reading under a good light.
c. Sitting in a good reading position.
d. Proper rest periods.
e. Eyedrops prescribed by a physician to reduce eyestrain.

**Can permanent damage to the eye result from overuse?**

No. The eyes will recover if properly treated.

**Why do people have different colored eyes?**

The color of the eyes depends on the amount of pigment in the iris. The less pigment there is, the bluer the eye; the more pigment, the browner the eye. The less pigment, the more sensitive the eye is to bright light.

**Is it natural for the pupils of children's eyes to be exceptionally large?**

Yes. As a child grows older, the pupil will appear smaller.

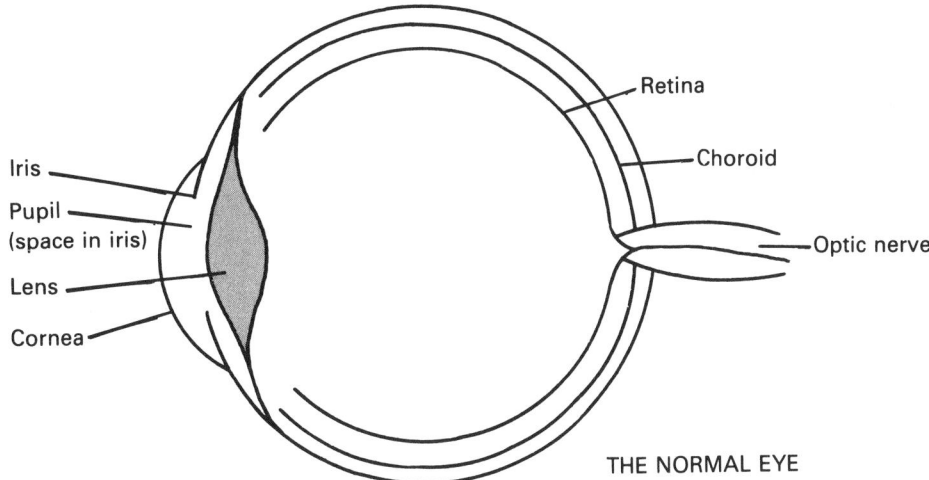

Iris
Pupil (space in iris)
Lens
Cornea
Retina
Choroid
Optic nerve

THE NORMAL EYE

**The Normal Eye.** *This diagram illustrates the mechanism of sight. Light rays pass through the pupil and through the lens, where they are bent so that they focus on the retina in the rear of the eye. This apparatus is almost exactly like a camera, with the pupil corresponding to the opening of the camera. The lens of the eye is similar to the lens of the camera, and the retina in the back of the eye is comparable to the photographic film in a camera.*

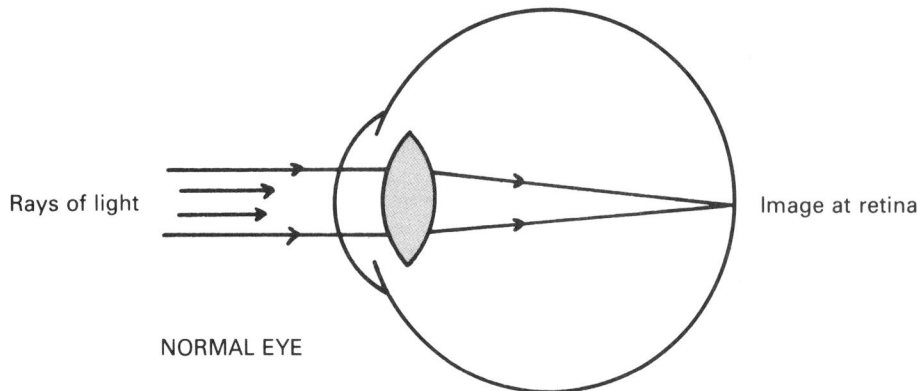

**The Normal Eye.**
*This diagram shows another view of the normal eye, with the light rays focusing exactly upon the retina in the back of the eye. When these rays hit the retina they are transmitted to the brain along nerve pathways and are interpreted by the brain as sight.*

### Is it significant if a person has one eye of a different color from the other?

No. This has no significance other than cosmetic, as long as no inflammation is present.

### What causes tearing of the eyes?

This may be due to irritation from excessively bright lights, allergies, a sharp wind, smoke, inflammation of the eye, a foreign body in the eye, or a blocked tear duct. It occurs more frequently in older people.

### What are the common causes for itching and swelling of the eyes and lids?

Itching may be due to an allergic condition such as hay fever or sensitivity to smoke or face powder or soap.

Swelling of the lids should be a signal to see a physician to make sure that kidney function is normal.

Slight swelling of the lids is sometimes caused by insufficient sleep.

### What causes red lid margins?

This condition may be caused by dandruff or seborrhea of the scalp, exposure to irritating smoke, dust, or wind, eyestrain, allergy, or chronic conjunctivitis. Children may develop red lid margins when they rub their eyes with dirty hands.

### What causes the spots that are seen floating in front of the eyes?

Spots are caused by opacities of protein matter that float in the internal portion (vitreous) of the eyeball. These opacities become visible as small spots or threads and are usually seen when a person looks at a bright background such as a clear sky or white paper. Usually they are of no significance unless associated with blurring of vision and/or flashes of light. If either should occur, consult an eye doctor for a thorough examination to rule out inflammation or disease of the retina.

### What causes bulging of the eyes?

Bulging or prominent eyes may be due to overactivity of the thyroid gland, inflammation, tumor behind the eye, or to excessive nearsightedness. In some people it is a normal anatomical feature and has no significance.

### How does one treat the so-called "black eye"?

An eye specialist should be consulted to make sure there has been no damage to the eyeball itself.

Then, for the first twenty-four hours, cold wet compresses should be applied to lessen swelling. After twenty-four hours, warm compresses should be used to hasten absorption of the blood clot.

## NEARSIGHTEDNESS
*(Myopia)*

### What is nearsightedness?

In nearsightedness, the eyeball is longer than it should normally be for that individual. Vision is better for near objects than for distant objects.

### How common is nearsightedness?

About one-third of all people who wear glasses are nearsighted.

### Are boys more likely to be nearsighted than girls?

No.

### Is nearsightedness inherited?

It often runs in families, particularly if both parents are nearsighted.

### Will wearing the proper eyeglasses lead to an improvement in nearsightedness?

No, but it will permit the eyes to function normally.

**Can anything be done to prevent nearsightedness?**

No.

**Does nearsightedness tend to get better by itself?**

No, except very occasionally.

**How early can children be fitted for eyeglasses for nearsightedness?**

Usually at three years, but if necessary, at one year of age.

**How can the doctor detect nearsightedness in small children?**

By shining a light in the eye and performing a test known as retinoscopy. Prior to the test, the pupils are dilated with eyedrops.

**Why does nearsightedness get worse as one matures?**

As the body grows, the eyeball gets larger while the optical system of the eyes remains unchanged.

**Should nearsighted people spare their eyes from excess reading?**

No. This is necessary only if the nearsightedness is very severe and associated with degeneration of the back of the eye.

**Does watching television have any adverse effect on the eyes of nearsighted people?**

None at all.

**What are contact lenses?**

These are molded plastic lenses that fit directly over the eyeballs and therefore disguise the fact that "glasses" are being worn.

**When are contact lenses recommended in nearsightedness?**

When the nearsightedness is of moderate severity, and the patient does not want to give the appearance of wearing glasses.

**Are contact lenses worn directly against the eyeball harmful?**

Not if they are well fitted.

**Are soft contact lenses advisable?**

Yes, for many people they represent a considerable improvement over the rigid lenses. However, they do not provide clear vision for people with astigmatism. (See the section on Astigmatism in this chapter.)

**Is there any medication to help nearsightedness?**

No, although certain eyedrops are being tried with some apparent success.

**Is there any surgical procedure that can help nearsightedness?**

In extreme cases of nearsightedness associated with weakening of the walls of the eyeball, implants of fibrous tissue are sewn to the weakened areas. Recently, a new operation on the cornea known as keratomileusis—an operation involving a change in the curve of the cornea—has been devised. This procedure can benefit both nearsighted and farsighted patients. Although the operation is still in the experimental stage, it has been used successfully on patients who have also had cataract operations, Keratomileusis may do away with the need for heavy spectacles or contact lenses among this group of patients.

**How effective are the newer operations for nearsightedness?**

Although the number of cases in which they have been performed is relatively small, first reports are that if patients are properly selected for these procedures, results are successful in a fair number of instances.

**Is there any surgical procedure that can arrest or decrease nearsightedness?**

In a few selected cases, operations to shorten the eyeball can be performed. These operations have just been developed recently and have not yet been perfected. They consist of taking out crescentic portions of the eyeball along the inner and outer aspects. This will shorten the length of the eyeball and thus bring the lens closer to the retina, overcoming

*Nearsighted Eye (Myopia). The diagram of the nearsighted eye shows the image focusing in front of the retina. When this defect is corrected by eyeglasses, the image is made to focus exactly upon the retina.*

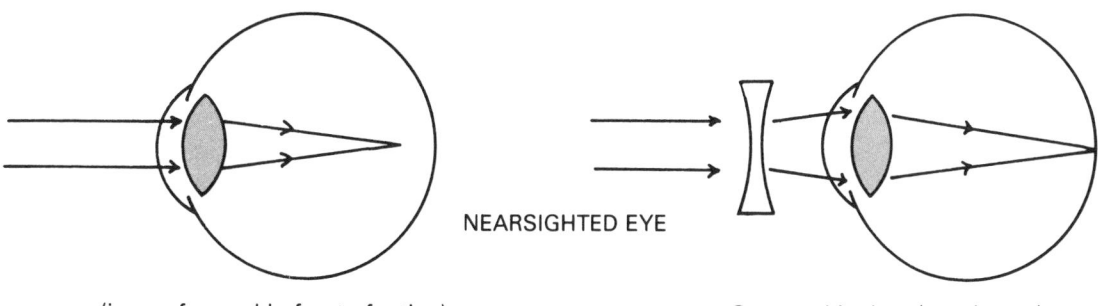

(image focused in front of retina)          NEARSIGHTED EYE          Corrected by lens (eyeglasses)

some of the nearsightedness. In addition, surgery upon the cornea to change its optical properties has been tried recently. (See above.)

### Does nearsightedness ever lead to blindness?

In the very rare case, nearsightedness may lead to degeneration—with or without detachment of the retina—with some loss of vision. (See the section on Detached Retina in this chapter.)

## FARSIGHTEDNESS
### (Hyperopia)

### What is farsightedness?

In farsightedness, the eyeball is shorter than it should normally be for that individual. Vision is better for distant than for near objects. In marked cases, vision is also blurred for distant objects.

### How common is farsightedness?

About one-third of all people who wear glasses are farsighted.

### Are boys more likely to be farsighted than girls?

No.

### Is farsightedness inherited, or does it tend to run in families?

Yes, in some cases.

### Can anything be done to prevent farsightedness?

No.

### Does farsightedness tend to get better by itself?

No, but in growing children, farsightedness may change into nearsightedness.

### Will wearing the proper eyeglasses lead to an improvement in farsightedness?

It will not bring about a cure but will improve the vision.

### Is it ever bad to wear eyeglasses for farsightedness?

No.

### How early can children be fitted with eyeglasses for farsightedness?

Usually at three years of age.

### How can the doctor detect farsightedness in small children?

By a special examination known as retinoscopy.

### Why does farsightedness get worse as one gets older?

As one gets older, the lenses of the eye grow more rigid and the patient is less able to compensate for his defect by muscle contraction.

### Should farsighted people spare their eyes from excessive reading?

This is not necessary if the patient wears proper eyeglasses.

### Does watching television have any harmful effect on the eyes of farsighted people?

No.

### When are contact lenses recommended for farsightedness?

When the farsightedness reduces vision enough to require constant use of spectacles and when it is desirable to avoid the latter for cosmetic, occupational, or athletic reasons.

### Is there any medication that can be given to help farsightedness?

No.

### Is there any surgical procedure that can help farsightedness?

Yes, keratomileusis.

### Does farsightedness ever cause blindness?

No.

## ASTIGMATISM

### What is astigmatism?

A defect in the curvature of the cornea and/or lens whereby there is an inequality preventing the light rays

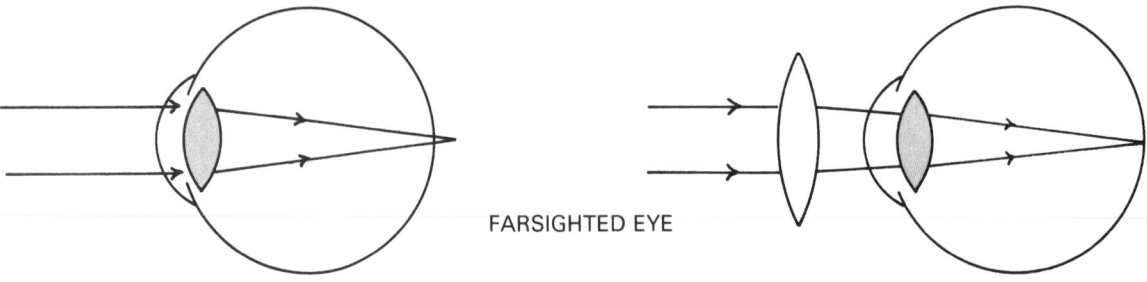

*Farsighted Eye (Hyperopia). This diagram of the farsighted eye shows the image focusing beyond the retina. This too can be readily corrected by appropriate eyeglasses.*

(Image focused beyond retina)          FARSIGHTED EYE          Corrected by lens (eyeglasses)

from hitting the retina at a point of common focus.

### What produces astigmatism?

The manner in which the eyeballs grow. This is inherited.

### How does a person know if he has astigmatism?

Astigmatic people are more prone to eyestrain and blurred vision. They soon become aware that something is wrong.

### What is the treatment for astigmatism?

The wearing of proper corrective glasses will relieve the symptoms and improve vision greatly.

### Does astigmatism ever get better by itself?

No.

### Can astigmatism lead to blindness?

No.

## CONJUNCTIVITIS

### What is conjunctivitis?

An inflammation of the conjunctiva, the thin membrane that covers the white part of the eyeball and the inner surface of the eyelids.

### What can cause conjunctivitis?

An injury, an infection, or an allergy. Injury can be caused by exposure to sunlight, dust, or wind. Infection may be caused by a streptococcus, staphylococcus, gonococcus, or any other bacteria.

### What are the symptoms of conjunctivitis?

The symptoms of the traumatic (injury) type are redness, itching, burning, and tearing of the eyes. The symptoms of the infectious type are the same as for traumatic conjunctivitis, plus the fact that there is a pus discharge from the eye. The symptoms of the allergic type are redness, burning, tearing, and itching of the eyes and lids, often accompanied by symptoms in the nose and throat.

### What is the treatment for conjunctivitis?

For the traumatic type, mild astringent eyedrops. For the infectious type, antibiotic eyedrops. For the allergic type, antihistamine or cortisone eyedrops.

### Is conjunctivitis contagious?

Only the infectious type is contagious.

### How can one prevent the spread of the contagious type of conjunctivitis?

By isolating the patient and having him use his own soap and towel.

### How long does it take for conjunctivitis to get well?

Usually two to four days if there are no complications and proper treatment is instituted.

### Does permanent damage to eyesight result from conjunctivitis?

No, unless there are complications.

### What is the most common complication of conjunctivitis?

An ulceration of the cornea, which may leave a scar obscuring vision to a greater or lesser degree.

### If conjunctivitis is due to a gonorrheal infection, can it be cured?

Yes, by proper use of an antibiotic medication, usually penicillin.

### What is the treatment for gonorrheal conjunctivitis?

The use of penicillin eyedrops.

### What are the preventive measures to avoid gonorrheal conjunctivitis?

If one has gonorrhea, strict personal hygiene is essential! The hands must be kept away from the eyes, and penicillin eyedrops should be used prophylactically.

### What is "pinkeye"?

"Pinkeye" is a very contagious type of infectious conjunctivitis caused by special bacteria.

### What are the symptoms of pinkeye?

The same as for any infectious conjunctivitis.

### How is pinkeye treated?

By eyedrops that will bring about a cure in two to three days.

### Can pinkeye permanently injure the eyes?

No.

## LACERATIONS, ABRASIONS, ULCERATIONS, AND FOREIGN BODIES OF THE CORNEA

### What is the first-aid treatment for a scratch or foreign body in the eye?

The use of anesthetic eyedrops and a bandage to cover the eye. After anesthetizing the eye, a foreign body can usually be wiped away with sterile, moist cotton on a stick.

### What should one do if this occurs late at night when the eye doctor is not available?

The use of the anesthetic drops and a patch will relieve the patient of pain and keep the eye clean until the patient can consult an eye doctor in the morning. However, it is much wiser to go to the emergency room of the nearest hospital than to leave a foreign body in the eye overnight.

### Can serious damage to the eye result if one waits several hours before receiving medical treatment?

No, but one should not wait more

than twelve hours before seeing a doctor.

### What is the treatment for an abrasion (scratch) or ulcer of the cornea?

The use of an antibiotic and cortisone eyedrops or ointment and a bandage to keep the eye covered. See your eye doctor.

### Can a laceration of the cornea be successfully sutured?

Yes. This is done when there has been a deep or extensive laceration.

### Is there any serious danger to the eye from a foreign body such as a small cinder or piece of steel?

If the foreign body is on the surface of the eye, there is usually very little danger. If the foreign body has penetrated the eyeball, there is serious danger to the eye.

### Do abrasions and lacerations tend to heal by themselves?

Small abrasions will heal by themselves. Lacerations usually have to be treated.

### How does one prevent scar tissue from forming when abrasions or lacerations heal?

By the use of cortisone eyedrops and the use of warm compresses to the eye.

### Is impairment of vision often found after an injury of this type?

If a corneal abrasion is superficial and does not become infected, there is usually no impairment of vision. Intraocular foreign bodies very often result in impairment of vision.

### How long do corneal abrasions take to heal?

With proper treatment, two to four days.

### How long do corneal lacerations take to heal?

Usually two to three weeks.

### What causes chronic ulceration of the cornea?

Chronic ulceration of the cornea occurs when the patient's resistance is low, as in diabetes or other debilitating illnesses. Infection of an abrasion can produce the same result.

### What is the treatment for chronic or recurrent ulcers of the cornea?

The use of antibiotics, cauterization of the ulcer, and a bandage to keep the eye covered and safe from possible external contamination.

### Is it possible to replace a cornea that has been damaged irreparably by scars?

Yes. Corneal transplants have recently been used for this purpose with great success. There are now eye banks in which normal corneas are preserved for long periods of time, to be used for purposes of transplanting to other individuals.

### Do corneal transplants usually survive?

Yes, in the great majority of cases a cornea transplanted from one human to another will live and will function normally.

### Is it possible to restore vision through a corneal transplant?

Most certainly, yes. There are now thousands of people who were formerly blind but can now see because they have received a corneal transplant.

### If one operation with corneal transplantation fails, is it possible to reoperate?

Yes. Every once in a while a transplanted cornea will fail to survive. In such cases, success may follow a second operative procedure.

### Can all blind people be helped by corneal transplants?

Unfortunately, no. It is estimated that approximately 5 percent of those who are blind have lost their sight because of scarring of the cornea. It is this small group that can be benefited by a corneal transplant.

### Can an entire eye be transplanted?

No.

## STYES AND CYSTS OF THE EYELIDS

### What causes recurrent styes of the eyelids?

a. Lowered body resistance due to poor health.
b. Conjunctivitis (inflammation of the covering of the eye).
c. Blepharitis (inflammation of the eyelid).
d. Lack of cleanliness.

### What is the treatment for styes?

Warm compresses and mild antiseptics will usually cause most of them to heal. Occasionally it is necessary for the eye surgeon to open them. Severe cases are treated with antibiotic drugs.

### How long does it take for the usual stye to disappear?

About five to eight days.

### What causes cysts of the eyelids (chalazion)?

An inflammation of one of the small glands in the lid with a clogging of its opening to the surface.

### What are the symptoms of a stye or cyst of the eyelid?

A markedly painful swelling and redness of the lid.

### What is the treatment for chalazions?

Most of them will respond to warm compresses and eyedrops. If they do not subside by themselves, they must be opened and removed under local anesthesia in the ophthalmologist's office.

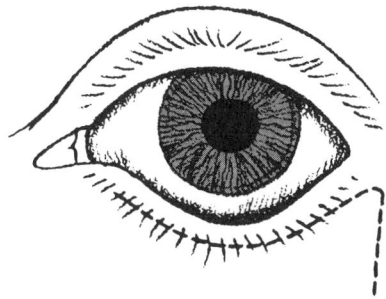

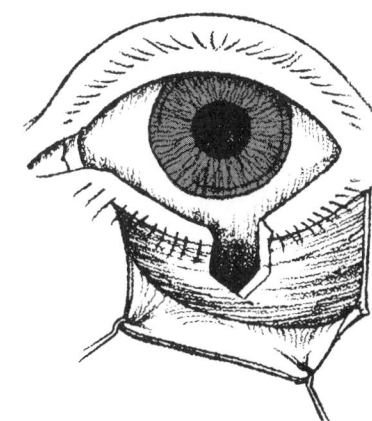

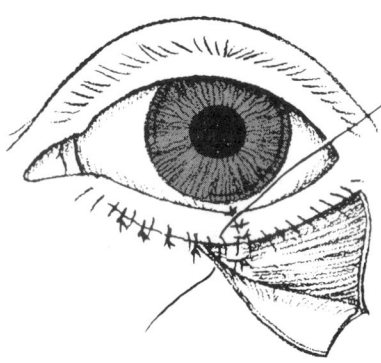

*Above:*
**Operation for Ectropion.** *The top diagram shows the line of incision. In the center, a wedge-shaped piece has been cut out of the lid. Below, the shortened eyelid is sutured.*

### Do these cysts have a tendency to recur once they are cured?

No, but there is a tendency for people who have developed one cyst (chalazion) to develop others.

## ENTROPION AND ECTROPION

### What is entropion?

It is a condition in which the margin of the upper or lower eyelid turns in, causing eyelashes to rub against and irritate the eyeball.

### What causes entropion?

It usually develops as a result of scarring consequent to an old inflammation of the eyelid. Occasionally it results from an injury with scarring. Another type is caused by overdevelopment of the muscle that closes the eyelids. This is the result of excessive squeezing of lids, particularly in older, high-strung people.

### Is it important to operate to repair an eyelid with entropion?

Yes, because the continued rubbing of the eyelashes against the eyeball will lead to permanent scarring and loss of vision.

### What operation is performed to correct entropion?

It is a simple plastic procedure, carried out under local anesthesia, in which a portion of the inside of the eyelid is cut away in such a manner as to cause the lid to bend outward.

### Are the results of operation for entropion successful?

Yes.

### What is ectropion?

It is a condition in which the margin of the upper or lower eyelid turns outward.

### Who is most likely to develop ectropion?

Older people whose elastic tissue of the eyelid is replaced with fibrous tissue.

### What is the most common cause for ectropion?

With advancing age there is a loss of elastic tissue within the eyelid, allowing it to fall away from the eyeball. Other cases are caused by scarring secondary to inflammation or injury.

### What are the symptoms of ectropion?

Since the eyelid—usually the lower one—has fallen away from the eyeball, tears run out onto the cheeks rather than into the tear duct.

*Below:*
**Operation for Entropion.** *The lashes are shown rubbing against the eye in the diagram at the top. Center, a wedge from the upper lid is inserted. The lengthened lid, with the lashes drawn away from the eye, is shown at the bottom.*

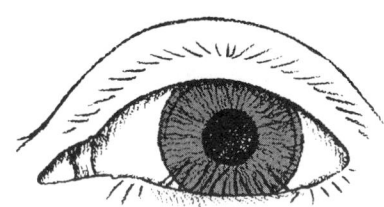

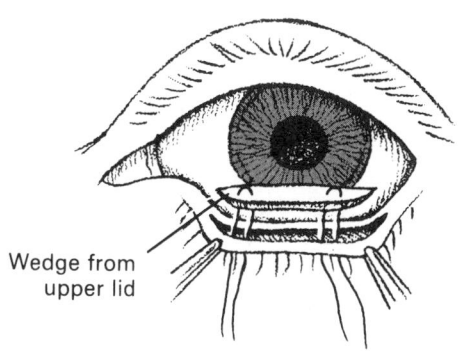

Wedge from
upper lid

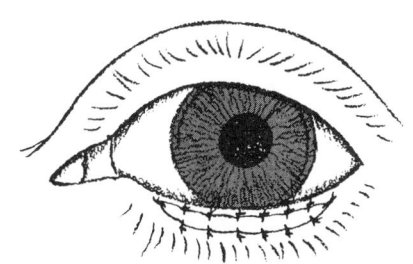

## Can ectropion be corrected surgically?

Yes, by a simple operative procedure a portion of the inside of the eyelid is excised so as to cause the lid to turn inward.

## How successful are operations for ectropion?

They are very successful in most cases.

# DACRYOCYSTITIS

## What is dacryocystitis?

Dacryocystitis is an inflammation of the tear sac of the eye.

## Who is most likely to develop dacryocystitis?

It is a common condition in infants under a year or two of age. It also occurs sometimes in elderly people whose tear ducts tend to become clogged or to be narrowed by fibrous tissue.

## What causes dacryocystitis?

Dacryocystitis is usually secondary to a blocked tear canal.

## What are the symptoms of dacryocystitis?

Pain and swelling of the inner corner of the eye, sometimes extending down toward the nose.

## What is the treatment for dacryocystitis?

The use of antibiotics and an incision for drainage of pus.

## Is recurrence frequent after cure of this condition?

Yes, unless the blockage of the tear canal is released by probing or by surgery.

## How long does it take for someone with dacryocystitis to get well?

Usually about a week.

# IRITIS

## What is iritis?

An inflammation of the iris, the colored part of the eyeball.

## What causes iritis?

Iritis may be caused by an immunological response to local infection, tuberculosis, syphilis, or other generalized diseases.

## What are the symptoms of iritis?

Pain, redness, and tearing of the eye, with inability to tolerate light.

## What is the treatment for iritis?

The treatment will depend upon the cause of the disease. It will consist, usually, of eyedrops containing atropine and cortisone.

## Is recovery possible after iritis?

Yes.

## Is the eyesight frequently damaged after iritis?

In some cases, a severe iritis may leave permanent damage to vision.

## How long does it take for iritis to get well?

In some cases, one to two weeks. In others, it may last for months and even years.

## Do some cases of iritis affect the deeper structures of the eye?

Yes, and if it involves the choroid, the inflammation may extend all the way back to the retina. In severe cases, vision may become greatly impaired, or even lost.

# GLAUCOMA

## What is glaucoma?

A condition in which the pressure within the eyeball is elevated above normal.

## What causes glaucoma?

The cause is unknown in most cases. Injury, hemorrhage in the eyeball, and/or displacement of the lens cause this condition.

## How often does glaucoma occur?

Two percent of all adults over the age of forty will develop glaucoma.

## Is it more common in males than in females?

No.

## Does it occur in children?

There is a rare form of glaucoma in children that is present from birth. This is called congenital glaucoma.

## Does glaucoma tend to run in families or to be inherited?

Yes.

## What are the harmful effects of glaucoma?

If untreated, it will cause serious decrease in vision and may result in blindness.

## What are the symptoms of glaucoma?

In the acute type, there is severe pain in the eye, redness of the eye, vomiting, and blurring of vision. In the chronic type, the patient may have no symptoms whatever until late in the course of the disease, when it is either difficult or too late to treat.

## How can one tell if he has glaucoma?

In the acute type, he will know very quickly because of the severe pain and blurring of vision. In the chronic type, it may be discovered on routine eye examination by the ophthalmologist.

## Is there any way to prevent getting glaucoma?

If the eye doctor suspects the patient of being a potential glaucoma case, he may prescribe prophylactic eyedrops, which will protect against the disease. Also, such patients require constant supervision.

## What tests are performed to make the diagnosis of glaucoma?

a. Taking the pressure of the eyeball with an instrument known as a tonometer.
b. Checking the visual fields.
c. Performing provocative tests.

## Should people be tested regularly for pressure of the eyeball?

Yes, this is an extremely simple test, and all adults should have it performed as part of their annual eye examination.

## Is it painful to have pressure of the eyeball tested?

There is no pain whatever.

## Does glaucoma usually affect both eyes at the same time?

Yes, except in an acute case. A patient who has developed the condition in one eye is more prone to develop it in the other eye at some later date.

## What is the treatment for glaucoma?

In the acute type, eyedrops and medications given by mouth or intravenously are used to reduce the intraocular pressure. If the pressure cannot be reduced after eight hours, surgery is indicated. In the chronic type, eyedrops may be continued for years as the sole means of treatment provided the pressure remains controlled; otherwise surgery is necessary.

## Is hospitalization necessary, or can the patient be satisfactorily treated at home?

Hospital care is necessary if surgery has to be done. Otherwise the patient may stay at home, but only if he maintains contact with his eye specialist.

## Is surgery always necessary?

It depends upon the pressure and the visual fields. If these can be controlled by eyedrops, surgery will not be necessary.

## What will happen if surgery is not performed when indicated?

Blindness will result.

## What will happen if the eyedrops are not used when indicated?

The patient may eventually lose the sight of the involved eye.

## Does glaucoma clear up by itself without treatment?

Usually not.

## Is the surgery for glaucoma dangerous?

No, but results are not always as good as one might wish. However, it is more dangerous in many cases *not* to operate.

## What are the chances for recovery after surgery?

In the acute type, the chances are excellent. In the chronic type, the earlier surgery is done, the better the chances for a good result.

## What kind of operation is performed?

An iridectomy, wherein a small piece of the iris is removed to allow drainage and to lessen the pressure within the eyeball. The actual procedure varies from case to case, depending upon whether the surgeon is dealing with an acute or a chronic glaucoma.

## What anesthetic is used?

Local or general anesthesia.

## How long a hospital stay is necessary?

Usually three to six days.

## Are special private nurses required after surgery?

No.

## Is there a visible scar after glaucoma operations?

No, except that one can see where a small piece of iris has been removed.

## Does glaucoma recur after it has been operated upon?

Usually not in the acute type. In the chronic glaucoma, it may recur.

## What limitations on activity are imposed after a succesful glaucoma operation?

a. Exceptional cleanliness must be maintained.
b. Water should be kept out of the eye if a *filtering* operation has been performed to cure the glaucoma.

## How soon after the operation can one do the following:

Bathe:
　One week.
Walk out in the street:
　One week.
Walk up and down stairs:
　One week.
Perform household duties:
　Two weeks.
Drive a car:
　Two weeks.
Resume sexual relations:
　Two weeks.
Return to work:
　Two weeks.
Resume all physical activities:
　Four weeks.

## Is it necessary to return for periodic examinations after an attack of glaucoma?

Yes. The physician will pay particular attention to the health of the uninvolved eye.

## CATARACT

## What is a cataract?

An opacity or a clouding of the lens.

## Where is the lens of the eye?

It is located inside the eye, just behind the pupil.

### What is its function?

To focus the image onto the retina in the back of the eye.

### What happens when a patient has a cataract?

The opaque lens does not allow light to enter the eyeball. Vision is thereby decreased.

### What causes cataract?

The cause is usually unknown. Sometimes, however, it may be due to diabetes, a glandular disorder, an infection within the eyeball, radiation, drugs, or a direct injury to the lens. The tendency to develop cataracts increases with age.

### Do cataracts tend to run in families or to be inherited?

Frequently, one finds that a tendency toward cataract formation is inherited.

### What harm results from leaving a cataract untreated?

As cataracts progress, vision decreases. If a cataract of long standing is not removed, it will become overripe, causing a severe inflammation and possible loss of the eyeball.

### How can one tell if he has a cataract?

Cataracts should be suspected if there is blurring of vision that cannot be improved by glasses. In the later stages it is possible to see the cataract as a white opacity in the pupil.

### Do cataracts usually affect both eyes at the same time?

Not often, but a person who has had a cataract is more prone to develop one on the other eye at some later date.

### Can people who have been operated upon for cataracts tolerate contact lenses?

Yes. They are advisable in many cases rather than standard eyeglasses.

### What is an intraocular lens?

It is a plastic lens that is sewn into the eyeball after the natural lens containing the cataract has been removed. The intraocular lens does away with the need for unsightly cataract eyeglasses and for contact lenses.

### Are intraocular lenses used routinely after cataract surgery?

No. At the present stage of development there is too great an incidence of serious complications, including infection followed by loss of vision.

### When are intraocular lenses most suitable?

a. When there is a cataract in one eye only. In such cases it does away with double vision.
b. In people in their eighties.

### How much greater is the risk of serious complication when intraocular lenses are employed?

The risk is approximately ten times greater when this type of lens is used after cataract removal.

### Are the new *continuous-wear* contact lenses valuable for use after a cataract removal?

Yes, although some problems still exist concerning their use by all patients. Nevertheless, they are much safer than intraocular lenses, and many patients tolerate them well.

### Is there any way to prevent getting cataracts?

No.

### What tests are performed to make a positive diagnosis of cataracts?

By using an instrument called an ophthalmoscope, the opacity of the lens can be seen readily.

### What is the treatment for cataracts?

Surgical removal of the lens.

### At what stage should a cataract be removed?

When it disables the patient. This usually does not take place until the vision in the involved eye is markedly diminished.

### Do cataracts ever disappear by themselves?

No.

### What are the chances for recovery following cataract surgery?

In over 90 percent of cases, good results are obtained.

### What kind of operation is performed?

An incision is made at the margin of the cornea and the white of the eye. Through this incision the surgeon inserts a probe, freezes it to the lens, and removes it.

### How long does an operation for removal of cataracts take to perform?

Forty to sixty minutes.

### What are the newer methods of cataract removal?

a. The use of cryosurgery, or lens removal through freezing. A "cryoprobe" freezes the probe to the lens, and the lens is lifted out. This method has largely replaced the technique of taking a forceps, grasping the lens, and lifting it out.
b. The employment of an ultrasound device to fragment, destroy, and suck out the lens. (Some people erroneously label this a laser device; it is not.) This method is reserved mainly for use in the treatment of cataracts in children.

### What anesthetic is used?

Usually a general anesthetic, but local anesthesia can be used, too.

### How long a hospital stay is necessary for a cataract operation?

In uncomplicated cases, five days.

### Are special private nurses required after surgery?

No, except for patients who are unable to care for themselves.

**Are special preoperative examinations necessary before a cataract operation?**

It is important to know that the patient is in good general health and free from infection, diabetes, etc. Poor general health or a distant focus of infection will interfere with the result of a cataract operation.

**Is the postoperative period especially painful?**

No.

**What is the postoperative treatment following cataract surgery?**

The patient is kept on his back for the first twenty-four hours with the operated eye bandaged. After this, the patient is allowed out of bed and the bandage is removed from the operated eye.

**What are possible complications of cataract surgery?**

Infection or hemorrhage within the eyeball.

**How are these complications treated?**

Infections are treated by the use of antibiotics and by washing out the eye. Hemorrhage is treated by applying a pressure bandage to the eye ball and keeping the patient quiet in bed. Certain drugs may also help to stop hemorrhage.

**How long does it take for the wound to heal after the usual cataract operation?**

Six weeks for thorough healing.

**What kind of scar remains?**

The scar is practically invisible.

**Do cataracts ever recur once they have been removed?**

Occasionally a membrane may form and obscure vision. However, this can be removed by a rather simple operation, and good vision usually will result.

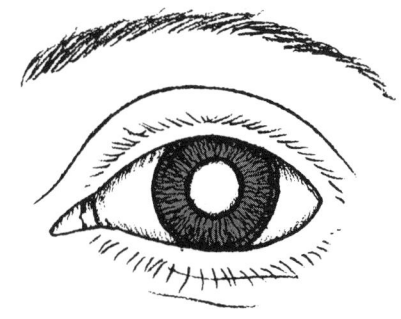

Eye with cataract

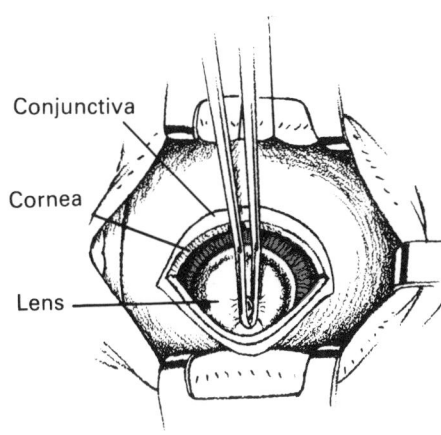

Conjunctiva

Cornea

Lens

Removing cataract

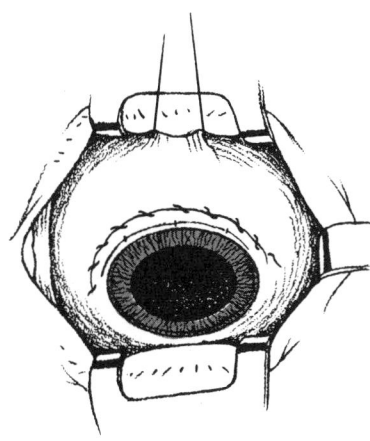

Eye with lens removed

*Cataract Operation. An eye with a cataract is shown at the top. In the center, the lens and cataract are being removed through an incision made in the cornea. At the bottom, the eye, with the lens removed, has been sutured.*

**How soon may a patient obtain glasses after a cataract operation?**

Within one month. If vision in the unoperated eye is good, it is sometimes not possible to use glasses for the operated eye as the patient may see double unless a contact lens is used.

**What postoperative precautions must be followed?**

The patient should not bend over or do strenuous work for about a month to six weeks after a cataract removal.

**After recovery from a cataract operation, does one return to a completely normal existence?**

Yes.

**How soon after the cataract operation can one do the following:**

Bathe:
   Two weeks.
Walk in the street:
   One week.
Walk up and down stairs:
   Two weeks.
Perform household duties:
   Four weeks.
Drive a car:
   Six weeks.
Resume sexual relations:
   Six weeks.
Return to light work:
   Two weeks.
Return to heavy work:
   Eight weeks.
Resume all physical activities:
   Eight weeks.

## STRABISMUS *(Crossed Eyes)*

**What is strabismus?**

A condition in which the eyes are not straight but are crossed. One or both eyes may turn in or out. The condition may be inconstant or constant.

**What causes strabismus?**

When strabismus is noticed at birth, it is due either to small brain hemorrhages or to abnormal attachments of the muscles of the eyeball. When it occurs after the first or second year of life, it is usually due to a weakness of the "fusion center" in the brain. It may also be associated with a weak or paralyzed eye muscle.

Convergent strabismus, where the eye turns in, is usually associated with farsightedness. Divergent strabismus, where the eye turns out, is often associated with nearsightedness.

### Does strabismus tend to run in families or to be inherited?

Yes.

### What is meant by "a cast in the eye"?

This is another term for crossed eyes.

### Is it more difficult to cure eyes that turn out than eyes that turn in?

Yes, but not always.

### How early in life can crossed eyes be recognized?

Often at birth; definitely at some time during the first three years of life. It may, however, start after the first three years.

### What percentage of crossed eyes can be cured with medical treatment alone?

About 40 to 50 percent.

### What is the medical treatment for strabismus?

a. The regular performance of special eye exercises known as orthoptics.
b. The regular performance of special eye exercises known as pleoptics. The latter is used to restore vision to a "lazy" eye.
c. The wearing of corrective eyeglasses and the use of eyedrops that constrict the pupil.
d. Placing a patch over the good eye to encourage vision in the crossed eye.

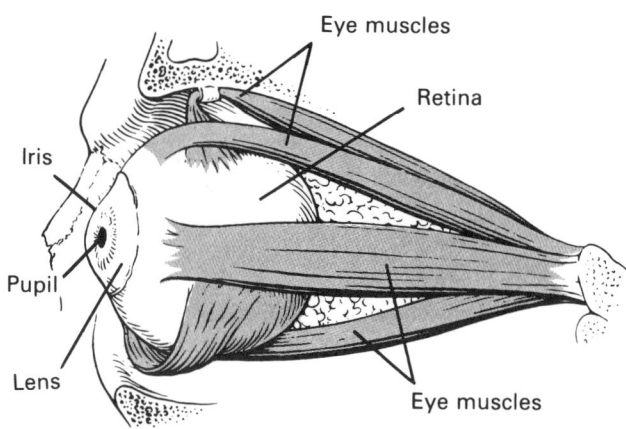

*Eye Muscles.* *This diagram shows the muscle attachments to the outside of the eyball. When these muscles fail to function normally, the eyes may become crossed or they may diverge. Both conditions can be helped greatly by surgery.*

*The surgeon will either shorten or lenghten the muscles in order to bring the eyes into proper alignment. Such an operation, although delicate, is not very complicated and may be performed safely on small children.*

e. The use of eyeglasses to correct farsightedness.

### How long must one wear glasses before the eyes straighten?

If the eyes are going to straighten, they will straighten immediately, but the glasses will have to be worn for many years.

### Why does strabismus sometimes not improve even after glasses are worn?

Because it is due to some factor other than nearsightedness or farsightedness such as faulty attachments of the muscles surrounding the eyeballs or to faulty nerves going to the muscles.

### What is the earliest age at which a child will be able to wear glasses for crossed eyes?

Two years of age.

### What harm results from strabismus?

It is disfiguring and can produce deep psychological harm. Convergent strabismus, if not treated, may result in poor vision or even loss of

vision in the eye that turns in. This is referred to as a "lazy eye."

### Is there any way to prevent strabismus?

Yes. If the patient shows signs of developing strabismus, the wearing of proper eyeglasses will often straighten the eye.

### Is there any way to prevent eyes that turn in from developing poor vision?

Yes. The patient wears a patch over the good eye, which forces him to use the weak eye. This will very often improve the vision in the weak eye. This method of treatment must be started at a very early age. After five or six years of age, this treatment is ineffective.

### Is surgery always necessary for strabismus?

No. If the strabismus is mild and inconstant, surgery is not necessary.

### Does strabismus ever get well by itself without treatment?

Yes. A mild case may get well by itself, but this is rare.

**What are the chances for a good result from surgery?**

The chances for a good result are excellent, but more than one operation may be necessary to obtain the desired result.

**What are the risks of surgery for strabismus?**

The risks are practically nil, but failure to correct the defect sometimes occurs.

**How long does it take to perform an operation for strabismus?**

This will depend upon the number of muscles that have to be operated upon. The average case takes one hour.

**What kind of operation is performed?**

This will vary with the type of strabismus. It may be necessary to strengthen a muscle. This is done by cutting off a piece of the muscle, or shortening it, and reattaching it to its original insertion on the eyeball. It may be necessary to weaken a muscle. This is done by detaching it from its insertion and reattaching it farther back on the eyeball.

**What anesthetic is used?**

For children, a general anesthetic. For adults, a local or general anesthetic.

**How long a hospital stay is necessary?**

Two days.

**Are special preoperative treatments necessary?**

In certain cases, orthoptics and/or patching is advisable.

**Are special private nurses required after surgery?**

No.

**Is the postoperative period exceptionally painful?**

No.

**What special postoperative procedures are carried out?**

Eyedrops and cold compresses are necessary following surgery. If the eyes are not absolutely straight, it may be necessary for the patient to take special eye exercises. These exercises are known as orthoptics.

**How long does it take for the wound to heal following a strabismus operation?**

About two to four weeks.

**Do patients ever see double after a strabismus operation?**

Yes, but this condition usually disappears within three to four weeks.

**What kind of scar remains after this operation?**

The scar is invisible.

**Does strabismus ever recur after it has been operated upon?**

Yes, in some cases.

**What can be done if the strabismus is not corrected by the initial surgery?**

Reoperation often brings about a cure.

**What postoperative precautions must be followed?**

For about a week after surgery, some patients should not read or watch television. Also, dirt must be kept away from the eye to avoid infection.

**Is it necessary for a patient to continue wearing glasses after surgery?**

If the patient was nearsighted or farsighted before the operation, it will be necessary for him to continue wearing glasses. Strabismus operations do not cure these eye conditions.

**After full recovery from a strabismus operation, can one use his eyes as much as he wishes?**

Yes.

**How soon after a strabismus operation can one do the following:**

Bathe:
As soon as one wishes.
Walk in the street:
Immediately.
Walk up and down stairs:
Immediately.
Resume some physical activity:
Immediately.
Perform light household duties:
One week.
Perform heavy household duties:
Two weeks.

## DETACHED RETINA AND RETINAL TEARS

**Where is the retina located and what is its function?**

The retina lines the inside of the back two-thirds of the eyeball. It is the sensitive part of the eyeball that transforms the light impulses into nerve impulses and transmits them to the brain. The retina is analogous to the film of a camera.

**What is a retinal tear?**

A rip in the retina, often caused by an injury.

**Is a retinal tear frequently followed by detachment of the retina?**

Yes.

**Can retinal detachment be prevented by prompt treatment of a retinal tear?**

Yes, in many cases.

**What are the symptoms of a retinal tear?**

Light-flashes and spots before the eyes. These symptoms are similar to those of a retinal detachment.

**What is the treatment for a tear in the retina?**

The tear is sealed by photocoagulation, using a laser beam.

## What is detachment of the retina?

A condition in which the retina is pulled away from its attachments to the inside of the eyeball.

## What causes detached retina?

It may be caused by a tear in the retina following an injury, inflammation, extreme nearsightedness, or a tumor of the choroid (a portion of the eye lying beneath the retina).

## Does detached retina occur more often among men than women?

No.

## Does it tend to run in families or to be inherited?

No.

## What harm results from a detached retina?

A detached retina, if not treated, may result in blindness.

## How can one tell if he has a detached retina?

A detached retina may be suspected if there is a veil or spots before the eyes or blurred vision in one portion of the eyeball. Light-flashes resembling lightning are a suspicious symptom.

## Is there any way to prevent getting a detached retina?

Exceptionally nearsighted people should be particularly careful to guard against injuries to the head. Also, a tear in the retina should be sealed off promptly.

## What tests are performed to make a positive diagnosis of detached retina?

The eye specialist will examine the eye with an ophthalmoscope, which allows him to see the retina. In the early cases, where the detachment is slight, or where the detachment is not centrally located, several examinations may be required before a definite diagnosis can be made.

## What surgical procedures are performed for detachment of the retina?

a. Light coagulation of the detached portion with the laser.
b. Freezing (cryotherapy) of the sclera over the area of the retinal detachment.
c. Shortening procedures of the eye in which portions are removed to cause buckling of the eyeball, thus allowing the retina to flop back into place against the back of the eyeball.
d. If there is a malignant tumor causing the detachment, it will be necessary to remove the eye.

## What will happen if surgery is not performed?

The eye will become blind and may even have to be removed.

## What are the chances of recovery of vision after surgery for retinal detachment?

This will depend upon the type of operation performed and the extent of the detachment. The recovery of vision and repair of the detachment takes place in about 90 percent of those patients who have undergone coagulation; the chances of successful results are about 75 percent when a buckling or shortening operation has been performed; with the use of the laser light coagulation, approximately 95 percent of tears in the retina can be sealed off.

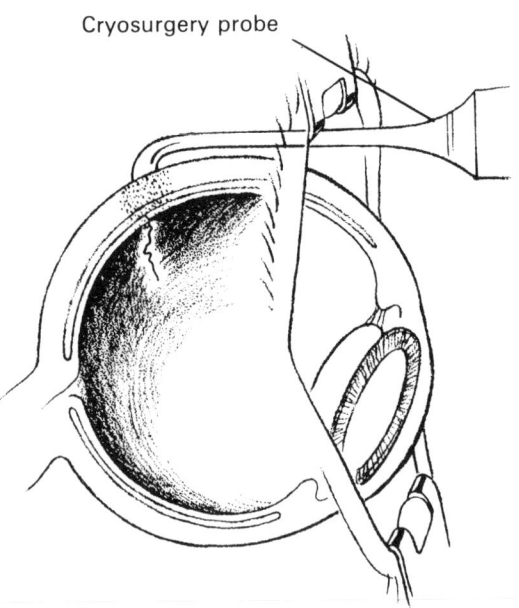

Cryosurgery probe

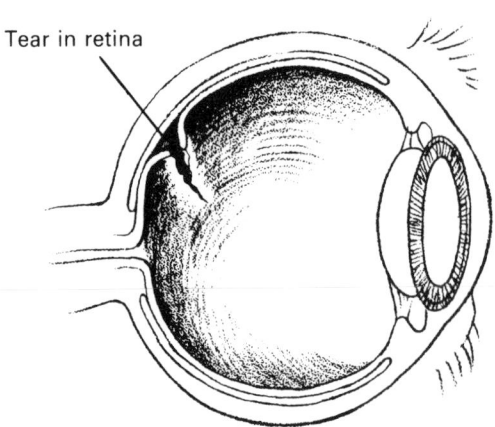

Tear in retina

**Retinal Detachment and Surgery.** *At left, the arrow points to the detached part of the retina. In the drawing above, a cryosurgical probe has frozen the detached retina to the eyeball.*

**How often is a detached retina caused by an underlying tumor?**

In only 1 percent of cases.

**How long does it take to perform an operation for detached retina?**

Approximately one to three hours.

**What anesthetic is used in surgery for retinal detachment?**

General anesthesia.

**How long a hospital stay is necessary?**

One to two weeks.

**Is the postoperative period exceptionally painful?**

No.

**What special postoperative treatments are carried out?**

a. The operated eye is bandaged for a few days.
b. The patient can be out of bed in one to four days.
c. Eyedrops are used for varying periods of time.

**How long does it take for the wound to heal?**

Three to six weeks.

**Are postoperative precautions necessary?**

Yes. The patient must limit physical activity for one to two months.

**Does detachment ever recur after it has once been successfully treated?**

Yes. This is not an infrequent occurrence.

**After full recovery from a detached retina, can one return to a completely normal existence?**

Yes.

**When should one return for a checkup after an operation for detached retina?**

Once a month for the first three months; thereafter, every four to six months.

**How soon after surgery for detached retina can one do the following:**

Bathe:
Three weeks.
Walk out in the street:
Two weeks.
Walk up and down stairs:
Four to six weeks.
Perform light household duties:
Six weeks.
Perform heavy household duties:
Eight weeks.
Resume all physical activities:
Eight weeks.

## DIABETES MELLITUS

**Does diabetes affect the eyes?**

Yes. Variations in the blood sugar can cause variations in vision. Diabetics who wear eyeglasses may require frequent changes in their prescriptions.

**Can diabetes cause blindness?**

Yes. It is one of the leading causes of blindness.

**How can partial or complete loss of vision be prevented in the diabetic?**

a. By regular periodic visits every four months to one's eye specialist.
b. By an immediate visit to one's eye specialist if a change in vision is noted.
c. By laser beam coagulation of areas of hemorrhage in the retina.

**Does leakage of blood from tiny vessels in the retina cause loss of vision in the diabetic?**

Yes, and the areas of leakage must be promptly treated with laser coagulation.

**Can vision be restored by use of laser coagulation?**

Yes, in a great many cases.

**Can vision ever be restored to an eye that has been blind for months or years?**

Yes, in some patients in whom hemorrhage has taken place within the inner gel (the vitreous) of the eye. To help these people, an operation known as a *vitrectomy* is performed in which the blood is washed out of the vitreous.

**Do cataracts occur more frequently, and at an earlier age, in diabetic patients?**

Yes.

## TUMORS OF THE EYE

**How common are tumors within the eyeball?**

They are rare.

**What are the common types of tumors within the eyeball?**

a. Melanomas, which arise in the choroid.
b. Gliomas, which arise in the retina.

**What age groups are most prone to develop these tumors?**

The glioma of the retina usually occurs in children under the age of five. It occurs in one eye in most cases, but sometimes occurs in both eyes. The melanoma of the choroid usually occurs in adults between the ages of forty and sixty and involves one eye only.

**What are the symptoms of glioma in children?**

If the child is very young, he may not complain at all. The parent, however, may notice a peculiar yellow color in the pupil. Older children may complain of blurring of vision, and in some cases the eye may turn in or out. In adults there may be blurring of vision. However, some patients may have no symptoms, and the condition is recognized only on routine examination.

## What is the treatment for glioma when only one eye is involved?

The eyeball should be removed as soon as possible! If both eyes are involved, the eye with the larger tumor is usually removed, and the tumor in the other eye is treated with radiation.

## What will happen if the operation is not performed?

The condition will spread to other parts of the body and cause death.

## What are the chances of recovery in adults?

The chances for recovery are good, especially if the tumor is treated during the early stages of its development.

## What are the chances for recovery when children have eye tumors?

Eye tumors in children are very serious. However, the latest reports are encouraging, and more and more children are being saved.

## RETINAL THROMBOSIS

### What is retinal thrombosis?

A condition in which clots form within the retinal blood vessels. As a result, a hemorrhage of the retina takes place, and vision is blurred or lost.

### What causes retinal thrombosis?

It is associated with hardening or arteriosclerosis of the blood vessels.

### What are the symptoms of retinal thrombosis?

Abrupt blurring or loss of vision.

### What is the treatment for retinal thrombosis?

In mild cases, rest of the eyes is all that is required. In severe cases, medication to reduce the clotting of the blood may be necessary. Laser beam coagulation is sometimes used to seal off newly formed blood vessels and thus prevent serious hemorrhage in the eye.

### Does recovery take place after retinal thrombosis?

In mild cases, yes. Severe cases may result in blindness.

### How long is one sick with retinal thrombosis?

Several months to years.

## SYMPATHETIC OPHTHALMIA

### What is sympathetic ophthalmia?

A strange inflammation that affects the healthy eye after a penetrating injury to the other eye.

### What causes sympathetic ophthalmia?

The cause is unknown.

### How does one know if sympathetic ophthalmia is developing?

If a patient has an injured eye that is red and painful, and he then develops redness or blurring of vision in the opposite eye, he may be developing the condition.

### Is there any way to prevent sympathetic ophthalmia?

In the past, it was often necessary to remove the injured eye in order to save the vision in the opposite eye. Today the use of cortisone and the antibiotic drugs often prevents sympathetic ophthalmia in the uninjured eye.

### After sympathetic ophthalmia has set in, is there any chance for complete recovery?

Yes.

### Does removing the injured eye help once sympathetic ophthalmia has set in?

No.

## TRACHOMA

### What is trachoma?

A serious, specific chronic inflammation of the eyes. It involves the cornea, the conjunctiva, and the eyelids.

### What causes trachoma?

The cause of trachoma is unknown, but poor hygiene and diet seem to play a great part in its causation.

### Where is trachoma most likely to be encountered?

In eastern Europe and northern Africa. It is extremely rare in the United States.

### What are the symptoms of trachoma?

In early cases, the symptoms are redness and tearing of the eyes. If the cornea is involved, there will be pain and extreme sensitivity to light.

### What is the treatment for trachoma?

The use of the sulfa drugs has proved to be effective in the early stages of the disease.

### Does trachoma ever cause blindness?

In serious cases, yes.

### Can trachoma be cured?

Yes, in its early stages.

### How long does trachoma last?

The neglected cases may last a lifetime.

### How can trachoma be prevented?

a. By proper diet and good hygiene.
b. By avoiding contact with people with trachoma.
c. By prompt medical attention to any eye irritation in those who live in an area where trachoma is prevalent.

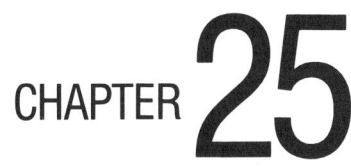

CHAPTER **25**

# THE FEMALE ORGANS

*(See also Chapter 3 on Adolescence Chapter 11 on Birth Control; Chapter 15 on Breasts; Chapter 55 on Pituitary Gland; Chapter 57 on Pregnancy and Childbirth; Chapter 64 on Sex; Chapter 69 on Sterility, Fertility, and Male Potency; Chapter 77 on Venereal Disease)*

## THE EXTERNAL GENITALS

### What is the vulva?

It is the area that surrounds the entrance to the vagina and is composed of the clitoris, the labia majora (major lips), the labia minora (minor lips), the opening of the urethra from the bladder, the hymen, the Bartholin glands, and the opening of the vagina.

### What is the clitoris and what is its function?

It is a small, knoblike structure on top of the vaginal opening where the lips of the vulva join together. The clitoris is a focal point of sexual excitement and plays an important part in sexual relations. The tissue structure of the clitoris is quite similar to that of the male penis.

### What is the hymen?

It is a fold of mucous membrane that partially or completely covers the vaginal opening. It is this membrane that is ruptured on first sexual contact.

### Are there many variations in the structure of the hymen?

Yes. In most girls, the hymen is not a complete covering but contains perforations that permit the exit of the menstrual flow. In some rare cases, these perforations are missing, and the hymen must be incised surgically in order to permit the exit of menstrual blood.

### What is a hymenotomy?

The surgical incision of the hymen in order to enlarge the vaginal opening.

### Why is hymenotomy performed?

a. For an imperforate hymen.
b. When a thickened or rigid hymenal ring makes sexual intercourse difficult or impossible.

### Is hymenotomy a major operative procedure?

No. It is a simple procedure performed under light anesthesia in the hospital.

### Is hymenotomy always necessary when intercourse is difficult?

No. Most cases of painful intercourse are due to vaginal spasm. This spasm is brought about by tension and fear of sexual relations. By proper advice and instruction, women can overcome many of their fears, thus controlling the spasm. Also, in many cases, stretching the hymen is all that is necessary. This procedure is performed in the gynecologist's office.

### Is difficulty in breaking the hymen a common occurrence?

No. It is relatively rare.

### How soon after hymenotomy can sexual relations be attempted?

About three weeks.

### What is the cause of painful intercourse in women who have been having normal relations for many years?

a. An emotional problem is often responsible for painful intercourse (dyspareunia) when it appears later in life.
b. Less commonly, there is an or-
ganic condition, such as an inflammation of the vagina or an inflammation of the pelvic organs, which is responsible for painful intercourse.

### What are the Bartholin glands?

They are two small bulblike structures located in the lower end of the lips, one on each side of the vagina. They are connected to the vaginal canal by a narrow duct.

### What is the function of the Bartholin glands?

They secrete a mucous substance, which acts as a lubricant for the inner surface of the lips of the vagina.

### What is a Bartholin cyst?

It is a swelling of the duct—or the duct and the gland—caused by a blockage at the vaginal end of the duct. These cysts may be as small as a pea or as large as a plum.

### What are the usual symptoms of a Bartholin cyst?

a. Pain on walking or during intercourse.
b. A swelling in the lips (labia).

### What is the treatment for a Bartholin cyst?

Either surgical removal or incision into the cyst and fashioning a new opening ("marsupialization" operation).

### Is hospitalization necessary for this type of operation?

Yes, for approximately three days.

### What is a Bartholin abscess?

It is an infection of a Bartholin gland caused by bacteria.

### What is the treatment for a Bartholin abscess?

a. Antibiotic drugs, hot soaks, and sedatives for the relief of pain.
b. In the more severe case, it will be necessary to incise and drain the abscess or to create a new perma-

nent opening by performing a marsupialization operation.

### Is hospitalization necessary for incision and drainage of a Bartholin abscess?

Yes. This procedure must be carried out under general anesthesia and will require hospitalization for a few days. In some instances, under local anesthesia, incision and drainage are performed as an office procedure.

### What is vulvitis?

It is an inflammation or infection of the area about the external genitals.

It is most often associated with an infection within the vagina.

### What is leukoplakia of the vulva?

It is a disease of the skin of the vulva characterized by an overgrowth of cells and a tendency toward the formation of cancer. The areas of leukoplakia look grayish white and develop a parchmentlike appearance.

### What causes leukoplakia of the vulva?

The exact cause is unknown, but it is supposedly related to a decrease in the secretion of ovarian hormone, which takes place after menopause.

### Who is most likely to develop leukoplakia?

Women who have passed the menopause.

### Is leukoplakia of the vulva a common condition?

No. It is relatively infrequent.

### What are the symptoms of leukoplakia of the vulva?

Itching is the most striking feature of this condition. Scratching will often lead to secondary infection from surface bacteria and may lead to inflammation, swelling, pain, redness, and even bleeding from the vicinity.

### Does leukoplakia ever develop into cancer of the vulva?

Yes. Most cases of cancer of the vulva are preceded by leukoplakia. However, this does not mean that all women with leukoplakia will develop cancer.

### What is the treatment for leukoplakia of the vulva?

a. If infection is present, antibiotic drugs should be given locally and orally.
b. If itching is severe, anesthetic ointments should be applied.

### Does leukoplakia ever clear up by itself?

Temporary relief often results from medical management, but surgery is the only real cure for this condition.

### How long would it take for leukoplakia to develop into cancer?

This is a very slow process, which takes place over a period of years.

### Does cancer ever involve the vulva?

Yes. The clitoris, the lips, the Bartholin glands, or the opening of the urethra may sometimes be involved in a cancerous process.

### What is the treatment for cancer of the vulva?

Vulvectomy. This means the surgical

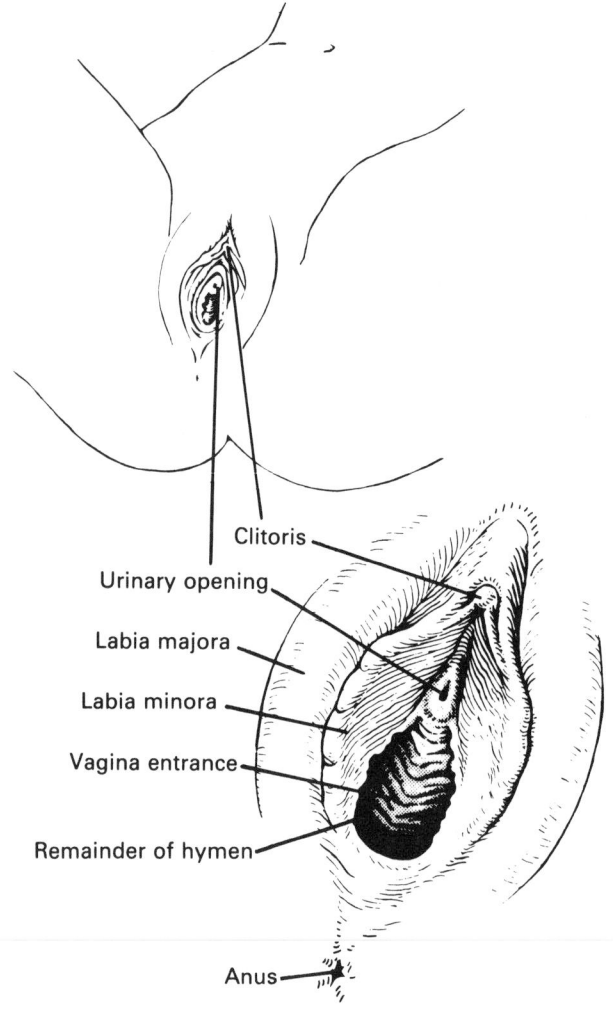

Clitoris
Urinary opening
Labia majora
Labia minora
Vagina entrance
Remainder of hymen
Anus

*The External Female Genitals. This diagram shows the external female genitals, including the clitoris, the lips of the vagina, and the vagina. It is amazing how few females are familiar with their own bodily construction in this region.*

removal of all those structures comprising the vulva. The lymph glands in the groin are also removed in performing a radical vulvectomy for the eradication of an extensive cancer of the vulva.

### Is cancer of the vulva curable?

Yes, if treated properly in its early stages by vulvectomy. It is estimated that more than 60 percent of cancers of the vulva can be cured permanently.

### What is the incidence of cancer of the vulva?

It is a rare disease.

### How is the diagnosis of cancer of the vulva made?

A piece of tissue is surgically removed and submitted to microscopic examination.

### Who is most likely to develop cancer of the vulva?

Women beyond sixty years of age.

### Is vulvectomy a serious operation?

Yes, but operative recovery takes place in almost all cases.

### What is the vagina?

It is a tubelike canal approximately three to four inches in length, extending internally from its opening at the vulva to the cervix of the uterus. It is lined by a mucous membrane, which has many folds and great elasticity.

### What are the functions of the vagina?

a. It is the ultimate female organ of intercourse.
b. It is a receptacle for the deposit of male sperm.
c. It is the outlet for the discharge of menstrual fluid.
d. It is the passageway for delivery of a baby.

### Should women douche regularly?

Some gynecologists do advocate douching for purely hygienic pur-

poses; others recommend it only for specific medical conditions.

### What is the best solution with which to douche?

An acid douche containing white distilled vinegar or lactic acid is adequate. Other commercially prepared douches are also effective. The latter should be prescribed by a physician.

### Are strong antiseptic douches harmful?

Yes. Strong chemicals can cause vaginal ulcers or burns.

### Should women douche if they have a vaginal discharge or unpleasant odor?

Not without a gynecologist's specific instructions.

### Should women douche following sexual relations or after the conclusion of a menstrual period?

Yes, as it will often prevent unpleasant odor or discharge. However, douching is not essential.

### Is cancer of the vagina very common?

No. This is a very rare disease.

### What is the treatment for cancer of the vagina?

Wide surgical excision of the vagina or radium implantation.

### What other growths may affect the vagina?

a. Polyps.
b. Cysts.
c. Benign tumors, such as fibromas of the vaginal wall.

### What is the treatment for benign growths of the vagina?

Simple surgical removal will bring about a cure in all of the above conditions.

### What is prolapse of the uterus?

It is an abnormal descent of the uterus and cervix into the vagina. It

is often associated with disturbance of the bladder and the rectum.

### What causes prolapse of the uterus?

Most cases occur as a result of stretching or tears that have been incurred during labor and delivery. Women who have had several children may suffer stretching or tearing of the ligaments and muscles that ordinarily support the uterus and the vagina.

### Is prolapse of the uterus caused by poor obstetrical management?

No. Tears of supporting ligaments may take place despite excellent obstetrical care.

### Are there various degrees of prolapse?

Yes. There may be just slight descent of the uterus and cervix into the vagina, or the entire cervix and uterus may come down so far that they appear outside the vaginal opening.

### What are the symptoms of prolapse of the uterus?

There is a feeling of fullness in the vagina and a sensation that something is falling down. These symptoms are aggravated after walking or lifting a heavy object. The prolapsed structures may interfere with sexual intercourse, and a disturbance in urination and bowel function may be present. Symptoms will depend largely upon the degree of prolapse.

### Can prolapse of the uterus be prevented?

Good obstetrical care will tend to minimize the incidence of prolapse, but it often cannot prevent it.

### What is the treatment for prolapse?

The treatment is surgical. It will require a plastic operation upon the vagina to reconstruct the ligaments and muscles, or, in a woman past the menopause, it may require the removal of the uterus and cervix (vaginal hysterectomy).

## Are operations for prolapse serious?

They are considered major surgery, but the risks are not great and recovery will take place.

## How long a period of hospitalization is necessary for prolapse operations?

Approximately ten to twelve days.

## Is there any medical treatment for prolapse?

Yes. The insertion of a pessary will help to keep the uterus and cervix in normal position. However, this form of treatment will not bring about a cure and should not be used as a substitute for surgery unless for some reason the patient cannot undergo an operative procedure.

## Why isn't the use of a pessary prolonged indefinitely?

a. It does not cure the underlying deficiency.
b. It may lead to an ulceration of the vagina, an inflammation of the vaginal wall, or secondary infection.
c. The wearing of a pessary requires frequent douching and frequent visits to the gynecologist.
d. A pessary requires monthly visits to the doctor's office for removal, cleansing, and replacement.

## What is a cystocele?

It is a hernia of the bladder wall into the vagina. Cystoceles may vary in degree from a mild bulge into the vagina to a maximum descent in which almost the entire bladder protrudes through the vaginal opening.

## What is a rectocele?

It is a hernia of the rectal wall into the vagina. Again, the degree of herniation varies markedly from case to case.

## What causes cystoceles or rectoceles?

They are caused by the same type of injury that causes a prolapse, that is, a tear of supporting ligaments as a result of childbirth.

## How often do cystocele, rectocele, and prolapse occur?

These are common conditions. The incidence is greater in women who have had many children. Also, women past forty are more likely to develop these conditions as their supporting ligaments begin to weaken and stretch.

## Do cystocele, rectocele, and prolapse tend to occur together?

Yes, in a great number of instances. However, it is entirely possible to have a prolapse without a cystocele or rectocele, or to have a cystocele without a rectocele, or vice versa.

## What are the symptoms of a cystocele?

The most common symptoms are frequency of urination, loss of urine on coughing, sneezing, laughing, or physical exertion. There may also be a sensation of a bulge into the vagina.

## What are the symptoms of rectocele?

A feeling of pressure in the vagina and rectum, with difficulty in evacuating the bowels.

## Do cystocele or rectocele and prolapse ever lead to cancer?

No.

## What is the treatment for cystocele and rectocele?

A vaginal plastic operation in which the torn ligaments and muscles are repaired and stretched or excess tissues excised.

## Are operations for cystocele and rectocele serious?

No, but they demand the attention of an expert gynecologist who understands the anatomy and function of the region.

## How long a period of hospitalization is necessary following vaginal plastic operations?

Seven days.

## Are the results of operations for cystocele, rectocele, and prolapse satisfactory?

Yes. Cure can be accomplished in almost all cases.

## Can cystocele, rectocele, or prolapse be corrected medically?

No, but temporary relief can be obtained with the use of rings or pessaries. Such appliances do not bring about a cure.

## When is surgery necessary for cystocele, rectocele, or prolapse?

When the symptoms mentioned previously are sufficient to interfere with normal happy living, or when bladder or bowel function becomes impaired.

## What are the chances of recurrence after surgery?

After competent surgery, the chances of recurrence are less than 5 percent.

## Are there any visible scars following vaginal plastic operations?

No.

## What type of anesthesia is used for these procedures?

Spinal, epidural, or general anesthesia.

## How long do these operations take to perform?

A complete vaginal plastic operation may take anywhere from one to two hours.

## Are private nurses necessary after these operations?

Not usually, although they are a

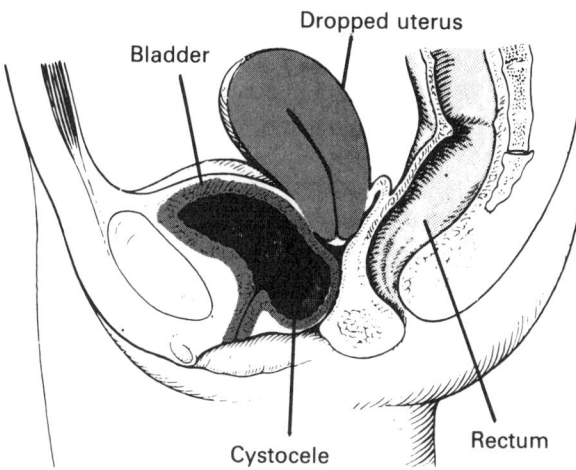

Bladder Dropped uterus

Cystocele Rectum

*Left:*

**Cystocele.** *Due to stresses and strains often occuring during childbirth, a tear of the muscles and ligaments that support the urinary bladder may take place and may result in a hernia of the bladder down toward the vagina. Loss of bladder control may follow, and when this happens, surgical repair should be undertaken.*

*Below:*

**Rectocele.** *When the tear in the supporting muscles and ligaments takes place in the posterior portion of the vagina, the rectum may protrude into the vagina. A rectocele is often accompanied by symptoms of marked constipation. Fortunately, this condition too can be repaired readily by surgery.*

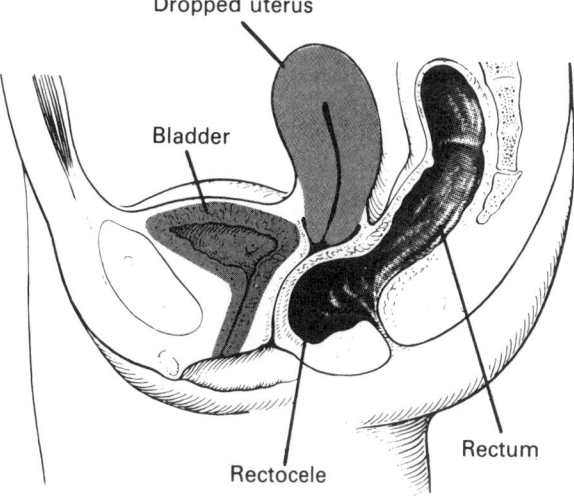

Dropped uterus

Bladder

Rectocele Rectum

great comfort if the patient is able to afford them for a few days.

### Are operations upon the vagina very painful?

No.

### How soon after vaginal operations is the patient permitted to get out of bed?

On the day following surgery.

### Are any special postoperative precautions necessary?

Yes, a catheter may be placed in the bladder for a few days to aid restoration of bladder function.

### What is the effect of vaginal plastic operations upon the bladder and rectum?

Occasionally, for the first week or two, there may be difficulty in urinating. Also, in operations for rectocele, there may be difficulty in moving one's bowels for a similar period. These complications are temporary and will subside spontaneously.

### Do stitches have to be removed after these operations?

No. The stitches are absorbable and do not have to be removed.

### Is it common to bleed a great deal after operations upon the vagina?

No.

### How soon after a vaginal plastic operation can one do the following:?

Shower:
  One to two days.
Bathe:
  Four weeks.
Walk in the street:
  One to two weeks.
Perform household duties:
  Three weeks.
Drive a car:
  Four weeks.
Resume sexual relations:
  Eight weeks.
Return to work: Six weeks.
Douche: Six weeks.

### Do vaginal plastic operations interfere with sexual relations?

No. When the tissues have healed, intercourse can be resumed. This usually takes six to eight weeks.

### Can women have babies after surgery for a cystocele or rectocele?

Yes, but delivery may have to be performed by Cesarean section, as surgery may have interfered with the ability of these structures to stretch and dilate sufficiently. Also, vaginal delivery might bring on a recurrence of the cystocele or rectocele.

### Can pregnancy take place after surgery for prolapse of the uterus?

Yes, if only the cervix has been removed. Here, too, delivery should be by Cesarean section. Of course, if a hysterectomy has been performed in order to cure the prolapse, pregnancy cannot take place.

### When is it best to undergo plastic repair?

After one has completed having children.

## What is vaginitis?

It is an inflammation of the vagina.

## What causes vaginitis?

a. Infections such as *Trichomonas*.
b. Fungi such as *Monilia*.
c. Common bacterial infections with staphylococcus, streptococcus, etc.
d. Changes due to old age (senile vaginitis).
e. As a complication of the administration of antibiotic drugs that destroy certain useful vaginal bacteria, vaginitis is occasionally encountered.

## Does the healthy vagina contain bacteria?

Yes, and most of these bacteria are beneficial and are not the cause of disease.

## What causes *Trichomonas* or fungus infections of the vagina?

A change in vaginal acidity, which permits these organisms to outgrow the other organisms that are normally present.

## Can *Trichomonas* infections be transmitted through sexual intercourse?

Yes. Men as well as women can have *Trichomonas* infections.

## What lessens acidity of the vagina?

Menstrual blood will often lessen the acidity and allow harmful organisms to grow and multiply and produce the symptoms of vaginitis.

## What are the symptoms of vaginitis?

This will depend upon the cause of the infection. Parasitic, fungus, or bacterial vaginitis usually produces the following symptoms:
a. Itching of the vulva.
b. Vaginal discharge.
c. Pain on intercourse.
d. Pain and frequency of urination.
e. Swelling of the external genital structures.

## What are the symptoms of senile vaginitis?

Itching, but very little vaginal discharge. There is also pain on intercourse and, rarely, vaginal bleeding.

## What tests are performed to determine the type of vaginitis that is present?

A smear of the vaginal discharge is taken and is submitted to microscopic examination. This will demonstrate whether the infection is caused by *Monilia, Trichomonas,* or bacteria.

## What is the treatment for vaginitis?

This will depend upon its cause:
a. Fungus infections are now treated successfully by giving various antifungal medications by mouth as well as local applications into the vaginal canal.
b. *Trichomonas* infections are treated by giving both the female and male a drug known as Flagyl. This medication is taken orally for seven to ten days.
c. Bacterial vaginitis is treated with one of the antibiotic medications, administered orally or locally.
d. Senile vaginitis is treated by the administration of a local cream containing an estrogenic substance.

## Is there a tendency for vaginitis to recur?

Yes. Many types of vaginitis do have this tendency. For this reason, treatment must be continued over a prolonged period of time. It is common for people to discontinue treatment too quickly because of early relief of symptoms.

## What is the most common time for a vaginitis to recur?

Just before or after a menstrual period and during the later months of pregnancy. This strongly suggests that hormone changes in the vaginal lining play an important role in these conditions.

## Does vaginitis ever occur in children?

Yes, vulvovaginitis is not uncommon in young girls from two to fifteen years of age. The infection is transmitted by poor hygiene, poor toilet habits, or by a foreign body the child might have inserted into her vagina.

## What is the treatment for vaginitis in children?

Specific medications should be given for the specific infection. These may include the administration of medications orally and the application of ointments locally.

## What causes gonorrhea in women?

In almost every instance it is caused by sexual intercourse with an infected male. Very rarely, gonorrhea may be transmitted from contaminated fingers or bathroom equipment.

## What structures in the female genitals are affected by gonorrhea?

The vulva, Bartholin glands, the urethra, the vagina, and the cervix of the uterus are almost always involved in the infection. If the infection extends, it goes up through the cervix into the uterus, out into the Fallopian tubes to the ovaries, and finally to the abdominal cavity, where it causes gonorrheal peritonitis.

## What are the symptoms of gonorrhea in the female?

There may be no symptoms at all, or the first symptoms might be slight discomfort in the vagina, vaginal discharge, burning, frequency of urination, and abdominal pain. These symptoms progress and become more marked for the first few days of the disease.

## How is the diagnosis of gonorrhea made?

Microscopic examination reveals the specific causative germ, the gonococcus. *A definite diagnosis is never made unless the actual germ can be seen under the microscope.*

### What is the treatment for gonorrhea in the female?

The administration of antibiotic drugs. *If treated promptly, all the harmful permanent effects of gonorrhea can be avoided.* All too often the shame of having a social disease restrains young women from seeking early treatment. The result is that the harmful results have taken too firm a hold before active treatment is instituted. If this has happened, infection of the tubes, ovaries, and abdominal cavity cannot be obliterated completely even with the use of the antibiotic drugs.

### Does gonorrhea ever require surgical treatment?

Yes, under the following conditions:
a. When the Bartholin glands are involved, they may have to be incised or removed.
b. When the Fallopian tubes or ovaries are chronically infected, they may have to be removed.

### Does gonorrhea interfere with childbearing?

Untreated gonorrhea, or chronic gonorrhea that has affected the tubes and ovaries, will definitely be a factor in the causation of sterility.

There is a very high incidence of sterility in women with chronic gonorrhea.

### Does complete recovery take place if treatment for gonorrhea is carried out promptly and adequately?

Yes.

### How does syphilis affect the female genital organs?

A painless chancre (syphilitic sore) may appear anywhere in the vulva or vagina.

### How is the diagnosis of syphilis made in a female?

It is diagnosed by direct examination of a suspicious lesion. A scraping from the sore is taken and is examined under a microscope. The diagnosis is then further confirmed by taking a blood test for syphilis.

### What is the usual method of transmission of syphilis?

Through sexual intercourse with an infected male.

### What is the treatment for syphilis?

See Chapter 77, on Venereal Disease.

### Can syphilis interfere with childbearing?

If the syphilis has been treated adequately and promptly, cure can be brought about so that childbearing will probably not be affected. Years ago, when syphilis was more prevalent, it caused miscarriages and stillbirths.

## MENSTRUATION

### What is menstruation?

It is a bloody discharge from the vagina occurring at more or less regular intervals throughout the childbearing period of a woman's life. Each month the womb (uterus) prepares itself for pregnancy by certain changes in its lining membrane. If a fertilized egg does not implant itself into the wall of the uterus, its lining disintegrates and is discharged from the uterus in the form of the menstrual flow.

### When does menstruation begin?

Sometime between the ages of eleven and sixteen years. This will depend upon factors such as climate, race, and general health. In rare instances, normal menstruation may commence before the eleventh year or after the sixteenth year.

### How long does menstruation last?

It usually continues until age forty-five to fifty-five.

### What is the normal interval between menstrual periods?

The normal menstrual cycle occurs approximately every twenty-eight days. However, this is highly variable, and some women may develop a cycle with intervals of twenty-one, thirty, thirty-five, or even forty days. A woman who menstruates every twenty-eight days and then changes to a twenty-one-day cycle or a thirty-five-day cycle should consult her physician.

### What are common conditions, other than pregnancy, that will cause a woman to miss a period?

a. A sudden change in climate.
b. An acute emotional upset.
c. An acute infection or illness.
d. Hormone imbalance or poor function of the endocrine glands.
e. A cyst or tumor of the ovary.
f. Poor nutrition or vitamin deficiency.
g. Marked anemia.
h. Chronic debilitating diseases, such as tuberculosis, cancer, etc.
i. The onset of menopause (change of life).

### How soon after a period has been missed can it be determined if pregnancy exists?

A pregnancy test can give this information approximately fourteen days after a period has been missed.

### Can medications, or other artificial measures, be used successfully to bring on a menstrual period when it has been skipped because of pregnancy?

No. Hot baths, laxatives, or patent drugs will not bring on a period if pregnancy exists.

### Are there harmful effects from taking medications to bring on a menstrual period when it is late?

Yes. The patient should never try to treat herself to bring on a menstrual period artificially. There is definite danger from the use of such medications. Moreover, if a pregnancy exists, the embryo may be injured.

## How long do menstrual periods usually last?

Approximately four to five days. Here again, the length of time may vary from one to seven or eight days. The important consideration is a deviation from the usual duration.

## What is the natural appearance of menstrual blood?

Normal menstrual blood is a pink to dark red color and does not clot. The presence of clots, or pieces of blood, or marked change in the amount of flow or the duration of the period warrants medical consultation.

## Is there a detectable odor to normal menstruation?

No.

## Is it normal for some women to have slight swelling of the face, neck, breasts, and abdomen during the menstrual period?

Yes. This is often due to retention of body fluids. Many physicians prescribe diuretic tablets to relieve this condition.

## What is the significance of scant menstruation?

a. If pregnancy is not a likelihood, then a single instance of scant menstruation should be disregarded as insignificant.
b. Repeated, persistent, scant menstruation is often due to a failure of the bleeding mechanism caused by an upset in the glands that regulate menstruation, such as the pituitary or the ovaries or the thyroid.
c. In women in their forties or early fifties, scant menstruation may be the forerunner of change of life (menopause).

## What is the cause of failure of onset of menstruation?

This is almost always caused by a disturbance in glandular function. Less frequently a mechanical block, such as an imperforate (closed) hymen, may be responsible.

## Should lack of menstruation in a girl in her middle or late teens warrant investigation by a physician?

Yes. Proper treatment can frequently correct this condition.

## What is the treatment for scant menstruation?

During the childbearing age, scant menstruation requires no treatment if there is evidence that the woman is ovulating regularly. This means that she is producing a mature egg from an ovary each month. If ovulation is not taking place, further medical investigation is indicated. This should include an evaluation of the activity of the various endocrine glands. Where a deficiency in the secretion of a particular hormone is discovered, specific treatment is directed toward replacing or correcting such deficiency.

## Does the giving of the appropriate hormone usually correct scant menstruation or absent menstruation?

When properly administered, hormone treatments will usually bring about regulation of the normal cycle.

## Does scant menstruation prevent pregnancy from taking place?

Only when it is associated with lack of ovulation. If ovulation is present, scant menstruation will not interfere with pregnancy.

## Does scant menstruation often indicate the beginning of menopause in a woman in her late forties or early fifties?

Yes.

## What is the significance of irregular menstrual bleeding?

Its significance varies with the type of irregularity. Most women have a slight variation of one to two days, either in onset or in length of flow. Marked changes in the time of onset, in the length of the flow, the amount of bleeding, or the presence of bleeding not associated with menstruation requires investigation by the gynecologist. The appearance of "staining" just before or just after menstruation should also be investigated.

## What are some of the more common causes of irregular menstruation?

a. Infection within the female genital system.
b A benign tumor of the uterus or ovaries.
c. A malignant tumor of the uterus or ovaries.
d. Imbalance of the endocrine glands (pituitary, thyroid, or ovaries).
e. Ectopic pregnancy (a pregnancy that takes place outside of the uterus, usually in the Fallopian tubes).
f. Other nongynecological conditions, such as hepatitis, pneumonia and other infections, or stress, often affect the menstrual cycle.

## What is the significance of excessive menstrual bleeding?

Excessive bleeding during the period is not normal and should be investigated. It may be indicative of infection, glandular upset, or the presence of a tumor within the uterus or the ovaries.

## What is the treatment for excessive menstrual bleeding?

This will depend entirely upon the cause; each cause will be discussed separately in other sections of this chapter.

## What is dysmenorrhea?

This term applies to painful menstruation.

## What causes dysmenorrhea?

In some patients, particularly those who have not had pregnancies, the cause may be associated with a narrow cervical canal (mouth of the womb). Excessive fluid retention within the body is also associated with painful menstruation. Various emotional conditions are seen in conjunction with dysmenorrhea, especially in patients who have a low threshold for pain.

Organic conditions such as cysts or tumors of the ovaries, tumors of the uterus, endometriosis (see the questions on Endometriosis in this chapter), and adhesions from previous infections or surgery in the pelvic area are also common causes of painful menstruation.

## What is the medical treatment for dysmenorrhea?

a. Pain-relieving and antispasmodic medications.
b. In many cases, the administration of birth control pills are very helpful.
c. Diuretic medications to get rid of excess water retention.

## Is surgery ever helpful in treating painful menstruation?

If the dysmenorrhea is so severe that it becomes disabling, surgery may be contemplated. This will consist of dilatation of the cervical canal to widen the opening. If the dysmenorrhea is due to disease of the tubes, ovaries, or uterus, these conditions must be remedied surgically.

## Will a pregnancy tend to relieve painful menstruation?

After a woman has borne a child, dysmenorrhea is often relieved.

## What is premenstrual tension?

It is the periodic appearance of disturbing anxieties occurring about the middle of the menstrual cycle and increasing in intensity as menstruation approaches. This tension subsides when menstruation begins.

## What causes premenstrual tension?

The exact cause is unknown, but this phenomenon is attributed to a change in the amount of hormones that are secreted at various times throughout the menstrual cycle and the amount of fluids that the body retains.

## What are some of the symptoms of premenstrual tension?

There may be personality changes, irritability, emotional instability, episodes of crying, etc. Physical symptoms such as backache, severe abdominal cramps, breast pain and tenderness, headaches, and swelling of the legs are some of the more definable features.

## What is the treatment for premenstrual tension?

Simple measures will include:
a. Restriction of salt intake prior to menstruation.
b. The giving of medications to increase the output of urine and the reduction of tissue fluids.
c. The taking of birth control pills.

## Will a woman who is taking birth control pills continue to menstruate regularly?

Yes, but menstruation will not be accompanied by ovulation (the shedding of an egg by the ovary).

## Are tampons that are inserted into the vagina harmful to use?

Not for the great majority of women. However, in a small number of cases, a serious infection called "toxic shock syndrome" has resulted following their use.

## What are the symptoms of toxic shock syndrome?

High fever, chills, nausea, and diarrhea.

## How common is toxic shock syndrome?

Tens of millions of women use tampons; only a few dozen cases of toxic shock syndrome have been reported.

## How is toxic shock syndrome treated?

By intensive antibiotic therapy carried out in a hospital.

## Can toxic shock syndrome be overcome?

Yes, in most instances, if treated early and intensively.

## What is the cause of toxic shock syndrome following the use of tampons?

It is thought that the condition occurs because of leaving the tampons in too long, thus allowing bacteria to grow and enter the body through the uterus.

## Should a young child of ten or eleven years be told about menstruation?

Yes. Preparing the girl for menstruation is a very important parental duty. Children should not be permitted to reach the age of menstruation without adequate advance information.

## Is it true that if a mother has painful menstruation her child will develop it?

Painful menstruation is not inherited, but a child unconsciously tends to mimic her mother's reactions. It is wise, therefore, for the mother to minimize the discomfort of menstruation.

## Can a shower be taken with safety during a menstrual period?

Yes.

## Is it dangerous to go swimming or to take a bath during a menstrual period?

No.

## Are sexual relations dangerous or harmful during menstruation?

No.

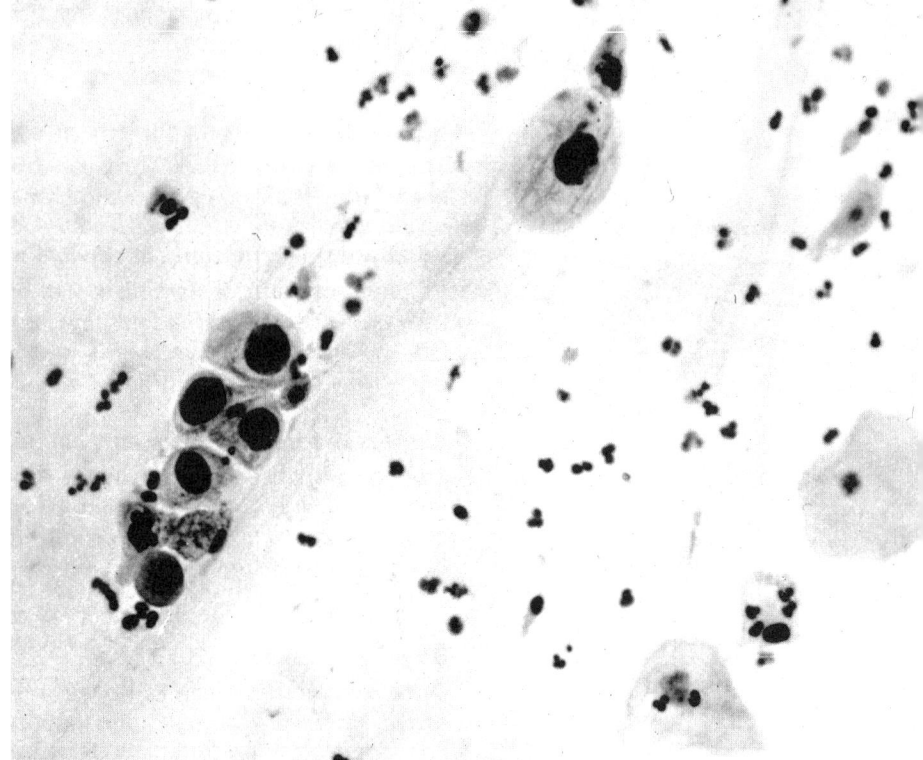

*Cancer Smear.* In this photomicrograph of a Papanicolaou smear, the very darkly stained cells are cancer cells, which have been extruded from the surface of the cervix. Such findings often enable the surgeon to make the diagnosis of cancer in its very earliest stage, thus increasing the chances for cure of this form of cancer. All women should have a Papanicolaou smear taken every year.

## THE CERVIX

### What is the cervix?

The cervix, or neck of the womb, is that portion of the uterus that appears in the vagina. It is a small, firm, muscular organ with a canal through its center (the cervical canal), extending from the vagina to the interior of the body of the uterus. The cervix is the only portion of the uterus that can actually be seen during the course of a pelvic examination.

### How is the cervix examined?

A special instrument known as a speculum is inserted into the vagina.

### What is the function of the cervix?

a. It guards the cavity of the uterus from invasion by bacteria or other foreign particles.
b. It allows for the passage of sperm into the cavity of the uterus.
c. It protects the developing embryo during pregnancy.
d. It opens during labor to allow for the passage of the baby.

### What is cervicitis?

It is an inflammation of the cervix.

### What are the causes of cervicitis?

a. Bacteria, fungi, parasites.
b. Injury secondary to delivery or surgery.
c. A congenital deficiency in the normal covering layer of the cervix.

### What are the symptoms of cervicitis?

a. The most pronounced symptom is vaginal discharge. The appearance of the discharge may vary from a colorless mucus to a whitish or yellowish discharge.
b. Bleeding after sexual intercourse.
c. In severe cases, menstrual bleeding may be heavier than normal or may be preceded or followed by staining for a day or two.

### Does cervicitis ever interfere with the ability to become pregnant?

Occasionally. In such cases it is necessary to clear up the cervicitis before pregnancy can take place.

### What is the treatment for cervicitis?

a. If an infection is present, it must be eradicated by appropriate, specific medication.
b. Douching helps to keep local infection under control; an acid douche may prevent the recurrence of an infection caused by a fungus or parasite.
c. Treatment by cauterizing with silver nitrate applications or by electrocauterization.

### How is electrocauterization of the cervix performed?

It is an office procedure in which incisions are burned into the cervix by means of an electrically heated, metal-tipped instrument. The burning incisions, of which many are made, cause the eroded or infected tissue to die and fall away from the underlying healthy cervical tissue. In time, the healthy tissue is able to grow again and to cover the entire cervix.

### Is cauterization of the cervix a painful procedure?

No. It is accompanied by relatively little discomfort. There may be a feeling of warmth in the vagina and some cramps may follow, but it does not produce any disability.

### How long does cauterization take to perform?

In the hands of a competent gynecologist, only a few minutes.

### What precautions should be taken after cauterization of the cervix?

The patient should abstain from intercourse and douches for twelve to fourteen days.

**Is it necessary to take douches at any time following cauterization?**

Yes. After the slough has been expelled—in about twelve to fourteen days—douches and antibiotic creams are used to prevent reinfection. These measures should be continued for approximately three weeks, except during the menstrual period.

**How long does it take for healing to be complete after cauterization?**

Approximately six weeks.

**Is there a tendency for cervicitis or cervical erosion to recur?**

Yes. If it recurs, treatment should be started again. It is not unusual for a slight recurrence to take place, but it will respond if treated promptly.

**Does the gynecologist always examine the cervix for cancer?**

Yes.

**What is a cancer smear (Papanicolaou smear)?**

It is a method of collecting surface cells from the vagina and cervix and examining them, with special staining techniques, for cancer. It concerns itself with examining those very superficial surface cells that are thrown off (desquamated).

**Is a "Pap Smear" the same as a Papanicolaou smear?**

Yes.

**What is the value of the cancer smear?**

It can reveal cancer cells at a *very early* stage of their development, thus allowing for extremely early treatment.

**Should all women have a cervical cancer smear?**

All women past the age of eighteen years should have a routine vaginal smear taken every year. Also, a smear should be taken at any time when a lesion is suspected.

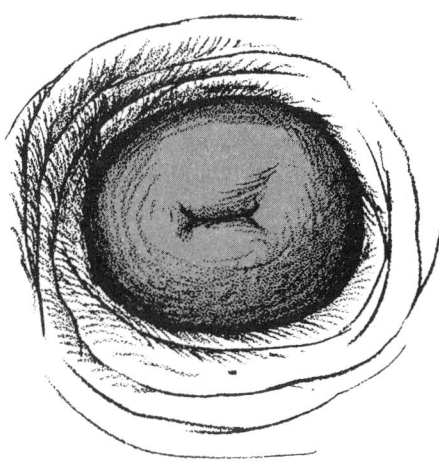

Normal cervix

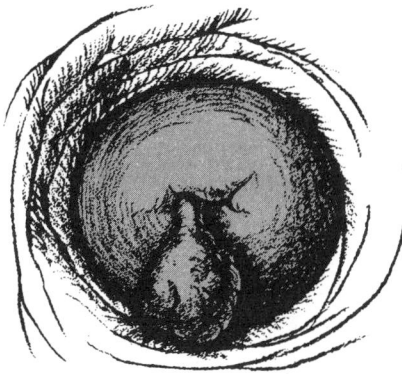

Polyp

*Cervical Polyp.* At the top is a normal cervix. Diagram at right, a polyp protrudes from the cervix. In the side view at the bottom, the cervical polyp is shown protruding into the vagina.

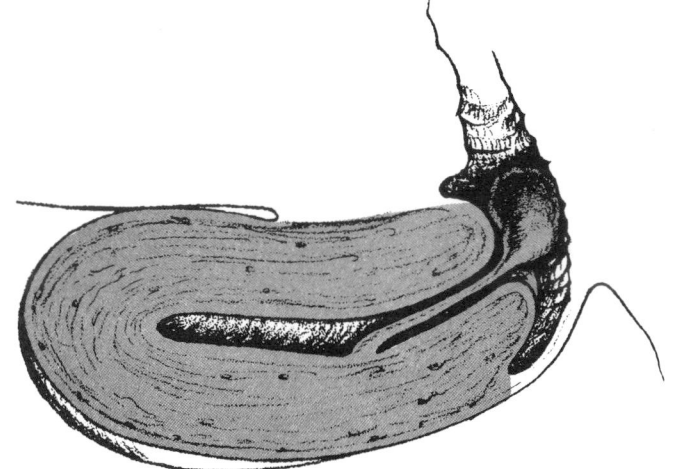

**Is it painful to take a cancer smear?**

Absolutely not. The entire procedure takes no more than a few seconds and is performed by merely swabbing the surface of the cervix and the vagina.

**What is a cervical polyp?**

It is a small benign tumor arising from the cervix. It usually has a thin stalk and assumes the size and shape of a pea, cherry, or grape.

**What causes cervical polyps to grow?**

The cause is unknown. They can oc-

cur at any time during the years that a woman menstruates.

**What are the symptoms of cervical polyps?**

Vaginal discharge, staining between periods, pre- and post-menstrual cramps. One or all of these symptoms may appear, or there may be no symptoms whatever.

**What is the treatment for cervical polyps?**

They should be removed in the office of the gynecologist or, under certain circumstances, in the hospital. This is considered a minor operative procedure and is accompanied by little discomfort.

## Do polyps tend to recur?

Once a polyp has been removed, it will not regrow. However, women who have developed one polyp do have a tendency to form others. These, too, should be removed.

## Are polyps of the cervix ever malignant?

Rarely.

## Do polyps interfere with pregnancy?

Usually not.

## Is cancer of the cervix a common condition?

It accounts for 25 percent of all cancer found in women!

## What causes cancer of the cervix?

The exact cause is unknown.

## At what age is cancer of the cervix usually encountered?

It can occur at any age, but it is seen most often in women between thirty and sixty years of age.

## Who is most likely to develop cancer of the cervix?

a. Women who began sexual intercourse at an early age.
b. Women who have had many different sexual contacts.
c. Women who have had children at a very early age.
d. Women who are married to, or have frequent sexual contacts with, uncircumsized men.
e. Women who have viral infections of the genitals, such as herpes.

## Is it wise to seek early treatment for any abnormal condition of the cervix in an attempt to prevent cancer?

Definitely, yes. Many component gynecologists feel that erosion, laceration, inflammation, or benign growths of the cervix may predispose toward cancer formation.

## Can cancer of the cervix be prevented?

Cancer prevention is not actually possible, but a *late cancer* can be avoided through early treatment. Thus, periodic examinations will uncover many cancers in their early curable stages.

## What are the early symptoms of cancer of the cervix?

Very early cancer may cause no symptoms whatever. This is one of the main reasons for periodic vaginal examinations, including Pap smears. Later on, there may be vaginal discharge, bleeding after intercourse, bleeding after douching, or unexplained bleeding between periods.

## Can early cancer of the cervix be detected by a cancer smear?

Yes.

## What is noninvasive cancer of the cervix?

This is a condition, also called *in situ* cancer of the cervix, in which the cancer is limited to the most superficial layer of cells, and there is no spread to the deeper tissues. This term is used to distinguish it from invasive cancer, in which the spread has extended beyond the superficial layers of cells into the deeper tissues, including the lymph channels and the bloodstream.

## How accurate is the cancer smear in diagnosing cancer?

A positive cancer smear is accurate in about 97 percent of cases.

## Does a positive cancer smear consitute sufficient investigation of cancer of the cervix?

No. Whenever a cancer smear is positive, a biopsy and cutterage should be taken to make the diagnosis and location absolutely certain.

## What procedures are carried out to further investigate whether a cancer of the cervix is present?

A more extensive biopsy, known as a *cone biopsy,* is taken. This involves removing the entire lining of the cervical canal (the entrance to the uterus). Examination of this large piece of tissue will not only reveal the presence of a cancer, but will show the extent of its invasiveness.

## Can a cancer of the cervix ever be cured by a cone biopsy?

Yes, if it happens to be a superficial *in situ* cancer. The cone biopsy must, on microscopic examination, show that the cancer has been completely removed.

## What is the treatment for cancer of the cervix?

This will depend entirely upon the stage of development of the cancer at the time it is discovered. There are three ways of treating this disease:
a. By the use of radium and x ray.
b. By wide surgical removal of the cervix, uterus, tubes, ovaries, and all the lymph channels draining the area.
c. By a combination of radium, x ray, and surgery.

## Who will determine what form of treatment should be administered?

The gynecologist will know which form of treatment to institute after the extent of the cancer has been determined.

## What are the chances of recovery from cancer of the cervix?

Early cancer of the cervix can be cured in almost all cases—by either radium, x ray, or surgery. As the extensiveness of the disease increases and the operative procedures become more involved, recovery rates are lower.

## Is it painful to insert radium?

No. This procedure is carried out in the hospital, under anesthesia.

**Does radium remain inside the body permanently?**

No. The radium is usually applied in capsules, and after a sufficient number of radioactive rays have been tranmitted, the capsule is removed.

**How long does radium usually remain within the genital tract?**

Anywhere from 72 to 110 hours, according to the specific dosage indicated.

**How long a hospital stay is necessary when radium is inserted?**

Anywhere from two to six days.

**Is the application of radium followed by postoperative discomfort?**

Yes, because extensive packing is inserted into the vagina when radium is being used. This is controlled by use of sedatives.

**Is x-ray treatment often given after radium treatment?**

Yes. This is given in the weeks after radium implantation to reach parts not reached by the radium.

**Are there any postoperative symptoms following radium implantation?**

Yes. Disturbance in bowel function and burning and frequency of urination are quite often complications of radium treatment of the cervix.

**Does cancer ever recur after radium treatment for cancer of the cervix?**

Not very often. Some cancers are resistant to radium or inaccessible to it. Recurrence will depend upon the stage of the disease at the time radium treatment was given.

**Can a patient return to normal living after radium treatment for cancer of the cervix?**

Yes.

**Can a patient become pregnant af-**

**ter radium treatment for cancer of the cervix?**

Because ovarian function will have been destroyed by the radium treatment, pregnancy cannot take place. Menstruation will also cease as a result of radium therapy.

**What type of surgery is performed for cancer of the cervix?**

a. Hysterectomy for *in situ*, or noninvasive, cancer.
b. Radical hysterectomy for most invasive cancers.
c. Exenteration for extensive and advanced cancer.

**What is meant by an exenteration operation for cancer of the cervix?**

This is an extremely radical operative procedure in which the entire uterus, cervix, vagina, tubes, ovaries, lymph glands, bladder, and/or rectum are removed for extensive cancer. Artificial openings are made for the passage of urine and stool. Fortunately, this procedure is not often necessary since the disease is usually detected in an earlier stage of its development.

**What is the future outlook for those afflicted with cancer of the cervix?**

Earlier detection can lead to a substantially higher cure rate in years to come. The advent of the cancer smear now permits the diagnosis to be made at earlier stages in the development of the disease.

## THE UTERUS

**What is the uterus?**

The uterus, or womb, is a pear-shaped muscular organ lying in the middle of the pelvis. It is approximately three inches long, two inches wide, and one inch thick. It consists of a smooth outer covering, a middle layer composed of thick muscle tissue, and an inner cavity lined with endometrial cells. The cavity of the uterus connects with the vagina

through the cervix and connects with the abdominal cavity through the Fallopian tubes. The hollow Fallopian tubes open within the abdominal cavity near the ovaries. The uterus is supported and suspended by several ligaments.

**What is the exact position of the uterus?**

It lies just above the pubic bones, behind the urinary bladder, in front of the rectum, and above the vagina.

**What are the functions of the uterus?**

a. To prepare for the reception of a fertilized egg.
b. To nurture and harbor the embryo during its development.
c. To expel the baby when it is mature and ready for delivery.

**What influences the uterus to prepare for pregnancy?**

Hormones that are secreted by the ovaries and the other endocrine glands. If the fertilized egg is not forthcoming, menstruation ensues, and the uterine lining is shed. This process is repeated each month, from puberty to menopause, unless there is a glandular upset or, of course, unless pregnancy exists.

**What is the significance of a tipped womb?**

Ordinarily, this condition has no significance.

**What symptoms are caused by a tipped womb?**

Usually none. In rare instances, backache and a dragging sensation in the lower pelvic region may occur with the finding of a womb that is tipped markedly in a backward direction.

**What is the treatment for tipped womb?**

The great majority of cases require no treatment whatever. (The large number of operations for "straightening out" the womb that were performed years ago have now been abandoned as unnecessary operative procedures.) In rare instances, a vaginal pessary is employed to maintain a forward position of the uterus.

**Does a tipped womb interfere with pregnancy?**

Definitely not.

**Does a tipped womb interfere with intercourse?**

No.

**What is an infantile uterus?**

This is a term formerly used to describe a smallsized uterus.

**What is the significance of an infantile uterus?**

None, providing the uterus functions normally. In other words, if menstruation is normal and pregnancy can take place, a small-sized uterus is of no significance.

**Do women with an infantile uterus have difficulty in becoming pregnant?**

Not if their menstrual function is normal.

**What is a curettage?**

This is an operation performed upon the cavity of the uterus through the vagina. It consists of scraping out the lining membrane of the uterus. Special instruments are used to dilate the cervix and to scrape out the uterine cavity.

**Why is curettage performed?**

a. For diagnostic purposes.
b. For therapeutic purposes.
c. A curettage is often diagnostic and therapeutic at the same time, as in cases of hyperplasia or polyps of the uterus.

**When is a diagnostic curettage performed?**

a. In cases of unexplained uterine bleeding.

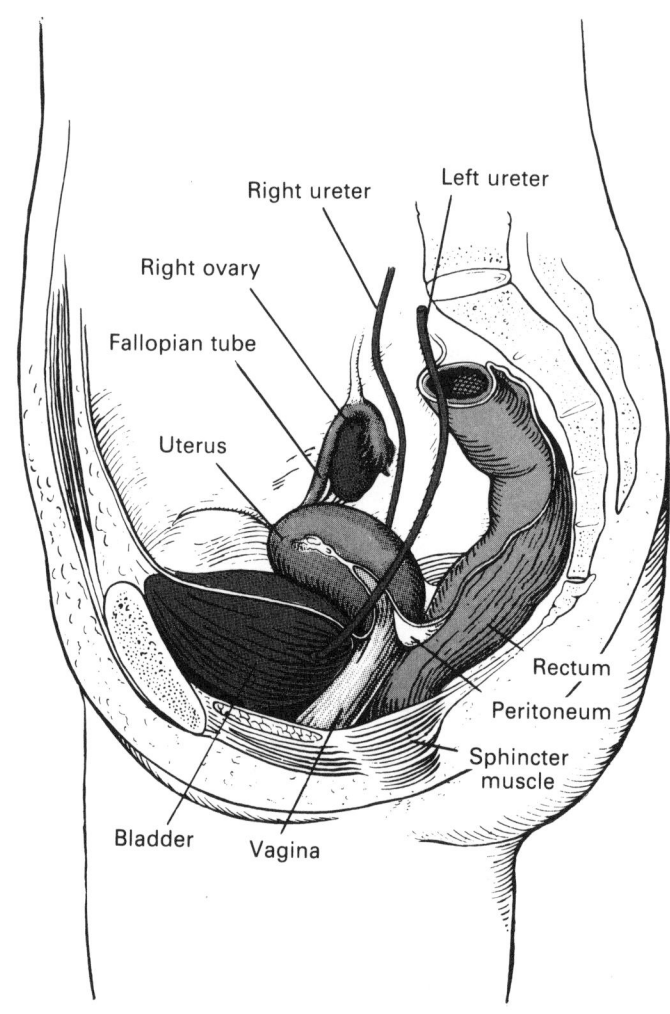

**The Female Organs.** *This diagram shows the female reproductive organs: the uterus, the Fallopian tubes, and the ovaries. Note the relation of the female reproductive organs to the surrounding structures in the pelvic region.*

b. In cases in which a polyp of the uterine cavity is suspected.
c. In cases in which a cancer of the body of the uterus is suspected.

**When is a therapeutic curettage performed?**

a. When a disorder such as a polyp of the lining membrane of the uterus has already been diagnosed, curettage may result in a cure.
b. When an overgrowth of the lining membrane of the uterus (endometrial hyperplasia) has been diagnosed, a curettage will often bring about a cure.
c. Following a miscarriage, when

parts of the fetus or placenta remain behind. Curettage in such instances will clean out the cavity and thus restore normalcy.

**What is another name for curettage?**

It is commonly called a "D and C" operation. This stands for dilatation and curettage.

**Is a D and C a painful operation?**

No. It is performed under general anesthesia in the hospital.

**How long a hospital stay is necessary following curettage?**

Approximately one to two days.

**Are there any visible incisions following curettage?**

No. It is done completely through the vagina.

**How soon after curettage can one return to work?**

Within a week.

**What restrictions must be followed after curettage?**

Douching and intercourse must not be performed for two weeks.

**Can normal pregnancy take place after a curettage?**

Yes, A curettage performed by a competent gynecologist in a hospital will not interfere with subsequent pregnancies.

**What is endometritis?**

It is an infection of the lining of the uterus.

**What causes endometritis?**

a. Bacterial infections such as gonorrhea.
b. It may follow a miscarriage or abortion.
c. It may follow normal delivery where an accidental infection of the uterus has taken place.

**What are the symptoms of endometritis?**

Irregular bleeding, vaginal discharge, pain and tenderness in the lower abdomen, a feeling of weakness, fever, urinary distress, etc.

**What is the treatment for endometritis?**

The first step is to determine the exact cause. If there has been an incomplete miscarriage, the uterine cavity must be emptied by the performance of a curettage. If the endometritis has been caused by bacterial infection, antibiotic drugs should be given. If the infection has extended beyond the lining membrane into the wall of the uterus, it may be necessary to remove the uterus in order to effect a cure.

**Does endometritis ever heal by itself?**

Yes, in certain cases. More often, the infection will spread outward to involve the deeper layers of the uterus, the tubes, the ovaries, and even the abdominal cavity.

**What is an endometrial polyp?**

It is a growth arising from the lining of the uterus and extending into the uterine cavity. Often there are multiple polyps.

**What are the symptoms of an endometrial polyp?**

In some cases there are no symptoms. In others, there is cramplike menstrual pain, staining between periods, excessive menstrual bleeding, and vaginal discharge.

**How is the diagnosis of an endometrial polyp made?**

By diagnostic curettage or by the performance of a hysterogram.

**What is a hysterogram?**

It is an x-ray investigation of the cavity of the uterus performed by injecting an opaque dye through the cervix into the uterine cavity. When films are taken, they will show the outline of the cavity.

**Do endometrial polyps ever become malignant?**

Yes, occasionally.

**What is the treatment for endometrial polyps?**

They are removed by curettage. When they protrude through the cervix into the vaginal canal, they can be removed with an instrument through the vagina. If there is any evidence of malignant change within the polyp, a total hysterectomy with removal of the tubes and ovaries must be performed.

**What is endometrial hyperplasia?**

It is a benign overgrowth of the lining of the uterus.

**What causes endometrial hyperplasia?**

It is usually associated with excessive and prolonged production of female sex hormone (estrogen) by the ovaries. Frequently, an ovarian cyst or tumor is present and may be responsible for the production of excess estrogen.

**What are the symptoms of endometrial hyperplasia?**

It is characterized by completely irregular and unpredictable bleeding, varying from total lack of menstruation to more frequent periods than normal, and from slight staining to profuse bleeding. Characteristically, endometrial hyperplasia results in painless bleeding.

**Does endometrial hyperplasia have anything to do with the inability to become pregnant (infertility)?**

Yes. Women with endometrial hyperplasia often do not ovulate and therefore cannot become pregnant.

**How is endometrial hyperplasia diagnosed?**

By microscopic examination of tissue that is taken from the lining of the uterus by endometrial biopsy. Also, by examination of tissue removed by curettage.

**Where and how is an endometrial biopsy performed?**

This is an office procedure and is performed simply by the insertion of a special instrument through the vagina and cervix into the uterine cavity. A small piece of tissue is removed and is examined microscopically.

**Is endometrial biopsy a painful procedure?**

No. It is a simple office procedure accompanied by a minimal amount of discomfort.

**What is the treatment for endometrial hyperplasia?**

This depends upon the age of the

patient, the type of hyperplasia found on microscopic examination, and the presence or absence of accompanying ovarian growths. In young females still in the childbearing age, simple hyperplasia is treated by curettage and by use of estrogen and progesterone (ovarian hormones) to simulate the normal menstrual cycle. This is called cyclic therapy.

After menopause, and depending upon the type of hyperplasia, the treatment varies from simple curettage to hysterectomy. If the hyperplasia recurs or shows a preponderance of certain types of cells, and if the patient is past childbearing age, hysterectomy will probably be the best treatment. In the presence of an enlarged ovary, hyperplasia must be suspected as being related to a tumor of the ovary. In these cases, an abdominal operation should be performed and the ovaries and uterus removed.

### Is there any connection between endometrial hyperplasia and cancer of the uterus?

In women past childbearing age, it is thought that certain types of endometrial hyperplasia may be associated with development of cancer of the uterus. For this reason, more intensive treatment is advised for older women with endometrial hyperplasia.

### Should women who have endometrial hyperplasia return for frequent periodic examinations?

Yes. Any irregularity in the menstrual cycle of a woman still in the childbearing age should stimulate a visit to the gynecologist.

### What is the treatment of choice for recurrent hyperplasia in young women?

a. Repeated curettage or cyclic hormone therapy for a prolonged period.

b. If symptoms of hyperplasia cannot be controlled, it may be necessary to perform a hysterectomy even in a young woman. Fortunately, this is rarely necessary.

### What is the incidence of cancer of the body of the uterus?

It is the second most common cancer of the female genital tract. However, cancer of the cervix is five times more frequent than cancer of the body of the uterus.

### Who is most likely to develop cancer of the uterus?

It occurs at a later age than cancer of the cervix. It is most prevalent in women past fifty.

### Is there a tendency to inherit cancer of the uterus?

No.

### What is the difference between cancer and sarcoma of the uterus?

Cancer arises from the lining membrane of the uterus, while sarcoma (an equally malignant tumor) arises from the muscle layer of the uterus.

### What are the symptoms of cancer of the uterus?

a. Irregular vaginal bleeding in women still having menstrual periods.
b. Bleeding after menopause.
c. Enlargement of the uterus.

### How is cancer of the uterus diagnosed?

By performing diagnostic curettage. Any bleeding in a woman past her menopause must be looked upon with suspicion and must be investigated by curettage to rule out cancer.

### What treatment is advocated for cancer of the uterus?

Application of radium in most cases, followed in four to six weeks by a total hysterectomy.

### Is this a serious procedure?

Yes, but recovery from surgery will take place in almost all cases.

### What is the rate of cure for cancer of the body of the uterus?

If the cancer is detected before it has extended beyond the confines of the uterus, approximately four out of five cases can be cured. In cases where spread has already gone beyond the uterus, only about one out of eight can be cured.

### Is it possible to prevent cancer of the uterus?

It cannot be prevented, but it *can* be detected earlier if women seek medical help as soon as they notice abnormal vaginal bleeding.

### What are fibroids (leiomyoma) of the uterus?

Fibroids are benign tumors composed of muscle tissue. They tend to be round in shape and firm in consistency.

### What is the incidence of fibroids?

Almost 25 percent of all women have fibroids of the uterus. The majority of such growths cause no symptoms and demand no treatment.

### What causes fibroids?

Although the exact cause is unknown, it has been found that certain ovarian hormones play an important role in the speed of growth. Thus, after menopause, when very little ovarian hormone is being secreted, fibroids stop growing and may even shrink.

### When are women most likely to develop fibroids?

During the later stages of the childbearing period, that is, between the ages of forty and fifty years. However, they may be found occasionally in women in their early twenties or in those past menopause.

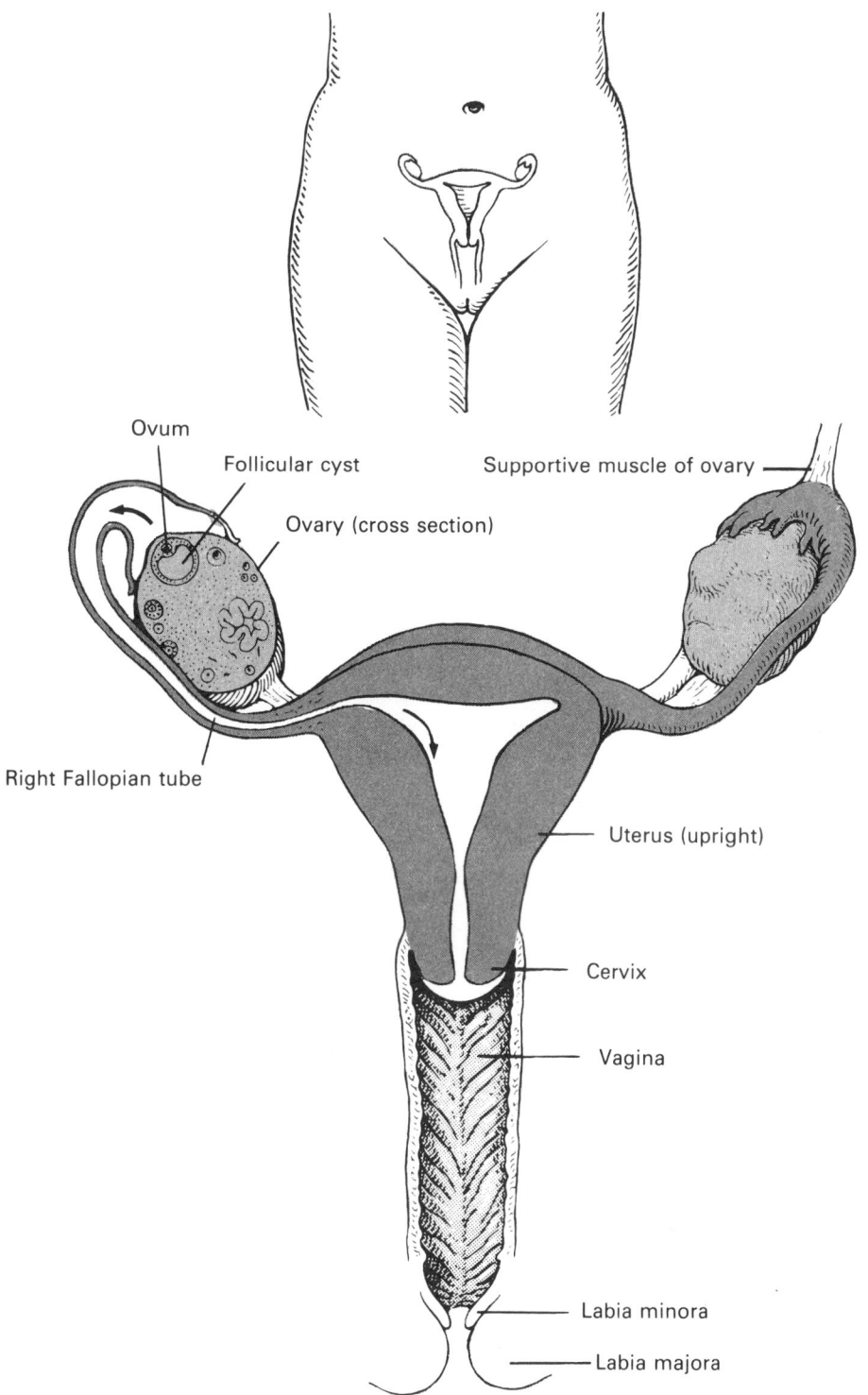

**The Female Organs.** *This frontal diagram of the female reproductive organs gives another view of these anatomical structures. Young women should be made familiar with the normal structure of their bodies so they can better understand problems that arise concerning them.*

### Do fibroids tend to run in families?

There is no actual inherited tendency, but since one in four women have fibroids, it is not uncommon to find more than one member of a family with this condition.

### What are the various types of fibroids?

a. Subserous; those growing beneath the outer coat of the uterus.
b. Intramural; those growing in the muscular layer of the uterus.
c. Submucous; those growing beneath the lining membrane of the uterine cavity.

### Do fibroids vary greatly in size?

Yes. They may be as small as a pinhead or as large as a watermelon. They are almost always multiple.

### What are the symptoms of fibroids?

a. Many fibroids cause no symptoms and are found inadvertently on routine pelvic examination.
b. If the fibroid is submucous in type, it may cause prolonged heavy menstruation.
c. Intramural and subserous fibroids may cause excessive menstrual bleeding but may produce no symptoms at all.
d. There may be frequency of urination and difficulty in bowel function if the fibroids grow to a large size and press upon the bladder or rectum.
e. Backache or lower abdominal pain occurs occasionally.
f. Infertility may ensue if the fibroid distorts the uterine cavity.
g. They may be the cause of repeated miscarriage.

### How is the diagnosis of fibroids made?

By manual pelvic examination. Such a vaginal examination will reveal the size, shape, and other features of the tumor. A hysterogram may help to diagnose small submucous fibroids. A

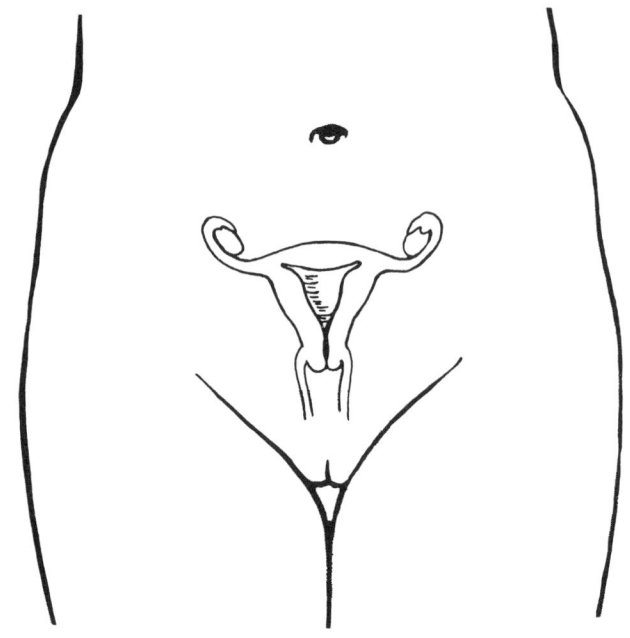

Position of organs in body

**Fibroids of the Uterus.** *This diagram shows various forms of fibroid tumors of the uterus and where they are located. These tumors are not malignant but can cause serious symptoms, such as bleeding between menstrual periods or, if they grow large enough, pressure upon the urinary bladder or rectum. When symptoms are pronounced or when the tumors grow very large, the surgeon may recommend their removal.*

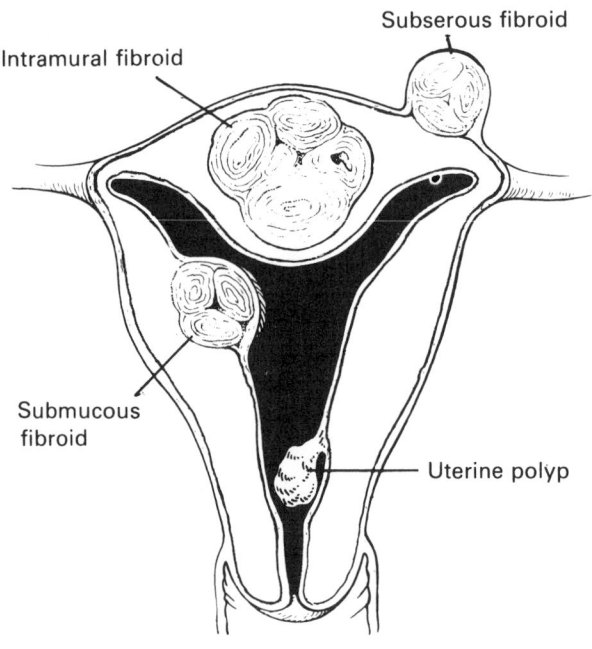

sonogram, too, often may reveal the presence of fibroids.

### Is a fibroid of the uterus a malignant tumor?

Definitely not. Fibroids are benign growths!

### Do fibroids become malignant?

Not frequently. Occasionally, cancer develops in a uterus containing fibroids, but the presence of the fibroid does not predispose toward the development of the cancer. Sarcoma, a malignant growth of the uterus, may develop from a fibroid in rare instances.

### Are fibroids found in association with other conditions within the uterus?

Yes. There is a high incidence of endometrial polyps and endometrial hyperplasia in those patients who have fibroids.

### What is the best treatment for fibroids?

If the fibroids produce symptoms or grow rapidly, they should be removed surgically.

### What operative procedures are performed for fibroids?

When only the fibroids are removed, it is called a myomectomy. When the entire uterus is removed, it is termed a hysterectomy.

### How does a gynecologist decide whether to do a myomectomy or a hysterectomy?

This will depend upon the age of the patient and her desire to have children. If the patient desires children, an attempt will be made to preserve the uterus, and a myomectomy will be performed.

### Are there methods of treating fibroids other than myomectomy or hysterectomy?

Yes. Some small submucous fibroids can be removed by simple curettage when they develop into polyplike growths.

### Do fibroids have a tendency to recur?

Ten percent will recur following myomectomy. Of course, if the entire uterus is removed, fibroids cannot recur.

### Must all fibroids be operated upon?

No. A fair proportion require no treatment whatever.

### What are the indications for surgical removal of fibroids?

a. Increased, prolonged, and more frequent menstruation.
b. Episodes of severe bleeding.
c. Pressure symptoms causing continued urinary or rectal discomfort.
d. Rapid increase in the size of a fibroid.
e. Any fibroid larger than the size of a three-month pregnancy should be removed even if it causes no symptoms.
f. Acute pain due to degeneration of a fibroid or to a twist in a fibroid.
g. Repeated miscarriage or sterility.

### Do fibroids ever occur during pregnancy?

Yes. When present, they may increase in size as the pregnancy grows.

### Should a fibroid be treated during pregnancy?

No. It is best to postpone treatment until after the baby is born.

### Is the surgical treatment of fibroids usually successful?

Yes, a cure is the result in almost all cases.

### Can a woman become pregnant after surgery for fibroids?

If a myomectomy has been performed, subsequent pregnancy is possible. In such cases, the baby may have to be delivered by Cesarean section.

### Is there any satisfactory nonsurgical treatment for fibroids?

No.

### Is myomectomy considered a major operation?

Yes, since it involves an abdominal incision. However, recovery takes place. Hospitalization for seven to ten days is usually required.

### Does menstruation return to normal after myomectomy?

Yes.

### How long does it take to recover from the effects of myomectomy?

Approximately six weeks.

### How long should a woman wait after myomectomy before attempting pregnancy?

Three months.

### What is a hysterectomy?

An operation for the removal of the uterus.

### What are the various types of hysterectomy?

a. Subtotal or supracervical hysterectomy; removal of the body of the uterus leaving the cervix behind.
b. Total hysterectomy; removal of the body of the uterus and the cervix.
c. Radical hysterectomy; this includes removal of a good portion of the vagina, the tubes and ovaries, the supporting tissues and lymph glands along with the body and cervix of the uterus.
d. Porro section; removal of the uterus at the time of delivery of a baby by Cesarean section.
e. Vaginal hysterectomy; removal of the uterus and cervix through the vagina instead of through an abdominal incision.

## What are some of the indications for hysterectomy?

a. Symptomatic fibroids.
b. Chronic, incurable inflammatory disease of the uterus, tubes, and ovaries, such as gonorrhea or tuberculosis.
c. Severe recurrent endometrial hyperplasia.
d. Cancer of the uterus or cervix.
e. Cancer of the tubes or ovaries.
f. Chronic disabling endometriosis.
g. Uncontrollable hemorrhage following delivery of a baby.
h. In certain cases where the ovaries must be removed for cysts or growths, the uterus should also be removed.
i. Rupture of the uterus during pregnancy.

## Is hysterectomy a major operative procedure?

Yes. However, it is not considered a dangerous operation, and operative recovery occurs in almost 100 percent of the cases.

## Does a woman menstruate after hysterectomy?

No.

## Can a patient become pregnant after hysterectomy?

No.

## Must the ovaries always be removed when hysterectomy is performed?

If the disease for which the hysterectomy has been performed is cancerous in nature, the tubes and ovaries must be removed. If the condition is benign and the woman is still under forty years of age, one or both ovaries may be left in place so that the uncomfortable symptoms of change of life do not ensue. Every attempt is made to leave the ovaries in place when the patient is young. They are usually removed when the patient is past the menopause. If the ovaries are inflamed or abscessed, or if endometriosis is present, the ovaries are removed when performing a hysterectomy.

## Do the symptoms of menopause (change of life) always follow hysterectomy?

No. If one or both ovaries are left behind, menopause will not follow. Menopause occurs only when both ovaries have been removed.

## Can the symptoms of menopause be controlled after hysterectomy?

Yes. There are excellent means of combating the symptoms of menopause by the judicious administration of female hormones.

## Does the removal of the uterus affect one's sex life in any way?

No. The removal of the uterus, with or without the removal of the ovaries, does not affect sexual ability or sexual desire. As a matter of fact, some women state that they are happier in their sexual relations after hysterectomy than before.

## Are the external genitals altered during hysterectomy?

No. The vagina and other external genital structures are unaffected by hysterectomy.

## Will hysterectomy cause changes in the physical appearance of a woman?

No. This is a common misconception. Women do not tend to become fat or to lose their feminine characteristics because of hysterectomy! It must be remembered, though, that most hysterectomies are performed in the fifth and sixth decades of life, when women ordinarily show signs of aging. It is the removal of the ovaries that sometimes causes weight gain.

## Is the scar from hysterectomy disfiguring?

No. It is a simple line on the abdomen. If a vaginal hysterectomy has been performed, no scar will be visible.

## What are the indications for the performance of a vaginal hysterectomy?

When there is prolapse of the uterus along with a cystocele and rectocele, it is sometimes advisable to remove the uterus through the vagina so that a vaginal plastic operation can be performed at the same time. This cannot be done if the uterus is enlarged to such an extent that it cannot be delivered through the vagina. Vaginal hysterectomy is not indicated when an invasive malignancy is suspected.

## Is vaginal hysterectomy a dangerous operative procedure?

No. It carries with it the same risks as hysterectomy performed through an abdominal incision.

## Is hysterectomy a painful operation?

There is the same discomfort that follows any abdominal operation. Most pain can be controlled readily by medication.

## How long does it take to perform the average hysterectomy?

From one to two hours.

## How soon after hysterectomy can a patient get out of bed?

Usually, the day following the operation.

## How long a hospital stay is necessary following hysterectomy?

Seven to ten days.

## What postoperative symptoms follow hysterectomy?

There may be vaginal bleeding or discharge for a week or two. There may also be difficulty in passing urine or in moving the bowels for a week or more after hysterectomy.

**How soon after hysterectomy can one do the following:**

Shower:
   One week.
Bathe:
   Four weeks.
Walk in the street:
   Eight to ten days.
Drive a car:
   Four to five weeks.
Perform all household duties:
   Six weeks.
Resume sexual relations:
   Eight weeks.
Return to work:   Eight weeks.
Resume all physical activities:
   Three months.

**What is endometriosis?**

A condition in which the lining cells of the uterus (endometrial cells) are found in abnormal locations. These cells may be found deep within the wall of the uterus, on the outer coat of the uterus, the Fallopian tubes, the ovaries, the uterine ligaments, bowel, bladder, vagina, or in other places within the abdominal cavity.

**How do these endometrial cells exist in abnormal positions?**

They implant upon the surface of other structures and grow as small nests of cells. They vary in size from that of a pinhead to the size of an orange. They often form cysts, which contain a chocolate-appearing fluid that represents old, bloody menstrual-like material.

**What abnormal conditions are produced by these endometrial implants?**

They may cause firm adhesions between the tubes and the ovaries or the bladder, the bowel, or the uterus. They may form cysts. These cysts may twist or rupture, causing acute abdominal pain and distress.

**Do these endometrial implants function like normal uterine cells?**

Yes. They become distended and engorged with blood as each menstrual period approaches, and they bleed when menstruation takes place.

**What causes endometriosis?**

The exact cause is unknown. One theory is that the lining cells of the uterus are expelled through the Fallopian tubes by a reverse peristaltic action in the tubes during menstrual periods. Another theory is that these cells are dislodged following surgery upon the uterus.

**What are some of the symptoms of endometriosis?**

a. It may cause no symptoms whatever and be discovered accidentally at operation for another condition.
b. There may be marked pain before and during the menstrual period.
c. There may be marked pain on urination, defecation, or during intercourse.
d. Menstrual bleeding may be markedly increased.
e. Inability to become pregnant is a complication of extensive endometriosis.

**What can happen if endometriosis is permitted to go untreated?**

The symptoms may become progressive and debilitating. If the endometriosis involves the bowel or intestinal tract, obstruction of the bowel may take place. In certain cases, endometrial cysts will grow so large that they will create pressure on other organs and will demand surgery. Endometrial cysts sometimes twist or rupture, thus requiring immediate surgical intervention.

**What is the treatment for endometriosis?**

a. Treatment is usually medical and will include the administration of enough female hormones to temporarily stop menstrual periods.
b. In persistent cases of endometri-

osis with marked symptoms, hysterectomy may have to be performed, This is reserved for women past the childbearing age or for those whose symptoms are so severe that they demand treatment.
c. In young women in the childbearing age, pregnancy causes temporary relief since the cyclic influence that causes the symptoms of endometriosis is interrupted.

**Does endometriosis lead to cancer?**

No.

## ABORTION *(Miscarriage)*

**What is an abortion?**

It is the expulsion of the products of conception from the uterus during the first six months of the pregnancy. Abortion applies to loss of pregnancy at a time when the fetus is unable to maintain life on its own.

**Does the term "abortion" always mean the pregnancy has been artificially interrupted?**

No. Among medical people, abortion refers only to the fact that the pregnancy has ended at a time when the fetus is not yet sufficiently developed to be able to maintain life.

**What are the various kinds of abortion?**

a. Spontaneous abortion, where no artificial means have been used to bring it on.
b. Induced abortion, where instrumentation, medication, or operation have been used to bring about the termination of the pregnancy.

**Are there various types of spontaneous abortion?**

Yes, They are threatened abortion, inevitable abortion, incomplete abortion, complete abortion, infected abortion, and missed abortion.

### Are there various types of induced abortion?

Yes. They are therapeutic abortion and voluntary abortion.

### What are some of the common causes of spontaneous abortion?

a. Defects in the egg, the sperm, the fertilized egg, or the placenta.
b. Disease of the uterus, such as an infection or a fibroid tumor.
c. Upset in the glandular system associated with ovarian, thyroid, or pituitary dysfunction.
d. Constitutional diseases, such as diabetes, malnutrition, syphilis, tuberculosis, etc.
e. Exposure to excessive x-ray radiation, the taking of poisons, etc.

### What is a threatened abortion?

It is a state during early pregnancy in which there are vaginal staining and abdominal cramps, but the cervix remains undilated and the products of conception are not expelled.

### What is inevitable abortion?

It is a state in which bleeding and dilatation of the cervix are so advanced that nothing can be done to prevent expulsion of the fetus from the uterus.

### What is incomplete abortion?

This refers to a condition in which there has been only partial expulsion of the products of conception.

### What is a complete abortion?

It is a state wherein the entire fetal sac and placenta have been fully expelled from the uterus.

### What are the symptoms of spontaneous abortion?

a. In the early stages of threatened abortion, staining is the only positive sign. Slight cramps or backache may then develop. This state often continues for days or even weeks.
b. In inevitable abortion, bleeding is heavier, cramps become regular, severe, and progressive, and the cervix begins to dilate.
c. In incomplete abortion, cramps and bleeding are marked, pieces of tissue or clots are passed, and the cervix is dilatated.
d. In complete abortion, after increasingly severe cramps and passage of clots, a large mass is expelled from the vagina. On examination, it will be found to contain all the products of conception.

### What is the treatment for inevitable abortion?

When it is obvious that abortion is inevitable, the uterus should be emptied. The evaluation of the inevitability of an abortion is difficult to make, but all gynecologists will give the patient every opportunity to maintain the pregnancy. When it is obvious that this is impossible, it is best to empty the uterus completely by curettage.

### What is the treatment for incomplete abortion?

A curettage should be performed in order to clean out the cavity of the uterus completely. If a great deal of bleeding has been associated with the miscarriage, blood transfusions should be given.

### What is the treatment for complete abortion?

No treatment is necessary unless severe blood loss has taken place. In that event, transfusions should be given. If there is evidence of infection, antibiotic drugs should be prescribed.

### What is a missed abortion?

This is a state of pregnancy wherein the fetus has died and has been separated from the uterine wall but, instead of being expelled, is retained within the uterine cavity. In certain cases, medications are given to bring on the onset of labor. However, the safest course may often be to wait for the uterus to empty itself spontaneously.

### What is habitual abortion?

This is a term applied to women with no children who have had four or more spontaneous abortions.

### What are thought to be the causes for habitual abortion?

a. Hormonal imbalance involving the pituitary, thyroid, or ovaries.
b. Uterine abnormalities.
c. Genetic abnormalities in the chromosomes of the embryo.

### Can habitual abortion ever be helped by medical treatment?

Yes, but it demands thorough investigation into all its aspects and intensive treatment by the physician.

### When does abortion require hospitalization?

When the bleeding is profuse or when abdominal cramps become severe and persistent.

### What are the greatest dangers associated with abortion?

a. In incomplete abortion, bleeding may be so profuse as to threaten life. In such cases, prompt transfusions are lifesaving.
b. Infection following abortion is an occasional complication, especially when abortion is performed under less than ideal conditions. Infection will require active, strenuous treatment with antibiotic drugs.

### What are the consequences of improper treatment of abortion?

a. Infection may set in and may necessitate removal of the uterus, tubes, and ovaries.
b. Sterility may ensue.

**Can infection follow any type of abortion?**

Yes, but it is rare when performed in a hospital operating room by a qualified gynecologist.

**What restrictions are imposed following miscarriage?**

a. Rest for one to two weeks.
b. No douches or tub baths for two weeks.
c. No sexual relations for two weeks.

**What laws now govern the performance of abortion?**

Up to the fourth month of pregnancy, a woman can voluntarily undergo abortion in all states. After the third month, states may regulate conditions under which abortions may be performed. These laws vary from state to state, some permitting abortion at any time up to the sixth or seventh month of pregnancy.

**Does the Supreme Court ruling obligate a doctor to perform an abortion?**

No. The attending physician may decide that in his opinion an abortion is not indicated. Under such circumstances, his patient's desire for an abortion may not sway him to perform the procedure. Also, some doctors do not believe in termination of pregnancy merely because the patient wishes it. A doctor may disapprove of abortion on moral and religious grounds and thus may decline to carry out the procedure.

**Does the Supeme Court ruling consider the matter of termination of pregnancy during the final ten weeks?**

Yes. It states specifically that a state may pass a law prohibiting termination of pregnancy during this period unless the life of the mother is seriously endangered.

**Why is termination of pregnancy**

**considered specially during the last ten weeks?**

Because this is the period when the fetus is considered capable of maintaining life outside the womb.

**Is there danger of sterility following abortion?**

No, unless postabortion infection sets in. This is unusual today because of the new abortion laws that have resulted in most abortions being performed under sterile conditions in hospitals.

**What kinds of operative procedures are used in doing an abortion?**

1. Dilatation and curettage. This means dilating the cervix (the entrance to the uterus) and scraping out the interior of the uterus with a curette.
2. The suction method. This means dilating the cervix and inserting a specially designed suction apparatus that will suck out the embryo and lining of the uterus.
3. "Salting out." This method of abortion is used when the pregnancy is several months old. It involves injecting a concentrated salt solution or substances known as prostaglandins into the fluid surrounding the fetus, thus stimulating the uterus to expel it.

**Are there any pills that can bring on a spontaneous abortion?**

No, although there are drugs on the market that claim to be able to do so. Most of these pills contain a potentially dangerous drug called ergot. Overdose of these drugs may lead to serious, irreversible damage to blood vessels.

**Will taking birth control pills for a long time make a woman more susceptible to miscarriage?**

No. Statistics have shown that women who have become pregnant after long use of birth control pills

have no greater tendency to miscarry.

**Is there any safe method of self-abortion?**

No! Attempts to produce abortion upon oneself are associated with a huge incidence of infection, hemorrhage, and fatality.

**Should a couple abstain from sexual relations if there is any vaginal staining or bleeding?**

Yes. If there is any evidence of a possibility of a miscarriage, sexual relations should be avoided.

**Is sexual intercourse conducive to miscarriage?**

No.

**Does emotional shock or severe stress predispose to miscarriage?**

There is no evidence that this happens.

**Is work or physical activity conducive to miscarriage?**

No.

**Is lower abdominal pain an indication that abortion or miscarriage might be imminent?**

In some instances, cramplike abdominal pains may signify that there is a possibility of miscarriage. If these pains persist, the obstetrician should be notified.

## THE FALLOPIAN TUBES
### (*The Uterine Tubes*)

**What are the Fallopian tubes?**

They are two hollow tubelike structures that arise at the upper end of the borders of the uterus and extend outward to each side of the pelvis for a distance of three to four inches. Each tube is the width of a lead pencil and at its most distant point is funnel shaped. The tubes are composed of an outer layer of muscle and an inner lining membrane covered with hairlike projections. These projections have a swaying, sweeping motion, which helps send the egg down toward the uterus and may aid the sperm in coming up through the tube to reach the egg.

### What is the function of the Fallopian tubes?

To transport the egg that has been discharged from the ovary down to the uterine cavity. To permit sperm to pass from the uterine cavity up toward the egg.

### What is salpingitis?

A bacterial infection of the Fallopian tubes.

### What are the most common causes of infection within the Fallopian tubes?

a. Gonorrhea, which has ascended via the vagina, cervix, and uterus.
b. Staphylococcus, pneumococcus, or streptococcus infections.
c. Tuberculosis, usually secondary to a primary infection elsewhere.
d. The presence of an intrauterine device (IUD).

### Is salpingitis a common condition?

Yes, but with the advent of the antibiotic drugs and the discovery of medications to control tuberculosis, inflammation of the tubes is much less frequently encountered than it was ten, twenty, or more years ago.

### What harm may result from an infection within the Fallopian tubes?

a. Sterility.
b. Tubal pregnancy (ectopic pregnancy).
c. The formation of a chronic abscess involving the ovary as well as the tube.
d. Spread of the infection out into the abdominal cavity, thus causing peritonitis.

### What treatment must often be in-

stituted in order to cure chronic infection of the Fallopian tubes?

Surgery, with removal of the uterus, tubes, and ovaries.

### What are the symptoms of acute salpingitis?

Lower abdominal pain, fever, chills, difficulty on urination, nausea and vomiting, vaginal discharge, increased menstrual bleeding, vaginal bleeding between periods, pain on intercourse, etc. Some or all of these symptoms may be encountered in salpingitis.

### What is the best way to prevent salpingitis?

Of course, women should avoid contact with infected men. However, whenever vaginal discharge develops following intercourse, it should be treated promptly by a gynecologist. This can, in the great majority of cases, prevent the spread of the infection through the uterus into the Fallopian tubes.

### What is the treatment for salpingitis once it has developed?

Acute salpingitis is treated with antibiotics. The patient is put to bed and given medications to relieve pain. If an abscess has formed and it persists, surgery, with removal of the tube, may be necessary.

### Is surgery usually performed during the acute phase of salpingitis?

No. The gynecologist will make every attempt to bring the inflammation under control by medical means. Immediate surgery may be necessary when an abscess within the tube is threatening to rupture and produce peritonitis.

### Is hospitalization necessary for all cases of salpingitis?

No. In the early stages of the disease, treatment can be carried out at home with safety. However, if response is inadequate, hospitalization is indicated.

### Does salpingitis ever clear up by itself?

No. All cases must be treated intensively.

### What are the chances of recovery from salpingitis?

Very few women die of salpingitis, but the chronic form of the disease can be cured only by removal of the tubes. In the acute stage, salpingitis can be cured if treatment is started quickly and is pursued vigorously.

### Can the antibiotics cure a chronic or persistent abscess within the Fallopian tubes?

Usually not. Once a chronic abscess has formed, the only satisfactory method of treatment is the removal of the tube.

### What kind of surgery is performed for salpingitis?

In disease restricted to one tube, simple removal of that tube is carried out. In more advanced disease, it may be necessary to remove both tubes, the tubes and the ovaries, or both tubes along with the ovaries and the uterus.

### Is operation for the removal of an inflamed tube a major operative procedure?

Yes. It is performed through an incision in the lower abdomen under general or spinal anesthesia.

### How long a hospital stay is necessary after an operation upon the tube?

Approximately five to nine days.

### How soon after an operation upon the tubes can a patient get out of bed?

The day following surgery.

### How long does it takes these wounds to heal?

Approximately ten days.

## Does recurrence of salpingitis ever take place after surgery?

Where surgery has been performed with the removal of the tubes, a recurrence will not take place. Where only one tube has been removed, it is possible for inflammation to return and involve the adjacent ovary or the other tube and ovary.

## Is there a tendency for salpingitis to recur when it is treated medically?

Yes.

## How often is salpingitis limited to one tube?

This situation occurs infrequently. In the majority of cases, the inflammation affects both tubes. However, removal of both tubes is not always necessary, as it is sometimes possible to salvage one tube.

## Will removal of the Fallopian tubes interfere with normal sexual relations?

No.

## Does removal of the Fallopian tubes cause change of life (menopause)?

No. It is only when the ovaries are removed along with the tubes that menopause follows.

## How soon after an operation for the removal of one or both tubes can a patient do the following:?

Shower:
  One week.
Bathe:
  Four weeks.
Perform household duties:
  One week.
Drive an automobile:
  Six weeks.
Resume sexual relations:
  Six weeks.
Douche:
  Six weeks
Return to work:
  Six weeks.

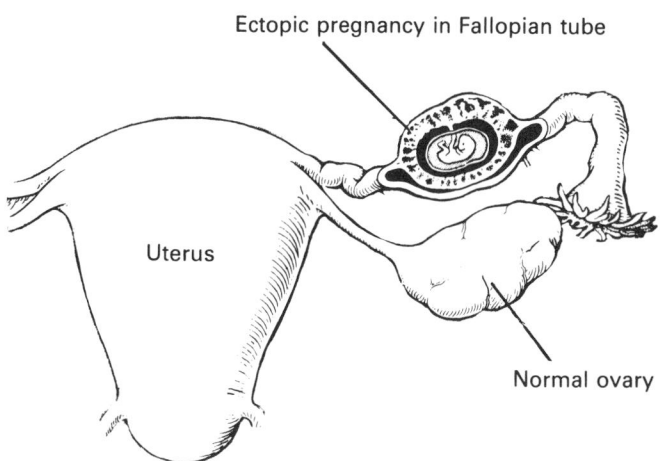

Ectopic pregnancy in Fallopian tube

Uterus

Normal ovary

*Ectopic Pregnancy. An ectopic, or tubal, pregnancy usually lasts only a few weeks, terminating in rupture of the tube and severe hemorrhage, which will require immediate emergency surgery. When ectopic pregnancy is diagnosed before rupture, the surgeon will operate and remove the involved Fallopian tube.*

## What is an ectopic (tubal) pregnancy?

It is a condition in which a fertilized egg implants in the wall of the Fallopian tube and starts to grow.

## What causes tubal pregnancy?

a. Previous inflammation of the tube is by far the most common cause of ectopic pregnancy. Approximately 25 percent of all cases occur in women who have had previous salpingitis.
b. Infection following abortion or infection following the delivery of a child.
c. Ovarian or uterine tumors that have produced mechanical compression, distortion, or blockage of a tube.
d. Previous peritonitis (inflammation of the abdominal cavity), which has created adhesions of a tube and has distorted its channel.
e. A birth deformity of the tube.
f. Unknown causes in women who are otherwise perfectly normal.

## How often does tubal pregnancy occur?

In approximately one out of every three to four hundred pregnancies.

## How soon after the egg is fertilized can a tubal pregnancy occur?

Two to four days after fertilization.

## How soon after a tubal pregnancy has taken place can a diagnosis be made?

Usually within four to six weeks.

## What are the symptoms of a tubal pregnancy?

In the early stages of an unruptured tubal pregnancy, the patient usually misses a menstrual period but does have slight vaginal staining. Some pain develops in the lower abdomen, particularly after intercourse. All of the signs seen during early pregnancy, including morning sickness, breast enlargement, etc., may be present.

When an ectopic pregnancy ruptures, the above symptoms may be followed by severe shock, fainting, marked pallor, abdominal pain, pain in the shoulder region, and pressure in the rectum.

## What causes the symptoms when a tubal pregnancy ruptures?

There is actual rupture of the tube

accompanied by great loss of blood into the abdominal cavity.

## What is meant by the term "tubal abortion"?

This is a situation in which the fertilized egg or young embryo is expelled from the end of the tube into the abdominal cavity. In many of these cases, the symptoms are not as severe as in a ruptured ectopic pregnancy, for the tube itself does not rupture, and there is much less blood loss and shock.

## Is a pregnancy test always positive in tubal pregnancy?

No. There are many cases in which the pregnancy test will be negative. This will depend upon whether the pregnancy is still viable (alive).

## How does the gynecologist make the diagnosis of tubal pregnancy?

a. By noting the appearance of the symptoms described above associated with the presence of a pelvic mass in the region of the Fallopian tube. A positive pregnancy test will also help to establish a diagnosis.
b. In suspected cases, a needle may be inserted into the pelvic cavity through the vagina to note the presence of blood within the pelvic cavity. Or an instrument can be inserted from the vagina into the pelvic cavity to visualize the tubes.
c. A sonogram will often demonstrate the presence of a tubal pregnancy.

## What is the best method of treatment when a tubal pregnancy is suspected?

If the diagnosis cannot be determined positively, the safest procedure is to operate and examine the tubes under direct vision. Although this involves an abdominal operation, it is much safer to follow this procedure than to permit a patient to progress to a stage where the tube will rupture.

## Is there any known method of preventing tubal pregnancy?

No, except to treat all disease within the pelvis prior to permitting the patient to become pregnant.

## What is the treatment for tubal pregnancy?

a. When a definite diagnosis has been made, the patient should be operated upon immediately and the tube removed.
b. Blood transfusions should be given rapidly if there has been marked blood loss.
c. Suspected cases should be watched carefully and advised to call the physician should there be any change in their condition.

## Are the ovaries removed when operating for tubal pregnancy?

No, unless they are found to be diseased.

## What is the greatest danger in tubal pregnancy?

Hemorrhage!

## What are the chances of recovery following tubal pregnancy?

When modern facilities are available and prompt surgery is performed, practically all cases recover.

## Is the operation itself a serious operation?

No more serious than the removal of a tube for any other reason.

## What anesthesia is used?

General anesthesia.

## How long a hospital stay is necessary after an ectopic pregnancy?

Seven to nine days.

## What treatments are given prior to operating upon a patient with a ruptured tubal pregnancy?

Transfusions are given to get the patient out of shock and thus permit surgery.

## Is it possible for someone to have a normal pregnancy after a tubal pregnancy?

Yes. The removal of one tube or ovary does not prevent a subsequent pregnancy, nor does it necessarily mean that another tubal pregnancy will occur.

## Are women who have had one tubal pregnancy more prone to develop a second ectopic pregnancy?

Yes.

## How soon after operation for a tubal pregnancy can one become pregnant again?

Two months.

## How soon after a tubal pregnancy will menstrual periods return?

Usually in six to eight weeks.

## Does cancer ever take place within the Fallopian tubes?

Yes, but it is an extremely rare condition.

## What is the treatment for cancer of a Fallopian tube?

It is treated like any other pelvic cancer, by complete removal of the uterus, tubes, and ovaries.

## Can a cure take place after cancer of a tube?

Yes, provided the disease has been eradicated before it has spread to other organs.

# THE OVARIES

## What are the ovaries?

They are a pair of almond-shaped glandular structures about one and a half inches by one inch in diameter. They are located in the pelvis on either side of the uterus and are suspended from the posterior wall of the pelvis in close proximity to the funnel-shaped openings of the Fallopian tubes. Each ovary consists of an outer capsule, which is grayish white in color, a cortex, or main substance, and a hilum, or stalk, through which the blood vessels enter and leave.

## What are the functions of the ovaries?

a. The periodic production and discharge of a mature egg. The cortex of each ovary contains several thousand immature eggs, one of which matures and is discharged into the funnel-shaped opening of a Fallopian tube each month. *This process is called ovulation.* If the egg is fertilized by the male sperm, the process halts. If fertilization does not take place, menstruation follows. The interval between ovulation and menstruation is approximately fourteen days.

b. The ovaries manufacture and secrete sex hormones into the bloodstream. These hormones are called estrogen and progesterone. They regulate ovulation and menstruation, help to maintain pregnancy when it exists, and are responsible for the development of female characteristics. Thus they are responsible for breast development, the female distribution of hair, the female figure, and the feminine voice.

## Are both ovaries necessary for normal ovarian function?

No. Only one ovary, or part of an ovary, is necessary to maintain normal function.

## At what age does the ovary begin to function?

From the onset of puberty, at approximately twelve to fourteen years of age.

## Is the ovary ever the site of inflammation or infection?

Yes. Because of its close proximity to the Fallopian tube, disease of that structure will frequently spread to the ovary.

## What are the symptoms of an inflamed or infected ovary?

They are the same as those involving disease of the Fallopian tube (salpingitis).

## What is meant by the term "ovarian dysfunction"?

It is a state in which there is disturbed ovarian hormone production or imbalance, characterized by upset in the menstrual cycle and in the ability to become pregnant or maintain pregnancy. Such disorders may originate within the ovary or they may be secondary to disturbed function within other endocrine glands, such as the pituitary or thyroid.

## What are some of the symptoms that may develop with prolonged dysfunction of the ovaries?

a. Complete upset in the menstrual cycle and in the character and nature of menstruation.

b. Obesity.

c. The development of extra hair upon the body (hirsutism).

d. Overgrowth of the lining membrane of the uterus (endometrial hyperplasia).

e. Infertility (inability to become pregnant).

## What is the treatment for ovarian dysfunction?

First, the exact cause of the imbalance must be determined. Hormone studies of the blood and urine are carried out in an attempt to find the seat of the difficulty and to determine whether it originates in the ovary, the thyroid, or the pituitary gland. Endometrial biopsy and vaginal smears are also performed as an aid to a precise diagnosis.

a. When cysts accompany ovarian dysfunction, an operation with removal of a wedge-shaped section from each ovary often helps correct the disturbance.

b. When thyroid or pituitary gland dysfunction is found to be the cause of the ovarian disorder, the condition must be remedied by appropriate medication before the ovarian dysfunction can be corrected.

c. Cyclic therapy, the giving of regulated doses of estrogen and progesterone hormones, in a manner simulating the normal cycle, may prove beneficial.

d. More recently, cortisone has been found successful in certain cases in restoring normal ovarian function.

## Does disturbed ovarian function ever subside by itself?

Yes. This occurs frequently without any treatment whatever.

## At what age may ovarian dysfunction occur?

It can take place at any age from puberty to menopause but is seen most often during the first years of adolescence or early adulthood.

## Can pregnancy follow ovarian dysfunction?

If ovarian dysfunction is accompanied by lack of ovulation, pregnancy will not take place. However, once the dysfunction is corrected, pregnancy may take place.

## Are there medications that can help a woman who fails to ovulate?

Yes. There are several medications that can correct this condition. In some instances, these drugs have not only encouraged ovulation and pregnancy but have been associated with multiple births such as twins, triplets, quadruplets, etc.

## What are follicle cysts?

These are small, fluid-filled sacs appearing on the surface of an ovary. They arise from the failure of the egg-producing follicle to rupture. Thus, the cyst persists instead of being absorbed.

## To what size do follicle cysts grow?

They may vary from the size of a pea to that of a plum.

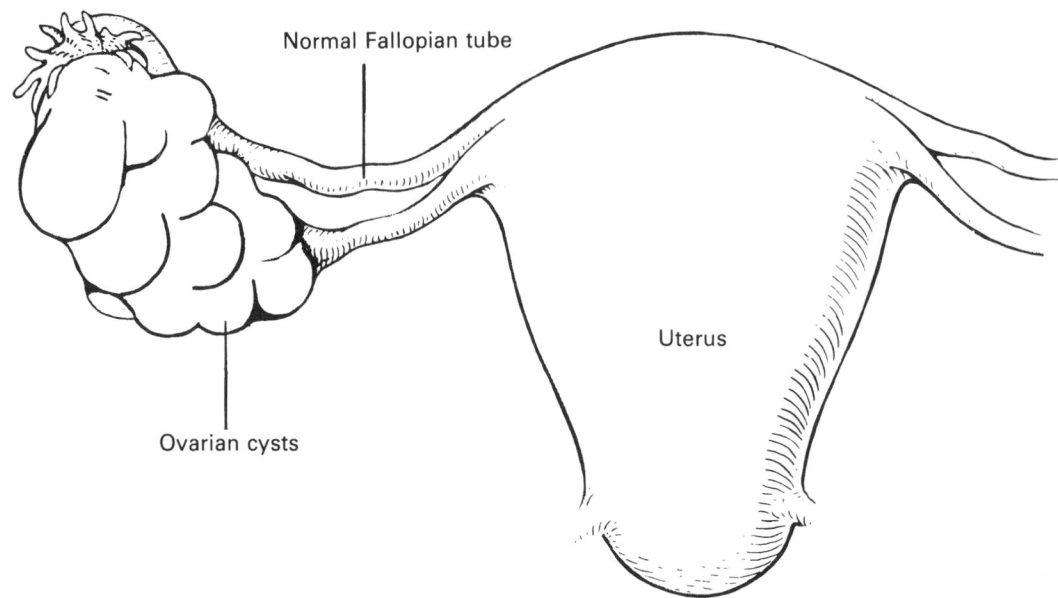

**Ovarian Cysts.** *This diagram shows an ovary involved in cyst formation. When ovarian cysts become larger than the size of a lemon or an orange and persist for any length of time, they are best treated by surgical removal. If the opposite ovary is normal, completely normal menstrual and reproductive functions will be maintained. A pathological enlargement of an ovary can be felt on pelvic examination.*

**What are the causes of follicle cysts?**

a. Previous infection that has produced a thickening of the outer coat of the ovary.
b. Disturbance in ovarian function.

**What symptoms do follicle cysts cause?**

They may cause no symptoms, or they may result in ovarian dysfunction as described above. The larger, solitary follicle cysts sometimes cause lower abdominal pain, urinary distress, pain on intercourse, and menstrual irregularity.

**Do follicle cysts ever rupture?**

Yes. When this happens, it may be accompanied by severe pain in the lower abdomen, tenderness on pressure, nausea, vomiting, or even a state of shock. It is often difficult for the gynecologist to distinguish a ruptured follicle cyst from appendicitis or from a tubal pregnancy.

**What is the treatment for follicle cysts?**

Treatment is seldom required for the simple, small, or multiple cysts that are associated with no symptoms. Multiple cysts that cause symptoms and are associated with ovarian dysfunction should be treated by surgery with the removal of wedge-shaped sections of the ovaries. If rupture or twist of a solitary cyst takes place and the symptoms do not abate within a day or two, surgery may be necessary.

**Do follicle cysts of the ovaries ever disappear by themselves?**

Yes.

**Is there a tendency for follicle cysts to recur?**

Yes. Patients who have had follicle cysts require periodic observation by their gynecologists.

**How is the diagnosis of an ovarian cyst or tumor made?**

a By pelvic examination.
b. By sonography (ultrasound test).
c. By laparoscopy (the insertion of a metal tube, with a light at the end, through the navel and into the abdominal cavity).

**What is a corpus luteum cyst of the ovary?**

After the egg has broken out of the ovary, the follicle is supposed to undergo shrinkage and disappear. In some cases, instead of disappearing, the follicle develops into a cyst (sac). Such a cyst may be filled with blood and may enlarge to the size of a lemon, orange, or even larger.

**What are the symptoms of a corpus luteum cyst?**

It may cause no symptoms, or if it is large, it may cause pain, delay in menstruation, or painful intercourse. If the cyst ruptures, there may be acute onset of pain, nausea, vomiting, urinary disturbance, and severe pain in the lower abdomen. This may give the appearance of an acute surgical condition such as appendicitis or ectopic pregnancy and may demand surgery.

**When is it necessary to operate upon a ruptured corpus luteum cyst?**

If the symptoms persist or if there has been a great deal of blood loss.

**Are there other types of ovarian cysts?**

Yes. There are many types, including simple solitary cysts and cystic tumors.

**Are tumors of the ovary very common?**

Yes.

**Do these cysts ever grow to a large size?**

Yes. Some of them may fill the entire abdominal cavity and reach the size of a watermelon.

**What is the treatment for these cysts?**

Surgical removal as promptly as possible.

**What types of tumors affect the ovary?**

a. Benign solid or cystic tumors.
b. Malignant solid or cystic tumors.
c. Hormone-producing tumors.

**Why is the ovary so often the seat of tumor or cyst formation?**

The eggs within the ovaries contain all the basic primitive cells that go into the formation of a new human being, and it is not surprising that some of these may undergo abnormal growth. Also, the ovary itself is subject to so many wide and varied fluctuations in function that it is not difficult to appreciate that things might go wrong and lead to tumor growth.

**Do tumors of the ovary occur in women at any age?**

Yes. They occur from earliest childhood to the latest years of life.

**What is a dermoid cyst of the ovary?**

This is a tumor occurring in women usually between the ages of twenty and fifty. It is frequently found in both ovaries and may grow to be as large as an orange. It is composed of many types of cells and may even in-clude hair, bone, and teeth. Dermoid cysts have also been found to contain other tissues that resemble organs in a primitive stage of development.

**Are dermoid cysts malignant?**

The great majority are not malignant, but some will become malignant if they are not removed.

**How is the diagnosis of a dermoid cyst made?**

By pelvic examination, sonography, and laparoscopy.

**What is the treatment for a dermoid cyst of the ovary?**

In the childbearing age, resection of the dermoid cyst. Past the childbearing age, removal of the ovary, or ovaries, and uterus.

**What are hormone-producing tumors of the ovaries?**

These are tumors that manufacture either female or male sex hormones in great excess. Thus, a tumor of the ovary that produces a male-type hormone will cause the patient to assume male characteristics, such as growth of hair on the face and chest, deepening of the voice, and loss of feminine appearance.

**Are hormone-producing tumors of the ovary very common?**

No.

**What is the treatment for hormone-producing tumors of the ovary?**

Age plays an important role. Surgical removal of the diseased ovary is indicated in some cases; in older women, the uterus should also be removed.

**Will altered characteristics disappear after removal of a hormone-producing ovarian tumor?**

Yes.

**What are fibromas of the ovary?**

These are solid tumors constituting about 5 percent of all ovarian growths. They are commonly associated with fluid secretion in the abdominal cavity, and, because of their similarity to certain malignant growths of the ovary, they must be very carefully analyzed after being removed.

**Does endometriosis affect the ovary?**

Yes. In about one out of eight cases of endometriosis, the condition is found in the ovary. It is almost always associated with endometriosis elsewhere.

**Is cancer of the ovary a common condition?**

Unfortunately, yes. Cancers will appear as either solid or cystic growths, and they may arise from one or from both ovaries. Cancer of the ovary may also develop from benign tumors of the ovaries, such as dermoid cysts.

**Does secondary cancer ever affect the ovary?**

Yes. This is quite common and occurs from the spread of a cancer of the stomach, bowel, breast, or uterus.

**At what age does cancer most commonly affect the ovary?**

The highest incidence occurs in the years between thirty-five and forty-five, although it is sometimes found in young girls and in elderly women.

**How does one make the diagnosis of cancer of the ovary?**

By pelvic examination, sonography, and laparoscopy. Fluid in the abdominal cavity is a frequent finding suggestive of an ovarian malignancy.

**What is the treatment for malignant tumors of the ovary?**

The present mode of treatment involves surgery with total and complete removal of the uterus, both tubes, both ovaries, and the ligaments and tissues surrounding these structures. Surgery is often followed by chemotherapy and, in some instances, by radiation.

**What are the possibilities of cure of cancer of the ovary?**

If the patient is operated upon early—before there has been spread to other structures or organs—the chances are fairly good. Surgical recovery takes place in almost all cases, as these operations are not excessively dangerous.

**What is the best method to prevent cancer of the ovary?**

Frequent, periodic pelvic examinations will reveal the presence of abnormality in the ovary and alert the patient to the need for possible surgery. If surgery is performed early for suspicious tumors, many patients can be saved before the tumor has become malignant or before it has spread to other structures.

**What is the best treatment for any ovarian cyst or tumor?**

If it persists or shows signs of growth an operation should be performed to evaluate the exact nature of the lesion. In this way, many ovarian tumors can be removed that might have become malignant at some future date. Also, early removal of a persistently cystic or enlarged ovary will prevent it from twisting or rupturing.

**Is medical treatment ever preferred to surgical treatment in tumors of the ovaries?**

No.

**What are some of the exact criteria for advising surgery for ovarian conditions?**

a. Any ovarian mass more than two inches in diameter that persists on repeated examination should be removed.

b. Any rapid growth of an ovarian tumor should be operated upon.

c. The presence of free fluid within the abdominal cavity in the presence of an ovarian tumor should indicate surgery.

d. The appearance of weight loss, anemia, and weakness in the presence of an ovarian tumor should warrant surgery.

**Is it possible to determine while the patient is on the operating table whether a tumor of the ovary is malignant?**

Yes. A pathologist will take a frozen section of a tumor and examine it under the microscope while the patient is on the operating table. This will determine whether or not the tumor is malignant and will suggest to the surgeon how extensive his operative procedure should be.

**How soon after operations upon the ovaries can one do the following:?**

Shower:
  One week.
Bathe:
  Two weeks.
Drive an automobile:
  Four weeks.
Resume household duties:
  Six weeks.
Return to work:
  Six weeks.
Resume sexual relations:
  Six weeks.
Douche:
  Six weeks.

**Do ovarian tumors ever occur during pregnancy?**

Yes. Cysts of the ovary occasionally occur during pregnancy.

**Do cysts that occur during pregnancy harm the embryo?**

No.

**Do ovarian cysts or tumors ever create an acute abdominal condition?**

Yes, there is a great tendency for cysts or tumors of the ovary to twist upon their stalks. This will cause all of the signs of an acute abdominal condition and will require immediate surgery.

**Do cysts of the ovary ever rupture?**

Occasionally this happens, and when it does, emergency operation is indicated.

**Does the removal of the ovaries alter one's sexual desires?**

Not in the slightest.

**Can a woman become pregnant after the removal of one ovary?**

Yes. This does not reduce her chances for pregnancy at all.

**Does a patient with only one ovary menstruate regularly?**

Yes.

**Does removal of both ovaries always bring on change of life (menopause)?**

Yes, unless the woman has already passed the menopause.

## THE MENOPAUSE
*(Change of Life)*

**What is the menopause?**

It is that period in a woman's life during which ovulation (the production of mature eggs) and menstruation come to an end. It is commonly called the "change of life." In other words, menopause represents the natural aging process.

**When does menopause occur?**

In most women between the ages of forty-five and fifty, but it may occur as early as thirty-five and as late as fifty-five years of age.

## What is meant by the term "artificial menopause"?

It is a state created by the surgical removal of the ovaries or by x-ray treatments to the ovaries that cause them to cease ovulating.

## What produces menopause?

A decrease and eventual stoppage in the secretion of hormones by the ovaries.

## What are the reactions to menopause?

These vary widely. They may be absent or minimal; they may be marked and disabling. The most important factor in menopause is a woman's psychological attitude toward it. Women who for one reason or another wish to suffer, may unconsciously have severe menopausal symptoms. It is not uncommon for a woman to mimic her mother's reaction to menopause. If women are properly oriented and informed as to the menopause, and if they are emotionally stable, they will probably react mildly.

## What are the usual general symptoms of menopause?

a. Hot flashes.
b. Cold sweats.
c. Headaches.
d. A feeling of fatigue.
e. Nervousness and a feeling of emotional strain and tension.
f. Depression and a feeling of inadequacy.

## What are early specific symptoms of menopause?

Irregularity of menstrual periods and a diminished flow.

## How can one distinguish between irregular bleeding due to menopause and that which is due to a tumor or other disorder within the pelvic organs?

If there is any doubt as to the cause of the irregularity of the menstrual flow, the gynecologist will investigate it by doing vaginal smears or by taking a biopsy of the tissue from the uterus or cervix. Frequently, the doctor will recommend a curettage in order to determine the exact nature of the condition.

## What is the usual duration of menopause?

It may last anywhere from a few months to a few years.

## What is the treatment of menopause?

a. The most important step in the treatment of menopause is to reassure the patient and to inform her fully as to the nature of the condition.
b. If the symptoms are not severe, the best treatment is no treatment.
c. Hormone replacement is often administered when symptoms are severe. Such therapy should not be given longer than necessary, as it increases the chances of developing cancer of the uterus.
d. Tranquilizing drugs and sedatives have proven helpful in relieving symptoms in some instances.

## Can relief from the symptoms of menopause be obtained by the giving of ovarian hormones?

Yes. This form of treatment, however, should be carried out only under the constant supervision of a gynecologist.

## Are the tranquilizing drugs efficient in relieving the symptoms of menopause?

Yes, but in mild cases only.

## Is there a changing attitude toward giving hormones to women who are past the menopause?

Yes. Formerly, continued ovarian-replacement therapy was advocated by many gynecologists. Today this is not advised routinely because there is a suspicion that it increases the chances of developing cancer of the uterus.

## Do the symptoms of menopause always subside after the passage of time?

Yes, within a few months to a few years.

## Is it natural for emotionally disturbed women to have more severe and longer menopause?

Yes.

## Does the desire for sexual relations change with the menopause?

No. After cessation of menstruation, sexual desire continues as previously.

## Should there be any change in a woman's personal feminine hygiene after menopause?

No.

## Is it natural for the voice to deepen and for hair to grow on the face and body with menopause?

Absolutely not.

## Can pregnancy occur after the menopause?

No. When ovulation and menstruation have ceased, pregnancy will not take place.

## For how long a period after the onset of menopause can pregnancy take place?

It is possible for pregnancy to take place during the first six months to one year of menopause.

## What is the significance of vaginal bleeding after the menopause has been well established?

Bleeding that occurs a year or more after the periods have stopped should always be looked upon as possible evidence of a tumor within the cervix or uterus. This must be investigated thoroughly.

**Are there any structural changes in the appearance of the ovaries or uterus following menopause?**

They tend to undergo slight shrinkage in size, but this change is not significant.

**Are a woman's abilities to think clearly and to be mentally alert just as great after the menopause as they were before?**

Yes.

**Is it common for women to lose their youthful appearance after the menopause?**

No, except that one must realize that the menopause occurs at an age when the youthful appearance tends to wane. The loss of female hormone secretions, however, has very little to do with the physical appearance of a woman.

**Will the giving of ovarian hormone drugs restore the youthful appearance of a patient past menopause?**

No, despite many reports to the contrary.

**Is there a tendency to inherit early menopause or late menopause?**

No.

**Can ovarian hormones delay the aging process in menopausal women?**

They may, but only to a limited extent and for a limited period of time. The aging process, unfortunately, is inevitable.

**Does an early menopause indicate that the life span will be short?**

Definitely not. The menopause is no indication whatever of a woman's ability to live a long life.

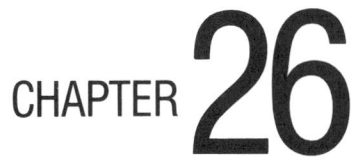

# CHAPTER 26
# FIRST AID IN EMERGENCIES

*(See also Chapter 2 on Abscesses and Bacterial Infections; Chapter 14 on Bones, Muscles, Tendons, and Joints; Chapter 29 on Heart; Chapter 71 on Throat)*

## BITES

### Animal or Human Bites

**What is the first-aid treatment for animal or human bites?**

These injuries usually consist of puncture wounds, jagged lacerations, or bruises. They should be treated quickly and thoroughly in the following manner:

a. Scrub and cleanse the wound with water and any mild soap for a period of five to ten minutes.

b. Apply a sterile bandage, or if this is not immediately obtainable, a clean handkerchief.

c. Any animal bite that has punctured the skin should be treated immediately by a physician so that he may give tetanus antitoxin and antibiotics and recommend antirabies injections if indicated.

**Are human bites particularly dangerous?**

Yes, because the germs in the human mouth frequently produce very severe infections, often much worse than those caused by animal bites.

**Should antiseptic solutions, such as iodine, be used in the first-aid treatment of animal or human bites?**

No. Strong antiseptics may damage the tissues further and should not be used.

**Are bites always sutured (stitched) by the physician?**

No. In some instances, for fear of infection, such wounds are left wide open to drain and are not sutured until several days later. Wounds of the face are usually sutured after thorough cleansing.

## Insect Bites

**Are bites dangerous from such insects as fleas, sandflies, mosquitoes, wasps, hornets, bees, or chiggers?**

If someone is allergic to the sting of these insects, such bites can be serious injuries requiring immediate treatment with antivenin.

**What is the first-aid treatment for insect bites?**

a. If a sting has been left in place, it should be gently plucked out. It is important not to break it in attempts at removal.

b. If a person is known to be allergic to a particular type of bite and is bitten on an extremity, it might be well to place a tourniquet above the bite on the extremity so that the absorption of the poison will take place more slowly. It is important not to allow a tourniquet to remain in place for more than twenty minutes at a time. Release it for ten minutes and then reapply.

c. Medical advice should be obtained if a great degree of swelling takes place. The physician will give an antiallergic medication or will take other measures to counteract the effect of the bite. Antivenin extracts are available in many hospitals for those who are extremely allergic to insect bites.

d. It is important not to scratch a bite, as this will cause secondary infec-

tion and will lead to greater absorption of the poison.

**Is a bite from a black widow spider a serious injury?**

Yes, particularly when it affects young children. Occasional fatalities have been reported. Bites from these spiders are characterized by severe abdominal pain and board-like stiffness of the abdominal muscles.

**How can one recognize a black widow spider?**

It has a rounded, jet black body with a red marking on its belly in the shape of an hourglass. This is the female of the species and the one to be avoided. The black widow male does not bite.

**What is the first-aid treatment for a black widow spider bite?**

a. It should be treated just like a snake bite, by making a crossed incision over the bite and sucking out the poison.

b. A tourniquet should be applied above the bite just tight enough to cut off the return circulation. The pulse should still be obtainable.

c. Medical consultation should be sought quickly as there are counteracting medications to the bite of a black widow spider.

d. Physical exertion should be avoided as much as possible.

**What should be done for the bites of other spiders, poisonous centipedes, scorpions, or tarantulas?**

These should be treated similarly to a black widow spider bite.

**Are the stings of centipedes, scorpions, or tarantulas very serious?**

Usually not. The only time a sting from these insects endangers life is when it happens to a young infant or when the bite is on the face or neck. However, stings from these insects may produce severe temporary symptoms and great discomfort.

## Snake Bites

### What is the first-aid treatment for a snake bite?

Since it is not always possible to tell whether the snake is poisonous, precautions should be taken in all cases of snake bite. The following procedures should be carried out:

a. A tourniquet should be placed just above the site of the bite. This should be only tight enough to stop venous flow and must not cut off the pulse. Anything, such as a handkerchief, tie, or belt, can be used as a tourniquet. The tourniquet must be released every twenty minutes for a ten-minute interval.

b. A crossed incision should be made over the site of the bite, and the bite should be sucked out.

c. The patient should be put at absolute rest and should undergo as little physical exertion as possible.

d. Have the patient transported to the nearest hospital and, if possible, ascertain the type of snake that caused the bite.

### What are some of the poisonous snakes commonly found in the United States?

The coral snake, the rattlesnake, the copperhead, and the moccasin.

### Is alcohol a good remedy for a snake bite?

Absolutely not.

### Are the bites of poisonous snakes always fatal?

On the contrary, the majority of adults recover from snake bites. This is especially true if they can be admitted to a hospital promptly for the administration of the appropriate antivenin. The danger is greater in children, as the snake poison is apt to be more overwhelming.

## BURNS AND FROSTBITE

### How are burns usually classified?

a. First-degree burns. These involve only the superficial layers of the skin and evidence themselves by mere reddening. Most sunburns are first degree.

b. Second-degree burns. These burns involve not only the superficial layers but also the deeper layers of the skin. They are characterized by blisters and by the discharge of serum. Severe sunburns may fall into this category.

c. Third-degree burns. These burns involve all of the layers of the skin and usually have caused complete skin destruction.

d. Fourth-degree burns. These burns not only destroy all layers of the skin but involve the tissues beneath the skin, such as the subcutaneous tissues, muscles, tendons, blood vessels, bone, etc.

### Are all burns caused by excessive heat?

No. There are many other types of burns, such as those caused by chemicals, alkalis, extreme cold, or strong acids. Also, some burns are caused by electricity or radiations such as x ray, radioactive substances, etc.

### What is the proper first-aid treatment for burns?

a. First-degree burns can be treated by any of the usual ointments that relieve pain and prevent the skin from drying or cracking. Most first-degree burns can be self-treated and do *not* require the advice of a physician unless the general health of the patient is also affected.

b. Second-degree burns must be treated by a physician. First-aid measures will include:
1. Immersing the burned area in running cold water for approximately ten minutes.
2. Covering the area with a sterile dressing.
3. Seeing that the patient maintains a large intake of fluids.
4. Cleansing the burned areas with large quantities of water and a mild soap.
5. Avoiding the use of ointments.

c. Third-degree burns should never be self treated. As a preliminary measure, dirt should be gently washed off with water and a clean dressing applied. Large quantities of fluids should be given by mouth, and if the patient is in shock, he should be immediately transported to a hospital on a stretcher. Ointments should *not* be applied to the burned area.

d. Fourth-degree burns should be treated in the same manner as third-degree burns.

### Should the blisters of a second-degree burn be opened by the patient himself?

No. A physician should treat these blisters. Some physicians open them while others allow them to dry up by themselves.

### Should people apply ointments to burns?

It is perhaps best not to apply an ointment to anything but a mild first-degree burn. There are various ways of treating a burn, and many physicians do not believe in the application of ointments. Furthermore, the ointment that the patient prescribes for himself may not be the one the doctor may want used. It then becomes difficult to remove it in order to apply the proper medication.

### Do chemical burns require special treatment?

Yes. It is wise to wash any chemically burned area thoroughly with large quantities of water in order to dilute the chemical and eliminate that which may still be in contact with the skin.

### What should be done about the shock that accompanies burns?

Shock demands immediate treatment. (See the section on Shock in this chapter.)

**Is any special first-aid treatment indicated for burns of the eye?**

Yes. These burns should be irrigated thoroughly with water to dilute the agent that has produced the burn. Medical care should then be sought immediately.

**Should butter or homemade remedies or greases be used on burns as a first-aid treatment?**

No.

## Frostbite

**What is frostbite?**

It is a burn caused by exposure to excessive cold.

**What is the first-aid treatment for frostbite?**

a. Treat the general condition of the patient by warming him and by giving him warm foods to eat and warm liquids to drink.

b. The patient must be thawed out gradually and not suddenly placed from a very cold into a very warm atmosphere.

c. Give medications to relieve any pain that may exist. Tylenol or similar medications are usually adequate.

d. The affected part should be brought back to use slowly and should be exercised, but should in no event be vigorously massaged or rubbed.

e. The frostbitten part should be covered with a dry, clean dressing.

**How warm should a frostbitten part be made?**

Immerse the part in lukewarm water (100° to 103°F.).

**Should snow be rubbed into a frozen part?**

No.

**Should antiseptics be applied to frozen areas?**

No. They may cause further burn.

**Are any medications helpful in aiding a part to return to normal circulation?**

Yes, but they must be administered by a physician.

**Can one determine the extent of the damage resulting from frostbite soon after it has occurred?**

No. It may take several days to several weeks to discover the full extent of the damage.

## CHOKING

**Do some people have a greater tendency to choke than others?**

Yes. People who eat rapidly and those who talk with food in their mouths are much more likely to choke than those who eat slowly and keep their mouths closed while chewing.

**Are children particularly prone to choking?**

Yes, because they do not observe the cautions described above. Also, they frequently put coins or other foreign bodies in their mouths.

**Do elderly people have a tendency toward choking on food?**

Yes, because the swallowing mechanism in older people doesn't often work as well as it does in younger people.

**What normally prevents choking on food?**

The epiglottis in the throat moves to close over the entrance to the trachea (windpipe) during the act of swallowing. This prevents liquids and solids from gaining access to the trachea, bronchial tubes, and lungs.

**What are common causes of the epiglottis not working during the swallowing process?**

A sudden cough or sneeze may prevent the epiglottis from shutting off the trachea, thus allowing food or liquid to enter it.

**Do most people recover spontaneously from choking?**

Yes. In the great majority of instances they cough out the liquid or food that has "gone down the wrong way."

**What first-aid measures should be given someone who is choking on food or some other ingested object?**

a. Strenuous coughing should be encouraged.

b. A few sharp slaps on the back of the chest may aid in the expulsion of the food.*

c. If the victim is a child, hold him upside down and give him a few sharp slaps on the back.*

d. If the obstructing object is not expelled, place an index finger in the back of the victim's mouth and sweep it around the back of the throat. This frequently dislodges the foreign body.

e. If the above measures fail, the Heimlich maneuver should be carried out promptly.

Time should not be wasted in repeating the above measures if they are not immediately successful.

**How is the Heimlich maneuver performed?**

a. The victim is raised to his feet.

b. The first-aider stands behind him and places both arms about the victim's waist at a level just below the rib cage.

c. The right fist is placed high up in the abdomen, just below the breastbone.

d. The right fist is firmly grasped with the left hand. The victim is held tightly.

e. With a sudden inward and upward

---

* Although the Red Cross recommends sharp slaps on the back, Dr. Henry J. Heimlich (the originator of the Heimlich maneuver) believes this is of no value and may even be harmful.

thrust, the grip on the victim is tightened as forcefully as possible. This will cause a sudden, tremendous increase of pressure within the victim's chest cavity and will force air—along with the foreign body or food—out of the windpipe.

f. If the first thrust fails to clear the windpipe, repeat the maneuver. Remember, the thrust must be a quick, instantaneous one. Release your grip once the thrust has been carried out.

### Does the Heimlich maneuver work?

Yes, in the vast majority of cases.

### Is a tracheotomy ever indicated if all other methods fail to relieve the choking?

Yes, but it should not be done by an inexperienced layman. If a physician is available, or an experienced paramedic is the only one available, it may be performed on a victim who is obviously choking to death.

### How can one tell if a victim is choking to death?

If he is unable to breathe at all, has turned blue, and his heart action becomes irregular, he will probably die within a few minutes.

### What is done when the patient *can* breathe but has not expelled the obstructing food or other object?

He should be transported as soon as possible, in a semisitting position, to the nearest doctor or hospital.

## CONVULSIONS AND "FITS"

### What is the first-aid treatment for someone who has had a convulsion or "fit"?

a. See that the patient does not further injure himself by striking his head or other parts of his body against hard objects.

b. Allow the patient to lie down and give him plenty of freedom. Do not attempt to restrain him.

c. Open a tight collar at the neck to allow easier breathing.

d. Lift up the chin to improve the breathing airway.

e. If it can be done easily, place a folded handkerchief between the patient's teeth to prevent tongue biting. (Do not place your fingers between the patient's teeth, as you may be bitten.)

### Should cold water be thrown on people who are having convulsions or fits?

No. This is improper treatment.

### Do most people recover from convulsions or fits?

Yes, particularly if the convulsions are epileptic in origin. Convulsions due to a brain hemorrhage or tumor may lead to death.

### Should small children with convulsions be immersed in water?

No. It is much better to allow these children to remain comfortably in bed.

### Should a parent pick up a child having a convulsion and run with him to a physician?

No. Recovery takes place in almost all cases of childhood convulsions. The best treatment is to allow the child to lie in bed unmolested.

### Is there any way to find out how to aid a person having a convulsion?

Yes. In many instances people subject to convulsions will carry instructions in their clothing concerning their condition. Diabetics may carry instructions on what to do for them if they go into insulin shock. Epileptics often carry explicit instructions as to how they should be treated if they have a seizure.

### What aftertreatment is necessary

for people who emerge from a convulsion or fit?

It usually takes quite a little time before they reestablish their normal thinking processes. Therefore, they should not be abandoned as soon as the convulsion has subsided. Many of these people will need quite a few minutes to know where they are and to realize what has happened. Stay with them until they regain their normal state completely.

## DROWNING

### What are the first-aid measures to be taken in cases of drowning?

After the patient has been removed from the water, he should be given artificial respiration if he is not breathing. The mouth-to-mouth breathing method is advocated and should be used instead of other methods.

### How does one carry out mouth-to-mouth artificial respiration?

a. Stretch out patient on his back; loosen any tight clothing around the neck, chest, or waist.

b. Lift up chin and tilt head back as far as possible. (This straightens out the windpipe and improves the airway to the lungs.)

c. With your fingers, pinch the patient's nostrils so that they are closed.

d. Place your mouth tightly over patient's mouth and blow as hard as you can.

e. Take your mouth away to permit air to be expelled from the lungs.

f. Repeat this every five to six seconds.

g. Continue this maneuver so long as there is any pulse or heartbeat. It may take as much as several hours to revive someone.

h. When you tire, have someone substitute for you.

i. If the patient seems to have water or mucus in his throat or chest, tilt him on his side to permit such fluid to run out the mouth.

j. Wipe out patient's mouth with your fingers if mucus or other material collects there. (A nonbreathing person will never bite.)

k. If you are squeamish about direct mouth-to-mouth contact, you may blow through an opened handkerchief. (This may not prove to be as effective as direct contact.)

l. Discontinue artificial respiration only when you are certain there is no pulse or heartbeat for several minutes. Listen carefully with your ear to patient's left chest region and feel for pulsations in the neck.

m. If patient is revived, keep him warm and do not move him until the doctor arrives, or at least for a half hour.

## MOUTH-TO-MOUTH ARTIFICIAL RESPIRATION

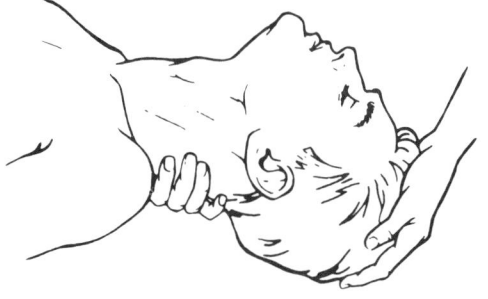

*Tilt head far back and elevate the chin* before beginning mouth-to-mouth breathing. This will straighten the windpipe and will provide a good air passage. If foreign matter is present in victim's mouth, it should be removed.

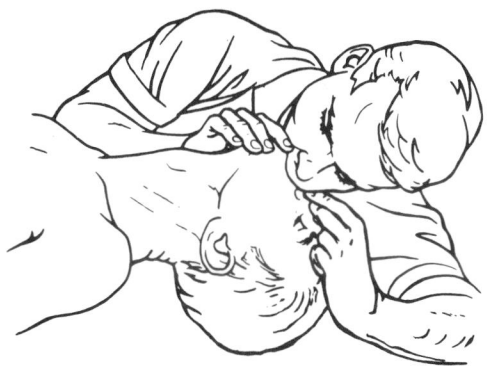

*Pinch nostrils shut with one hand* and keep the chin elevated with the other. Place mouth directly over victim's mouth and blow air until his chest rises. Repeat about twelve to twenty times a minute until spontaneous breathing resumes.

**Should mouth-to-mouth artificial respiration be used in all cases where breathing has stopped—whether due to drowning, suffocation, poisoning, electric shock, etc.?**

Yes.

**Is the mouth-to-mouth breathing method of artificial respiration beneficial in cases of drowning?**

Yes, but it is easier for the victim to expel water from the lungs when he is in a prone position. After water has been expelled, mouth-to-mouth breathing can be started.

**Is drowning always caused by too much water in the lungs?**

Not always. Many cases of drowning are caused by spasm of the larynx and can be relieved by overcoming the spasm. There are many cases on record in which life has been saved by the performances of a tracheotomy below the point of the laryngeal spasm.

## Three Basic Techniques

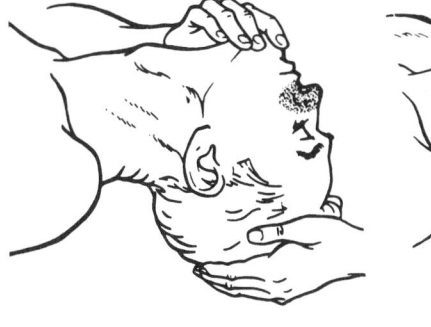 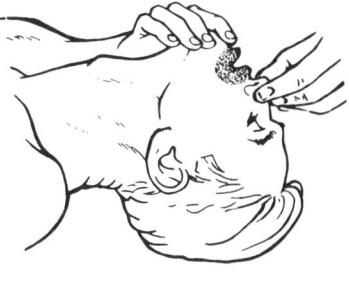 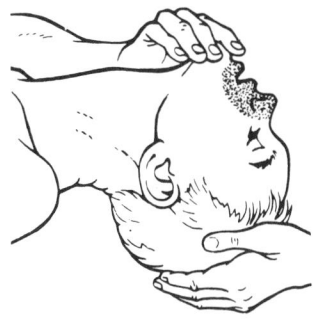

*Mouth-to-nose breathing* (left). Inflate lungs by holding victim's mouth tightly closed and blowing hard into his nostrils. In *mouth-to-mouth breathing* (center) hold nostrils closed and blow air into mouth. *Nose-and-mouth breathing* (right) is useful on children. Place mouth firmly over victim's nose and mouth and blow gently.

**Should a tracheotomy be performed by a first-aider?**

No, unless it is almost certain that medical attention cannot be obtained or that the patient will die before it arrives.

**Does it help to turn a drowning person upside down and to hold him in this position?**

Usually not. He will bring up water from his lungs if merely permitted to lie in a prone position.

**When should artificial respiration be abandoned?**

When the patient no longer has a heartbeat and is obviously dead.

## ELECTRIC SHOCK

**What is the first-aid treatment for electric shock?**

Do not touch a person who is still in contact with an electric wire! This may cause your death as well as his. The patient should be removed from electric contact as quickly as possible. This may be accomplished by cutting off the current that is going to the patient or by disconnecting the patient from the wire contact by use of a dry stick or rope that is thrown around him. An axe may be available to cut the wire that is causing the contact with the patient. When using an axe, be sure that your hands are dry and that the wood handle of the axe is dry.

**What treatment should be carried out for electric shock after the patient has been disconnected from electric contact?**

a. Artificial respiration should be instituted as soon as possible.
b. The patient should be kept quiet and warm and supplied with oxygen if this is available.
c. The burned area, which is often present at the site of contact, must

be treated in the same manner as any burn.

## FAINTING, DIZZINESS, AND VERTIGO

**What is the first-aid treatment for fainting, dizziness, or vertigo?**

a. Place the patient in a lying-down position with his face up and his head at body level or slightly lower than the level of the rest of his body.
b. Raise the legs slightly above the level of the rest of the body.
c. If there is a tight collar or tie, loosen it so that the patient can get plenty of air.
d. If breathing is shallow, it can be improved by artificial respiration.

**How long should a patient be kept in a supine position after he has fainted or after an attack of vertigo has taken place?**

Until he is fully recovered and feels himself again.

**Is it common for people to faint a second time soon after they have recovered?**

No, but they should be observed for a considerable time before being permitted to proceed on their own.

**Do people ever die in a faint?**

This almost never takes place unless a person has struck his head violently in the process of fainting and has sustained a fatal head injury.

**Should cold water be thrown upon people who have fainted?**

No.

**Do people who faint or who have attacks of dizziness or vertigo usually recover by themselves?**

Yes, without any treatment other than being permitted to lie down for several minutes.

## FOREIGN BODIES

**What should be done in the way of first-aid treatment for foreign bodies?**

a. Eyes. Only the most superficial foreign bodies should be removed from the eyes by nonphysicians. If medical care is not readily available, the eye should be irrigated with lukewarm water, or a moist piece of cotton can be used to brush out the foreign body. A little bit of mineral oil instilled into the eye will relieve most of the irritation. Avoid rubbing the eye and avoid trying to scrape out a foreign body with any hard object.
b. Nose. If one can get the patient to sneeze, the foreign body will often be extruded. This can be accomplished by having him inhale some pepper through his nostrils or by tickling the opposite nostril.
c. Ears. Foreign bodies in the ear should not be attacked by lay people, as damage may result to this delicate structure. The best first aid is to place some olive oil, mineral oil, or castor oil into the ear and let it stay there for a few minutes. This will usually bring out the foreign body. No great harm will result from a foreign body remaining in the ear until medical attention is obtained.
d. Splinters. Only those splinters that can be grasped firmly by a protruding end and can be gently withdrawn should be attacked by laymen. Soft splinters or broken-off splinters should be treated by physicians. If a piece of a foreign body is allowed to remain in the skin, it will usually become infected. If medical care is not available, warm soaks for a period of a few days will often bring a splinter to a position where it can be withdrawn with a pair of tweezers.
e. Stab wounds (knives, shrapnel, or other weapons). Protruding objects of this type should usually be left in place until medical care can

be obtained. Removal by nonphysicians may result in severe hemorrhage. The best first aid is to place a sterile dressing over the area and transport the patient to the nearest hospital.

### What should be done about pieces of clothing or dirt that have gotten into an abrasion or laceration?

Thorough washing with soap and water will usually dislodge such foreign bodies. This should be done as soon as possible after the injury. The injured area should then be covered with a clean dressing, and medical attention should be obtained.

## FRACTURES, DISLOCATIONS, SPRAINS

### What is the first-aid treatment for fractures?

a. Keep the patient quiet and do not move the injured part until the extent of the injury has been determined.
b. Immobilize or splint the damaged extremity before moving the patient.
c. Always move the patient to a hospital in a lying-down position. Never sit the patient up or bend or move the injured part any more than is absolutely necessary.

### What should one do if a splint is not available?

There is always a piece of wood or a stick or some straight, firm object that can be used as an improvised splint. Furthermore, a fractured arm can be splinted against the body, and a fractured leg can be splinted against the other leg.

### Should the splint be padded before being placed alongside a fractured extremity?

Yes. A piece of clothing placed between the injured extremity and the splint will prevent injury from undue pressure.

### How should a splint be kept in place?

By tying handkerchiefs at various places along the splint or by tearing up a shirt and using it as a bandage.

### Before applying a splint, what should be done with the fractured limb?

Try to place it in as straight a position as possible. Do it gently so as not to hurt the patient.

### What are the best positions in which to splint an arm?

In a straight position; or the arm can be strapped to the side of the body. In this way, the body itself acts as a splint.

### What is the best way to splint a leg?

The opposite leg can be used as a splint so that the injured leg can be straightened and attached to the other leg. This will form an excellent splint in most instances.

### Are special first-aid measures needed in the treatment of compound fractures?

a. Yes, the wound must be covered with a clean dressing or, if none is available, a clean handkerchief.
b. If there is severe hemorrhage from a compound fracture, it may be necessary to apply a tourniquet temporarily. If bleeding can be controlled by direct pressure over the wound, a tourniquet should not be applied.
c. The limb should be splinted, but no attempt should be made to alter the position of the broken fragments.

### How long can a tourniquet be safely left in place?

A tourniquet should be released every twenty minutes for a few minutes to restore circulation. During this time, pressure with one's fingers should be applied over the bleeding artery.

### What special first-aid treatment is necessary for a fractured skull?

a. The patient should be placed on his back with his head flat.
b. The patient should be kept still and not allowed to move about.
c. The patient should be kept warm and transported to the hospital as soon as possible.

### Should whiskey or pain-killing drugs be given to a patient with a possible fractured skull?

No. This may do definite harm.

### Should fractures of the bones of the face be treated as potential fractured skulls?

Yes. A fractured bone in the face is often accompanied by a fractured skull.

### What is the best first-aid treatment for a fractured jaw?

a. Close the mouth so that the teeth come together as closely as possible.
b. Tie a handkerchief so that it circles the head from under the chin to the top of the head.
c. Allow the patient to remain in a sitting-up position.

### What is the best first-aid treatment for a fractured shoulder or a fractured collarbone?

Place the hand on the chest in a comfortable position and tie a shirt or necktie around the entire body, keeping the arm and hand close to the chest wall. This will act as a splint and prevent motion in the fractured area.

### Is it safe to immobilize a fractured limb in the position that is most comfortable for the patient?

Yes. This is safer than forcibly attempting to straighten out an extremity.

**Should people with severe injuries to a lower extremity be permitted to walk or bear weight on the extremity?**

No. When in doubt as to whether a fracture exists, do not put weight on the extremity.

**How can one distinguish between a severe sprain and a fracture?**

It is not always possible to make this distinction. It is wisest, therefore, to treat all severe injuries as if they were fractures.

**What is the first-aid treatment for a dislocation?**

Nonphysicians should not try to correct dislocations but should immobilize the affected part and take the patient to a hospital as soon as possible.

**Is it safe to pull or stretch a dislocated shoulder or finger?**

This should be done only if medical attention is unavailable.

**What special first-aid treatment is indicated for neck injuries?**

If there is a severe neck injury, the patient should be transported, flat on his back, on a board, to the hospital. It is important to avoid twisting the body or bending the neck.

**Is it necessary to keep the head rigid and not allow flexing of the neck if there is an injury in this area?**

Yes. This is absolutely essential in order to prevent movements of the vertebrae. Movement may press upon the nerves in the spinal cord and cause paralysis.

**What is the best way to avoid neck movement?**

Someone should hold the head rigid by placing the palms of his hands firmly against the sides of the injured person's face and head.

**What special first aid is required for a possible fracture of the back?**

People with back injuries should be transported to a hospital lying flat, face downward. A board should be obtained, or a blanket can be used as a stretcher.

**Is it safer to keep a patient at the scene of an accident until medical attention arrives, or should immediate transportation to a hospital be attempted in the case of a severe fracture?**

If possible, wait for medical help before moving the patient, as serious damage can result from improper methods of transportation.

## GAS POISONING

**What is the first-aid treatment for gas poisoning?**

a. Shut off the gas and open the windows.
b. Get the patient out into the open where he can breathe fresh air.
c. Mouth-to-mouth breathing should be applied if the victim is not breathing on his own.
d. Loosen any tight collars or tight clothing.
e. Call for an emergency squad so that pure oxygen can be administered.

**For how long a period should artificial respiration be continued if the victim is not breathing?**

For as long as there is the slightest evidence of a pulse or heartbeat. Feel for the pulse in the neck.

**Do people who recover from gas poisoning require careful observation?**

Yes. There may be serious mental disturbance as a consequence of the effect of the gas poisoning upon the brain cells.

## HEAT STROKE AND HEAT EXHAUSTION

**What is heat stroke?**

It is sunstroke, caused by overexposure to sun and extremely high temperatures.

**Who is most likely to be affected by heat stroke?**

Older people and those who are not in good health; men seem to be more readily affected than women.

**What are the characteristic symptoms and results of heat stroke?**

The patient runs an extremely high fever, which may cause extensive damage to important structures such as the brain, the liver, or the kidneys.

**What is the first-aid treatment for heat stroke?**

a. Place the patient in a tub of cold water, preferably containing ice. This will reduce the body temperature.
b. Wrap the patient in cold, wet sheets or towels.
c. Give an enema containing iced water.
d. Summon the doctor as quickly as possible. People whose temperatures remain much above 106° F. for prolonged periods usually do not recover.

**What is heat exhaustion?**

This is a condition caused by excessive exposure to heat, not necessarily in the sun, in which the patient perspires, becomes weak, and may faint or lose consciousness. Heat exhaustion is more common in women than in men.

**What is the first-aid treatment for heat exhaustion?**

a. People suffering from heat exhaustion should be cooled quickly by being placed into a tub of cold water.
b. Salt tablets should be given. Ten

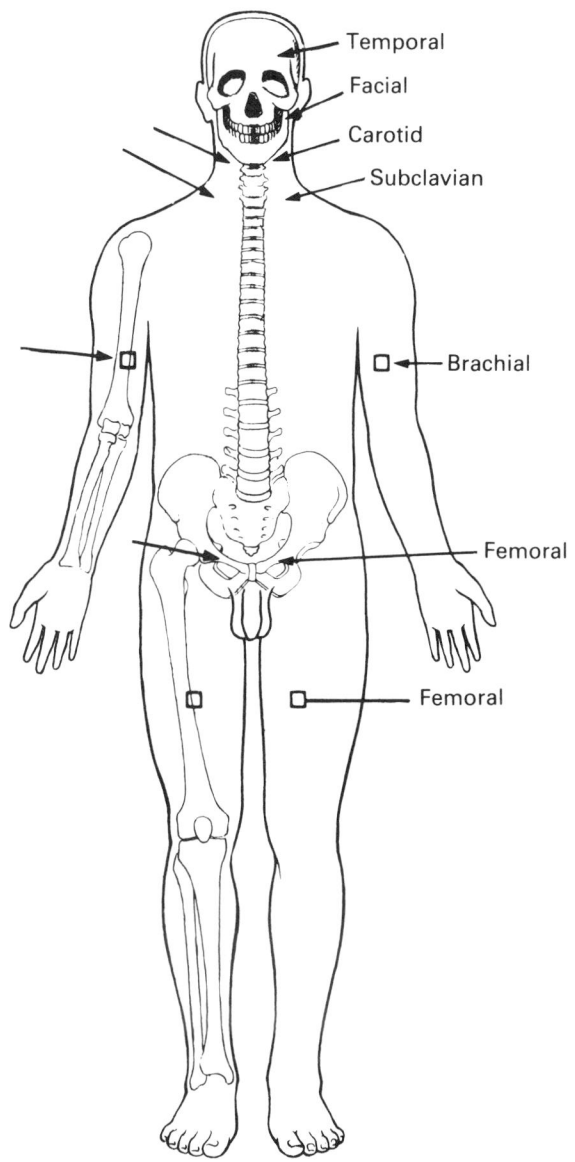

Temporal
Facial
Carotid
Subclavian
Brachial
Femoral
Femoral

Rectangles = *Points of application of tourniquets*

Arrows = *Digital pressure points*

***Pressure Points to Stop Bleeding from Major Arteries.*** *These pressure points can be located by noting the pulsations of the arteries at various spots throughout the body.*

grains three times a day is sufficient. (Heat exhaustion is always accompanied by free perspiration and loss of body salt.)

c. The patient should be kept in bed and allowed to rest until body fluids and salt have had time to be absorbed.

## HEMORRHAGE

### What is the best first-aid treatment for hemorrhage?

This will depend on the type of hemorrhage. If there is severe internal bleeding, such as may occur from an ulcer or tumor within the intestinal tract or hemorrhage secondary to the coughing up of large quantities of blood, the patient should be placed in a lying-down position and transported as quickly as possible to a hospital.

### Are there any medications that should be given to a patient to stop bleeding from the intestinal tract or from the lungs?

This does not constitute first-aid treatment. Such people should receive expert medical care, and it is perhaps best not to attempt to treat them before such care can be obtained.

### What is the best treatment for external hemorrhage?

a. Place pressure directly on the wound! This can be accomplished by placing a sterile gauze dressing or a clean handkerchief on the bleeding points and pressing firmly with the flat of one's hand or with one's fingers.

b. If the bleeding is secondary to a very severe laceration in the arm or in the leg, a tourniquet may be required. This should be applied only as a last resort if the bleeding cannot be controlled by direct pressure. The tourniquet is placed just above the site of the injury. It should be remembered that tourniquets must be loosened every ten minutes to allow the circulation to return.

### How near to a wound should a tourniquet be applied if it is needed?

As close as possible and just tight enough to stop the bleeding. If a tourniquet is applied too loosely, it will increase the amount of bleeding. If applied too tightly, it may unnecessarily damage tissues.

### Does bleeding always start again after a tourniquet has been loosened for a few minutes?

No. It is often found that when a tourniquet has been in place for some minutes, it can be removed permanently without resumption of hemorrhage.

### Should a tight pressure dressing or tourniquet be applied in the region of the neck?

No. The best way to stop bleeding from the neck is to constrict the bleeding vessel with one's fingers.

### Do people often bleed to death from external wounds?

No. Hemorrhages from the scalp, the face, or from one of the extremities usually look much worse than they are. It is rare for someone to bleed to death from the ordinary scalp or extremity wound, and most of these lacerations will stop bleeding by themselves within a few minutes.

### In what position should people who have hemorrhaged be transported?

Usually lying flat or with the feet elevated. This will tend to combat shock by causing blood to gravitate toward the head.

### Should alcohol or coffee be given to people who have had a severe hemorrhage?

It is perhaps best not to give any stimulants to those who have hemorrhaged. All efforts should be concentrated on getting the patient to the hospital.

## LACERATIONS, ABRASIONS, AND CONTUSIONS

### What is the first-aid treatment for lacerations, abrasions, and contusions?

a. Thorough cleansing of the wound with soap and water for five to ten minutes.

b. Direct pressure with a clean dressing to stop bleeding.
c. The application of a clean dressing and transportation of the patient to the nearest hospital or physician.

### Should antiseptics such as alcohol, iodine, etc., be poured over abrasions, contusions, or lacerations?

No. It has been found that these substances do more harm than good. The best insurance against infection is a thorough cleansing for a period of five to ten minutes with ordinary soap and tap water.

### Will the application of ice to a bruise or contusion tend to lessen the amount of hemorrhage into the tissues?

Yes, but it should be remembered that damage can result if the ice is applied for too long a period of time. Ice should be applied for no longer than twenty minutes at one time and then discontinued for a similar period.

## POISONS

### What are the best first-aid treatments for swallowed poison?

a. Call the Poison Control Center in your area. The number is in the front of the telephone book. Give them all the details, including the name of the poison or drug, if known, and the quantity you believe has been swallowed. The Control Center will instruct you on how to obtain medical help quickly. If you can't locate the Poison Control Center, call 911 or dial 0.
b. If the swallowed poison is an overdose of a medication or drug, vomiting should be induced.
c. If the swallowed poison is a petroleum product such as gasoline, kerosene, or oil, or if it is a

strong acid or alkali, vomiting should *not* be induced.
d. If vomiting is not being induced, the poison should be diluted by giving the victim a glass of water or milk. Repeat this, but if nausea ensues, discontinue the process.
e. If the victim vomits, save the vomit for subsequent analysis.
f. If respirations cease or are shallow and irregular, give the victim mouth-to-mouth artificial respiration.
g. If the heart stops, give the victim CPR (cardiopulmonary resuscitation).

### Why is it bad practice to cause vomiting when someone has swallowed a petroleum product or a strong acid or alkali?

a. When one vomits a petroleum product, some of it may get down into the lungs and cause pneumonia.
b. When one vomits a strong acid or alkali, the substance may result in further burning of the esophagus (foodpipe) and mouth.

### What are the best ways to cause vomiting?

a. Tickle the back of the throat with your finger.
b. Give the victim a glass or two of warm water containing salt, soap, or mustard.
c. If you have syrup of ipecac on hand, give the victim a tablespoonful.

### If vomiting is indicated, is it advisable to cause more than one episode?

Yes. The stomach may not completely empty itself the first time one throws up.

### After the stomach has been emptied, what should be given to drink?

Tea, milk, or the whites of several eggs. These will act as antidotes to many poisons.

**Should activated charcoal be given to one who has swallowed a poison?**

Yes. This is a good substance to have on hand in the household as it tends to bind (deactivate) the poison.

**How can one tell whether a strong acid or alkali has been swallowed?**

In many cases there will be obvious burns around the lips or in the mouth.

**How can one tell whether a petroleum product has been swallowed?**

Often one will be able to smell gasoline, kerosene, or oil on the victim's breath.

**What poisons are most apt to interfere with breathing?**

One of the most common causes of depressed breathing is an overdose of barbiturates or other sleeping pills. Also, morphine and heroin cause deep depression of respirations when taken in large doses.

## RADIATION EXPOSURE

**What are the chances of being overexposed to nuclear radiation?**

Although one or two accidents have threatened people living in the vicinity of nuclear plants, governmental authorities are moving toward minimizing possibilities of the release of radioactive substances. To date, there are no proven cases of harmful effects to people living near nuclear plants.

**What would be the first-aid treatment should radiation exposure actually take place?**

a. People threatened with radiation exposure should evacuate the area in a quick, orderly manner. Local authorities will give specific instructions on how best to do it.
b. People already exposed should remove and discard all clothing that was worn at the time of the exposure and should wash their bodies thoroughly for a prolonged period of time in a shower.
c. Medical advice should be sought promptly. Evacuation and admission to a hospital out of the area of radiation may be advised.

## SHOCK

**What are the symptoms of shock due to injury?**

a. There may or may not be loss of consciousness.
b. The skin becomes a dull gray color and is cold and clammy to the touch.
c. The patient's body is covered with a fine perspiration.
d. The pulse is weak and rapid.
e. The pupils of the eyes are dilated.
f. Respirations are rapid and shallow.
g. The patient is apprehensive and complains of weakness and excessive thirst.

**What is the first-aid treatment for shock?**

a. Place the patient on his back with his feet higher than his head.
b. If there is any active bleeding contributing toward the shock, it should be stopped. (See the section on Hemorrhage in this chapter.)
c. The patient should be kept warm. Supply him with adequate blankets or other covering.
d. If there is severe pain that can be relieved by the first-aider, this should be done immediately. Pain is one of the strongest contributors toward the development of shock. If a fracture is present, it should be splinted.
e. If it can be determined that there is no injury or wound to the abdo-
men, the patient may be given warm fluids to drink.
f. The patient should be transported to a hospital as soon as possible.

**Should tea or coffee be given to people who are in shock?**

No. In the time it takes to obtain tea or coffee, the patient should really have had provisions made for transportation to a hospital where specific treatment can be instituted.

**Should alcohol be given as a stimulant to patients who are in shock?**

No. This will only serve ultimately to increase the state of shock.

## SUFFOCATION OR STRANGULATION
*(See also the section on Choking in this chapter)*

**What is the best first-aid treatment for suffocation or strangulation?**

a. The patient should be placed in the open air.
b. If there is anything about the neck that might obstruct breathing, it should be loosened immediately.
c. Elevate the chin; this will give the patient a better airway.
d. If strangulation is due to a foreign body that has lodged in the windpipe, grasp the victim around the waist from behind with both hands and tighten your grip with a sudden, forceful inward and upward thrust. This will usually cause him to cough up the foreign body.

## CPR *(Cardiopulmonary Resuscitation)*

**What is CPR?**

CPR is an abbreviation for cardiopulmonary resuscitation, a series of maneuvers to bring back to life a person whose heart has stopped beating. It is a combination of closed cardiac massage and mouth-to-mouth artificial respiration.

**What is cardiac arrest?**

Heart stoppage.

**Can a patient ever be saved once the heart has stopped beating?**

Yes. Although the majority of people whose heart has stopped beating do die, it is possible to save a considerable number of them if prompt CPR is instituted.

**How soon after cardiac arrest must CPR be started?**

It must be begun *immediately.* Unless CPR is instituted within a few minutes, the patient will succumb.

**How can a first-aider know that CPR should be carried out?**

a. He notes an unconscious patient.
b. He feels for a pulse in the neck and does not find it.
c. He listens with his ear over the heart and hears no beat.
d. He looks for respirations and finds none.

**Is CPR indicated when there is a heartbeat but no obvious breathing?**

No. In such cases only mouth-to-mouth artificial respiration is indicated.

**Does the heart ever stop beating and respirations continue?**

No. Once the heart stops, breathing stops.

**Can anyone carry out CPR?**

Yes, but it is much better if a trained person does it. Civilians are being trained all over the country in the techniques of this lifesaving procedure.

**What is closed cardiac massage?**

The pumping of blood throughout the body by intermittent thrusts upon the breastbone (sternum) overlying the heart. By pushing down every second against the breastbone, it is possible to expel blood from the heart so that it will circulate throughout the body. Closed cardiac massage is an essential part of CPR.

**How hard should one press against the breastbone in performing CPR?**

Sufficiently enough to depress the breastbone about one to two inches.

**What steps should be carried out after it has been definitely determined that cardiac arrest exists?**

a. The first-aider kneels alongside the head of the victim.
b. The left hand is placed under the victim's neck, thus raising his chin and opening the air passage.
c. The right hand pinches off the victim's nostrils.
d. The first-aider then places his mouth firmly against the victim's mouth and artificial respiration is begun. The first-aider blows hard into the victim's mouth twice.
e. The first-aider then locates the lowest extent of the sternum (the xiphoid process), measures up about one-and-a-half inches, places the heel of one hand on the breastbone and his other hand over it, and begins the intermittent thrusts in a downward direction. The thrusts are continued for fifteen strokes, after which the first-aider again pinches off the nostrils and blows hard once into the victim's mouth.
f. Cardiac massage is resumed for fifteen more strokes and then mouth-to-mouth respiration is given again.
g. These maneuvers are continued indefinitely until the first-aider notes the resumption of a heartbeat and spontaneous respirations.

**Is CPR best carried out with two first-aiders?**

Definitely, yes! One will concentrate on the cardiac massage; the other on mouth-to-mouth artificial respiration. The cardiac massage should consist of a downward thrust upon the breastbone every second. The person giving artificial respiration should employ it after every five thrusts of the person performing the cardiac massage.

**Should the two first-aiders change places when doing CPR?**

Yes. Usually the person performing the cardiac massage tires first. He should then exchange duties with the one performing the mouth-to-mouth breathing.

**How long should CPR be continued?**

At least a half hour. By this time, some kind of heartbeat should be restored if the first aid is going to be successful.

**Should CPR be continued indefinitely if the slightest evidence of an occasional heartbeat is noted?**

Yes. Occasional heartbeats often signify that a rhythmic beat can be restored.

**Does regular breathing come back before a heart beat is restored?**

No. Heart actions come before resumption of breathing.

**How long does it take to learn CPR?**

The average intelligent individual can learn the technique in several hours of instruction.

**Where can one get instruction in CPR?**

Call your local Red Cross.

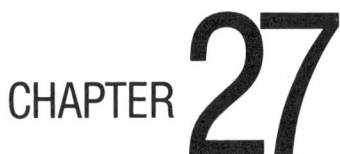

# CHAPTER 27

# GALL BLADDER AND BILE DUCTS

*(See also Chapter 40 on Liver; Chapter 70 on Stomach and Duodenum)*

**Where is the gall bladder and what is its function?**

The gall bladder is a pear-shaped sac attached to the underside of the liver beneath the ribs in the upper right part of the abdomen. Its function is to receive bile produced and secreted by the liver and to store and concentrate it for use when needed in the processes of digestion.

**For what types of food is bile particularly necessary for digestion?**

Bile is essential for the digestion of fats and fat-like substances.

**How does bile reach the intestinal tract?**

Through a system of ducts or tubes. The cyctic duct leads from the gall bladder into the common bile duct. The common bile duct is the result of the joining of the two hepatic ducts, which originate in the liver. Bile from the liver and the gall bladder travels down the common bile duct and enters into the intestine at the ampulla of Vater in the second portion of the duodenum.

**If the liver produces and secretes bile, what is the special function of the gall bladder?**

To store and concentrate bile so that an additional supply can be secreted

into the intestine when it is needed after the eating of a meal.

**What foods often disagree with the individual who has a gall bladder disorder?**

Any fried and greasy foods, French fried potatoes, heavy sauces, gravies, chicken or turkey skins, eggs fried in lard, turnips, cabbage, cauliflower, sprouts, radishes, certain raw fruits, etc.

**Are disorders of the gall bladder and bile ducts very common?**

It is generally agreed that disease of the gall bladder and malfunction of the sphincter at the end of the common duct constitute the most common causes of indigestion.

**Is it necessary to operate upon the gall bladder very often?**

Surgery for removal of a diseased gall bladder is the most frequently performed abdominal operation in people past middle life and is one of the most common indications for surgery in all age groups.

**What causes gall bladder disease?**

a. Infection with bacteria. This may result in an acute or chronic inflammation in the same manner that infection involves the appendix, tonsils, or any other organ.

b. A functional disturbance in which the gall bladder fails to empty when it is called upon to secrete bile.

c. A chemical disturbance causing stones to precipitate out from the bile. These stones may create an obstruction to the passage of bile along the ducts and into the intestinal tract.

**Are gallstones always caused by an upset in chemistry within the gall bladder?**

No. Gallstones may result from a chemical disturbance, or they may form as a result of infection within the gall bladder.

**How prevalent are gallstones?**

It is estimated that approximately one out of four women and one out of eight men will develop gallstones at some time before reaching sixty years of age.

**Is there a special type of person who is most likely to develop gall bladder disease?**

Yes. It is thought that the heavyset type of person who eats a large amount of fats and greases is most likely to develop gall bladder disease. However, the condition is seen in all ages and in all types of people.

**At what age does gall bladder disease usually develop?**

In the thirties and forties, although it is occasionally seen in younger people.

**Does childbearing predispose one to the formation of gallstones?**

Yes. Pregnancy often produces a disturbance in fat and cholesterol metabolism. This is often followed by stone formation within a few months after the pregnancy has terminated.

**Does gall bladder disease often take place *during* pregnancy?**

Not very frequently. (It is seen most commonly in women who have had one or two children.)

**Does gall bladder disease tend to run in families or to be inherited?**

Only insofar as there is a tendency to inherit the type of body configuration, the type of chemical metabolism, and the type of eating habits that one's parents maintain.

**What takes place when the gall bladder becomes acutely inflamed?**

The blood supply to the wall of the gall bladder may be interfered with, and the gall bladder may become filled with pus, or its walls may undergo gangrenous changes as the result of inadequate circulation.

**What causes most acute inflammations of the gall bladder?**

A stone blocking the cystic duct, the outlet from the gall bladder.

**What takes place when there is a chronic inflammation of the gall bladder?**

Stones, resulting either from previous inflammation and infection or from an upset in chemistry within the gall bladder, will be associated with a thickening and chronic inflammation of the gall bladder wall. This will lead to poor filling and emptying or even to nonfunctioning of the gall bladder.

**What takes place when there is a functional disorder of the gall bladder or bile ducts?**

This condition is characterized by failure of the gall bladder to empty and secrete bile when it is called upon to do so. Or there may be spasm at the outlet of the common bile duct, which interferes with the free passage of bile into the intestinal tract. The patient has indigestion, heartburn, and an inability to digest fatty foods, greases, and certain raw fruits and vegetables.

**Are functional disorders of the gall bladder usually accompanied by the formation of gallstones?**

Not necessarily.

**Is there any way to prevent gall bladder disease or the symptoms of a poorly functioning gall bladder?**

Moderation in one's diet—with the eating of small quantities of fats, fried foods, and greases—will cut down on the demands made upon the gall bladder and may lessen the chances of symptoms due to inadequate function.

**How can one tell if he has gall bladder disease?**

a. Acute gall bladder disease (acute cholecystitis) is accompanied by an elevation in temperature, nausea, and vomiting, along with pain and tenderness in the upper right portion of the abdomen beneath the ribs. An x ray or sonogram (see Chapter 67, on Sonography) of the gall bladder may reveal a nonfunctioning organ or may demonstrate the presence of stones. A blood count may show the presence of an acute inflammation.

b. Chronic gall bladder disease (chronic cholecystitis) when accompanied by stones may cause excruciating attacks of colicky pain in the upper right portion of the abdomen. This is usually due to a stone being stuck in the cystic duct or bile duct. The pain often radiates to the right shoulder or through to the back. There is nausea, vomiting, and tenderness in the abdomen, which may cease abruptly within a half hour or so if the stone drops back into the gall bladder or passes through the obstructed duct. X-ray studies in chronic gall bladder disease usually show a nonfunctioning gall bladder and sometimes demonstrate the presence of gallstones.

c. Functional disturbances of the gall bladder evidence themselves by chronic indigestion, inability to digest fats, greases, and certain raw fruits and vegetables, and heartburn. X-ray studies in these cases may show poor filling and poor emptying of the gall bladder.

**Are there tests that can make a diagnosis of gall bladder disease?**

Yes. An x-ray test known as a cholecystogram. This is done by giving the patient a specific dye in the form of pills. Some hours later, x rays of the gall bladder are taken, and if the organ is normal, the dye will fill it up and outline its contours smoothly. The x ray will also show emptying after the ingestion of a fatty meal. Sometimes, instead of giving the dye by mouth, it is injected into the veins prior to taking the x ray. Failure of the gall bladder to show upon x ray usually indicates the presence of disease. In other instances, stones are seen as negative shadows on the cholecystogram x rays.

A sonogram is also a good test to show presence or absence of gall bladder disease. This test is carried out by recording ultrasound waves that echo over the region of the gall bladder. Irregularities in the recording of the waves may demonstrate the presence of gallstones.

**What is the significance of a gall bladder not showing on gall bladder x-ray film?**

Almost invariably this shows that the gall bladder is not functioning. Often, if the gall bladder fails to visualize with the dye, a second and larger dose of dye is given. Should the gall bladder not show with a double dose of dye, it is clearcut evidence that the gall bladder is diseased or, in rare instances, that advanced liver disease is present.

**Do gallstones always show on x-ray examination?**

No. In some cases there may be many stones present, and still they will not show on x ray.

**Can x rays show stones in the bile ducts?**

Yes. A new diagnostic process called intravenous cholangiography will demonstrate stones in the bile ducts. This is performed by injecting the dye directly into a vein of the patient's arm and taking x rays immediately thereafter.

**Is this type of test dangerous?**

No, except in the very rare case where an allergy to the dye exists.

**How does a physician decide whether to advise medical or surgical treatment for gall bladder disease?**

The functional disorders of the gall bladder, when not accompanied by

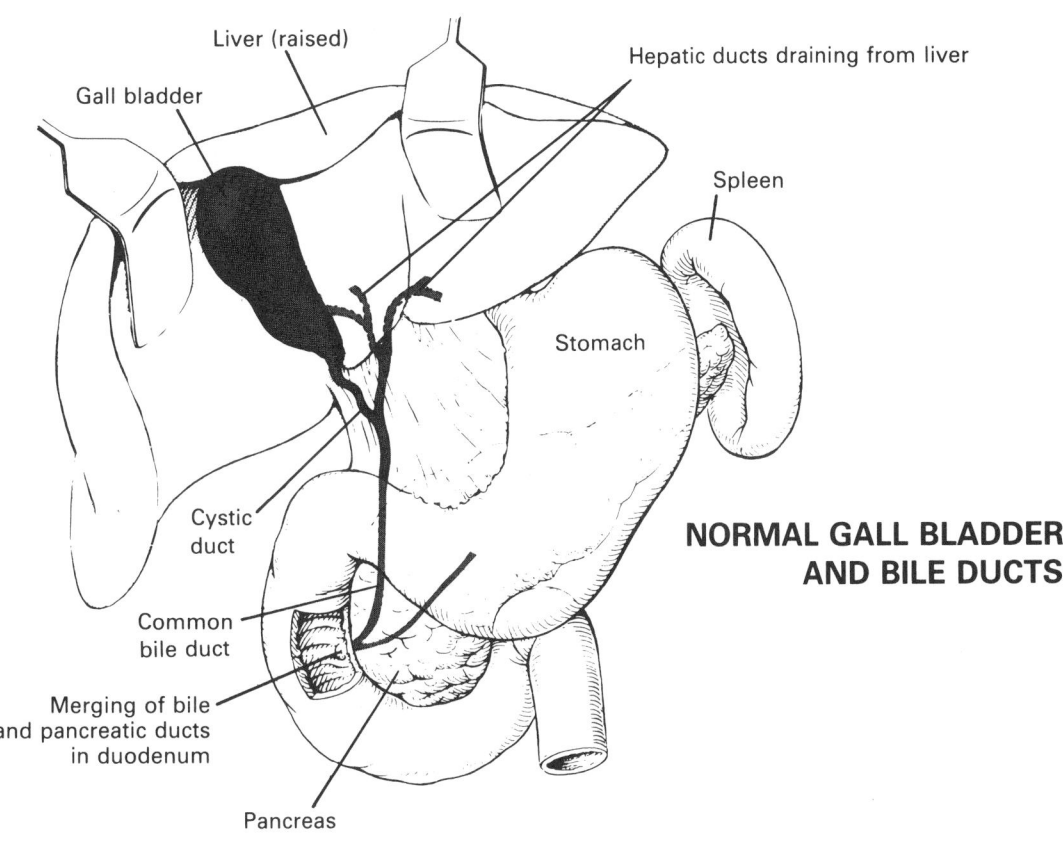

Liver (raised)

Gall bladder

Hepatic ducts draining from liver

Spleen

Stomach

Cystic duct

Common bile duct

Merging of bile and pancreatic ducts in duodenum

Pancreas

**NORMAL GALL BLADDER AND BILE DUCTS**

**GALL BLADDER CONTAINING STONES**

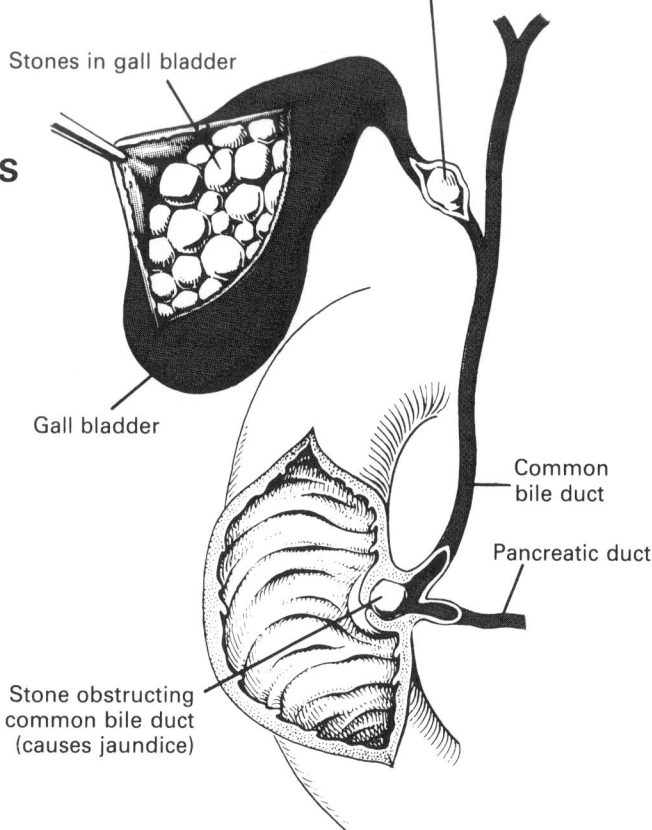

Stones in gall bladder

Stone in cystic duct

Gall bladder

Common bile duct

Pancreatic duct

Stone obstructing common bile duct (causes jaundice)

*The Gall Bladder and Bile Ducts.* *The top diagram shows the anatomical relations of a normal gall bladder and bile ducts. It is seen that the bile ducts and gall bladder are connected to the liver and to the intestinal tract. The lower diagram shows a gall bladder containing stones, a stone jammed in the cystic duct, and one in the common bile duct leading into the intestine. When a stone obstructs the common bile duct, jaundice ensues. People with gallstones should have them removed surgically since they never dissolve by themselves.*

stone formation, are best treated medically. All other disturbances of the gall bladder are best treated surgically.

## Is the medical management for functional disorders of the gall bladder very helpful?

Yes, when the patient cooperates by adhering closely to a sensible diet and when medications are taken as advised.

## Does a patient with gallstones always have to be operated upon?

Not in all instances. There are many people who have stones in their gall bladder that produce no symptoms. However, if gallstones cause any symptoms whatever, it is safer to operate than not to operate.

## When is a gall bladder operation mandatory?

a. When the organ is acutely inflamed.
b. When the patient is suffering from repeated attacks of severe colicky pain due to the presence of stones.
c. When the gall bladder is known to have stones and the patient is suffering from chronic indigestion, nausea, flatulence, and occasional pains in the abdomen.
d. When jaundice (yellow discoloration of the skin) occurs as a result of a stone obstructing the bile ducts.

## What is the medical management for gall bladder disease?

a. The avoidance of those foods that produce indigestion, such as fats, greases, sauces, stuffings, and certain raw vegetables and raw fruits.
b. The eating of a bland, well-rounded diet, with no large meals.
c. The use of certain medications to relieve spasm of the bile ducts and to reduce excess acidity in the stomach.

## Does surgery always relieve the symptoms caused by a functional disorder when the gall bladder is known to be free of stones?

Although a certain percentage of these patients are benefited by gall bladder removal (cholecystectomy), others are not.

## What can happen if an operation upon the gall bladder is not performed when indicated?

a. An acute inflammation of the gall bladder may progress to gangrene, with rupture of the organ. This may lead to peritonitis and possible death.
b. Recurring attacks of colic due to an obstructing gallstone may lead to the stone being passed into the common bile duct, where it will obstruct the passage of bile and cause jaundice.
c. If jaundice takes place because of an obstructing stone and surgery is not performed, the patient may die from liver damage and the toxic effects of prolonged bile obstruction.

## Is jaundice always produced by gallstones?

No. There are many other causes for jaundice. The most common is hepatitis, an inflammation of the liver.

## How can one tell whether jaundice is caused by an obstructing gallstone or some other cause?

There are many tests that help make a conclusive diagnosis as to whether the jaundice is obstructive or is inflammatory in nature. A thorough history and physical examination, x-ray examinations, and several blood chemical tests will usually reveal the correct diagnosis.

## Do stones predispose toward the formation of cancer in the gall bladder?

Yes. Approximately 1 to 2 percent of those who have stones in the gall bladder will eventually develop a cancer. This is an important reason for advocating surgery upon gall bladders containing stones, regardless of the presence or absence of symptoms.

## Is removal of the gall bladder (cholecystectomy) a dangerous operative procedure?

No. It is no more dangerous than the removal of an appendix.

## Can gallstones be dissolved with medications?

Recently, the administration of concentrated bile salts over a period of many months has resulted in dissolving some gallstones. However, this method of treatment is still in the experimental stage and is not a substitute for surgical removal of the stones.

## When operating upon the gall bladder, does the surgeon remove the entire organ or just the stones?

In almost all cases, the gall bladder is removed. However, there are occasional cases where the organ is so acutely inflamed and the patient so sick that the surgeon may decide merely to remove the stones and place a drain into the gall bladder. This procedure takes less time to perform and carries with it less risk.

## Are the bile ducts removed when operating upon the gall bladder?

No. There must be a free passage of bile from the liver into the intestines. The bile ducts are therefore left in place.

## How does the surgeon remove stones from the bile duct?

He makes a small incision into the duct, picks out the stone or stones with a specially designed instrument, and then drains the duct with a rubber tube (T tube). This tube is removed anywhere from a few days to a few weeks later, depending upon the subsequent tests and x-ray findings.

**How long does it take to perform a cholecystectomy?**

From three-quarters of an hour to one and a half hours, depending upon the severity of the inflammatory process.

**What type of anesthesia is used for gall bladder operations?**

A general inhalation anesthesia.

**Is it common practice to remove the appendix while operating primarily for a gall bladder condition?**

This used to be done quite often, but since appendicitis has become so rare, the practice has been discontinued by most surgeons.

**What special preparations are necessary prior to gall bladder surgery?**

Usually none for the patient being operated upon for a simple chronic inflammatory condition without jaundice. However, patients who have acute inflammation or who are suffering from jaundice require considerable special preoperative preparation.

**What are the special preoperative measures used in these cases?**

a. The passage of a tube through the nose to make sure the stomach is empty at the time of surgery.
b. The giving of intravenous medications before operation in the form of fluids, glucose, and certain vitamins, particularly Vitamin K in the presence of jaundice to protect against possible postoperative hemorrhage.
c. The giving of antibiotics to the patient who has an acutely inflamed gall bladder or an inflammation of the bile ducts.

**Are blood transfusions given in gall bladder operations?**

Not usually; only in the most seriously sick and complicated cases.

**Are private nurses necessary after gall bladder operations?**

If the patient can afford it, a private nurse for two or three days will add greatly to his comfort.

**How long a hospital stay is required?**

Approximately nine days.

**How soon after surgery can the patient get out of bed?**

For the ordinary case, on the first or second postoperative day.

**Where are the incisions made for gall bladder disease?**

Either a longitudinal incision in the upper right portion of the abdomen or an oblique incision beneath the rib cage on the right side is carried out for a distance of five to seven inches.

**Are drains usually placed in gall bladder wounds?**

Yes. One or two rubber drains will be inserted following surgery. These will stay in place anywhere from six to ten days.

**Are gall bladder operations especially painful?**

No. There may be some pain on deep breathing or coughing for a few days after surgery, but the operative wound is not exceptionally painful.

**What special postoperative measures are carried out?**

a. In the ordinary operation for a chronically inflamed gall bladder with stones, there are few special postoperative orders. The patient may eat the day after surgery, but fats, greases, raw fruits and vegetables should not be included. Antibiotics may be given if there is fear of infection. A stomach tube is passed through the nose and kept in place for the first day in order to avoid discomfort from distention.
b. The patient operated upon for an acute gall bladder inflammation or

for jaundice will probably receive intravenous solutions, drainage of the stomach through a tube inserted through the nose, medications with Vitamin K to counteract jaundice, and large doses of antibiotics for a few days. Occasionally, blood transfusions are also given.

**How long does it take the average gall bladder wound to heal?**

Anywhere from twelve to fourteen days.

**Can a patient live a normal life after removal of the gall bladder?**

Yes.

**What takes over the function of the gall bladder after it has been removed?**

Bile continues to flow from the liver directly into the intestinal tract. The bile ducts take over many of the duties of the gall bladder.

**Is it common for indigestion to persist for several weeks after removal of the gall bladder?**

Yes.

**Should a woman whose gall bladder has been removed allow herself to become pregnant again?**

Yes, if she so desires.

**Is it necessary to follow dietary precautions after gall bladder removal?**

Yes. The patient should stay on the same kind of diet he followed before surgery, that is, a bland, low-fat diet.

**How soon after the removal of a stone from the common bile duct will jaundice disappear?**

Within several weeks.

**Do symptoms of gall bladder disease ever persist or recur after surgery?**

Yes. Approximately 10 percent of patients who have been operated upon for gall bladder disease will continue to have symptoms after surgery. These symptoms are thought to be caused by spasms of the lower end of the common bile duct (biliary dyskinesia).

**Do patients ever form stones again after they have once been removed?**

If the gall bladder has been removed, they cannot re-form stones in the gall bladder. However, a very small percentage of patients may re-form stones in the common bile duct or in the stump of the cystic duct that has been left behind.

**What treatment is carried out when stones are inadvertently left behind in the common bile duct or when stones re-form in the common bile duct after initial surgery?**

Attempts are made to remove left-behind stones in one of the following ways:

a. A specially designed metal instrument with a basket attached to its end is passed through the channel leading from the skin into the bile duct. When this instrument, as determined by x ray, has gone beyond the stone in the common bile duct, the basket is opened and the instrument is withdrawn. As the instrument is withdrawn, the stone is snared by the basket and comes out of the body with the instrument.

b. By endoscopy. This entails passing a specially designed tube through the mouth and down through the stomach into the duodenum. The opening of the bile duct into the duodenum is then dilated, thus permitting the stones to fall out into the duodenum where they will do no harm.

c. If the above methods fail, reoperation to remove the stones is necessary.

**Can any doctor pass a tube down into the duodenum to retrieve stones from the bile duct?**

No. This is a very specialized procedure carried out by highly trained physicians known as *endoscopists.*

**Is there any way to prevent stones from reforming?**

Not really, except that one should guard against infection and follow a sane, sensible, bland, lowfat diet.

**Does gall bladder removal affect the life span?**

Not at all.

**What are the chances of recovery from a gall bladder operation?**

The mortality rate from gall bladder surgery is less than 1 percent. A fatality occurs mainly in the very complicated case or in people who have neglected to seek treatment early.

**How soon after a gall bladder operation can one do the following:**

Bathe:
   In about eleven to twelve days.
Walk out in the street:
   Two weeks.
Walk up and down stairs:
   Ten to twelve days.
Perform household duties:
   Four weeks.
Drive a car:
   Six weeks.
Resume sexual relations:
   Four to five weeks.
Return to work:
   Five to six weeks.
Resume all physical activities:
   Six weeks.

**How often should one return for a checkup after a gall bladder operation?**

About six months after surgery and then again a year after surgery.

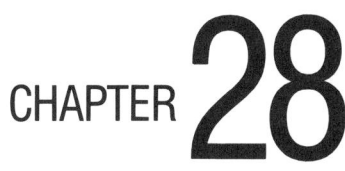

# CHAPTER 28
# THE HAND

*(See also Chapter 10 on Arthritis; Chapter 14 on Bones, Muscles, Tendons, and Joints; Chapter 26 on First Aid in Emergencies; Chapter 62 on Rheumatic Fever)*

## How common are hand injuries and other conditions affecting this vital structure?

Approximately a third of all accident victims suffer from hand-related injuries, and millions of others are afflicted with painful arthritis and inflammatory disorders of the hand. The importance of normal hand function cannot be overstated. Deformities and impairment cause enormous socioeconomic and psychological problems for all peoples and age groups. Due to the magnitude of the problem and the need for expert care, hand surgery has now evolved into a comprehensive medical specialty. The hand, a magnificently designed organ, is extremely complex in structure, function, and repairs. The hand surgeon requires special training in order to afford proper treatment.

## What is the most common hand injury?

The fingertip injury.

## Is this a minor injury?

No. There is no such thing as a minor injury to the hand. Without proper treatment, poor healing, painful scars, swelling, loss of sensation, joint stiffening, and infection may lead to a severe disability of the entire hand.

## What are common problems with fingertip injuries?

a. Loss of the skin and the fingertip pad.

b. Loss of the nail and damage to the nail bed.

c. Fractures of the bone and joint.

All of the above may require surgical treatment. Skin grafting, repair of the nail bed, and reduction and fixation of the fracture are frequently necessary.

## Do amputated fingertips grow back?

No. However, young children have the peculiar ability to heal and remodel tissues in a way that can compensate for small losses.

## Are nerve and tendon injuries common?

Yes, particularly with deep cuts in the wrist, palm, and finger.

## With a nerve injury, is the finger always completely numb?

No. There are two nerves in each finger. If only one is injured, some feeling is still present.

## With a tendon injury, is all finger motion lost?

No. There are two flexor tendons and one extensor tendon in each finger. If only one tendon is cut, some movement will still be present.

## Can nerves be repaired?

Yes. Using microsurgery, the nerves may be accurately repaired. However, under the best circumstances, the nerves may not regenerate, or heal, completely.

## When should a tendon be repaired?

Formerly, flexor tendons cut in the finger were not repaired immediately. Most hand surgeons now feel that better function will result if the tendons are repaired soon after injury.

## What is the major problem following tendon repairs?

Scar tissue that binds the tendon and prevents its movement.

## What is required for successful tendon repair?

Delicate surgery and a cooperative patient pursuing a carefully planned postoperative hand therapy program. By special exercises and splinting, the patient must actively break up the scar tissue to regain good tendon function.

## What is tendon grafting?

A surgical technique in which a "spare" tendon is taken from another part of the body and is used to replace a damaged tendon in the hand.

## What is a "jammed" finger?

This is a nonspecific term that refers to a joint, bone, or tendon injury of the fingers. These are often neglected and lead to permanent and disabling finger deformities. Each injury should be carefully examined with x rays. Examples of the jammed finger are the baseball finger, boutonniere finger, and the skier's thumb.

## What is a "baseball" finger?

A bent fingertip, which results from a tendon rupture. This is also called a "mallet" finger and is usually caused by a direct blow to the fingertip from a baseball, football, volleyball, etc.

## What is a boutonniere, or buttonhole, deformity?

This is a bent finger caused by a tendon rupture. Here the middle finger joint buttonholes through the ruptured tendon.

## How does one treat the mallet and boutonniere deformities?

By splinting for about six weeks.

## Is a dislocated finger a minor injury?

No. The dislocation is often "popped" in by the patient with no further treatment. However, this is frequently followed by prolonged pain, swelling, and stiffness. Each injury requires followup, evaluation with x rays, and, in most cases, the finger is splinted.

### What is a skier's thumb?

This is a torn ligament of the thumb, which can happen to anyone but is particularly common among skiers. A completely torn ligament requires surgical repair.

### What is a fracture?

A fracture, crack, or chip all mean a broken bone. The hand is the most common site for fracture in the entire body.

### What are the common signs of a fracture?

Painful swelling and deformity in the region of the bone.

### What is a "boxer's" fracture?

This is a fracture near the knuckle of the little finger. It usually results from the fist striking a hard object.

### How are fractures treated?

Most should be splinted or placed in a cast for three to four weeks. If the fracture is out of place, the bone fragment must be accurately placed in proper position.

### Do most fractures heal rapidly?

Yes, with one exception: fractures of the scaphoid bone. This is a small bone in the wrist located deep in the anatomical snuffbox on the thumb side of the hand. It is possibly the most difficult bone in the body to heal and usually requires three to four months of casting. Some cases may require surgery.

### Is the anatomical snuffbox area in the wrist a common area for pain?

Yes. Arthritis, fractures, and tendon inflammations frequently cause pain in this area.

### What is de Quervain's disease?

A painful tendon inflammation in the anatomical snuffbox. The tendons that straighten the thumb are caught or squeezed in a narrow tunnel at the side of the wrist.

### What is a "trigger" finger?

Painful clicking or snapping occurs when the finger moves. The flexor tendons are caught or squeezed in a narrow tunnel at the base of the finger.

### Is there effective treatment for de Quervain's disease and trigger finger?

Yes. Local injections may give some relief. Surgical unroofing of the tunnel gives permanent relief. These are simple operations followed by good results.

### What is the most common cause of pins and needles or numbness in the fingers?

The so-called carpal tunnel syndrome.

### What is the carpal tunnel syndrome?

It is a condition in which there is numbness and weakness of the thumb, index, and middle finger along with pain, especially at night. The condition is caused by a pinched nerve in the wrist.

### What causes the pinching of the nerve in the carpal tunnel syndrome?

A tightness of the carpal ligament, which stretches across the front of the wrist. This tightness presses upon the median nerve as it courses through the narrowed tunnel from the wrist to the hand.

### What is the treatment for the carpal tunnel syndrome?

An incision is made on the anterior surface of the wrist, and the carpal ligament is cut. This enlarges the tunnel and takes the pressure off the pinched nerve.

### Are operations to relieve the carpal tunnel syndrome very successful?

Yes.

### What is the most common cause of numbness in the little finger?

A pinched nerve at the elbow.

### Are there other causes for numbness and pain in the hand?

Yes. Neck and shoulder problems, as well as diseases such as diabetes, may cause these symptoms.

### How does one diagnose a pinched nerve?

By examination and special electrodiagnostic tests.

### Is surgery necessary for a pinched nerve?

Yes, if the pain and numbness are progressive or constant and if there is evidence of nerve damage.

### Is nerve surgery safe?

Yes. It is delicate, but with little risk to the patient. In most cases, the severe pain is relieved almost immediately.

### What is Dupuytren's contracture?

Thickening of the tissue beneath the skin of the palm. This tissue is called fascia. The thickened tissue may cause the finger to contract toward the palm.

### Is medication helpful in preventing Dupuytren's contracture?

No. The only treatment of value is surgery.

### Is surgery necessary for all cases?

No. Surgical excision of the fascia is reserved for those cases in which deformities are present.

### Is the hand a common site for tumors?

Yes. However, the vast majority are benign and do not threaten either life or function. Surgery is necessary only if the tumor is painful, enlarging, or interferes with function.

### What is a ganglion?

It is a benign tumor or cyst usually arising on the back of the wrist.

### Where do infections commonly occur in the hand?

At the fingertips and along the tendons. A paronychia is an abscess around the nail, and a felon is an abscess in the pad of the fingertip.

### What is the proper care for infections?

Antibiotics, elevation of the infected part, rest, saltwater soaks, and incision and drainage if an abscess is present. Infections of the hand tend to be underestimated and neglected. Unless properly treated, they may rapidly spread and destroy normal tissues.

### Are human bites serious injuries?

Yes. These often lead to extremely serious infections in the knuckle joints. The most common cause of human bites is a fight in which a fist strikes an opponent's mouth. Hospitalization is generally required for proper care.

### What is the cause of birth deformities of the hand?

In most cases, the cause is unknown; in others, a family history of such deformities can be elicited. (See Chapter 35, on Genetic Medicine.)

### What are the common birth deformities of the hand?

Webbing of the fingers, called syn-dactyly, and extra fingers, called polydactyly. With surgery, the webbed fingers can be separated and the extra fingers removed.

### When should surgery be performed?

Generally anytime after one year of age. It is wise to complete all surgery during the preschool years.

### Can absent fingers be replaced?

There are no normal substitutes for missing fingers. Unrealistic surgery should be avoided. In most cases the child will adapt quite well to an absent finger. However, when a thumb is missing, it is frequently beneficial to fashion a thumb from one of the other fingers. This is a major operative procedure (pollicization), but results are often very rewarding.

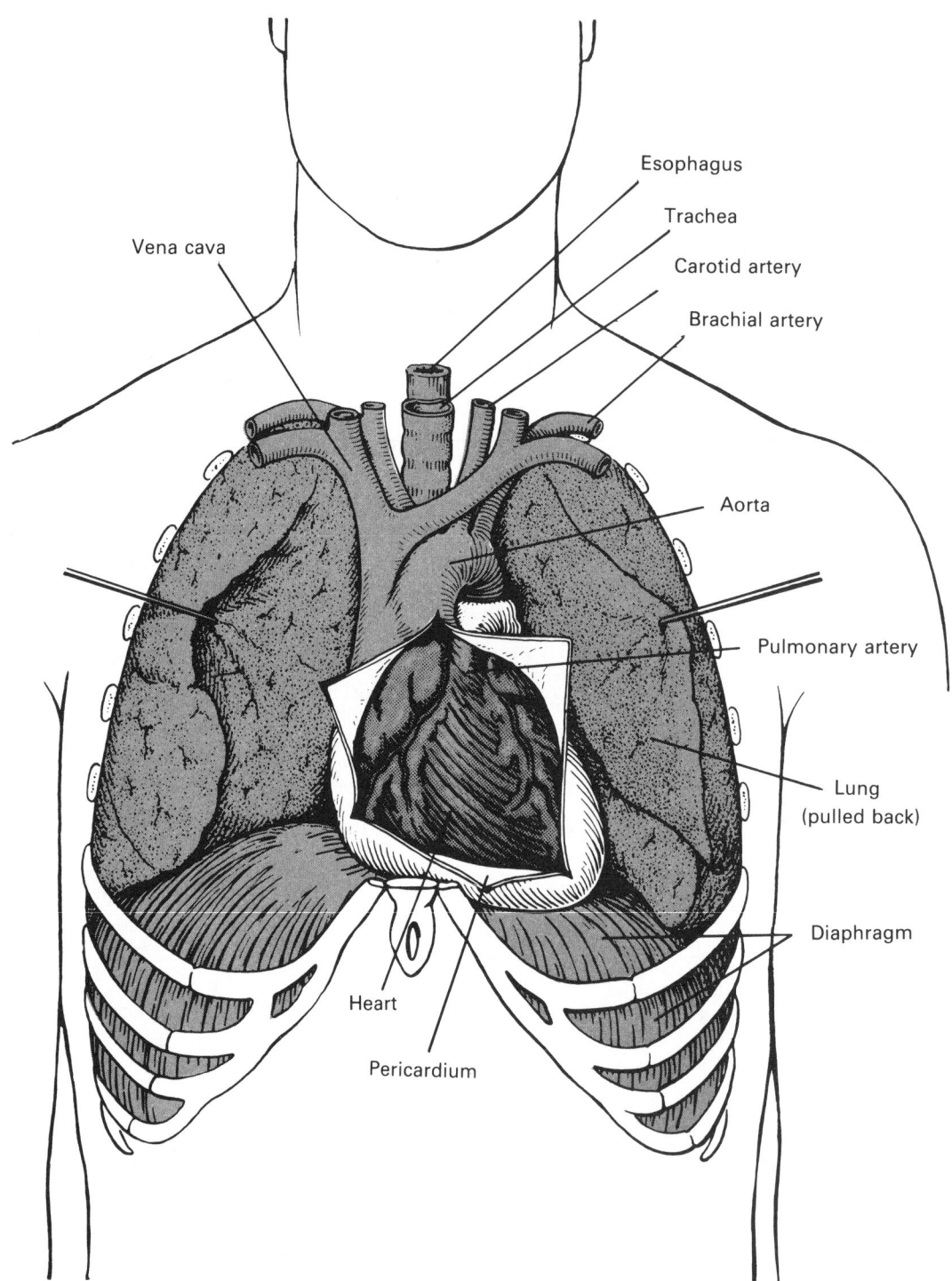

Vena cava

Esophagus

Trachea

Carotid artery

Brachial artery

Aorta

Pulmonary artery

Lung
(pulled back)

Diaphragm

Heart

Pericardium

**Position of Heart in Chest Cavity.** *The normal heart is shown in relation to surrounding organs. Contrary to popular belief, the heart tends to be more in the middle of the chest than on the left side, and a part of it actually extends over into the right chest cavity.*

# CHAPTER 29
# THE HEART

*(See also Chapter 5 on Aging; Chapter 13 on Blood Vessels and Blood Vessel Surgery; Chapter 62 on Rheumatic Fever; Chapter 73 on Transplantation of Organs)*

### What is the structure of the heart?

The heart is a hollow, globular, muscular organ composed of four compartments. It is divided into a left side and a right side, each of which has two connecting chambers—an atrium and a ventricle.

The right atrium receives blood supplied to it by two great veins—the inferior and superior vena cavas. These vessels carry to the right atrium the blood from all the veins of the body. This venous blood is dark red in color, having a low proportion of oxygen and a high proportion of waste carbon dioxide and other products absorbed from the intestinal tract or manufactured by the tissues. From the right atrium, passing through a valve called the tricuspid valve, this blood travels to the right ventricle. From there blood passes through another valve called the pulmonic valve and then enters the blood vessels of the lungs. Here the oxygen supply of the venous blood is replenished, and the waste carbon dioxide is passed out into the exhaled air. From the lungs, the reoxygenated blood passes on to the left side of the heart, first entering the left atrium. From there it passes through another intervening valve called the mitral valve and enters the powerful and muscular left ventricle. The left ventricle contracts forcefully and expels this fresh blood through the aortic valve into the largest artery of the body—the aorta. From there on, the reoxygenated blood is distributed to all the blood vessels and tissues of the body.

### What is the function of the heart?

The heart is the motor, or main source of energy, that supplies the propelling force to keep the bloodstream in motion through all the blood vessels of the body. This organ, hardly larger than a fist, pumps an average of six thousand quarts of blood a day and can multiply its efforts manyfold when necessary. It beats incessantly during life, contracting at an average rate of seventy-eight times per minute, or approximately a hundred and ten thousand times daily.

Poor heart action leads to poor circulation, which in turn leads to derangement and impairment of the function of the vital tissues of the body.

### How can a doctor tell if a patient has a "good heart"?

He evaluates the heart on the basis of the patient's clinical history, the physical examination, and by other tests, such as fluoroscopy, x ray, and electrocardiography, which are carried out when additional investigation is indicated.

### What is meant by the expression a "strong heart"?

Any heart that is normal in structure and that functions efficiently can be "strong."

### What is meant by the expression a "weak heart"?

A heart that functions inefficiently because of underlying disease or defect in structure.

### Does heart trouble tend to be inherited or to run in families?

While certain conditions that attack the heart may tend to run in families, heart disease, by and large, is *not* inherited. The fact that one member of a family suffers from a heart ailment should not alarm related individuals about the condition of their own heart. However, it should serve as an additional incentive for these individuals to visit their physician regularly so that he may outline a preventive program if indicated.

### Does a patient with a "poor heart" ever develop a "strong heart"?

This depends upon the age of the individual as well as the primary cause of the heart condition. Many types of heart trouble can be treated effectively, and in certain cases complete cure can result.

### Do children with heart trouble ever outgrow it?

The term "outgrow" is one that physicians no longer use. The thought that a condition will clear up without treatment often encourages a negligent attitude rather than a positive approach to a heart problem. Strictly speaking, heart trouble is not outgrown.

The popularity of this term had its origin in the fact that some heart murmurs heard in childhood were found to disappear later on in life. In actuality, these murmurs were not really indicative of true heart disease but were innocent, atypical heart sounds. A true murmur indicative of an actual organic heart disease almost never disappears spontaneously.

### Is strenuous physical exertion bad for someone with a normal heart?

Strenuous physical exertion probably has no significant harmful effect upon a normal heart.

### Is strenuous physical exercise dangerous for someone with a "weak heart"?

Patients who suffer from heart disease should not indulge in strenuous physical exercise! This does not mean that such patients should make complete invalids of themselves. Rather, they should function within the range of limitations dictated by their own particular heart condition. The specific advice of their physician should be followed carefully.

## What effect does smoking tobacco have upon the heart?

It is now generally agreed among most doctors that smoking is harmful to the heart. It causes constriction of small and large arteries, which supply the muscle of the heart, and thus deprives the heart of much-needed oxygen. In some patients, smoking manifests itself by causing spasms of the coronary artery, by creating irregularities in the rhythm of the heart, or by elevating the blood pressure. It is estimated that heart attacks are much more common among smokers than among non-smokers. Certainly, people with heart disease should discontinue smoking.

## Is drinking of alcohol bad for the heart?

Not particularly, unless drinking is excessive and prolonged. Recent studies have shown that under the latter conditions, definite injury to the heart muscle can occur.

## Is it harmful to the heart to take aspirin?

No.

## What medications in common usage are harmful to the heart?

Most of the commonly prescribed medications have no effect at all upon the heart.

## Is excessive emotional strain bad for the heart?

Yes, but the normal heart tolerates acute emotional, as well as physical, strain remarkably well. Chronic emotional strain may eventually cause heart disease. Also, exceptional strain caused by a life crisis may precipitate an acute heart attack in an otherwise normal heart. Clearly, prolonged emotional strain is

deleterious to a heart whose function is already impaired by primary, underlying disease.

## How can one tell if pain in the heart region is due to a heart condition or is due to trouble in some other organ?

Heart pain is an extremely variable symptom. It requires the skill of an experienced physician to evaluate whether a particular ache or pain actually arises from the heart. Frequently, he must resort to procedures such as electrocardiogram or x ray to reinforce his clinical opinion.

## Is there such a thing as a "broken heart"? In other words, can the heart be affected by grief or disappointment?

The term "broken heart" is, for all practical purposes, a purely poetic expression.

## Do people with normal hearts tend to outlive those who have heart trouble?

Other things being equal, yes.

## How often should people have their heart examined?

People without a specific history of heart disease should not think in terms of having their heart checked. Rather, they should think in terms of a periodic, comprehensive physical examination.

The patient with heart disease should have his heart examined at regular intervals, as advised by his physician. These intervals may vary greatly from patient to patient.

## Do men have heart trouble more often than women?

Men have a much greater tendency toward diseases of the coronary arteries and therefore are more prone to develop angina pectoris or coronary thrombosis. Other forms of heart disease are equally distributed between the sexes.

## Do thin people tend to get heart conditions less frequently than obese people?

Statistically, the incidence of coronary artery disease is definitely greater among overweight people. Other forms of heart disease do not appear to be appreciably greater among the obese. But it should be remembered that obesity places an additional burden upon an already weakened or impaired heart.

## Can doctors predict length of life by listening to the heart and making heart tests?

No. A doctor can merely determine whether a heart is functioning properly or whether it is diseased. However, in spite of all modern medical advances, it is impossible to make more than a rough guess as to the life span of the patient with a diseased heart. Certainly, there is no basis whatsoever for predictions of longevity in the patient with an apparently normal heart.

## IMPAIRED HEART FUNCTION AND HEART DISEASE

## What are some of the common causes of impaired heart function and heart disease?

a. The heart muscle itself may be weakened so that it cannot contract with sufficient force. This may be caused by poor nourishment to the heart muscle tissue (as in disease of the arteries supplying the heart). Also, infection, inflammation, toxins, hormonal disorders, or blood-mineral imbalance may weaken the muscle tissue of the heart.

b. The heart valves may not function properly—either because they do not open and close adequately or because they were defectively formed or absent as a result of a developmental birth deformity.

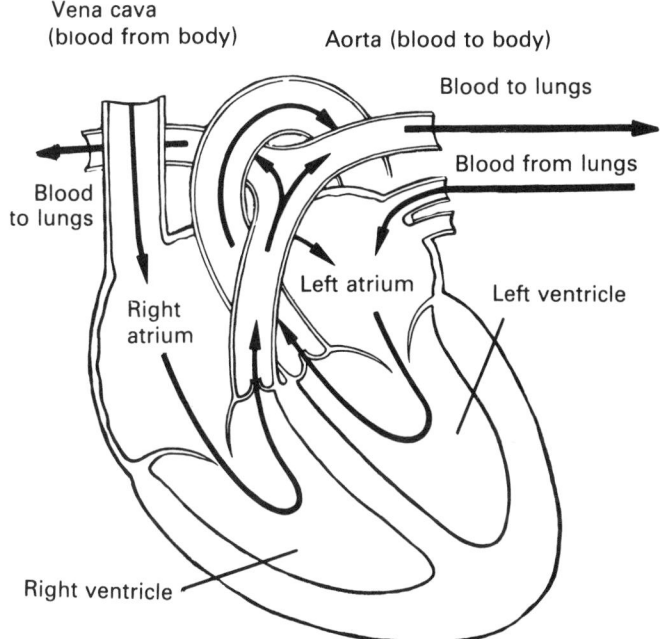

Vena cava (blood from body)

Aorta (blood to body)

Blood to lungs

Blood from lungs

Blood to lungs

Left atrium

Left ventricle

Right atrium

Right ventricle

**Heart Chambers.** *This diagram illustrates the four chambers of the heart; the arrows indicate the direction of blood flow through the heart.*

Heart valve disorders may also be caused by acquired disease, the most common of which is rheumatic fever. Other less common causes of heart valve dysfunction are syphilis, bacterial infection, or diseases of the cell-cementing substance.

c. The heart muscle may be weakened if it has been overworked because of high blood pressure, chronic lung disease, endocrine gland disorders, anemia, abnormal connections between arteries and veins, or the above mentioned valvular disorders.

d. Congenital (inborn) defects in the wall dividing the right and left side of the heart, as well as a great variety of bizarre inborn abnormalities of the heart and connecting great blood vessels. Fortunately, these birth deformities are quite rare.

e. Inflammatory diseases of the heart muscle and sheath of the heart may be caused most likely by viral infections known as myocarditis and pericarditis.

f. Structural abnormalities of the chest cage and spine.

g. Disorders of the rhythmicity of the heart. Instead of beating regularly, the heart may adopt any of a variety of disorderly or abnormal rhythm patterns. As a result of these rhythm disorders, the heart is sometimes unable to pump blood efficiently.

h. Tumors of the heart may seriously interfere with good heart function. These tumors may arise in the heart tissue itself, or they may spread to the heart from other organs. (Such tumors of the heart are a rare cause of cardiac impairment.)

**What are the more common causes of heart disease?**

a. Coronary artery disease. (The coronary arteries are the blood vessels supplying the blood to the heart muscle.)

b. High blood pressure.

c. Chronic lung disease.

d. Congenital (inborn) heart abnormalities.

e. Rheumatic fever.

## HEART FAILURE

### What is heart failure?

Heart failure, medically known as cardiac decompensation, may be caused by one or more of the conditions enumerated above. The term is applied when the heart is no longer able to accommodate to the normal circulatory requirements of the body.

Ordinarily, the human heart has sufficient reserve strength to compensate for most ordinary handicaps in the course of the above-mentioned disorders. However, as the disorder increases in severity and as the heart muscle becomes more and more fatigued, the heart becomes increasingly incapable of meeting its obligations.

### What are the symptoms of heart failure?

a. Easy fatigability.

b. Shortness of breath, increased by mild exertion.

c. Swelling of the feet, ankles, and legs, usually increasing toward the end of the day and improving overnight.

d. Inability to lie flat in bed without becoming short of breath, thus requiring several cushions to prop up the head and chest.

e. Blueness of the lips, fingernails, and skin.

f. Accumulation of fluid in the abdomen, chest, and other areas of the body.

g. Sudden attacks of suffocation at night, forcing the patient to sit up or get out of bed and gasp for air.

h. Distention of the veins of the neck.

### How long does it take a damaged or strained heart to go into failure?

The time required is extremely variable from patient to patient. The heart has an amazing capacity to do its work under great handicaps for a period of many years and will continue to do so provided the obstacles do not become overwhelming.

### Once the heart begins to decompensate (fail), does it mean the patient will die?

No. A decompensating heart may be bolstered for many years with proper care such as limitation of activity, salt restriction, digitalis therapy, diuretics (drugs that increase the elimination of water and salt by the kidneys), or surgery in specially indicated instances.

### How does a physician evaluate the cardiac status of a patient?

a. By taking a careful history of symptoms and past illnesses.

b. By listening to the heart through a stethoscope.

c. By fluoroscoping or x raying the heart.

d. By taking an electrocardiogram.

e. By other, more exhaustive tests, such as the stress test.

### What is an electrocardiogram?

The heart muscle generates a feeble, though characteristic, electrical current when it contracts and relaxes. This current can be picked up and recorded on paper by a very sensitive instrument known as an electrocardiograph. Variations in amplitude and direction of the current may give important information concerning the heart's function and state of health.

### Are electrocardiographic findings

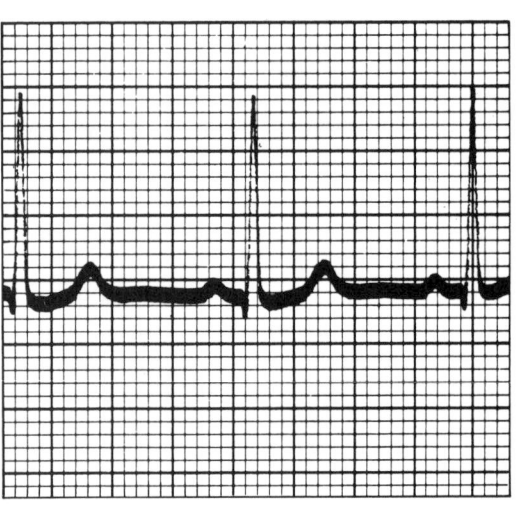

*Left:*
**Normal Electrocardiographic Tracing.** *Cardiologists interpret variations from normal tracings and thereby diagnose heart disease.*

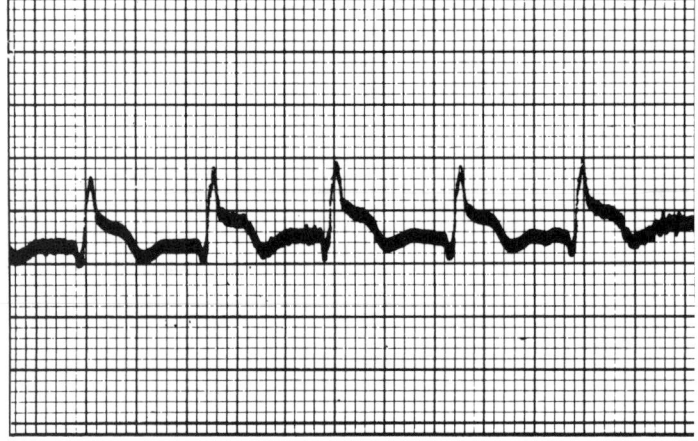

*Below:*
**Coronary Thrombosis.** *This electrocardiographic tracing shows that the patient has had an acute cornonary thrombosis. It is not difficult to note the variation in this tracing from the normal electrocardiographic tracing shown at left.*

**in themselves sufficient to establish a patient's cardiac status?**

No. They give only supplementary information. The electrocardiogram may be completely normal in the presence of a serious heart disorder. On the other hand, it may demonstrate abnormalities at a time when the physical examination is essentially normal.

### What is an exercise *stress test*?

For certain patients, heart function is normal at rest but not during exercise. The response of the heart rate and electrocardiogram to measured exercise will help find those patients whose activities must be limited.

### What is an echocardiogram?

It is a test in which sound waves are directed at the heart, and echoes reflected from these waves are recorded. The pattern seen on the recording gives important information on the health of the heart muscle and heart function. The test is completely without risk.

### What are radionucleotide studies of the heart?

Radioisotope substances are injected into the patient's arm vein, and energy emitted from these radioactive isotopes is measured. From these measurements one can obtain information about damage to the heart muscle and heart function. This test can be performed easily and without risk.

### What is cardiac catheterization?

There are a number of situations in the evaluation of a patient's heart in which the methods listed above do not yield enough information. In such instances, cardiac catheterization may be performed. This consists of passing and threading a long, narrow, hollow plastic tube into the blood vessel of one of the extremities until it reaches one or more chambers of the heart. Pressure recordings are made through the tube, and blood samples are withdrawn. This is not a routine procedure and requires the skill of a specially trained physician. (Cardiac catheterization has become an important research tool, adding immensely to our knowledge concerning the working of the heart.)

### What is angiocardiography?

Primarily, angiocardiography is used for the same reasons as cardiac catheterization and under similar circumstances. However, it does impart a somewhat different type of information. It consists of injecting a chemical into the bloodstream that is opaque to x rays. X rays of the heart are taken in rapid progression as this chemical passes through the various chambers. Like cardiac catheterization, this procedure is not employed routinely and requires specialized skills and training. However, in recent years, it has contributed greatly to our knowledge of heart function.

## BLOOD PRESSURE

### What is blood pressure?

Blood pressure is the force created by the contracting heart to keep the blood circulating adequately and constantly through the blood vessels of the body. In order to overcome the resistance that is present in miles of narrow blood vessels, and in order for the blood to finally arrive at the tissues with enough residual pressure to effect an interchange of chemicals, the heart must maintain a certain minimal level of pressure within the circulatory system.

### How is blood pressure measured?

A tubular rubber cuff is strapped around the upper arm. The cuff is connected to an apparatus that measures pressure, and it is inflated with air while the physician listens to the arterial pulse in the crook of the elbow. The air pressure in the cuff is raised until the pulsation can no longer be heard. After this the cuff is deflated until the physician begins to hear the pulse beat return. This is known as the systolic pressure. The cuff is gradually deflated further until the pulse beat again disappears. The pressure at this point is called the diastolic pressure.

### What causes high blood pressure?

It is thought that narrowing of the smaller arteries throughout the body causes the heart to pump harder to get the blood to the various tissues. When the heart pumps harder, blood pressure is elevated.

### Is there a hereditary tendency toward high blood pressure (essential hypertension)?

Yes, but it should be stated that the presence of high blood pressure in a parent does not necessarily imply that the offspring will have hypertension.

### Does overweight tend toward elevated blood pressure?

Yes.

### Is high blood pressure caused by eating red meat, salt, or spices?

No.

### Is there a variation in the way different individuals react to high blood pressure?

Yes. Females are able to withstand continuous high blood pressure levels much better than males. Also, there is a great variation in reaction among different people.

### Why may high blood pressure be harmful?

a. A greater-than-average strain is placed upon the heart. If it is prolonged, the heart may become enlarged and damaged.
b. Greater wear and tear is placed upon all the blood vessels since blood courses through them at greater pressure. Eventually, vital damage may be inflicted upon vessels. This in turn causes impairment of function of the tissues and organs that they supply. Organs particularly susceptible to such damage are the heart, brain, kidneys, and eyes.

### Is high blood pressure curable?

Not really, but modern methods of medication make it possible to keep the pressure under control, thereby minimizing serious potential injury.

In addition to medication and a sensible pattern of living, reduction of overweight and constant surveillance also contribute substantially toward the control of high blood pressure.

On the other hand, there are other less common causes of hypertension—such as certain tumors, kidney diseases, and endocrine disturbances—which can actually be cured, providing the underlying cause is detectable and can be eradicated.

### Can high blood pressure (essential hypertension) be prevented?

No, but the above measures can in many instances lead to its control.

### Do emotion and temperament affect the blood pressure?

Yes. Imprudent living and extravagant emotional excesses can raise blood pressure. Such extremes of conduct are thought not to be the basic cause for hypertension but, rather, aggravating influences.

### Can a patient with high blood pressure feel healthy and be unaware of its presence?

Many people have high blood pressure for years without being aware of it.

### What are the usual symptoms of high blood pressure?

Actually, there are none specifically attributable to the elevated pressure. The headaches and hot flashes complained about are usually due to other conditions.

### What is the normal blood pressure level?

There is no such thing as a set, normal blood pressure. There is a wide range of pressures considered normal for the average adult. The upper limit of normal systolic pressure is about 150 to 160mm. of mercury, and the upper limit for the diastolic pressure is from 90 to 100mm.

### What is low blood pressure?

The common or garden variety of low blood pressure is not a disease. It refers to a state in which blood pressure readings are found to be in the lower level of the normal range. This is usually a healthy situation for it means that the heart and blood vessels are not being put to undue strain.

### Is low blood pressure ever an evidence of true disease?

In certain rare diseases, persistent low blood pressure is found as a constant sign.

### Does the common form of low blood pressure give rise to symptoms such as fatigue or lethargy?

Only rarely. Unfortunately, low blood pressure has become a psychological hat rack upon which many individuals hang a variety of unrelated complaints.

### Does low blood pressure require treatment?

Rarely, if ever.

### Can one have "temporary" high blood pressure?

Yes. Often the excitement of an examination or the circumstances surrounding an examination may give rise to abnormally high pressure readings. Later examination under more relaxed conditions may yield a perfectly normal result. Also, exceptional emotional stress may cause elevated blood pressure for a period of several days or weeks. This will usually return to normal when the strain is eased.

## CONGENITAL HEART DISEASE

### What types of congenital heart conditions are there?

a. Abnormal communications between the right and left sides of the heart, so that blood from the veins passes into the arterial circulation.
b. Abnormalities in the structure and function of the heart valves, which separate the various chambers of the heart.
c. Abnormalities in the heart muscle itself.
d. Abnormalities in the inner and outer linings of the heart.

### What causes congenital heart conditions?

Defects in prenatal development due to a variety of causes not yet fully understood. Recent evidence has illustrated that the incidence of congenital heart disease is much greater if the mother has contracted German measles in the first three months of pregnancy. Other viral diseases during this stage of pregnancy have been suspected but not yet substantiated. Certain drugs (such as thalidomide) have been shown to have the potential to develop cardiac as well as other abnormalities in the embryo. It is therefore advisable to avoid any and all drugs in the first three formative months unless recommended by the physician. Also, a variety of poorly understood changes in the genes have been shown to lead to congenital heart abnormalities.

### Are congenital heart conditions hereditary?

Most often, no. However, in a small but definite percentage of cases, certain heart abnormalities have been shown to be hereditary.

### Can abnormalities of the heart be detected immediately after the child is born?

Some may be detected by listening with a stethoscope at birth or noting the blue color of the baby. Other conditions remain obscure until much later in childhood or even until adulthood.

### How common are congenital heart conditions?

They occur approximately three times in every thousand births.

### Are congenital heart conditions serious?

Yes, because they often lead to impairment of heart function and circulation and produce situations in which the tissues receive an insufficient quantity of oxygen.

### What is a "blue baby"?

A baby born with a condition in which oxygen-poor blood from the veins passes directly from the right side of the circulatory system to the left, or arterial, side. This blood bypasses the lungs and is therefore deficient in oxygen.

### Can congenital heart abnormalities be cured?

In the past few years tremendous strides have been made surgically in the treatment of these conditions. Some abnormalities can be cured completely through surgery; others may be helped considerably. (See the section on Heart Surgery in this chapter.)

## CORONARY ARTERY DISEASE

### What are the coronary arteries?

They are the blood vessels that course through the wall of the heart and nourish the heart muscle. They are the first blood vessels to branch off from the aorta as it leaves the heart.

## What is coronary artery disease?

Since the heart muscle expends a huge amount of energy in its ceaseless work, it naturally demands a good supply of blood. Any impairment of these blood vessels that interferes with adequate blood flow is known as coronary artery disease.

## What is the most frequent cause of coronary artery disease?

Arteriosclerosis (hardening of the arteries).

## What is coronary insufficiency and angina pectoris?

If the blood flow through the coronary arteries is significantly diminished, the heart cannot function at maximum efficiency. The heart then signals its plight by registering pain or discomfort in the chest—usually under the breastbone. Often, however, the discomfort or pain may be manifest in more remote regions of the body, such as in the back, arms, neck, jaw, or upper abdomen. The registering of such pain, with or without exertion, is called angina pectoris. The pain subsides when the patient rests and stops any physical exertion.

## What is coronary occlusion?

It is the complete interruption of blood flow through one of the branches of the coronary artery. As a result, a portion of heart muscle may be destroyed from lack of nourishment. This is called myocardial infarction. If a large main artery is blocked, a large portion of heart muscle is damaged. If a small subsidiary branch is blocked, a smaller portion of muscle is damaged. The term "heart attack" is commonly used to allude to this sequence of events.

## What is the cause of coronary occlusion?

The most common cause is the blockage of the coronary arteries by the formation of a blood clot. This is termed coronary thrombosis. It usually occurs at a site where the artery was previously damaged by arteriosclerosis.

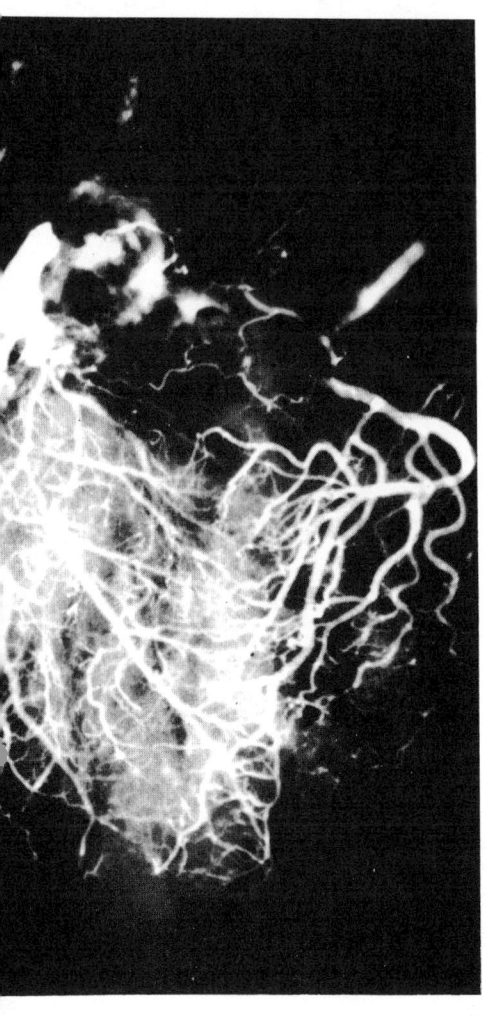

*The Coronary Arteries. This illustration shows a heart specimen in which the coronary arteries have been injected with dye. It demonstrates that the coronary arteries supply blood to the wall of the heart itself. Blockage of these arteries causes serious heart damage and may result in sudden death.*

## What are some of the factors that govern the outcome of a heart attack?

a: The amount of previous heart damage.

b. The size of the area of heart muscle damaged by the particular attack.

c. The amount of remaining normal heart muscle.

d. The degree to which the coronary obstruction spreads toward other branches of the artery.

e. The occurrence or absence of disorders in the rhythm of the heart.

f. The presence or absence of blood clots on the inner wall of the heart that may break off and travel to other parts of the body.

g. The possibility of rupture of the weakened heart wall.

## What are the chances of recovery from an initial coronary thrombosis?

Approximately four out of five people recover.

## What is the significance of coronary insufficiency or angina pectoris?

Angina pectoris is a term applied to the chest pain caused by coronary insufficiency. There are many degrees of angina pectoris and many degrees of coronary insufficiency. Mild degrees are compatible with all but the most strenuous activity. Severe degrees may completely incapacitate a patient.

## Can attacks of angina pectoris be prevented?

To a certain extent; that is, a more orderly, regulated life with the deletion of excessive work and excitement, plus the taking of certain medications, may control attacks of angina pectoris. In some cases, they can be avoided completely.

## Is angina pectoris compatible with a normal life span?

Yes. However, the individual outlook

*Normal Coronary Artery.* This photomicrograph shows a cross section of a normal coronary artery. Note how wide and open the passageway is in the middle of the vessel.

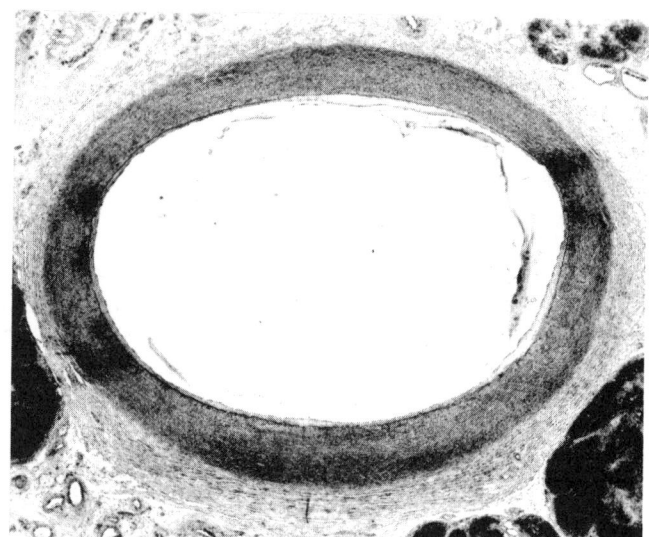

*Coronary Thrombosis.* This photomicrograph shows a cross section of an arteriosclerotic coronary artery in which thrombosis (a clot) has taken place. Naturally, no blood can flow through such an artery, and the heart muscle wall supplied by such an artery will be severely damaged from lack of circulation.

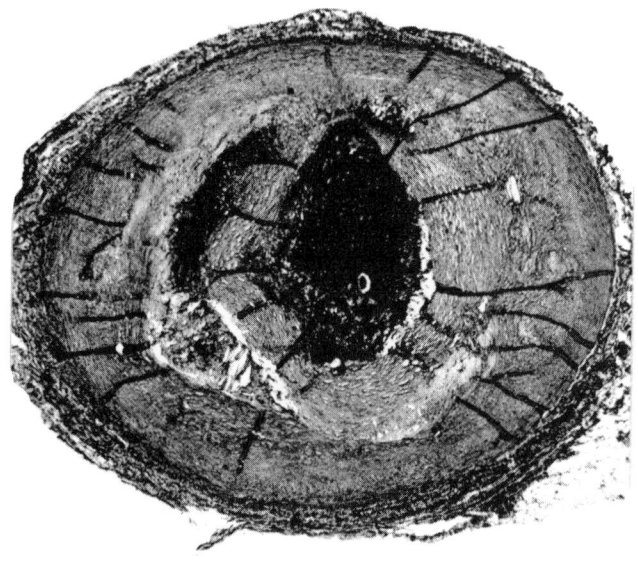

depends on many factors that vary from patient to patient.

### Do all people with angina pectoris eventually develop coronary occlusion?

No, though it is true that such patients are definitely more prone to such heart attacks.

### What is the treatment for coronary thrombosis?

The mainstay of treatment is careful monitoring, twenty-four hours a day, for cardiac arrhythmias (heartbeat irregularities) and prompt treatment should they arise. Oxygen is administered for several days following onset of an attack. Formerly, anticoagulant drugs were given during the acute phase of a coronary attack, but now these medications are reserved for long-term use after the acute attack has subsided. Drugs to strengthen the heart, such as digitalis, may at times be given, and drugs to correct irregular heart rhythm may be prescribed. Medications to relieve pain are also of considerable benefit.

### Is surgery helpful in coronary artery disease?

Yes. The coronary bypass operation has helped a considerable number of people with coronary disease. Also, an operation in which the passageway of the coronary artery is restored by removing obstructing arteriosclerotic plaques of tissue gives promise of being helpful.

### Why are bed rest and limited physical activity important?

The less active the individual, the less the heart has to work to supply the necessary circulatory support. It may not seem so, but there is a tremendous difference in the amount of energy expended by the heart during absolute rest and ordinary activity.

### How long must a patient with coronary thrombosis stay in bed?

This depends upon the extent and progress of the illness. If there is no shock, heart failure, or serious irregularity of the heart, patients are gotten out of bed in a week.

### How long must a patient with coronary thrombosis stay in the hospital?

The average hospital stay in uncomplicated acute cases is approximately three weeks.

### How long must a patient who has had a coronary occlusion stop working?

On the average, most patients may return to work two to three months after the onset. It is wise that these people increase their activity in a gradual fashion rather than plunge right in. It is also important that the patient provide for modification in his occupation if it is unduly taxing. Most patients who have had a heart attack *can* and *should* return to work, but they must avoid emotional as well as physical strain.

**What percentage of people who have had coronary thrombosis can make a good recovery and return to work?**

Statistics show that most patients who have had a heart attack make an excellent recovery and return to their usual occupation.

**What are anticoagulant drugs?**

They are chemical compounds that decrease the normal clotting ability of the blood. (Heparin and dicumarol are two of the most frequently used.)

**Why are anticoagulant drugs used in treating coronary thrombosis?**

a. To prevent the clot in the artery from spreading, thus further impairing the blood supply to the heart muscle.
b. To prevent clots from forming on the inner lining of the heart and in the leg veins, since the clots may break loose and travel in the bloodstream (embolism).

**Is it possible to predict the onset of a heart attack?**

Not always. It often occurs without warning to people who have been in apparent good health and who may have had a normal electrocardiogram just prior to the attack. There are instances, however, where warning signs—such as chest pains—may have occurred for weeks or months prior to an acute attack.

**Can periodic electrocardiograms give advance information as to the possibility of a future heart attack?**

Only to a very limited extent.

**What age group is most susceptible to a heart attack?**

People between forty and sixty years of age.

**Are men more susceptible to heart attack than women?**

Yes. They are approximately three times more prone to coronary artery disease. However, after fifty years of age, the incidence of coronary thrombosis increases markedly in women.

**Can a patient who has had a heart attack look forward to many years of life?**

Yes. Patients who have had serious heart attacks often live twenty-five to thirty or more years thereafter.

**Is there a hereditary susceptibility to coronary artery disease?**

There sometimes appears to be a hereditary predisposition, but this is not an exclusive determining factor in the causation of the disease.

**How important is emotional strain in the production of a heart attack?**

It is thought to be a contributing factor, although it is usually not the sole, or the main, causative agent.

**What influence does physical exertion have upon the immediate or future occurrence of coronary heart disease?**

Generally speaking, physical exertion is not a highly significant factor in the cause of heart attacks. However, there have been instances of heart attacks having occurred concomitantly with, or shortly after, severe physical exertion. The consensus is that most of these people had quiescent underlying disease of the coronary arteries, which predisposed them to attacks.

**What conditions predispose one toward the development of coronary artery disease?**

Diabetes, high blood pressure, excessively high cholesterol levels in the blood, obesity, and heavy smoking.

**What is the influence of diet on coronary artery disease?**

A number of factors in the diet have been indicted as contributing to coronary artery disease, e.g., saturated fatty acids derived from animal meats and dairy foods such as milk and cream; common table sugar, known as sucrose; and foods with a high cholesterol content.

**What is the influence of smoking upon coronary artery disease?**

At the present time it is the consensus of opinion that the more one smokes, the more likely is coronary artery disease to develop, all other factors remaining equal. Certainly, an individual who already has coronary artery disease should not smoke at all.

## HEART IRREGULARITIES
### (Cardiac Arrhythmia)

**What is cardiac arrhythmia?**

An irregularity in the rhythmic beat of the heart.

**What causes cardiac irregularity?**

Some cases are caused by true heart disease; others are associated with normal hearts that for one reason or another go "off beat." The physician can usually distinguish between the various causes for such irregularities.

**Do irregularities of the heart interfere with its function?**

An occasional extra beat or skip (extrasystole) has little effect upon heart function. Other cardiac arrhythmias may seriously interfere with circulation.

**Can cardiac irregularities be treated successfully?**

In the great majority of cases, cardiac irregularities will respond to treatment with certain heart drugs.

**What is a skipped beat or premature beat?**

This is an occasional irregularity of the heart in which the patient is aware of a peculiar ("butterfly") sensation in the chest or a fleeting, sinking, or empty sensation in the chest.

Technically, it is known as an extrasystole.

### What is the significance of a skipped beat?

In the vast majority of cases, there is no serious significance to this, although at times it may be annoying.

### What causes skipped beats?

A variety of conditions, among which are exhaustion, the unwise taking of drugs, nervousness, irritability, an acute infection, etc. Less commonly, the cause may be underlying heart disease.

### Is the use of tobacco ever a cause for extrasystoles?

Yes, this is one of the commonest causes for cardiac irregularity.

## ATHLETE'S HEART

### What is "athlete's heart"?

This term has been used erroneously in most instances to refer to enlargement of the heart in people who had overexerted themselves during days of strenuous athletics. At present it is felt that these hearts were, in effect, basically unsound to begin with. There is no sure evidence that indulgence in athletics produces heart disease in a normal heart.

## PALPITATION OF THE HEART

### What is meant by "palpitation of the heart"?

This is a nonmedical expression often used to denote consciousness of a rapid and exceptionally forceful heartbeat. Occasionally this feeling of palpitation is associated with irregularities of the heartbeat.

### Does palpitation denote heart disease?

Usually not. It occurs most often in people who are suffering from undue tension and anxiety.

## PAROXYSMAL ARRHYTHMIA

### What is paroxysmal arrhythmia?

This is a condition in which the heart suddenly and abruptly goes into another rhythm, often becoming extremely rapid. These attacks may come on suddenly, at frequent or infrequent intervals, without warning.

### How long do attacks of paroxysmal arrhythmia last?

Anywhere from a few minutes to a few days.

### Do these attacks occur only in diseased hearts?

No. Often the heart is completely normal.

### What causes episodes of paroxysmal arrhythmia?

a In organic heart conditions, it is usually a disease of the "rhythm centers."

b. In normal hearts, the cause is usually unknown.

### What is the treatment for paroxysmal arrhythmias?

In most cases, these episodes can be controlled by medications such as quinidine. Occasionally, the treatment of choice is the use of electronic heart-shocking devices.

## HEART BLOCK

### What is heart block?

Complete heart block is a condition in which the electrical impulse from the atrium (which initiates heart contractions) is not transmitted to the ventricle. As a result, there can be complete cardiac standstill, cessation of heartbeat, and death, or there can be temporary cardiac standstill with loss of consciousness and strokelike manifestations. On the other hand, the ventricles can set up their own focus of activity and operate independently of the atrium. Another type of heart block is known as incomplete heart block, where every second or third beat may not be transmitted from the atrium to the ventricle. The manifestations of this phenomenon are not as dramatic as complete heart block.

### Is heart block usually associated with a disease of the heart?

Yes.

### How is the diagnosis of heart block usually made?

By physical examination corroborated by electrocardiographic study.

### Is heart block compatible with life?

This depends on the severity of the condition. Such a patient is constantly threatened with the possibility that the ventricles may cease to beat at all or react in such a way as to be life threatening.

### What can be done when heart block becomes a life-threatening situation?

Either temporary or permanently implanted electronic devices can be instituted surgically. These devices electrically stimulate the ventricles of the heart to beat regularly and effectively. These devices are known as pacemakers.

## FIBRILLATION OF THE HEART

### What is auricular atrial fibrillation?

It is a condition in which there is complete disorder, originating in the auricles, in the rhythmic beat of the heart.

### What causes auricular atrial fibrillation?

It is commonly seen in long-standing

rheumatic heart disease, arteri-osclerotic heart disease, and in hyperthyroidism (a disease in which there is overactivity of the thyroid gland).

## What is the significance of auricular atrial fibrillation?

An irregularly beating heart is usually not as efficient as one that beats regularly, and it therefore pumps blood to the tissues in an inefficient manner.

## What complications may occur with chronic auricular atrial fibrillation of the heart?

a. Because of too rapid and irregular contractions, the output of the heart may be inadequate and may lead to heart failure or decompensation.
b. A fibrillating heart may develop clots of blood on its inner wall. If these should break off and travel to other organs of the body, they can cause severe damage (embolization).

## Can a fibrillating heart be brought back to normal rhythm?

In many instances this can be accomplished by either medication or by electronic heart-shocking devices. Very often the results are temporary, and the heart reverts to auricular fibrillation.

## HEART MURMURS

## What is a heart murmur?

An abnormal sound produced by the beating heart.

## How can a physician make a diagnosis of a heart murmur?

By listening with a stethoscope.

## Do heart murmurs cause symptoms?

No. The patient is usually unaware that a murmur exists.

## Do all murmurs indicate heart disease?

No. A high percentage of murmurs are produced by normal hearts and are of no clinical significance.

## What is a functional heart murmur?

One not associated with heart disease.

## What is an organic murmur?

A murmur associated with heart disease.

## Can a doctor tell the difference between an organic and a functional murmur?

Usually it is quite simple for the physician to determine the difference by the location and position of the murmur, by the heartbeat cycle, and by other distinctive features. A small percentage of murmurs remain in question, and diagnosis is quite difficult.

## HEART VALVE INFECTION
*(Bacterial Endocarditis)*

## What is bacterial endocarditis?

Heart valves previously damaged by rheumatic fever, congenital heart disease, or other pathology, are particularly susceptible to bacterial infection. This is called bacterial endocarditis. This complication is an extremely serious one and unless promptly treated causes irreparable destruction of the valves. In addition, bacteria are carried by the bloodstream to other organs of the body, which in turn may also be seriously damaged.

## Is bacterial endocarditis curable?

At the present time, successful treatment is available for the majority of these cases.

## What is the treatment for bacterial endocarditis?

The prolonged and intensive administration of antibiotics.

## Is bacterial endocarditis preventable?

To a degree, yes. Any infection in the body should be promptly and vigorously treated lest bacteria break through the tissue barriers, enter the bloodstream, and become implanted upon a heart valve.

## What other measures should be taken to prevent the onset of bacterial endocarditis?

All people suffering from rheumatic heart disease should be particularly careful about surgical procedures. For instance, the extraction of a tooth should be preceded and followed by antibiotic therapy.

## HEART SURGERY

## What conditions can be helped through heart surgery?

a. Congenital heart conditions:
1. Patent ductus arteriosus—the persistence of a blood vessel that ordinarily closes by the time the child is born.
2. Septal defects—abnormal opening and connections between the various chambers of the heart.
3. The condition that causes blue babies, the tetrology of Fallot—abnormal position and connections of major blood vessels leading to and from the heart.
4. Pulmonic stenosis—a condition in which there is either an underdeveloped pulmonary artery leading from the heart to the lungs or a constricted pulmonary valve opening.
5. Coarctation of the aorta—a narrowing of the aorta in the chest.
b. Acquired heart conditions:
1. Rheumatic heart disease—a condition in which there is constriction or other deformity of the heart valves secondary to rheumatic fever.
c. Coronary artery disease.
d. Pericarditis—an inflammatory

## HEART DEFECTS THAT CAN BE CORRECTED SURGICALLY

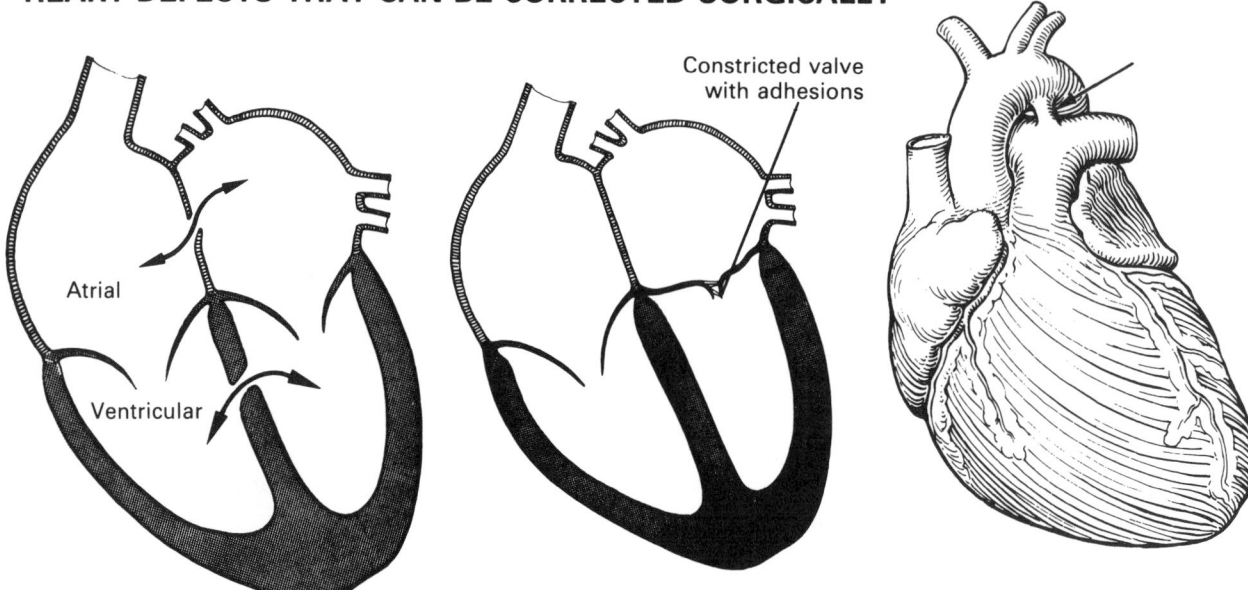

Constricted valve
with adhesions

Atrial

Ventricular

*Clockwise:*

**Septal Defects.** *This diagram shows defects in the walls between the various heart chambers. newer advances in heart surgery have made it possible to open the heart and repair septal defects. During the operation the patient's circulation is conducted with the help of a heart pump so that the heart is bypassed until the surgical repair is completed.*

**Mitral Stenosis.** *This illustration shows one of the most common of all heart conditions, mitral stenosis. This disease is characterized by a narrowing of the valve between the left atrium and the left ventricle of the heart. Mitral stenosis is the end result of a severe attack of rheumatic fever.*

**Patent Ductus Arteriosus.** *This diagram shows a common congenital heart deformity known as patent ductus arteriosus. This can be surgically corrected by tying off the artery. People born with this abnormality can now be cured by a simple, safe heart operation.*

**Mitral Commissurotomy.** *Overgrowths and adhesions on the constricted mitral valve are freed by finger in this operation. This is usually done by sight during open heart surgery.*

**Coarctation of Aorta.** *This diagram shows a birth deformity of the vessels of the heart known as coarctation of the aorta. With newer surgical techniques, it is now possible to remove this constricted portion of the aorta and to reshape it to allow for normal circulation.*

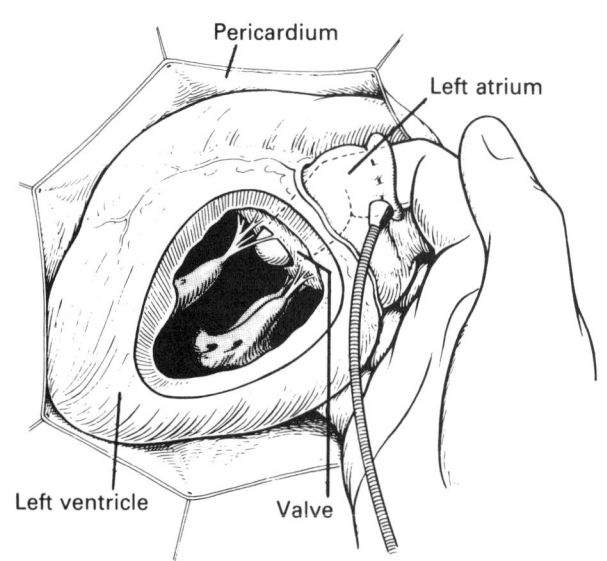

Pericardium

Left atrium

Left ventricle

Valve

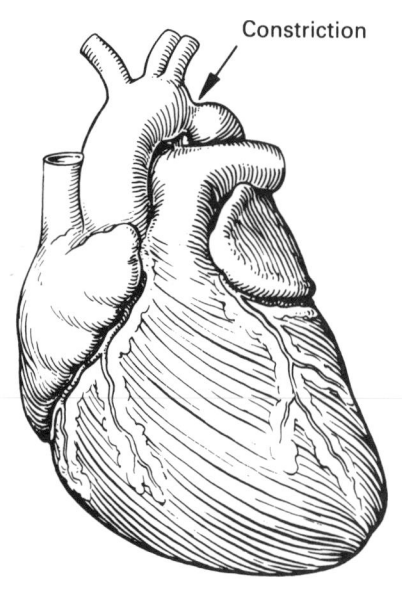

Constriction

condition of the sheath (pericardium) that surrounds the heart.

e. Heart injuries:
  1. Stab wounds or gunshot wounds.
  2. Aneurysm of the heart—in which there is a bulge of the muscle wall secondary to damage caused by a previous coronary thrombosis.

f. Heart block due to inadequate transmission of impulses from the atrium to the ventricle.

## Are operations upon the heart dangerous?

Refinements in the techniques have reduced the dangers of heart surgery remarkably, so that it is fast approaching the degree of safety obtained in some of the other major fields of surgical endeavor.

## Can all people with heart disease be operated upon?

No. Only certain types of heart conditions lend themselves to surgical help.

## Is it difficult to approach the heart surgically?

No. Incisions into the chest cavity make the heart readily available to the surgeon.

## How successful are heart operations for congenital defects?

Almost all of those suffering from a patent ductus arteriosus can be cured; approximately 85 to 90 percent of those with coarctation of the aorta can be cured; and approximately 75 percent of the blue babies can be cured. Septal defects, utilizing a heart pump and open heart surgery, can be controlled either by patching the defects with a Dacron graft or, if the hole is very small, by direct suturing. These operations are successful in well over 90 percent of cases.

## Can patients with congenital heart defects that have been successfully operated upon look forward to a more normal life?

Yes. Many children who were labeled heart cripples can now look forward to near-normal lives after heart surgery.

## Do congenital defects often come back once they have been corrected?

No.

## Is surgery for rheumatic heart disease successful?

Yes. Most of those who have defects of their valves can be helped tremendously through surgery. There are many cases now on record in which the heart valve has been repaired surgically through open heart surgery or has been replaced by an artificial valve.

## What percentage survive of those operated upon for rheumatic heart disease?

Approximately 90 to 95 percent.

## What percentage are benefited by such surgery?

Almost all of those who are operated upon.

## Do all patients with rheumatic heart disease require surgery?

No. Surgery is limited to those whose lives are severely handicapped by the disease.

## Is life expectancy improved by operations upon hearts that have been affected by rheumatic fever?

Yes.

## Do these patients often return to normal living?

Yes.

## What operations are performed upon those with coronary artery disease?

Several operations have been devised, but the most popular procedure involves using a patient's leg vein as a graft to bypass coronary artery obstruction. This is known as a coronary bypass operation. Another one consists of transplanting the internal mammary artery from beneath the breastbone into the heart muscle. An older procedure, in which talcum powder was instilled into the sac surrounding the heart, has been discarded.

## What is the benefit of a coronary bypass operation?

It carries the blood, through the vein graft, from the aorta (the large artery leading away from the heart) back to the heart muscle at a point *beyond* the obstruction in the coronary artery. As a result, the heart muscle receives blood that would otherwise not be able to pass through the obstructed, arteriosclerotic portion of the coronary artery.

## Are coronary bypass operations done very frequently?

Yes. It is estimated that more than a hundred thousand such operations are performed every year in this country.

## Are coronary bypass operations carried out with the use of only one graft from the aorta to the coronary artery?

Ordinarily, several grafts are used, thus bypassing several obstructed areas in the various branches of the coronary arteries. As many as five grafts are not unusual.

## Does the bypass operation often relieve the angina pectoris (heart pain) suffered so often by people with coronary artery disease?

Yes. The great majority are relieved of their pain.

## Will the performance of a coronary bypass operation prolong one's life span?

Most specialists in the field believe that the life span is extended by this operation.

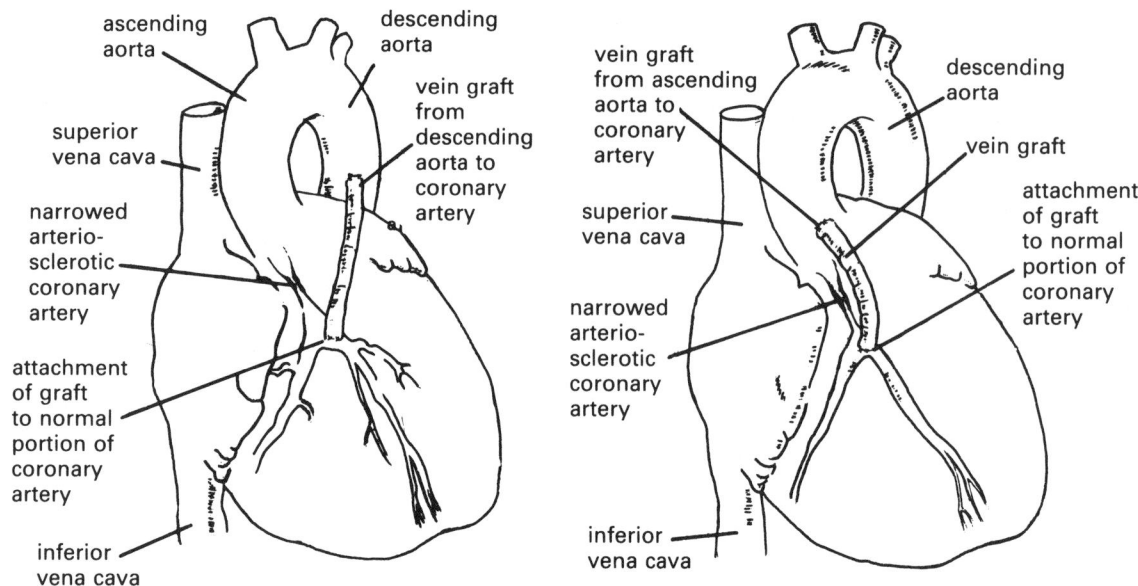

ascending aorta
descending aorta
vein graft from descending aorta to coronary artery
superior vena cava
narrowed arterio-sclerotic coronary artery
attachment of graft to normal portion of coronary artery
inferior vena cava

vein graft from ascending aorta to coronary artery
descending aorta
vein graft
attachment of graft to normal portion of coronary artery
superior vena cava
narrowed arterio-sclerotic coronary artery
inferior vena cava

**Coronary Bypass Operation.** *This diagram illustrates how the narrowed arteriosclerotic segment of the coronary artery is bypassed by placing a vein graft from the aorta to a normal portion of the artery.*

### Can one do physical exercise after a coronary bypass operation?

Yes. As a matter of fact, it is advisable to exercise as this increases the flow of blood to the heart muscle. Of course one should avoid violent exercise and other stressful situations.

### Are there any other operations for coronary artery disease?

Yes, although some of them are still in an experimental stage. Some surgeons have cored out the narrow channel of the diseased coronary artery in an attempt to restitute its passageway. This operation is quite dangerous and is carried out while the patient is on the heart pump. Also, the coronary bypass operation has proved helpful to some patients with acute coronary thrombosis, if performed within six to eight hours after the onset of the acute attack.

### Are the results of surgery for coronary artery disease satisfactory?

The bypass operation has had remarkably satisfactory results in the great majority of cases. However, many people who have had coronary thrombosis do not, at the present time, lend themselves to this surgical procedure.

### What anesthesia is used for heart operations?

An inhalation anesthesia given through a tube placed in the trachea.

### Where is the incision made for heart operations?

Between the ribs that overlie the left side of the chest.

### Have methods been devised that permit bypassing of the heart during surgery?

Yes, there are heart pumps that can take the place of the heart during the time that it is undergoing surgery. This permits the surgeon to open the heart and operate upon it under direct vision and in a bloodless field.

### What is meant by "hypothermia" in heart surgery?

This means cooling the patient's body so that his heart action is slowed down markedly. This permits the surgeon to work upon the heart while it is more at rest and when blood flow is greatly curtailed.

### When will physicians recommend heart surgery?

a. When it is felt that the ultimate chances for survival are greater with surgery than without surgery.
b. When a person is leading an invalided, useless life and desires the chance for more normal living through heart surgery.
c. When a reasonable chance for cure or improvement exists through heart surgery and when the patient or his family fully understands the risks involved.

### Are heart operations lengthy?

Yes. Some heart operations take several hours to perform.

### Are heart operations painful?

No. Patients are usually quite comfortable during recovery from a heart operation.

### Do heart conditions tend to recur once they have been benefited by heart surgery?

No. The majority of successful results in heart surgery are of a permanent nature.

**Do all of the heart valves lend themselves to surgical repair?**

Yes. Formerly, only the mitral valve was operated upon when it was found to be damaged. Now the other major valves—such as the pulmonic, aortic, and the tricuspid valves—have been repaired or replaced successfully through surgery.

**Does the surgeon ever purposely stop the heart from beating while it is being repaired?**

Yes. This procedure can be carried out only when the patient is on the heart-lung pump so that there can be continued circulation of blood. The heart is sometimes stopped temporarily to allow more rapid and accurate repair of defective structures.

**Can people who have undergone successful heart operations return to a completely normal life?**

It may be necessary for some to restrict their physical activity even though the operation may have been extremely successful.

**Is it ever possible to reoperate upon a patient who has had a poor result from heart surgery?**

Yes. Many of those who underwent mitral valve surgery for rheumatic fever in the early days of this type of treatment have developed recurrences of their disease. These patients can now be successfully reoperated on, and the damaged valve can be repaired under direct vision with the heart open, or the valve can be replaced with an artificial valve. Patients whose coronary bypass grafts have closed down can frequently be reoperated with successful results.

**Are heart transplants practicable?**

The actual technique of heart transplantation is not very difficult and has been performed several hundred times at various cardiac surgery clinics throughout the world.

**Are heart transplants usually successful?**

Because of the rejection phenomenon most patients who have successfully undergone a heart transplant operation have not survived more than a few months or a year to two. However, better matching procedures and methods of combating the rejection reaction have been found. As a consequence, much better results have been achieved.

**Are heart transplants being done at the current time?**

Yes, but only upon patients who would not survive more than a few weeks or months unless they were operated. There are a few surgical clinics throughout the world where encouraging results are now being attained.

**What are the chances of surviving a heart transplantation?**

In one of the most expert cardiac surgical clinics, 50 percent of those operated upon have survived for a year, and some have lived for more than five years. It must be remembered, however, that *none* would have lived for more than a few weeks or months had they not received a new heart.

## CCU (Cardiac Care Unit)

*(See also Chapter 36 on ICU)*

**What is a CCU?**

A CCU is essentially an Intensive Care Unit (ICU) for patients with acute, serious heart ailments. In many hospitals, the CCU is located adjacent to the ICU, and some of the staff, especially nurses and technologists, serve both units. In most large hospitals, however, the units are separate.

**Do CCUs usually serve all types of cardiac patients who have acute problems?**

Yes, but by far the greatest number are those who have experienced an acute coronary thrombosis. Most of the other patients suffer from various degrees of heart failure.

**What are some of the other heart conditions that might be treated in a CCU?**

a. Pericarditis, an inflammation of the outer covering of the heart.
b. Acute myocarditis, an inflammation of the muscle wall of the heart.
c. Heart valve disease.
d. Endocarditis, an inflammation of the inner lining of the heart.
e. Injuries to the heart.
f. Uncontrollable irregularities in the heartbeat.

**How many beds are in a CCU?**

This will depend upon the size of the hospital and whether it has a large heart surgery service. Naturally, the larger the hospital and the more cardiac surgery that is performed, the more beds will be needed for the CCU. A general hospital of five hundred beds will probably have six to eight beds in its CCU.

**What are the advantages of a CCU over ordinary hospital care?**

In no other illness is it more essential to monitor patients constantly. Changes in heart action are so abrupt that response on the part of the medical and nursing staff must be instantaneous. Such a response is not possible except in a unit staffed twenty-four hours a day by specially trained personnel.

**Should a physician always be on duty and physically present in a CCU?**

Yes.

**What special equipment is in a CCU?**

a. An apparatus that connects the patient to a cardiogram and constantly records the electrical impulses on a video screen. The slightest change in these electrocardiographic tracings will be noted immediately by the physician and nursing staff so that immediate corrective treatment can be started.

b. An alarm system that alerts the CCU staff to changes in the patient's heartbeat or in the transmission of electrical impulses through the heart.

c. Electrical equipment to "shock" the heart back to a normal rhythm should a dangerous irregularity, or even cardiac arrest, develop.

d. Equipment and medications to combat sudden heart irregularities or cardiac arrest. This will include respirators, endotracheal tubes, apparatus for instituting cardiac massage, etc.

e. An intravenous line is always kept going in a patient in a CCU so that medications can be given directly into the bloodstream at anytime without waiting.

f. Catheters for insertion into veins, arteries, or even into the heart itself.

g. Apparatus to measure the *cardiac output.* (A failing heart is unable to pump sufficient blood through the body.)

h. Apparatus to take samples of blood for laboratory testing. This is important so that the blood gases and body chemistries can be monitored, and treatment can be begun for abnormalities if present.

**Have many lives been saved through establishment of the CCU?**

Yes. Tremendous numbers of cardiac patients owe their lives to their sojourn in a CCU.

**What determines when a patient may be transferred from the CCU to an ordinary hospital room?**

When the physicians responsible for the patient's care decide that his condition is *stable* and that he can sustain life without minute-to-minute monitoring and support. Stability would include a satisfactory blood pressure, a regular heartbeat, and evidence that the heart is mending. However, before the decision to transfer is made, the patient must maintain a satisfactory condition for a few days *without* the supportive measures that are available only in the CCU.

# CHAPTER 30

# HERNIA

## What is a hernia?

A hernia is a defect in a body compartment (cavity) that permits a structure to leave its normal confines and extend into a region where it does not belong. As an example, in a hernia of the diaphragm, the stomach may leave the abdominal cavity and enter the chest cavity through the diaphragmatic defect.

## What other name is used for hernia?

The word "rupture" is frequently used to denote a hernia.

## What causes hernias?

The great majority of hernias are caused by defects or weaknesses in the muscular and connective tissue structures that separate the various compartments or cavities of the body, such as the chest from the abdomen, or the abdomen from the limbs. Other hernias result from an injury that tears the muscular or connective tissue barriers at various exit points of the body compartments.

## Are many hernias present at birth?

Yes. A sizable number of children are born with hernias because of defects in development. These are commonly noted in the region of the navel (umbilical hernia) or in the groin (inguinal hernia).

## At what specific areas in the body are hernias most likely to occur?

At the various points where large structures—such as blood vessels or portions of the intestinal tract—leave or enter the various body cavities. At these sites there are loose tissues that, when placed under great strain, may separate and tear.

## What types of strain or injury are most likely to lead to a rupture?

a. Lifting heavy objects.
b. Sudden twists, pulls, or muscle strains.
c. Marked gains in weight, which cause an increase in intraabdominal pressure.
d. The growth of a large abdominal tumor, which displaces the organs.
e. Pregnancy, with its accompanying increase in intraabdominal pressure.
f. Chronic constipation, with its associated straining at stool.
g. Repeated attacks of coughing, which create sudden increases in intraabdominal pressure.

## How common are hernias?

Hernias are one of the most common of all conditions requiring surgery.

## Are men more prone than women to develop hernias?

Yes, if it is the type that results from physical strain and effort, such as hernia in the groin (inguinal hernia). Women are more likely to get hernias of the umbilical region (navel) as a result of pregnancy.

## Do hernias tend to run in families or to be inherited?

No, but the kind of muscular development that one possesses does tend to be inherited.

## What are the most common types of hernia?

a. Inguinal hernia. This is the most prevalent type of hernia. It occurs in the groin, often developing on both sides of the body. Such ruptures are called bilateral inguinal hernias.
b. Femoral hernia. This type is located just below the groin and occurs alongside the large blood vessels that extend from the trunk into the lower limbs.
c. Ventral hernia. This type usually occurs in the midline of the abdomen below the navel and often takes place as a result of the separation of the muscles of the abdominal wall following pregnancy.
d. Epigastric hernia. This type is located in the upper midline of the abdomen above the navel. Such hernias probably exist from birth but only become apparent in adult life.
e. Umbilical hernia. This is one of the most common forms of hernia and takes place in the region of the navel. Newborns and women who have had many pregnancies appear to be particularly prone to develop umbilical hernias.
f. Incisional hernia. This type of hernia occurs through an operative scar, either because of poor healing power of the wound or because infection has caused the tissues to heal inadequately. A hernia of this type can be located anywhere on the abdominal wall.
g. Recurrent hernia. About one in ten hernias will recur after surgical repair. This is called recurrent hernia.
h. Diaphragmatic hernia. This is an extremely common defect and takes place most frequently alongside the point where the esophagus (foodpipe) passes through the diaphragm from the chest into the abdomen. Other diaphragmatic hernias result from lack of development of the diaphragm or from rupture of the diaphragm due to an injury. These hernias of are characterized by abdominal organs—such as a portion of stomach, small intestine, or large bowel—entering the defect and lodging in the chest cavity. Hernias alongside the entrance of the esophagus into the abdominal cavity are known as *hiatus hernias*.

*(continued)*

i. Internal hernia. This is an unusual type of rupture in which an internal abdominal organ, usually the small intestine, enters crevices or subdivisions of the abdominal cavity where it does not belong.

j. Gluteal and lumbar hernias. These hernias are extremely rare and are due to defects in the musculature of the buttocks or back. The herniated organs will appear as bulges posteriorly in either the buttocks or the back.

**When is medical, rather than surgical, management advocated in the treatment of hernias?**

a. If a hernia has recurred two or more times after surgery and the patient's tissue structures appear to be poor, it is probably best not to attempt surgical repair a third or fourth time, as it will be met with failure in a large percentage of cases.

b. Patients who are markedly overweight should not be operated upon until they reduce, as repairs in these people are notoriously unsuccessful.

c. People with serious medical conditions, such as active tuberculosis or serious heart disease, are probably best treated without surgery.

d. People with small hernias who are in their seventies or eighties are perhaps best treated medically unless the hernia causes severe symptoms.

**What is the medical treatment for hernias?**

The wearing of a support or truss to hold the hernial contents within the abdominal cavity.

**As a general rule, should trusses be worn for prolonged periods of time before surgery is carried out?**

No. Trusses tend to weaken the structures with which they are in constant contact. Therefore they should not be worn for more than a few weeks prior to surgery.

**Why isn't the wearing of a truss advised—rather than surgery—in all hernias?**

Because trusses do not cure her-

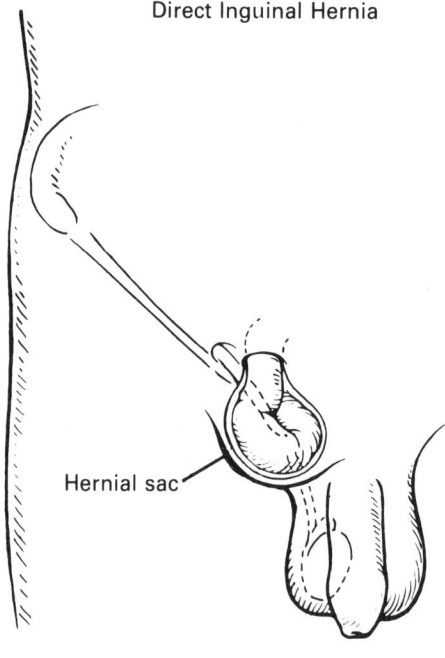

Direct Inguinal Hernia

Hernial sac

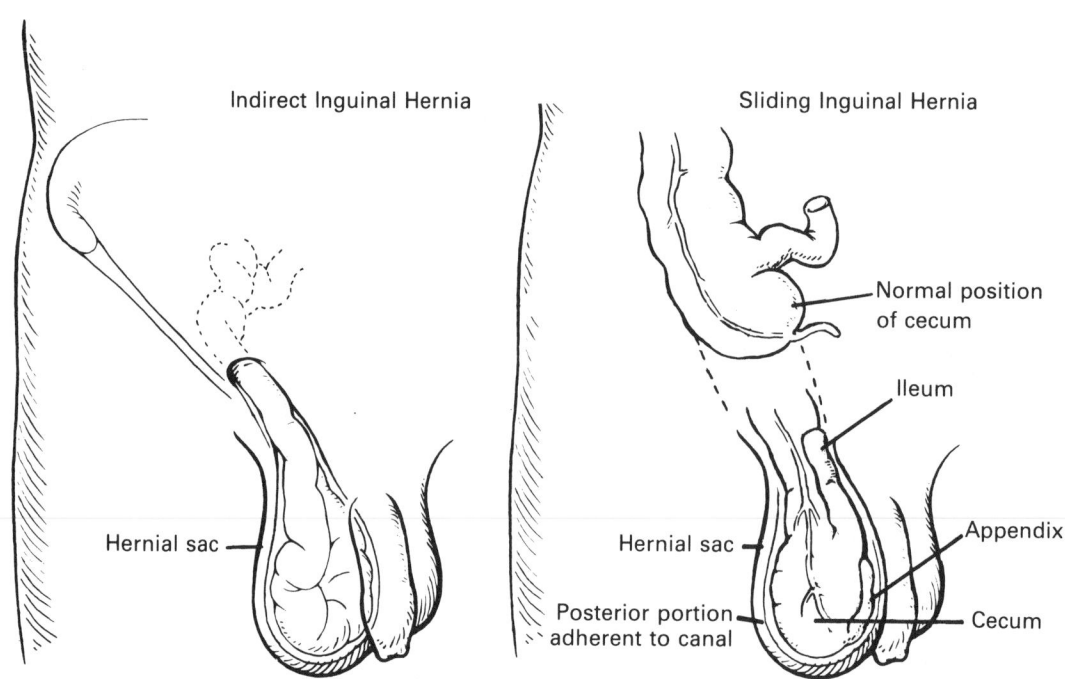

**Inguinal Hernia.** *The accompanying diagrams on this and the opposite page show various types of inguinal herniae, or hernias, which are located in the groin. If the patient is in satisfactory general health, surgery should be performed for their repair. Failure to undergo surgery may result in a loop of bowel becoming caught within the hernial sac, thus producing bowel strangulation, a very serious condition.*

Indirect Inguinal Hernia

Hernial sac

Sliding Inguinal Hernia

Normal position of cecum

Ileum

Appendix

Hernial sac

Cecum

Posterior portion adherent to canal

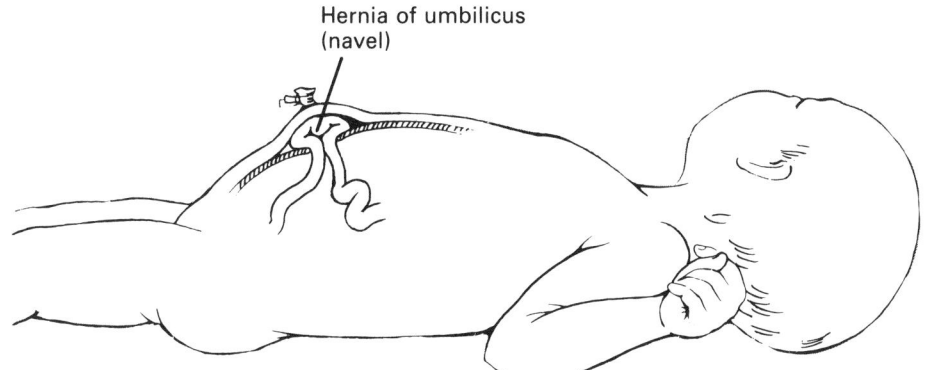

Hernia of umbilicus (navel)

*Umbilical Hernia or Hernia of the Navel. Many children are born with small umbilical hernias. The majority of these will heal by themselves within the first year of life. If the hernia persists, it is advisable to have it repaired surgically. The operation for repair of an umbilical hernia is a simple, safe procedure.*

nias. They merely hold the hernial contents in place. As people get older and hernias enlarge, trusses work less satisfactorily.

**Are any dangers involved in neglecting to operate upon hernias?**

Definitely, yes. The chance of strangulation of bowel is always present, and such a situation is dangerous to life.

**Is the injection treatment satisfactory in the treatment of hernias?**

No. This method has been abandoned as dangerous and ineffectual.

**Do hernias tend to disappear by themselves?**

No. The only hernias that ever disappear by themselves are the small hernias of the navel seen in newborns, and an occasional small inguinal hernia in a newborn.

**How effective is surgery in the treatment of hernias?**

The vast majority of hernias can be repaired successfully by restoring and reinforcing the torn structures, replacing the extruded structures into their normal anatomical location, and by removing the outpouching of abdominal tissue (peritoneum), which makes up the hernial sac.

**When is the best time to operate upon hernias?**

Hernia operations are usually elec-

tive procedures, and the time for their repair can be chosen by the patient to suit his convenience. It must be remembered, however, that most hernias tend to enlarge; the larger the hernia, the more difficult it is to repair and the greater the chance of subsequent recurrence.

**When is a hernia operation an emergency procedure?**

When the hernia strangulates, a condition in which an organ such as the intestine or bowel is caught in the hernial sac and its blood supply is interfered with. Under such circumstances, the patient must be operated upon immediately! Failure to do so will lead to gangrene of the strangulated hernial contents and possible death from peritonitis.

**Will surgeons delay operations in elective cases if the patient is overweight?**

Yes. If the patient is too stout, the repair of the hernia is similar to an attempt at stuffing too much clothing into a small valise. If such a valise does close, the great pressure from within is likely to pop it open!

**Are hernia operations dangerous?**

No. They are rarely followed by complications, except when the operation has been carried out for strangulation. In such cases, gangrenous bowel or intestine may be encountered, and this will entail extensive serious surgery for removal of the gangrenous portions.

**What procedure is carried out when gangrenous intestine or bowel is found in a hernia?**

The gangrenous portions of bowel are removed. This is a most serious and complicated operation with many dangers. The mortality rate in these cases has been lowered remarkably by improved surgical techniques and the use of antibiotic drugs, but the procedure still constitutes one of the most formidable in abdominal surgery.

**Are hernia operations particularly painful?**

No, except for pain in the operative region for a few days after the surgery has been performed.

**Are operations for diaphragmatic hernias particularly dangerous?**

No, but these are more extensive procedures than those for hernias in the abdominal region.

**How are diaphragmatic hernias repaired?**

Through an abdominal incision, one of three procedures may be carried out:
a. Closure of the opening of the diaphragm with sutures.
b. Wrapping the fundus (top portion) of the stomach around the lower end of the esophagus. This is known as *fundal plication.*
c. Insertion of a silicone ring, shaped like a doughnut, around the lower end of the esophagus so as to plug the opening in the diaphragm.

**Is repair of a diaphragmatic or hiatus hernia usually successful?**

Yes, in the great majority of cases.

**How long do hernia operations take to perform?**

The simple inguinal hernias can be repaired in a half to three-quarters of an hour. The more extensive hernias, such as the diaphragmatic or the incarcerated ones, in which the herniated organs are firmly attached to the sac wall, may take several hours to repair.

**What kind of anesthesia is used?**

For hernias below the level of the navel, general, epidural, local, or spinal anesthesia is most often employed. Diaphragmatic hernias and hernias in the upper abdomen are operated upon only under general inhalation anesthesia.

**How soon after the operation can the patient get out of bed?**

In most cases, the patient can get out of bed on the day of, or the day following, surgery.

**How long does one have to stay in the hospital following an ordinary hernia operation?**

Approximately four days. However, it is possible for some patients to leave the hospital a day or two after surgery; others who are older or who had a complicated hernia repair may require seven to ten days of hospitalization.

**What is the "Canadian" method of hernia repair?**

It is a slight variation in the technique used in numerous other types of hernia repair.

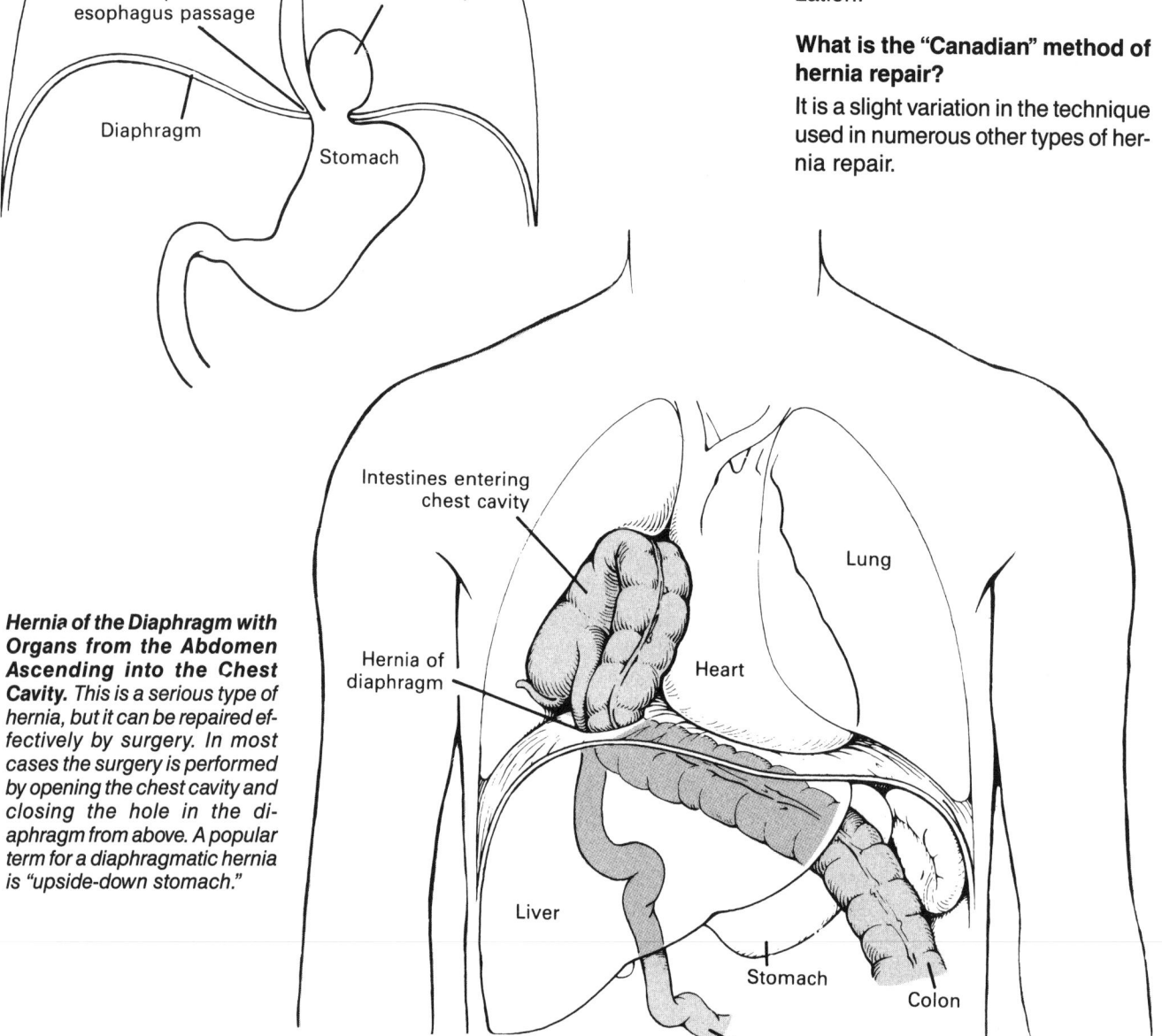

*Hernia of the Diaphragm with Organs from the Abdomen Ascending into the Chest Cavity. This is a serious type of hernia, but it can be repaired effectively by surgery. In most cases the surgery is performed by opening the chest cavity and closing the hole in the diaphragm from above. A popular term for a diaphragmatic hernia is "upside-down stomach."*

**Are results of the "Canadian" operation superior to other methods?**

The results are excellent provided the repair is carried out on an appropriate patient and that it is done carefully. Other methods, performed carefully on appropriately selected patients, obtain the same good results.

**How soon after the "Canadian" type of hernia repair can the patient leave the hospital?**

In many cases, the day following surgery. However, it must be kept in mind that if a patient has heart disease, difficulty with his respiratory tract, problems in urinating postoperatively, or other complications, he may have to be hospitalized for several days or longer.

**Can coughing or sneezing cause a recurrence of the hernia?**

No, despite the fact that patients often feel as though they have ripped open all of their stitches when they cough.

**What are the chances of recurrence following surgery?**

More than 90 percent of hernias are cured permanently after surgery. Most recurrences are seen in elderly people or in those who have particularly fragile muscle and connective tissues.

**How long does it take for the average hernia wound to heal?**

Seven days.

**What precautions should be taken to prevent hernia recurrence?**

a. The patient should not permit himself to gain a large amount of weight.

b. Pushing, pulling, or lifting heavy objects (those over forty to fifty pounds) should be avoided whenever possible.
c. All strenuous exercise should be avoided for a period of four to six months.

**If hernias do recur, what procedure is indicated?**

About four out of five recurrent hernias can be cured by reoperation.

**Should patients who have been operated upon for hernias wear trusses or abdominal supports?**

No. Surgical repair is sufficient protection.

**Is it common for patients to have slight pain, numbness, or tingling in the wound or along the scrotum for several weeks or months after hernia operations?**

Yes. This happens occasionally but will disappear spontaneously.

**Is sex life affected by the repair of an inguinal hernia?**

No. The testicles and the other genital structures are not interfered with when hernia repair is carried out.

**How soon after birth can an infant have a hernia repaired?**

Newborns withstand surgery exceptionally well. If the hernia is large or if there is a danger of bowel strangulation, it is preferable to operate upon these children during the first few weeks or months of life.

**Do hernias in the newborn tend to occur in both groins?**

Yes. It is a common practice to operate upon both sides in these children, even though a hernia may be felt on only one side. Two out of three infants who have a hernia on one side will also have one on the other, though the second hernia may not be discovered on physical examination.

**Will operating on both sides increase the risk of surgery?**

No.

**Can normal physical activity ever be resumed by someone who has undergone a hernia repair?**

Most certainly, yes!

**Can a woman permit herself to become pregnant after a hernia operation?**

Yes, within a few months after surgical recovery.

**How soon after a hernia operation can one do the following:**

Bathe:
    Seven days.
Walk out on the street:
    Seven days.
Walk up and down stairs:
    Seven days.
Perform household duties:
    Three to four weeks.
Drive a car:
    Five to six weeks.
Resume sexual relations:
    Four weeks.
Return to work:
    Six to eight weeks.
Resume all physical activities:
    Three to six months.

**How often should one return for a checkup following a hernia operation?**

Approximately every six months, for a period of two years.

CHAPTER 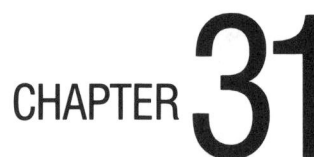 **31**

# IMMUNIZATIONS AND VACCINATIONS

*(See also Chapter 7 on Allergy; Chapter 18 on Contagious Diseases; Chapter 34 on Infectious and Virus Diseases; Chapter 38 on Laboratory (Pathology) Tests and Procedures; Chapter 74 on Tuberculosis)*

**What is active immunity?**

t is the protection afforded by having the disease or by receiving an injection of a substance that stimulates the body to produce long-lasting, protective antibodies.

**What diseases afford permanent immunity after one has had them?**

Measles, scarlet fever, diphtheria, German measles, mumps, chickenpox, and whooping cough. Typhoid fever, smallpox, and poliomyelitis also give permanent immunity if one has had them.

**What is meant by passive, or inherited, immunity?**

This is the type of immunity one inherits at birth if the mother has had the disease sometime previously. The immunity is passed through the placenta and into the child's bloodstream. This type of immunity lasts only a few months. Passive immunity can also be accomplished by the injection of convalescent serum from someone who has just recently had the disease or by the injection of gamma globulin for selected illnesses. Breast milk also confers limited passive protection against certain conditions.

**Is gamma globulin effective in preventing measles, German measles, infectious hepatitis, or polio if one has been exposed to these diseases?**

Unfortunately, gamma globulin does not often give protection, but it may cause the disease to be milder if it is contracted.

**How long does passive, or inherited, immunity usually last?**

About three to six months. In some instances, as long as nine months.

**What is the reason for creating passive immunity if it lasts for only a short time?**

It will tide the patient over a period when an epidemic may be in progress and thus spare him from contracting the disease.

**Are convalescent serums useful in treatment of contagious diseases?**

In general, no. However, convalescent serum does have some effectiveness in the treatment of whooping cough.

**What is the best immunization schedule for infants?**

It is best to give the triple vaccine (DPT) against diphtheria, whooping cough, and tetanus at the second, fourth, and sixth month; polio oral vaccine also at the second, fourth, and sixth month; and measles, mumps, and German measles vaccines at fifteen months. Smallpox vaccination is no longer advocated or required.

**Can this immunization schedule be changed without adversely affecting the child?**

Yes. It is often varied at the doctor's discretion.

**What are so-called "booster shots?**

These are additional injections given a year or two after the original immunization in order to maintain immunity.

**Is the effectiveness of these injections lost if the interval is prolonged because of an illness the child may have?**

In general, no. The intervals may be prolonged for several weeks or even months without affecting the value of immunizations.

**Should inoculations against disease be given if the child is sick from another cause?**

No. Injections should be postponed when the child has another illness.

**What are the reactions to injections against these contagious diseases?**

Usually there are none, or they are very mild. Occasionally, one notices irritability, fever, restlessness, lack of appetite, or vomiting. These symptoms do not last for very long.

**Are there any local reactions in the area where injections are given?**

In some cases, there is redness and swelling in the area, but this usually passes within a day or two.

**Is it common for a small lump to appear at the site where an injection was given?**

Yes, but this has no significance and will disappear within a few days.

**What is the treatment for reactions to immunization in children?**

A small dose of aspirin or similar medication as prescribed by your doctor.

**On what part of the body are injections usually given?**

In young infants, on the outer thigh; in older children, on the upper arm.

**Who usually gives immunization injections?**

Your physician or his regular nurse-assistant.

**If there is a marked reaction to an injection, is it wise to inform your physician?**

Yes. This information may influence him to reduce the dose of the next injection or to spread the series of injections over four to five injections instead of the usual two or three.

**Is it ever necessary to discontinue immunization injections entirely?**

If the child is highly allergic to the material on which the live virus is grown, it is wise to skin test the child before administering the virus.

**Are there ever any harmful effects from immunization injections?**

Just one or two patients among millions may have a serious reaction. The beneficial effects far outweigh any possible harm that may come from immunization injections.

**Can allergic people be given immunization injections?**

Yes, but smaller amounts may have to be given at each injection.

**Is there any modification of this schedule for older children or adults?**

Yes. In older children, a special vaccine containing only the diphtheriaand tetanus vaccine is used instead of the DPT vaccine. Also, when boosters are given to older children who have already had DPT vaccine, the boosters should contain only DT vaccine, with no pertussis.

## THE SCHICK TEST

**What is the Schick test?**

This is a test to determine whether a child is immune or has developed an immunity (by injections) to diphtheria. The Schick test is rarely done nowadays.

**How is the Schick test done?**

A small amount of toxin is injected into the skin of the forearm, and the

reaction is noted two to four days later. If nothing appears on the arm, the test is called negative, and the child is judged to be immune to diphtheria.

**What is a positive Schick test?**

If there is an area of redness and thickening of the skin the size of a dime, it is called a positive Schick test and shows that the child is not immune.

**Does the Schick test cause the child to become sick in any way?**

No.

**What should be done if there is a positive Schick test?**

The child should be given the complete course of injections against diphtheria.

## THE TUBERCULIN TEST

**What is the tuberculin test?**

It is a test done to find whether the child has any tuberculosis germs in his body.

**What tuberculosis tests are available?**

a. The intradermal, or Mantoux, test.
b. The tine test.
These tests determine sensitivity to the germ of tuberculosis. They tell whether there have been any germs in the body, not necessarily whether they have done any damage. Only a chest x ray can do that.

**How is the tine test done?**

With a small instrument consisting of a plastic handle that has four small points, or tines, coated with testing material. These points are pressed against the forearm for a second or two. A few days later the doctor will look at the arm to see if there is swelling where the test was given.

**Is this test painful?**

No.

**What does the test show?**

If the test is negative, there will be no swelling. This means there are no tuberculosis germs in the child's body.

**What if the test is positive?**

Then a chest x ray should be taken to show whether or not the tuberculosis germs have done any harm to the body. In a very young child, a positive test usually means active tuberculosis requiring treatment. This is not so in an older child.

**At what age should the test be done?**

The first test may be done at twelve months of age, then every year or two thereafter. It is important to recognize the disease early, when it can be cured and prevented from spreading to other parts of the body.

**What about the family of a child with a positive test?**

The other members of the family should be checked to make sure no one has tuberculosis.

## SMALLPOX VACCINATION

**Should all children in this country be vaccinated against smallpox?**

No. Smallpox vaccinations are no longer recommended, as the risk of complications from the vaccine has become greater than the risk of contracting smallpox. The disease has been almost eradicated from the earth. Of course, vaccination should be carried out if an outbreak of smallpox occurs in the vicinity.

**Where is smallpox vaccine best given?**

It is best to vaccinate on the outer surface of the upperarm, usually the left arm, near the shoulder.

**Can people be vaccinated on the thigh?**

Yes, but there is more danger of contamination by stool or urine in that area.

**Is there any immediate reaction to smallpox vaccination?**

No.

**When does the positive reaction to smallpox vaccination set in?**

In four to five days a red spot will appear and become larger and will form a blister. At about the eighth to ninth day, the blister is quite large and is surrounded by an area of redness the size of a quarter or half-dollar. Thereafter the blister dries up, leaving a crust, and the redness begins to subside and disappear within about two weeks after the original vaccination.

**Is smallpox vaccination accompanied by fever and other signs of illness?**

Yes, during the second week, when the vaccination reacts and is at its height. Temperatures as high as 103° to 104°F. may be recorded.

**What is the treatment for the vaccination reaction?**

It is wise to give aspirin in doses recommended by your doctor. Cool sponges to the body may be given if the temperature is high.

**Are there any other signs of severe vaccination reaction?**

Yes. There may be swelling in the armpit near the site of the vaccination. This does not necessarily indicate that an infection has set in.

**If the vaccination seems to be exceptionally red, swollen, and painful, should the patient see his doctor?**

Yes.

**Does the patient ever develop a rash from smallpox vaccination?**

In a small percentage of cases, a mild rash may appear. This will disappear as the reaction subsides.

**Is it necessary to keep a dressing on the vaccination?**

No. In fact, it is preferable not to have a dressing.

**Should a vaccination shield be used?**

Definitely not.

**Should the vaccination area be bathed?**

No. It is preferable to keep the area dry until the inflammation has subsided completely and a firm crust has formed.

**Can a child be bathed and the arm wet when the scab on a vaccination is dry?**

Yes.

**Does one ever encounter secondary vaccinations?**

Yes. Sometimes there may be a small blister near the original large vaccination. This will cause no harm.

**How long does it usually take for the scab to fall off?**

Between two and three weeks. It is best to allow it to fall off by itself.

**Does it do any harm if the vaccination scab is rubbed off accidentally?**

No.

**Does the vaccination usually leave a large scar?**

No.

**What should be done if the smallpox vaccination does not "take"?**

It should be done over again, after a wait of two to four weeks from the original vaccination.

**Is it necessary to continue vaccinations until there is a positive "take"?**

Yes, if vaccination is a requirement for travel.

**Should a baby be vaccinated when he has a cold?**

No.

**Should a baby with eczema be vaccinated?**

No. Even if the child has had a rash or a skin condition for a period of months or years, the vaccination should be delayed. *Never* vaccinate a child while he has a rash!

**Should a baby be vaccinated if another child in the family has eczema?**

No. It is easy for the virus to be transmitted from the baby to the other child, with possible serious consequences.

**Do vaccinations often become infected?**

No. This is a common misconception.

**Are there ever any convulsions from vaccination?**

Rarely. They are caused by the high fever accompanying some vaccinations.

**What are the chances of encephalitis (inflammation of the brain) from smallpox vaccination?**

This is extremely rare, occurring perhaps once in 500,000 vaccinations.

**Does this encephalitis occur in young infants?**

Not usually. It occurs more often in children who are vaccinated for the first time after they are five years of age.

**Do adults ever get encephalitis as a result of smallpox vaccination?**

No.

**Should schools permit children to enter who have not been vaccinated?**

In this country, schools no longer require vaccination prior to admission. This, however, is not the case in certain other countries.

**How effective is smallpox vaccination?**

If there has been a positive "take," it

will protect completely against this disease.

## POLIOMYELITIS VACCINATION

**Should polio vaccination be given if a patient is ill?**
No. It is best to wait until he has recovered from any illness.

**Is polio vaccine safe?**
Yes. It is completely safe.

**Can polio vaccine produce poliomyelitis?**
No!

**How effective is polio vaccination?**
It is considered to be tremendously effective and will prevent the disease in more than 95 percent of those vaccinated. Those who may get it despite vaccination will get a very mild form of the disease, often without paralysis.

**Can allergic people be given polio vaccine?**
Yes. There have been no serious effects in allergic patients.

**Are there usually reactions to polio vaccination?**
No.

**Are any special precautions necessary after polio vaccination?**
No.

**Does polio vaccine contain penicillin?**
No. The Salk-type vaccine used to, but the Sabin oral vaccine does not. Today the Sabin vaccine is used almost exclusively.

**Should people who are sensitive to penicillin be given the oral polio vaccine?**
Yes.

**Is it permissible to give polio vaccine at the same time as other vaccines?**
Yes.

**Is it permissible to vaccinate against polio at any time of the year?**
Yes.

**How soon after a full course of oral polio vaccine does immunity develop?**
Within a period of several weeks.

**Is it necessary after the three oral doses of polio vaccine to repeat the course within the next year or two?**
No. It is thought that the full course of oral vaccine will produce a permanent immunity. However, just to be safe, some pediatricians do prescribe a second course of vaccine a year or two after the original one.

**Should older children and adults be given the polio vaccine?**
Yes. Only in this way can the disease be totally and permanently eradicated as an epidemic menace.

**If a person has already had polio, will he benefit from vaccination?**
Yes. The vaccine will increase his immunity. Also, he may also have immunity to only one strain of the polio virus; the vaccine will give him immunity to other strains as well.

**Should polio vaccination be withheld if the child is going to have his tonsils removed?**
No.

**Is there any way to tell if someone is immune to polio before the vaccine is given?**
Yes, but the procedure is not practical for everyday use. It is a very expensive test and takes a long time to perform. Also, there are only a few laboratories in the country equipped to perform such a test.

## MEASLES VACCINATIONS

**Are there satisfactory methods of immunizing against measles?**
Yes, measles vaccine is effective in well over 90 percent of cases.

**At what age should measles vaccination be carried out?**
When the child is about fifteen months old. Older children who have never had measles should receive the vaccine no matter what their age.

**How long does the immunity to measles last?**
Permanently.

**How is measles vaccination carried out?**
By injection of a weakened (attenuated) live virus.

**What is the reaction to measles vaccination among children?**
In about one out of ten cases, a fever, upper respiratory congestion, and a slight rash appear within seven to twelve days after vaccination. Recovery is prompt within two to three days.

**Are there any children who may not be suitable for measles vaccine?**
Yes. Those who are allergic to egg may develop a severe reaction. They should undergo skin testing before attempting vaccination.

**What should be done if a child does have a reaction to the measles vaccine?**
Small doses of aspirin or a similar medication may be given for a day or two.

**May the vaccine be given when a child who has not had the disease is exposed to a case of measles?**
Yes. It would be wise under such circumstances to give the live vaccine along with the gamma globulin. In that way the attenuated virus may give immunity and prevent the growth of the virus caught from the

other child. In any event, the gamma globulin would insure that the disease would be very mild even if the active caught virus did gain the ascendancy.

### Is it necessary to give measles vaccine to a child who has had measles?

No. If you are sure the child has had the disease, he is permanently immune. However, if there is any doubt, there is no harm in giving him the measles vaccine.

## GERMAN MEASLES IMMUNIZATION

### Should people be vaccinated against German measles?

Yes. German measles vaccine is very effective. It should be given to all children and to women of child-bearing age who have not had the disease. Women must not be pregnant at the time of vaccination, and they must be warned to avoid becoming pregnant for two months after being vaccinated with the German measles vaccine. The main purpose of immunization is prevention of birth defects in the unborn child.

## MUMPS IMMUNIZATION

### Is there any vaccine against mumps?

Yes. A very effective mumps vaccine is available and should be given to all children who are not allergic to eggs.

## TYPHOID FEVER VACCINATION

### When is typhoid fever immunization given?

When the child or adult is going into an area where there is danger of exposure to typhoid fever. This applies particularly to certain foreign countries.

### What is the routine immunization against typhoid fever?

A series of three injections into the skin or beneath the skin, given one to two weeks apart.

### What vaccine is used?

Usually a vaccine containing the dead typhoid and paratyphoid germs.

### Are injections against typhoid fever effective?

Yes.

### Are there any reactions to typhoid immunization?

Yes. The arm may become very red and swollen, and there may be fever for a few days.

### What is the best treatment for the reaction to typhoid immunization?

Aspirin and bed rest.

### Are booster injections necessary after typhoid immunization?

Yes. One injection a year of a small dose of the vaccine should be given if a patient is again going to an area where there is danger of contracting typhoid.

## OTHER IMMUNIZATIONS

### Are there any effective immunizations against the common cold?

No.

### Is there any immunization against tuberculosis?

Yes, there is a vaccine called BCG. (See Chapter 74, on Tuberculosis.)

### Is vaccination against tuberculosis effective?

There is great controversy on this subject; the vaccine is not generally used in this country.

### When is tuberculosis vaccination advised?

In certain situations when the in-

dividual has been exposed for long periods of time to a known case of tuberculosis, it will be advised.

### Is there an effective immunization against rabies?

Yes.

### When is vaccination against rabies given?

When an individual has been bitten by any animal that is suspected of being rabid, such as a dog, cat, fox, squirrel, rabbit, rat, wolf, etc.

### Are rabies immunization injections given in every case of a dog bite?

No. They are given when the dog is known or suspected of being diseased. The dog must be sent to a place where he can be held and examined for a few days to note whether he develops rabies. If the dog is found to be healthy, no immunization is necessary.

### If the animal that has caused the bite cannot be found, should the injections be given?

Yes, as a safeguard.

### How is rabies inoculation carried out?

By daily injections for fourteen days.

### Is there any effective treatment for rabies once it has developed?

No. There is a very high mortality rate once a child or adult has developed the disease.

### What is the best local treatment for a dog bite?

Thorough washing of the area with soap and water for at least five to ten minutes.

### If the skin has not been broken by a dog bite, is there any danger of infection?

Not usually, but the area should still be washed thoroughly with soap and water for ten to twenty minutes.

**Should a dog bite be reported to the authorities?**

Yes. In almost all communities, it is the law that such bites be reported to the police or to the board of health.

**Does it make any difference where the animal has bitten the patient?**

Yes. The closer to the head the bite is, the more serious it is.

**Are there any dangers from giving rabies inoculations?**

No, but it is a painful process to have to endure.

**Are there any effective vaccinations against typhus fever, cholera, yellow fever, and the plague?**

Yes. There are very effective vaccinations against all of these diseases.

**When should vaccinations against typhus fever, cholera, yellow fever, or the plague be given?**

Only when one is traveling to an area where there is danger of contracting these diseases.

**What immunization procedures are necessary for travel to foreign countries?**

If one is traveling to Europe or well-developed countries in the Orient such as Japan, no special immunization procedures are now mandatory. Formerly, it was necessary for a traveler to be vaccinated against smallpox, typhoid and paratyphoid fever, and tetanus prior to departure for a foreign land. However, the general level of public health in most developed countries today is as high as it is in the United States. Therefore these vaccinations are not essential. To be perfectly safe, however, it is wise to check with the local department of health for the most recent requirements. And in terms of reentry, the United States no longer requires a smallpox vaccination unless one is returning from an area where cases of smallpox have been reported.

**Where can one get additional information on immunizations necessary for foreign travel?**

The United States Department of Health and Human Services and the Public Health Service issue a booklet giving exact details of immunization procedures advisable for travelers. The World Health Organization issues a standard certificate that can be filled in by your physician. It lists the injections and the dates on which they have been given.

## IMMUNIZATION CHART
**Present accepted ideal schedule for infants and children**

| | |
|---|---|
| 2–3 months | First DPT (diphtheria, pertussis, tetanus) and Sabin oral vaccine |
| 4–5 months | Second DPT and second Sabin vaccine |
| 5–6 months | Third DPT and third Sabin vaccine. If desired, the DPT may be given along with the polio vaccine, or the polio vaccine may be given separately |
| 12 months | Tuberculin test |
| 15 months | Measles, mumps, and German measles vaccinations |
| 18 months | DPT, polio vaccine boosters |
| 4–6 years | DPT booster and tuberculin test |

**Additional boosters:** Tetanus—after injury from rusty object or one contaminated by dirt. Such additional boosters may be advisable for any suspicious injury causing a puncture wound if the last tetanus immunization is more than three years old.

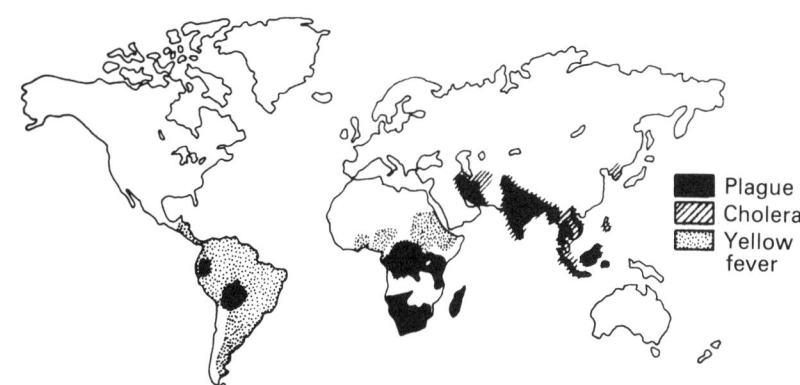

**Areas of Plague, Cholera, and Yellow Fever.** *If one intends traveling to places where these diseases are prevalent, it is necessary to be immunized against them. Statistics were unavailable for the People's Republic of China at the time this chart was prepared.*

## IMMUNIZATION AND VACCINATION CHART

| Disease | Material Used | When Given | Number of Injections | Spacing of Injections |
|---------|---------------|------------|----------------------|----------------------|
| MUMPS | Mumps vaccine | 15 months of age | 1 | . . . |
| CHICKENPOX | None | . . . | . . . | . . . |
| INFECTIOUS HEPATITIS | Gamma globulin | Exposure to case of infectious hepatitis | 1 | . . . |
| SCARLET FEVER | Penicillin | Exposure to case of scarlet fever | Oral medi- cation | . . . |
| RABIES | Rabies vaccine | Following suspicious animal bite | 14 | Daily |
| CHOLERA | Cholera vaccine | *For foreign travel | 2–3 | 1 week |
| TYPHUS FEVER | Typhus vaccine | *For foreign travel | 2–3 | 1 week |
| YELLOW FEVER | Yellow fever vaccine | *For foreign travel | 1 | . . . |
| PLAGUE | Plague vaccine | *For foreign travel | 2–3 | 1 week |
| INFLUENZA | Influenza vaccine | During epidemics | 2 | 1 week |
| ROCKY MOUNTAIN SPOTTED FEVER | Rocky Mountain spotted fever vaccine | For persons exposed to tick in suspicious areas | 3 | 1 week |
| DIPHTHERIA | Diphtheria fluid toxoid | Infancy and childhood, or upon exposure | 3 | 1 month apart |
| WHOOPING COUGH | Pertussis vaccine | Infancy and childhood, or upon exposure | 3 | 1 month apart |
| TETANUS | Tetanus fluid toxoid | Infancy and childhood, or after injury | 3 | 1 month apart |
| SMALLPOX | Cowpox virus | Infancy, childhood, and adulthood | 1 | . . . |
| POLIOMYELITIS | Sabin polio vaccine | 2, 4, and 6 months of age | No injections; 3 oral doses | 2 months apart |
| TYPHOID FEVER | Typhoid, paratyhoid vaccine | At any age when traveling to suspicious area | 3 | 1–4 weeks |
| MEASLES | Measles vaccine | 9–12 months, or any time thereafter | 3 of killed virus—1 of live virus | 1 month apart |
| GERMAN MEASLES | German Measles vaccine | Childhood, and adult- hood for females of child- bearing age | 1 | . . . |

*Needed only in traveling to countries where these diseases are present—as in Asia, Africa, and some parts of Europe, Central and South America.

| Reactions | Duration of Immunity | "Recall" or Booster Injections | Remarks |
|---|---|---|---|
| **Not to be given to egg-sensitive people | Probably lifelong | ... | ... |
| ... | ... | ... | ... |
| None | 4–6 weeks | None, except where exposure is prolonged | ... |
| None | ... | Same procedure if re-exposed | May give penicillin only in adequate dosage |
| Slight | 3–6 months | If bitten again after 3 months | May not need full series if dog is found not infected |
| Slight | Short | Every 6–12 months | ... |
| Slight | Short | Annually | ... |
| **May be moderate | Long | Every 6 years | ... |
| Slight | Short | every 6–12 months | ... |
| Slight | Short | ... | ... |
| **Moderate | Short | Annually | ... |
| None to slight | Varies | First booster—after 1 year; second booster at 4–6 years; then every 10 years. | All three (diphtheria, tetanus, and whooping cough) may be combined in a single injection—in young children only. After 6 years of age, only diphtheria and tetanus (DT) are given |
| Slight to moderate | Varies | | |
| None to slight | Varies | | |
| Moderate | Several years | Every 5 years for foreign travel | Smallpox vaccination no longer required in most countries |
| None | ... | Not necessary | ... |
| Moderate | 1–3 years | Every 1–3 years | ... |
| None, or very slight | Long | None | May be given with or without gamma globulin |
| None | Probably lifelong | None | Females of childbearing age must not be pregnant or become so for 2 months after vaccination. |

**Must be careful of reactions in allergic people sensitive to eggs.

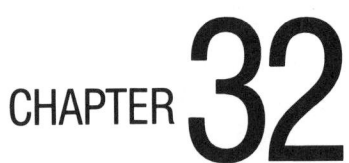

CHAPTER 32

# INFANT AND CHILDHOOD DISEASES

*See also Chapter 17 on Child Behavior; Chapter 18 on Contagious Diseases; Chapter 33 on Infant Feeding; Chapter 47 on the Newborn Child)*

### What is croup (catarrhal laryngitis)?

It is an inflammatory disease of the respiratory passage involving the larynx, or voice box, and occurring mostly in children between the ages of one and five.

### What causes croup?

It is caused by a virus infection in most cases. Bacterial organisms also may be the causative agent.

### Does diphtheria cause croup?

Yes. There is a type of diphtheritic croup in which a membrane is formed in the larynx and trachea.

### How can croup be recognized?

The first symptoms are difficulty in breathing, hoarseness or loss of voice, coughing, crowing, and a barking sound similar to that made by a seal. There is a slight elevation of temperature in the average case, but it may be considerably elevated in the severe case.

### When does croup usually start?

At night. It tends to subside during the day and then to become worse again the next night.

### How long does the average case of croup last?

About one to three days.

### What is the treatment for croup?

a. Steam inhalations or a cold mist vaporizer.
b. Keeping the room moist with a vaporizer.

### Is there any way to prevent croup?

No.

### Does croup tend to recur?

Yes. Children who have once had an attack of croup may have repeated attacks with each respiratory infection during the next two to three years.

### Do the severe forms of croup require special treatment?

Yes. It is imperative that children with severe croup be seen by a doctor immediately, because in the severe case there is a great tendency toward obstruction of breathing.

### What should be done in severe cases of croup?

Where there is obstruction to the breathing that is not relieved by mist, it may be necessary for the doctor to admit the child to the hospital for an immediate tracheotomy.

### What is a tracheotomy?

It is an opening made into the windpipe to allow the child to breathe.

### Is there any other treatment for severe croup?

Yes. Many cases will be benefited by giving oxygen.

### What special diet should be given to a child with croup?

It is preferable to give increased fluids and soft foods.

### Are antibiotics effective against croup?

No.

### Is there any effective vaccine against croup?

No.

### Are there permanent aftereffects of croup?

Usually not. The great majority of cases make a complete recovery.

### Is it necessary to quarantine a child with croup?

No, but the disease is somewhat contagious, and the same precautions should be taken as for any ordinary upper respiratory infection.

### Does croup tend to occur more often in allergic children?

Yes.

### Does it occur more often during ons particular season?

Yes. It occurs more frequently in the winter and fall months.

### When may the child be allowed out of doors after recovery from croup?

When fever abates and the child returns to his usual level of activity.

## CELIAC DISEASE

### What is celiac disease?

It is a disturbance of the digestive system chiefly involving the digestion of starches and fats.

### What causes this disease?

A failure or deficiency of some of the enzymes involved in the digestive process. It has been found that the digestion of gluten products is impaired, particularly the gliadin protein. This is found in wheat and rye products.

### How often does celiac disease occur?

About one in a hundred children has this condition.

### Does it tend to run in families?

Yes.

**Is there any relationship to allergies?**

Yes. We seem to find more of these cases in families that have a history of allergies. Some of the children with this condition later manifest allergic symptoms as well.

**When does celiac disease become evident?**

Usually during the first year of life. The baby may appear to be normal at first and then begin to show signs of this condition between six and eighteen months of age.

**How does this condition manifest itself?**

By alternate periods of diarrhea and constipation, with large, bulky, foul-smelling stools. The infant fails to gain weight and may even lose weight. The abdomen becomes large and distended, the buttocks become small and flabby. The appetite is poor, and occasionally there may be some vomiting. Also, the infant is subject to frequent colds and bronchitis and may have a chronic cough.

**Are there varying degrees of severity of celiac disease?**

Yes. There are very mild cases, which are difficult to diagnose, and severe forms, which can be easily recognized.

**What tests can be done to make a positive diagnosis?**

The stool is examined for the presence of undigested fats and starches and for the presence of trypsin, one of the digestive enzymes. There are also certain tests to determine the absorption of Vitamin A, gelatin, and glucose into the blood from the stomach and duodenum.

**Will x rays help in the diagnosis of this condition?**

Yes, sometimes gastrointestinal studies will help in the diagnosis.

**What is the treatment for celiac disease?**

The child must be kept on a special diet for a long time. The diet will be high in proteins, low in fat, with no starches or sugars (other than natural fruit sugar). No wheat or rye products are to be given. These are the greatest offenders in causing a flare-up of the disease as they contain a large amount of gluten.

**What milk is used?**

Ordinary cow's milk is usually well tolerated.

**What solids are tolerated by the child with celiac disease?**

All foods except those containing gluten (gliadin).

**Can the baby have the usual vitamins?**

The water-soluble multivitamin preparations are given, usually in increased amounts because of the difficulty in absorption.

**How long does the infant stay on this diet?**

About six months to two years, until gliadin is tolerated.

**Is recovery usually complete in celiac disease?**

Yes.

**Can the child take a full diet later in life?**

Yes, most can. Some children may still require a gliadin-free diet.

**Are there any setbacks during the treatment?**

Yes, when offending foods are eaten.

**How does this diet affect the child's disposition?**

Some children take the diet well and eat avidly without any disturbance. Others seem to get bored by the diet, so the mother must use her ingenuity to get the child to eat the foods prescribed.

**Can celiac disease be treated satisfactorily at home?**

Yes. Hospitalization may be necessary only in the beginning of the disease or for thorough investigation and diagnosis.

**Does the baby have to stay in bed with this condition?**

No, except during an acute illness.

**Will celiac disease clear up without treatment?**

No. If the baby stays on a full diet, the stools become worse, weight loss increases, and severe infections are more apt to occur.

**Does celiac disease tend to recur?**

In some cases it may be necessary to continue modified dietary care for several years. Otherwise there may be relapses or recurrences, especially when infections occur.

**Is the pancreas involved in this condition?**

No.

## CYSTIC FIBROSIS

**What is cystic fibrosis?**

It is a disease somewhat similar in its manifestations to celiac disease, but it is more severe in nature and tends to have more complications, such as lung infections.

**How often does it occur?**

About one in five to six hundred babies has this disease.

**When does it start?**

It starts earlier than celiac disease, usually from birth to six months of age.

**Does it tend to run in families?**

Yes.

**Does heat affect these children inordinately?**

Yes. They lose a great deal of salt in

the sweat secretions and may go into collapse on a hot summer's day.

## Do some children die with cystic fibrosis?

Yes. Some children may die during a heat spell, others may die of pulmonary complications, and still others from malnutrition. About 50 percent die before the age of five.

## What is the treatment for cystic fibrosis?

Diet similar to that in celiac disease, adequate salt intake, large amounts of vitamins, constant use of antibiotics to prevent infections, and the giving of pancreatic extracts.

## How long does treatment have to be continued to maintain these children?

For several years, and often through adolescence.

## What causes cystic fibrosis?

The exact cause is not known, but investigations have shown that there is a basic defect in the function of many organs of the body, such as the pancreas, the liver, the lungs, and the intestinal tract. There seems to be an underlying disorder in the production of enzymes and in the mucous production of the various organs.

## Was it formerly thought that cystic fibrosis was a disease limited primarily to the pancreas?

Yes. This concept has been discarded within recent years as it has become evident that the organs mentioned above are also involved in the disease process.

## Is cystic fibrosis often associated with excess mucous production and excess viscosity (thickness) of mucus that is secreted in the lungs and in the intestinal tract?

Yes, this is one of the most characteristic findings in cystic fibrosis.

## If there is a case of this disease in

the family, should the parents plan to have other children?

Yes. They may have additional children, but they should be told that there is a one in four chance that another child will have the same condition.

## Are there any special tests for this disease?

Tests of the sweat to determine the salt content are specific for this condition. Recently, other tests of saliva, nails, and hair show this same particular increase in sodium.

## Is it easy to differentiate this condition from celiac disease?

In very frank cases, the two can be differentiated, but in mild ones it may be difficult to tell them apart.

## What is the outlook for a child with cystic fibrosis?

The outlook is improving as more and more is being discovered as to the cause of this condition. Also, the protection of the child against frequent upper respiratory infections has been shown to reduce the chances of permanent damage to the lungs. Finally, many children are now being saved by the continued use of various antibiotics, both prophylactically and in the treatment of infections.

# HIRSCHSPRUNG'S DISEASE (Megacolon)

*(See also Chapter 66 on Small and Large Intestines)*

## What is Hirschsprung's disease?

It is a disease present from birth involving the large intestine, in which there is a contracted segment in the sigmoid colon on the left side with tremendous dilatation and enlargement of the remainder of the bowel above the constricted portion.

## How common is Hirschsprung's disease?

It is a relatively rare condition, seen more often among males, and constitutes about one out of every ten thousand hospital admissions.

## What causes Hirschsprung's disease?

It is thought to be due to a developmental deformity in which certain nerves are lacking in the contracted portion of the bowel (sigmoid colon). This lack prevents the involved segment of bowel from relaxing and dilating. In order to propel the feces forward, the bowel above the constriction enlarges, and because it is difficult to get gas and feces beyond the contracted area, the bowel above dilates tremendously.

## How is the diagnosis of Hirschsprung's disease made?

By characteristic findings on x-ray examination with the giving of barium to outline the bowel. Also, a biopsy of a small portion of the rectal muscle may show the absence of nerve cells.

## What is the course and treatment of this condition?

Mild cases tend to improve and get well with medical management over a period of years. The majority of severe cases will require the surgical removal of the constricted portion of large intestine.

## Is surgery successful in curing Hirschsprung's disease?

Yes. Modern techniques have improved greatly, and the surgical treatment of this condition is now safe and can promise an extremely high rate of cure.

# NEPHROSIS

*(See Chapter 37 on Kidneys and Ureters)*

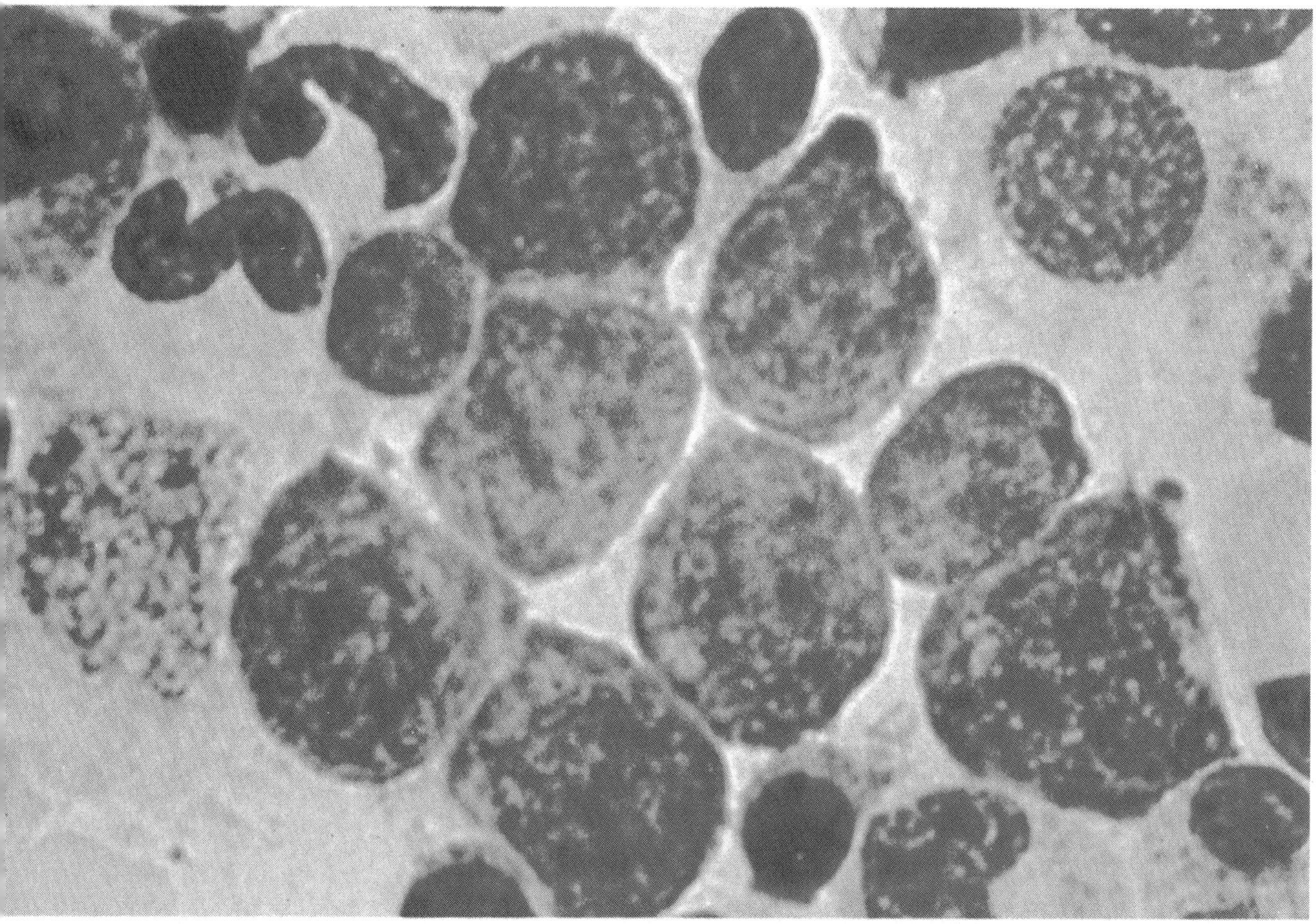

Blood cells are formed in the bone marrow, and diseases of the blood can often be diagnosed by studying a bone-marrow smear. The one above reveals an iron-deficiency anemia, the most common form of anemia.

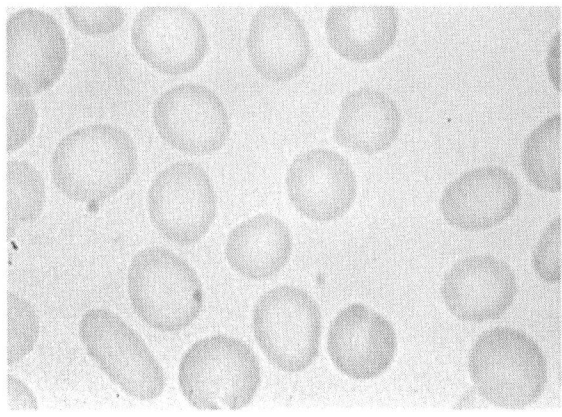

Iron-deficiency anemia is revealed by this smear of the circulating blood. The light-staining quality of the blood cells denotes lack of iron.

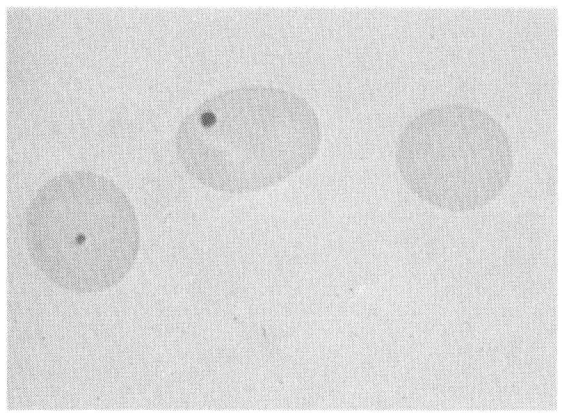

The red blood cells in a patient with pernicious (primary) anemia are few in number, larger than normal, and often contain the small black dots known as Howell-Jolly bodies.

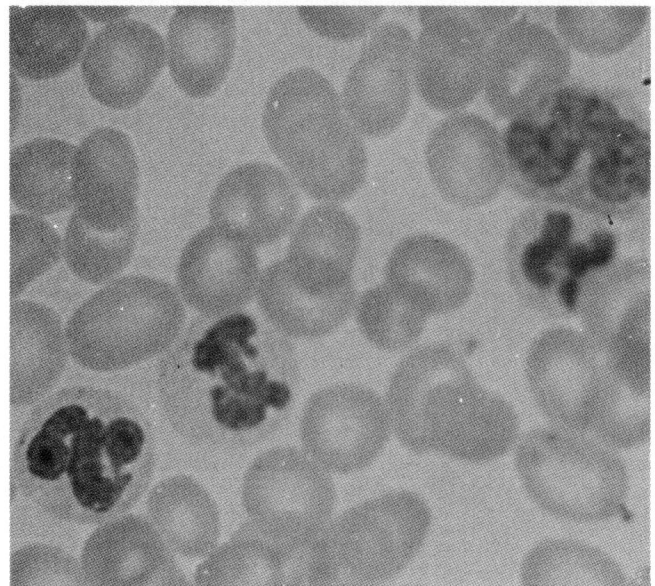

The white blood cells stain a characteristic bright pink in pernicious anemia, in which a gastric imbalance eventually prevents normal blood-cell formation.

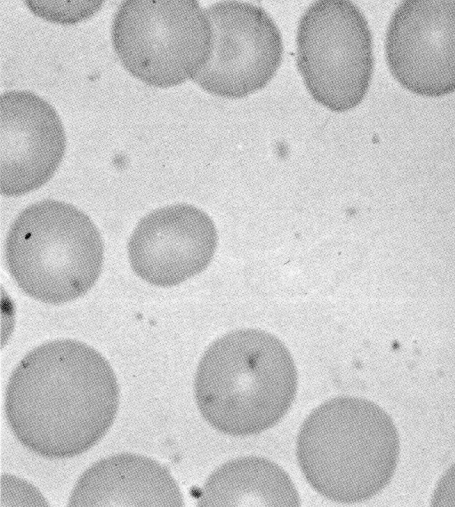

In cases of aplastic anemia, caused by a defect in the bone marrow, the red blood cells (*above*) are low in hemoglobin and fewer than normal in quantity.

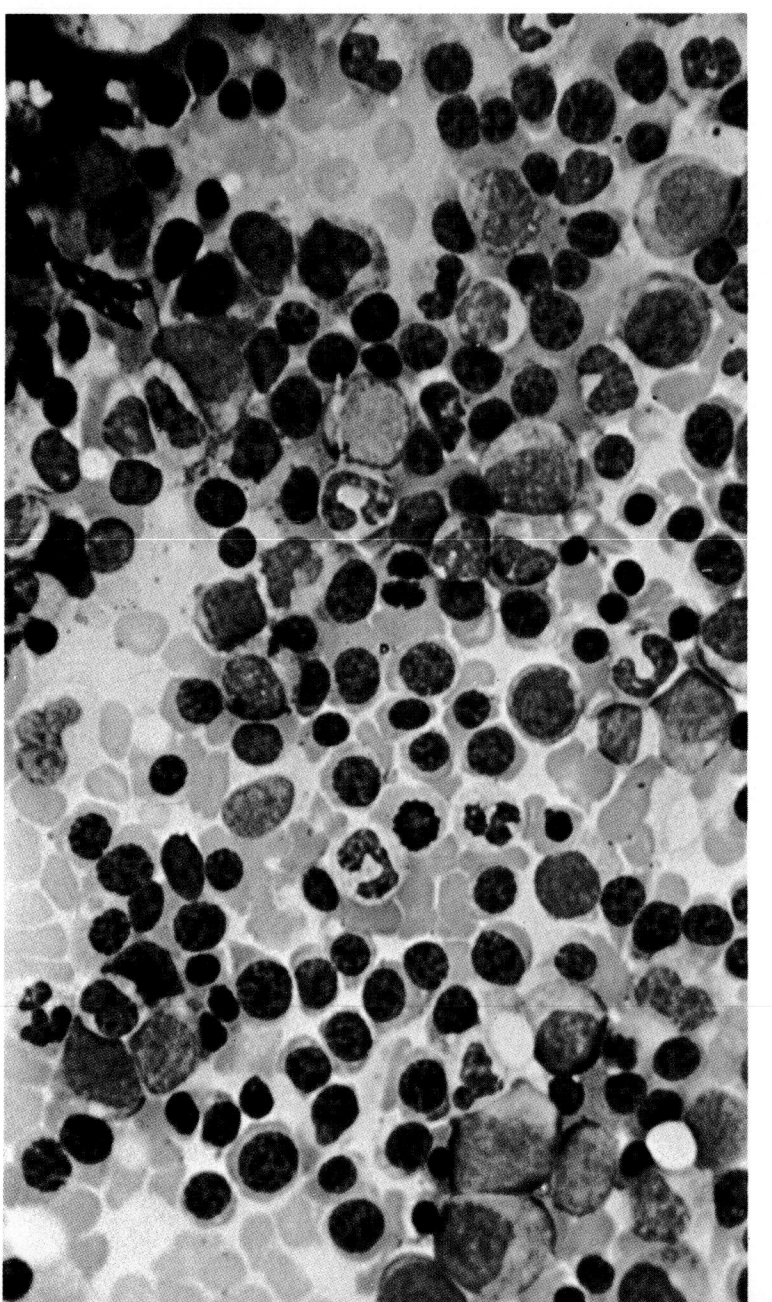

The bone marrow smear at the left is typical of hemolytic anemia, in which there is abnormal destruction of red blood cells.

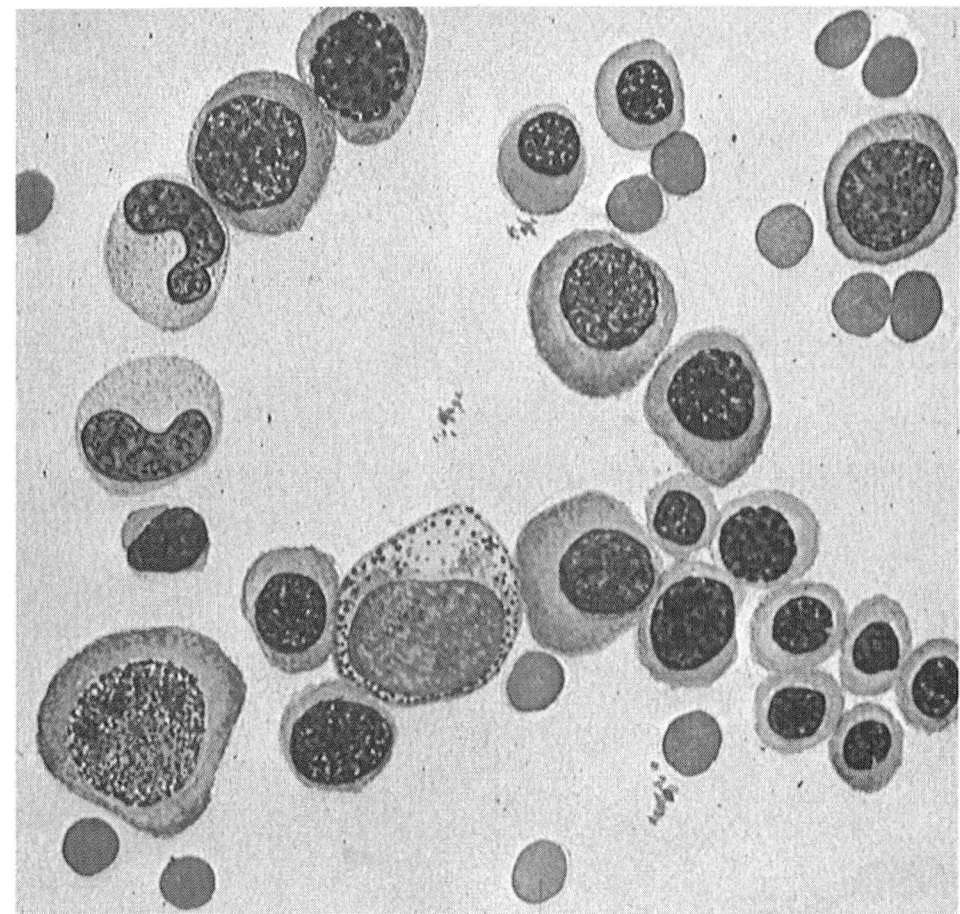

The sparse number of red blood cells in this smear is typical of hemolytic anemia; it can be due to an inherited defect in the blood as well as a destructive agent.

The smear below is from the circulating blood of a patient with hemolytic anemia; the destruction of red blood cells is usually caused by an infection, a toxin, or a poison.

In sickle-cell anemia, an inherited condition, some of the red blood cells are sickle-shaped instead of round, and some contain small specks of dark-staining material known as inclusion bodies.

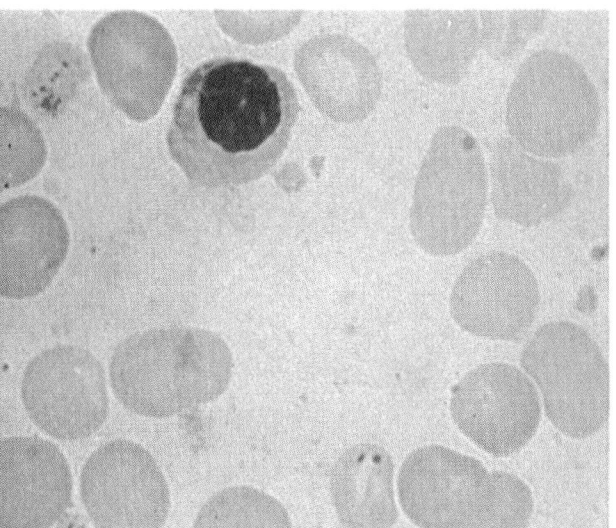

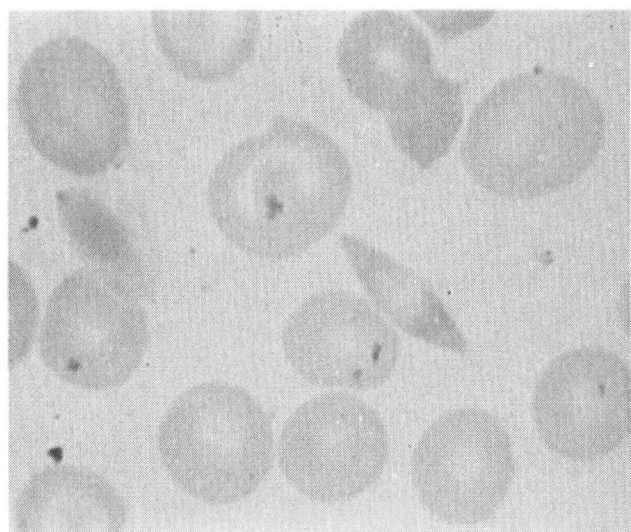

# HEMANGIOMAS

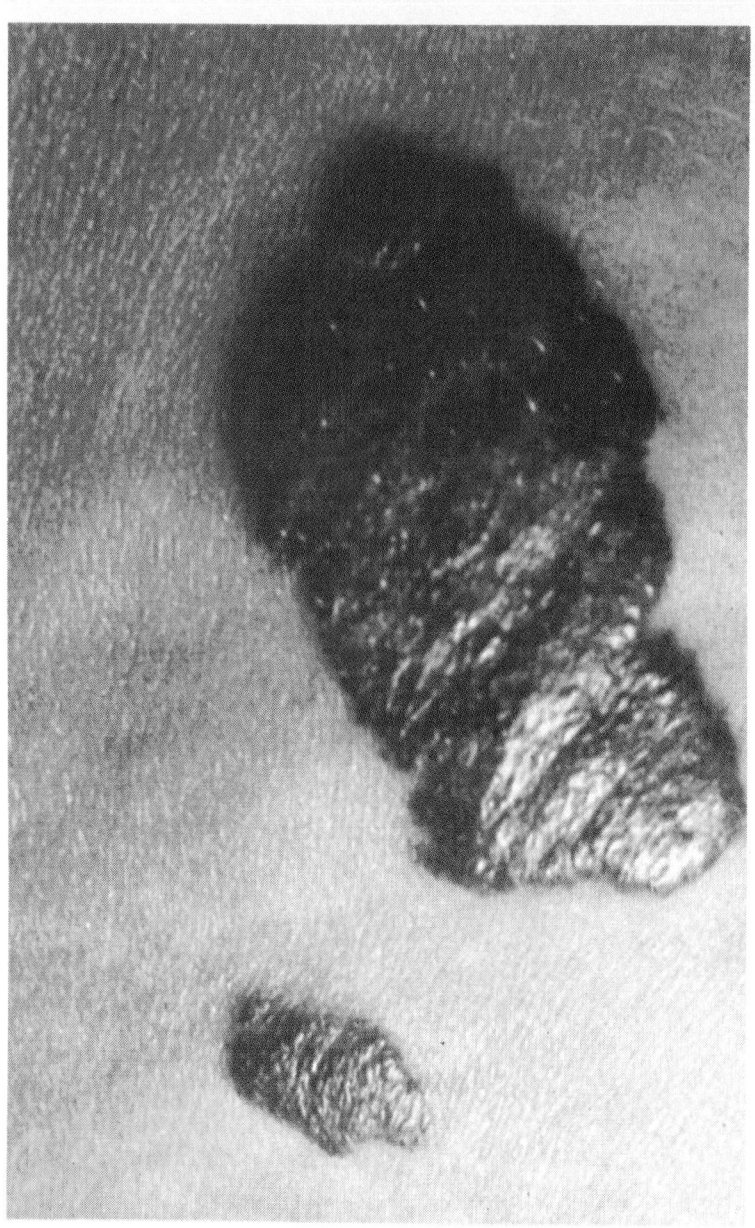

Hemangiomas which have a knobby appearance rather than the usual smooth surface are called tuberous hemangiomas.

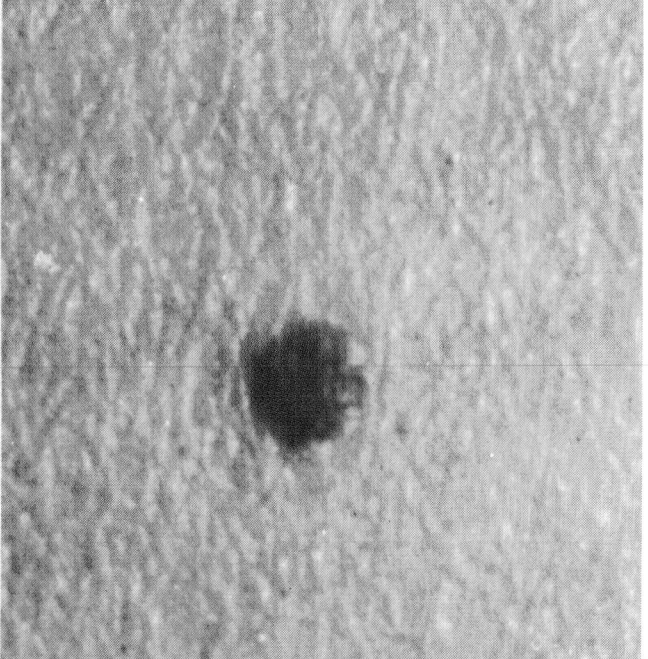

Small, discrete blood vessel tumors, known as senile angiomas, sometimes develop on the skin of elderly people.

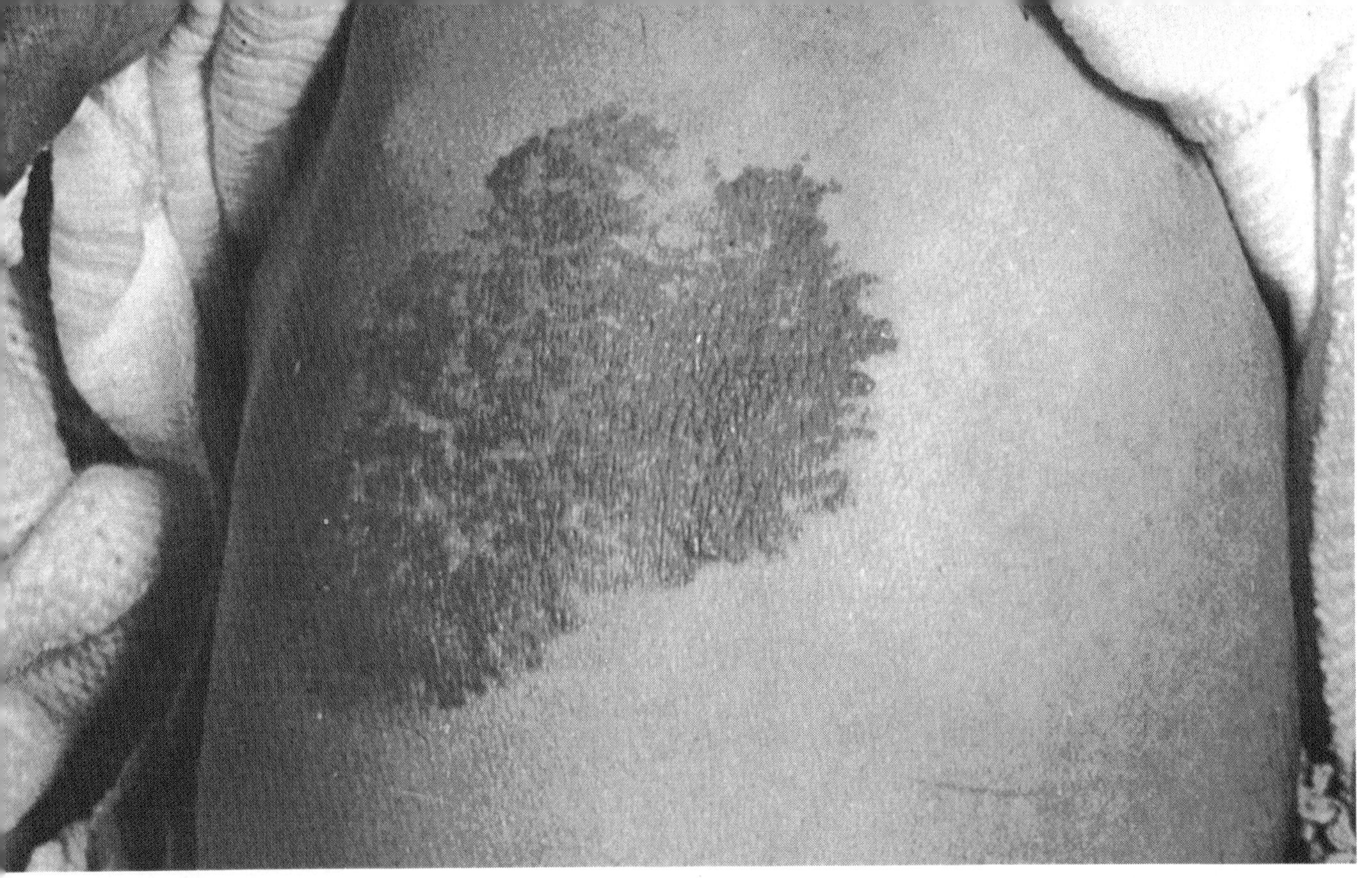

When hemangiomas are almost flush with the skin surface, they are known as flat hemangiomas.

The lips and gums are common locations of hemangiomas. These benign tumors, composed of dilated blood vessels, often occur in young children as well as in adults.

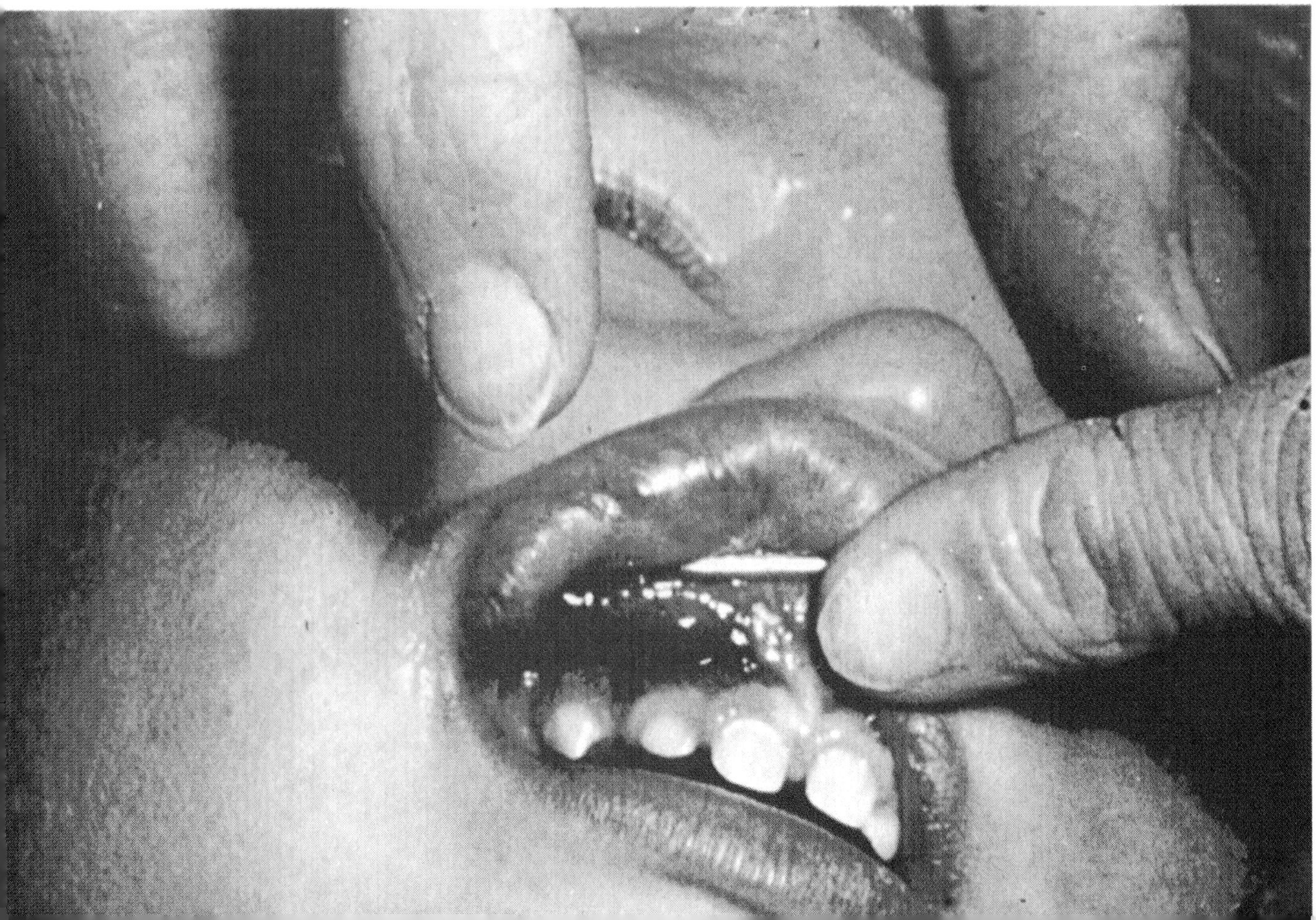

## ALLERGIC REACTIONS

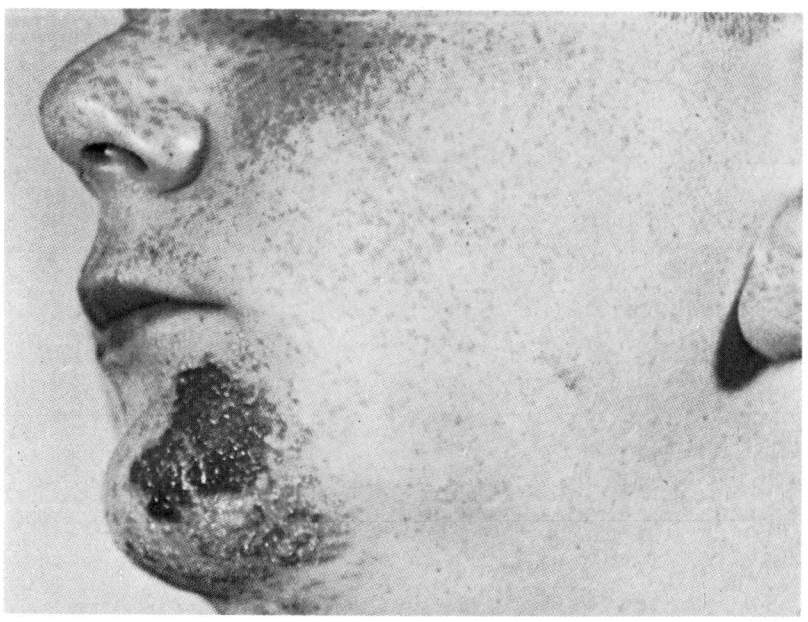

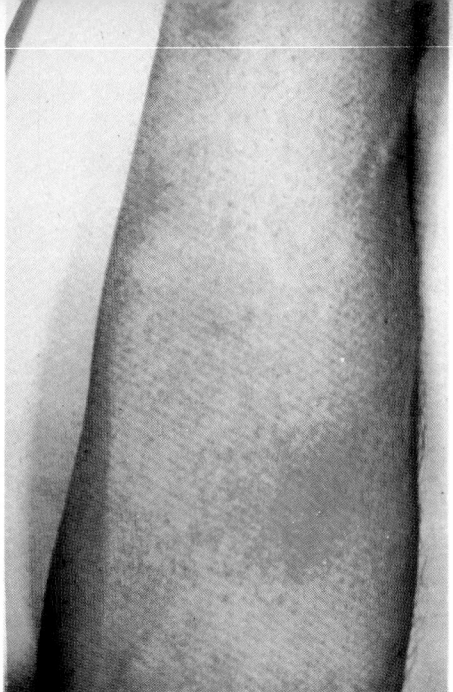

People can be allergic to many different things; the rash shown above is a reaction due to a caterpillar that walked along the patient's forearm.

Hypersensitivity to metal is a common cause of contact dermatitis. The wrist of the allergic patient has broken out in a rash owing to direct contact with the metal watch and watchband.

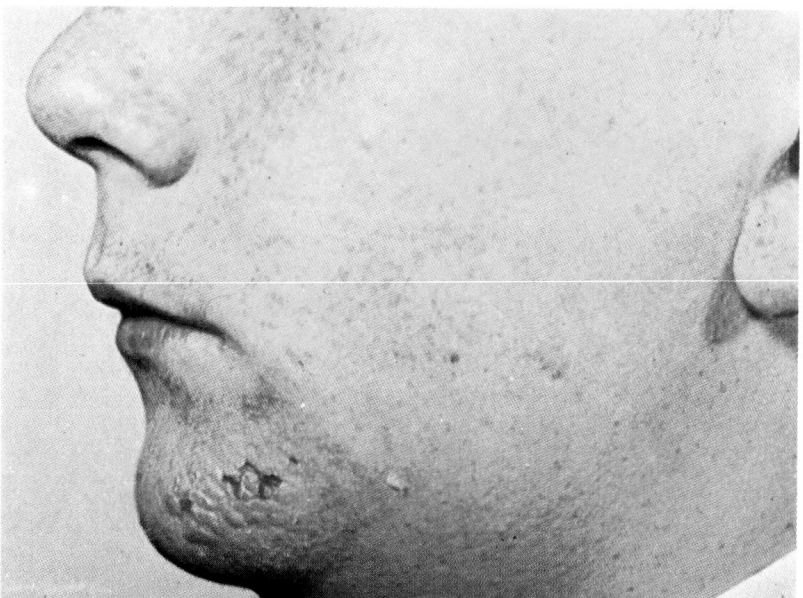

Contact dermatitis, one of the most common allergic reactions, caused by exposure of the skin to a substance to which one is hypersensitive, often resembles herpes, with its characteristic oozing, swelling blisters and crusts (seen in two typical stages of this condition, *above*).

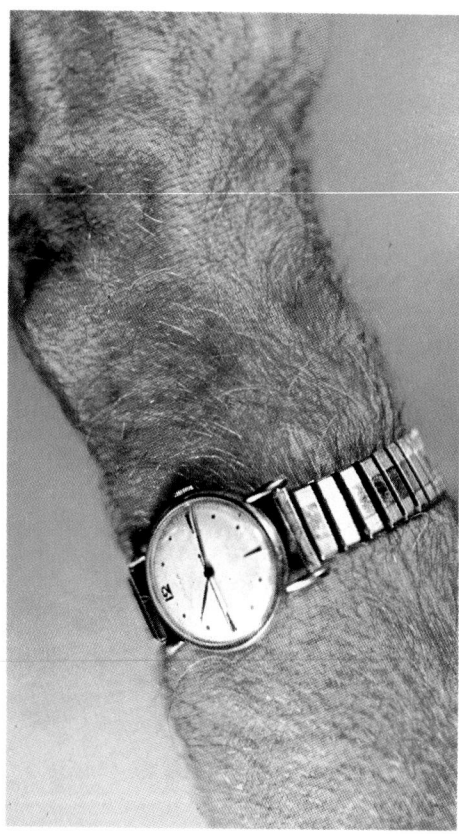

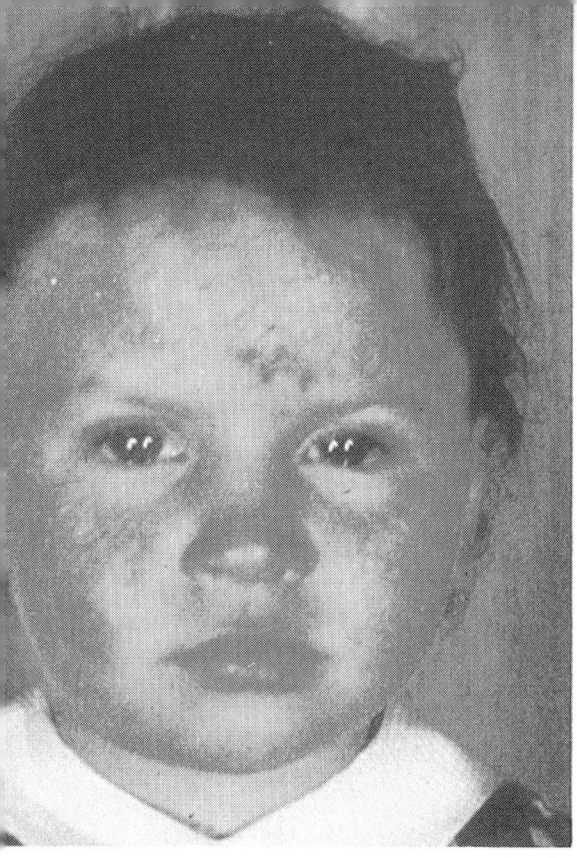

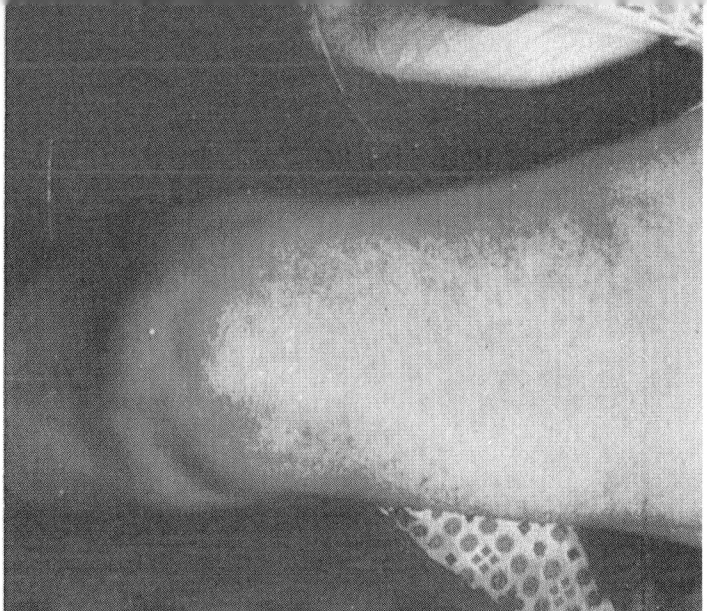

Certain materials, particularly wool or nylon, may produce contact dermatitis in people who are sensitive to them. The rash on this patient's thigh is due to the wearing of nylon stockings.

Atopic eczema, an inflammatory disease of the skin, frequently occurs in infants and small children as a result of a food sensitivity. It appears often in children with family histories of allergy.

The characteristic rash, swelling, and itching following insect bites have affected the face of the child below. Such a reaction is actually a form of allergic response.

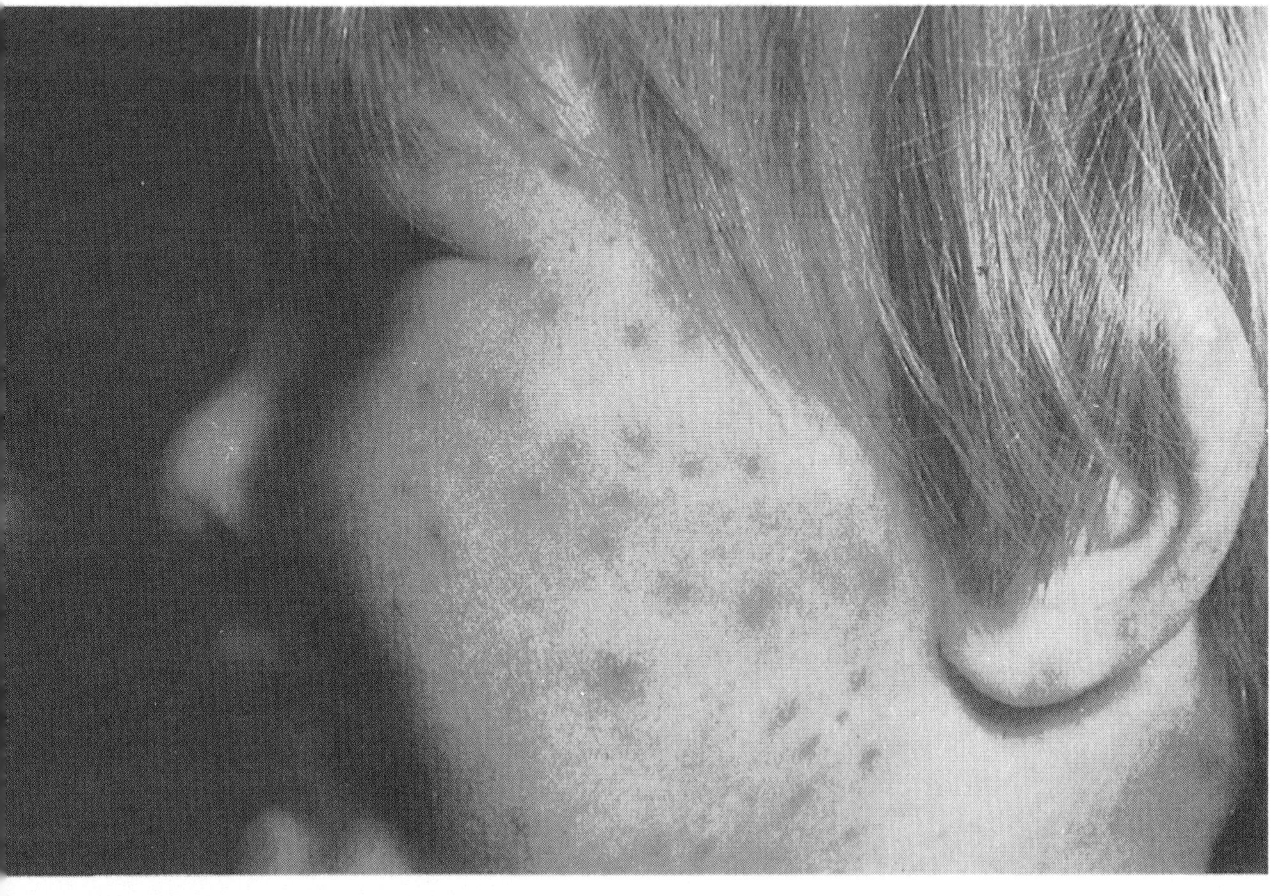

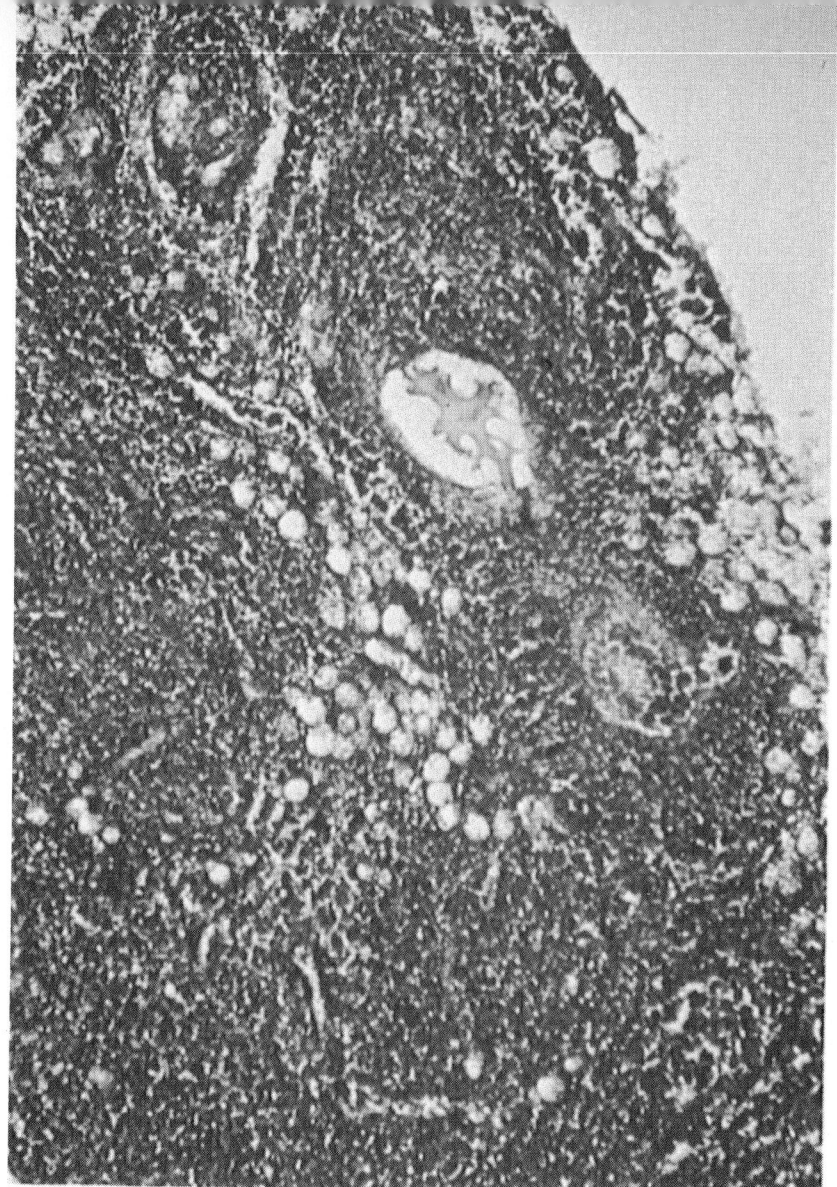

Lymphocytic leukemia is a type of leukemia characterized by enlargement of the lymph glands and by a large number of lymphocytes in the circulating blood. The microscopic appearance and the gross appearance of lymph glands involved in this condition are shown here.

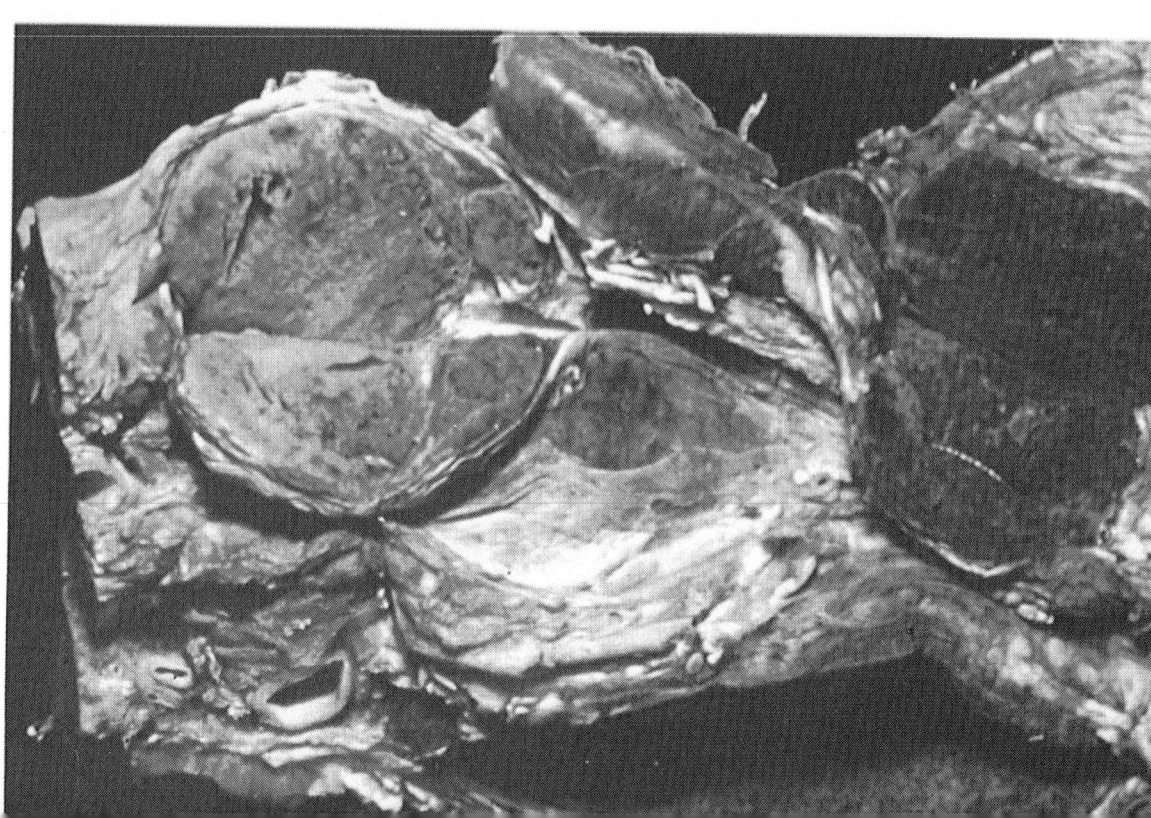

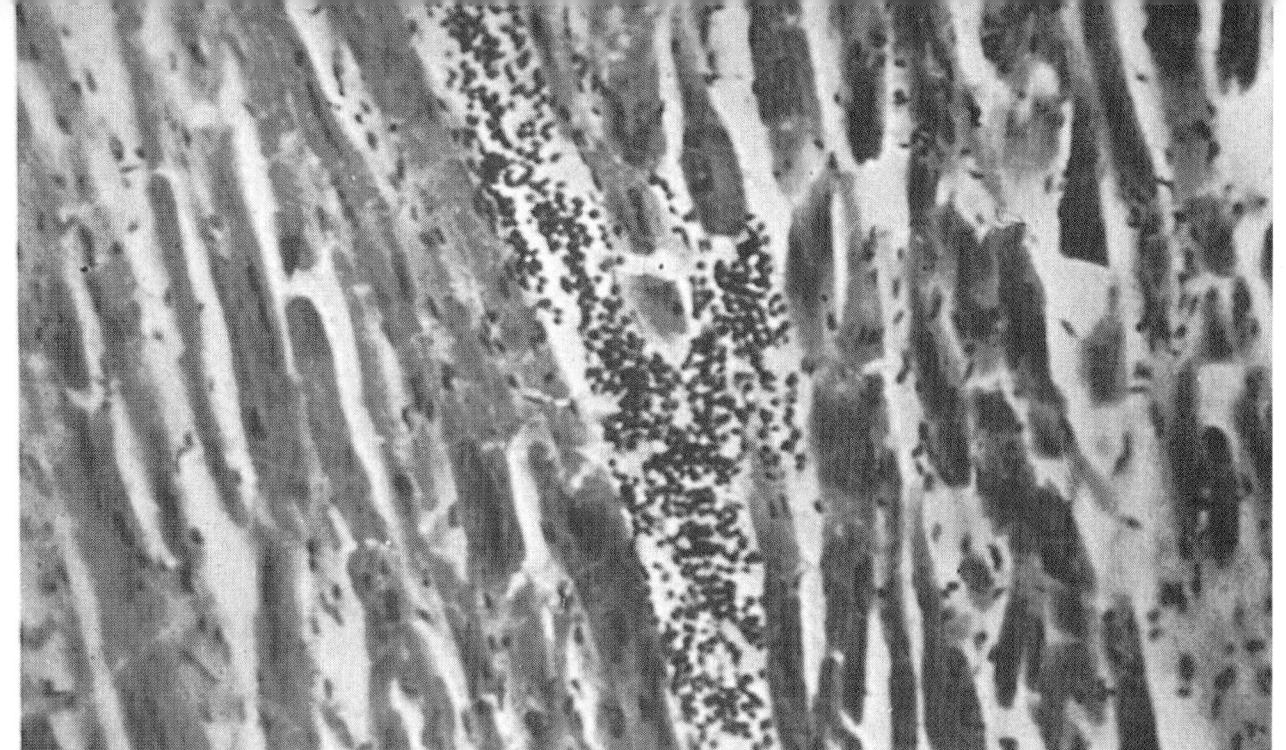

The spreading nature of lymphocytic leukemia may be observed in this photomicrograph of heart muscle which shows the invasion by the leukemic cells, the dark-stained material.

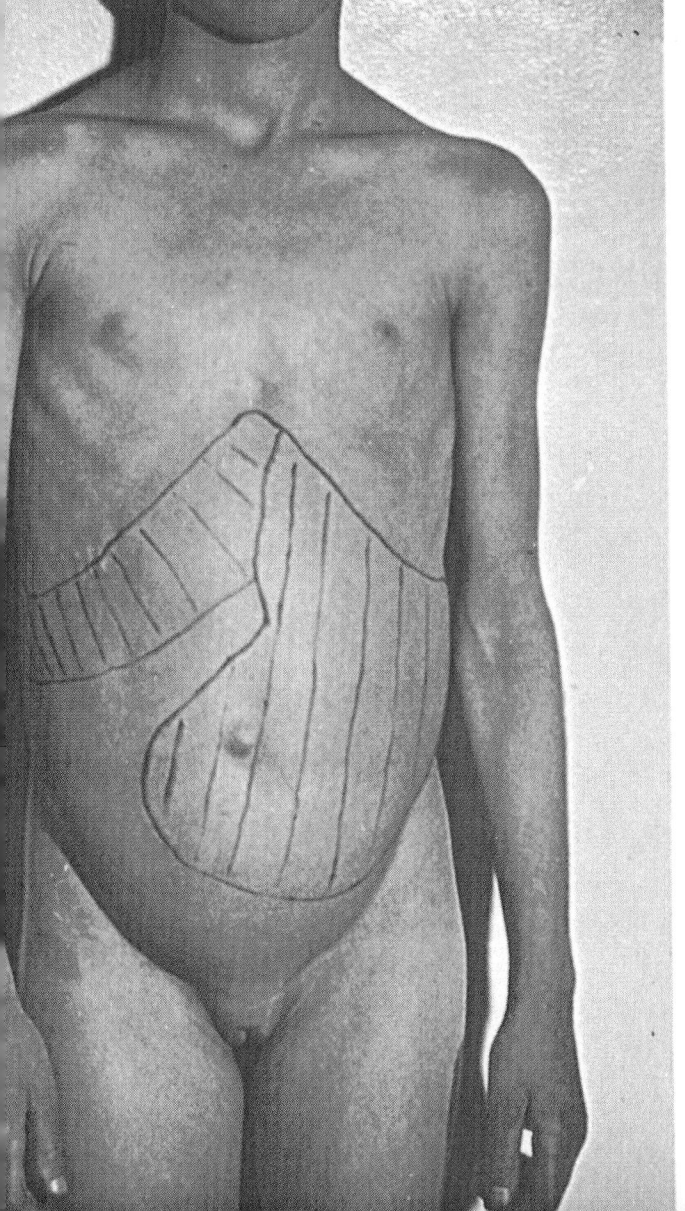

Myelocytic leukemia commonly involves the liver and spleen, as well as the lymph glands. The drawing on this patient's abdomen outlines the area of liver and spleen enlargement.

## BONE ANATOMY AND PATHOLOGY

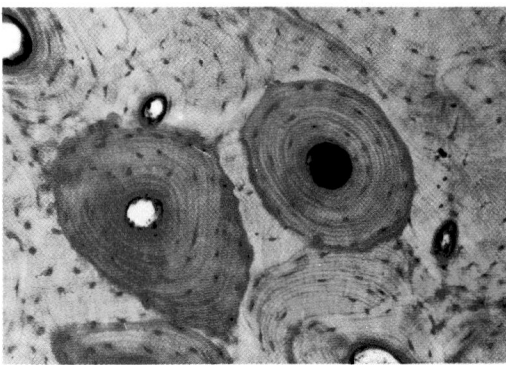

The conformation of compact bone with nourishing blood vessels and connective-tissue cells appears in this cross section.

Normal bone cells appear as elliptical, nucleated structures in this microscopic lateral section of bone substance.

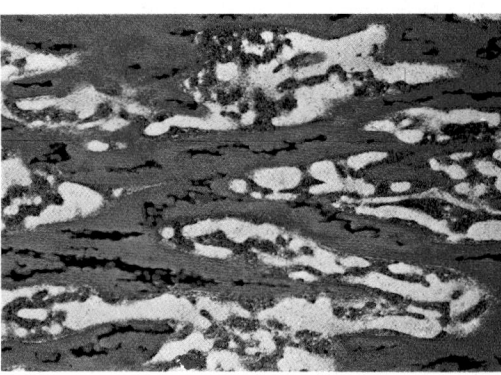

This photomicrograph (*above*) shows the microscopic structure of spongy bone. The spaces in between the bone tissue are occupied by bone marrow.

This photomicrograph (*below*) shows blood vessels and bone-forming cells beginning to form new tissue in areas which were originally cartilaginous.

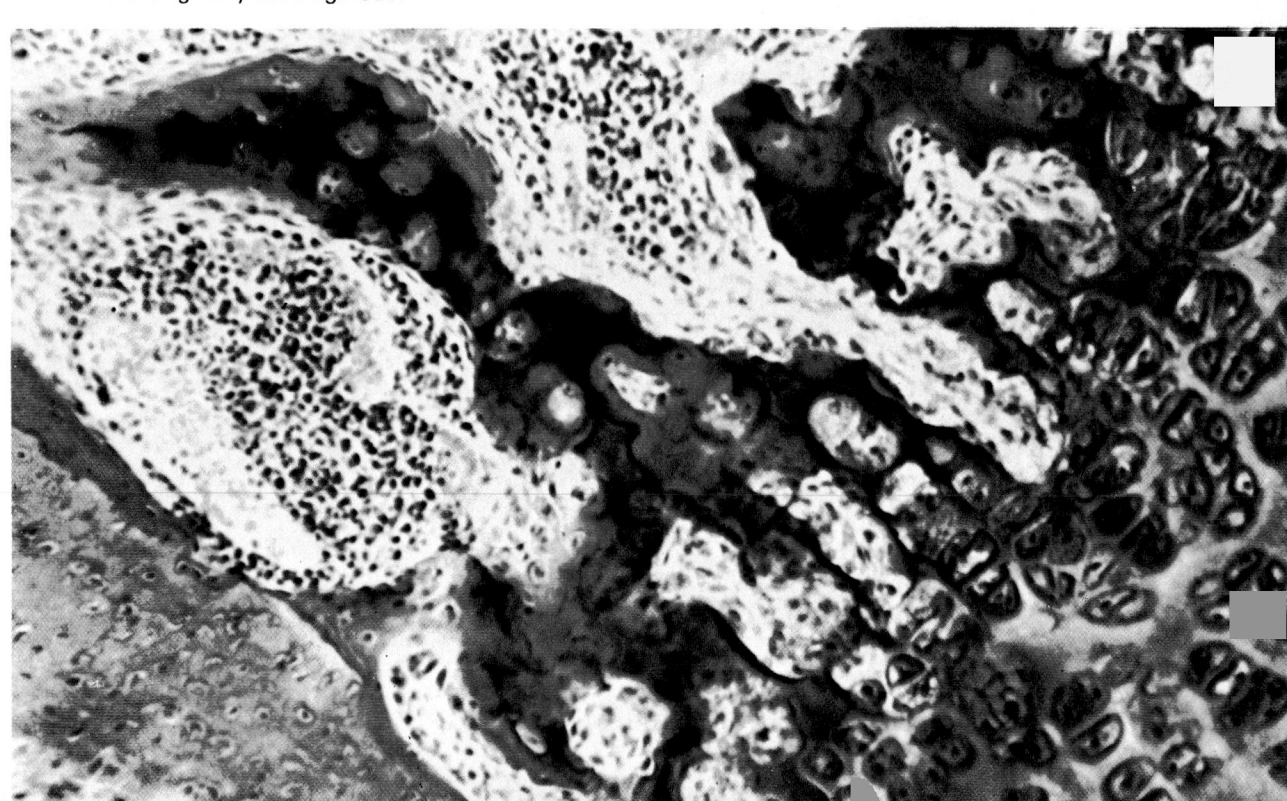

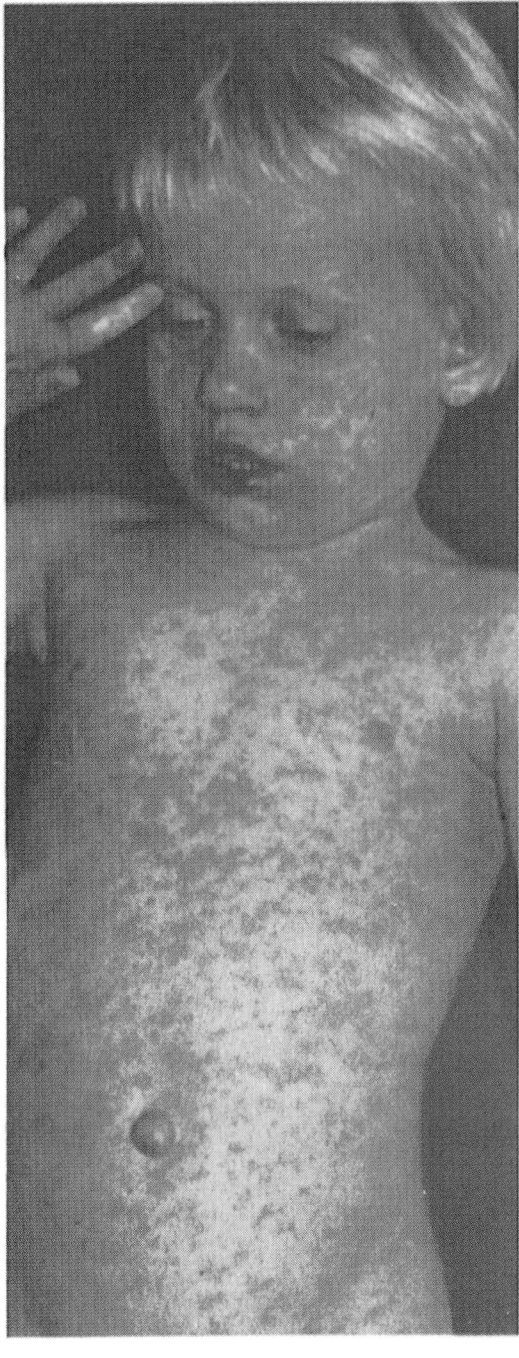

Although the measles rash may resemble that of German measles or scarlet fever, the generalized symptoms of the disease differ considerably. Measles is accompanied by typical Koplik spots in the mouth, a high fever, and by an inflammation of the mucous membranes of the eyes, nose, and throat. The diffuse nature of the German measles rash is shown at the right. This disease is much milder than measles and rarely causes a high temperature or toxicity.

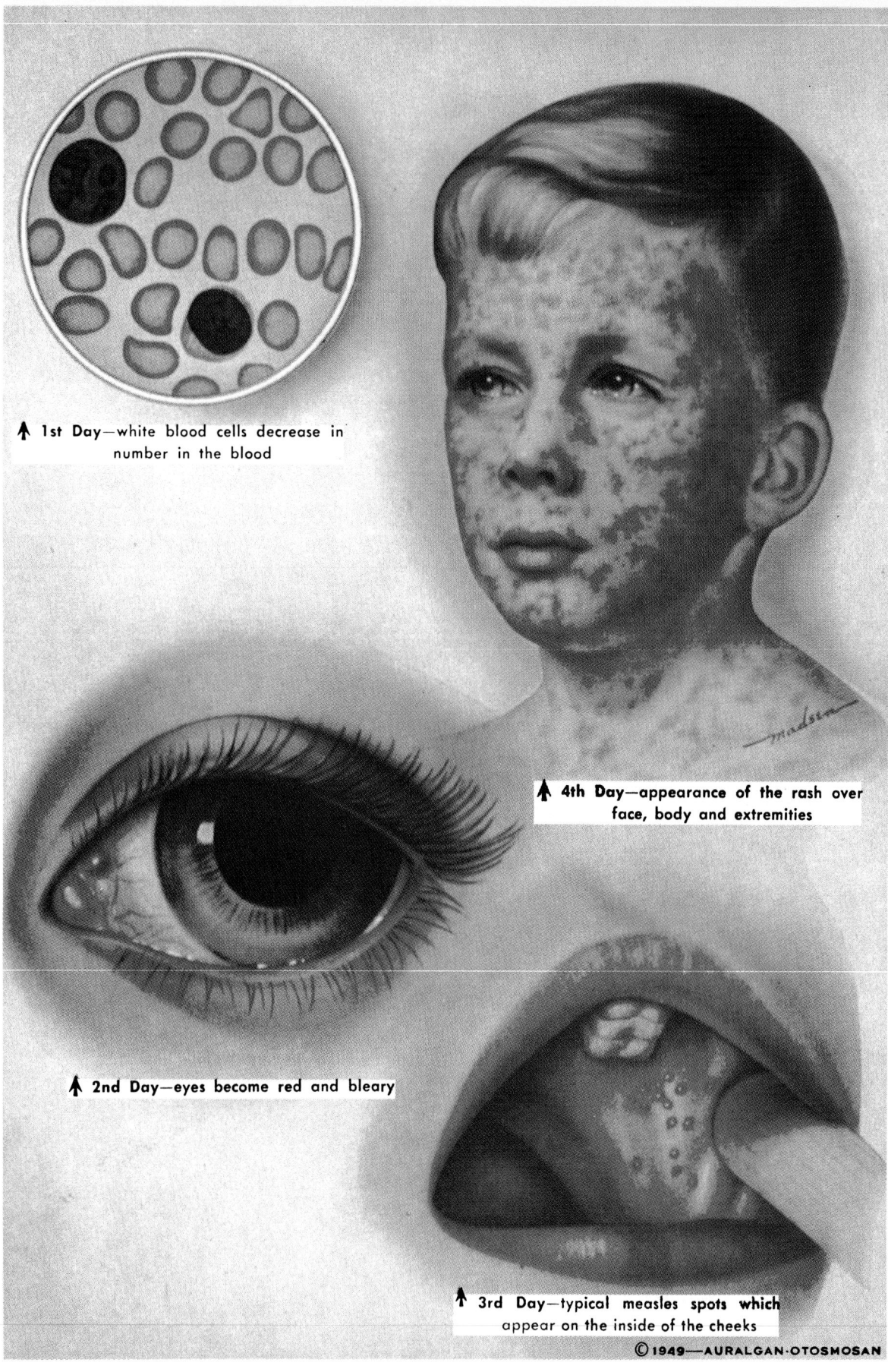

↑ 1st Day—white blood cells decrease in number in the blood

↑ 4th Day—appearance of the rash over face, body and extremities

↑ 2nd Day—eyes become red and bleary

↑ 3rd Day—typical measles spots which appear on the inside of the cheeks

Typical measles rash. The rash of measles is usually much more pronounced than that of German measles. Measles can be a severe disease, so the child should be kept in bed and watched carefully until temperature and all other symptoms have subsided. In occasional cases measles may affect the brain, causing encephalitis. This is a serious condition, although recovery takes place in the great majority of instances.

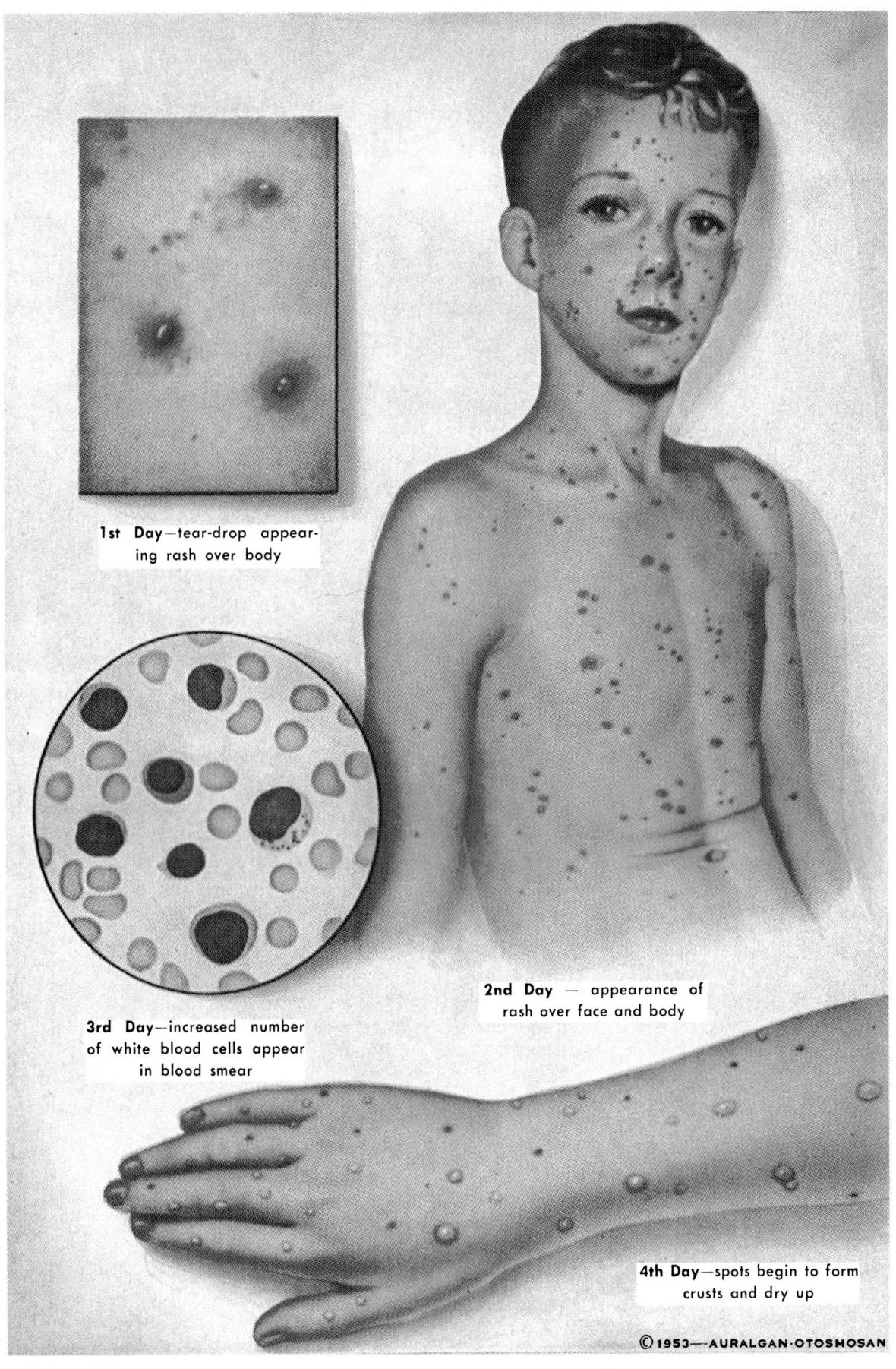

1st Day—tear-drop appearing rash over body

3rd Day—increased number of white blood cells appear in blood smear

2nd Day — appearance of rash over face and body

4th Day—spots begin to form crusts and dry up

© 1953—AURALGAN·OTOSMOSAN

Typical chickenpox rash. Although chickenpox is by no means a dangerous disease of childhood, it can often cause disfiguring scars if the child is permitted to pick at the scabs. During the period when scabs have formed, it is important to keep the child's fingernails clipped, and if he is old enough to understand, he should be urged not to to scratch the pockmarks.

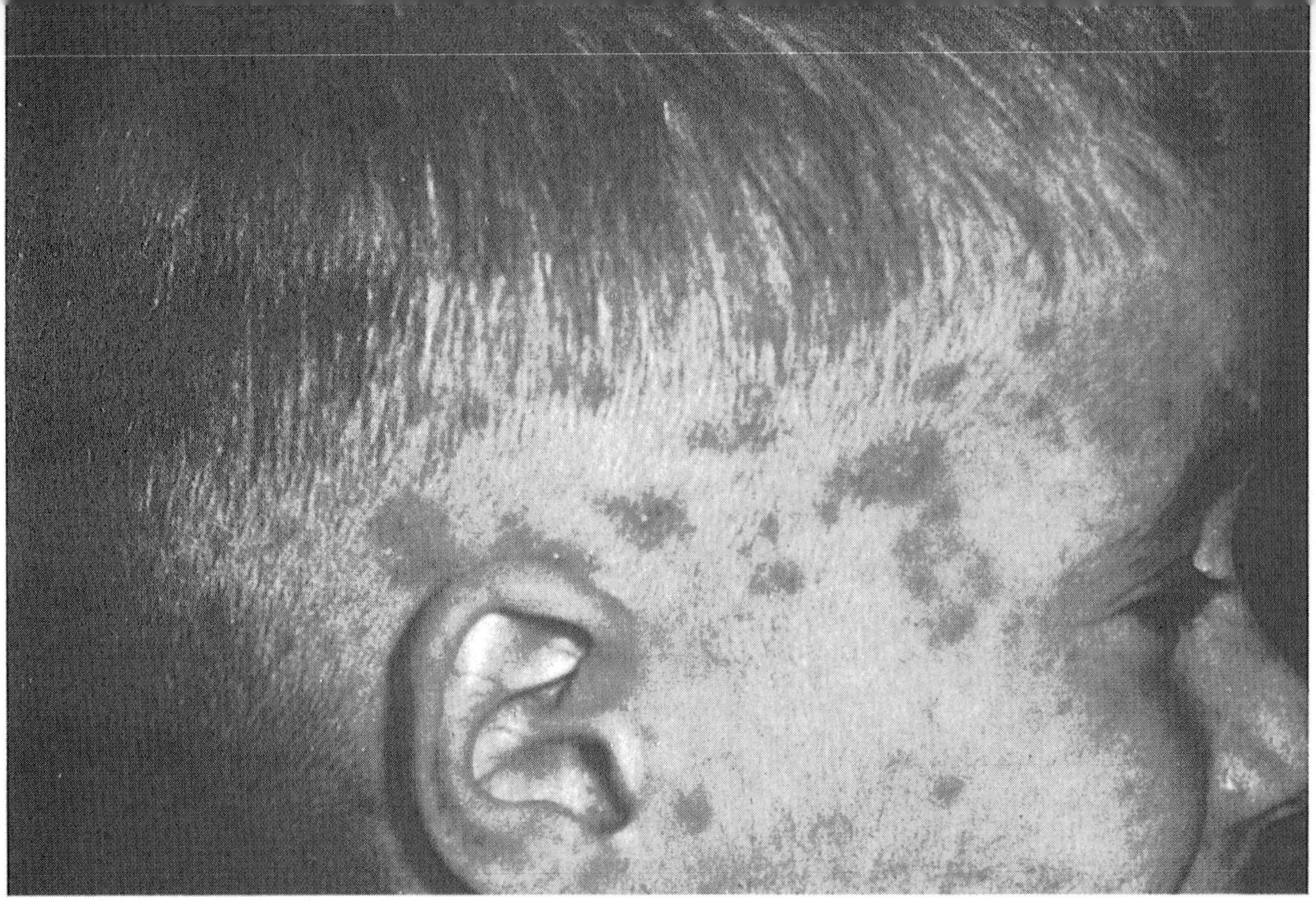

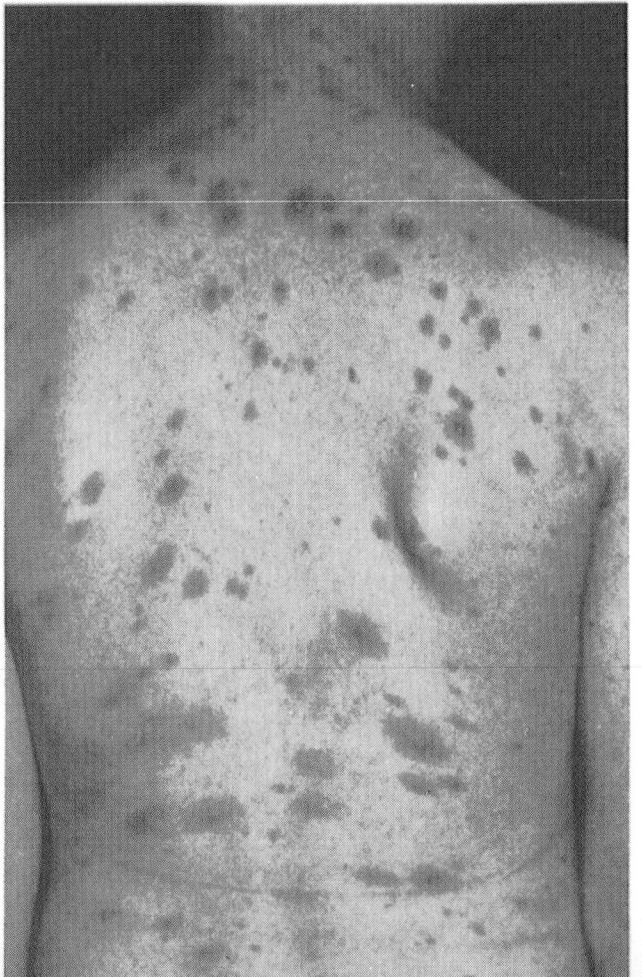

The chickenpox rash sometimes occurs on the scalp where it causes a good deal of itching and discomfort.

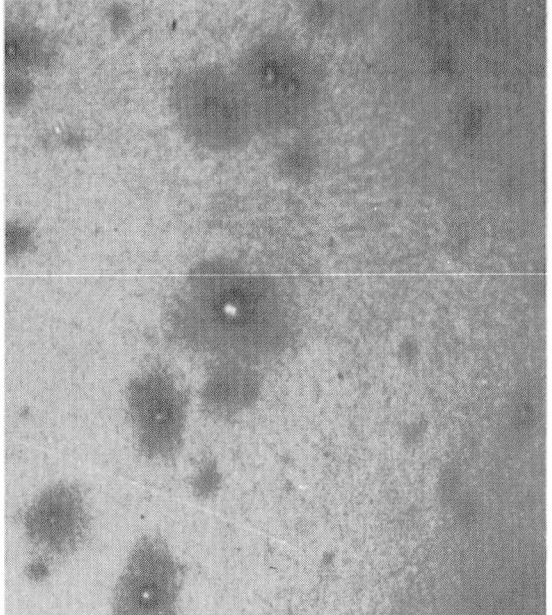

During the earliest stage of chickenpox there may appear on the body an area of diffuse, flat redness. Within 24 to 48 hours thereafter, the typical rash of raised pustules (*above*) will appear over the entire body (*right*). Although the pox are isolated and sharply demarcated, scratching may cause the area of redness to extend beyond the area of the individual pustule.

# NORMAL VACCINATION REACTIONS showing typical "take"

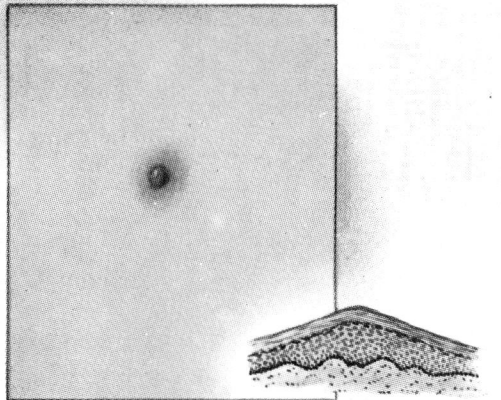

**4th Day**—showing hard, red, round, raised area

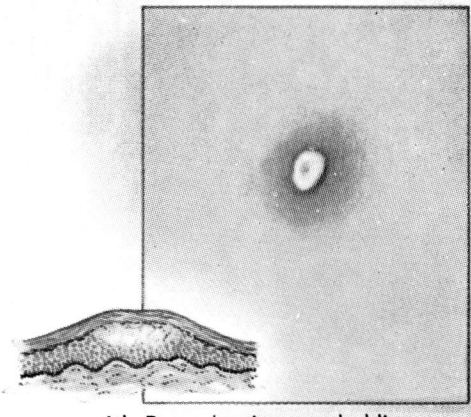

**6th Day**—showing pearly blister surrounded by red area

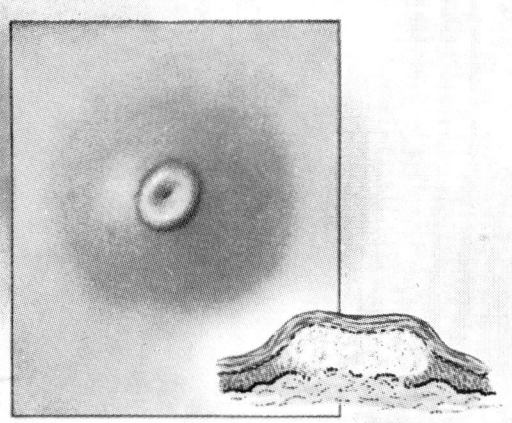

**8th Day**—showing larger blister and wider area of redness

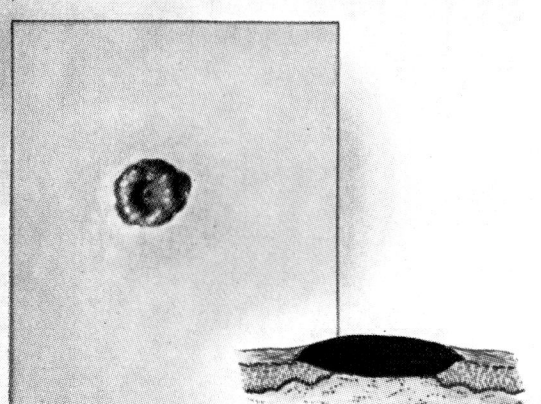

**12th Day** — showing dried blister which has formed a brownish scab

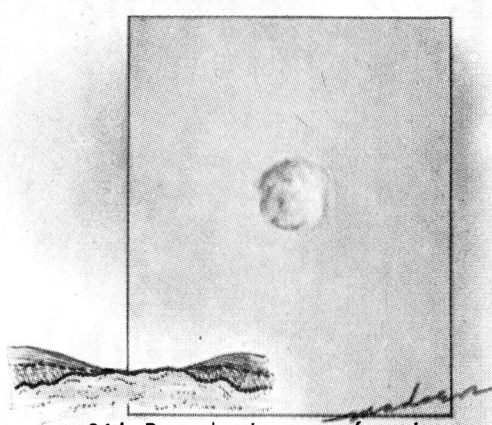

**24th Day**—showing scar of vaccination which is beginning to turn white

Smallpox vaccination reactions. It is a common misconception that only young children need to be vaccinated against smallpox. Before traveling to areas where smallpox exists, it is wise to be re-vaccinated. Many adults will have positive reactions if they have not been vaccinated for many years.

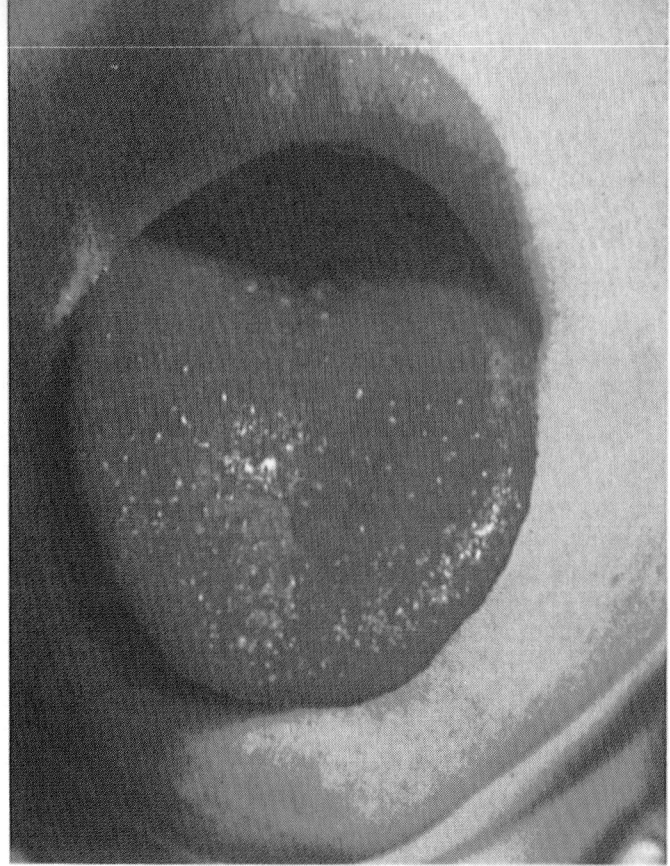

The tongue in patients with scarlet fever has a characteristic strawberry-red appearance. Fortunately, this serious disease is much milder today than it was a few decades ago.

Erysipelas is an acute inflammatory condition of the skin, caused by a streptococcus germ. It is accompanied by high fever and signs of great toxicity. Fortunately, the disease can be controlled by intensive antibiotic therapy.

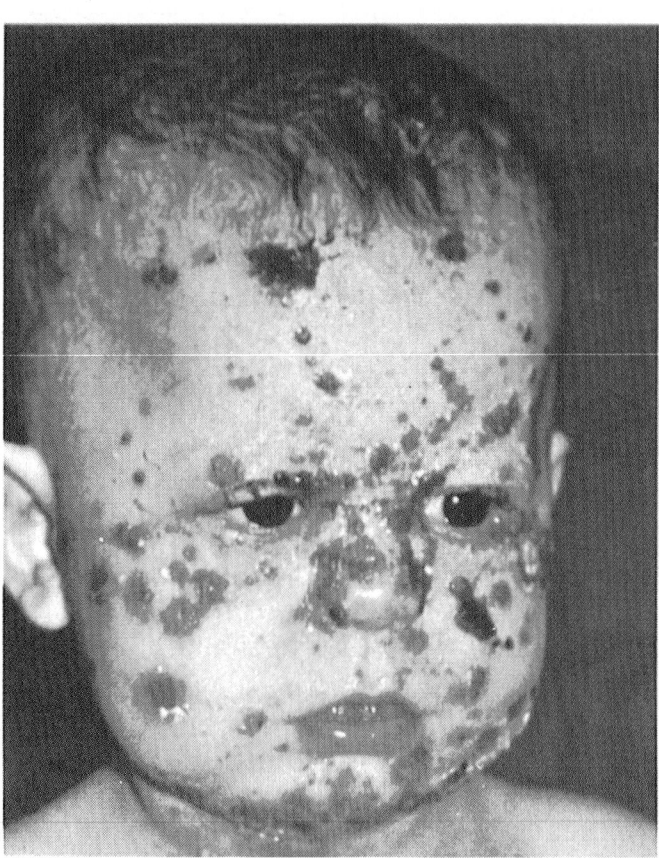

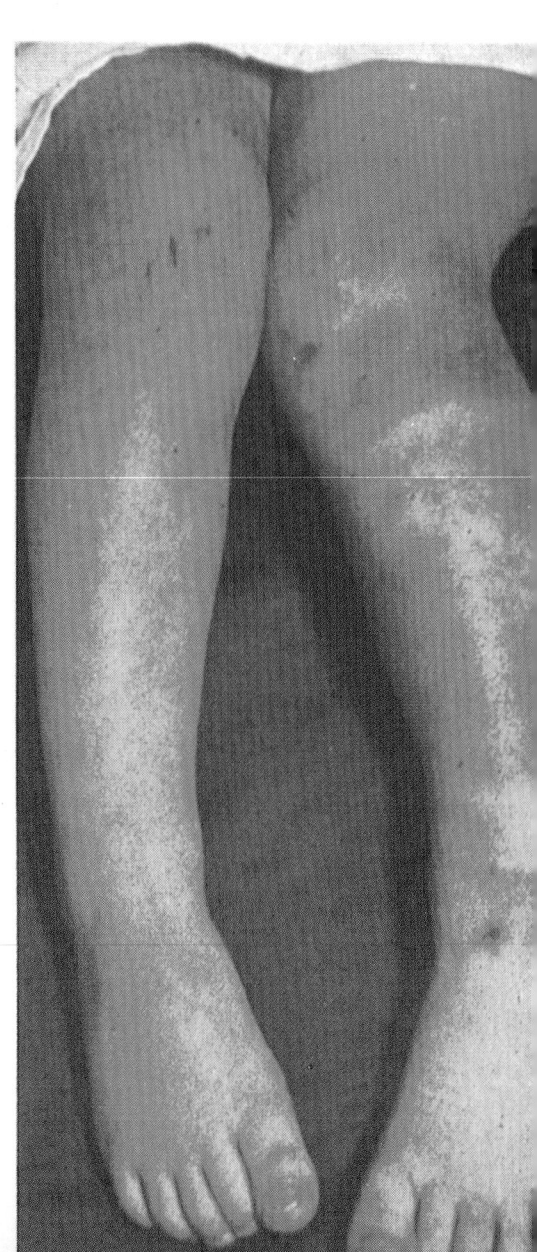

Impetigo is a highly contagious pustular condition resulting from a staphylococcal or streptococcal infection. It occurs most often on the faces of young children, although older children and adults are not immune.

# RHEUMATIC FEVER

*(See Chapter 62 on Rheumatic Fever)*

# ERYTHROBLASTOSIS

### What is erythroblastosis?

Erythroblastosis, also called Rh-factor disease, is a condition in which the red blood cells of the embryo or newborn are destroyed because of an incompatibility between the mother's and the child's blood.

### What are other names for erythroblastosis?

a. Rh-factor disease.
b. Erythroblastosis fetalis.
c. Severe jaundice of the newborn.
d. Severe anemia of the newborn.
e. Hemolytic disease of the newborn.

### What is meant by the "Rh-factor"?

All people are either Rh-positive or Rh-negative. This means that the blood contains a substance (Rh substance) in Rh-positive people that is not present in Rh-negative people.

### What percentage of people are Rh-positive?

Eighty-five percent. The other 15 percent are Rh-negative.

### Are these blood factors transmitted from parent to child?

Yes.

### Under what circumstances will an embryo or newborn have no Rh problem?

a. If the mother is Rh-positive.
b. If the father and mother are both Rh-negative.

### Will all babies born of an Rh-negative mother and an Rh-positive father develop erythroblastosis?

No, only a small percentage will develop it.

### What brings about this condition?

An Rh-negative mother carries an Rh-positive baby in her uterus. Some of the Rh-positive baby blood substance gets into the mother's circulation and produces Rh-positive antibodies. These antibodies in turn will later get into the baby's circulation and destroy the baby's own blood cells.

### How does this affect the newborn infant?

By producing anemia due to destruction of the infant's red blood cells, thus producing jaundice (yellow skin and eyes).

### How is the jaundice produced?

The infant's liver is unable to clear all the destroyed cells from the circulation, causing an overflow of bile into the circulation.

### How can this condition be recognized?

The infant becomes pale and jaundiced during the first twenty-four hours of life. In addition, the liver and spleen are found to be enlarged. Blood tests will show the presence of the antibodies in the infant's blood.

### How does the jaundice in the Rh-factor disease differ from normal newborn jaundice?

By its very early development, in the first twenty-four hours, and its severity.

### Is there any way to determine during the pregnancy whether the baby may have this disease?

Yes. Every mother should be tested in advance to determine whether she is Rh-positive or Rh-negative. If she is Rh-negative, her blood should be tested frequently during the latter weeks and months of her pregnancy for the presence and amount of these specific antibodies. If they are present, the baby may develop this disease.

### What is the treatment for erythroblastosis?

As soon after birth as possible, an exchange transfusion should be done. More recently, children with erythroblastosis have been subjected to special lights to reduce jaundice. This treatment is called *phototherapy.*

### What is meant by an "exchange transfusion"?

An attempt is made to remove all, or nearly all, of the baby's blood and replace it with blood from a donor—blood that does not contain these dangerous antibodies. This procedure will require the services of an expert in the field.

### Is it ever necessary to give more than one exchange transfusion?

Yes. In some cases, the jaundice may reappear in two to three days, necessitating a second and, in rare cases, even a third exchange transfusion.

### Can an exchange transfusion cure erythroblastosis?

Yes. If done early enough, it will cure almost every case.

### What can happen in an untreated case of erythroblastosis?

The baby may die in a few days because of the extreme blood destruction, or the intense jaundice may permanently injure certain parts of the brain.

### What is the nature of this brain injury?

It may produce spasticity or extreme drowsiness in the baby and may later be the cause of mental retardation, convulsions, and a form of cerebral palsy.

### Can an exchange transfusion prevent brain injury?

Yes. By removing the antibodies and the jaundice producing substance, it will prevent brain injury. It must be done very early, however, and may need to be repeated if jaundice recurs.

## Does Rh-factor disease ever produce stillbirths before the baby is delivered?

Yes. In some cases it is a cause of death in the uterus or just before birth. In some Rh-negative women, there may be a history of repeated stillbirths due to this disease. Physicians are now trying to prevent such stillbirths by giving the baby a transfusion through the mother's abdomen before the baby is born.

## Is there any way to treat an unborn child who is being carried by an Rh-negative mother and is therefore more likely to be born with Rh-factor disease?

Yes. It is possible to give such a child blood transfusions while still in the mother's womb.

## Is it possible to have a live baby in such cases?

Yes. If the condition is recognized during pregnancy, the live infant may be taken prematurely by Cesarean section or by prompting premature labor. An exchange transfusion is done immediately after birth, or the prenatal transfusion may be used if it is expected that the baby will be stillborn.

## Is there any way to prevent the development of sensitizing antibodies in an Rh-sensitive mother so that subsequent pregnancies will not result in erythroblastosis?

Yes. It is now possible to immunize an Rh-negative mother against the Rh-positive factor of the embryo. A substance known as RhoGAM can be injected into an Rh-negative mother within seventy-two hours after a child is born. Mothers so injected prior to a second pregnancy will not have subsequent children born with Rh-factor disease.

## May a child who has recovered from erythroblastosis be breast-fed?

Yes. There was a time when the possible introduction of these antibodies (some of which may be present in the breast milk) into the baby's stomach was feared. It is now known that they cause no harm when introduced in that manner.

## Are firstborn babies ever affected with erythroblastosis?

Not ordinarily. It usually affects later pregnancies. It may affect a firstborn infant if the mother has been given a transfusion or blood injection with Rh-positive blood some time prior to her first pregnancy. Then her blood may contain the dangerous antibodies as a result of the previous blood injection.

## Is there any other mechanism that can produce erythroblastosis besides the Rh-factor?

Yes. In a number of cases of so-called ABO incompatibility, in which the mother's blood group is "O" and the baby's group is "A" or "B," a form of this disease may be produced.

## What proportion of cases is caused by ABO incompatibility?

About 5 to 10 percent.

## How long does the baby have to stay in the hospital after an exchange transfusion?

For about a week, to make sure that there is no recurrence of anemia or jaundice. No other special treatments are required.

## AMAUROTIC FAMILIAL IDIOCY
### (Tay-Sachs Disease)

## What is amaurotic familial idiocy?

It is a fatal disease of young infants associated with blindness and mental retardation.

## What are the manifestations of this disease?

A baby will progress normally until about six months of age, then he will stop in his develop about six months of age, then he will stop in his development and regress. He will show signs of blindness, apathy, weakness of his muscles, and later spasticity and convulsions.

## What causes this condition?

The infant is unable to utilize certain fatty substances in his food. These substances then accumulate in the brain, causing destruction of the normal brain cells.

## What is the nature of the deficiency?

It has recently been found that certain enzymes are missing in the baby's blood. These enzymes act on one of the forms of sugar in its metabolism.

## How is the diagnosis of this condition made?

By examination of the eyes with an opthalmoscope, A characteristic abnormal "cherry-red spot" will be seen on the retina.

## Does this disease run in families?

Yes. If a family has one baby with this condition there is a one in four chance that another baby born to these parents will have the same condition. We have also found that the parents may have a partial deficiency of the enzyme. If both parents have a partial deficiency, then there is a one in four chance that they will have a baby with this condition.

## Is there any way of preventing Tay-Sachs disease?

Yes. It is now possible to test the parents for a tendency toward passing on this condition to an offspring. If one parent has a deficiency of the enzyme that is associated with this disease, then one in four children may be born with the condition. If both parents are found to have a deficiency of the enzyme, the chances are even greater that another offspring will be born with the condition.

### Does amaurotic familial idiocy occur only in Jewish families?

Almost exclusively. About 95 percent of the cases occur in Jewish families. This condition occurs in about 1 in 6,000 Jewish births and in about 1 in 600,000 non-Jewish births.

### If both parents have a deficiency of the enzyme, should they risk having a child?

No, because the chances of the child having this fatal disease are too great.

### How long can a baby live with this condition?

About two to three years. The baby's nutrition goes steadily downhill, there is loss of weight and increasing spasticity, until the baby eventually dies.

### Is it necessary to put a child with this condition in a hospital?

No, as there is little that can be done in a hospital that cannot be done at home. However, in certain instances, it may be wiser to place the baby in a chronic-disease hospital or institution so as not to excessively encumber the home environment. The presence of such a baby in a home may have a bad psychological effect upon the parents and other children.

## NIEMANN-PICK DISEASE

### What is Niemann-Pick disease?

It is similar to Tay-Sachs disease, with the added element of a large spleen and liver. It, too, involves blindness, the cherry-red spot in the eye, and mental retardation.

### Is this also familial, and does it tend to occur in Jewish families?

Yes.

### Is this also fatal before three years of age?

Yes.

## DOWN'S SYNDROME
### (Mongolism)

### What is mongolism?

It is a form of mental retardation occurring in three out of every thousand newborns. It is properly called Down's syndrome.

### How is Down's syndrome recognized?

By the appearance of the child. In Down's syndrome, the head is usually small, the muscles are flabby, and the face has a characteristic appearance: eyes slanting upward and outward, a wide nasal bridge, and a protruding tongue. The hand is broad and spadelike, the palmar creases are not normal, the neck is short and broad, and there may be an abnormal heart condition present.

### What causes Down's syndrome?

It is due to a defect in the chromosomes. The normal infant has forty-six chromosomes. An infant with Down's syndrome has forty-seven chromosomes.

### Is Down's syndrome hereditary?

No.

### Does it occur more often with older mothers than with younger ones?

Yes.

### Does it occur more often after several normal babies than as a first baby?

Yes.

### Is there any special test that will make the diagnosis?

Yes. Chromosome studies will show the presence of this condition.

### Can Down's syndrome be diagnosed before the child is born?

Yes, by performing amniocentesis. This involves withdrawing some fluid from the pregnant uterus.

### Is there any treatment for Down's syndrome?

No.

### Is there any way of preventing it?

No.

### Do children with Down's syndrome grow to maturity?

Yes.

### What level of intelligence do these people reach?

They usually require supervision all their lives. However, the range of disability ranges from mild to severe, with some Down's syndrome people being able to work at simple jobs.

### What is the usual disposition of children with Down's syndrome?

There are many stereotypes, but personalities vary widely, as in normal children.

### Can children with Down's syndrome be cared for at home?

Yes, in most cases. Institutionalization should be avoided whenever possible. When home care is not possible because of parental objection, foster care in a family setting should be found.

### Can children with Down's syndrome be educated?

Yes. It is a federal law that they must be educated.

### Can they be taught a trade?

Yes. Most can be taught tasks and simple occupations.

### Can they be made self-supporting?

Rarely, though many can be taught an occupation and can become useful citizens, though requiring support.

### Why was this condition formerly called mongolism?

Because of the facial appearance and the upward slant of the eyes.

### Does Down's syndrome occur only among Caucasians?

No. It occurs in all races.

## RETROLENTAL FIBROPLASIA

### What is retrolental fibroplasia?

This is a form of blindness which used to occur in very small premature babies who developed lung problems and required large amounts of oxygen.

### What causes this disease?

Until recently, the cause was unknown. It has now been ascertained that retrolental fibroplasia was caused by *oxygen poisoning!*

### Oxygen is a beneficial, lifesaving gas; how can there be "oxygen poisoning"?

Too much oxygen, when given to very small premature babies, interferes with normal eye development and can lead to blindness in some cases.

### How much oxygen is used now for premature babies?

Enough to support life, but not excessive quantities.

### Do all premature babies require extra oxygen?

No, only those who appear to have difficulty in breathing.

## HYALINE MEMBRANE DISEASE
### (Respiratory Distress Syndrome)

### What is hyaline membrane disease?

It is a disease of premature babies and some Cesarean babies in which there is an interference with the normal breathing mechanism. It is also called the Respiratory Distress Syndrome.

### When does it develop?

Usually within six to twenty-four hours after birth.

### Are babies born with hyaline membrane disease?

It is difficult to tell at birth. These infants seem normal at birth and for several hours thereafter. Then they start having difficulty in breathing.

### What are the manifestations of this disease?

The baby's breathing becomes labored and grows progressively worse until death from suffocation ensues in about one to three days.

### What causes this condition?

The cause is unknown, but it is suspected that changes in the surface tension overlying the air cells of the lungs may prevent oxygen from gaining ready access to the bloodstream.

### Does this disease always terminate fatally?

No, a considerable number of infants can be saved.

### What is the treatment for hyaline membrane disease?

Oxygen inhalations and increased moisture in the incubator. Some cases may require assisted breathing.

### If an infant recovers from this condition, can it be normal?

Yes, especially when it has been cared for in a modern neonatal care center.

### Does the oxygen act in a harmful way in these cases, as in retrolental fibroplasia?

Not necessarily, because the oxygen concentration is not too high. In any event, the eyes are examined closely.

### Is there any way to prevent this disease?

The best preventive is to try to avoid a premature birth. Recently it has been discovered that the giving of cortisone to a mother who may give birth to a premature baby will prevent the onset of hyaline membrane disease.

## ATELECTASIS OF THE NEWBORN

### What is atelectasis of the newborn?

This is a failure of expansion of some parts of the baby's lungs. These areas contain no air or oxygen and do not function properly.

### What is the cause of atelectasis?

It may be due to obstruction by mucus or amniotic fluid in the respiratory passages, or it may be caused by an immaturity of the lung tissue with failure of this tissue to develop the ability to expand.

### What are the manifestations of atelectasis?

The infant will have rapid, shallow breathing, may have a grunt while breathing, may become bluish because of lack of oxygen, and may display a pulling-in of the chest wall at its ribs and near the neck when attempting to breathe in.

### Is there any way to make a definite diagnosis of this condition?

Examination of the chest will reveal that air is not entering certain parts of the lungs. In addition, an x ray of the chest will show that air has not entered these areas.

## What is the treatment for atelectasis of the newborn?

If there is any obstructive fluid in the respiratory passages, it must be sucked out. Sometimes, bronchoscopy is necessary in severe cases to remove any obstruction. In addition, the infant is kept in an incubator with high humidity and high oxygen content. It is important to stimulate the baby to breathe deeply by making it cry frequently, every few minutes, if necessary.

## What is the outcome in these cases?

If the atelectasis is mild, it will clear up in a few days with normal lung expansion. If it is extensive, it may cause lack of oxygen to the brain and damage to the brain cells. In very severe cases, it may be fatal in one to two days.

# HEMORRHAGIC DISEASE OF THE NEWBORN

## What is hemorrhagic disease of the newborn?

This occurs about the second to fifth day of life and is manifested by bleeding into the skin, the mucous membranes, the navel, and occasionally by bleeding from the rectum or vagina. There may be blood in the urine or in the vomit.

## What causes this type of hemorrhagic disease?

It is believed to be caused by a deficiency of one of the components in the blood-clotting mechanism and by a deficiency of Vitamin K.

## What is the treatment for hemorrhagic disease of the newborn?

Vitamin K is given by injection to all newborns to prevent the condition.

# TETANY OF THE NEWBORN

## What is tetany of the newborn?

It is a condition that occurs during the first week or two of life, associated with irritability, extreme restlessness, twitchings, and occasionally convulsions.

## What causes tetany?

It is caused by a diminished amount of calcium in the blood. It may be brought on by impaired function of the parathyroid glands or the kidneys, or by feeding the child milk that has a higher proportion of phosphorus to calcium than is normal.

## Does tetany occur in breast-fed infants?

It occurs less frequently in breast-fed than in bottle-fed infants, because breast milk has the proper proportions of phosphorus and calcium.

## What test can help to make a positive diagnosis?

A blood test for determination of the amount of calcium in the blood.

## What is the treatment for tetany of the newborn?

Calcium solution is given intravenously, followed by the addition of a calcium-containing solution to the formula.

## What can happen if the treatment is not given?

The infant will become more restless and will develop convulsions. These may be serious if calcium is not given quickly.

## Can tetany be prevented?

Yes, by feeding breast milk or by putting calcium into each bottle the infant takes.

# SEPSIS OF THE NEWBORN

## What is sepsis of the newborn?

It is a bloodstream infection or poisoning occurring usually during the first week of life.

## What is the cause of sepsis in newborns?

Bacteria entering the blood by way of the skin, mucous membranes, nose, mouth, or by way of the umbilicus.

## Do these germs enter before birth or after birth?

The bacteria may enter the body at either time and then gain access to the bloodstream.

## What are the manifestations of this sepsis?

Failure to take feedings, vomiting, diarrhea, loss of weight, restlessness, high fever, and occasionally convulsions.

## How can the diagnosis be established definitely?

Blood cultures are taken to determine whether bacteria are present in the bloodstream.

## What is the treatment for sepsis of the newborn?

Prompt administration of the appropriate antibiotic in adequate doses.

## Are there any complications of sepsis (blood poisoning)?

Yes. Pneumonia, meningitis, peritonitis, abscesses of various organs, or skin abscesses may appear.

## What is the outlook in this condition?

With prompt and early recognition and treatment, the outlook is good. If not recognized early or if the infection is a severe, overwhelming one, it will lead to death of the infant within a short period of time.

## Can sepsis be prevented?

If there is any evidence of infection in the mother before or during delivery, the baby should be given antibiotics prophylactically. If the baby shows any evidence of skin or navel infection, treatment with antibiotics should be instituted promptly.

## THRUSH

### What is thrush?

It is a disease of the tongue and mouth, usually occurring toward the end of the first week of life.

### What is the cause of thrush?

It is caused by a yeast organism.

### Where does this organism come from?

Usually from the mother, who may have a mild yeast infection of her vagina. During the birth passage, the infant becomes infected with this same yeast. It takes about a week for the yeast to grow. It may also come from contamination by rubber nipples and other equipment that may have been in contact with another infant who has thrush.

### What are the manifestations of thrush?

There is a heavy whitish coating on the tongue, which may spread to the gums, lips, and mucous membranes inside the mouth.

### Is thrush serious?

No, and it is quite common.

### What is the treatment for thrush?

The use of an antibiotic called nystatin. It is applied locally to the infected areas and is also given to the infant to swallow.

### Does it take long to clear up thrush?

No. In about a week to ten days the condition will have cleared.

### Can thrush be prevented?

If the mother is known to have a vagi-nal infection with discharge, she should be treated for it during pregnancy.

### In the nursery, should an infant with thrush be isolated?

Yes. In this way the spread from one infant to another can be prevented. The isolation should apply to all utensils used in the care of the infant.

## OMPHALITIS

### What is omphalitis?

It is an infection in the region of the navel (umbilicus) occurring during the first week of life.

### Is omphalitis a serious infection?

Usually it will clear up promptly with adequate treatment. It may be serious if it spreads to a bloodstream infection.

### What is the treatment for omphalitis?

a. Local applications to control the infection.
b. Antibiotics in adequate doses given internally.

## CONGENITAL LARYNGEAL STRIDOR

### What is congenital laryngeal stridor?

It is a noisy breathing, usually on inspiration, and especially pronounced with crying.

### What is the cause of this condition?

It is usually caused by a flabbiness of the tissues around the larynx, particularly the epiglottis.

### Are there ever any more serious causes for congenital laryngeal stridor?

Yes. In some cases there may be a malformation of the larynx or structures adjacent to it. Foreign bodies that have been inhaled, growths on the larynx, or an abnormality of the aorta that may be pressing on the trachea—all may be the underlying cause for this condition.

### When is congenital laryngeal stridor first noticed?

Usually at birth—and it may persist until the child is about twelve to eighteen months of age, when it gradually disappears.

### Is any treatment necessary in the usual case of congenital laryngeal stridor?

No. It is a self-limited condition. As the infant grows older, the flabbiness of the laryngeal tissues disappears.

### How are the more serious deformities in this region recognized?

By looking into the larynx with a laryngoscope. If the physician finds a cyst or web or other cause for obstruction, he will treat it at that time.

### Is there need for special care in feeding infants with congenital laryngeal stridor?

Yes. These infants must be fed more slowly and carefully to prevent aspiration of the food into the windpipe. Sometimes these babies may find difficulty in sucking from a nipple and may need spoon-feeding.

### Is the usual case of congenital laryngeal stridor serious?

No. It may sound very annoying to the parents, but it is usually not serious. It is important that the parents be reassured that the condition will eventually clear up spontaneously.

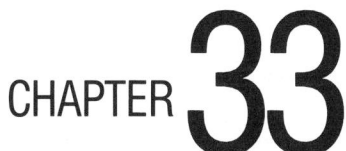

CHAPTER **33**

# INFANT FEEDING AND BOWEL FUNCTION

*(See also Chapter 15 on Breasts; Chapter 17 on Child Behavior; Chapter 47 on Newborn Child; Chapter 78 on Vitamins)*

## BREAST-FEEDING

**Is breast-feeding preferable to bottle-feeding?**

Yes.

**Why is breast milk best for the newborn child?**

It has all the proper elements for the baby's best growth and development; it is clean and sterile; it is of the proper temperature. Also, immune substances are contained in the mother's milk, which help protect the newborn child against disease.

**Are there psychological advantages to nursing?**

Yes, for both the mother and the child. The closeness, the cuddling, etc., are important for both the baby and the mother.

**Does a nursing mother require any special diet?**

She should eat a full, balanced diet, being sure to include plenty of fluids, milk, eggs, meat, fruits, vegetables, and cereal.

**Should the nursing mother avoid certain foods?**

No. However, she may want to avoid

gassy foods such as cabbage, broccoli, rhubarb, garlic, etc.

**Do nursing mothers supplement their diet with vitamins?**

Yes. Most nursing women take supplemental vitamins and calcium.

**Do drugs or medications that the mother takes affect her milk?**

Consult your physician on this matter. Most medicines do show up in the mother's milk but do not affect the baby.

**What general precautions should the nursing mother take?**

She should:
a. Get plenty of rest.
b. Get plenty of relaxation.
c. Avoid tension and anxiety.
d. Avoid excessive smoking.
e. Avoid excessive drinking of alcoholic beverages.

**Will nursing adversely affect the mother's teeth?**

No. However, she should take an adequate supply of calcium in her diet every day.

**Is nursing ever harmful to the mother?**

Only if she is emotionally disturbed by the act. Those women who become tense or who find nursing exceedingly disagreeable should not be forced to nurse.

**If the mother is ill or has a chronic debilitating disease, should she nurse?**

No.

**When is it wisest not to breast-feed a child?**

When the child is very small or weak, or is premature, or has a cleft palate or harelip.

**How soon after birth can nursing be started?**

The very first day.

**Is there any milk in the mother's breast during the first few days after delivery?**

No, but the nursing child does obtain a substance known as colostrum.

**What is colostrum, and what is its value?**

Colostrum is a substance secreted by the breasts before the milk fully comes in. It contains many immune substances, which may help to protect the baby during its first few days of life.

**Does the nursing child obtain sufficient nourishment the first two or three days of life, before breast milk begins to flow?**

Yes.

**When does real milk start to flow?**

About the third or fourth day after birth, but this varies from the second to the fifth or sixth day.

**What starts the flow of milk into the mother's breast?**

Certain hormones in the mother's body. Also, the baby's sucking will accelerate the flow of milk.

**At what intervals should the baby breast-feed?**

Normal healthy babies may nurse every two and a half to three hours.

**If the baby seems to need it, is it permissible to nurse more often?**

Yes, but not more often than every two hours. Consult your doctor about frequency of feedings.

**Should the baby nurse on one or both breasts?**

In general, it is best to nurse at both breasts.

**How long should each nursing last?**

Starting slowly, about five minutes on each breast. As the infant gets larger, each feeding can take up to fifteen to twenty minutes on each breast.

## What should be done if the baby falls asleep during nursing?

Gentle stimulation may help to wake him. He should be permitted a rest of five minutes during nursing, but no longer. Following such a rest he may resume sucking at a normal rate.

## In what position should the mother nurse the baby?

In any comfortable position that avoids strain on the mother's elbow or shoulder.

## Should water be given to the baby between nursings?

This is not necessary in most instances, but if the baby seems to be thirsty and cries, he may be given a few ounces of water.

## Is it permissible to skip nursings if the child has not awakened?

Within the first few days it is best not to skip nursings. Later on the baby may be permitted a longer sleep and have a bottle to substitute for a nursing during the middle of the night.

## What is the treatment for "cracked" nipples?

A mother with cracked nipples should skip a few nursings or alternate breasts. The use of a nipple shield helps protect the breast and helps it to heal more quickly. A soothing ointment may be applied after each nursing, but it must be washed off before the baby is again put to the breast.

## What special care should be given the nipples?

Cleanliness is the most important objective. The nipples should be washed before and after each nursing. A comfortable, well-fitting uplift brassiere should be worn.

## What is the treatment for "caked" breasts?

A good supportive brassiere and medicines to relieve pain.

## Should nursing be stopped if an infection of the breast occurs?

Only if it is too painful or if an abscess must be drained.

## If it is necessary to stop nursing because of a breast condition, can nursing be resumed at a later date?

Yes, but only if the breasts have been pumped regularly and the milk flow has continued to flow.

## How long should breast-feeding be continued?

As long as a woman wishes to continue.

## Can a woman stop breast-feeding after three to four months?

Yes, or at any time she wishes to stop it.

## Is weaning a difficult process?

No. Most babies are given a supplementary bottle during the early months of life and therefore will not resist the change to bottle-feeding later on. Some babies are weaned directly to a cup.

## How soon can a supplementary bottle be started?

Whenever one wishes.

## What can be done if the mother must be away from the child for two or three days?

The breasts can be pumped so that the milk supply will not diminish. This will enable the mother to resume nursing when she returns.

## If the mother and child are to be separated for more than a few days, is it wiser to discontinue nursing completely and to start bottle-feeding?

Yes.

## Is sudden, abrupt weaning harmful?

No. Most children take the change from breast-feeding to bottle-feeding without difficulty.

## Are vitamins and solid foods given to children who are breast-fed, just as they are given to bottle-fed children?

Yes. There is no variation in these supplementary substances.

## What does the mother do when she stops nursing?

She usually wears a tight breast binder or brassiere. It is also advisable to limit her intake of fluids for several days. If breasts are not emptied periodically, they will not refill. The baby's sucking and breast emptying are the greatest impetus to milk formation.

## Is it permissible for the mother to take pain-relieving medications when she stops nursing?

Yes.

# BOTTLE-FEEDING

## If the mother cannot nurse, is bottle-feeding almost as satisfactory?

Yes. There are many excellent preparations of formulas that give the newborn child all he needs in the way of nourishment.

## How soon after birth can a child start getting his formula?

Within eight to twelve hours.

## How much formula is given at first?

About a half-ounce during the first day, increased to an ounce at each feeding the second day, one and a half to two ounces on the third day, and increased gradually as the baby needs it thereafter.

## How can a mother know what equipment is needed to prepare a formula?

Your child specialist (pediatrician) will supply you with this information. Also, many hospitals give lectures to mothers about formula preparation before they leave the hospital.

**From whom will a mother receive instructions about methods of sterilization?**

a. From the pediatrician or physician.

b. From the hospital.

c. From the baby's nurse or from a nursing agency.

**What types of bottles and nipples should be used?**

There are many excellent ones on the market. It makes very little difference which kind is used, as long as it functions well. The small or large nipples are equally effective.

**Is it safe to use plastic bottles?**

Yes.

**How can a mother tell if the nipple is good?**

Turn the bottle upside down; the milk should come through the nipple openings freely, a drop at a time.

**Is it permissible to enlarge nipple openings?**

Yes, with a sterile needle.

**What should be done if too much milk flows through the nipple?**

Discard that nipple and use another one.

**What are the basic ingredients of most baby formulas?**

Most formulas are manufactured with care from modified cow's milk protein. It is not necessary to use evaporated milk formula. Consult your pediatrician.

**When can the formula be changed to whole milk?**

When the child is about five to seven months of age.

**Is it necessary to add any other substances to the prepared formulas?**

No. They are usually made with adequate amounts of all necessary ingredients. Also, these preparations come with complete and simple instructions.

**Can it harm the baby if the proportions of the various ingredients are varied slightly?**

No.

**How many bottles are made from the formula?**

In the beginning, divide the formula into six or seven bottles of three and a half or four ounces each. Later, four to six ounces are put into each bottle. As the baby grows older and takes fewer feedings, the thirty-two-ounce formula may be divided into five bottles.

**How often should a baby be given his bottle?**

Most pediatricians recommend a modified demand approach, that is, a baby is fed whenever hungry with variable intervals, usually totaling six to eight feedings a day.

**Should the baby be made to adhere to a rigid feeding schedule?**

No, especially in the beginning. It is best to feed the baby as often as he needs it. This is called the "self-demand schedule." As he grows older, he will adopt a more definite pattern.

**What should be done if the baby wants to be fed every two hours?**

Let the baby have his formula every two hours.

**How soon after birth do children start regulating their own schedule?**

Most babies will develop a fairly regular schedule at about four to six weeks of age, some a little earlier, some later.

**Should a baby be forced into a rigid schedule?**

No. Let the baby, within reason, decide his own schedule. Gentle persuasion into a regular schedule can be carried out. However, much depends on the mother's time schedule as well as on the baby's requirement.

**Should milk or formulas be heated before being given to an infant?**

No. Infants adapt readily to milk or formulas whether they are cold, room temperature, or heated.

**Is there any harm in letting the baby's feedings go beyond the four-hour interval?**

No.

**Should the baby be awakened for a night feeding?**

No. It is preferable to wait until he awakens. However, if the baby tends to awaken at an inopportune hour, such as 4:00 or 5:00 A.M., it may be wiser to awaken him earlier. Some mothers find it best to wake the baby between 11:00 and 12:00 P.M. while they are still awake, so that the baby will sleep through until 6:00 or 7:00 A.M.

**How soon do most babies skip their night feedings?**

Many babies skip the 2:00 A.M. feeding when they reach two to three months of age. There are great variations, all of which fall into the category of normal.

**What are the best hours for feeding the baby?**

This depends on the family pattern of living. Some babies will thrive on a 6:00 A.M., 10:00 A.M., 2:00 P.M., 6:00 P.M., 10:00 P.M., 2:00 A.M. schedule. In other families, the hours can be varied to 7:00 A.M., 11:00 A.M., 3:00 P.M., etc.

**How much of the formula should the baby take?**

This will vary according to each baby's needs. In the early months, he will take two to four ounces, later on, four to six ounces, and still later six to eight ounces at each feeding. The average total daily intake during the first month of life will be twenty to twenty-five ounces; later it increases to twenty-five to thirty-two ounces, and in some instances the baby may require as much as forty ounces of formula. As solid foods are added, most babies will take less formula.

## Do most babies take the same amount at each feeding?

No. There may be great variations from feeding to feeding.

## Should each bottle contain the same amount of formula?

Yes. However, it is usually best to let the baby set his own pattern, as he may develop the habit of taking more at one feeding than at another.

## Should the baby be expected to drain each bottle?

No.

## Can the amounts in the bottles be varied?

Yes, if the mother gets to know how much the baby takes at certain feedings.

## What should be done with the milk the baby does not take?

Discard it.

## What should be done when the baby takes only an ounce of milk at one feeding and wants more an hour later?

For a time it is permissible to allow this habit to develop. In such instances, the formula should be put into the refrigerator and rewarmed for the remainder of the feedings.

## How long should it take for a baby to drain his bottle?

Most babies will fulfill their requirements within ten to fifteen minutes. If the baby dawdles, discard the remainder of the bottle, for he has probably finished feeding.

## Should a baby be permitted to spend an hour at his feeding?

No. Some babies develop the daw-

dling habit; this should be discouraged.

## Should the baby be permitted to cry for his feeding if he awakens too early?

On the self-demand schedule, the baby is usually permitted to eat whenever he wishes. However, sometimes it is necessary to vary that procedure, and it does no harm to permit a baby to cry for a little while before he gets his feeding. It is never necessary to rush to feed the baby when he cries. It should also be remembered that sometimes he may only want water.

## Should babies be given water between feedings?

Most infants won't require extra water. However, one to three ounces may be given occasionally, especially in warm weather.

## Do babies often take too much of their formula?

In general, babies stop when they are satisfied. Occasionally, a baby will take too much and will usually vomit the excess. There is no harm in this.

## When are vitamins added to the diet?

Vitamins are usually present in prepared formulas. Breast-fed babies start vitamins at one month of age.

## What vitamin preparations are usually used?

A multivitamin drop, usually one that contains Vitamins A, $B_1$, $B_2$, $B_6$, $B_{12}$ C, D, and E. Most vitamin preparations on the market contain all of these vitamins.

## How are these vitamins given?

Practically all of these preparations are soluble in water, milk, or fruit juices. They can either be dissolved in these liquids, or they may be dropped directly on the infant's tongue.

## How much of the vitamins is given?

Start with one to three drops for the first few days and then increase gradually up to fifteen drops a day. Most vitamins come with medicine droppers that are marked with accurate instructions on how much to give.

## Can the droppers hurt the baby's tongue?

No. Today most droppers are made of plastic material.

## What is the maximum amount of vitamins to be given each day?

Fifteen drops, or 0.6cc. This amount should be given every day.

## Should vitamins be given in the summertime?

Yes, in the same amounts as during the other months.

## Is there any great harm if the child doesn't finish the bottle into which the vitamins have been dissolved?

It is not harmful if the child skips an occasional feeding in which the vitamins are given.

## Is it possible to give too much of a particular vitamin?

Not ordinarily. There is a great deal of leeway in the amount the body can tolerate. However, on occasion, an excess has been given with harmful results. This is a rare occurrence.

## Can the vitamins occasionally cause a rash?

Yes.

## What is done for rashes caused by vitamins?

It may be necessary to stop giving the vitamins entirely for a while or to substitute a preparation containing only Vitamins A, C, and D. Some physicians prefer to start with an A, C, and D preparation.

## At what age is orange juice started?

Usually at about six months of age.

### How is orange juice given?

Start with a teaspoonful, dilute it with an equal quantity of boiled water. Increase gradually up to one ounce each of juice and water.

### Is it necessary to use fresh orange juice?

No. Frozen or canned orange juice is adequate.

### Do all babies tolerate orange juice?

No. Some babies will vomit or develop a rash from orange juice. In that event, do not give it.

### Is there any harm if the baby does not tolerate orange juice?

Not if the baby is getting a multivitamin preparation containing Vitamin C.

### Can juices other than orange juice be added?

Yes, but be sure they have an adequate supply of Vitamin C.

### Can cod-liver oil be given instead of vitamin drops?

Yes, but only to supply Vitamins A and D. In that case, it is essential to add Vitamin C in the form of orange juice or Vitamin C drops.

### Can various fish-liver oil preparations be used?

Yes, but again it is necessary to add Vitamin C.

### Is it necessary to add Vitamin B when giving drops other than the multivitamin preparations?

Yes. It is advisable to add a Vitamin B preparation when using cod-liver oil or fish-liver oil only.

### When may the baby be given solid foods?

Solid foods are not necessary for the first four to six months. However, some physicians start the baby on solid foods considerably earlier.

### Which solids are given first?

Either cereal or fruit. Rice or barley cereals are excellent, too. Applesauce and mashed ripe banana are also frequently given as first foods.

### How much of these foods is given?

Always start with a teaspoonful of a new food and increase the amount gradually, depending on how well the baby takes to it, until half a jar or several tablespoons of each food can be given.

### Should solid foods be given before or after the formula?

In the beginning, it may be necessary to give a few ounces of the formula first and then introduce the solid food. Later on, it is better to give the solid food first and allow the baby to take the milk later.

### At what feeding should the solids be given?

This does not matter. In general, cereal may be given at the 10:00 A.M. and 6:00 P.M. feedings; fruit at the 2:00 P.M. feeding.

### Do all babies readily take solid food?

No. If the baby spits out the solid food, try it again and again, until he gets used to it. If the baby definitely cannot manage solid foods, stop attempts at giving them for a week or two and then start over.

### How should solids be fed?

With a small spoon.

### Can solids ever be given through a bottle?

Yes, but this is not recommended.

### What cooked cereals can be used?

Farina, Cream of Wheat, or oatmeal may be used well cooked. This usually means cooking for twenty to thirty minutes. Precooked cereals now on the market are much easier to prepare.

### When can any cereal be given?

At two to four months of age.

### Can prepared fruits out of cans be given?

Yes. These preparations are all adequate.

### How are solids usually added to diets?

This varies widely according to each physician's custom and also according to the child's individual taste. The following schedule is often utilized:

| Age | Add |
| --- | --- |
| 4 months | Cereals (barley and rice). Fruits (applesauce and mashed banana). |
| 5 months | Other cereals and fruits. |
| 6 months | All foods eaten by adults in proper consistency and quantity, either from jars or home prepared. |

### What are good diets for children of eight, ten, twelve, and twenty-four months of age?

SAMPLE DIET SCHEDULE FOR BABY: *EIGHT MONTHS OLD*

**On Arising:**
Vitamin drops and orange juice.

**Breakfast:**
Cereal—any cooked or precooked cereal with milk.
Egg—coddled, soft-boiled, or hard-boiled.
Bottle.

**Noon Meal:**
Vegetables—all prepared, strained vegetables or combinations.
    Fresh vegetables, cooked and strained.
    Potato, baked or boiled with butter added.
Meats—chicken liver, broiled and mashed or strained.
    Chicken, minced or shredded.
    Beefsteak patty, finely ground and broiled.
    All strained meats.
Desserts—any prepared fruits or fruit combinations.
Bottle—if baby wants it.

*(continued)*

**3:30 P.M.**
Bottle, with arrowroot cracker or cookie.
(Some babies prefer a morning bottle on arising. In that case give vitamin drops and orange juice at this time.)

**Evening Meal:**
Cereal—as at morning meal—or
Baby soup—any of the prepared baby soups mixed with a little milk.
Egg—if not given in the morning.
Dessert—banana or any of the baby fruit combinations with a little milk or cream. Jello, junket, custard, chocolate, or tapioca pudding.
Bottle.

NOTE: The baby may not take all these foods. This is a menu from which to select the foods. Do not insist upon giving the baby any food not desired. Feeding, diets, and menus are highly individual. The main thought should be *not to overfeed.* Fat babies are not necessarily healthy babies.

NEW FOODS THAT MAY BE ADDED TO DIET LIST: *AT TEN MONTHS*

STARCHY FOODS: Spaghetti, noodles, pastina.
(These may be well cooked and strained.)
Rice, sweet potato.
CREAM: Sweet or sour cream.
CHEESE: Cream cheese, cottage or pot cheese. (These may be mixed with a little cream or milk.)
BACON: Crisp.
JUICES: Other fruit juices, in addition to orange juice.

NOTE: At this age the baby may refuse certain foods, or may refuse milk. This is not unusual. He may even go on jags—all milk, no solids, or the reverse, for periods. Do not be disturbed by this.

DIET LIST: *ONE YEAR OLD*

**Breakfast:**
Any cooked or precooked cereal with milk.
Egg—coddled, poached, soft-boiled, or hardboiled.
Strip of bacon may be added.
Bread or toast. Milk.
Vitamin drops and orange juice may be given during the morning or at mealtime.

**Noon Meal:**
Meats—chicken, chicken liver, calf's liver, lamb chop, lamb stew, beef-steak patty, chopped meats.
Fish—broiled or boiled. No mackerel, salmon, or salty fish.
Vegetables—all the prepared, strained vegetables or combinations of them. Strained, cooked fresh vegetables. When the baby is ready for chopped foods, these may be used.
Dessert—all prepared baby fruit desserts.

**Midafternoon:**
Milk with crackers, cookies, or toast and butter.

**Evening Meal:**
Any one of the baby soups, plain or creamed.
Spaghetti, noodles, or pastina.
Cheese—cream, cottage or pot cheese. Sweet or sour cream.
Raw vegetables—chopped carrot or tomato.
Dessert—banana and sweet cream, junket, Jello, custard, chocolate or tapioca pudding; fruit desserts.
Milk.

Occasionally egg or cereal may be omitted from the morning meal and given in the evening. Other fruit juices may be substituted for orange juice.

DO NOT FORCE THE BABY TO TAKE ANY FOOD OR MILK NOT DESIRED.

DIET LIST: *TWO YEARS OLD*

**Breakfast:**
Fruit—orange, grapefruit, apple, prunes, cooked pears, peaches, or apricots; any fruit juice.
Cereal—any cooked or dry cereal with milk or cream.
Eggs—may be given in any form.
Bacon may be added.
Bread or toast and butter.

**Noon Meal:**
Soup—any clear broth or creamed vegetable soup.
Meat—chicken or chicken liver, beef or calf's liver, lamb chop or lamb stew, ground beefsteak patty or roast beef, diced meats.
Fish—any fresh fish, broiled, baked, or boiled.
Vegetables—all cooked vegetables, preferably fresh or frozen. Prepared, chopped vegetables may be used. Raw vegetables occasionally.
Potato, rice, spaghetti, macaroni, or pastina.
Dessert—any raw or cooked fruit, custard, junket, Jello, puddings, ice cream.

**Midafternoon:**
Milk with crackers, cookies, or toast and jam.

**Evening Meal:**
Any fruit or vegetable juice, or soup if not given at noon.
Salad of cooked or raw vegetables.
Cheese—cream, cottage or pot, Swiss, or American.
Sour cream.
Spaghetti or noodles.
Eggs—if not given at breakfast.
Dessert—banana or berries and cream or other desserts as listed above.
Bread and butter. Milk.

NOTE: The vitamin drops may be given at any mealtime.
Do not give any fried or canned fish; no salted, pickled, or smoked foods; no highly seasoned sauces or gravies; no pastries or rich cakes.

The above list does not represent all the foods that must be given. It is only a suggested list from which to start the menu for the day.

NEVER FORCE THE CHILD TO EAT ANY FOOD OR TO DRINK MILK.

### Is it harmful if the baby tends to take too much solid food and cuts down on his liquids?

No. It is common for the child to drink less formula or milk as he takes more solids. This will vary from child to child.

### Does the amount of solids in the formula the child takes vary from day to day?

Yes.

### How should new foods be introduced into the diet?

Always try to introduce one new food at a time. Always start new foods with a very small amount and increase gradually on successive days.

### Can babies eat the foods safely from a jar or can?

Yes. Foods as they are processed today do not spoil as long as the container is unopened.

### How long can leftover foods in a jar or can be used?

After opening, they can be kept in a refrigerator for about a day or two without spoiling.

### Is it necessary to use canned foods?

No. Many mothers prefer to prepare their own fruits, vegetables, soups, or meats. They should be well cooked, well pureed, and put through a strainer so they may be digested easily.

### Can small amounts of salt or sugar be added to the foods for seasoning purposes?

Yes.

### Which should be the heaviest meal of the day?

Preferably the noon meal.

### When can the child be permitted to feed himself?

Some babies will start finger-feeding at nine to eleven months of age. This may be quite messy, but the child should be allowed to do it. It represents a step toward self-sufficiency.

### When are chopped or junior foods introduced into the diet?

When the baby is about ten to twelve months of age.

### When should cup training be started?

When the baby is about ten to twelve months of age.

### When can the bottle be eliminated?

Babies vary a great deal in this matter, as they do in all feeding matters. Some will allow themselves to be fed from a cup at twelve to fifteen months of age. Others will take juice from a cup but insist upon milk from a bottle until eighteen months of age. Do not be insistent in eliminating the bottle. Some children may require a bottle until two years of age. This will do no harm.

### Is sterilization of nipples and bottles necessary?

The nipples may be sterilized, but all the bottles require is washing thoroughly with soap and hot water.

### How should the baby be held during feeding?

It is best to hold him in a semierect position in the curve of your arm. In this way the air bubble he swallows during feeding will rise to the top of his stomach and will come up as a "burp" more easily. In addition, the baby will not bring up any of the milk with the burp.

### Is it permissible to feed the baby in a semierect position on a small pillow?

Yes.

### Is it permissible to feed the baby lying down?

Yes, but he should be picked up once or twice during the feeding to bring up the air bubble.

### What can be done to help the baby bring up the air bubble?

The mother puts him over her shoulder and holds him there for several minutes. Sometimes stroking his back or gently patting him will help.

### How soon after feeding can the baby be put down in a lying position?

It is best to keep him upright for ten to fifteen minutes after a feeding.

### At what age can the child be fed in a high chair?

When he is able to sit up comfortably for about ten to fifteen minutes. This will be somewhere between four and six months of age.

### What is the significance of hiccups?

They are spasms of the diaphragm and have no special significance. They occur normally.

### What should be done for hiccups?

In most cases, nothing should be done. A small drink of water may help end them more quickly.

### Is it normal for infants to spit up or regurgitate some of their feedings?

Yes. "Burping" often brings up a little of the formula. It may occur from changing the child's position or when he is taking a little too much food.

### Is vomiting serious?

Occasional vomiting is not serious. It may be caused by the same factors that cause slight regurgitation. Repeated or persistent vomiting should lead you to consult your physician.

## COLIC

**What is colic?**

It is a pain in the baby's abdomen due to spasm of the intestines.

**What are the symptoms of colic?**

Excessive crying, especially in the evening hours, and drawing up of the child's legs as if he were in pain; sometimes these symptoms are accompanied by extreme irritability.

**What causes colic?**

The exact cause is unknown. However, the following may be factors:
a. Underfeeding and hunger.
b. Excessive carbohydrates in the formula.
c. Too much butterfat in the formula.
d. Swallowing air and failure to burp.
e. Intolerance to cow's milk.
f. Immaturity of the baby's nervous system.
g. Improper feeding technique.
h. Fatigue.

**How is colic prevented?**

By finding out which of the above factors is the cause and by correcting it. It is often necessary to obtain the doctor's help in this matter.

**What is first-aid treatment when the child is crying with severe colicky pain?**

Be calm. Hold the baby erect, close to your body, and keep something warm near his abdomen. (Do not burn him with a hot water bottle.) Placing the child on his abdomen on a warm pad may also help to relieve the colic.

**Should medicines for colic be given without a doctor's advice?**

Never.

**How long does colic last?**

Some babies have colic for two to three months and then it disappears spontaneously.

**Are second and third children in the family less colicky?**

Not necessarily.

**Is colic dangerous?**

No.

## BOWEL MOVEMENTS

**How many bowel movements a day are normal for a newborn child?**

Anywhere from one to five movements a day. Breast-fed babies may have more bowel movements than bottle-fed infants. Occasionally, the baby will have a movement with each feeding. As long as the consistency of the stool is good, the number of stools per day does not matter too much.

**What is the normal consistency of stools?**

They should be mushy or pasty or even somewhat firmer. They should have a fairly sweetish odor.

**What is the normal color of an infant's stool?**

Golden yellow. It may also be greenish or turn greenish-brown after standing for some time. This is normal.

**Is constipation serious?**

Ordinarily not. If the baby has one firm stool per day, nothing need be done about it as long as the infant is not uncomfortable.

**Is it normal for some infants to strain at stool?**

Yes. This will disappear as the child grows older, unless he is unusually constipated.

**Can the mother help the child when he is straining at stool?**

Yes. Flexing the legs on the abdomen frequently helps.

**Should suppositories be given if the baby is constipated?**

Only on the doctor's advice.

**Is it ever necessary to stretch the anus when children are constipated?**

Occasionally, but not often.

**Are there ever a few streaks of blood in a constipated stool?**

Yes. The hard stool stretches the anal opening and may cause a small scratch on the surface. This in itself is not serious. This can often be helped by a suppository or by making the stool softer.

**How can the stools be made softer?**

a. Increase the baby's water intake.
b. Increase the carbohydrates added to the formula.
c. Reduce constipating foods such as banana, Jello, junket, chocolate, cheese, oatmeal, apples.
d. Increase laxative foods such as cooked fruits and cooked vegetables.
e. Give prune juice or cooked prunes.

**Can mineral oil ever be given to soften the stools?**

Yes, but only on a doctor's prescription.

**Are there any other medications that can soften the child's stool?**

There are many medications on the market that will perform this function, but they must be given only on a doctor's prescription.

**Is it permissible to use laxatives to soften the stool?**

Usually not. The eagerness to remedy constipation may produce a diarrhea in a baby. This is a much more serious condition and a much more difficult one to control.

# DIARRHEA

### What is diarrhea?
Too frequent stools. In an infant this may mean ten to twelve or fifteen per day.

### Is the character and color of the stools usually changed in infant diarrhea?
Yes. The stools may show undigested material and may be greenish or greenish brown in color and may have a foul odor.

### Are diarrheal stools irritating to the child?
Yes. They may cause a rash on the buttocks.

### What is the significance of blood or mucus in the stools?
The appearance of blood or mucus is due to prolonged irritation of the mucous membrane lining of the intestinal tract and is an indication that the child needs medical treatment.

### What are the causes of infant diarrhea?
a. Faulty technique in preparation of the formula.
b. Excessive carbohydrates in the formula.
c. Allergy to cow's milk.
d. Introduction of a new food that is irritating.
e. Excessive amounts of laxative foods.
f. Infection within the intestinal tract.
g. Infection elsewhere within the body.

### How long does diarrhea last?
It may be a very short-lived, temporary digestive upset, or it may persist for some time and be a symptom of a more serious general condition.

### What is the treatment for infant diarrhea?
a. Skip one or two feedings to give the intestinal tract a rest.
b. Give only boiled water in small amounts until feedings are resumed.
c. Start feedings with more dilute formulas, preferably with less carbohydrates and fat.
d. Give smaller amounts during the first few feedings, perhaps only one to two ounces per feeding for a day or two. Supplement the lack of formula with boiled water.
e. Add a bland, constipating food such as mashed ripe banana, raw, scraped apple, and a little pot cheese that has been thinned with boiled water.

### Can paregoric or other medicines be used to stop diarrhea?
These medications should be given only under a doctor's direction.

### Should a laxative be given to stop diarrhea?
No. This is incorrect treatment.

### When can a normal diet be resumed after an attack of diarrhea?
When the child has had several hard, firm movements for a period of two to three days. At first, small amounts of the baby's normal diet should be given, and then the amounts should be increased gradually.

### What should be done if the diarrhea is persistent and severe?
Contact your physician and get instructions from him. Stop all feedings until he calls.

### Is vomiting serious when associated with diarrhea?
Yes. The baby will then lose fluids and minerals from his body tissues, which must be replaced quickly.

### Can milk be resumed after diarrhea?
If the baby has been on a formula, the formula should be resumed gradually. If he has been on whole milk, use diluted boiled milk until his stools have returned to normal. Slowly return to full strength, unboiled milk if that is what the baby was taking prior to the diarrhea.

### Do cases of diarrhea have to be treated in the hospital?
Serious cases should be; mild cases may be treated at home.

### What treatment is carried out in the hospital for severe cases of diarrhea?
Oral feedings are discontinued, and the baby is given the proper amounts of nourishment and fluids through the veins.

### What is the outlook for severe cases of infant diarrhea?
If treated early in their course, practically all cases recover. The serious cases and deaths from infant diarrhea that used to occur many years ago are now a thing of the past, owing to improved methods of treatment.

### Were these cases of diarrhea once called "summer complaint" or "summer diarrhea"?
Yes.

### For how long a period is hospitalization necessary in a case of severe infant diarrhea?
Approximately seven to ten days. The child must be hospitalized until the diarrhea and vomiting have stopped, the infection has cleared up, and the infant has returned to his normal diet schedule.

### Are special formulas used for diarrheas?
Yes. In some cases, the infant is not put back on his original formula but is given a new formula containing skimmed milk or a fat-free mixture. Some physicians use a milk-free or soy-based formula.

### How long are these special formulas continued after an attack of diarrhea?
For a few weeks.

### Are episodes of diarrhea ever recurrent?

Occasionally. In these instances it is necessary to find the underlying cause and treat it strenuously.

### What are the common causes for recurrent diarrhea?

a. An allergy.
b. An infection in the intestinal tract.
c. A form of celiac disease. (See Chapter 32, on Infant and Childhood Diseases.)
d. An abnormality within the intestinal tract.

### Is allergy to cow's milk a common condition among children?

A very small percentage of children cannot take cow's milk because they are allergic to it.

### Is there often a history of allergy in the family of a child who is allergic to cow's milk?

Yes. A careful history will often reveal another member of the family with a food allergy.

### How can one tell if an infant is allergic to cow's milk?

Usually there will be vomiting, colicky pains, loose stools, or mucus in the stools. Occasionally there will be a rash, particularly on the face. There may also be failure to gain weight or actual weight loss.

### What is the treatment for an allergy to cow's milk?

Do not give the child cow's milk.

### What substitutes may be used for cow's milk?

A prepared synthetic milk produced from soybean.

### Is this substitute for milk satisfactory?

Yes. It contains all the elements necessary for the infant's growth and development.

### hould other milk products be excluded from the diet of an allergic baby?

Yes. Cheeses, butter, etc., should not be given.

### Can a child allergic to cow's milk ever take milk?

Yes. Usually after the child is a year or eighteen months of age, he will lose this allergy and can then be put back on regular milk. This must be done slowly after testing the child with small amounts.

### When the child is allergic to cow's milk, should vitamins and juices be given?

Yes. These are added in the usual way.

### If a child is allergic to cow's milk, is it possible that he will demonstrate other allergies?

Yes. For this reason it is important to be cautious in adding any new food to the diet of such an infant.

### Can allergy to milk be a serious condition in children?

There are occasional children who may go into collapse when given cow's milk. In such a case, make sure to avoid giving cow's milk again.

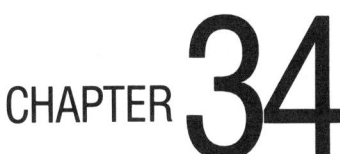

CHAPTER **34**

# INFECTIOUS AND VIRUS DISEASES

*(See also Chapter 12 on Blood and Lymph Diseases; Chapter 18 on Contagious Diseases; Chapter 50 on Parasites and Parasitic Diseases; Chapter 75 on Upper Respiratory Diseases)*

## What are the causes of infectious diseases, and what are examples of each?

a. Bacteria (typhoid fever, pneumonia, etc.).
b. Protozoa (amebic dysentery, malaria).
c. *Rickettsia* (typhus fever, Rocky Mountain spotted fever).
d. Virus (influenza, smallpox, measles).
e. Fungus (athlete's foot, blastomycosis).

## What is the difference between bacteria and viruses?

Bacteria may be seen under the ordinary microscope; viruses are too small to be seen except under a very high-powered electron microscope. Bacteria are too large to pass through certain earthenware filters, whereas viruses are small enough to pass through these filters.

## Do bacteria and viruses require living cells for their growth and multiplication?

Bacteria do not. They can be grown, and they multiply, on nonliving substances; viruses, however, cannot grow or multiply except in the presence of living tissue cells, either animal or human. New tissue culture techniques have resulted in the identification of large numbers of new viruses, some of which produce syndromes now recognized as distinct diseases.

## How are viral diseases spread?

By contact, by droplet infection in the air, and by intermediates (vectors) such as mosquitoes, lice, ticks, etc.

## Do bacteria and viruses respond to antibiotic and chemical agents in the same manner?

No. Many bacteria are killed or inactivated by the antibiotic and chemotherapeutic drugs (penicillin, the mycin group, the sulfa group, etc.), but viruses are not so affected.

## Does one attack of a virus disease protect the individual against further attack?

Not always. In many instances, as in smallpox, measles, polio, etc., this does hold true. But there are other diseases, such as the common cold, influenza, etc., that can occur many times in the same person.

## How can immunity against virus diseases be obtained?

By the development and use of vaccines made from dead or weakened viruses. Poliomyelitis and influenza vaccines are examples. Measles vaccine (from both live and attenuated viruses) and vaccines for German measles and mumps are other examples.

## Is there an effective vaccine for the common cold?

Not as yet. Recent work, however, seems to hold hope for the future development of such a vaccine.

# TYPHOID FEVER

## What is typhoid fever, and how is it transmitted?

Typhoid fever is a generalized disease caused by the typhoid bacillus. It is transmitted from infected food, milk, or water (usually contaminated by sewage). It can be spread by flies but also by direct contact with infected material.

## What is a "typhoid carrier"?

This is a "healthy" person who had typhoid fever at one time, who recovered from it, but still harbors the live germs in his body. He can act as a source of widespread contamination in a community, especially if he has anything to do with the handling of food.

## What are the methods of preventing the spread of typhoid fever?

Purification of water supplies and pasteurization of milk are essential measures. Typhoid carriers, when discovered, must be prevented from handling food that is to be used by other people. Typhoid fever must be recognized early, and the patient must be isolated from healthy people. All of the typhoid patient's belongings and all of his excretions must be sterilized and kept from contact with other people.

## Is vaccination against typhoid fever effective?

Yes, small "booster" doses are effective in maintaining immunity even if taken only every three or four years. Typhoid vaccine should be taken under the following circumstances:

a. When traveling in a country where the water purity is doubtful and where the disease is known to exist.
b. During typhoid epidemics.
c. When there has been contact with a patient who has the disease.

## How is a positive diagnosis of typhoid fever made?

There is a special blood test that becomes positive during the second week of the disease. This is called the Widal test. Also, the germ can be grown in the laboratory from the patient's blood, urine, or stool, usually during the first week of the disease.

## How common is typhoid fever in the United States today?

With the establishment of pure water supplies, the proper handling of food supplies, and the proper isolation of the occasional case, this disease is now quite a rarity in the United States. Also, the advent of the newer antibiotic drugs can kill the typhoid germs readily and thereby prevent the patient from spreading the disease. Only about eight hundred cases per year have been reported in recent years.

## What is the incubation period for typhoid fever?

Approximately ten to fourteen days.

## How long does it take for the disease to run its course?

Usually, about four to six weeks.

## Are there any serious complications of typhoid fever?

Yes. Rupture of the intestines and intestinal hemorrhage are the two most serious complications, but they do not occur very often.

## How soon can the typhoid patient be allowed out of bed?

He can sit up in bed after his temperature has been normal for one week. He may get out of bed about three or four days later.

## How can one tell when the typhoid patient is cured?

When repeated stool examinations and cultures are negative for the typhoid germ. This will insure the fact that the patient is not a typhoid carrier.

## What is the present-day treatment for typhoid fever?

a. Bed rest.
b. Intravenous fluids to combat the dehydration caused by diarrhea.
c. Large doses of Ampicillin or Chloromycetin, both of which are effective antibiotic medications.

# VIRUS PNEUMONIA
*(See Chapter 41 on Lungs)*

# MALARIA

## What is malaria?

It is an infectious disease caused by one of four different types of parasites. It is transmitted by the bite of an infected mosquito or by the transfusion of blood from a malarial blood donor.

## Does malaria occur in the United States?

Yes. There are not too many cases, except in the southeastern states. Most cases occur in tropical countries where there are many swamplands in which the mosquitoes breed readily. It is difficult for people in the United States to comprehend that malaria is still one of the world's greatest health problems—particularly in the tropics.

## How is the diagnosis of malaria made?

By the finding of a malarial parasite in the blood cells of the patient. The disease may be suspected whenever there are periodic chills and high fever in a person who has recently been in a malarial area.

## Is there a vaccine to prevent malaria?

No.

## How can the disease be prevented?

a. By eliminating or controlling the mosquitoes' breeding places, by the use of adequate mosquito netting and screens in an area of infected mosquitoes, and by placing protective screening around the malarial patient so that he will not be bitten by a mosquito that will then spread the disease to a healthy individual.

b. By taking a drug known as chloroquine in doses of 300mg. per week.

## Is there an effective treatment for malaria?

Yes. Most cases respond well to drugs such as primaquine and chloroquine, which are now used instead of the old standby remedy, quinine. A more resistant form of malaria caused increasing difficulty among our armed forces in Viet Nam, requiring searches for new drugs and new treatment regimens.

## Do malarial attacks tend to recur over a period of years if the disease has not been completely eliminated by treatment?

Yes. Formerly, patients often would have malaria on and off for many years.

# YELLOW FEVER

## What is yellow fever, and how is it transmitted?

It is a disease caused by a filtrable virus and transmitted by the bite of a female mosquito *(Aëdes aegypti),* which has previously fed upon the blood of a yellow fever patient.

## Is yellow fever ever seen in the United States?

No. The last epidemic occurred in New Orleans in 1905. It is prevalent, however, in Western Africa and in certain parts of South America.

## Why is the disease of importance today?

Because of the widespread air travel to areas in which yellow fever is prevalent. Great caution must be taken not to introduce even a single case from an infected area. It is also important that travelers from this country remember to be vaccinated against yellow fever before traveling to infected regions. The disease may masquerade as typhoid, malaria, influenza, dengue, or some form of hepatitis.

## DENGUE FEVER

### What is dengue fever?

It is one of the tropical fevers—also called breakbone fever—caused by a virus and transmitted by the bite of a mosquito.

### Can dengue fever be prevented?

Yes, by controlling or eliminating the mosquito that transmits the disease. DDT must be sprayed over the area of the mosquitoes' breeding places.

### Is there a vaccine that will prevent dengue fever?

No, but studies are in progress to produce a live attenuated vaccine against this condition.

### Does dengue fever occur in the United States?

Occasional cases do occur in the southeastern states.

## RELAPSING FEVER
## (Recurrent Fever or Tick Fever)

### What is relapsing fever, and how is it transmitted?

It is a disease characterized by bouts of fever with periods of apparent recovery that are followed by recurring bouts of fever. It is caused by a spirochete germ and is transmitted by the bites of lice or ticks.

### Where is relapsing fever found?

The louse-borne type is common in Europe, Africa, and India. The tick-borne type is common in the United States.

### Is there a vaccine that will protect against relapsing fever?

No.

## TULAREMIA
## (Rabbit Fever)

### What is tularemia, and how is it transmitted?

It is an acute disease caused by a bacillus and characterized by the appearance of a skin sore or ulcer, and it is accompanied by fever that resembles typhoid fever. It is a disease of wild animals, especially rabbits, and is spread among animals by the bites of bloodsucking insects. During the past ten years, the incidence of tularemia has exceeded that of tetanus.

### How do humans get tularemia?

Most human cases occur in hunters, butchers who skin rabbits or other animals, and farmers and laboratory workers who handle or breed infected rabbits.

### How can tularemia be prevented?

By being extremely careful with the handling of wild rabbits and rodents. Care must be exercised in removing ticks from the fur of such animals, and proper clothing must be worn to avoid tick bites. Any wild game that is to be eaten must be very thoroughly cooked.

### What is the treatment of tularemia?

Streptomycin, tetracycline, or Chloromycetin usually cure the disease within a short period of time.

## THE RICKETTSIAL DISEASES

### What are the rickettsial diseases, and how are they transmitted?

They are a group of infectious diseases, with fever, caused by *Rickettsia,* which are germs smaller than bacteria but larger than viruses. They are transmitted to man by the bites of lice, fleas, or mites, or by the attachment of ticks to the skin.

### Which diseases are caused by the *Rickettsia?*

Epidemic typhus fever, Rocky Mountain spotted fever, South American spotted fever, Q fever, scrub typhus, trench fever, and rickettsialpox. Brill's disease is a type of typhus fever seen in America and probably represents a flare-up of a former attack of epidemic typhus fever in a patient who may have had that disease when he lived in Europe, many years prior to the present attack.

### How may these diseases be prevented?

By the eradication of fleas, mites, body lice, ticks, and by the control of their breeding places. In tick-infested areas, it is important to inspect the body at frequent intervals to discover any tick attachments to the skin. At night it is important to use netting to keep insects out.

### Are vaccines effective against any of these diseases?

Yes, against typhus fever and Rocky Mountain spotted fever. However, tetracycline and Chloromycetin are of value in the treatment of these diseases if administered promptly. Control of Q fever in man depends upon control of the disease in animals, especially those raised for meat and milk.

### Are the rickettsial diseases serious?

Yes, particularly Rocky Mountain spotted fever and certain types of typhus fever, which may lead to death in a rather high percentage of cases if not treated properly.

## INFECTIOUS OR EPIDEMIC JAUNDICE
## (Spirochetal Jaundice or Weil's Disease)

### Is infectious jaundice the same disease as infectious hepatitis?

No. This disease is caused by a

spirochete germ and is transmitted by contact with rats, either by eating or drinking food or water that has been contaminated by rat feces or urine, or occasionally by a rat bite.

### Where is infectious jaundice most commonly found, and who is most apt to develop the condition?

It is most common around wharves, mines, and sewers, because rats are more apt to be found in these places. Miners, sewer workers, and wharf men are therefore more apt to contract the disease.

## BRUCELLOSIS
### (Undulant Fever, Malta Fever, Mediterranean Fever, Gibraltar Fever)

### Is brucellosis primarily a disease of humans?

No. It affects animals, usually cattle, swine, and goats. It is caused by a germ called *Brucella.* It is transmitted to man by contact with the secretions and excretions of the above animals and by the drinking of contaminated milk.

### Is brucellosis contagious from man to man?

No.

### Who is most apt to contract brucellosis?

It is considered an occupational disease among veterinarians, meat packers, butchers, dairy farmers, and livestock producers.

### What are the symptoms of brucellosis?

Fever, chills, body aches and pains, profuse sweating, and loss of weight. The fever is usually intermittent with long periods of normal temperature. These symptoms may go on for as long as a year or more, and if brucellosis becomes chronic and is untreated, the symptoms may go on for many more years.

### Is there an acute form of this disease?

Yes. This lasts only about two to three weeks and must be differentiated from typhoid fever, malaria, or tuberculosis.

### How can brucellosis be prevented in man?

By pasteurization of milk. Also, people who handle meat must protect themselves by wearing rubber gloves. All skin lesions should be properly cared for in these people. Infected animals should be detected and destroyed.

### What is the treatment for brucellosis?

Tetracycline has been found to be most effective in this disease.

## PLAGUE
### (Black Plague, Bubonic Plague)

### What is plague?

It is a serious disease, which occurred in huge epidemics throughout Europe and Asia in ancient times and in the Middle Ages. It was known as the Black Death. The last great epidemic occurred in India in the early 1900s.

### Is plague very common today?

No. There have not been any great epidemics since extensive programs for its extermination have been carried out.

### How is the plague transmitted?

The bacteria that cause plague are found in fleas on the bodies of rats. Thus the fleas from rats get onto the bodies of humans and transmit the disease.

### How does one prevent the plague?

By the extermination of rats.

### What are the symptoms of plague?

Fever, severe chills, vomiting, great thirst, morning diarrhea, blood spots on the skin, and enlargement of the lymph glands.

### What is pneumonic plague?

This is a form of the disease that involves the lungs. It can be transmitted from person to person by droplet infection.

### Is plague a serious disease?

Yes. It formerly carried with it a tremendous mortality, but today, with streptomycin and tetracycline used together, the mortality has been reduced from over 90 percent to less than 20 percent.

## LEPROSY

### What causes leprosy?

It is believed to be caused by a germ called Hansen's bacillus.

### Is leprosy very contagious?

No. This is a very common misconception. Leprosy is only mildly contagious, and its method of transmission is relatively unknown.

### Is leprosy found in the United States?

Yes, mostly in the southern and Gulf states, but the number of cases is small.

### What are the symptoms of leprosy?

There may be lumps and thickening of the skin, loss of hair, deformities of bones and joints, and loss of sensation in various areas of the body due to nerve involvement.

### What is the outlook in cases of leprosy?

It depends upon the extent and type of involvement. In some cases, after a certain amount of damage has been done, there may be spontaneous disappearance of symptoms that return at a later date. Other cases go on for twenty years or more.

**Is there any effective treatment for leprosy?**

Yes. Several sulfone drugs have been used with favorable results. Treatment is carried on in the National Leprosarium, a special government hospital in Louisiana. With early diagnosis and well-planned treatment, the prognosis for arrest or cure of leprosy is now favorable.

## INFECTIOUS MONONUCLEOSIS (Glandular Fever)

**What is infectious mononucleosis or glandular fever?**

It is an infectious disease, probably caused by a virus, which often occurs in mild epidemics among children and young adults in schools, colleges, and other institutions.

**How is infectious mononucleosis transmitted?**

Probably by air-borne droplet infection.

**After exposure, how long does it take for infectious mononucleosis to develop?**

Anywhere from five days to two weeks.

**What are the main symptoms of infectious mononucleosis?**

Fever, headache, generalized aches and pains, and swelling of the lymph glands in the neck, armpits, and groin. The spleen becomes enlarged, and certain changes occur in the blood cells. A very prominent symptom at the onset of the disease may be a sore throat.

**How can the disease be definitely established?**

By certain specific blood examinations.

**What is the usual course of infectious mononucleosis?**

It is a self-limited disease with recovery in one to three weeks. The outlook for complete recovery is excellent except in very rare instances. A certain small number of cases may be prolonged for several months.

**What are the complications of infectious mononucleosis?**

There are not too many, but they may be serious. They include:
a. Throat infection.
b. Liver involvement, with jaundice and hepatitis.
c. Rupture of the spleen.
d. Involvement of the nervous system, with meningitis or encephalitis. This occurs rarely.

**What is the specific blood test that clinches the diagnosis of this disease?**

The heterophile agglutination test.

**Is there any specific treatment for infectious mononucleosis?**

No. Antibiotics have been used to prevent secondary bacterial infections, but there is no known cure for the disease itself. Bed rest is very important during the period of fever and for a few days thereafter and should be prolonged in cases in which liver involvement is suspected. Even though there is no specific treatment, it must be remembered that almost all cases get well by themselves.

**Is infectious mononucleosis transmitted by kissing?**

It is thought that this occurs, particularly among young adults.

**If someone has the type of I.M. (infectious mononucleosis) that persists for several weeks, or even months, must he remain isolated and stay in bed?**

No. If his temperature is normal, he may be permitted to return to school or work. But such a person should avoid close contact with others, as he may still be capable of transmitting the disease.

## RABIES (Hydrophobia)

**What is rabies, and how is it transmitted?**

It is an acute infectious disease of animals, especially dogs and cats, caused by a virus, which affects the nervous system. The virus is present in the saliva of infected animals and is transmitted by the bite of the animal to another animal or to a human.

**What is the incubation period of rabies?**

Usually about two weeks, but prolonged periods up to two years following an animal bite have been recorded in rare instances.

**What are the symptoms of rabies?**

Fever, restlessness, and depression. The restlessness leads to uncontrollable excitement and convulsions. There is excessive salivation and painful spasms of the throat muscles. Death occurs in three to five days. Because of the spasms of throat muscles, there is fear of drinking or swallowing, thus the term "hydrophobia."

**What should be done to a dog or other animal that bites a human being?**

It should be kept under observation for about two weeks. If it does not become ill or die in this period of time, its bite may be considered harmless, and the animal can be released to its owners. If the animal becomes ill, it should not be killed but allowed to die naturally, since this will make the diagnosis easier. An autopsy should then be performed and the animal's brain examined to obtain positive proof that the animal had rabies.

### Can rabies be prevented and controlled?

Yes, by the impounding and destruction of stray dogs and cats and by the mass inoculation of licensed dogs and cats against rabies.

### What is the local treatment for a dog or cat bite?

Thorough washing with soap and water for a period of five to ten minutes is sufficient. Cauterization is no longer considered to be good treatment.

### Is there an effective vaccine against rabies, and when should it be used?

Yes. Antirabies vaccine is very effective in preventing the disease, but it must be used cautiously as it sometimes has toxic effects. When the animal that caused the bite is known to have the disease or cannot be examined because it cannot be located, immediate vaccination against rabies should be begun. In cases in which the dog is thought to be healthy and can be observed, the animal should be watched for fourteen days. If the animal remains healthy, it is not necessary to vaccinate the human. If the dog becomes ill and dies, immunization of the bitten person should be started at once. Recent attempts to actively immunize high-risk groups such as veterinarians, mail carriers, and speleologists (cave explorers) with a new duck embryo vaccine have been very successful.

### Can rabies be prevented if one waits several days after the bite before starting the vaccination?

Yes. It is safe to wait and see what happens to the animal before starting to give rabies vaccination.

### If a human being once develops rabies, what is the outcome?

Rabies is fatal in almost 100 percent of cases, and there is no known treatment of any value.

## TETANUS (Lockjaw)

### What is tetanus, and what causes it?

It is an acute infectious disease causing spasm of muscles and convulsions. The spasm of the jaw muscles accounts for the name "lockjaw." The disease is caused by a bacillus that can survive in extreme heat or cold for many years because it forms inert "spores" that may become activated after they enter the body of a human.

### How is tetanus transmitted?

The germ is distributed widely throughout the world, especially in soil that has been contaminated or fertilized by animal or human feces. Wounds, especially deep puncture wounds that are contaminated, form excellent sites for the development of tetanus. The germ forms a toxin, which acts upon nerves in the brain and spinal cord and leads to muscular spasms and convulsions.

### What is the incubation period of tetanus?

Between five and ten days, but it may vary from two days to two months.

### How is the diagnosis of tetanus made?

A history of recent injury or operation is given. The wound appears infected, and upon taking cultures of the pus, the tetanus germ is found. The symptoms must be distinguished from those of meningitis, rabies, or other conditions.

### How can tetanus be prevented?

By the use of:
a. Tetanus toxoid—for active immunization of people liable to injuries, such as gardeners, farmers, soldiers, mechanics, children, athletes. Immunity with toxoid is prolonged but is best "recalled" by boosters given about every four years and also at the time of injury.
b. Tetanus antitoxin (TAT)—for pas-

sive immunization. Once an injury has occurred, this will afford protection of short duration.

### What is the outlook once tetanus has developed?

It depends upon the promptness with which treatment is begun. The mortality rate is very high, especially in the very young and very old. The mortality rate varies from 30 to 100 percent. If the patient survives the first nine or ten days, his chances for full recovery are considered improved.

### What is the treatment for tetanus?

a. Huge doses of antibiotics.
b. The giving of large doses of tetanus antitoxin.

## ANTHRAX

### What is anthrax, and how is it transmitted?

It is a highly infectious disease of animals, which is caused by the anthrax bacillus and can be transmitted to man directly or indirectly. It occurs chiefly in goats, cattle, sheep, horses, and hogs. Thus, people who have contact with these animals are prone to develop the disease.

### How do humans develop anthrax?

The germs usually enter the skin through a small cut or laceration on the hands of people who habitually handle the animals mentioned above. Also, by breathing in anthrax germs, the lungs may become infected. Or if infected material from the animals is swallowed, intestinal involvement may develop.

### What is the treatment for anthrax?

Antiseptic dressings and antibiotics should be applied to local wounds, and antianthrax serum should be given in large doses.

**What is the outlook once anthrax has developed?**

Four out of five people will recover if properly treated.

**Is anthrax common?**

Not anymore, because people who handle animals that have anthrax sores are now fully aware of the possibility of catching the infection. Such people now take proper precautions. No potent vaccine is as yet available for human use in preventing the disease in people who handle infected animals.

## ECHO VIRUS DISEASE

**What is ECHO virus disease?**

It is a contagious viral infection affecting the intestinal, respiratory, and nervous systems and is seen most often in young children and, occasionally, in adults. It frequently occurs in large epidemics.

**What are the symptoms and course of ECHO virus disease?**

Fever, headache, pain and stiffness in the neck and back, vomiting, sore throat, abdominal cramps, and diarrhea. The usual course is spontaneous with complete recovery within three to five days.

**Are specific medications necessary to cure ECHO virus disease?**

No. Usually aspirin for the aches and pains and drugs to relieve the vomiting and diarrhea are sufficient. Antibiotics are not indicated.

**Is ECHO virus disease serious?**

No, but it is sometimes erroneously diagnosed as polio or meningitis, thus alarming the family.

## CHOLERA

**What is cholera?**

It is a disease affecting the intestinal tract and caused by a bacterium usually transmitted by water through fecal contamination.

**Where does it occur?**

Mostly in Asia, especially in India and Bangladesh. No cases have occurred in the Americas for about fifty years.

**What are the symptoms?**

Severe diarrhea with "rice-water stools," followed by extreme dehydration.

**How serious is the disease?**

Until recently it carried a 30 to 60 percent mortality rate.

**What are the most effective methods of prevention?**

a. Effective quarantine of known cases.
b. Careful hygiene and general sanitation to prevent contamination of water supplies.
c. Vaccination of all individuals traveling to or through areas where there is danger of endemic or epidemic cholera.

**What is the treatment for cholera?**

a. Prompt administration of huge amounts of fluids containing salt. This is to combat the great dehydration so characteristic of cholera. If the fluids cannot be given intravenously, the patient should drink large quantities of saltwater.
b. Administration of the antibiotic tetracycline.

**How effective is treatment in cholera?**

Very effective if started early in the course of the disease. Mortalities have been reduced markedly.

## AIDS

**What is AIDS?**

AIDS (Acquired Immune Deficiency Syndrome) is caused by a virus called HTLV-III/LAV that attacks and destroys T-cell lymphocytes. T-cell lymphocytes are white blood cells that protect the body against infections. When they are present in insufficient numbers, the body's ability to overcome bacterial, viral, or other harmful invaders is diminished.

**How is AIDS transmitted?**

AIDS is transmitted through exchange of body fluids during sexual contact or by direct contact with blood from infected persons. Most cases are found among promiscuous male homosexuals. Some cases occur from ordinary penis-vaginal heterosexual contacts, but the number is small. Other cases are found among intravenous drug users who share a needle with someone infected with the virus, or who use unsterile needles. (Now that donor blood is tested for the AIDS antibodies before being used, cases of transmission via transfusion have been virtually eliminated.)

**How is the disease transmitted by male homosexuals?**

Mainly through anal intercourse, since the virus is present in the semen (the fluid ejaculated during orgasm). Sex with multiple partners increases the chances of exposure to someone who has AIDS or who has been exposed to the virus. AIDS is not common in homosexuals who have only one partner.

**Why is anal intercourse more likely to spread AIDS than vaginal intercourse?**

It is thought that the mucous membranes of the anus and rectum are more likely to tear and permit the virus to enter the body than the vaginal mucous membranes.

**Do most people exposed to the AIDS virus develop the disease?**

No, the majority do not develop the disease, but they should monitor their health carefully. Some persons develop a milder form of the disease called AIDS Related Complex (ARC), which may or may not develop into AIDS.

**Does AIDS come about from an occasional nonsexual contact such as shaking hands or eating with someone who might have AIDS?**

AIDS is not transmitted by handshakes or sneezes, or even light social kisses. It is not transmitted in swimming pools or spas, or from drinking vessels or toilet seats.

**Can deep kissing transmit AIDS?**

It is theoretically possible since the saliva occasionally contains the virus, but this form of transmission has not been documented.

**How is AIDS transmitted through heterosexual contact?**

Mainly through an infected male who is both homo and heterosexual (bisexual), or who is an intravenous drug user. Also, sexually active heterosexuals who have many contacts, especially with prostitutes, are at a higher risk of acquiring AIDS.

**Do newborn children ever have AIDS?**

The AIDS virus can be transmitted by an infected mother to her offspring during pregnancy, even if the mother is not ill. Such infected mothers usually have been intravenous drug users or Haitian.

**Can someone be tested to see if he or she is harboring the AIDS virus?**

Yes. Certain blood tests will tell. The most commonly used test, the HTLV-III/LAV antibody ELISA (enzyme linked immunosorbant assay), is an extremely sensitive test that detects antibodies in blood created by the immune system when the HTLV-III/LAV virus enters the body. Because of its extreme sensitivity, it reacts to other conditions besides the presence of HTLV-III/LAV antibody. Consequently, it is not a test for AIDS itself and probably only a small number of persons who test positive will develop AIDS.

However, they may be infectious to others.

**Can someone get AIDS from being a blood donor, or from receiving a transfusion of blood, or from products obtained from blood?**

No. All needles used in taking blood for a transfusion are sterile and are used only once and then thrown away. Since blood is tested to make sure it is free from possible AIDS virus contamination, transfusions and blood products are unlikely to be routes of transmission in the future.

**What are the main symptoms and signs of AIDS?**

Loss of appetite and weight; persistent unexplained fatigue and weakness; unexplained fever; enlarged lymph glands; infections that stubbornly resist treatment; dry, persistent cough that is not related to smoking or a cold; blue/black discolorations on or under the skin or white spots in the mouth. Eventually, infections such as pneumonia or blood poisoning overwhelm the body and the patient dies. Other patients develop malignancies, especially of the lymph glands and skin.

**How long does it take to contract the symptoms and signs of AIDS?**

It is thought that it usually takes anywhere from two to seven years after infection with the virus before signs of the disease develop.

**Is AIDS curable?**

Not at present. Treatment consists only of combating the infections as they arise.

**Do most people with AIDS eventually die of the disease, and how quickly does AIDS kill?**

Yes, at present most people die. Patients usually have the active disease for one or more years before an overwhelming infection carries them away. But there is hope for the future.

**What can male homosexuals do to avoid AIDS?**

Shun promiscuity; avoid intercourse if they are aware that they harbor the AIDS virus; use a condom during anal intercourse.

**What can heterosexuals do to avoid AIDS?**

Shun sexual contacts with promiscuous partners; use a condom to minimize exchange of body fluids; avoid sexual contacts with people who are at a high risk for AIDS, such as those who are drug addicts.

**Is the number of AIDS cases likely to increase within the next few years?**

Yes, for the following reasons:
1. Many hitherto unreported cases are now being reported.
2. Many people who were infected with the virus during recent years have not yet shown active symptoms of the disease.
3. Drug addiction has not diminished significantly. However, the fear of contracting AIDS may alter ihe incidence of new cases by changing the sex habits of male homosexuals. A high percentage of male homosexuals now limit their activity to just one partner.

**How long do physicians think it will be before satisfactory measures will be available to combat AIDS?**

Most researchers think that an effective vaccination against the AIDS virus will not come about until 1990, or later.

# CHAPTER 35

# INHERITED AND CONGENITAL CONDITIONS

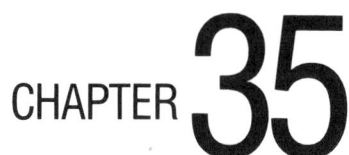

*(See also Chapter 18 on Contagious Diseases; Chapter 43 on Medications and Drugs; Chapter 57 on Pregnancy and Childbirth; Chapter 79 on X ray)*

## What is meant by an inherited characteristic?

It is a trait or bodily characteristic that is passed on from one generation to another. Such a trait or characteristic is determined by units within the nucleus of the germ cells called chromosomes or genes.

## What is DNA?

It is the basic substance, found in the nucleus of cells, responsible for transmitting hereditary characteristics.

## What is deoxyribonucleic acid?

It is the full name for DNA.

## What is meant by a congenital condition?

A trait or bodily characteristic with which one is born, usually as a result of something that happens to the embryo during its development or at birth. For example, if the mother develops German measles during the early weeks of pregnancy, this is likely to affect the growing embryo and produce blindness, heart disease, and other conditions. Under such circumstances, these conditions would be regarded as congenital, since they occurred during the formation of the embryo and were *not* inherited.

## Do inherited characteristics tend to follow any pattern of inheritance?

Yes. The Mendelian law governs inheritance.

## What is the difference between a dominant and a recessive characteristic?

A dominant characteristic is much more likely to appear in the offspring than a recessive one. For instance, with one brown-eyed and one blue-eyed parent, the chances are that more of the children will be brown-eyed, as brown eyes are the dominant characteristic. When a child has parents with black hair but is born with red hair, red hair is the recessive characteristic.

## Are most inherited defects and deformities dominant or recessive characteristics?

Most of them are recessive characteristics and will appear in only a small percentage of cases.

## Do inherited characteristics sometimes skip generations and appear in subsequent generations?

Yes.

## If someone has an inherited deformity, is there a tendency for his children to have this deformity?

Yes, but it must be remembered that inherited defects occur in only a small percentage of offspring. However, a family with known inherited defects has a much greater chance of having children with these defects than does a family in which there are no known inherited abnormalities.

## Is it safe for two people, each of whom has a family history of inherited deformities, to marry one another?

Yes, but they must carefully consider the possibility of passing on an abnormality to their children. It is wise for such a couple to seek expert advice before having children.

## Is it safe to marry a blood relative?

It is safe to marry a relative, but it is wise not to have children when the relationship is close. This is apt to bring out undesirable recessive traits.

## Is it safe to marry into a family in which there is known insanity?

Yes. Insanity is not inherited, although the tendency to inherit personality disorders may occur in some families. Environmental factors are usually much more important.

## What are some of the common inherited traits and abnormalities?

Color blindness, skin color, eye color, hair color, harelip, clubfoot, cleft palate, twinning or other multiple birth tendencies, body build, mental deficiency, hemophilia, etc. Also, certain allergies and tendencies toward development of other diseases may be inherited.

## Is cancer inherited?

No, although the tendency toward the development of tumors might be inherited.

## Can paternity be determined accurately?

Yes. By means of certain blood studies, it can be determined with a good degree of accuracy.

## Can events in the life of a pregnant woman alter the physical development of the unborn child?

Illness in the mother may produce a defect in the development of her embryo. Also, excessive drinking, smoking, and use of drugs can cause physical and developmental defects. Emotional upsets that affect the mother during her pregnancy will *not* influence the child.

**Can x-ray radiation or exposure to radioactive substances alter the characteristics of offspring or produce abnormalities?**

Excessive exposure to x rays or radioactive substances during the early weeks of pregnancy might influence and disturb the normal development of the embryo. Also, it is now thought that excessive x-ray radiation in the region of the ovaries may cause alteration of some of the cells so that an abnormality might crop up in a child or grandchild. This entire subject is now undergoing very intensive investigation.

**Can the taking of certain medications and drugs during the early months of pregnancy alter the physical or mental characteristics of the offspring?**

Yes. It has been found recently that there are many drugs that can injure and cause malformations in the embryo during the first few weeks or months of its life. For this reason, mothers are cautioned never to take any medicines except those that are precisely prescribed by the attending physician.

**Is it possible to avoid having children who will inherit abnormalities from their parents?**

This question is related to the general problem of preventive medicine in relation to hereditary disease. First, it might be well to avoid having children with a mate whose family is known to have inherited diseases. Second, relatives who marry one another should seriously consider the advisability of having children. This relationship, called consanguinity, may bring out undesirable, latent hereditary traits. Further, couples in whose families inherited diseases exist should seek genetic counseling before having children. Parents can now be tested for a sickle-cell trait and for a tendency toward passing on Tay-Sachs disease. If both parents exhibit these tendencies, it is perhaps best if they do not have children.

**Are intellect and intelligence inherited?**

It is difficult to assess the relative roles of heredity and environment in this connection. It is known, however, that intelligent people have a greater tendency to have intelligent children. How much of this is due to their environment we cannot now state. It is known that mental retardation is often inherited or may result from a birth injury or infection.

**Should people who have one abnormal child risk having other children?**

Many abnormalities are now known to be the result of conditions that occurred during pregnancy or at birth and therefore would not affect subsequent children. Of the inherited conditions, many are recessive, and the chance of other children being affected is small. Expert medical advice is available and should be sought in such cases.

**Should people with inherited defects marry and have children?**

They may marry, but they should consider carefully whether they ought to have children, and the advice of medical experts should be obtained. Some inherited conditions are recessive and will affect only a few scattered members in a family tree. Other inherited disorders run a dominant pattern, and the chances of their appearance in the children are great. In such cases it might be wiser for a couple to adopt a child rather than have their own.

**Should people who have had defects such as clubfoot or harelip, etc., exercise more than the usual care in the selection of a mate?**

Yes. They ought to avoid having offspring with anyone with a similar family history of defects.

**Is longevity inherited?**

No, but the tendency toward longevity may be inherited. (See Chapter 5, on Aging.)

**Should one exercise caution in marrying into a family in which there are several members who have had epilepsy or mental disorders?**

Yes.

**Are weight and height characteristics inherited?**

Height is much more likely to be inherited than weight. Weight will depend upon one's eating habits.

**Is it serious if a pregnant woman develops German measles?**

Yes. If it occurs during the first few months of pregnancy, it may lead to blindness, deafness, heart disease, or mental retardation in the offspring.

**Are personality traits inherited?**

Heredity may play a role in the development of personality, but it is probably a small one. The most important contribution to personality development is the environment in which the child grows up.

**Is there any truth to the statement that a "black sheep" is one who has inherited certain unfavorable characteristics from an ancestor?**

No.

**Are criminal tendencies inherited?**

No.

**Is there any such thing as inheriting a "weak character"?**

No.

**Are many diseases inherited?**

No. Your physician will be able to inform you precisely as to which diseases are inherited. They are relatively few in number.

## INHERITED OR CONGENITAL CONDITIONS ASSOCIATED WITH MENTAL AND PHYSICAL RETARDATION

**What are some of the factors associated with inherited and congenital diseases that are accompanied by mental and physical retardation?**

a. The inheritance of defective genes.

b. The development of chromosome abnormalities as in mongolism, Klinefelter's syndrome, and Turner's syndrome.

c. Inherited defects in metabolism.

d. Defects secondary to skull or brain malformations.

e. Conditions that affect the mother during her pregnancy, such as German measles, syphilis, or other infections.

f. Extremely poor nutrition of the mother during pregnancy.

g. The ingestion by the mother of certain harmful drugs during the early weeks and months of her pregnancy.

h. Exposure of the mother and the young embryo to excess radiation.

i. Difficulties during childbirth, especially those associated with the delay in the baby's breathing.

j. Marked jaundice of the newborn baby, as in erythroblastosis (Rh-factor disease).

k. Causes after the child has already been born, such as meningitis, encephalitis, severe head injuries, lead or other type poisonings, etc.

**What are some of the more commonly encountered metabolic disorders causing mental retardation?**

a. Phenylketonuria, otherwise known as PKU disease.

b. Galactosemia.

c. Maple syrup urine disease.

d. Tay-Sachs disease.

e. Wilson's disease.

**BROWN EYES**

**BLUE EYES**

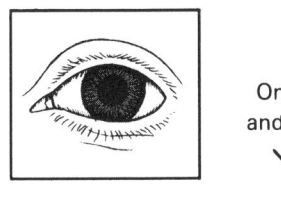
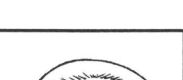

PARENTS:

One pure brown eyes and one pure blue eyes

CHILDREN:

Eyes brown (dominant) with blue recessive

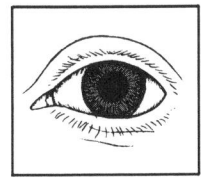
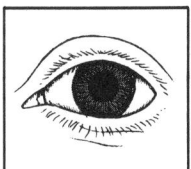

PARENTS:

with brown dominant and blue recessive

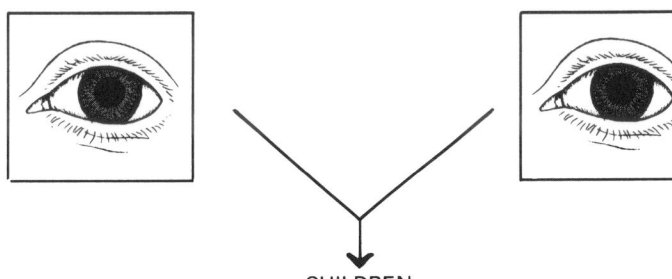

CHILDREN:

¼ will be pure brown     ½ will be brown dominant and blue recessive     ¼ will be pure blue

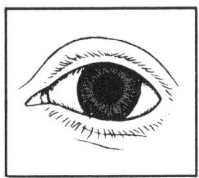
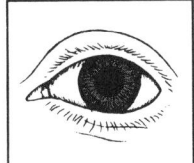
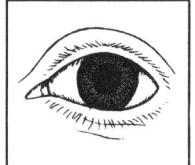
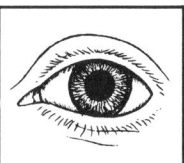

***The Mendelian Law.*** *The illustration above is a schematic representation of the Mendelian Law as it applies to the inheritance of eye color. The same law applies to the inheritance of other physical characteristics.*

### What causes PKU disease?

It is caused by the absence of an enzyme that acts on one of the protein elements in the food. Improper metabolism of this element accounts for the accumulation of abnormal metabolic constituents in the brain.

### Is PKU disease inherited?

Yes.

### Can PKU disease be recognized early in an infant's life?

Yes. There is a blood test (Guthrie test) that can be done on the baby's blood when the baby is three to four days old. There is also a urine test that can detect PKU disease when the baby is four to six weeks old. Many states in the country now have mandatory laws requiring that the Guthrie blood test be done prior to the newborn child's leaving the hospital.

### Can PKU disease be treated successfully?

Yes, if it is recognized early. It is first necessary to discover the particular protein that is not being metabolized properly. When this has been discovered, this protein is completely eliminated from the infant's diet. Under such circumstances, it is possible to avoid the ultimate brain damage that is associated with this condition.

### How common is PKU disease?

It occurs approximately once in every ten to twenty thousand births.

### What is galactosemia?

It is a disease characterized by a disturbance in the metabolism of the sugar present in milk. There is no disturbance, however, in fruit or cane sugar metabolism.

### Can galactosemia be detected early in an infant's life?

Yes. There is a blood test for the presence of the enzyme necessary in the metabolism of milk sugar. Also, one can test for the presence of sugar in the urine in very young babies.

### Can galactosemia be prevented or treated?

Yes, by eliminating milk sugar from the child's diet. This means that the child will have to have a milk substitute instead of regular milk.

### What is Tay-Sachs disease?

See Chapter 32, on Amaurotic Familial Idiocy.

### What is Wilson's disease?

It is a condition in which there is a disturbance in the metabolism of copper in the body that allows it to accumulate in the brain, liver, eyes, and other organs. Eventually, the accumulation of copper will interfere with the function of these structures.

### Is there any way to treat Wilson's disease?

Yes. There is a substance that can be given to the child that will aid in the removal of excess copper from the body.

### Are there any other forms of metabolic disorder that can produce mental retardation?

Yes, new conditions—most of them, fortunately, are very rare—are being discovered all the time.

## GENETIC MEDICINE

### What is meant by the term "genetic medicine"?

This is a new, rapidly developing science that deals with the circumstances and conditions influencing and surrounding inheritance. With the development of new high-powered microscopes, the actual chromosomes and genes can now be seen and studied microscopically.

### What is a karyotype?

The chromosomal characteristics of an individual. Karyotype charts are arranged so that chromosomes are paired and placed in order, from the largest to the smallest. By studying these chromosomes under a microscope, one may detect defects.

### Is it possible to determine defects in a newborn child by examining his chromosomes or genes?

It is now possible to examine a child's chromosomes by scraping a few cells from the inside of his mouth or by examining the cells in his blood. The chromosomes can be classified and sorted out, but this is not yet possible to do with the genes. A considerable number of defects have been uncovered by examination of chromosomes.

### What diseases can be spotted by examination of the chromosomes?

It has already been determined that Down's syndrome, Klinefelter's syndrome, and Turner's syndrome are caused by defects in the chromosomes.

### Is it possible that a day will come when one will be able to spot defects in the genes?

Yes. Recent advances in genetic medicine make it highly likely that the day is not far off when one will be able to note potentialities for health and disease through the study of the genes.

### Can birth defects sometimes be diagnosed before a child is born?

Yes, by a procedure known as *amniocentesis.* This is carried out by inserting a needle into the pregnant uterus through the abdominal wall. A small amount of the amniotic fluid surrounding the fetus is withdrawn and is examined under a high-powered microscope. It may reveal the presence of cells that contain abnormal chromosomes, thus denoting the presence of a defective fetus. Further studies of cells may reveal metabolic disorders that can cause

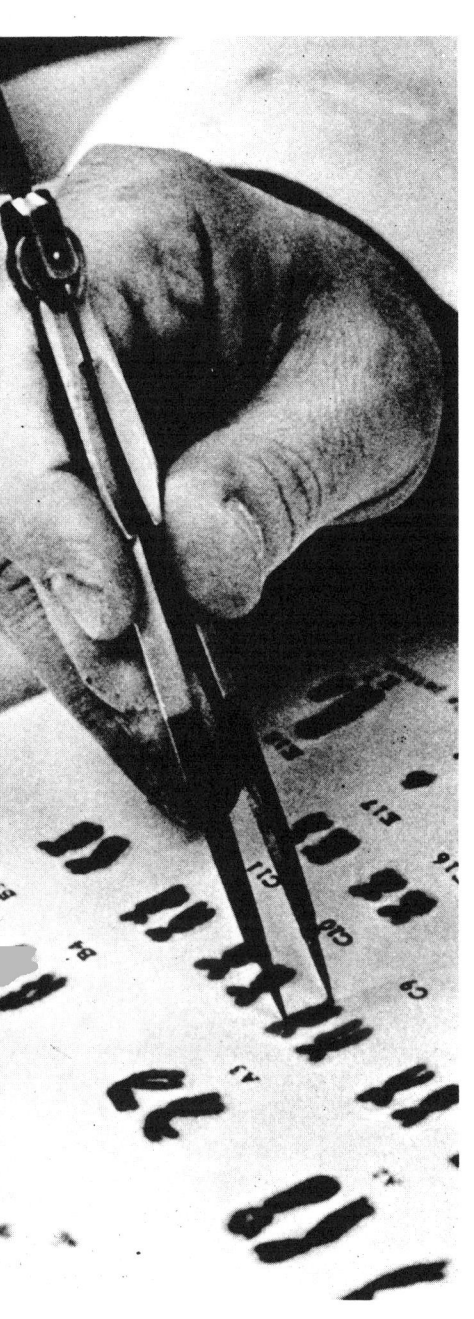

*Working on Karyotypes. A geneticist analyzes a karyotype and measures the matched pairs of chromosomes in the chart.*

any one of several diseases in the newborn child.

### Is it possible that in the future some diseases can be eliminated as a result of genetic studies?

Yes. A day may come when we will be able to discover certain characteristics within the genes or chromosomes that might lead to the development of such diseases as diabetes, cystic fibrosis, or even cancer. Once the basic abnormality creating these tendencies is discovered, ways may be found to eliminate them.

### What is meant by the term "genetic engineering"?

Genetic engineering is a new science that attempts to alter and improve the genes or to transplant them from one form of living matter to another.

### What is hoped to be accomplished by genetic engineering?

There are genes in people that tend to cause bad traits as well as good traits. By altering "bad" genes, scientists hope to be able to do away with some of the defects and illnesses caused by their inheritance.

### Is experimentation in the altering of genes now being carried out?

Yes. Under very strict control, much progress has been made in altering genes in bacteria. Alteration of human genes is still far in the future.

### What benefits might come from altering genes in bacteria?

Recent experiments have been carried out whereby genes from the human pituitary gland in the base of the skull have been implanted in bacteria, resulting in those bacteria producing the human growth hor-

mone. Other experiments in gene transfers have resulted in bacteria producing insulin and a cancer-fighting substance known as interferon.

### Are there certain dangers to genetic engineering?

Yes. New forms of bacterial or animal life may be created through genetic engineering. As a consequence, if not strictly controlled, new forms of harmful bacteria to which we have no immunity may be brought into being.

### What is genetic counseling?

It is a service that physicians trained in genetic medicine should give to all people who fear that their offspring might inherit certain diseases or defects.

### Can genetic counselors predict with any degree of accuracy whether a particular couple will produce a healthy or defective child?

Yes. If one looks over the list of inherited diseases discussed in this chapter, he will find many conditions whose inheritance can be predicted with considerable accuracy.

### Who is most likely to have children with inherited defects?

a. Couples who have a history of an inherited defect or disease in both sides of the family. Thus, a male and female who both have diabetes will have children with a very great chance of being diabetic.

b. Certain inherited defects and diseases are known to be dominant in character. These conditions are much more likely to be inherited than defects or diseases that are recessive in character.

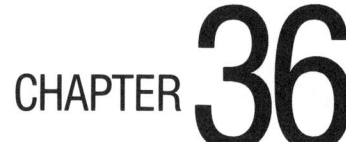

# CHAPTER 36

# THE INTENSIVE CARE UNIT (ICU)

*(See also Chapter 8 on Anesthesia; Chapter 26 on First Aid in Emergencies; Chapter 29 on Heart; Chapter 58 on Preoperative and Postoperative Routines)*

### What is an ICU?

An ICU, or Intensive Care Unit, is an area in a hospital where specialized care is given to the desperately sick patient. In the ICU, the patient is monitored constantly and receives a great deal more attention from physicians and nurses than could possibly be given in a ward or in a private or semiprivate hospital accommodation. A well-equipped ICU has sophisticated equipment, which permits moment-to-moment monitoring of the patient's condition. In addition, it is able to render immediate treatment when critical situations demand it. Most ICUs are staffed so that a physician is always present and on duty, and there is a nurse for every three patients.

### Does the ICU care for the terminally ill?

No. The ICU is a facility that ministers to those who are critically ill but are potentially curable.

### What specific advantages does an ICU have over ordinary, routine hospital care?

a. The constant presence of highly trained attending physicians and nurses.
b. Equipment to assist respiration, such as respirators, suction apparatus, oxygen, etc. Also, equipment to insert a tube into the trachea or, in extreme cases, instruments to perform a tracheostomy.
c. Cardiac monitoring equipment, which records every heartbeat for twenty-four hours each day. Then, if heart action appears to be failing, medications are always on hand to help support it.
d. Dialysis equipment, for use when the kidney function shows evidence of failing.
e. ICU patients have priority for any laboratory or x-ray test that may be required at any time of the day or night.
f. The patient in the ICU is supported by the presence of medical technologists to insure the proper maintenance of all therapeutic and monitoring devices.

### Is it important that laboratory tests be taken frequently on patients in the ICU?

Yes. It is essential to maintain the body's chemistry at normal or near-normal levels at all times. There is a great tendency for patients in shock, and among those who have severe impairment of their heart, lung, liver, or kidney function, to get into chemical imbalance. This may mean that their body fluids are too acid, or in some cases, too alkaline. If one of these abnormalities persists, the patient may not survive.

The monitoring of one's blood volume, blood gases, and blood components, such as the number of red blood cells and the quantity of hemoglobin in those red cells, is vital, too.

### Can imbalances in one's chemistry or deficiencies in one's blood be helped through treatment?

Yes. Intravenous medications can be given to improve chemical balance.

Blood transfusions can be given to replace blood loss.

### Do all hospitals have an ICU?

Accredited hospitals do have an ICU. However, the number of beds in the unit, the amount of specialized equipment available, and the ratio of physicians and nurses to patients will vary according to the size of the hospital. The larger the hospital, the more beds will be set aside for an ICU.

### What proportion of a hospital's beds should be designated for the ICU?

Approximately 5 percent.

### Do hospitals that specialize in cancer treatment or in heart surgery usually require more ICU beds than the ordinary general hospital?

Yes.

### Does the ICU accept only patients with specific illnesses?

No. Any critically ill patient is eligible for care in the ICU.

### Do some hospitals have separate ICUs for individual departments?

Yes, some of the very large hospitals may have a surgical ICU separate from a medical ICU.

### What are some of the newer devices in an up-to-date ICU?

a. Automatic respiratory devices to breathe for a patient who is unable to breathe on his own.
b. Electronic devices to monitor heart action.
c. Computerized multichannel devices to record on a visual screen various vital signs.
d. An alarm system to instantly alert the staff to any change in the patient's condition.

### Are the nurses on duty in an ICU specially trained?

Yes. Most have taken courses in the

recognition and treatment of critically ill patients. Their special training enables them to render treatments that the regular floor nurses do not perform.

### Are patients frequently referred to the ICU after serious operations?

Yes, but only if they are in a "high-risk" category for developing life-threatening, postoperative complications. Very elderly patients, patients with advanced heart or blood vessel disease, patients with serious chronic lung ailments, patients with advanced kidney disease, etc., are candidates for admission to the ICU after major surgery. Also, patients who have encountered serious complications during an operative procedure are often sent to the ICU.

### Are patients often sent to an ICU prior to surgery?

Yes, if they are in such poor condition that the risks of surgery are too great for them to survive. Treatment in an ICU may so improve their condition that surgery may become possible.

### Does care in an ICU substantially increase one's chances for survival?

Definitely, yes.

### When is an ICU patient transferred back to his room?

When the physicians in the ICU conclude that his vital signs are stable and that he needs no assistance to function on his own.

### How long may a patient remain in the ICU?

Some patients may require care in the ICU for only a few hours; others may need several days, or even weeks, until they can function without the special supportive measures given in the ICU.

CHAPTER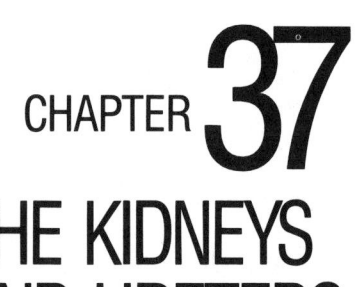

# THE KIDNEYS AND URETERS

*(See also Chapter 25 on Female Organs; Chapter 42 on Male Organs; Chapter 59 on Prostate Gland; Chapter 73 on Transplantation of Organs; Chapter 76 on Urinary Bladder and Urethra)*

## What is the location and structure of the kidneys?

The kidneys are two bean-shaped, reddish brown organs covered by a glistening, thin capsule. Each kidney measures approximately four inches in length, two inches in width, and approximately one and a half inches in thickness.

The kidneys lie on either side of the posterior portion of the abdomen, high up in the loin, behind the abdominal cavity, and beneath the diaphragm.

## How do the kidneys function?

The kidneys are composed of hundreds of thousands of tiny units known as nephrons, which empty into microscopic ducts known as tubules. Each nephron is a small, independent chemical plant that forms urine as the plasma of the blood passes through. The nephrons empty the urine they produce into collecting tubules and then on into the pelvis of the kidney; thence, via a tubular structure called the ureter, into the urinary bladder.

## What are the main duties of the kidneys?

Approximately one-fourth of the blood output of the heart is conveyed to the kidneys. The nephrons extract waste and toxic chemicals, excess minerals, and water from the blood, which passes through them. It is also the function of the kidney *not to extract* certain needed chemicals and substances from the blood.

## Can one live a normal, healthy life with only one kidney?

Yes, provided the remaining kidney functions normally.

## What happens when kidney function is damaged?

a. There is an excessive accumulation of chemical wastes and toxins in the bloodstream.
b. Excessive loss of essential chemicals from the bloodstream into the urine occurs.
c. As a result of impaired kidney function, the tissues of the body are supplied with blood and solutions with improper chemical components. Eventually, if kidney function deteriorates beyond a certain point, such a severe chemical upset occurs that life cannot continue.

## How can one tell if his kidney function is normal?

a. By analysis of the urine.
b. By chemical analysis of various constituents of the blood.
c. By x-ray examination of the kidneys and the rest of the urinary tract.
d. By special kidney function tests.

## Is urine analysis always a good test for kidney diseases?

No. There are occasions when a kidney may be seriously damaged and yet the urine specimen may appear to be normal. However, by and large, urine analysis is a simple, rapid, and inexpensive initial test for screening.

## Is diabetes a kidney disease?

No. Diabetes is essentially a disease of the pancreas, but the diagnosis is aided by examining the urine. (See Chapter 19, on Diabetes.)

## What are the common causes of impaired kidney function?

a. Any generalized severe infection or inflammation.
b. Mechanical obstruction of the outlet of the kidneys.
c. General abnormalities of the kidneys that have existed since birth.
d. Tumors of the kidney.
e. Poisons that have been taken into the body and that damage kidney structure.
f. Interference with blood circulation to the kidneys.
g. Metabolic or hormone disease.
h. Abnormal concentrations of minerals in the bloodstream or dehydration.

## Does swelling of the legs, the abdomen, and the face always indicate kidney disease?

Not necessarily. There are many other conditions that may cause this swelling.

## Is it necessary to drink large quantities of water to make the kidneys function normally?

Let your thirst be your guide. This will usually provide sufficient fluid for adequate kidney function.

## Are the advertised drugs that supposedly "flush the kidneys" beneficial?

No. Normal kidneys do their own flushing, and abnormal kidneys cannot be beneficially "flushed" by these drugs.

## Do backaches usually indicate kidney disease?

The majority are not related to kidney disease. Certain types of backaches may be symptoms of a kidney disorder, but the diagnosis requires an examination by a physician.

## What is the relationship between high blood pressure and kidney disease?

Long-standing high blood pressure over a period of years may eventually

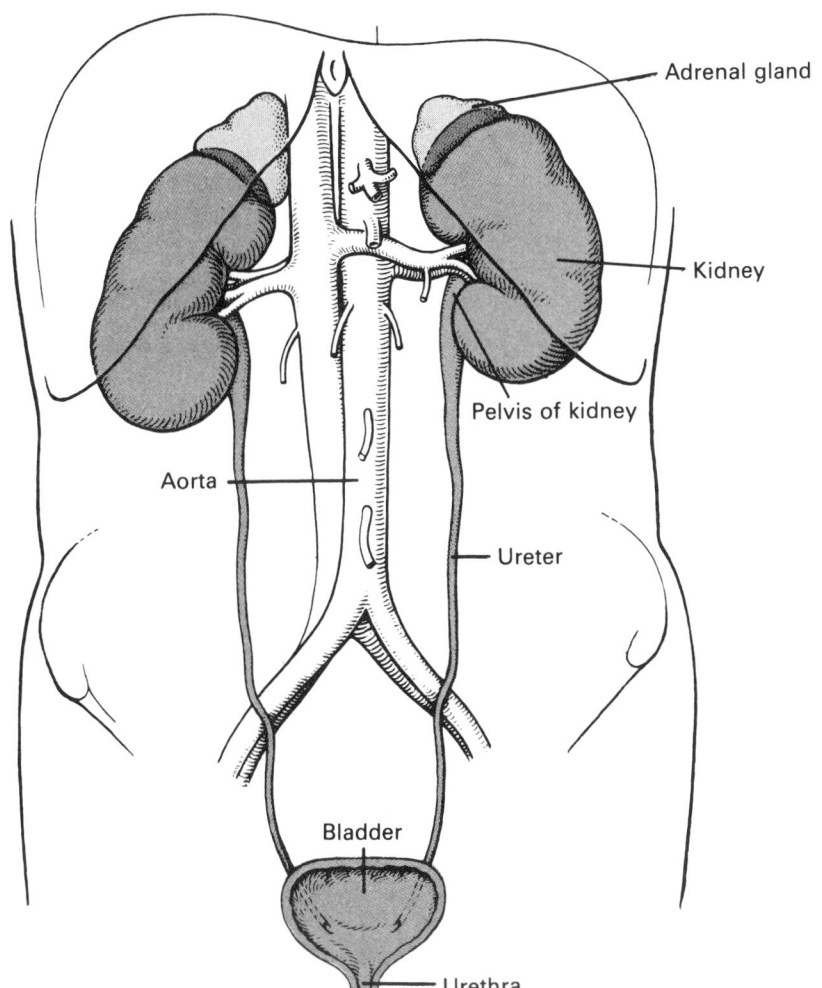

*Normal Kidneys and Ureters. The kidneys manufacture urine, which is secreted down through the ureters and into the urinary bladder. Obstruction to the flow of urine down the ureters may cause severe damage to kidney substance and may eventually result in total loss of kidney function on the obstructed side.*

cause kidney disease due to disturbance in the circulation of the kidney. Conversely, severe kidney disorders often lead to high blood pressure. It has been found within recent years that narrowing of the renal artery, the main artery to the kidney, can also cause high blood pressure.

**Is it ever possible to cure high blood pressure by surgery upon the blood vessels to the kidney?**

Yes. It can now be determined accurately by special x-ray techniques whether the major artery to the kidney is narrowed. If this condition is found to be present, plastic surgery upon the renal blood vessel can often be carried out successfully. If the narrowing is due to arteriosclerosis, the inner lining of the artery is reamed out, and a patch graft made of Dacron is applied. This will increase the blood supply to the kidney, in many instances eliminating the cause for the high blood pressure.

**Does albumin in the urine always indicate kidney disease?**

Not necessarily. However, the presence of albumin must be considered to be indicative of a kidney disorder until further testing and procedures prove otherwise.

**Does frequency of urination indicate kidney disease?**

Sometimes frequency of urination is caused merely by excessive drinking of fluids or by nervous tension. On the other hand, disorders such as diabetes or enlargement of the prostate may be the cause of frequency of urination. Repeated episodes of frequency of urination should lead to a thorough investigation by your physician to rule out disturbance in kidney function or disease of the kidneys.

**Does bedwetting indicate kidney disease or a weak bladder?**

No. Most cases have their origin in emotional disturbance or may be due to excessively deep sleep.

**Is salt restriction in the diet essential to a person with kidney disease?**

Only in certain types of chronic kidney disease, namely, when undue amounts of fluid are already being retained by the body.

**Can excessive eating of meats, eggs, or the intake of too much salt cause kidney disease?**

No, but these foods are often restricted in patients who have advanced kidney disease.

**Does smoking hurt the kidneys?**

It can affect them indirectly by causing decreased arterial circulation, and it may increase the incidence of cancer.

**Is drinking of alcoholic beverages injurious to the kidneys?**

Large quantities of alcohol may damage the kidneys, as it will all other tissues. It is well for a patient suffering from serious kidney disease not to drink alcoholic beverages.

**Is the taking of large amounts of spices and condiments injurious to the kidneys?**

Not usually. However, it can act as a temporary irritant when there already is disease in the urinary tract.

**What is the significance of blood in the urine?**

This should indicate that something is wrong somewhere in the urinary tract, and the patient should seek medical advice promptly.

**Does blood in the urine always indicate kidney disease?**

No. The source of the blood may be the ureter, the bladder, or the urethra leading from the bladder to the outside. Occasionally, blood may appear in the urine without any underlying disease. However, such patients should consult their doctor to be sure.

**Does cloudiness of the urine or pain on urination indicate kidney disease?**

Not necessarily, although it may indicate that there is some disturbance within the urinary tract. Patients with such symptoms should seek medical advice promptly.

**What is Bright's disease?**

This is an old term, named after a famous physician, which denotes a variety of kidney diseases. In most instances, it denotes glomerulonephritis.

**What is nephritis?**

This is also a broad descriptive term denoting a diseased functioning of the kidneys.

## GLOMERULONEPHRITIS

**What is glomerulonephritis?**

This is a specific disease that affects the nephrons of the kidney. It is caused by inflammation of the nephrons and may, if not checked, lead to scarring and destruction of these structures with consequent impairment of kidney function.

**What forms of glomerulonephritis are there?**

a. Acute glomerulonephritis.
b. Chronic glomerulonephritis.
The acute stage may last from a few days to a year or more; the chronic stage may last as long as the patient lives. There is also an intermediate stage known as subacute glomerulonephritis.

**How common a disease is acute glomerulonephritis?**

It is quite common, especially among children.

**What causes acute glomerulonephritis?**

Although the cause is not known, it usually appears shortly after a bacterial infection, most often after an infection caused by a streptoccocus germ, which is commonly the cause of sore throats, tonsillitis, and scarlet fever.

**What is the usual course of acute glomerulonephritis?**

It usually lasts for several weeks and then subsides spontaneously. It is estimated that in children with acute glomerulonephritis, 75 to 90 percent will get well without resultant kidney damage.

**Is acute glomerulonephritis ever fatal?**

Yes. In about one out of twenty cases, the patient may not survive this disease.

**What are the symptoms of acute glomerulonephritis?**

The patient may give a history of a previous acute infection, such as a severe sore throat. Blood and albumin may appear in the urine with varying degrees of elevation of the blood pressure and tenderness over the kidney region.

**At what age is acute glomerulonephritis most frequently seen?**

Seventy percent of all cases occur before age twenty-one.

**Is this type of nephritis hereditary?**

It is not thought to be hereditary, although there is a certain tendency for the condition to occur in families.

**Is there any way to prevent getting nephritis?**

All acute infections, especially sore throats, tonsillitis, and scarlet fever, should be treated promptly and thoroughly by a physician.

**Is there any specific treatment for acute glomerulonephritis?**

No. However, with proper rest and supportive measures, the majority of people will make a good recovery.

**Is there any specific treatment for chronic glomerulonephritis?**

No. However, people with chronic glomerulonephritis may live normal lives for many years if they take care of themselves by observing certain dietary precautions and avoiding acute infections.

## NEPHROSIS

**What is nephrosis?**

It is a general term relating to certain types of kidney disorder in which there is generalized water-logging and swelling of the body tissues. This swelling and water-logging may be visible in the face, abdomen, and legs. There is also a loss of large quantities of body proteins, elevation of certain of the fatty substances in the bloodstream, and a lowering of the basal metabolism of the individual. There are many different specific causes of nephrosis.

**Who is most likely to get nephrosis?**

Children between the ages of two and seven years.

**Is nephrosis a very common disease?**

It is relatively rare.

**What is the treatment for nephrosis?**

This depends upon the primary cause. General measures include diet and salt restrictions. Cortisone and related steroids are used in certain types of nephrosis with gratifying results.

**Is it necessary to restrict salt intake in treating nephrosis?**

Yes. Since retention of salt causes retention of water, it is important to restrict this substance.

**Is restriction of meat, eggs, and other proteins recommended in nephrosis?**

No.

**What is the recovery rate from nephrosis?**

In former years, about half the children with nephrosis would die. Today, with newer methods of treatment, three out of four will get well.

## UREMIA

**What is uremia?**

This term denotes the abnormal chemical changes in the blood as well as the associated symptoms that appear in the advanced stages of kidney failure, when the kidney is unable to eliminate waste products.

**Can a patient with uremia recover?**

Yes, provided the cause is found and is capable of being eliminated. As an example, if it is caused by an obstruction of the ureter or the kidney outlet and this is promptly relieved, the uremia will subside, and the patient will get well. If the uremia represents the terminal stage of chronic nephritis, the only cure may be through a kidney transplant. Dialysis, the use of the so-called "artifi-cial kidney," may keep these people alive until a kidney is available for transplant.

## PYELONEPHRITIS *(Kidney Infections)*

**What is pyelonephritis?**

A bacterial infection of the kidney including the outlet of the kidney.

**What causes pyelonephritis?**

It is caused by bacteria, which reach the kidney through the bloodstream, or by extension from other portions of the genitourinary tract, such as the bladder, the prostate, the cervix, the vagina, or the urethra.

**Who is most likely to develop pyelonephritis?**

Pyelonephritis is seen quite often in children as an acute infection, but is also quite common in adults. Females, especially pregnant women, are most likely to develop kidney infection, since they are more prone to develop bladder infections. Also prone are diabetics and people who are debilitated or who have certain neurological disorders.

**What are the symptoms of pyelonephritis?**

High temperature, possibly with intermittent chills, backache, tenderness over the kidney area, frequency of urination along with painful voiding and blood in the urine. Nausea, vomiting, and lack of appetite are common. Examination may reveal pus and bacteria in the urine and an elevated white blood cell count.

**Are both kidneys usually affected at the same time?**

No, but this can occur in some cases.

**What is the treatment for kidney infections?**

a. Drinking large quantities of fluids so as to flush out the pelvis and ureters of the kidneys.
b. Antibiotics to take care of the infecting organism.
c. Bed rest and a bland diet.
d. Medications for relief of pain.

**What is the usual course of kidney infections?**

If properly treated, almost all patients get well. It is important to discover whether there is an underlying obstruction of the ureter which might have caused the urine to dam up and become infected, and it is important to eradicate any infection elsewhere in the body that might have precipitated the kidney infection.

**How long is one usually ill with these infections?**

Anywhere from a few days to several weeks.

**Do antibiotics always prove effective in curing pyelitis or pyelonephritis?**

In almost all instances, provided the correct antibiotic drug is found for the particular bacteria causing the infection, and provided that other urinary tract defects are corrected.

**Is hospitalization necessary in kidney infections?**

The average case can be treated well at home. However, if the temperature is very high or if the pelvis of the kidney does not drain out its infected urine, then hospitalization is advisable.

**What special hospital treatments may become necessary if the case does not respond to ordinary treatment?**

The urologist may be called upon to pass a catheter (a long rubber tube) into the bladder and then up into the ureter in order to drain out any infected urine blocked in the pelvis of the kidney.

## Is surgery necessary for pyelitis or pyelonephritis?

Usually not. However, if an abscess forms in or around the kidney, operative drainage may be necessary. Similarly, if the kidney infection is secondary to some other kidney disease such as stones, surgery may be required.

## Do kidney infections have a tendency to recur?

Yes, if there was a delay in the treatment of the initial attack or if treatment was inadequate. In these cases, lasting damage to the kidney occurs, which may permanently impair its function.

## Will frequent follow-up visits to a physician aid in preventing recurrence of kidney infection?

Yes.

## Is it true that people with diabetes are more prone to develop kidney infection?

Yes.

## Does chronic kidney infection lead to the development of other diseases?

Yes. People with this condition often form stones, develop high blood pressure, and may eventually develop uremia.

## KIDNEY STONES

## What is the composition of kidney stones?

They are a combination of inorganic salts such as calcium, phosphorus, ammonium, etc., or they may be composed of organic compounds such as uric or amino acids.

## What causes the formation of kidney stones?

In certain instances the exact cause is known. For instance, in gout, there is a high concentration of blood uric

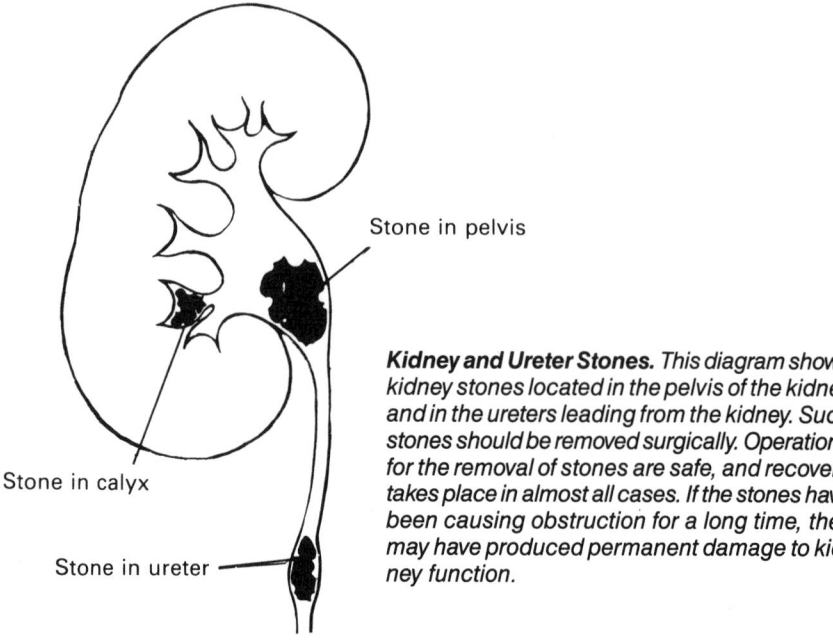

Stone in pelvis

Stone in calyx

Stone in ureter

**Kidney and Ureter Stones.** *This diagram shows kidney stones located in the pelvis of the kidney and in the ureters leading from the kidney. Such stones should be removed surgically. Operations for the removal of stones are safe, and recovery takes place in almost all cases. If the stones have been causing obstruction for a long time, they may have produced permanent damage to kidney function.*

acid and a high concentration of uric acid in the kidney excretions, causing the precipitation of uric acid stones. Similarly, in disorders of calcium metabolism, there is a precipitation out of calcium compound stones in the urine and in the kidneys. However, in most situations, the exact mechanism is not known, but there are many theories:

a. Improper diet.
b. Chemical imbalances in the urine, cause unknown.
c. Disorders of the endocrine glands, especially the parathyroid glands in the neck.
d. Vitamin deficiencies.
e. Infections within the kidney.
f. Poor drainage in one or more parts of the urinary tract.
g. Living in areas where hard water causes stones.

## Do kidney stones appear as frequently in both sexes?

No. They are somewhat more common in men.

## Do kidney stones occur at any age?

Yes, but they are much more common in adults during the fourth, fifth,

and sixth decades of life. Children do not get kidney stones very frequently.

## What symptoms are caused by kidney stones?

In some instances the stones are quiescent and cause no symptoms. This type may be discovered accidentally. Usually, they cause pain, blood and pus cells in the urine, and, not infrequently, they impair kidney function.

## Do kidney stones tend to be single or multiple?

They are more often single, but they may be multiple. When multiple stones are encountered, they may be found in both kidneys.

## Is there much variation in the size of a kidney stone?

Yes. They vary in size from tiny fragments like grains of sand to stones that form an outline or cast of an entire kidney (staghorn or coral stones).

## Must all kidney stones be removed surgically?

No. Many of them pass spontaneously. Some are quiescent, causing no pain, infection, or interference with kidney function. The latter may be left alone. The stones that should be removed are those that appear to be too large to pass, those that cause obstruction and infection, those that cause constant pain or periodic attacks of severe pain, and those that appear to be causing progressive damage to kidney function.

### Are there any *medications* that can be taken to dissolve kidney stones?

There are some dietary programs, such as low-phosphorus diet, an alkaline ash diet, or an acid diet, which may help to retard the growth of a stone or may help to prevent new stones from forming. There are also some drugs that have somewhat the same effect (Basaljel, acid salts, alkaline salts, etc.). New research gives promise that uric acid stones may be dissolved through medications.

### Are there any *solutions* that can be used to dissolve stones?

There are solutions that are helpful in reducing the size of stones, and in some cases they actually dissolve them. However, these solutions must be brought into direct contact with the stone for a sufficient length of time to permit this to take place. This means that if the stone is in the kidney, catheters must be put up to the kidney and left there for several days. This form of treatment is not universally applicable and cannot be used as a standard method. There have, in fact, been fatalities reported with improper use.

### Do kidney stones ever recur after they are once removed or passed?

Yes. However, dietary regulation, large fluid intake, the use of certain drugs, and the elimination of infection and obstruction of the urinary tract help to prevent their re-forming.

Despite all precautions, in a small percentage of cases, stones will form again.

### What are stones in the ureter?

The ureter is the tubelike structure connecting the kidney with the bladder. Stones rarely form primarily in the ureter, but kidney stones often pass down into the ureter and lodge there. When discovered there, they are known as ureteral stones.

### What symptoms accompany stones in the ureter?

The principal symptom is excruciating pain of a colicky type. This may be so severe as to defy the effect of the most powerful painkiller. If the stone causes blockage of the flow of urine from the kidney, fever may result. If the urine is infected, the fever may be very high and may be accompanied by severe chills. Nausea, vomiting, and constipation are also common symptoms. Urinary discomfort, urgency, and frequency may be present. Blood in the urine is found in most cases.

### What is the treatment for ureteral stones?

First, the pain must be controlled; next, if infection is present, it must be treated by the use of the antibiotic or sulfa drugs. If pain and infection cannot be controlled adequately, drainage of the kidney must be performed. This is done by passing a catheter beyond the stone through a cystoscope. If the catheter cannot be passed beyond the stone, then the stone must be removed surgically.

### Is surgery always necessary in the treatment of stones in the ureter?

No. Most stones in this location will pass spontaneously. If no infection supervenes, if the pain does not recur, and if the flow of urine is not blocked, then it is advisable to await the spontaneous passage of the stone. This may happen at any time

within a period of several days or weeks.

### When is surgery required for a ureter stone?

a. When the stone is obviously too large to pass.
b. If there is prolonged obstruction of urine.
c. If there are recurrent attacks of severe pain.
d. If infection persists.
e. If kidney function becomes impaired.

### Can a stone ever be grasped by an instrument passed through a cystoscope?

Yes, when the stone lies near the bladder, stone-grasping instruments are sometimes successful in bringing the stone down through the ureter. If this method fails, then surgery must be instituted.

### Is the surgical removal of a stone in the ureter a serious operation?

It is a major procedure but carries with it virtually no mortality.

### How long is the usual hospitalization period after surgery for a ureter stone?

Five to seven days.

### Will the patient be able to live a completely normal life after surgery for a kidney stone?

Yes.

### Should a patient who once had a kidney stone be checked periodically by his physician?

Yes. He should also follow all of the precautions mentioned previously to prevent re-formation of stones.

## KIDNEY TUMORS

### Who is most likely to get a tumor of the kidney?

Tumors of the kidney occur at any

age, in either sex. However, the majority occur after the age of forty. One special type, called Wilms's tumor, occurs in infancy and childhood.

### Are all kidney tumors malignant?

No, but the malignant tumors are seen more often than the benign ones.

### What is the technical name for the most common malignant kidney tumor?

The most common kidney tumor is a renal cell carcinoma.

### How can one diagnose the presence of a kidney tumor?

By physical examination and by special x rays of the kidneys, such as pyelograms, arteriograms, and CAT scans.

### What is an intravenous pyelogram?

It is an x-ray procedure in which a radiopaque solution is injected into the bloodstream. The solution is excreted by the kidneys, and as it is being excreted, it outlines the kidneys, which are visualized by taking an x ray.

### Is an intravenous pyelogram a painful or dangerous procedure?

No. However, if the patient is markedly allergic, special precautions must be taken before this procedure is carried out.

### Are pyelograms important in making a diagnosis in other kidney diseases besides tumors?

Yes. They will show the presence of many other abnormalities within the urinary tract. They are also valuable in making a diagnosis of prostate enlargement or the presence of stones in the prostate gland.

### What other diagnostic tests are valuable in making a diagnosis of kidney disease?

a. Angiograms, which show the outlines of blood vessels to the kidneys. Variations from normal often indicate the presence of kidney cysts or tumors.
b. Sonograms (ultrasound) frequently demonstrate kidney tumors or cysts.
c. CAT scans (computerized axial tomography) can often outline kidney cysts or growths.

### What symptoms and signs do kidney tumors produce?

a. Blood in the urine.
b. Pain in the loin over the kidney region.
c. The presence of a mass or lump in the kidney area.
d. Fever.

### What is the treatment for a kidney tumor?

Prompt removal of the entire kidney and surrounding tissue and lymph glands. Preliminary x-ray therapy and postoperative x-ray treatments are also advised in certain types of kidney tumor.

### Is the removal of a kidney a serious operation?

Yes, but if the opposite kidney is normal, the removal of one kidney will not adversely affect life.

### Is kidney removal (nephrectomy) a dangerous operation?

No. Recovery, with an uncomplicated postoperative course, is the usual outcome.

### How long is the patient in the hospital after an operation for removal of a kidney?

Eight to ten days.

## CYSTS OF THE KIDNEY

### What are some of the common forms of cystic disease of the kidney?

a. Solitary cysts of the kidney. This type usually does not impair kidney function.
b. Congenital polycystic kidneys. This is a condition with which one is born and is characterized by numerous large and small cysts, usually of both kidneys. Kidney function is impaired in this type of disease as the individual grows older. This condition occurs in families.

### What are the symptoms in polycystic kidney disease?

As the patient grows into adulthood, there may be pain in the kidney area, blood in the urine, infection, elevated blood pressure, and a large mass in the abdomen.

### What are the symptoms of a solitary cyst of the kidney?

Usually there are no symptoms. Occasionally, there may be pain and blood in the urine.

### What is the treatment for polycystic kidneys?

There is no effective treatment for cysts themselves. However, since the advent of the artificial kidney, these people can be kept alive until a time when a kidney is available for transplant.

### What is the treatment for a solitary cyst of the kidney?

The cyst itself is removed, leaving the remainder of the kidney in place. Once in a great while, a solitary cyst can be treated by withdrawing the fluid and injecting a solution that induces the cyst to close itself off. This is not, however, the most common method of handling solitary cysts.

## CONGENITAL DEFECTS OF THE KIDNEY (Birth Abnormalities)

### Is the kidney subject to many types of congenital abnormalities?

Yes. There may be only one kidney

instead of two; there may be one or two small additional kidneys; the kidneys may be in the wrong position in the body (ectopic kidneys); both kidneys may be on the same side of the body; the kidneys may be joined across the midline of the body (horseshoe kidney); the collecting portions of the kidney (pelvis) may be duplicated; the ureters may be duplicated.

An important abnormality is the presence of a narrowing or stricture at the kidney pelvis at the junction between the kidney and ureter. Such a condition may impede the normal flow of urine and eventually lead to obstruction of the kidney.

### Do most congenital abnormalities of the kidneys cause symptoms?

No, with the exception of the strictures that cause the symptoms listed above.

### Are these abnormal kidneys more prone to infection?

Yes.

### What is the treatment for the congenital obstruction at the junction between the kidney and the ureter?

Where there is advanced obstruction of the kidney or where the kidney function is impaired, surgery is indicated.

### What surgery is carried out for obstruction of the kidney at its junction with the ureter?

A plastic operation is performed to widen the passageway. Formerly, simple attempts to dilate the stricture with dilating instruments were made in some cases. But this frequently resulted in infection and added damage to the kidney.

### Are operations for obstruction at the kidney outlet serious?

Yes, but they are not dangerous. They may involve a long hospitalization, usually three to four weeks, and the patient may have to carry tubes

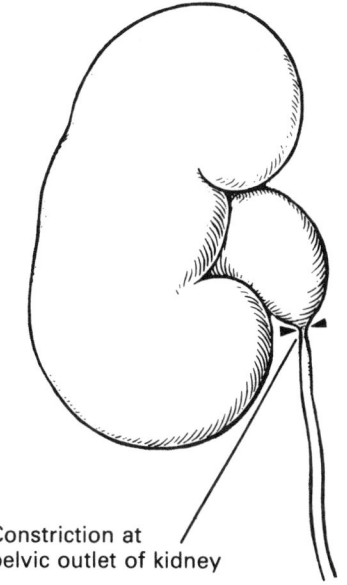

Constriction at
pelvic outlet of kidney

*Constriction at the Outlet of the Kidney. Such a condition often requires surgical reconstruction to relieve the obstruction to the flow of urine.*

that are inserted to splint and drain the area while healing takes place.

### Are the results of these operations successful?

Yes, in the great majority of cases.

## KIDNEY INJURIES

### What are the common causes for kidney injuries?

a. Automobile accidents.
b. Athletic events such as football or boxing.
c. A fall from a height with a direct blow to the kidney area.

### How can one tell if he has a kidney injury?

a. By noting pain and tenderness in the kidney region.
b. By noting blood in the urine.

### What is the treatment for kidney injuries?

For the minor injuries, which make up the great majority, bed rest is the main form of treatment. If the bleed-

ing is alarming and the x ray shows a badly damaged kidney, surgery may become necessary for removal of the organ or drainage of the blood and urine that have escaped from the injured kidney.

### Can a damaged kidney ever be restored surgically?

Yes. If the damage has not been too extensive, the kidney may be sutured instead of being removed.

### Is it often necessary to operate for a kidney injury?

The great majority will get well without surgery.

### How can one tell whether surgery is necessary?

By noting whether the urine clears and whether there is evidence of restored kidney function. If blood continues to appear in the urine and kidney function fails to return, or if the patient's general condition deteriorates and there is swelling in the loin, surgery is indicated.

## TUBERCULOSIS OF THE KIDNEYS
*(See Chapter 74 on Tuberculosis)*

### Is tuberculosis of the kidneys often a primary disease?

No. It is usually secondary to tuberculosis of the lungs.

### How does tuberculosis reach the kidneys?

The germs are carried to it through the bloodstream.

### What are the symptoms of kidney tuberculosis?

Frequent, painful urination and bloody urine compel consideration of tuberculosis among the possible diagnoses.

### How is the diagnosis of tuberculosis of the kidney made?

By finding the tuberculosis germs in

the urine. It is often necessary to inoculate animals (guinea pigs) with the urine to see whether they develop tuberculosis several weeks later. There are also characteristic x-ray findings that help to make the diagnosis. When tuberculosis has involved the bladder, cystoscopic examination will reveal a characteristic appearance. Findings in the scrotum and prostate also may suggest kidney tuberculosis.

### What is the treatment for tuberculosis of the kidney?

In the early stages, the disease may be arrested with the use of some of the newer antituberculosis drugs. If the disease is limited to one kidney and has already produced marked destruction, the use of drugs *and* surgical removal of the kidney may be indicated. Where both kidneys are involved, drug treatment is preferable. The drugs most often used are isoniazid, Myambutol, para-aminosalicylic acid, and streptomycin.

### If tuberculosis is limited to one kidney and that kidney is removed, can a cure be obtained?

We do not speak of cures in tuberculosis, but rather of *arrest* of the disease. If the disease is limited to one kidney, its removal will arrest the disease.

## "DROPPED KIDNEY" OR "FLOATING KIDNEY"

### (Nephroptosis)

### What is a dropped, or floating, kidney?

A kidney that has become detached from its moorings and drops to an abnormally low position in the body.

### What type of person is most likely to have a floating kidney?

Thin individuals, especially women.

### Is a dropped kidney more likely to be seen on the right side?

Yes.

### What are the symptoms of a dropped kidney?

If any symptoms are present, they will consist of backache and abdominal pain. The kinking of the outlet of the kidney may interfere with the ready outflow of urine. This may result in a so-called "renal crisis," with attacks of severe colicky pain in the kidney area.

### Is it necessary to treat a dropped kidney that causes no symptoms?

No.

### What treatment is indicated when the dropped kidney does cause symptoms?

a. Medical management, with a special diet to increase body weight and the wearing of a support or corset to keep the kidney in its proper position.
b. A surgical procedure in which the kidney is fixed by sutures into its normal position. Such an operation is called a nephropexy, but it is seldom found necessary to perform.

## TUMORS OF THE URETER

### Are tumors of the ureter very common?

No. They are extremely rare.

### What forms do tumors of the ureter usually take?

The great majority of them are malignant.

### What are the symptoms of tumors of the ureter?

Blood in the urine, obstruction to the passage of urine into the bladder, and eventual infection.

### How is the diagnosis of a tumor of the ureter made?

By x-ray studies of the urinary tract and by noting obstruction on attempted passage of a catheter up the ureter.

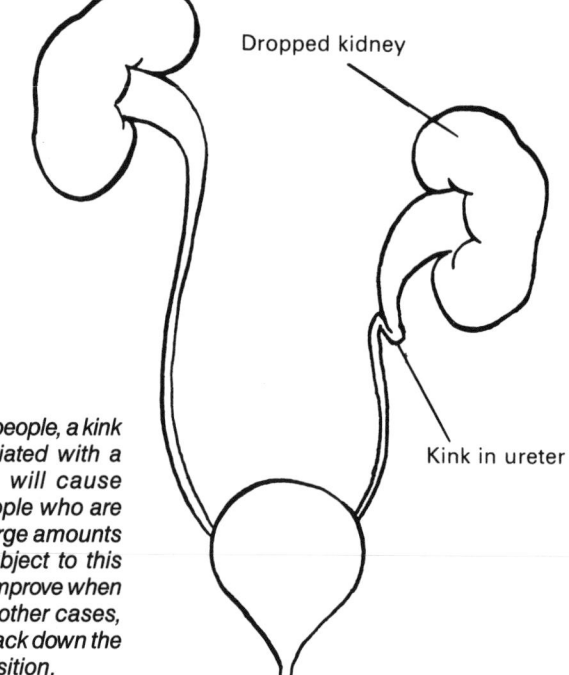

*Dropped Kidney. In certain people, a kink develops in a ureter associated with a dropped kidney, and this will cause marked pain in the loin. People who are very thin or who have lost large amounts of weight are especially subject to this condition. Symptoms often improve when the patient gains weight. In other cases, it is necessary to operate to tack down the kidney in a more normal position.*

## What is the treatment for a tumor of the ureter?

Removal of the ureter along with its kidney and a portion of the bladder surrounding the entrance of the ureter.

## Are operations of this type serious?

Yes, but recovery can be expected in the great majority of cases.

## Can tumors of the ureter be cured by surgery?

Yes, when they are discovered at an early stage and when the operation, as outlined above, is carried out.

## How long a hospital stay is necessary after operations of this type?

Eight to ten days.

# URETEROCELE

## What is a ureterocele?

A cystic formation at the bladder end of the ureter due to an abnormal opening of the ureter into the bladder. There is also a weakness in the wall of the ureter in its lowermost portion, probably the result of a birth deformity.

## What are the symptoms of a ureterocele?

There may be no symptoms at all, and the condition may be discovered accidentally during the course of a routine investigation for some other condition in the urinary tract. Ureteroceles can, however, be the cause of a chronic infection in the bladder and kidney and can also, by blocking the outflow of urine, damage the ureters and kidneys.

## What is the treatment for a ureterocele?

If it is a small one, it can be treated successfully by enlarging the opening of the ureter into the bladder. Some ureteroceles may be treated

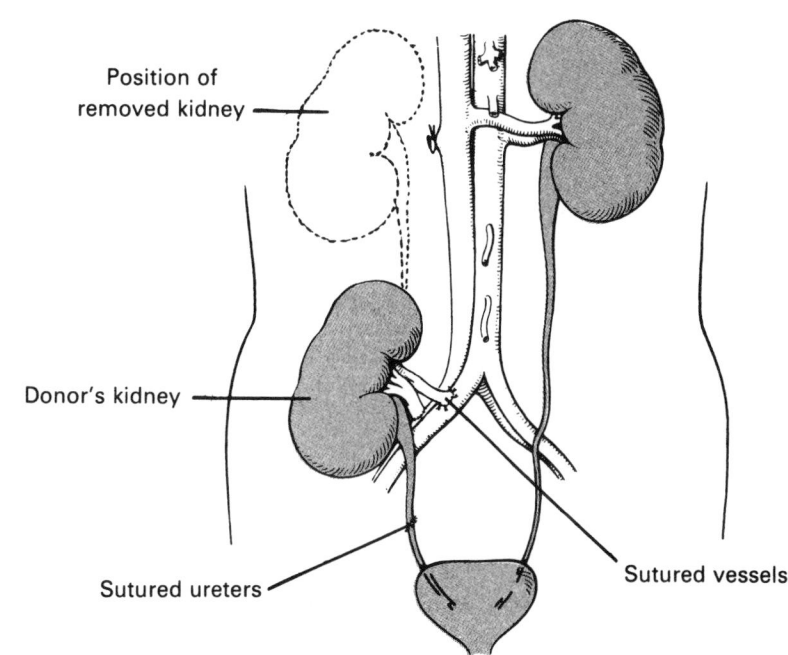

*Kidney Transplant.* The dotted outline shows where the diseased kidney was situated. The new, or donor's, kidney has been transplanted lower in the abdomen, creating a shortened ureter, which will be less likely to deteriorate.

through a cystoscope by either burning off a portion of the cyst or by shaving off a portion of it. If the ureterocele is large, it may be necessary to operate and remove it through an opening made in the bladder.

## Are operations for ureteroceles successful?

Yes.

## Are these operations dangerous?

No.

# TRANSPLANTATION OF KIDNEYS

## Can kidneys be successfully transplanted from one individual to another?

Yes. The technical procedure is perfectly feasible, as outlined in the accompanying diagram. However, difficulties following transplantation of a kidney often ensue when the rejection reaction sets in, and this may

occur anywhere from a few weeks to a few months after the operation has been performed.

## What causes a kidney to die after it has been successfully transplanted?

A phenomenon known as the *rejection reaction* takes place. All people have antibodies whose duty it is to protect against invading foreign bodies. Tissue cells from other animals or humans are judged by the host to be a foreign body, and the normal protective mechanisms of the host are mobilized to destroy them. Thus a transplanted kidney will be attacked by the white blood cells of the host, which will cause the grafted organ to die.

## When is kidney transplantation indicated?

It is performed only as a lifesaving measure in a patient who would otherwise die due to kidney failure. In this category, one would place conditions such as uremia, polycystic kidneys, chronic inflammation of the kidney due to multiple stones or overwhelming infection, or a malignant tumor of a kidney in a patient who only has one kidney.

### What kidney transplants are most likely to succeed?

It has been found that permanent survival of a grafted kidney is most likely to take place when the organ is transplanted from one identical twin to another. Also, survival is more apt to occur when matching of the donor and recipient through tissue typing occurs.

### Can anything be done to overcome the rejection reaction?

Yes. There are many measures that can be taken to tide the host over the period when the rejection reaction is at its height. Various drugs can be given to slow down or entirely stop the host from producing the antibodies that will kill the transplant.

### How successful are kidney transplants?

Kidney transplants have been carried out successfully in more than two out of three people upon whom the operation has been done. It is now possible to keep the transplanted kidney alive for many years in approximately half the patients who undergo this form of treatment.

### What can be done if the transplanted kidney fails to survive?

a. The patient can be placed on the artificial kidney (dialysis) temporarily.

b. The patient can be reoperated and a new kidney from another donor can be inserted.

### When a kidney transplant is carried out, is it usually placed in the normal position in the upper back?

No. It has been found that it is much better to place the kidney in the pelvic region and to attach the blood vessels of the kidney to the iliac vessels in the pelvis. In this position, there is the greatest chance of the transplant functioning satisfactorily. Also, the ureter in this position will be much shorter in length, thus enabling it to function more satisfactorily.

### Are operations for kidney transplantation serious?

Yes, they are. It must be realized that these procedures are only carried out on those who would otherwise succumb to kidney failure. A kidney is never transplanted to an individual who has at least one functioning kidney.

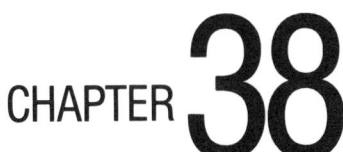

CHAPTER **38**

# LABORATORY (PATHOLOGY) TESTS AND PROCEDURES

*(See also Chapter 12 on Blood and Lymph Diseases; Chapter 19 on Diabetes Mellitus; Chapter 31 on Immunizations and Vaccinations; Chapter 34 on Infectious and Virus Diseases)*

### What is a pathologist?

A physician who specializes in the study of disease and in laboratory medicine and who works closely with other physicians as a consultant in the diagnosis, prognosis, and in some aspects of the treatment of disease.

### What are the usual duties of a pathologist?

To interpret laboratory tests performed upon patients, to examine human tissues that have been removed from patients, and to determine the cause of death in certain cases by making autopsy examinations. The hospital-based pathologist usually has additional duties of teaching and active participation in various hospital committees.

### In addition to the above duties, is the pathologist responsible for the operation of a clinical and pathologic laboratory?

Yes.

### What types of tests do these laboratories usually perform?

a. All types of tests on blood, such as blood chemistries, drug levels, hormone levels, enzyme levels, number and types of blood cells, levels of blood gases, blood cultures for bacteria, titers of antibodies, and levels of coagulation factors.

b. All types of tests on urine, such as routine urine analysis, urine chemistries, hormone levels (including pregnancy tests), drug levels, and urine culture for bacteria.

c. Stool analysis.

d. Sputum analysis.

e. Analysis of the stomach and duodenal contents (gastric analysis).

f. Bone marrow analysis.

g. Pus cultures.

h. Spinal fluid examinations.

i. Examination of fluid or material from various other cavities of the body, such as lung taps or abdominal taps.

j. Serologic tests to detect antigens or antibodies in serum, cells, or tissues.

k. Cytologic examinations, in which cells taken from the body are examined for malignancy.

### Why is it necessary for a patient to make a special appointment before going to a laboratory for a test or series of tests?

Appointments are advisable because it is often necessary for the patient to make special preparations, such as not eating for a certain number of hours before coming to the laboratory. Many tests cannot be carried out unless special instructions are given beforehand as to how to prepare for them.

### Is it usually best to have blood tests performed upon a fasting stomach?

Yes, especially for those blood tests concerned with the chemistry of the blood. In those instances, a twelve-hour period of fasting often precedes the test.

## HEMATOLOGICAL BLOOD TESTS

### What is a complete blood count, and how is it taken?

A complete blood count is usually obtained by passing a sample of venous blood through an automatic blood analyzer, which then prints out the number of red cells, white cells, hemoglobin content, and other blood indices calculated from this data. The test can be taken at any time and without special preparation.

### What is a differential blood count, and how is it taken?

This test is done by examining a blood smear on a glass slide under a microscope for the different cells present and obtaining a percentage of the various types of white cells present. A complete blood count and differential blood count will reveal diseases like anemia, leukemia, or infection.

### Is it painful when the vein is punctured for a blood test?

There is only very slight pain if a good sharp needle is used.

### How does the taking of a blood count show anemia?

By counting the number of red blood cells, noting the amount of hemoglobin in the cells, and noting the characteristic appearance of the blood under the microscope.

### Can a pathologist diagnose the varying types of anemia by examination of blood?

Yes. There are many types of anemia, and the treatment for each may be different.

### How does a blood count indicate an acute infection?

By an increase in the white cell count and an increase in the number of bands (white cells with nuclei containing no lobes).

**Is the taking of a white blood count frequently important in determining the seriousness of the illness and in determining whether or not an operation is necessary, such as in the case of a possible appendicitis?**

Yes. This is a most valuable test in helping to make a decision.

**What is hemoglobin?**

The iron-containing pigment in red blood cells that carries oxygen to the cells throughout the body.

**Why is it necessary to have a blood test before tonsils are removed?**

The tendency of the tissues to bleed and the blood to clot should be recorded before tonsils are removed. When these tests, known as bleeding time and clotting time, are normal, the surgeon can proceed without fear of hemorrhage due to an abnormal condition of the blood.

**Can anemia be successfully treated by blood transfusions?**

Blood transfusions may temporarily correct the deficiency, but they do not relieve the underlying cause of the anemia and therefore cannot produce a permanent cure. There is one exception, and that is when anemia has been caused solely by sudden hemorrhage. In this instance, blood transfusion can bring about a cure of the anemia.

**Can the taking of a blood count determine whether a child has lead poisoning?**

Up to a certain point, yes. In microscopic examination, the red blood cells usually show anemia and a characteristic stippled appearance. This disease was quite prevalent in the days when toys were coated with paint containing lead. The child would chew on the toys and develop lead poisoning. Even today, painters who use leaded paints in their work are subject to this disease.

**What is a sedimentation rate?**

This is a test performed after drawing a small amount of blood from a vein in the arm. The withdrawn blood is placed in a special glass tube containing an anticoagulant, and the blood cells are allowed to separate out from the plasma. The rate at which the blood cells drop to the bottom of the tube is called the sedimentation rate. It is a rough index of the presence or absence of inflammation somewhere in the body. The more rapid the sedimentation rate, the more likely that an inflammatory process exists.

## SEROLOGIC TESTS

**What is a serologic test?**

Serum is tested for the presence or absence of antigens and antibodies, which indicates the presence or absence of disease.

**What are antigens and antibodies?**

An antigen is a substance, usually a protein, which, when introduced into the body, stimulates the production of antibodies that react specifically with the antigen. Antibodies are protein substances produced by the immune system of the body and are part of the defense against attack by bacteria, viruses, parasites, and other antigens.

**Are there different blood tests to determine the presence or absence of syphilis?**

Yes. These serologic blood tests consist of two general groups of procedures: (1) the nontreponemal antigen tests (e.g., VDRL) and (2) the treponemal antigentest (e.g., the *Treponema pallidum* immobilization test). The second group of tests are highly specific and sensitive as compared with the first group of tests.

**What is a dark-field examination?**

This is a test whereby material is taken from an ulcer or other lesion suspected as being syphilitic and examined directly under a special microscope. The finding of typical spirochetes is diagnostic. The test should be performed only by individuals who have special training and experience in the technique.

**Is the diagnosis of syphilis made from the blood test alone?**

Never. The clinical history, physical examination, and findings are just as important as the results of the blood test.

## BONE MARROW ANALYSIS

**What is a bone marrow study?**

A test in which a small amount of marrow is obtained from the breastbone or some other bone by placing a needle into it. It enables the physician to see how well the blood is being formed and whether it contains tissues or cells that should not normally be present.

**Is a bone marrow test painful?**

There is only very slight pain, since a local anesthetic is used before the needle is inserted.

**Is a bone marrow study important in determining the presence or absence of blood diseases and various types of anemia?**

Yes. It is an extremely valuable test and should always be done whenever there is doubt as to the exact diagnosis.

**Who should perform a bone marrow test?**

A physician who has specialized in the diagnosis of diseases of the blood.

## BLOOD TRANSFUSIONS

**When are blood transfusions most valuable?**

a. When there has been an acute,

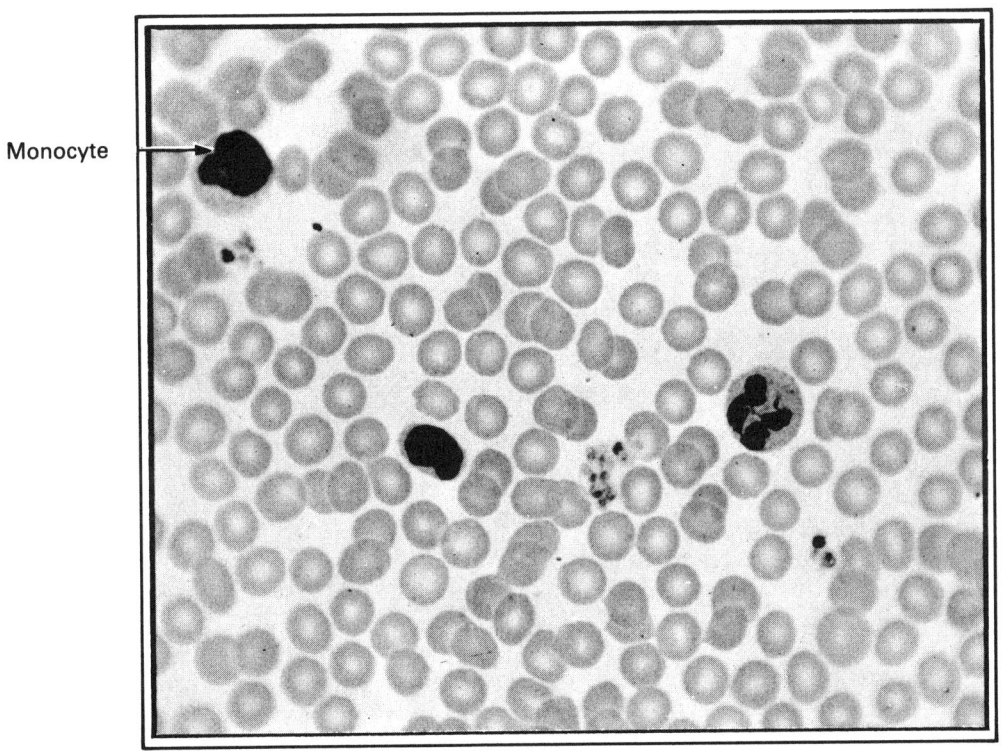

Monocyte

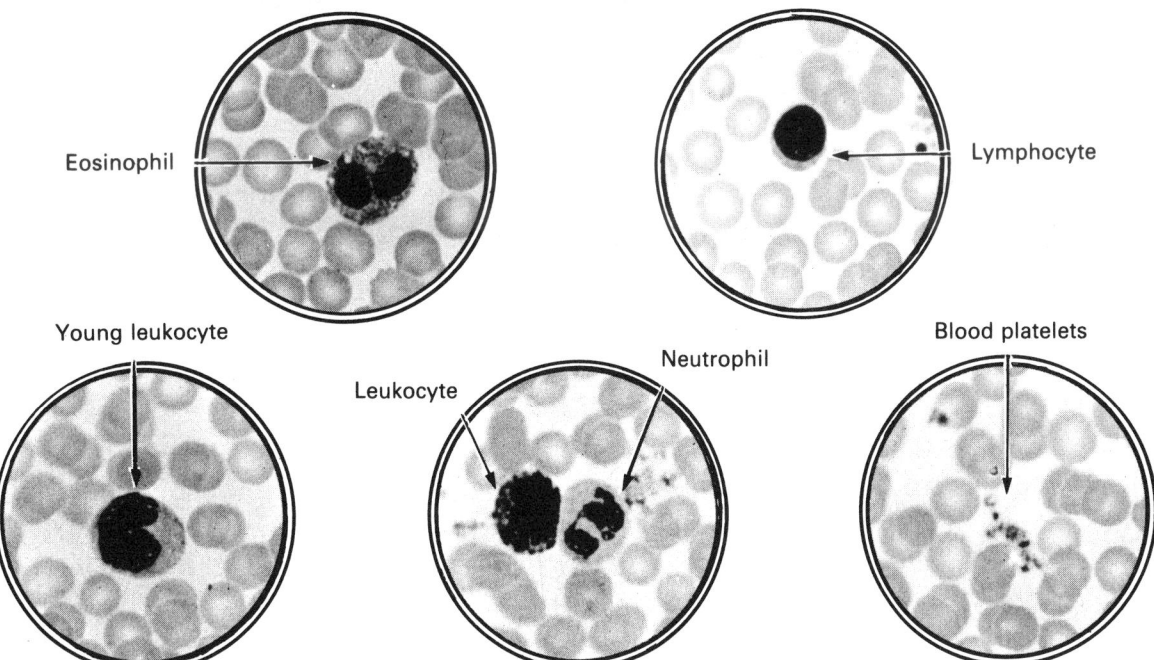

Eosinophil

Lymphocyte

Young leukocyte

Leukocyte

Neutrophil

Blood platelets

**Blood Smear.** *This photomicrograph shows what blood cells look like under the microscope. Variations in the size, shape, and number of blood cells are frequently diagnostic of specific diseases, and the pathologist also learns a great deal about all aspects of the patient's health merely by examining a sample of blood under the microscope.*

# CHEMICAL ANALYSIS OF BLOOD

| | Normal | Abnormal |
|---|---|---|
| **Urea nitrogen** | 12 to 15 milligrams per 100 cc. | Increased amounts may indicate kidney disease (nephritis, etc.). |
| **Glucose-sugar** | 80 to 120 milligrams per 100 cc. | Increased amounts may indicate presence of diabetes mellitus. |
| **Uric acid** | 4 to 8 milligrams per 100 cc. | Increased amounts may indicate presence of gout. |
| **Nonprotein nitrogen** | 25 to 45 milligrams per 100 cc. | Increased amounts may indicate kidney or genitourinary disorder. |
| **Creatinine** | 1 to 2.5 milligrams per 100 cc. | Increased amounts may indicate inability of kidneys to excrete urine (as in obstruction due to markedly enlarged prostate gland). |
| **Cholesterol** | 130 to 240 milligrams per 100 cc. | a. Increased amounts may indicate a tendency toward premature hardening of the arteries.<br>b. Increased amounts are also seen in some pregnant women and in disorders of the thyroid gland. |
| **Calcium** | 9 to 11 milligrams per 100 cc. | Increased amounts may indicate overactivity or a tumor of parathyroid glands in neck. |
| **Sodium** | 137 to 143 milli equivalents per liter. | Decreased amounts may occur from excess vomiting or loss of body fluids, thus endangering normal body processes. |
| **Chlorides** | 585 to 620 milligrams per 100 cc. | Decreased quantities usually result from loss of salt from the body. Excessive loss is incompatible with normal body function. |
| **Phosphorus** | 3 to 4.5 milligrams per 100 cc. | Variation in amounts may indicate functional disorder of the parathyroid glands in the neck. |
| **Potassium** | 4 to 5 milli equivalents per liter. | Marked alterations occur in many disease states and may cause disturbance in heart function. Potassium quantities must be in balance with sodium quantities. |
| **Bilirubin** | 0.1 to 0.25 milligrams per 100 cc. | Increased quantities may indicate jaundice, obstruction to normal flow of bile from liver, or liver disease. |
| **Phosphatase** | 1.5 to 4 units per 100 cc. | Increased quantities indicate obstruction to flow of bile, or jaundice. |
| **Icterus index** | 4 to 6 units. | Increased reading indicates presence of jaundice. |
| **Total protein** | 6.5 to 8.2 grams per 100 cc. | Decreased amounts are seen in debilitated states, in chronic illness. |
| **Serum albumin: Globulin** | 1.5 to 2.5 grams per 100 cc. 2.5 to 3.0 grams per 100 cc. | A reversal so that the ratio is below 1, indicates poor protein metabolism. |
| **$pCO_2$** | 35–45 mmHg. | Increase indicates acidosis; decrease alkalosis. |
| **pH** | 7.35–7.45 | Increase indicates alkalosis; decrease acidosis. |
| **$pO_2$ *(Arterial)*** | 95–104 mmHg. | Increase indicates alkalosis; decrease acidosis. |
| **Amylase** | 80–160 Samagyi Units. | Increase indicates pancreatitis. |
| **SGOT** | <40 I.U. | Increase may indicate liver disease, myocardial infarction, etc. |

sudden loss of blood due to disease or injury.

b. When an acute loss of blood is anticipated, such as when a major operation is to be performed.

c. To give the patient a temporary lift until his own bone marrow can resume the manufacture of blood, as after a prolonged or debilitating disease that has produced anemia.

**Should blood transfusions be given under the direct supervision of a physician?**

Yes, most emphatically. A transfusion means taking blood from a healthy individual and injecting it into a patient. This is a serious procedure and is sometimes associated with complications demanding expert knowledge.

**Who should perform the blood**

grouping (typing) preparatory to the giving of a blood transfusion?

A well-qualified laboratory employing expert technicians should always be used to type the patient's blood. Accidents occur if correct typing and crossmatching are not performed.

**What complications can occur from giving the wrong type of blood?**

Chills and fever, jaundice, or even death may ensue from giving improperly crossmatched blood.

**Should people know their blood groups (types) so that if an accident should occur they can be transfused more quickly?**

Yes. It is wise to know one's own blood group. The blood must always be reexamined prior to transfusion. The blood to be given must always be matched with the recipient's blood before transfusion.

**When given under proper supervision, are blood transfusions safe?**

Yes.

**What are some of the complications of blood transfusions?**

a. Chills and fever. This is a common complication.
b. Allergic reactions such as hives, asthma, etc. When this occurs, the transfusion is usually stopped.
c. Jaundice. This may occur as long as three to four months after the transfusion has been given.
d. Shock, from giving the wrong type of blood or contaminated blood. This is an extremely rare event.

**Can infants and children be given transfusions?**

Yes.

**Are there satisfactory methods for combating reactions to transfusions?**

Yes. Most reactions can be mitigated by proper medical treatment.

**What is meant by an "exchange transfusion"?**

This is a special type of blood transfusion usually performed on newborns who have a blood condition known as erythroblastosis. It attempts to exchange all or most of the infant's blood for new blood and thus gets rid of the blood causing the disease. This must only be performed by an expert in the field.

**What is meant by an "intrauterine transfusion"?**

Within recent years it has been found possible to transfuse the fetus while it is still in its mother's womb. This is done in cases where erythroblastosis (Rh factor disease) is suspected. By an ingenious procedure performed under fluoroscopic x ray, a needle is inserted through the mother's abdominal wall, through the wall of her uterus, and into the fetus. Blood is transfused directly to the fetus in this manner, thus protecting the child against the development of erythroblastosis.

**How successful have intrauterine transfusions been?**

When performed by an expert, the number of instances in which erythroblastosis has been prevented is quite large.

**What is a blood bank?**

There are special blood laboratories set up in large hospitals and institutions where blood is collected from donors and is stored. Blood may be kept for periods up to three weeks prior to use. It is an excellent idea, because the bank tries to maintain a supply of blood of all types to meet any emergency.

## BLOOD CHEMISTRY

**What is a blood chemistry?**

It is a test performed on blood to determine the amount of the various minerals and chemicals circulating in the body.

**What are some of the usual chemicals and minerals tested for when a blood chemistry is taken?**

a. Albumin.
b. Bilirubin, total.
c. Bilirubin, direct.
d. Blood urea nitrogen.
e. Calcium.
f. Carbon dioxide content.
g. Chloride.
h. Cholesterol.
i. Creatinine.
j. Inorganic phosphorus.
k. Iron.
l. Potassium.
m. Protein, total.
n. Sodium.
o. Triglyceride.
p. Uric acid.

**Are blood chemistries valuable in diagnosing the presence or absence of disease?**

Yes. In certain instances, the diagnosis cannot be made without a characteristic blood test.

**Are characteristic findings in the blood chemistry helpful in determining treatment for disease?**

Yes. The quantity of a certain chemical circulating in the blood is often an essential factor in deciding what form of treatment should be given.

**Does life ever depend upon the amount of certain chemicals circulating in the blood?**

Definitely, yes. An excessive amount of certain chemicals, or an excessive lack of certain chemicals, may throw the patient into shock, coma, and may eventually lead to death.

**Can blood chemicals be artificially replaced?**

Yes. One of the most common forms

of treatment for serious disease is to have certain of the chemicals, which may be lacking, given by mouth or by injecting them under the skin or directly into the bloodstream.

### Are blood tests valuable in determination of various types of jaundice?

Yes. A distinction can usually be made between obstructive jaundice, which is due to the prevention of outflow of bile from the liver, jaundice that is due to an inflammation or disease within the liver, and jaundice due to an excessive destruction of blood.

### Are blood tests valuable in detecting the quantity of cholesterol in the blood?

Yes. The presence of an increased amount of cholesterol in the blood is called hypercholesterolemia. Many investigators feel that hardening of the arteries is associated with an excessive amount of cholesterol in the body.

### Are there any blood tests that give information about metabolism?

Yes. A determination of thyroid hormones and thyroid-stimulating hormones gives information about metabolism. These tests aid the physician in determining the state of underactivity or overactivity of the thyroid gland.

### Are there any reliable chemical tests on blood specific for cancer?

No. However, the presence in blood of carcinoembryonic antigen, Alpha Feto protein, or the prostatic component of acid phosphatase is noted in some types of cancer. The presence of high levels of these substances in blood by themselves are not specific for the diagnosis of a particular cancer. They are useful aids in the diagnosis and the follow-up of cancer treatment.

## GLUCOSE TOLERANCE TEST

### What is a glucose tolerance test?

A test in which the fasting patient is given a known amount of glucose (sugar) by mouth, and the blood is tested at intervals thereafter to note the quantity of sugar in the blood. A curve is then constructed from which important information can be drawn.

### What will a glucose tolerance test curve show?

a. Whether the patient is a diabetic.
b. Whether the patient has too little sugar in his blood (hyperinsulinism).
c. Characteristic changes in certain other hormonal disturbances.

### Will blood tests in diabetic patients usually show an excessive amount of sugar?

Yes.

## BLOOD CULTURES

### Of what value are blood cultures?

In diseases in which one suspects that bacteria are circulating in the bloodstream, blood is taken to the laboratory and is cultured to see if bacteria will grow from the blood.

### What types of diseases may show positive blood cultures?

Cases of blood poisoning (septicemia).

## BLOOD GASES AND ACID-BASE STATUS

### What are blood gases?

When we inhale oxygen and exhale carbon dioxide, these gases are transported by blood between the tissues and the lungs. The oxygen and carbon dioxide content of blood can be determined along with the pH, base excess, and other data by passing a sample of blood through a blood-gas analyzer.

### What is meant by acid-base status?

Human metabolism generates the production of acids that are first buffered and then excreted mainly via the kidneys and lungs to maintain the neutrality of body fluids. These mechanisms maintain the neutral acid-base status of the body. Disturbances of acid-base status are broadly divided into two groups: (1) acidosis (acid excess relative to base) and (2) alkalosis (base excess relative to acid). Each is subclassified depending on whether it is primarily a respiratory or metabolic disturbance and whether the condition is compensated or noncompensated.

### What are the common causes of respiratory acidosis?

A respiratory acidosis occurs when carbon dioxide is poorly exchanged by the lungs due to an inadequate ability of the lungs to exhale the gas or due to an obstruction to the passage of the gas from the blood into the lungs. Some examples are: (1) chronic obstructive lung disease (chronic bronchitis and emphysema) and (2) severe restrictive lung disease (pulmonary edema and pulmonary fibrosis).

### What are the common causes of respiratory alkalosis?

When an excessive amount of carbon dioxide is exhaled by the lungs, usually as a result of hyperventilation, alkalosis occurs. Some examples are: (1) a severe decrease in the amount of oxygen that can pass through the lungs into the blood (2) a severe decrease in the oxygen-carrying capacity of blood and (3) excitement or anxiety.

### What are the common causes of metabolic acidosis?

When an excessive amount of acid

is produced by the body or an excessive amount of base is lost by the body, metabolic acidosis occurs. Some examples are: (1) diarrhea (2) diabetic acidosis and (3) renal failure (accumulation of acid in body fluids).

## What are the common causes of metabolic alkalosis?

When acid is lost by the body or a base is retained or ingested, then metabolic alkalosis occurs. Some examples are: (1) vomiting (loss of acid) (2) excessive ingestion of base, as in the "milk-alkali syndrome" and (3) prolonged gastric suction (loss of acid).

## Are the words "alkaline" and "base" synonymous?

Yes.

## URINE ANALYSIS

## When is it usually best to collect one's urine for testing?

Most urines, except for certain special tests, should be collected in a clean bottle as the first specimen passed in the morning.

## What are the substances usually tested for in a urine analysis?

a. Albumin.
b. Sugar.
c. Acidity or alkalinity.
d. Presence or absence of pus.
e. Presence or absence of blood cells, both red and white.
f. Presence or absence of bile pigment, as in cases of jaundice.
g. Presence or absence of casts (microscopic forms denoting kidney damage).
h. Presence or absence of crystals of certain chemicals.

## What can be learned from the presence or absence of these substances in the urine?

Examination of urine gives valuable information concerning the state of health of the kidneys or other portions of the urinary tract. In addition, it may suggest the presence of diabetes, liver disease, etc.

## Does the finding of abnormal substances in the urine always denote the presence of disease?

Not always. Sometimes these are transient findings. It is therefore important to repeat urine tests at regular intervals before making a diagnosis of disease.

## Is it often wise to double-check findings on urine analysis by testing the blood?

Yes. Urine analysis is a helpful test but not always a conclusive one.

## PREGNANCY TESTS

## Are pregnancy tests conducted on the urine?

Yes.

## How accurate are pregnancy tests?

Most laboratories report about 95 to 98 percent accuracy in their pregnancy tests.

## If the examination by the physician does not seem to coincide with the pregnancy test, is it wise to repeat the test?

Yes. It is occasionally necessary to repeat the urine pregnancy test several times before coming to a definite conclusion.

## How are pregnancy tests carried out?

Pregnancy tests are based on the detection of human chorionic gonadotropic hormone (HCG) in urine by using the principle of antigen-antibody reaction. The test is performed on a slide or in a test tube and requires a small quantity of urine. These tests have largely replaced tests using animals. There is also a reliable pregnancy test performed by examination of the serum in the blood.

## How long does it take to get the result of a pregnancy test?

Results can be obtained in a few minutes with some methods or in a few hours using other methods. The latter are usually more reliable.

## How soon after a woman thinks she is pregnant would a pregnancy test show a conclusive result?

For utmost reliability, a woman should not have the test performed before the tenth day following the day of the first missed menstrual period. In many early pregnancies, human chorionic gonadotropic levels may be so low as to yield negative results; these tests should be repeated within one to two weeks for conclusive results.

## Is the pregnancy test always positive if there is a pregnancy in the Fallopian tube?

No. The pregnancy test in tubal (ectopic) pregnancy is not nearly as important as the physical examination performed by the physician.

## R$_H$ TEST

## What is an Rh test?

An Rh test determines the presence or absence of the Rh factor in the blood. It is done whenever a person's blood is typed.

## Should all pregnant women have Rh-factor blood tests done upon them?

Definitely, yes.

## Why is the Rh factor important in pregnancy?

It is particularly important in pregnancy because Rh-negative women (those who lack the Rh factor), when married to men who are Rh-positive, may carry an embryo which is Rh-positive. These women may become sensitized to the Rh factor in the unborn child. Under ordinary circumstances, this does the mother no harm, but it may affect the baby.

### If a mother is Rh-negative, will her baby require a blood transfusion?

The baby will require a transfusion only if the mother has been sensitized to the Rh factor and antibodies produced by the mother affect the baby. The fact that the mother is Rh-negative does not in itself mean that her baby will require any treatment at all.

### What is erythroblastosis?

This is a condition in the newborn in which blood cells are destroyed in huge quantities because of difficulties with the Rh factor.

### Is erythroblastosis a dangerous condition?

Yes. If not treated promptly, it may lead to the death of the infant.

### Should the fact that a woman is Rh-negative influence her to avoid having more children?

No. An Rh-negative mother can be injected with a substance known as RhoGAM within seventy-two hours after a child is born. This injection will protect her next child from developing Rh-factor disease.

### Is it possible for an Rh-negative woman married to an Rh-positive man to bear an Rh-negative infant?

Yes.

### Is it possible for an Rh-positive woman to bear a child who will have complications due to other blood factors?

Yes. Other factors in the blood may at times cause trouble, but these are usually of far less importance and severity than the Rh factor.

### How can one predict whether an

unborn child will have trouble because of the Rh factor?

The mother's blood can be tested for anti-Rh antibodies during the course of her pregnancy. These afford a rough index of what may be expected when the baby is born.

### What are antibody studies?

These are tests to determine whether the body has produced antibodies.

### What is the danger of antibodies in a person sensitized to the Rh factor?

The antibodies have no effect on the person so sensitized unless they are transfused or get an injection of Rh-positive blood. In this case, a severe reaction may develop.

### Can a sensitized woman who remarries bear normal children?

Yes, if the new husband is Rh-negative or of a blood group other than the one that caused the original sensitization.

### Will an erythroblastotic baby be a normal baby if it survives?

If the damage to the baby incident to the disease is minimal, and this is usually the case, such a baby will almost always develop normally.

### Is there any difference between an erythroblastotic baby and a blue baby?

Yes. A blue baby is one who has a congenital disease of the heart or lungs. An erythroblastotic baby is one who suffers as a result of his mother's sensitization to the Rh factor in the blood.

### Is there any way of preventing the development of erythroblastosis in babies to be born to a mother known to have been sensitized to the Rh factor?

There are no injections or drugs known at present that will prevent the disease.

### Can the first child of an Rh-negative woman have erythroblastosis?

This is rare, but it can happen if she has previously been sensitized to the Rh factor by means of an injection or transfusion containing the Rh factor.

### What is the treatment for erythroblastosis?

Exchange transfusion to replace the baby's Rh-positive blood with the donor's Rh-negative blood.

## GASTRIC ANALYSIS

### What is a gastric analysis?

A test whereby the secretions of the stomach are removed, and the constituents are analyzed.

### What is looked for in a gastric analysis?

a. The presence or absence of hydrochloric acid, which should normally be secreted by the cells lining the stomach.
b. The presence or absence of lactic acid, a substance that should not normally be present in the stomach.
c. The presence or absence of blood, which should not normally be present in the stomach.
d. The presence or absence of cancer cells, which, by special tests, can be noted in the gastric secretions of those who have cancer of the stomach.

### In what conditions are gastric analyses most important?

a. In pernicious anemia. In this condition an absence of hydrochloric acid is found.
b. In an ulcer of the stomach or duodenum. In these conditions an excessive amount of acid is often found.
c. In tumors of the stomach. In such conditions, the presence of lactic acid or even the presence of actual cancer cells may be deter-

mined on analysis of the gastric content.

d. In tuberculosis, when it is suspected that sputum is being swallowed.

### How is a gastric analysis performed?

By placing a tube into the mouth or nose and passing it down into the stomach.

### Is this a very painful test?

Not at all, although it is somewhat unpleasant.

### How long does a gastric analysis take to perform?

This is determined by the purpose of the test. It may take only a few minutes, or it may require three hours to complete.

### Should a gastric analysis be performed on a fasting stomach?

Yes.

### Where are gastric analysis tests carried out?

Usually in the office of a well-equipped laboratory. Also, the test is frequently performed upon hospitalized patients.

### Is there any danger involved in having a gastric analysis test performed?

None whatever.

## PAPANICOLAOU TEST

### What is a Papanicolaou smear?

It is one in which cells are wiped from the surface of various organs, usually the uterine cervix or vagina, for the diagnosis of cancer. It has a high degree of reliability when performed by persons trained in cytology. These smears, generally known as Pap smears, can also be taken from cells found in the woman's sputum, urine, or discharges from the nipple.

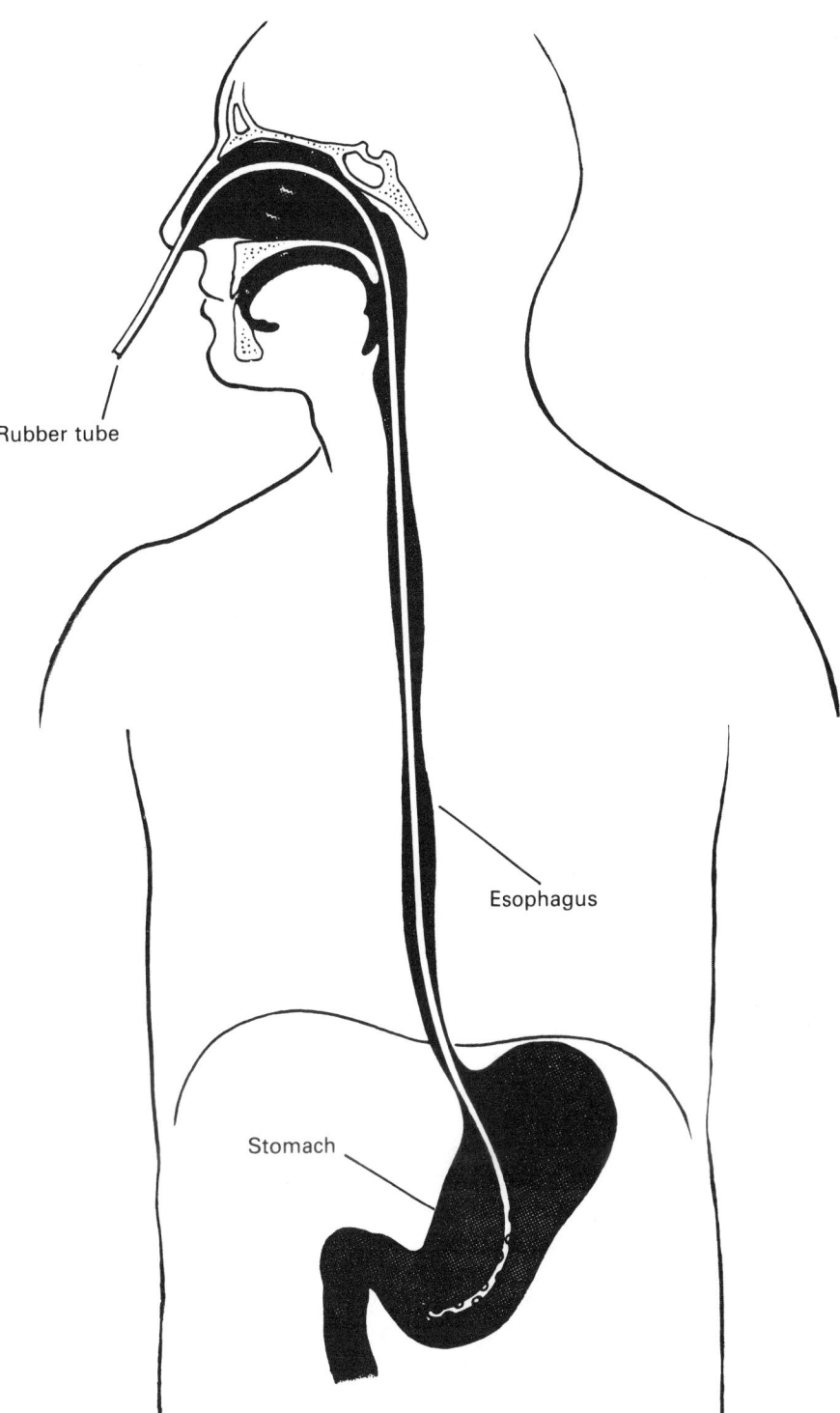

Rubber tube

Esophagus

Stomach

*Gastric Analysis. This diagram shows a rubber tube that has been inserted through the nose, down the esophagus, and into the stomach in order to perform an analysis of the stomach contents. The contents are analyzed for the presence or absence of acid, blood, and other substances. Gastric analysis, while uncomfortable, is not a painful procedure; most people undergo it without complaint.*

### How are Papanicolaou smears performed?

By taking a cotton swab and scraping off the superficial cells from the surface of the cervix or vagina. Cells from sputum, from urine, or from nipple discharge are also prepared by smearing them on a slide and examining them under a microscope.

### Is this a painful or unpleasant test?

Not at all.

**Who should take Papanicolaou smears from the cervix or the vagina?**

A gynecologist, any examining physician, or a specially trained nurse.

**Should all women undergo Papanicolaou tests?**

Yes. It is now advised that every adult female have a "Pap" test performed at least once every year. In this way, very early curable cancers can be discovered. Some of these early cancers, known as cancer *in situ,* are 100 percent curable through surgery.

**Can a woman who is virginal have a Pap test performed upon her?**

Yes, as it is only necessary to insert a small applicator with a swab of cotton into the vagina.

# BIOPSY

**What is a biopsy?**

It is the removal of tissue by a physician or surgeon, who sends it to a pathology laboratory where it is examined grossly and microscopically in order to make a diagnosis.

**Where are biopsies most likely to be taken?**

In hospitals or in physicians' offices.

**What is meant by a needle biopsy?**

This is a test whereby a needle is placed into a diseased area, and cells or contents are withdrawn and examined by the pathologist.

**Is a needle biopsy as accurate as an ordinary biopsy?**

Usually not, because the amount of tissue that can be obtained with the needle is so small that it makes interpretation difficult.

**What is an incisional biopsy?**

It means taking a scalpel and cutting into a diseased area and removing a portion. This fragment is subjected to gross and microscopic examina-tion by the pathologist, who then makes a diagnosis.

**What is meant by an excisional biopsy?**

This means removing the entire diseased area, which is then submitted to gross and microscopic examination by the pathologist.

**What is meant by a "frozen section"?**

This means taking tissue from the patient while the patient is on the operating table and having it immediately submitted to microscopic examination by the pathologist.

**Are frozen-section examinations infallible?**

No. The methods by which the tissues are frozen and subjected to immediate microscopic examination are not as accurate as the usual, more time-consuming methods of preparing tissues for examination in a pathology laboratory.

**What is the value of a frozen-section examination?**

It will tell the surgeon whether a diseased area is malignant or not, thus indicating whether or not a more extensive operation is necessary.

**When are frozen sections particularly useful?**

In determining whether a mass is cancerous. The pathologist will usually be able to make a diagnosis from this examination. If the frozen-section examination reveals that the mass is not cancerous, a less extensive operation is performed. However, if a cancer is diagnosed on frozen section, then the surgeon proceeds to do a more extensive operation. This extensive operation is withheld for a few days if the pathologist informs the surgeon that there is the slightest doubt regarding the diagnosis.

**Is the pathologist only asked to do frozen-section examination to determine the presence or absence of cancer?**

No. There are many situations in which the surgeon is operating to remove inflammatory tissue. He can learn through a frozen-section biopsy whether his operation has extended beyond the region of inflammation.

**Is the pathologist ever called into the operating room?**

Sometimes. Especially when it is necessary for the pathologist to see the entire tumor and decide what tissue is needed for examination to obtain a diagnosis.

**What are some of the tissues frequently submitted for frozen-section biopsy examination?**

a. Skin, to determine the presence or absence of a malignancy.
b. Tissue taken from the bronchial tubes or larynx.
c. Brain tissue and tissue from the spinal cord.
d. Thyroid tissue.
e. Parathyroid tissue.
f. Lymph nodes.
g. Tissue from the tongue or gums.
h. Tissue from the lungs.
i. Liver tissue.
j. Tissue from the spleen.
k. Tissue from the pancreas.
l. Kidney tissue.
m. Adrenal gland tissue.
n. Tissue from the ovaries or testicles.
o. Tissues from the cervix or lining of the uterus.
p. Bone tissue.
q. Bone marrow tissue.
r. Tissues from the fat or muscles of the body.

# SPUTUM ANALYSIS

**Why is sputum analysis carried out?**

a. For determining the presence or absence of the germ causing tuberculosis or other lung infections.

b. For analysis in certain cases of asthma.

c. For determining the presence or absence of malignant cells in possible cancer of the lung.

### How is the sputum analyzed?

Concentrated smears are made, and these are examined carefully under the microscope by the pathologist. Cultures are made to isolate the offending bacteria.

## STOOL ANALYSIS

### For what conditions is the stool analyzed?

a. For any of the diarrheal diseases, such as dysentery, etc.

b. In cases of sprue or celiac disease.

c. In cases of anemia if the cause has not been determined through other means.

d. For any condition in which parasitic invasion is suspected.

e. For conditions in which there is bleeding into the intestinal tract.

f. For colitis or any other infection involving the large bowel.

### Is it important for a fresh specimen to be analyzed?

Yes. The specimen has to be brought to the laboratory almost immediately after it has been passed; otherwise the bacteria, parasites, enzymes, etc., in the stool may be lost.

## PUS CULTURES

### Why are cultures made from pus?

It is very important when pus has been evacuated from the body to determine the particular germ that has produced the infection.

### How is this done by the pathology laboratory?

By growing the germs on appropriate culture media.

### What is the advantage of finding out the particular germ that has caused an infection?

The treatment rendered will be dictated by the exact nature of the germ that has caused the infection. Different germs vary in their susceptibility to drugs; the appropriate drug must be used to combat a given infecting organism.

## LUNG TAPS *(Thoracentesis)*

### Why is a lung tap performed?

a. To remove fluid that may have accumulated in the chest cavity.

b. To determine whether a germ has caused a pleurisy, and to identify it.

c. To determine the presence or absence of any malignant cells in a case of possible cancer of the lung or in the coverings of the lung.

### Are lung taps painful?

There is very little pain. A local anesthetic will probably be given before the needle is inserted.

### Where are the lung taps carried out?

Either in the laboratory, the doctor's office, or the hospital.

## ABDOMINAL TAPS *(Paracentesis)*

### Why are abdominal taps carried out?

a. To remove fluid that may have accumulated in the abdominal cavity.

b. To determine the presence or absence of bacteria that may have caused a peritonitis.

c. To determine the presence or absence of malignant cells.

### Is an abdominal tap painful?

The pain is not very great, as some local anesthesia will be given before the needle is inserted into the abdominal cavity.

## GUINEA PIG INOCULATIONS

### What are guinea pig inoculations used for?

Material is taken from a patient's body and is injected into a guinea pig in order to determine the presence or absence of tuberculosis.

### How long does it take for a report to be given when a guinea pig inoculation has been carried out?

It takes approximately six weeks.

## SPINAL TAPS

### What is a spinal tap?

It is a procedure wherein a needle is inserted in the back and into the spinal canal, and spinal fluid is withdrawn.

### Is a spinal tap painful?

No. It causes only slight discomfort, as it is common practice to inject Novocain into the sensitive structures prior to inserting the needle into the spinal canal.

### Why are spinal taps carried out?

a. To determine the presence or absence of infection within the spinal fluid and brain coverings.

b. To determine the presence or absence of increased pressure within the spinal canal, which may be caused by the presence of a tumor of the spinal cord or brain.

c. To instill air or opaque substances prior to examining the spinal cord and brain by x ray for the presence or absence of tumors or other disease.

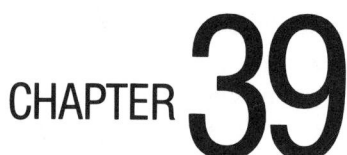

CHAPTER 39

# THE LIPS, JAWS, MOUTH, TEETH, AND TONGUE

*(See also Chapter 48 on Nose and Sinuses; Chapter 63 on Salivary Glands; Chapter 71 on Throat)*

## THE LIPS

**Why do the lips swell so much after even a slight injury?**

Because the tissues beneath the skin in this region are elastic and spongy, thus permitting the collection of large amounts of blood.

**What is the treatment for swollen lips due to bruises or other injuries?**

Apply cold applications and direct pressure as soon as possible after the injury. Most of the swelling will subside within a few days without treatment.

**Is it advisable to have a surgeon suture severe lacerations of the lip?**

Yes. Cuts about the lips should be stitched expertly, so that an ugly scar will not result.

**Are infections about the lips, such as boils, pimples, or carbuncles, dangerous?**

Yes, especially those around the nose, cheeks, and upper lip. These

are a source of danger, if improperly handled, because the blood vessels in this area of the face drain into veins at the base of the brain. Extension of an infection along this channel may lead to an infection within or surrounding the brain.

**What is the most important precaution in the treatment of an infection of the lip?**

Never open or squeeze an infected pimple or boil on a lip!

**What is the treatment for lip infections?**

Small pimples are best left alone. The larger infections are treated by giving the antibiotic drugs and by applying hot, wet compresses to the area. Infections of the lip, especially the upper lip, should be opened only by a surgeon.

**Can a syphilitic infection of the lip result from kissing an infected person?**

Yes. In former years, chancres of the lip were seen quite often.

**Should one avoid kissing a person with a sore on the lip?**

Definitely, yes!

**Are tumors of the lip common?**

Yes. They usually take the form of small, wartlike growths (papillomas), bluish blood vessel tumors (hemangiomas), small frecklelike moles (nevi) of the colored part of the lip, small firm nodules caused by fibrous tissue (fibromas), small retention cysts from one of the glands of the lip, or cancer.

**What is the treatment for tumors of the lip?**

All of the above-mentioned tumors, except cancer, are benign. They should be removed surgically if they are subject to constant irritation or if they show signs of growth. They are

variously treated by surgical excision, by being burned off with an electric needle, by the use of dry ice, or by the application of radium or x-ray therapy. The type of treatment will depend upon the kind of tumor encountered. It is very important that treatment be performed by an expert, so that a minimal scar will result.

**Is cancer of the lip common?**

Yes. It comprises 2 percent of all cancer in the body, about 30 percent of all cancer about the oral cavity.

**Who is most likely to be afflicted with cancer of the lip?**

Approximately 95 percent of all cases are in men, and the lower lip is involved in nine out of ten cases.

**What are thought to be major contributing causes of cancer of the lip?**

Smoking, particularly of pipes; lip biting; overexposure to the sun; overexposure to wind and adverse weather conditions. Also, any recurrent irritant, such as a jagged tooth, that comes into contact with the lip is likely to be a predisposing cause for the development of cancer.

**What is the appearance of cancer of the lip?**

It may look like a wart, a sore that fails to heal, or a cyst.

**What is the treatment for cancer of the lip?**

Any suspicious chronic sore or lesion of the lip should be removed and submitted for microscopic examination. If a frank cancer has been found, it should be widely excised by a wedge-shaped excision of the sore and surrounding normal tissue.

**Is x-ray therapy, radium treatment, or excision with an electric needle ever used instead of surgery?**

Yes, but only on rare occasions.

## What are the results of surgery for cancer of the lip?

When surgery takes place early, before spread to the glands in the neck, cure is the usual outcome. If spread has already reached the glands in the neck, a more extensive excision is carried out, and a radical neck dissection is performed with removal of all the lymph glands and surrounding tissues.

## Is cancer of the lip curable?

Definitely, yes, when discovered in its early stages. The great majority of cancers of the lip can be removed by wide local excision before they have extended to the glands of the neck. Even if the tumor has extended to the glands in the neck, competent radical surgery can produce cure.

## Is the local removal of a cancer of the lip disfiguring?

Not usually. It is surprising how little deformity results from even the removal of 30 to 40 percent of the lip. Of course, these procedures must be carried out by surgeons who understand the cosmetic aspects of this type of surgery.

## HARELIP

### What is harelip?

It is an open, or cleft, upper lip with which a child is born.

### Does the lower lip ever show a cleft?

Only in very rare instances.

### What causes harelip?

Failure of the two sides of the upper lip to fuse during the development of the embryo.

### How often does harelip occur?

About once in every thousand births.

### Does harelip tend to run in families?

Yes.

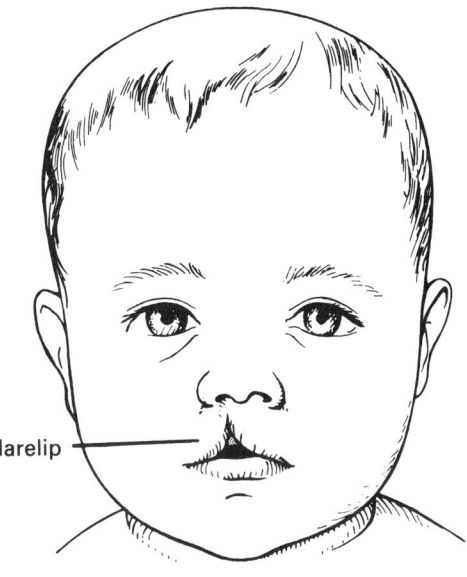

Harelip

*Harelip. This is a rather uncommon birth deformity. Fortunately, plastic surgery can repair this deformity so that it becomes barely visible. It is wise to operate soon after birth to enable the child to nurse normally.*

### What is the treatment for harelip?

Surgical restoration of the lip to normal appearance and function is performed as soon as the infant has shown evidence of gaining weight and is able to stabilize himself on a feeding formula.

### At what age can harelip operations be performed?

Preferably within the first few weeks of life. Because the presence of a harelip in an infant may have a bad psychological effect on other children in the family, it is advisable, if possible, to have the operation performed even before taking the baby home from the hospital.

### What is the actual surgical procedure for repair of harelip?

The meticulous and accurate suturing of the separated tissues, layer by layer, so that not only are the external skin surfaces stitched to one another but also the underlying tissues.

### What are the results of harelip operations?

They are almost always functionally excellent; cosmetically, they will leave a small, thin scar, which will tend to fade as the child grows older.

## CLEFT PALATE

### What is a cleft palate?

A malformation of the roof of the mouth of the newborn child that allows open communication between the nose and the mouth. The cleft, or separation, may extend through the hard and soft palate in the complete type or may involve only the soft palate.

### What causes cleft palate?

It is a malformation during the growth of the embryo, which is thought to take place somewhere between the sixth and twelfth week of development.

### Does cleft palate tend to run in families?

Yes, but present-day investigators feel that some diseases such as German measles, which the mother may develop during early pregnancy, is also a factor in the development of this and other deformities.

### Does cleft palate interfere with normal feeding?

Yes. Food and liquids are pushed through the defect up into the nose during the course of swallowing.

**How often does cleft palate occur?**

Possibly once in every thousand births.

**Will a cleft palate interfere with speaking?**

Yes. Normal sounds of speech cannot be developed, as there is a loss of the resonating factor of the closed palate.

**What is the treatment for cleft palate?**

Surgical correction to overcome the defective fusion of the palate and to develop normal function for speech and eating purposes. The operative procedures are often performed in successive stages for the more extended conditions and require very expert and special surgery.

**At what age should operations for cleft palate be performed?**

In an occasional case, it can be done as early as the first few months of life; other children should be operated on anywhere between the ages of one and a half to three years, or later in some cases.

**Who should perform operations for cleft palate?**

It is a team function and will often demand the cooperation of the oral surgeon, the plastic surgeon, and the dental surgeon.

**Is follow-up care essential after operations for cleft palate?**

Yes. Psychologists and speech instructors are often necessary to teach the child the normal use of his voice after operations of this type.

**Are operations for cleft palate successful?**

Yes, but failures of one particular operation are encountered often. It must be remembered that several operations may be necessary over a period of years to bring about an eventual cure.

## THE JAWS

**What are the common conditions affecting the jaws?**

a. Infection. Infections of the bones of the jaw are usually secondary to infected teeth. Such infections (osteomyelitis) are seen much less often since the advent of antibiotic drugs.

b. Fractures of the jaws.

c. Cysts or tumors of the jaws.

**What is the treatment for an infection of the jaws?**

Infection of the bones of the jaw, as mentioned above, occurs from abscessed teeth or, in rare instances, from an infected sinus. The treatment may involve the expert use of the antibiotic drugs and, in occasional cases, surgical drainage and removal of infected bone.

**Are bone infections of the jaws serious?**

Yes, but with newer methods, eventual recovery over a period of time will result.

**Are fractures of the jaw common?**

Yes, particularly with the increasing number of auto accidents taking place today.

**What are the symptoms of a fractured jaw?**

Pain, swelling, tenderness, difficulty in chewing, loose or missing teeth, and bleeding from the mouth. When the fragments of the fracture are displaced, the patient may find himself unable to close his mouth properly. In fractures of the upper jaw, air may become trapped under the skin, and the front of the face may become swollen, particularly under the eyes.

**When one notes a fracture of the jaw, is there often an accompanying fracture of the skull?**

Yes. The injury that has produced the jaw fracture has often produced damage to the bones of the skull as well.

**Where do jaw fractures usually take place?**

In the lower jaw they occur most commonly in the center at the level

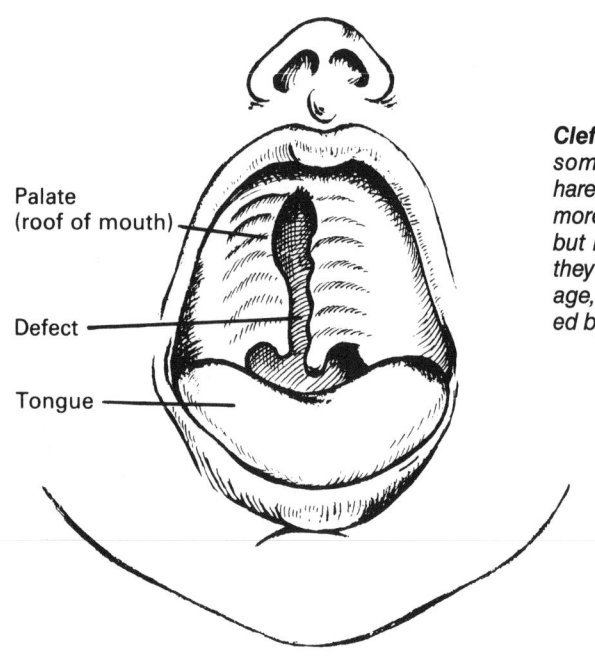

Palate
(roof of mouth)

Defect

Tongue

*Cleft Palate. This deformity is sometimes associated with harelip. Cleft palate is somewhat more difficult to cure surgically, but most children, by the time they are two to three years of age, can be successfully treated by surgery.*

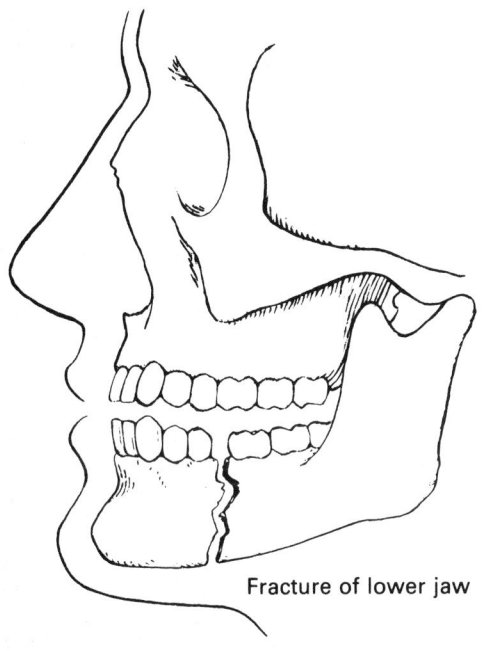

Fracture of lower jaw

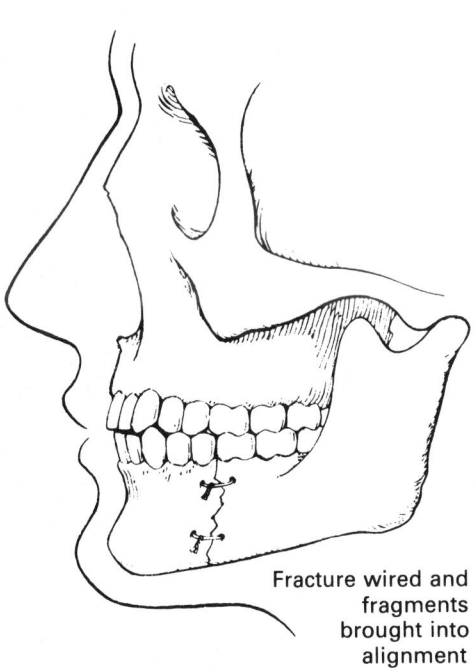

Fracture wired and
fragments
brought into
alignment

*Fracture of the Lower Jaw. The fracture has been wired, and the fragments have been brought into alignment. Most of these conditions are treated by an oral surgeon or by one who specializes in conditions about the face. Orthopedists do not usually treat fractured jaws.*

of the premolar teeth. The upper jaw usually breaks transversely, with loosening of the teeth, and also involves the maxillary sinus.

### Who should treat fractured jaws?

Oral surgeons, often in conjunction with nose and throat surgeons or plastic surgeons.

### What is the treatment for a fractured jaw?

In the uncomplicated case, first-aid treatment aims to immobilize the jaw, either with a handkerchief or bandage. Definitive treatment aims at immobilizing the jaws by wiring the teeth together after setting the deformity. The upper teeth are often wired to the lower teeth in order to keep the jaws splinted or closed.

### Is it ever necessary to operate for fracture of the jaw?

Yes. In the more complicated case, particularly in the compound fracture, it is often necessary to perform an operation within the mouth and to nail or pin the fragments together. Where bone has been lost, a bone graft may be taken, or a metal plate may be used to make up for lost fragments.

### How does a patient eat when the jaws are wired together?

It is often necessary to limit the patient to a completely liquid diet so long as the jaws are wired together.

### How long do fractures of the jaw take to heal?

Anywhere from four to six weeks.

### Is hospitalization necessary for fractured jaw?

The simple cases can be handled in the office of the oral surgeon, but severe cases must be hospitalized and anesthesia given if they require operative intervention.

### Are cysts of the jaws common?

Yes. Malformation of the teeth, with

failure of the tooth to emerge beyond the jaw margins, often leads to the formation of cysts. These are called dentigerous cysts.

### What is the treatment for cysts of the jaw?

The oral surgeon must open the bone overlying the cyst and remove the tooth. The cyst will then fill in with bone.

### Are malignant tumors of the jaw common?

No. When they are encountered, they require wide removal of the jaw bones. These procedures must be carried out by surgeons who specialize in this type of work (maxillofacial surgeons).

## THE MOUTH

### What causes bad breath?

The condition may be transitory and may develop after eating certain foods, taking certain medications, or after excessive smoking or drinking of alcoholic beverages. Under these circumstances, all one has to do is remove the inciting cause. Local disease within the mouth, such as infected or poorly cared-for teeth—or infected gums—may also cause bad breath. Generalized disease such as gastrointestinal illness or diseases of the lungs, liver, or kidneys may also result in bad breath.

### What is the treatment for bad breath?

Since there are innumerable possible causes, it requires a thorough investigation to eliminate the condition. Any local disease within the mouth should be corrected, and proper hygiene of the teeth should be instituted. A general examination by a physician is warranted in such cases to rule out general disease.

## What can be done locally to cut down on bad breath?

Oral hygiene should be maintained. Consult your dentist for treatment of any possible infected teeth or gums. The usual mouthwashes and other measures are usually of a temporary nature in helping to eliminate bad breath.

## What is pyorrhea?

An infection of the gums involving the margin of the teeth with the gums.

## What causes pyorrhea?

A bacterial infection of the mouth, frequently with a streptococcus. Local causes permitting infection to take place usually involve improper bite, poor dental hygiene, tartar formation, improper and infrequent brushing of the teeth, irritation by smoking, or the excessive use of alcohol. Certain deficiency diseases, such as the vitamin-deficiency diseases, may also be accompanied by pyorrhea.

## What are the signs of pyorrhea?

Redness and sponginess, with bleeding from the gums. Also, there may be frank yellow pus formation at the base of the teeth.

## What is the treatment for pyorrhea?

Treatment by a competent dentist is necessary in order to remove tartar and to correct any other dental defects. He will undoubtedly prescribe local medications that will help in obliterating the infection.

## Is pyorrhea curable?

Yes, but treatment is often prolonged and requires rehabilitation of the mouth cavity.

## What is trench mouth?

Trench mouth, or Vincent's angina, is a frequently encountered specific infection and inflammation of the lining of the mouth.

## How does one get trench mouth?

It is usually spread by direct contact with an infected person or by using articles, such as eating utensils, that have been used by a contaminated person.

## Can trench mouth be transmitted by kissing?

Yes.

## Does trench mouth ever affect the tonsils and the throat as well as the mouth?

Yes.

## What are the symptoms of trench mouth?

If it is localized, the patient may complain of a bad taste in the mouth, and those surrounding him may note a bad odor to his breath. There may be small, painful ulcerations on the tongue or inner aspect of the lips or gums that may produce some bleeding.

## Can trench mouth cause swollen glands in the neck?

Yes, and it may also cause fever.

## What is the treatment for trench mouth?

a. Avoid contact with others, as this is a highly contagious disease.
b. Antibiotics, particularly the proper usage of penicillin.
c. Local application of the proper medications to the ulcerations, and the local use of a mouthwash.

# LEUKOPLAKIA

## Is there any other name for leukoplakia?

Yes. It is frequently called smoker's tongue, smoker's patches, etc.

## What is leukoplakia?

The word means white plate. It is manifested as a disease appearing on the mucous membranes or lining of the oral cavity and presents itself as whitish or whitish blue thickenings on the inner aspects of the cheeks, palate, gums, tongue, wall of the pharynx, and sometimes the larynx. These patches are sometimes elevated, roughened, or barklike.

## What causes leukoplakia?

The exact cause is not known, but its high incidence among smokers suggests that local irritation in the mouth from smoking is a strong contributory factor. Also, roughened tooth edges, poorly fitting dentures, etc., are thought to predispose to leukoplakia.

## Who is most likely to be afflicted with leukoplakia?

It is seen more often in men than in women—particularly between the ages of twenty and sixty. However, since smoking has become so fashionable among women, the incidence of the condition is on the rise in that sex.

## What are the symptoms of leukoplakia?

Often there are none at all, and the condition may be noticed accidentally by the patient himself or by the dentist or physician. Occasionally there is burning and tingling and cracking in a leukoplakial plaque.

## What is the significance of leukoplakia?

It is of great significance because it supposedly can be a forerunner of cancer. This is one of the definite instances in medicine where a noncancerous condition (such as leukoplakia) can lead to malignant degeneration.

## What is the treatment for leukoplakia?

a. Stop smoking.
b. Remove all possible sources of local irritation, such as poorly fitting

dentures or roughened skin edges.

c. Removal of the leukoplakial patch either by an electric needle or by surgical excision of the area.

## Is hospitalization necessary for removal of areas of leukoplakia?

The great majority of these cases can be treated adequately in the surgeon's office by treatment with an electric needle. However, when patches must be removed from the throat or from the larynx, hospitalization is advised.

## Can successful treatment of leukoplakia avoid the development of cancer?

Yes. People with leukoplakia should be kept under constant supervision so that the progress of the disease can be noted.

# THE TEETH

## What causes cavities of the teeth?

The specific cause is not actually known, but it is thought that a chemical decalcification is stimulated by the action of certain acid-producing bacteria or germs that grow in the mouth. Improper diet and improper hygiene also predispose to cavity formation. Also, irritation of the teeth by poor bite or by poorly fitting dentures are thought to cause cavities.

## What is the best way to prevent cavities of the teeth?

Dental examination at regular intervals. Also, the maintenance of proper dental hygiene and attention to one's general health. The weight of evidence today is that fluoridation of water will cut down greatly on the incidence of cavities. It has been found that children living in areas where the drinking water has been fluoridated have a much lower incidence of tooth decay.

## Can the presence of diseased teeth affect the general health of a patient?

Yes. The teeth are part of the human body, and infection or disease within the teeth can spread to other parts of the body.

## How can one tell if he has an abscessed tooth?

Abscessed teeth are almost always accompanied by a local reaction involving swelling, pain, and redness in the area. A chronic abscess, however, may not be readily discernible by the patient.

## What is the treatment for an abscessed tooth?

See your dentist. He will usually prescribe antibiotics and, in most instances, will have to remove the infected tooth.

## Can bacteria affecting the teeth spread to other parts of the body?

Yes. This is particularly important to avoid in people who have disease of the heart. It is known that people with valvular disease of the heart may develop an infection on those diseased valves from infected teeth.

# THE TONGUE

## What is glossitis?

It is an inflammation of the tongue.

## Is the tongue often involved in an infection or inflammation or true abscess formation?

No. The tongue is peculiarly immune to the formation of abscesses. This may possibly be attributed to its very rich blood supply.

## What is the treatment for inflammations of the tongue?

Since glossitis is usually a sign or a symptom of disease elsewhere, the treatment will depend upon the causative factor. Whenever a local irritant is causing a change in the tongue, this must be eliminated.

## Is the tongue subject to many changes in its appearance?

Yes. The tongue has been used for generations by physicians to make various diagnoses of general diseases. The tongue may be swollen or reddened or whitish or smoother than normal, and may change its appearance from day to day.

## What local factors often produce changes in the appearance of the tongue?

Tobacco, alcohol, highly spiced foods, or excessively hot foods may cause a tongue to look red and irritated. The edge of the tongue may be irritated by rough, sharp edges of teeth or improperly fitted dentures. Also, the tongue may be affected by infections within the mouth, such as trench mouth, syphilis, etc. Vitamin deficiencies, too, as well as allergic reactions to antibiotic throat lozenges, may alter the appearance of the tongue.

## What general diseases of the body are most frequently reflected in changes of the appearance of the tongue?

Deficiency diseases, such as certain types of anemia (pernicious anemia). Also, generalized skin conditions will give a characteristic appearance to the tongue.

## What condition of the body is most closely reflected in the appearance of the tongue?

The state of hydration or dehydration. The tongue appears dry and coated whenever the patient lacks the proper amount of fluids within his body.

## Is the tongue often the site of tumor formation?

Yes.

## What are the common tumors of the tongue?

a. Leukoplakia. This is really not a true tumor but is a forerunner of tumor formation.
b. Blood vessel tumors (hemangiomas).
c. Wartlike tumors (papillomas).
d. Gland cell tumors (adenomas).
e. Connective tissue tumors (fibromas).
f. Cysts of the tongue occasionally caused by failure of the thyroid gland to develop fully (thyroglossal cysts).
g. Cancer of the tongue.

## Is cancer of the tongue a common condition?

Yes. It comprises about one out of five of all cancers within the oral cavity.

## Where is cancer of the tongue usually seen?

Along the tongue margins or at the edge of the tongue.

## What causes cancer of the tongue?

It is not definitely known, but it is thought that the common factor of chronic recurrent irritation may be a predisposing factor. It must be strongly emphasized that the greatest incidence of cancer of the tongue is seen among pipe smokers and heavy drinkers. The second most common predisposing cause of cancer of the tongue appears to be sharp edges of the teeth, poorly fitting dentures, and poor hygiene of the mouth.

## Does cancer of the tongue affect men more than women?

Yes—by a ratio of eight to one.

## At what age is cancer of the tongue most frequently encountered?

Between forty and sixty years of age.

## How is the diagnosis of cancer of the tongue made?

It has a characteristic appearance, which soon makes itself evident to the examining physician. The positive diagnosis is made by removing a small piece of the tissue and submitting it to microscopic examination.

## What is the treatment for tumors of the tongue?

Most benign tumors can be removed surgically or can be treated with surgery plus x ray or radium applications. All benign tumors of the tongue are curable. Early cancers of the tongue can be cured by wide local excision.

## Is it ever necessary to remove the entire tongue for cancer?

Usually, a portion of the tongue is left behind when a cancer is found. However, if the cancer has already spread to the glands in the neck, a wide radical excision of the tongue and the glands in the neck may produce a cure.

## Is surgery always the treatment of choice for cancer of the tongue?

No. There are certain types of cancer, particularly those that occur in the posterior portions of the tongue, which are better treated with radium or x ray.

## What are the chances of cure for cancer of the tongue?

More than half of those cases seen in their early stages can be permanently cured. However, all too often treatment is started late, and it is sad to report that cancer of the tongue is responsible for more deaths than any other tumor arising in the head and neck.

# CHAPTER 40

# THE LIVER

*(See also Chapter 6 on Alcoholism; Chapter 27 on Gall Bladder and Bile Ducts; Chapter 68 on Spleen; Chapter 73 on Transplantation of Organs)*

## What is the liver, and where is it located?

The liver is a very large glandular organ of reddish brown color located in the upper abdominal cavity beneath the diaphragm and ribs. It stretches across the upper abdomen for approximately eight inches and extends irregularly in shape for six or seven inches in a vertical direction from front to back. It is divided into two lobes, a right and left, the right lobe being about three times the size of the left lobe.

## What are the functions of the liver?

The liver is the most important structure in the body in the regulation of chemical reactions. It is not possible to enumerate all of its functions, but the main ones are:

a. To receive blood from the portal system. Such blood contains the nutritive substances absorbed from the intestines. This blood is transported through the portal vein, which receives tributaries from smaller veins arising in the intestines.

b. The production and storage of proteins; the regulation and control of the many by-products of protein metabolism.

c. The storage of sugar and the regulation of the amount of sugar circulating in the blood.

d. The neutralization of toxic and harmful substances in the body.

e. The utilization and storage of fats.

f. The manufacture of substances important to blood coagulation.

g. The manufacture of bile and bile salts, which are secreted through the ducts into the intestines and that aid in digestion.

h. The manufacture and storage of substances important to the production of red blood cells and other components of the blood.

i. The breakdown of drugs for eventual elimination from the body by the kidneys.

## Can a patient survive without a liver?

No. It is essential to life.

## What are the usual causes of impairment of liver functions?

a. Infection of the liver.

b. Parasite infestation of the liver.

c. Cancerous invasion.

d. Liver poisoning from the ingestion of poisons or certain medications, which may adversely affect the liver.

e. Prolonged obstruction of the bile ducts with obstruction to the outflow of bile.

f. Severe malnutrition.

g. Disturbance in the blood supply to the liver.

h. Replacement of its vital structure by abnormally produced substances such as amyloid.

i. Upset in liver chemistry.

j. Cirrhosis of the liver (replacement of liver substance by fibrous tissue).

## Are diseases of the liver very common?

Yes, but they are not very obvious because the liver has an extraordinary ability to fight off disease and to function satisfactorily despite disease.

## Can the liver continue to function satisfactorily when a large portion of its substance is involved in a disease process?

Yes.

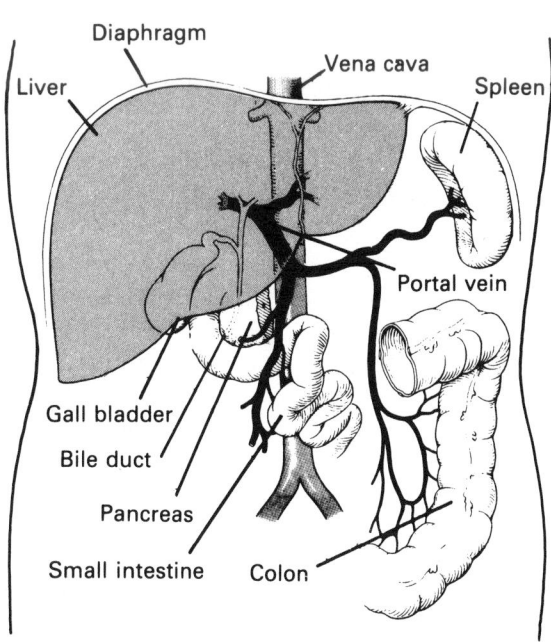

**Anatomy of the Liver and the Portal System.** *The portal vein collects blood from the intestinal tract and transports it to the liver. Through this portal system, food elements that have been absorbed from the intestines are brought to the liver, where their chemical components are extracted.*

### Is liver disease easy to diagnose?

Not always, because serious and progressive liver disease may exist for many years without giving any apparent signs or symptoms to the patient. This is because the liver has a great functional reserve.

### How does one go about discovering if there is liver disease?

By careful noting of the patient's history, careful physical examination, and by a variety of laboratory tests performed on the blood, stool, and urine.

### What is meant by the terms "biliousness," "torpid liver," and "liverish"?

These are terms used by lay people who believe they may have disease of their liver. More usually, the symptoms are not related to liver upset but are associated with indigestion, dietary indiscretions, emotional disturbance, or perhaps other diseases of the gall bladder or intestinal tract.

### What is jaundice?

Jaundice is a generalized yellowish discoloration of the skin and the white of the eyeball due to an abnormally high concentration of bile pigments in the blood.

### Does jaundice always indicate liver disease?

No. It may be due to excessive destruction of red blood cells by disease involving the blood itself. Or it may be due to the damming back of the bile into the bloodstream because of disease of the gall bladder, bile ducts, pancreas, or other organs adjacent to the liver. This latter type of jaundice is called "obstructive jaundice."

### What is acute yellow atrophy of the liver?

This term signifies rapid and progressive destruction of the liver as a result of infection or chemical poisoning. The condition is accompanied by a severe degree of jaundice and by a shrinking or death of many of the liver cells. Usually, this condition is rapidly fatal.

### Can heart disease affect the liver?

Yes. With a poorly functioning or failing heart, the liver may become enlarged and engorged with stagnated blood. If this situation persists over a prolonged period of time, permanent liver injury may result.

### Do gallstones ever cause liver damage?

Yes, by obstructing the bile ducts and the flow of bile into the intestines, the bile is dammed back into the liver substance. This may result in grave damage to liver function and to the liver cells themselves. Such a condition, if persistent, may cause biliary cirrhosis.

### Is the liver ever afflicted with bacterial infection?

Yes. Bacteria may set up infection within the liver, either generalized or in the form of an abscess or abscesses. This may occur as a complication of other diseases, such as pneumonia, typhoid fever, appendicitis, etc. These complications are relatively rare today because of the effective treatment of the primary disease with antibiotic drugs.

### Is the liver ever afflicted by other microorganisms?

Yes, by a protozoan known as *Entamoeba histolytica*, the cause of amebic dysentery. Quite often liver infection and abscess formation are complications of this type of dysentery.

### Can infectious mononucleosis (glandular fever) cause liver disease?

Yes. The patient may develop the same clinical picture as seen in infectious hepatitis. The condition usually clears up completely and leaves no residual liver damage.

### Do parasites ever infest the liver?

Yes. A wide variety of parasites may find their way to the liver, either through having been eaten in contaminated foods or water or by penetrating the skin of a person bathing in infested waters. This occurs much more frequently in tropical climates outside of the United States—in the Orient, Africa, the Philippine Islands, etc. Two of the most common types of infestation are caused by the *Echinococcus*, originating from infestation of dogs, and by the schistosome (blood fluke), originating from infestation of snails.

## CIRRHOSIS

### What is cirrhosis of the liver?

It is a general term meant to signify chronic generalized destruction and scarring of liver tissue, with impairment of liver function to a slight or greater degree.

### What causes cirrhosis of the liver?

Any disease process that involves the liver may eventually lead to cirrhosis, that is, destruction of liver cells and replacement by scar tissue.

### Can drinking alcohol over a prolonged period of time produce cirrhosis?

Yes. The association between people who drink alcoholic beverages excessively and the occurrence of cirrhosis is well known. It is thought that the liver damage results from the combined effects of the toxic action of the alcohol upon the liver and the poor nutritional intake usually associated with those who drink excessively.

### Will drinking in moderation cause cirrhosis of the liver?

No, but of course this involves a definition of the term "moderate drinking." An occasional highball or drink before dinner is not likely to cause liver damage, especially when the diet and food intake is adequate. However, the tolerance to the toxic effects of alcohol varies widely from one individual to another.

### What are the symptoms of cirrhosis?

These vary with the degree of liver destruction and liver reserve. Many cases go undetected and without symptoms for years. As liver function deteriorates, it may be accompanied by loss of appetite, anemia, nausea, vomiting, and weight loss. There may be abdominal discomfort, fullness in the upper abdomen, and indigestion. When the disease progresses, there may be a listlessness and weakness with loss of energy. When extensive liver destruction has taken place, the legs and abdomen may become swollen with fluid (dropsy), jaundice may come on, and the patient's mental state may become confused and disoriented. The final outcome may be coma and death.

### Is cirrhosis always fatal?

No. If it is detected at an early stage, and if proper treatment is carried out, a patient with cirrhosis may live his normal span of years.

### How is cirrhosis of the liver diagnosed?

By studying the patient's history and by physical examination, as well as by certain laboratory tests performed upon the blood, urine, and stool.

### How is cirrhosis of the liver treated?

First, it is important to remove any toxic influences, such as infection, obstruction to the outflow of bile, or liver poisons that the patient may be taking. Next, there must be a satisfactory dietary intake, with the proper amounts of minerals and vitamins. Finally, bleeding due to cirrhosis is treated by performing a mesocaval or portacaval shunt. (See Chapter 13, on Blood Vessel Surgery.)

### Is cirrhosis ever complicated by hemorrhage?

Yes. Varicosed veins within the esophagus will frequently bleed in cases of advanced cirrhosis. This is caused by these veins becoming swollen because they carry blood that would ordinarily have gone through the liver had it not been involved in cirrhosis.

### Is the liver always enlarged in cirrhosis?

No. During the later stages it may become shrunken and smaller than normal.

### Is the spleen often enlarged in cirrhosis of the liver?

Yes.

## FATTY LIVER

### What is a fatty liver?

A fatty liver is one that has many times the normal component of fat.

### What is the cause of fatty liver?

It is caused by malnutrition, alcoholism, marked anemia, diabetes, or chemical poisoning.

### What are the symptoms of fatty liver?

Usually there are none, except for enlargement of the liver. However, if the underlying cause is not removed, severe and progressive damage to the liver may occur.

### What is the treatment of fatty liver?

Elimination of the basic cause, then giving a well-balanced diet, with proper vitamin and mineral supplements.

## CANCER OF THE LIVER

### Is the liver ever involved in cancer?

Yes. There may be a primary cancer, in which the cells of the liver themselves originate the cancer; or there may be metastatic involvement of the liver, in which the cancer cells have originated elsewhere in the body.

### What causes primary cancer of the liver?

The cause is not really known, but it has been found that a considerable number of cases develop in those livers that have been previously cirrhotic. In addition, certain chemical toxins and parasitic infestations have been incriminated in a small percentage of these cases.

### Is it common for the liver to be involved in cancer that has originated elsewhere?

Yes. The liver is the organ most commonly involved in cancer that has spread from another organ, such as the stomach, pancreas, gall bladder, breast, kidney, or intestines.

### What are the symptoms of cancer of the liver?

These vary widely, depending upon the extent and nature of the involvement as well as upon how the other organs of the body are involved. Usually, there is loss of weight, weakness, loss of appetite, and nodular enlargement of the liver. Eventually, all the symptoms of typical severe liver damage ensue—such as jaundice, hemorrhage, swelling of the legs, with eventual coma and death.

### Can cancer of the liver ever be treated effectively by surgery?

Yes, in occasional cases in which there is involvement of but one segment of the organ. It is now possible to remove half of the liver surgically and for the patient to survive. There are also a few cases on record in which an entire liver has been removed and a whole liver transplant from another body has been inserted in its place.

# INFECTIOUS HEPATITIS

### What is infectious hepatitis?

This is a common type of infection of the liver that may occur in epidemics and is caused by a virus infection.

### Are there any other names for infectious hepatitis?

It is also called epidemic hepatitis, catarrhal jaundice, hepatitis A or B.

### What age groups are most likely to develop infectious hepatitis?

At any age, but young people seem to be most prone to this condition.

### Is infectious hepatitis very common?

Yes, and it has been increasing greatly in incidence within the past few years.

### What are thought to be some of the causes of an epidemic of infectious hepatitis?

Poor sanitation, contaminated food or water, crowding, malnutrition, the use of contaminated hypodermic needles, as in drug addiction.

### What are the symptoms of infectious hepatitis?

Over a period of a few days, the patient begins to feel ill, loses energy, loses appetite, feels nauseated, and develops a slight fever. There then ensues tenderness and enlargement of the liver, some pain in the upper right portion of the abdomen, and eventually—about the fifth or sixth day—onset of jaundice. There may also be a gastrointestinal upset, with vomiting and diarrhea.

### Does infectious mononucleosis ever cause hepatitis?

Yes. The course, clinical findings, and laboratory tests are often indistinguishable from infectious hepatitis. The true diagnosis is suspected when typical physical findings of infectious mononucleosis such as generalized lymph node en-

largements, are found; or when certain types of abnormal white blood cells are found in the blood smear; or, finally, when a specific type of laboratory test such as the heterophil antibody titer is found to be elevated and rising.

### Does jaundice always accompany infectious hepatitis?

No. In a small percentage of cases, actual jaundice does not occur.

### How is a diagnosis of infectious hepatitis made?

By noting the history and symptoms; by finding a tender, enlarged liver; by noting the presence of jaundice; and by characteristic findings on laboratory tests of blood, stool, and urine.

### Can infectious hepatitis be distinguished from other liver diseases by special laboratory tests?

Yes.

### How long is one usually ill with infectious hepatitis?

Anywhere from six to twelve weeks.

### Is it necessary for the patient with infectious hepatitis to spend a great deal of time in bed?

Definitely, yes. The liver is a large organ, and when it is inflamed and infected, it must have rest. This can be obtained only in bed.

### Does a relapse of infectious hepatitis ever take place?

Yes, in about one out of ten patients if the patient gets out of bed too soon or resumes activity before he has fully recovered.

### Are there any other causes for a relapse of infectious hepatitis?

Yes; poor diet or the drinking of alcoholic beverages.

### Are there any specific drugs or antibiotics that are of value in treating infectious hepatitis?

No. Rest and an adequate well-

balanced diet are the best forms of treatment.

### What are the chances for recovery from infectious hepatitis?

The chances are excellent, although a small percentage of patients—those who do not take care of themselves properly or who have other illnesses—may die. In a very small percentage of cases, this disease takes on a chronic form extending over many years with progressive destruction of the liver. The reason for this deleterious course is unknown. In rare cases, the disease may be rapidly fatal.

### Is infectious hepatitis classified as a contagious disease?

Yes. It can be spread by close contact with a patient who is ill with hepatitis. However, the degree of contagion is relatively mild.

### Does infectious hepatitis usually cause permanent liver damage?

No. In the vast majority of cases, complete recovery of liver function takes place.

### Is there a tendency toward getting another attack of hepatitis once a patient has fully recovered?

No.

### Can infectious hepatitis be prevented if one has been exposed to a patient who has the disease?

Yes, in many cases. Gamma globulin injection is believed to be effective in preventing the disease if given early enough after exposure. This protection lasts only four to six weeks.

### Can one be immunized against infectious hepatitis?

Recent research has developed a vaccine to prevent one type of hepatitis, but the vaccine is not yet generally available.

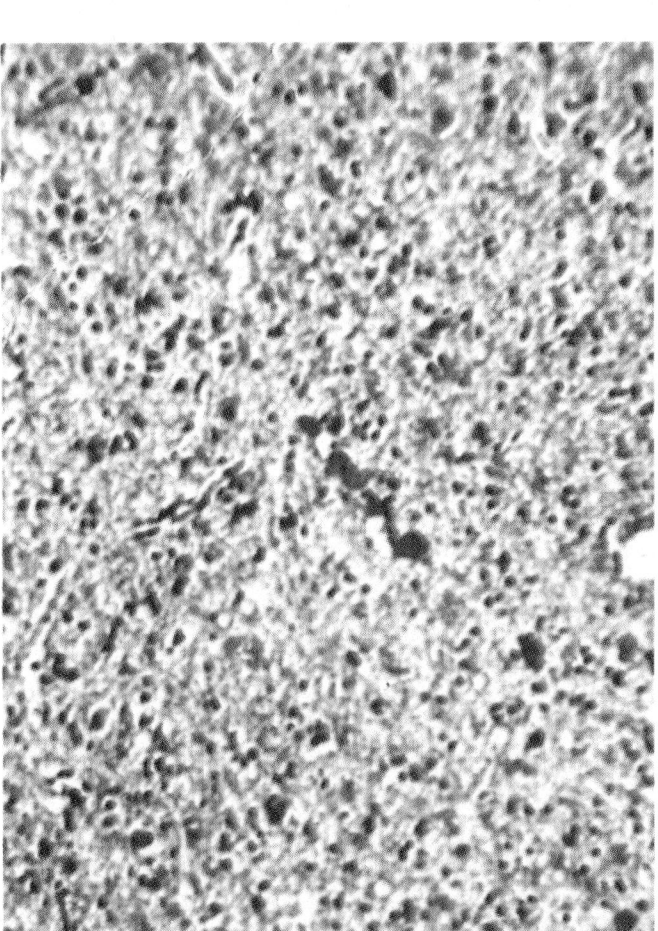

A fat embolism occurs when fat tissue cells travel through the bloodstream and obstruct a small artery. In the case of the obstructed brain tissue in this photomicrograph (*left*), the fat embolism originated from a fractured hip.

The dark-colored area in this photograph (*below*) is a portion of lung whose circulation has been cut off because of a pulmonary embolus. Such an area is called an infarct.

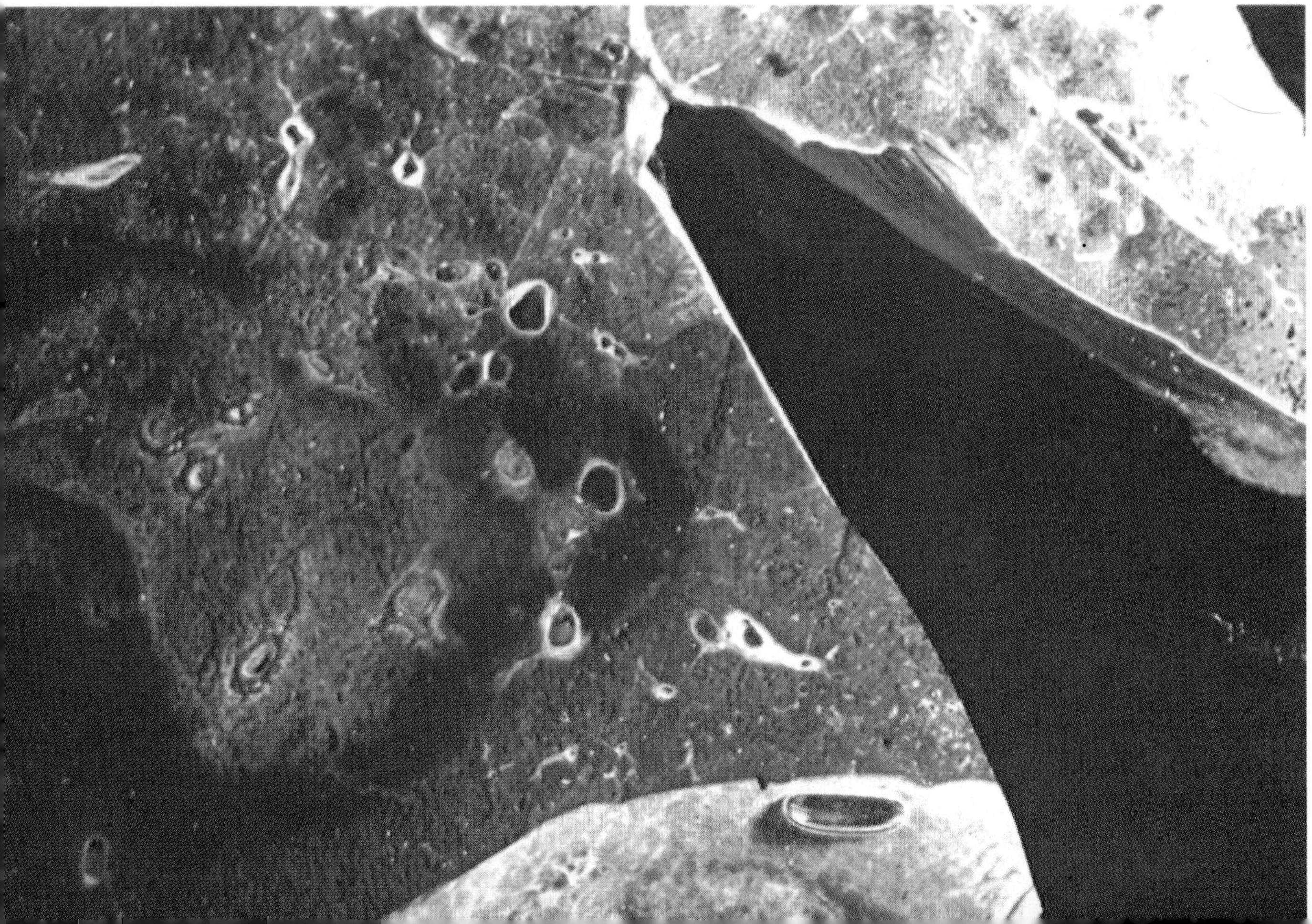

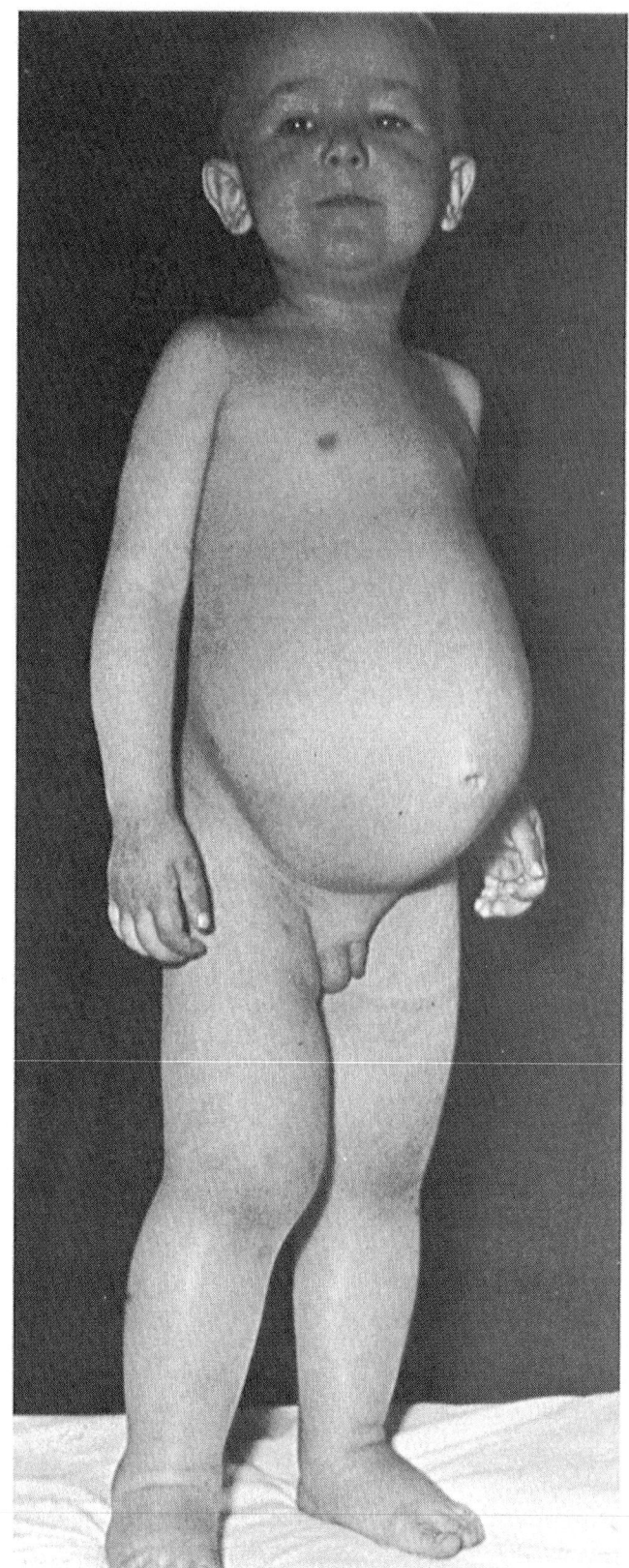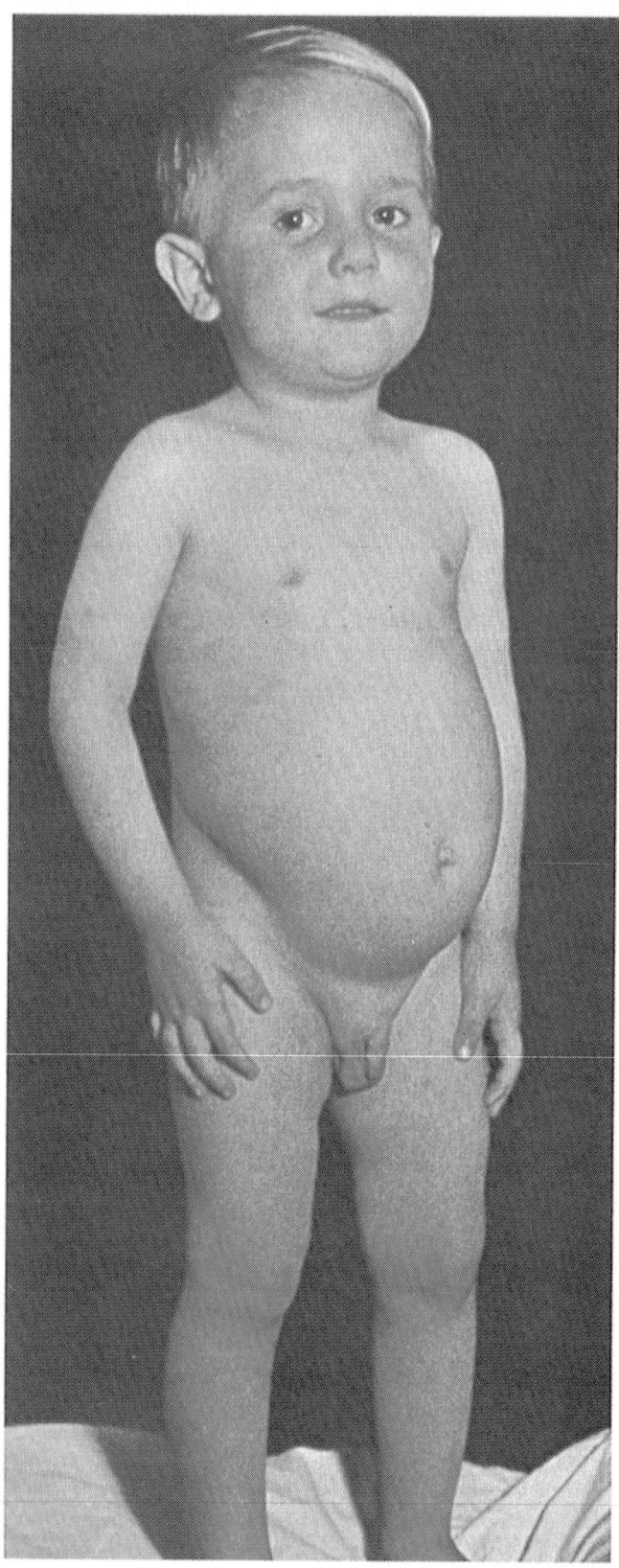

Nephrosis is a serious kidney disorder which manifests itself by a swollen, waterlogged appearance of all the tissues of the body and which results in impairment of kidney function. Until recently, most children with this condition died; today, with new methods of treatment, most survive. This child is shown both before treatment and during the healing phase of his disease.

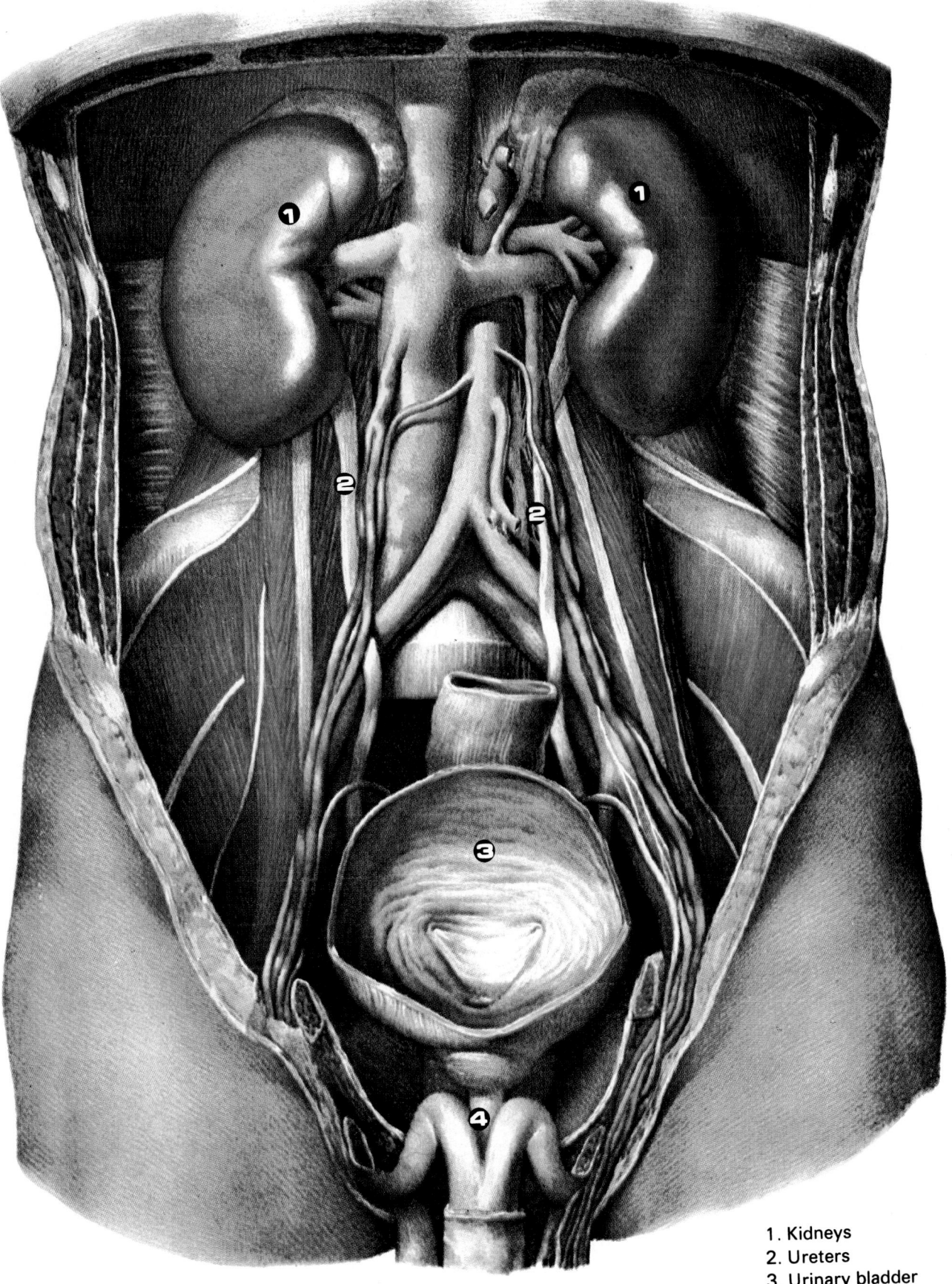

1. Kidneys
2. Ureters
3. Urinary bladder
4. Urethra

**THE MALE GENITOURINARY SYSTEM**

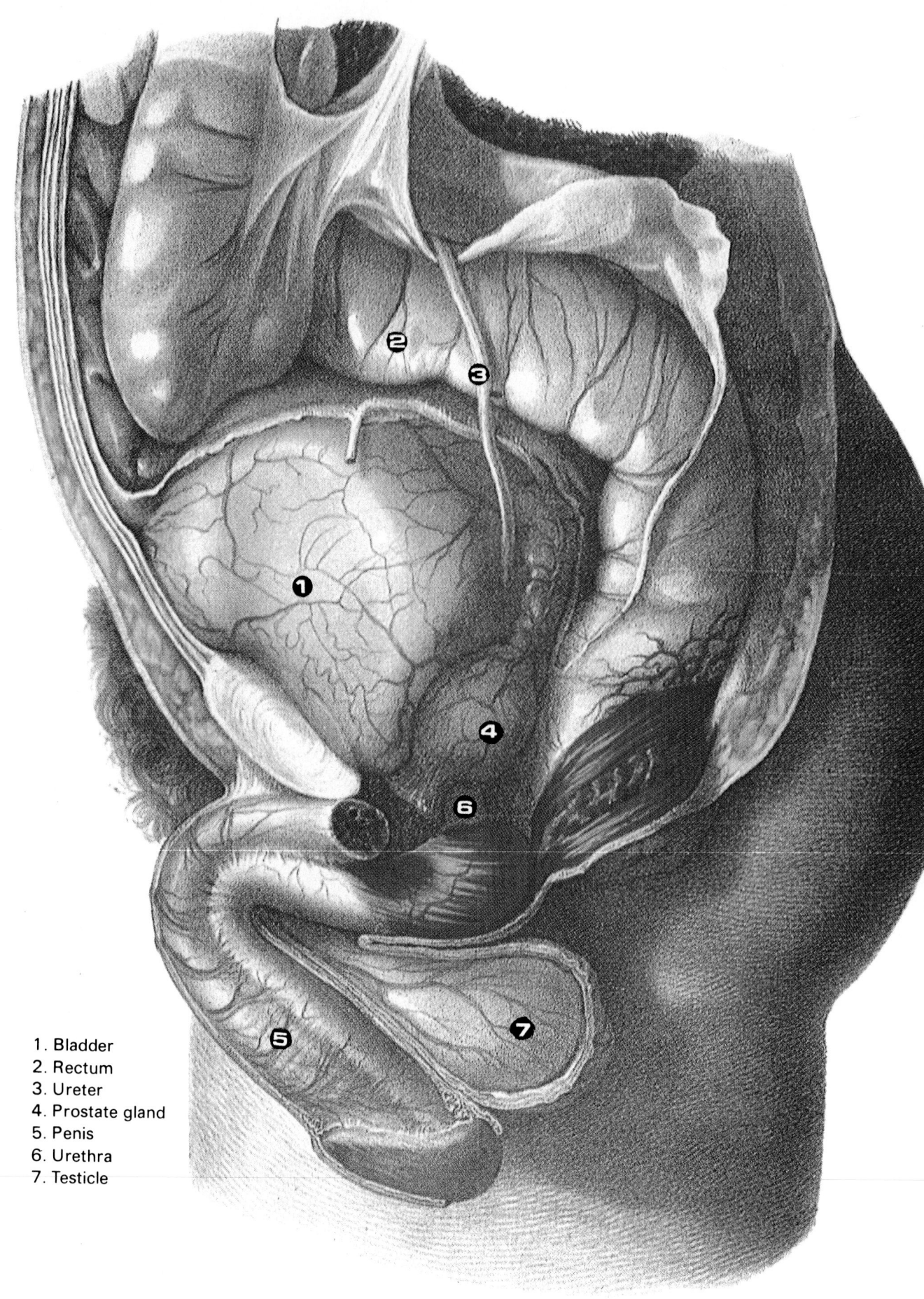

1. Bladder
2. Rectum
3. Ureter
4. Prostate gland
5. Penis
6. Urethra
7. Testicle

**GENITOURINARY ORGANS IN THE MALE—SIDE VIEW**

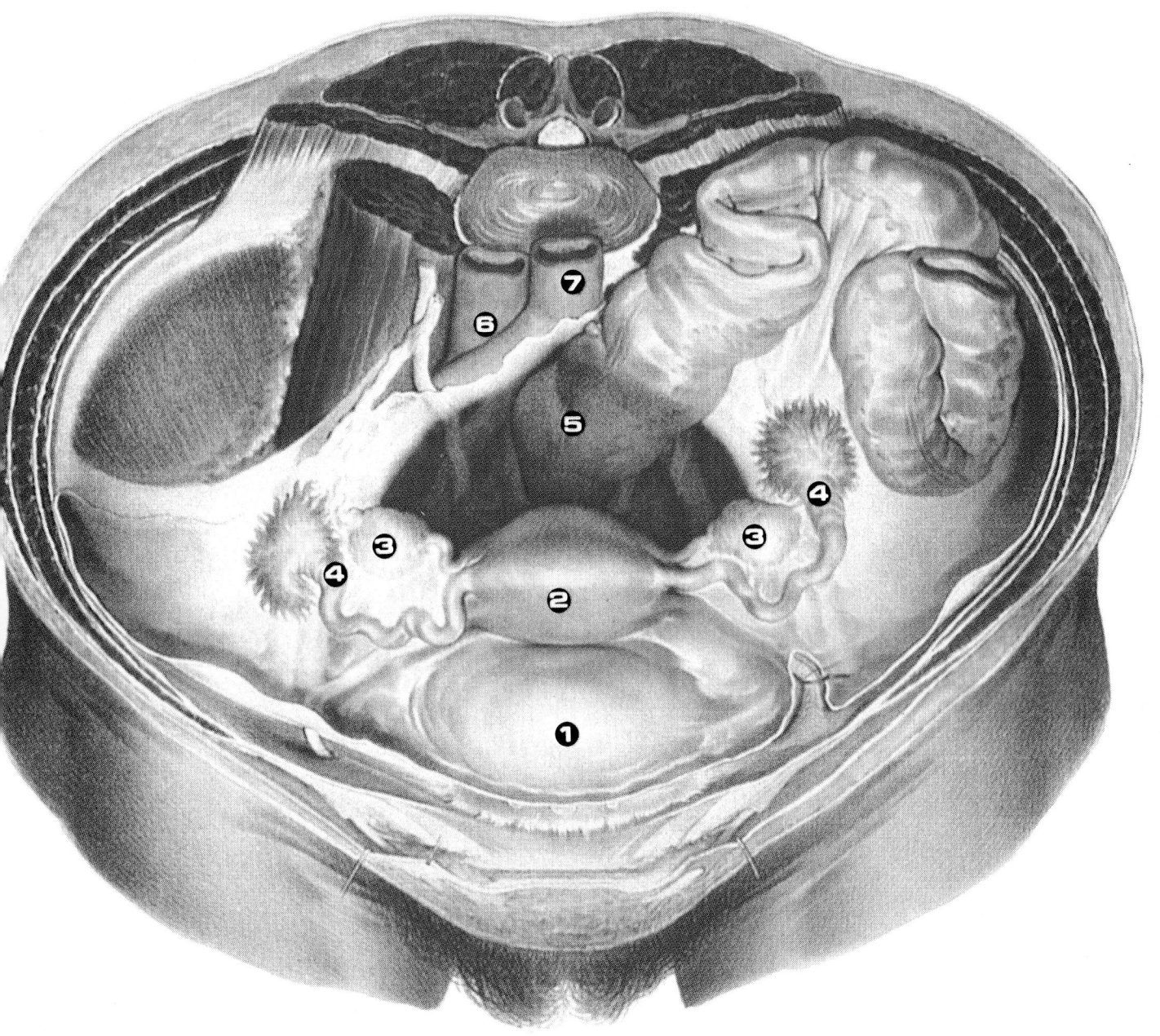

1. Urinary bladder
2. Uterus
3. Ovaries
4. Fallopian tubes

5. Rectum
6. Inferior vena cava
7. Aortic artery

**GENITOURINARY ORGANS IN THE FEMALE—TOP VIEW**

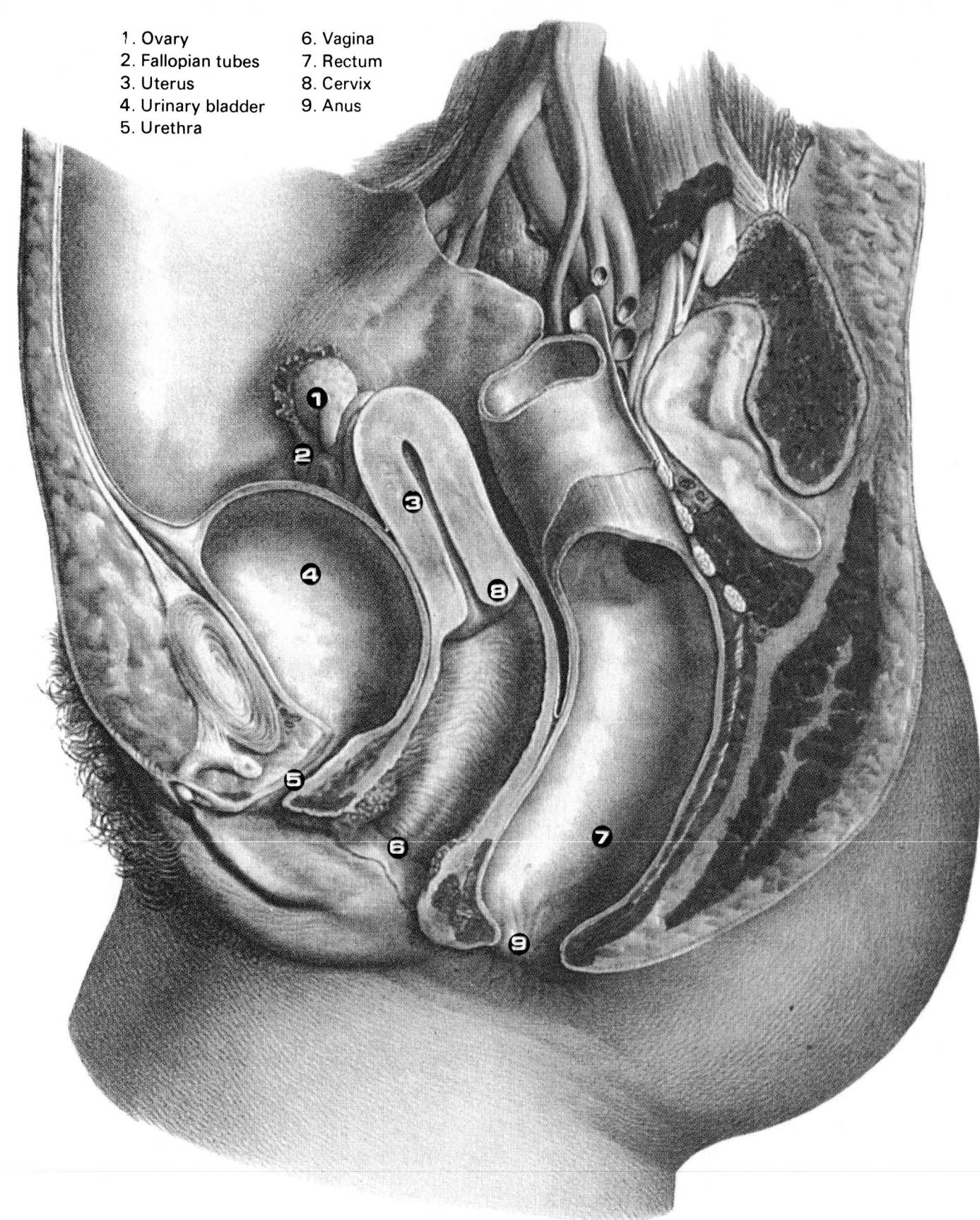

1. Ovary
2. Fallopian tubes
3. Uterus
4. Urinary bladder
5. Urethra
6. Vagina
7. Rectum
8. Cervix
9. Anus

**GENITOURINARY ORGANS IN THE FEMALE—SIDE VIEW**

# FEMALE GENITAL ORGANS

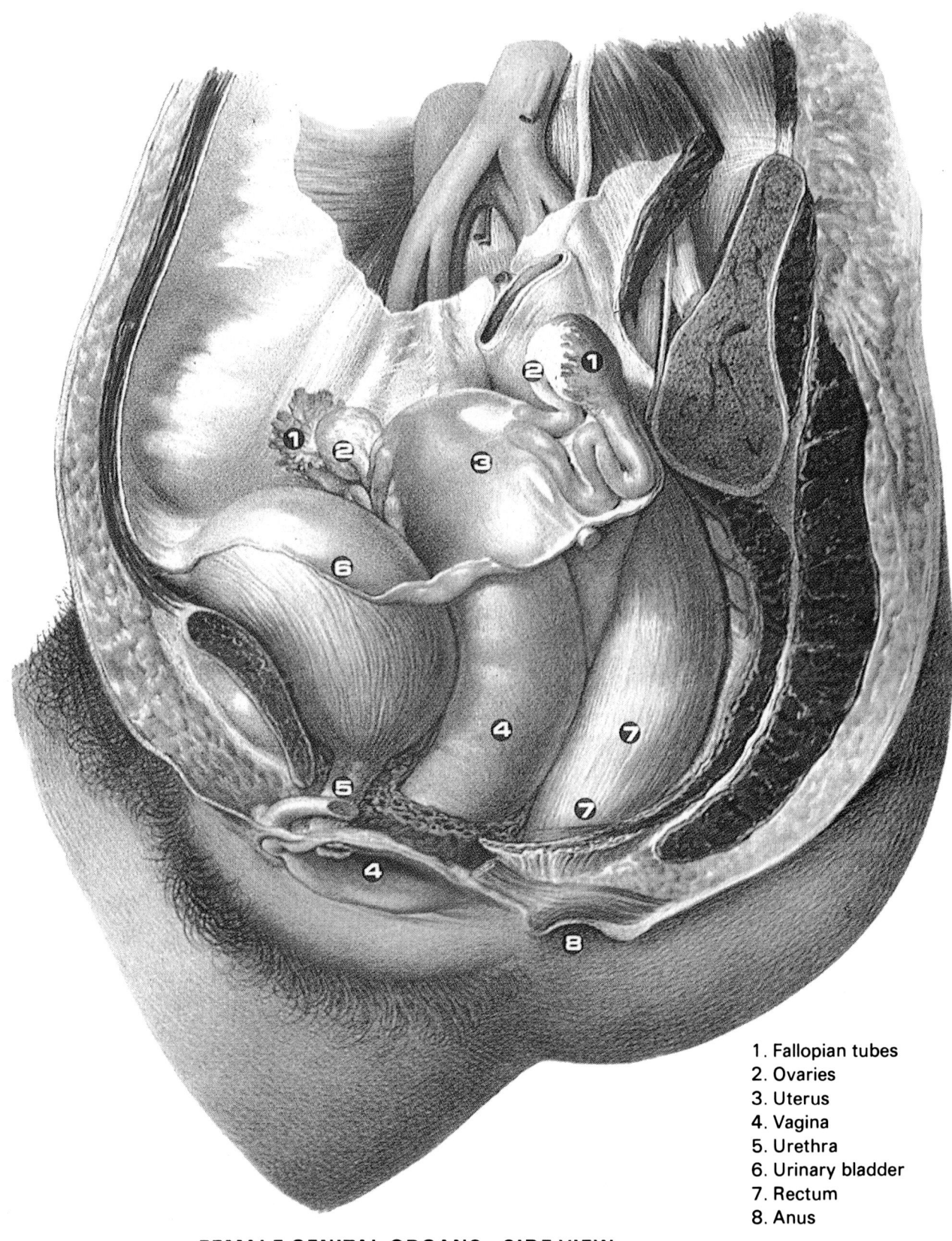

1. Fallopian tubes
2. Ovaries
3. Uterus
4. Vagina
5. Urethra
6. Urinary bladder
7. Rectum
8. Anus

**FEMALE GENITAL ORGANS—SIDE VIEW**

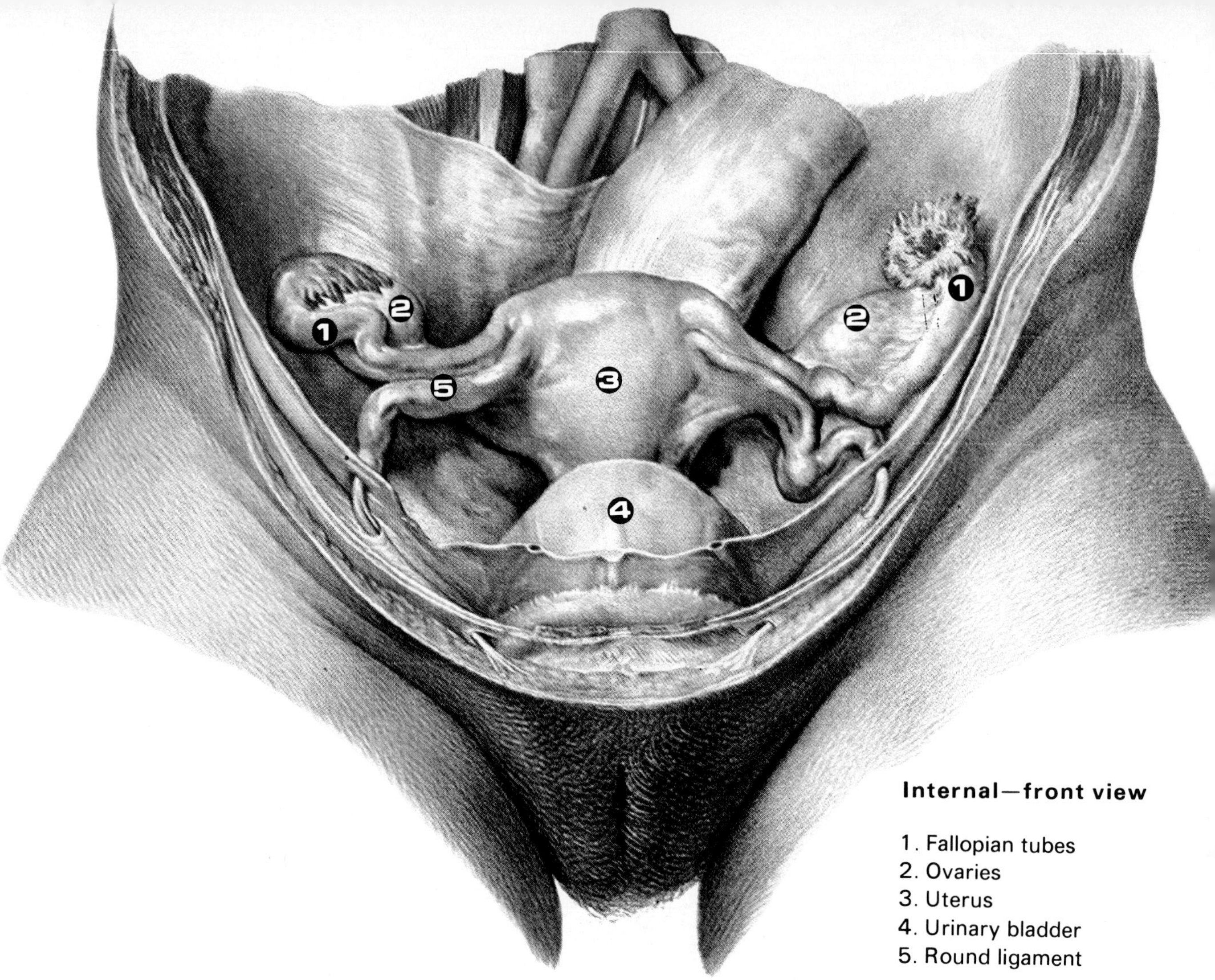

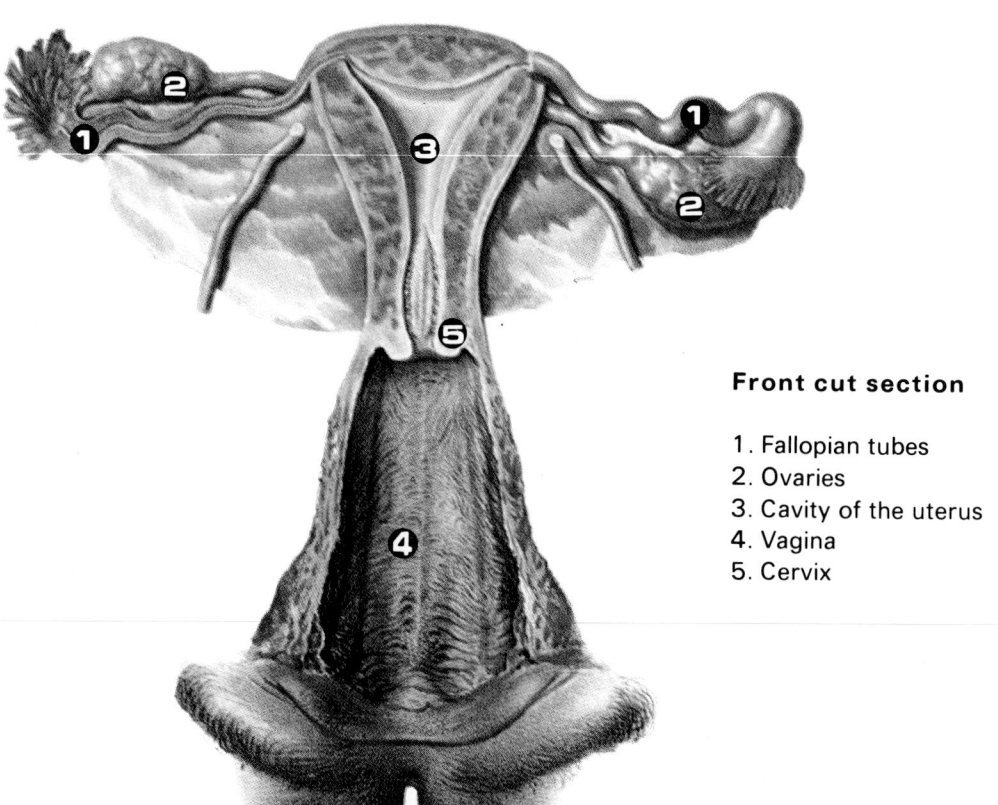

## Internal—front view

1. Fallopian tubes
2. Ovaries
3. Uterus
4. Urinary bladder
5. Round ligament

## THE FEMALE GENITAL ORGANS

## Front cut section

1. Fallopian tubes
2. Ovaries
3. Cavity of the uterus
4. Vagina
5. Cervix

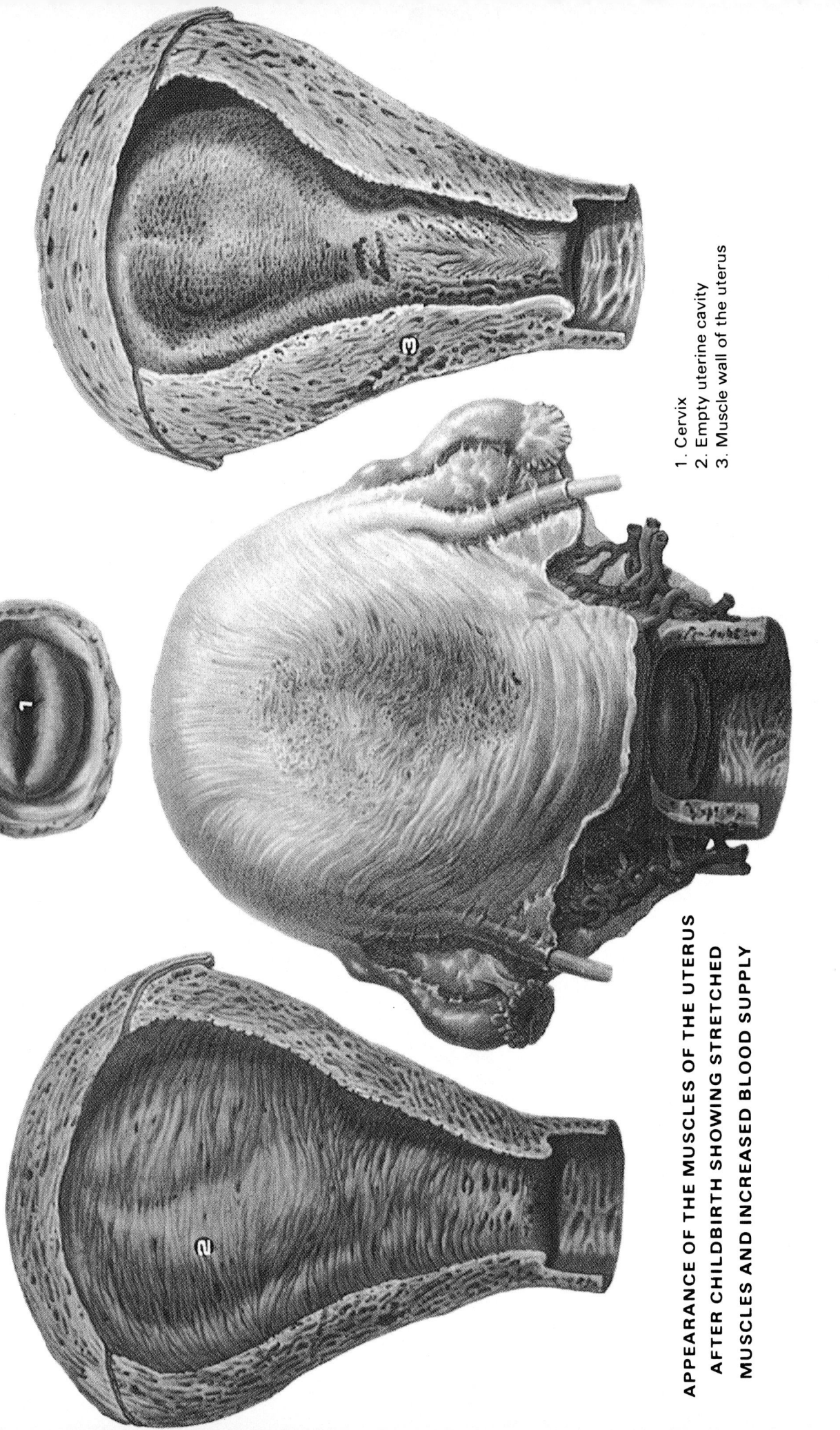

**APPEARANCE OF THE MUSCLES OF THE UTERUS
AFTER CHILDBIRTH SHOWING STRETCHED
MUSCLES AND INCREASED BLOOD SUPPLY**

1. Cervix
2. Empty uterine cavity
3. Muscle wall of the uterus

1. Pulmonary artery
2. Superior vena cava
3. Aorta

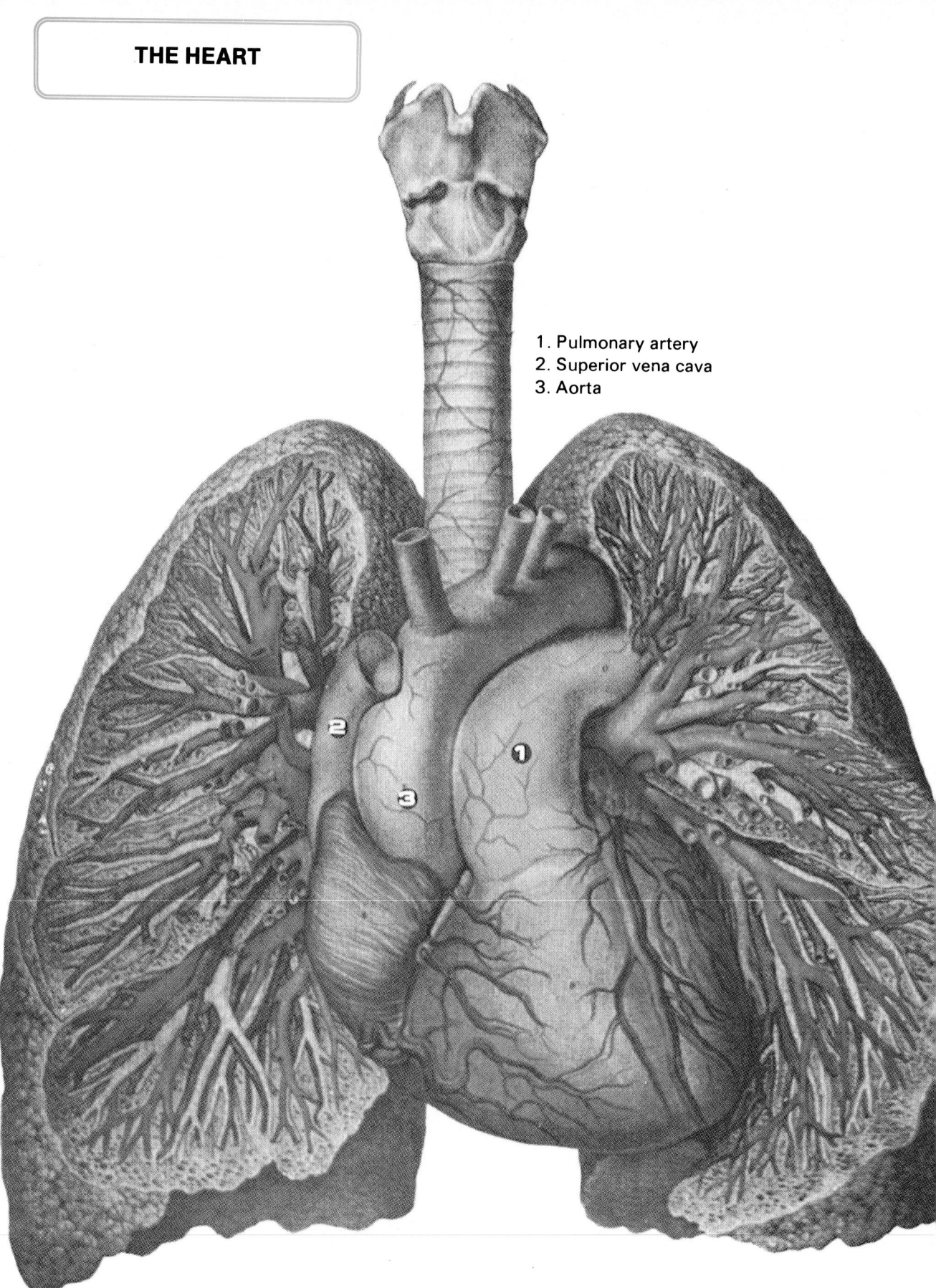

**THE HEART, LUNGS, AND GREAT BLOOD VESSELS—FRONT VIEW**

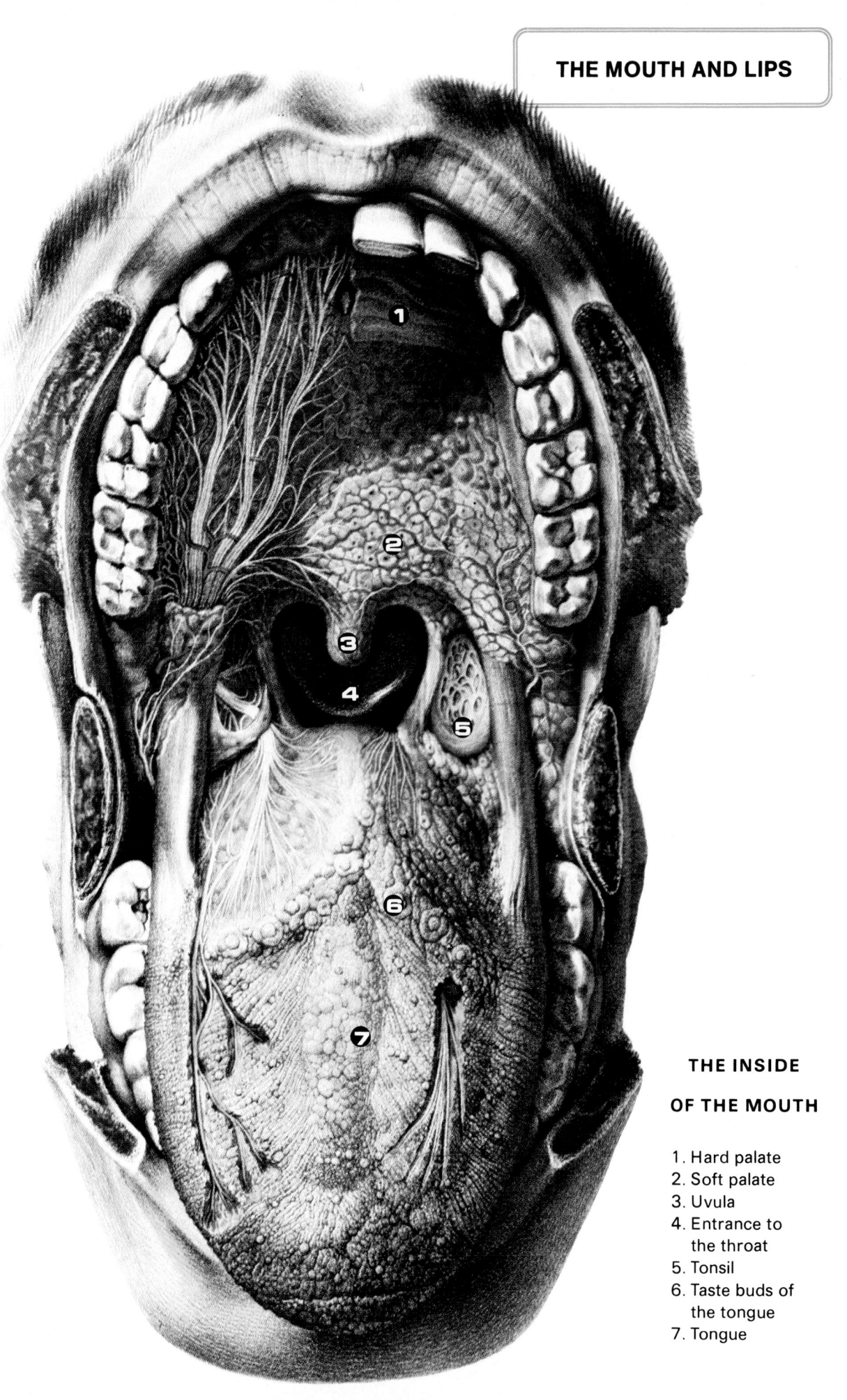

## THE INSIDE

## OF THE MOUTH

1. Hard palate
2. Soft palate
3. Uvula
4. Entrance to
   the throat
5. Tonsil
6. Taste buds of
   the tongue
7. Tongue

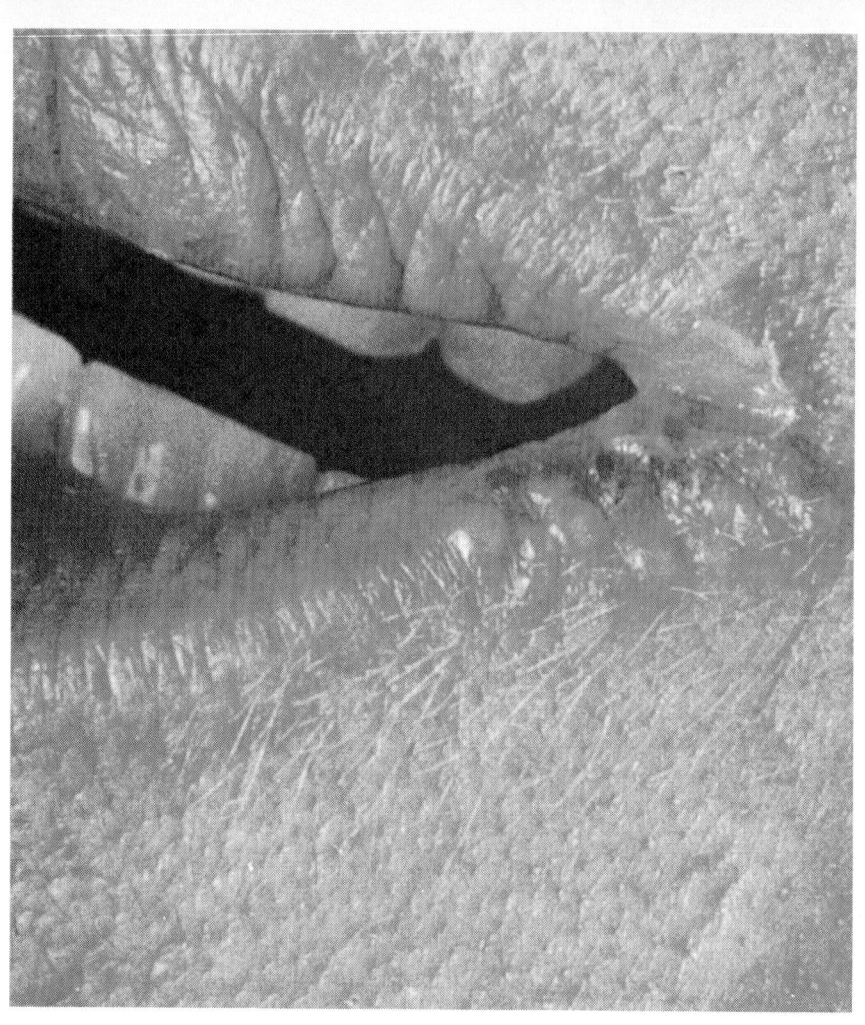

Herpes simplex, commonly known as "cold sore," is thought to be caused by a virus. Overexposure to sunlight or a high fever during an illness seems to activate these viruses.

The whitish overgrowth of mucous membrane on the lower lip of the man pictured below is leukoplakia. Such plaques, which may develop into cancer, occur most often in men who smoke pipes with hot stems.

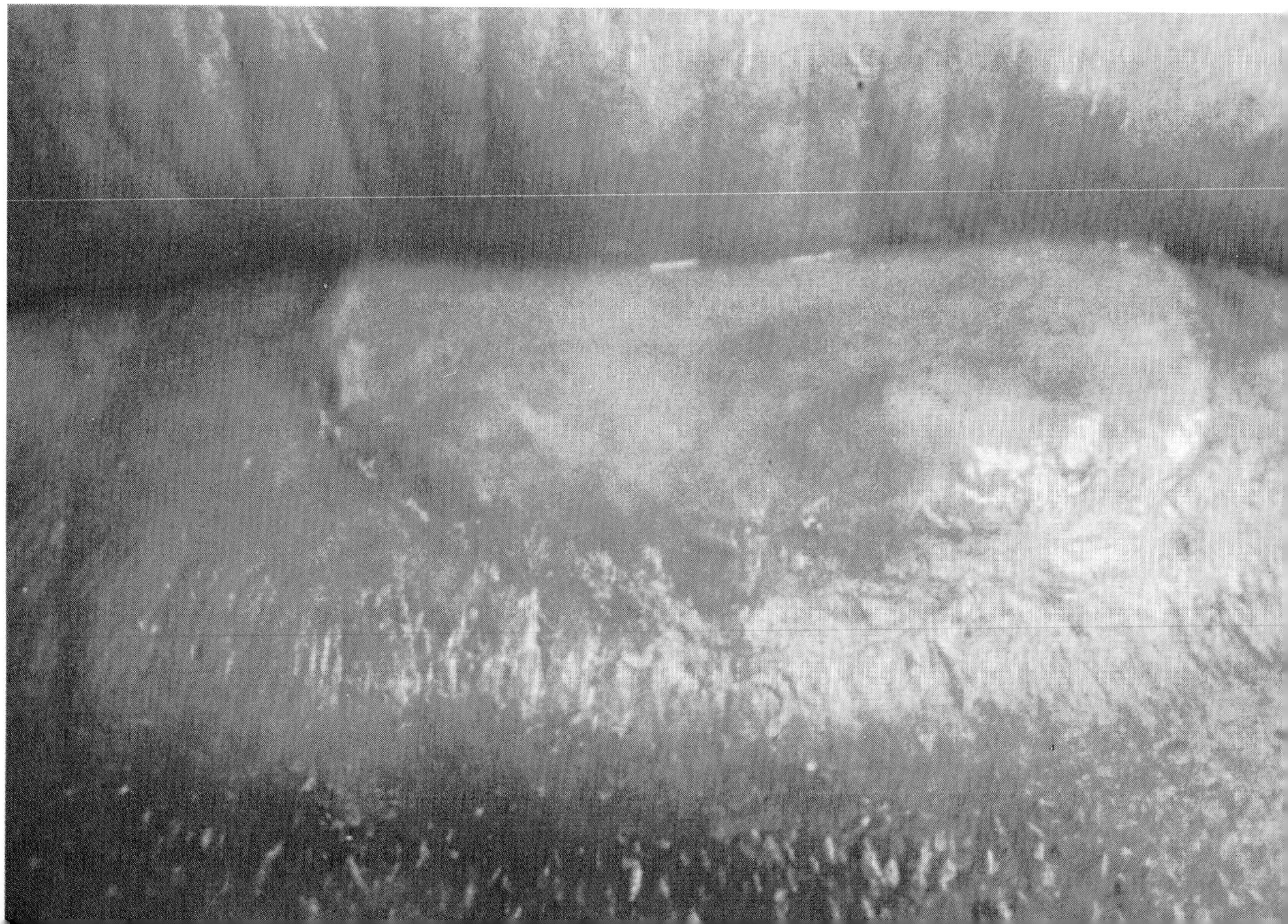

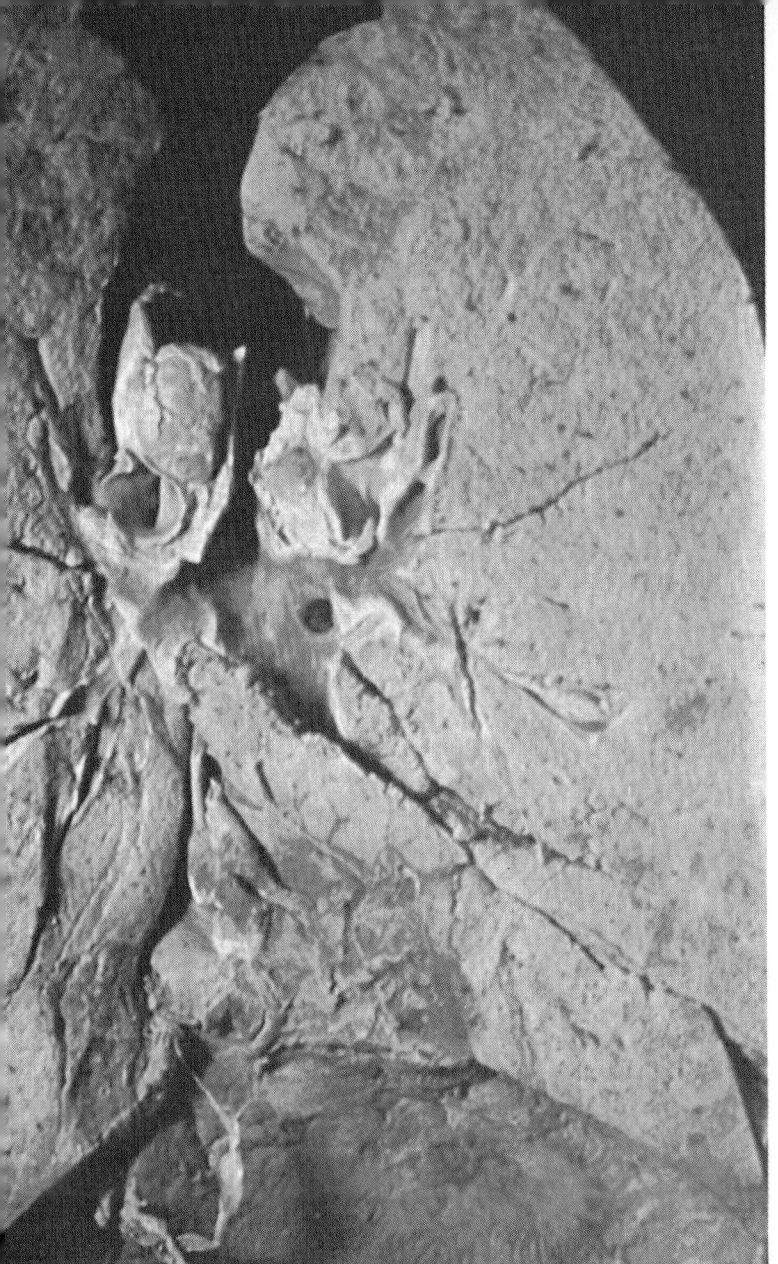

The lungs in patients with lobar pneumonia appear solid because the cells are filled with mucus and pus, rather than air.

In cases of bronchiectasis, many of the air cells are enlarged or ruptured. Such broken-down air cells form large sacs which tend to collect mucus and pus.

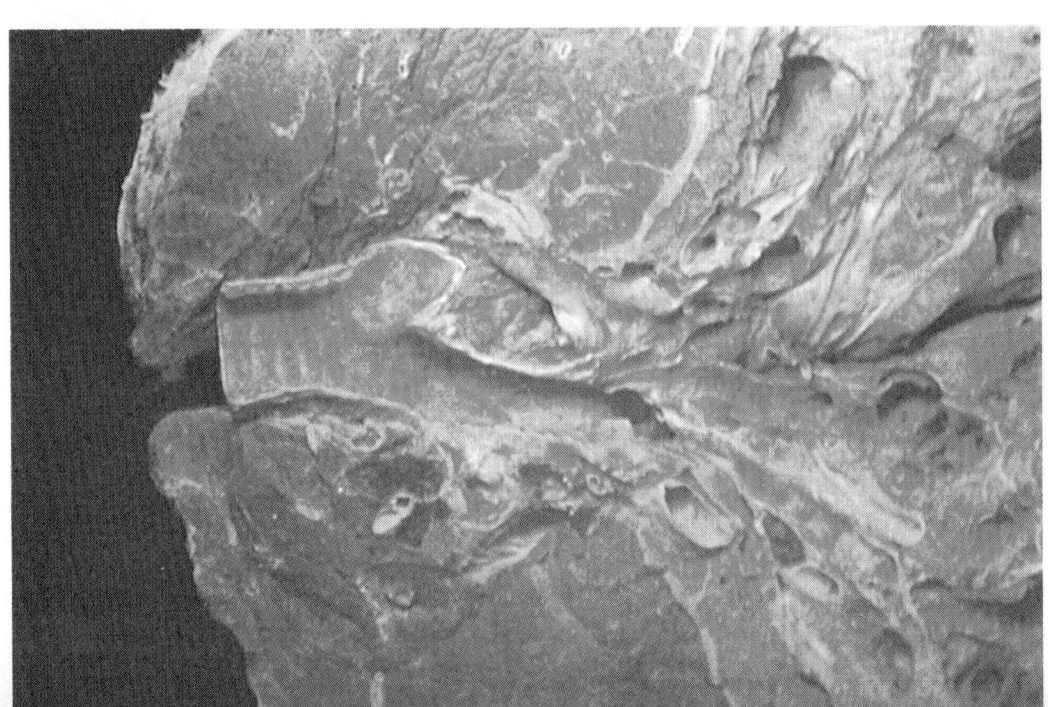

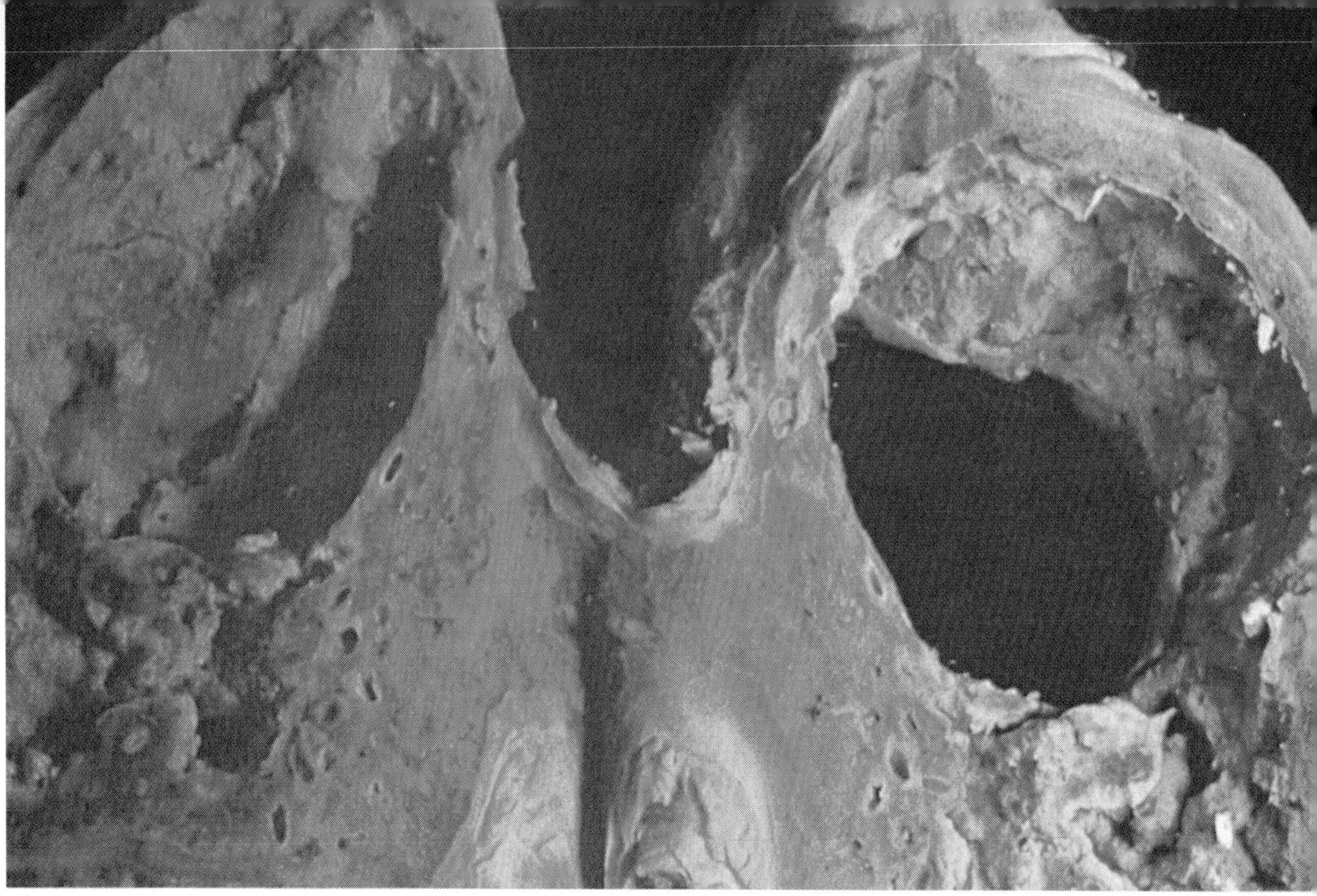

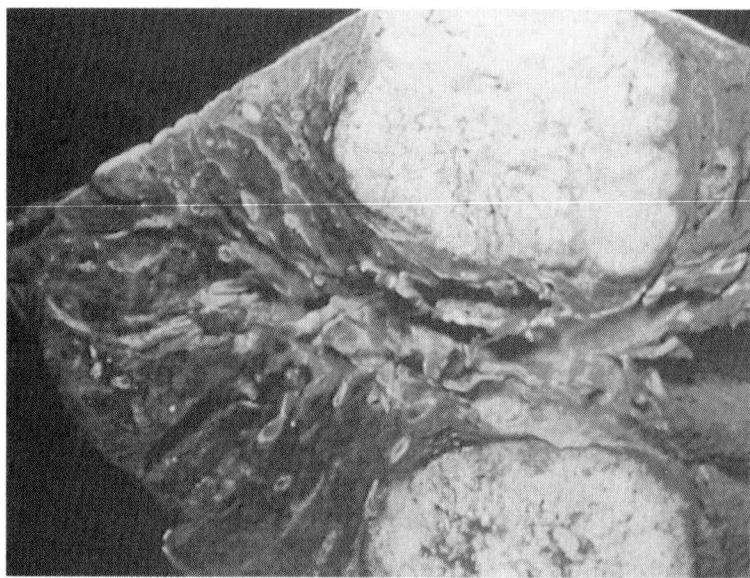

Large cavities in the lungs are typical in patients with advanced tuberculosis

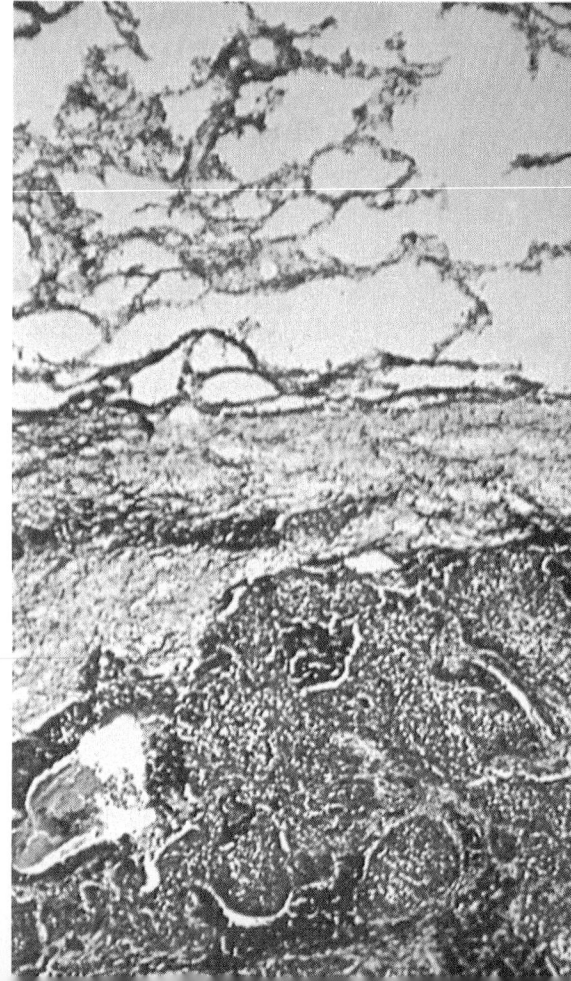

The rounded tumor seen above and in microscopic detail at right is a huge lung cancer. Such large tumors of the lung are often difficult to treat successfully because they have usually spread to the adjacent lymph glands.

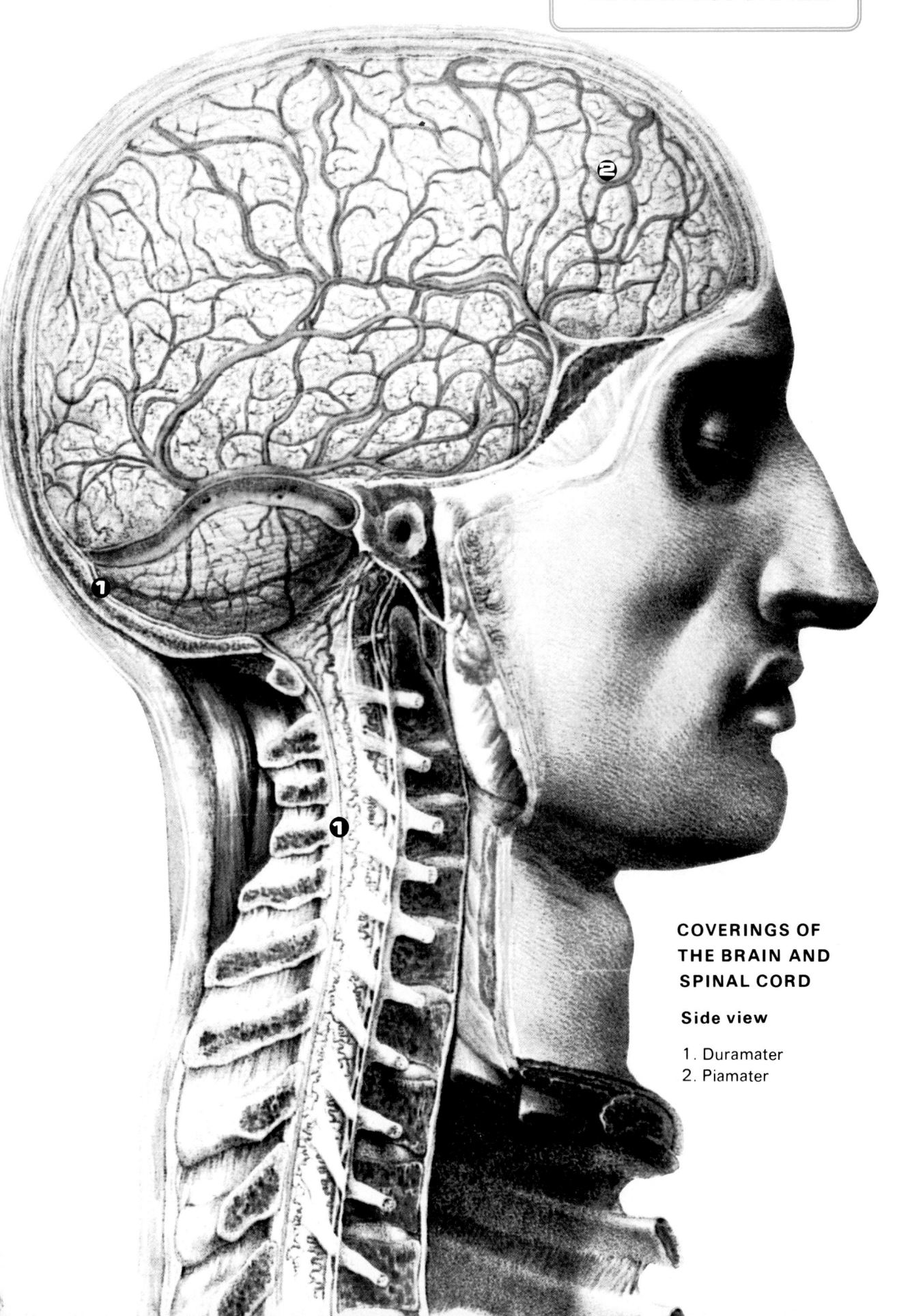

**COVERINGS OF
THE BRAIN AND
SPINAL CORD**

**Side view**

1. Duramater
2. Piamater

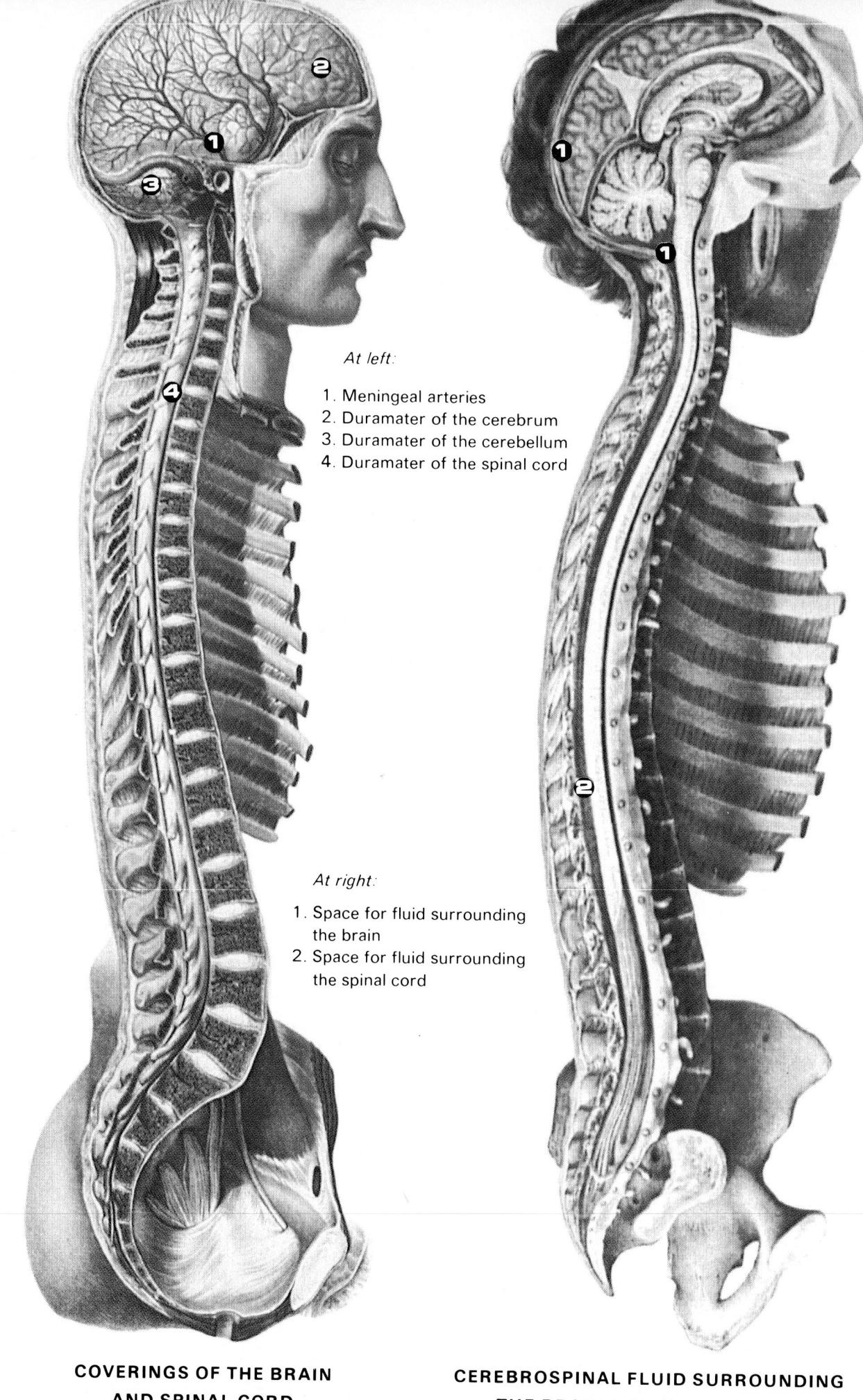

*At left:*

1. Meningeal arteries
2. Duramater of the cerebrum
3. Duramater of the cerebellum
4. Duramater of the spinal cord

*At right:*

1. Space for fluid surrounding the brain
2. Space for fluid surrounding the spinal cord

**COVERINGS OF THE BRAIN
AND SPINAL CORD**

**CEREBROSPINAL FLUID SURROUNDING
THE BRAIN AND SPINAL CORD**

## SERUM HEPATITIS
### (Homologous Serum Jaundice)

### What is serum hepatitis?

An infection of the liver caused by a virus presumably different from the germ causing infectious hepatitis.

### How does one contract serum hepatitis (homologous serum jaundice)?

It is transmitted through receiving a transfusion of blood or plasma, or by contamination from an infected hypodermic needle or syringe.

### Is serum hepatitis caused by transfusion of the wrong type of blood?

No.

### How long after receiving a blood transfusion or an injection can one contract serum hepatitis?

It takes anywhere from a few weeks to a few months to develop the disease after one has been inoculated with the virus.

### Is serum hepatitis preventable?

Only to a limited extent by the proper selection of blood donors, proper technique in storing and handling blood and plasma, by proper sterilization of needles and syringes, or by using only disposable needles and syringes. However, it must be stated emphatically that even after the above precautions are taken, it is not possible to eliminate entirely the risk of contracting serum hepatitis.

### What are the symptoms and course of serum hepatitis?

Practically the same symptoms and course as that of infectious hepatitis.

## TOXIC HEPATITIS

### What is toxic hepatitis?

It is a term used for liver injury caused by taking chemical poisons or drugs that adversely affect the liver.

### How does one contract toxic hepatitis?

It may develop rapidly after the inhalation or eating of significant amounts of chemical poisons or drugs, or it may develop gradually over a period of years as a result of prolonged consumption or inhalation of small amounts of these same toxic substances. There is a great individual variation in the susceptibility to such agents.

### Is toxic hepatitis curable?

It depends upon the extent to which the poison has already damaged the liver. If the damage has been mild and reversible, recovery will take place.

## SURGERY OF THE LIVER

### For what conditions is the liver operated upon?

a. Injuries, such as gunshot wounds, stab wounds, or rupture of the liver due to an accident.
b. Abscesses of the liver as a complication usually of some other disease within the abdominal cavity or elsewhere in the body.
c. Cysts of the liver, most common of which is the echinococcus cyst, which is caused by a parasite that infests dogs. Constant contact with a dog can transmit this infection to man.
d. Benign tumors, such as hemangiomas (blood cysts) or lymph tumors such as lymphangiomas.
e. Cancer of the liver, in the occasional instance where only one lobe (segment) is involved and can be removed surgically.
f. Cirrhosis of the liver.

### How can one diagnose an injury to the liver?

a. There will be signs of shock and internal hemorrhage.
b. There is a history of an external injury.
c. There may be swelling and tenderness in the abdomen.

### Is it always necessary to operate for an injury to the liver?

No. If the patient does not go into shock and if there is evidence that little bleeding has taken place, it is possible to withhold surgery and await developments.

### Is rupture of the liver a serious injury?

Yes. However, many of these patients can be saved by prompt surgery.

### Is it necessary to operate on all liver abscesses?

No, because the antibiotic drugs may permit the patient to get well without surgery. However, if there is a large collection of pus within the liver, it must be removed by surgical drainage.

### Does recovery usually take place after drainage of a liver abscess?

Yes.

### Is it possible to successfully remove benign tumors and cysts of the liver?

Great advances in surgical technique have been made so that tumors can now be removed from the liver satisfactorily. There are many cases in which an entire lobe of the liver has been successfully removed.

### Is it ever possible to help a patient whose liver is extensively involved with cancer?

Usually not.

### What is done surgically to help people with cirrhosis of the liver?

Many of these patients can now be helped largely through surgery. Because cirrhosis prevents much of the blood from coursing through the

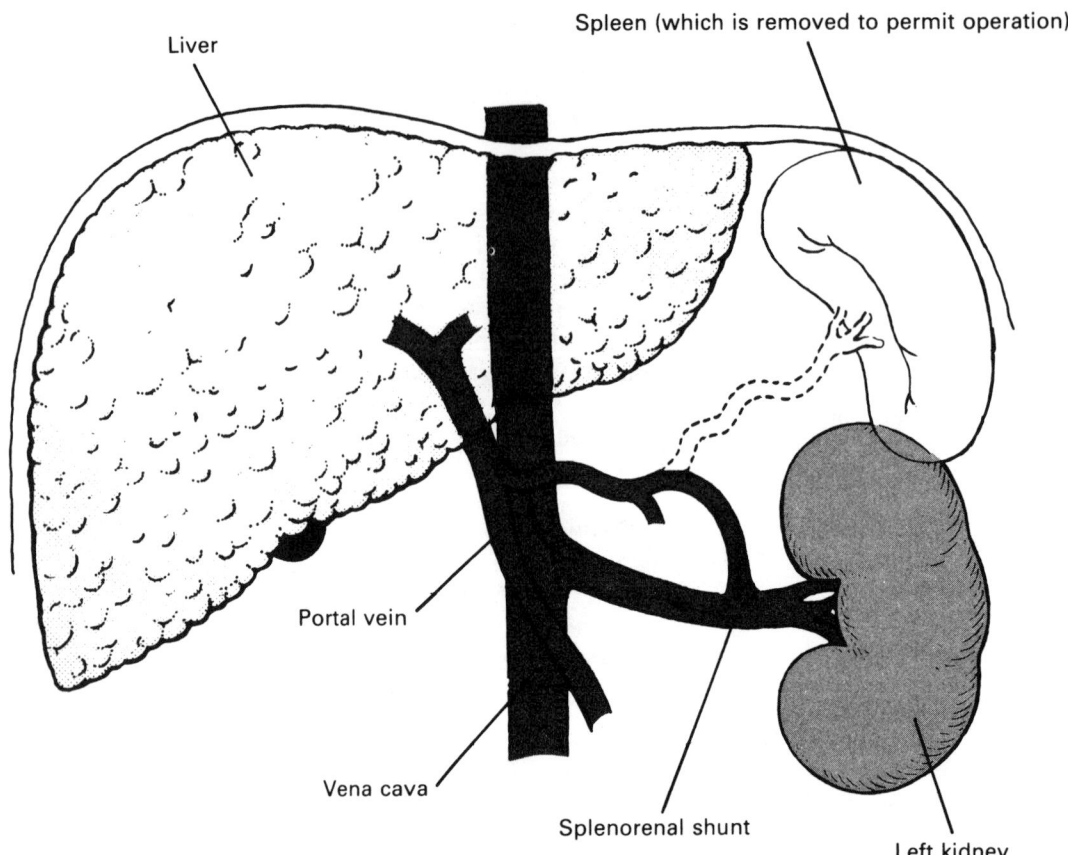

Liver

Spleen (which is removed to permit operation)

Portal vein

Vena cava

Splenorenal shunt

Left kidney

**Splenorenal Shunt Operation.** *This diagram shows an operation that joins the main vein of the spleen to the renal (kidney) vein, thus shunting blood away from the liver and into the general circulation. This procedure accomplishes the same purpose as the portacaval shunt.*

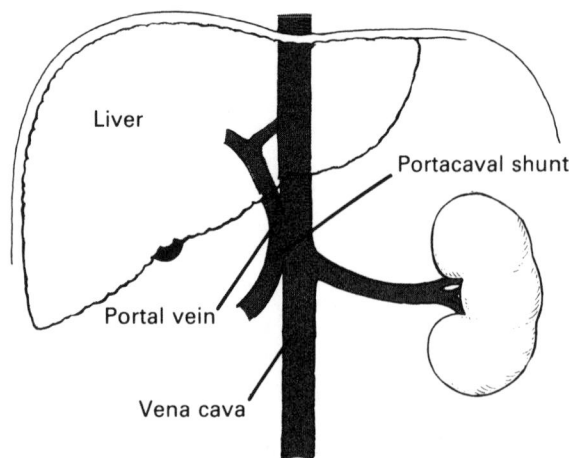

Liver

Portacaval shunt.

Portal vein

Vena cava

**Portacaval Shunt Operation.** *This diagram shows the joining of the portal vein to the vena cava, thus diverting blood that would ordinarily flow through the liver into the general circulation. This procedure is sometimes necessary for people who have advanced cirrhosis of the liver with obstruction of blood flow.*

liver, operations have been devised that shunt the blood around the liver and thus aid circulation. The three most common operations of this type are:

a. A portacaval shunt, in which the portal vein is stitched to the vena cava. This permits much of the blood to pass directly into the general circulation instead of being held up by a cirrhotic liver.

b. A splenorenal shunt, in which the vein from the spleen is stitched to the left kidney vein. This also allows much of the blood that would ordinarily have gone to the liver to be shunted directly into the general circulation.

c. A mesocaval shunt, in which a graft joins the superior mesenteric vein with the vena cava. The superior mesenteric vein carries blood from the small intestines to the liver. (See diagram in Chapter 13, on Blood Vessel Surgery.)

**Are operations for cirrhosis of the liver serious?**

Yes, but many excellent results have been obtained through these procedures.

**What are the chances for improving cirrhosis through these operations?**

More than half of these patients are benefited by the shunt operations.

**Is it necessary to protect the liver before operating upon diseases of the gall bladder or bile ducts?**

Yes. It is important to see that the liver has an adequate supply of sugar to protect it while these structures are being operated upon.

**Can one live a normal life after removal of part of the liver?**

Yes. Only about one-fifth of the liver substance is necessary to maintain normal function.

**Are there accurate tests to determine how badly liver function is impaired?**

Yes. There are many blood, urine, and stool tests that will give an accurate picture of what is going on within the liver.

# CHAPTER 41

# THE LUNGS

*(See also Chapter 8 on Anesthesia; Chapter 29 on Heart; Chapter 34 on Infectious and Virus Diseases; Chapter 74 on Tuberculosis; Chapter 75 on Upper Respiratory Diseases)*

### What is the structure of the lungs?

The lungs are the organs of breathing, which are located in the chest cavity. The right lung consists of three sections called lobes, while the left lung has but two lobes. The lungs are composed of spongy tissue surrounding treelike branches of the bronchial tubes. The lung tissue itself consists of approximately 300 million air sacs surrounded by a mesh of small blood vessels.

### What is the function of the lungs?

The lungs take out oxygen from the air that is inhaled and give up carbon dioxide, which has been brought to the lungs by the bloodstream. The carbon dioxide and a certain amount of water in the form of vapor are expelled when one exhales.

### Is there such a thing as someone having weak lungs?

No. This expression usually means that the person has some form of lung disease, such as bronchitis or tuberculosis.

### Is the tendency toward lung trouble inherited?

No. Lung trouble (usually tuberculosis) occurs in families because of spread from one member to another rather than by inheritance. The parent or grandparent who is not aware that he or she has tuberculosis can spread it to a child or grandchild.

### Is it healthier to live in the country where the air is pure than in the city where the air tends to be impure?

In general, yes. Irritating dusts and fumes are more prevalent in the cities and tend to produce respiratory difficulty in the nose, throat, and in the bronchial tubes.

### What conditions can be caused by breathing impure air?

The impurities in the air, such as smoke, fumes, smog, etc., cause irritation of the lining membranes and lower the resistance of these tissues to infection and possibly to tumor formation.

### How often should one have his lungs examined?

About once a year. Healthy adults should have chest x rays about every year or two unless there is some reason for more frequent x rays.

### Can lung disease always be diagnosed by x-ray examination?

For all practical purposes, yes. Sometimes it is necessary to have repeated examinations or films taken from several angles before a definite diagnosis can be made.

### What harm can result from tobacco smoking?

It can cause local irritating effects on the membranes of the nose, throat, larynx, bronchial tubes, and lung tissues. No doubt, heavy smoking predisposes one toward the development of chronic bronchitis, bronchiectasis, emphysema, and cancer of the lung.

### What is the significance of a chronic cough with expectoration of mucus?

It is indicative of irritation or inflammation in the larynx, windpipe, or bronchial tubes, and merits medical investigation.

### Should one swallow the mucus he has coughed up or should he spit it out?

It should not be swallowed as it may upset digestive processes. Also, if such material contains tuberculosis germs, it may cause an intestinal infection. Sputum should be expectorated into tissues or receptacles that can be discarded without spreading germs.

### What is the main significance of coughing up blood?

When a patient coughs up blood, it is most important to determine whether he has tuberculosis or a tumor of the lung. These are the most important conditions that cause coughing up of blood, but any small break in a blood vessel in the throat, larynx, or bronchial tubes can cause blood spitting. Thus, this symptom does not necessarily mean that tuberculosis or cancer exists.

### Can breathing of excessively hot air hurt the lungs?

The lining of the bronchial tubes and lungs can be burned seriously when hot steam is inhaled. This occurs occasionally in industrial accidents.

### Can exposure to extremely cold air hurt the lungs?

Deep breathing of extremely cold air, as in the polar regions or at very high altitudes, can produce "frostbite" of the lining of the windpipe and bronchial tubes, with subsequent development of pneumonia.

### Can one live a normal life with one lung nonfunctioning?

Yes, if the remaining lung has adequate function. Restriction of activity would depend upon the degree of impairment of the remaining lung.

## ATELECTASIS

### What is atelectasis?
A condition in which the lung tissue is collapsed and contains no air.

### What causes atelectasis?
Obstruction of a bronchial tube.

### What types of atelectasis are there?
a. Those occurring at birth, which are due either to a mucous plug in a bronchial tube or to a congenitally deformed and narrowed tube.
b. In later life, it may be caused by a blockage of a bronchus by mucus, pus, or blood. Also, foreign bodies such as peanuts, meat, or other foods that have gone down the wrong way, may obstruct a bronchial tube and produce atelectasis. The first indication of the presence of a tumor of the bronchus is frequently the discovery of an area of atelectasis (collapsed lung) caused by the obstruction of the bronchus by growing tumor tissue.

### What is massive atelectasis?
A postoperative complication in which there is a large amount of mucus plugging one of the main bronchial tubes. This may cause an entire lung to collapse.

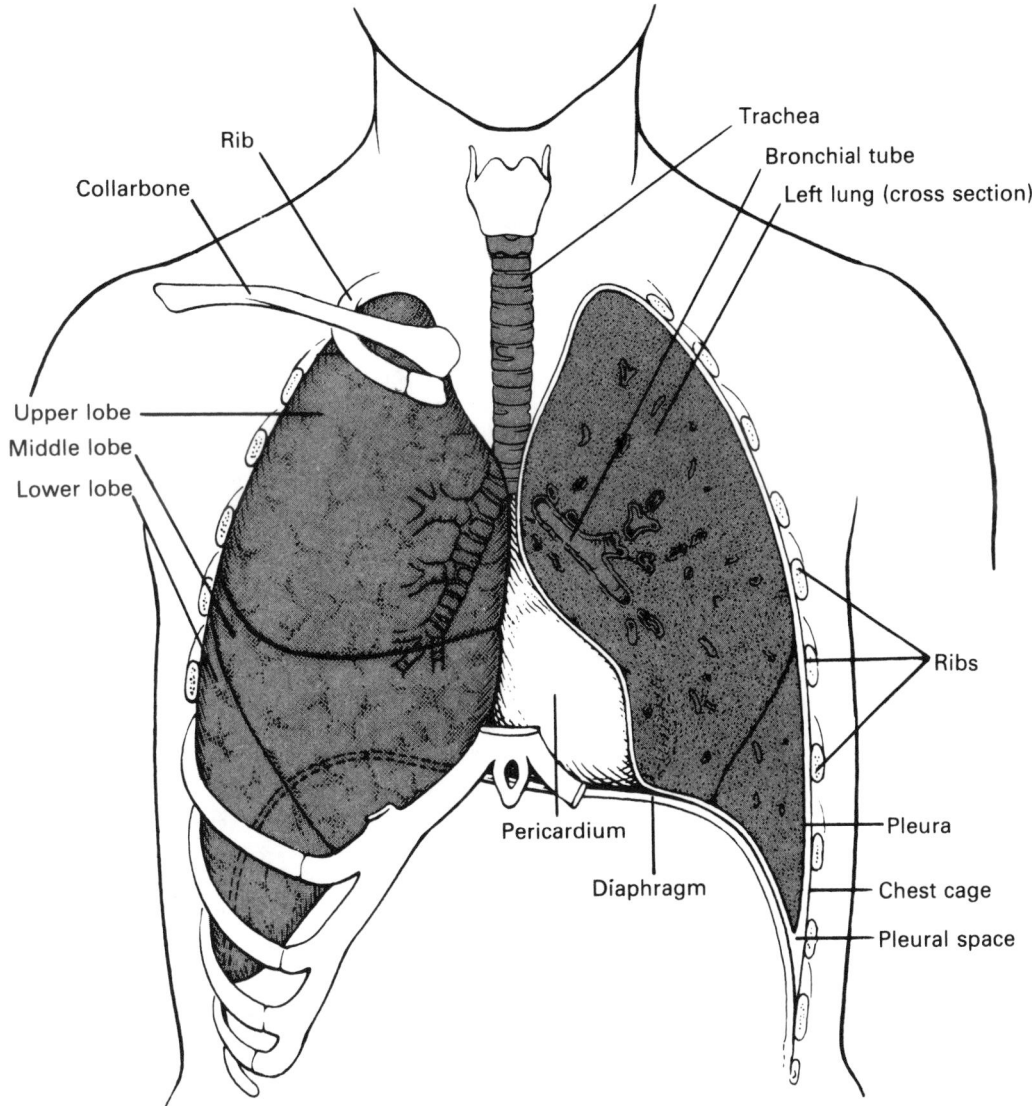

*The Lungs and Chest Cavity. This diagram shows the anatomy of the lungs with its bronchial tubes and air sacs.*

## What is the treatment for massive atelectasis?

A bronchoscope is passed into the trachea (windpipe), and the plug of mucus is sucked out with a suction apparatus.

## Is massive atelectasis very common?

Not since anesthesia methods have improved so greatly. Anesthetists today keep the bronchial passages clear by sucking them out during and after the giving of anesthesia through an endotracheal "airway," or tube, which is passed through the larynx into the trachea.

## Is massive atelectasis a serious condition?

Yes. It is accompanied by high fever and marked shortness of breath. This may complicate the recovery of a patient who has just undergone surgery.

## Is the present form of treatment effective in curing massive atelectasis?

Yes. The sucking out of the mucous plug and the giving of antibiotics will cure almost all cases of massive atelectasis.

## Is it always necessary to have a bronchoscope passed to cure massive atelectasis?

No. Frequently, by stimulating deep breathing, the giving of oxygen, and stimulating the patient to cough, he can be helped to expel the mucous plug by himself.

## EMPHYSEMA

## What is emphysema?

A condition in which the lung tissue loses its elasticity and becomes overstretched. It is usually associated with partial obstruction of the bronchial tubes, so that air is trapped within the lung. Thus, air can get into the lungs readily but cannot get out easily. If this process continues, lung tissue becomes like an overstretched balloon.

## In what condition is emphysema found most often?

Chronic bronchitis and asthma of long duration.

## What are the symptoms of chronic emphysema?

a. Increasing shortness of breath.
b. Coughing.
c. Gasping.
d. Cyanosis (blueness of the skin, lips, and nails due to lack of oxygen).
e. Decreased oxygen supply to the vital structures in the body.
f. Eventual heart failure.

## Does emphysema ever progress to heart failure and death?

It may, in severe cases.

## Is there any satisfactory way to prevent emphysema?

Yes, by the prompt treatment of conditions such as bronchitis, asthma, sinus infections, and bronchiectasis. Also, by the avoidance of exposure to irritating factors such as tobacco smoke, chemical fumes, and industrial dusts.

## Does the overstretched lung found in emphysema ever rupture?

Yes. A cyst or blister on the surface of the lung caused by emphysema occasionally ruptures, causing spontaneous collapse of the lung.

## What is another name for this sudden collapse of the lung?

Spontaneous pneumothorax.

## SPONTANEOUS PNEUMOTHORAX

## What are the symptoms of spontaneous pneumothorax, or collapse of the lung?

There is a sudden and dramatic occurrence of chest pain, shortess of breath, and, occasionally, severe shock and collapse.

## How does the physician make a diagnosis of spontaneous pneumothorax?

a. By noting the history of the onset.
b. By listening to the chest and noting the absence of breath sounds on that side.
c. By noting a marked increase in the resonant sound on tapping the chest with his fingers (percussion).
d. By taking an x-ray picture and discovering that the lung is collapsed.

## What is the treatment for spontaneous pneumothorax?

Because of sudden shock and the severity of the symptoms, immediate hospitalization is necessary. If the extent of the lung collapse is greater than 25 or 30 percent, or if the leak in the ruptured lung is not sealed off so that air continues to flow out into the chest cavity causing "tension pneumothorax," a tube must be inserted through an opening into the chest cavity. This will draw off the air and allow the lung to reexpand. Occasionally it is necessary to open the chest cavity and to remove the damaged portion of the lung.

## What other situations may produce pneumothorax?

A perforation of the chest wall, such as a stab wound, gunshot wound, or a blast injury, etc. Also, a fractured rib may puncture the lung, allowing air to escape from it to the chest cavity, and thus causing the lung to collapse.

## Is collapse of the lung ever a fatal condition?

Not if it occurs on one side only. However, some blast injuries or gunshot wounds may cause collapse of both lungs, and such a condition may lead to a fatality.

# PNEUMONIA

## What is pneumonia?

An infection, usually acute, of the air spaces and sacs of the lung.

## What types of pneumonia are there?

They are usually classified as to cause, that is, as to whether they are caused by bacteria, viruses, fungus infection, or other types of germs.

## What is lobar pneumonia, and how does it differ from bronchopneumonia?

Lobar pneumonia is an inflammation of an entire lobe or more than one lobe. It usually starts suddenly as a distinct illness, and causes, at its onset, chills and fever. Bronchopneumonia is an inflammation involving small patchy areas of lung tissue surrounding small bronchial tubes. It usually comes on more slowly than the lobar type and is seen most often as a complication of bronchitis or influenza.

## What is the most common variety of pneumonia seen today?

Pneumonia caused by a virus (virus pneumonia). Since the advent of antibiotic drugs, the lobar type has become much less prevalent.

## How do the antibiotics lessen the incidence of lobar pneumonia?

Since these drugs are so effective in the treatment of infections of the upper respiratory tract, they prevent the bacteria from gaining a foothold in the lungs.

## What are the predisposing causes of pneumonia?

Undernourishment, fatigue, neglect of upper respiratory infections, chronic alcoholism, and the aspiration of foreign material into the bronchial tubes.

## How long does pneumonia last?

With adequate treatment, it can usually be cured within five to fourteen days.

## What is the outlook for recovery from pneumonia?

Excellent. Years ago, almost one out of four people would die from a severe case of pneumonia. Today, a fatal termination is a great rarity except among very old or debilitated people.

## How long must one stay in bed and remain at home after recovery from pneumonia?

At least two to three days after the temperature has returned to normal and after the antibiotic drugs have been discontinued.

## Are there any unusual types of pneumonia that do not respond readily to treatment?

Yes; tularemic pneumonia, which is transmitted by rabbits; and psittacosis pneumonia (parrot fever), transmitted by birds. Also, some cases of pneumonia caused by uncommonly encountered bacteria are resistant to treatment.

## What is aspiration pneumonia?

An inflammation of the lungs caused by the inhalation of a foreign substance, such as vomit, poisons, oily nose drops, or food particles that have gained access to the lung tissue through the bronchial tubes. This material often becomes secondarily infected by the growth of bacteria or viruses.

## What is hypostatic pneumonia?

This type occurs in the course of certain chronic diseases, most often among elderly, weakened, bedridden patients. It is associated with a sluggish circulation within the lungs, which permits bacteria and viruses to gain a strong foothold.

## Can hypostatic pneumonia be prevented?

In many cases, yes, by controlling the underlying disease and by frequent changes of the patient's position in bed. These patients should be gotten out of bed at the earliest possible time.

# LUNG ABSCESS
*(See also the section on Surgery of the Lungs in this chapter)*

## What is a lung abscess?

An area of pus formation within the lung.

## What causes lung abscess?

It is usually caused by a blockage of a bronchial tube, with the development of infection beyond the point of obstruction. One of the most common causes is the aspiration of pus or infected mucus during an operation upon the nose, throat, or mouth.

## Do lung abscesses ever occur without a preceding operation?

Yes, an abscess can form whenever an area of inflamed lung, or an area affected by tumor tissue, breaks down due to localized death of tissue.

## How does one make a diagnosis of lung abscess?

a. The patient coughs up extremely foul-smelling pus.
b. There may be high fever, chills, and malaise during the early days of the illness.
c. There is a characteristic appearance of the lung on x-ray examination, and the abscess cavity itself can often be plainly seen on the film.

## Must lung abscess always be operated upon?

No. Many clear up completely with antibiotics, especially if any bronchial obstruction can be relieved.

# PULMONARY EMBOLISM AND INFARCTION

## What is pulmonary infarction?

The destruction of a portion of lung

tissue due to interference with its blood supply.

## What causes pulmonary infarction?

Usually an embolus (blood clot), which has traveled from another part of the body to a blood vessel within the lung. The blood vessel is obstructed by this blood clot, and the tissue beyond it is said to have become infarcted.

## Where do these emboli or blood clots usually arise?

From clotted blood in the deep veins of the legs or pelvic organs. These clots may form during the course of various disease processes, or they may form as a complication of a surgical operation. Portions of the clot that break off and are carried through the bloodstream are termed emboli. Some lung emboli originate from clots in the right side of the heart.

## Does pulmonary infarction follow in all cases where there has been clotting of the veins in the legs or pelvic organs?

No. In the great majority of instances, the clot stays where it is in the veins of the legs or pelvis. It is only rarely that it breaks off and produces an embolus.

## What are the symptoms of pulmonary infarction?

These vary with the size of the clot, the size of the vessel that has been plugged, and the suddenness of onset. There may be varying degrees of sharp chest pain, shortness of breath, cough, blood-streaked expectoration, and fever. In some cases, there may be severe shock or sudden death.

## Will a pulmonary infarct show on x-ray examination?

Yes, in some cases. However, the best way to discover the presence of a lung embolus is to perform a *lung scan*. This is a technique using a radioactive isotope, which, after injection into a vein, is picked up in the lungs and will show the area of infarct.

## Is there any way to prevent pulmonary infarction in patients who have phlebitis (inflammation) in a leg vein?

Yes. In most instances it is advisable to use anticoagulant drugs (heparin or similar medications). These drugs keep the clot within the veins as small as possible and tend to prevent it from spreading or extending. Also, the patients should wear elastic stockings as a preventive measure during periods after surgery.

## What is the outlook for recovery in pulmonary embolism?

The outlook is good in the majority of cases. Formerly, about 85 percent of those affected had nonfatal embolism, while about 15 percent of cases were fatal. Since the advent of the anticoagulant drugs, only about 1 percent of cases end fatally.

## How important is bed rest after a pulmonary infarction?

Very important. Once a clot has formed, the patient must be kept at complete rest so that no further clot formation takes place and so that the chances of a piece breaking off are minimized. It must be remembered, though, that too much bed rest following surgery is conducive to clot formation in the legs.

# DUST DISEASES
## (Pneumonoconioses)

## Does exposure to dust always cause lung trouble?

No. Dust and fumes of many varieties may be inhaled over long periods of time without causing any disease of the lungs.

## How does coal dust affect the lungs?

It produces "miner's lung," also known as "black lung," usually associated with cough, shortness of breath, and eventually pulmonary (lung) insufficiency and replacement of lung tissue by fibrous tissue (pulmonary fibrosis). Advanced stages of this condition are accompanied by crippling lung symptoms, with inability to work or perform anything effortful.

## Are anthracosis and silicosis the same as "miner's lung" and "black lung"?

Yes.

## Which are the most harmful dusts?

Those of silica (quartz), asbestos, talc, sugarcane, cotton fiber, and beryllium (dust from fluorescent light bulbs).

## Which are the most serious dust diseases?

Silicosis and asbestosis. They occur among miners, stonecutters, and workers in asbestos.

## How long must one be exposed to these irritants before symptoms are produced?

Anywhere from a few weeks (asbestos) to two years (mining).

## What are the symptoms of silicosis?

It causes progressive damage to lung tissue. This eventually leads to inflammation of the lungs; tuberculosis is a not infrequent eventual complication. There may be mild to severe shortness of breath, chronic cough, and impairment of lung function. The endurance for work is markedly curtailed in serious cases.

## How is the diagnosis of silicosis made?

By studying the patient's history, examining dust samples from the occupational site, and noting characteristic x-ray appearance of the lungs.

### Can silicosis be prevented?

Yes, by providing healthful working conditions and by providing masks and other protective equipment, such as vacuum blowers, etc.

### Is there any treatment for silicosis?

No. Once scarring has occurred and lung function is impaired, there is no way of reversing the process. These patients must be guarded against further exposure to dust, or additional damage will result.

### What harm can result from inhalation of asbestos fibers?

It has been found that cancer of the lung may ensue if one inhales large amounts of asbestos. The cancer may not ensue until many years after exposure. Those who do not develop cancer may have many of the same symptoms as those suffering from silicosis.

### What is byssinosis?

A disease of the lungs caused by inhaling cotton dust for a period of years. It is thought to be an allergic condition and produces cough and sputum, as in bronchitis.

### What is bagassosis?

A lung disease due to dust from sugarcane fibers that have been baled and stored for long periods of time. It may be an allergic reaction to moldy dusts.

### What is farmer's lung?

An acute lung disease caused in farmers by the inhalation of the dust of moldy hay.

### What is silo-filler's disease?

A disease of the lungs in farmers who inhale certain nitrogenous gases in storage silos.

## SARCOIDOSIS

### What is sarcoidosis?

It is a chronic disease involving many organs, but especially the lungs, which may contain many fine and coarse inflammatory nodules in its tissues.

### Is sarcoidosis ever confused with other diseases?

Yes, its appearance on an x-ray film is very much like that of tuberculosis and is often mistaken for it, although the course of the disease is entirely different from tuberculosis.

### What are two important points of difference between sarcoidosis and tuberculosis?

a. No tubercle bacilli are found in the sputum.
b. The tuberculin skin test is negative in sarcoidosis.

### Is sarcoidosis often disabling?

Not usually. Even with extensive involvement, the majority of patients carry on their work. Sufficient scarring may ensue, however, so that in the end stages of severe cases, lung insufficiency or heart failure may develop.

### What is the best method of establishing a diagnosis of sarcoidosis?

Biopsy of an accessible enlarged lymph node will reveal the characteristic microscopic appearance. There is also an effective skin test (Kveim test), but it is not widely used as the material is not readily available.

### Is there any specific treatment or prevention of sarcoidosis?

No, nor is its cause known. Some patients respond favorably to cortisone like drugs, but these drugs must be used carefully to avoid causing a flareup of any latent tuberculosis.

## MUCOVISCIDOSIS
### (Cystic Fibrosis)

### Why is this disease of importance in a discussion of the lungs?

Because, although it also involves other organs, it causes progressive, and sometimes fatal, bronchial disease in childhood. The disease affects mainly the mucous glands of the air passage.

### What causes mucoviscidosis?

It is a hereditary abnormality of the glands that secrete mucus, tears, sweat, saliva, and digestive juices. These secretions are much thicker than normal and cause obstruction of the gland ducts and small bronchial tubes. Obstructed bronchioles are particularly prone to infection.

### What are the complications and end results of mucoviscidosis?

In very early life, about 10 percent of infants with this condition die of intestinal obstruction. Those who survive may suffer from malnutrition and are subject to repeated respiratory infections, any one of which may be very serious. Those who survive often go on to adult life suffering from chronic bronchiectasis and emphysema.

### How is this disease detected?

a. Sweat is collected from the skin and is tested. It will reveal a salt content two to four times the normal amount.
b. X rays of the chest reveal increased bronchial markings, possibly with patchy areas of pneumonia.
c. The stools show an excess of undigested fat.

### How can the lung and bronchial effects of mucoviscidosis be prevented?

By early vaccination against influenza, whooping cough, and measles, and by the early use of appropriate antibiotics to combat respiratory infections.

# SURGERY OF THE LUNGS

**What are the various lung conditions for which surgery is sometimes required?**

a. Infections.
b. Injuries to the lungs or chest cavity.
c. Cysts of the lungs.
d. Benign or malignant tumors of the lungs.

**Are operations upon the lungs or chest cavity safe to perform?**

Modern advances in surgical techniques and in anesthesia methods have made operations upon the chest practically as safe as those upon the abdomen.

**How does a patient breathe when the chest cavity has been opened surgically?**

Endotracheal anesthesia is utilized. By this method, oxygen can be supplied to the lungs without the necessity for active breathing by the patient. The endotracheal tube is inserted into the windpipe, and the anesthetist, by compressing the rubber breathing bag, controls the amount of gas that goes to the lungs.

# INFECTIONS

**Which types of lung infection may require surgery?**

a. Lung abscess. The great majority of abscesses are now brought under control successfully with the antibiotics, but there are still a certain number of cases that require surgical drainage. In former years, lung abscess was accompanied by a high mortality, but with modern methods of surgery and antibiotic therapy, practically all cases now get well.

b. Bronchiectasis. This is a condition in which the small bronchial tubes become widened and are partially destroyed. This makes them particularly susceptible to infection. When chronic infection sets in as a result of bronchiectasis, it is occasionally necessary to operate and remove that portion of lung. This procedure, known as lobectomy, can be carried out safely and gives great promise of cure.

c. Empyema. This is a condition in which pus forms in the space between the lung and the chest wall (the pleural cavity). It was encountered often in bygone days as a complication of pneumonia. Today it is a relatively rare condition, since pneumonia is controlled so effectively with antibiotics. However, when a case of pneumonia has been neglected or has been treated inadequately, empyema may develop. An incision into the chest cavity with drainage of the pus is the treatment of choice and results in a cure in the great majority of cases.

d. Tuberculosis. (See Chapter 74, on Tuberculosis.) Formerly there were many surgical procedures carried out for the cure of tuberculosis of the lung. These included removal of an involved lobe or of an entire lung. Such procedures are called lobectomy or pneumonectomy. They were usually advocated only when the opposite lung was uninvolved in the tuberculous process. Thoracoplasty was advised in a certain number of cases, In this procedure, the ribs surrounding a tuberculous lobe of a lung are removed, thus allowing the chest cage to collapse and to permit the underlying lung to rest. Another procedure, known as phrenic nerve crush, was occasionally recommended. This was carried out by making a small incision in the base of the neck, isolating the nerve, and crushing it with a clamp. The phrenic nerve supplies the diaphragm, and when it is crushed, the diaphragm rises and becomes inactive, thus decreasing the size of the chest cavity and allowing the lung to collapse partially and to rest. Fortunately, the advent of the antituberculosis drugs has eliminated the need for surgery in all but a few cases of tuberculosis.

# INJURIES TO THE LUNGS OR CHEST CAVITY

**Are injuries to the lungs or chest cavity seen very often?**

Yes, particularly in our mechanized society; accidents involving injuries to the chest wall and to the lungs are increasing at an alarming rate.

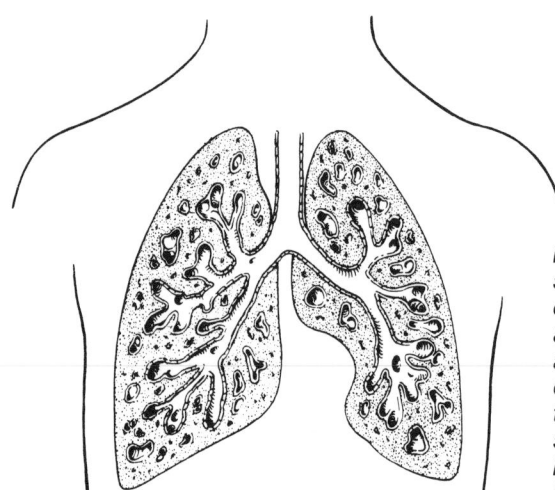

Dilated bronchioles

*Bronchiectasis. This diagram shows a chronic condition, bronchiectasis, in which the air sacs and small branchioles are enlarged and irregularly shaped. This disease is serious, as mucous secretions tend to stagnate in the air sacs, and this leads to chronic lung infection. Bronchiectasis can often be cured by removing the diseased portions of lung.*

**What are the most common injuries to the chest wall or lung?**

a. Severe contusion of the chest cage.

b. Fractured ribs or fractured breastbone (sternum).

c. Laceration of a lung caused by the sharp edge of a broken rib being driven into the lung.

d. Air, blood, or both in the pleural cavity surrounding a lung. This may come about as a result of lung puncture or as a result of a foreign body penetrating the chest wall.

e. Collapse of a lung secondary to spontaneous rupture or to hemorrhage.

f. Stab wounds or gunshot wounds of the chest.

**Is it possible to save people who have received serious chest or lung injuries?**

Yes. Contrary to general belief, the great majority of these people can be saved by proper surgical treatment.

**What is the treatment for injuries to the chest cavity and lungs?**

a. The first thing to treat is the shock that usually accompanies such injuries. Blood transfusions, inhalations of oxygen, and the giving of narcotics are a few of the immediate measures to be started.

b. If a gaping hole or sucking wound of the chest wall is present, the wound should be covered immediately so that air cannot enter the chest cavity from the outside. Tight bandaging of such a wound with gauze dressings and adhesive tape (or even with a torn shirt, if necessary) should be carried out as an emergency procedure whenever a sucking chest wound is encountered.

c. If hemorrhage from the lung into the chest cavity is severe, the chest cavity should be tapped by inserting a needle and withdrawing the blood. If the bleeding continues despite this procedure, then surgery should be performed, and the bleeding brought under control by tying off the bleeding vessels, suturing the lung, or removing that part that is damaged.

d. Air may have collected around the lung (pneumothorax). This is withdrawn by inserting a needle or small rubber tube into the chest cavity and attaching it to underwater drainage. The lung will then expand and function again.

e. An extensively lacerated lung may have to be removed surgically.

**Should people with severe lung injuries be transported lying down?**

No. Injuries to the chest may create considerable difficulty in breathing, and it is therefore best to transport these patients in a semisitting position.

## CYSTS OF THE LUNGS

**When are lung cysts encountered?**

They are usually birth deformities and are characterized by thin-walled sacs filled with air or fluid. Some lung cysts produce no symptoms, while others create pressure and cause collapse of surrounding lung tissue.

**Do lung cysts ever become infected and form abscesses?**

Yes. Others may burst and permit air to escape into the chest cavity.

**What is the treatment for cysts of the lungs?**

Those cysts that are causing symptoms should be removed surgically. Such an operation involves removal of the cyst and surrounding lung tissue (segmental resection).

**Are operations for removal of lung cysts successful?**

Yes. The great majority of these patients make a complete recovery.

## LUNG TUMORS

**Are all lung tumors cancerous?**

No. Benign tumors (adenomas of the lung) do occur, but, unfortunately, they are not encountered as frequently as the malignant growths.

**What is the treatment for benign lung tumors?**

Since it is almost always impossible to distinguish the benign from the malignant tumor preoperatively, the same surgical treatment is carried out for the noncancerous growth as for the cancerous tumor.

**Is lung cancer a common condition?**

Yes. It is one of the most frequently encountered cancers in men and is fast becoming one of the most frequent in women.

**Are cigarette smokers more prone to develop cancer of the lung than are nonsmokers?**

Most definitely, yes! It is estimated that cancer of the lung is ten times more common among heavy cigarette smokers than among nonsmokers.

**What are the early signs of lung cancer?**

a. Persistent cough.

b. Chest pain.

c. Spitting of blood.

d. Characteristic findings of a shadow in the lung on x-ray examination.

**Is there any way to tell if one is developing lung cancer?**

The best protection is to undergo a yearly x-ray examination of the chest.

**What is the treatment for cancer of the lung?**

Surgical removal of the diseased portion of the lung (lobectomy), or removal of the entire lung (pneumonectomy).

**Can a patient breathe normally after the removal of a lobe of the lung?**

Yes, but his ability to engage in strenuous physical exercise is limited.

**Can a patient live a normal life and breathe normally after the removal of an entire lung (pneumonectomy)?**

Such people must refrain from strenuous physical exercise, but they can carry on most normal activity. Breathing is normal if they do not overexert themselves.

**What fills in the empty space in the chest cavity after removal of a lobe of a lung or an entire lung?**

The chest wall tends to collapse, the diaphragm ascends into the chest, and the empty space fills in with scar tissue.

**Are the scars of operations upon the chest cavity or upon the lung very disfiguring?**

There is a long twelve- to fourteen-inch incision coursing from the back to the front of the chest. However, this usually heals as a thin line and creates relatively little disfigurement.

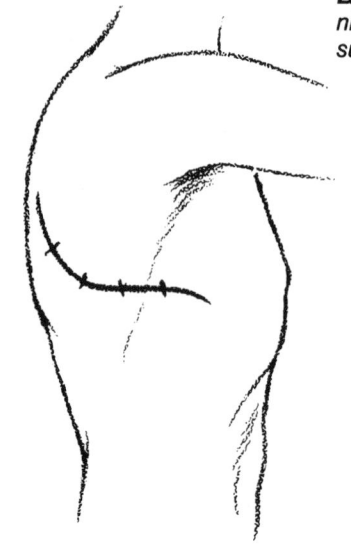

*Lung Surgery.* The long, curved scar, running from the chest to the back, is the result of surgery on the lung.

**Is the chest cavity badly deformed after the removal of a lobe of a lung or an entire lung?**

No. When the patient is fully dressed, it is impossible to note that such a procedure has been carried out.

**Is the chest markedly deformed after thoracoplasty (removal of several ribs)?**

No. Such deformity is noticeable only when the patient is undressed.

**Is anesthesia an important consideration in chest surgery?**

Yes. It is vital to have good anesthesia during chest operations.

**How long a hospital stay is necessary for removal of a lung or a portion of a lung?**

Approximately two weeks.

**Can patients get out of bed soon after major chest operations?**

Yes, within two to three days.

**What are the chances of ultimate cure following surgery for the following:**

a. Tuberculosis: Excellent, with the great majority being cured.
b. Lung cysts: Excellent. Almost all cases will recover completely.
c. Lung tumors: For the benign tumors, the chances for permanent recovery are excellent. In cancer of the lung, more and more patients are being cured as the result of earlier diagnosis and improved operative techniques.

# CHAPTER 42

# THE MALE ORGANS

*(The Penis, Scrotum, and Testicles)*

*(See also Chapter 50 on Prostate Gland; Chapter 64 on Sex; Chapter 69 on Sterility, Fertility, and Male Potency; Chapter 76 on Urinary Bladder and Urethra)*

### What is the structure of the penis?

It is composed of three tubular structures made of erectile tissue. Two of these are located on its upper aspect, and the third is on the lower aspect of the organ. The urethra, which transports the urine and seminal fluid, passes through one of these tubular structures.

All three tubular structures, called corpora, are made up of spongy tissue, and when filled with blood they become rigid, thus producing an erection. The head of the penis, or glans, is covered at birth by the foreskin. The latter structure is removed when circumcision is performed.

### What is the function of the urethra?

a. To transport urine.
b. To transport seminal fluid containing the sperm.

## CIRCUMCISION

### What is circumcision?

The removal of the foreskin.

### Why is circumcision recommended universally?

Because it is almost certain insurance against the development of cancer of the penis, since this condition rarely occurs in circumcised males. It is also recommended because it is more hygienic and permits easier cleansing of the penis.

### Is it true that women who are married to circumcised men are less likely to get cancer of the cervix or uterus?

Some investigators hold the theory, which seems to be borne out by recent statistics, that some of the material in an uncircumcised penis may act as an irritant when in contact with the cervix of certain women, and that, therefore, women who are married to circumcised men are less likely to develop cancer of the cervix.

### When is the proper time to circumcise a newborn child?

Before he leaves the hospital, between the third and fifth day.

### Is anesthesia necessary when performing circumcision in a newborn?

No.

### Is anesthesia necessary when circumcising older children or adults?

Yes.

*Circumcision. These diagrams show one method for performing circumcision. Most male infants born today are submitted to circumcision because it is a safguard against the development of cancer of the penis. Furthermore, a circumcised penis is much easier to keep clean than one that has not been circumcised.*

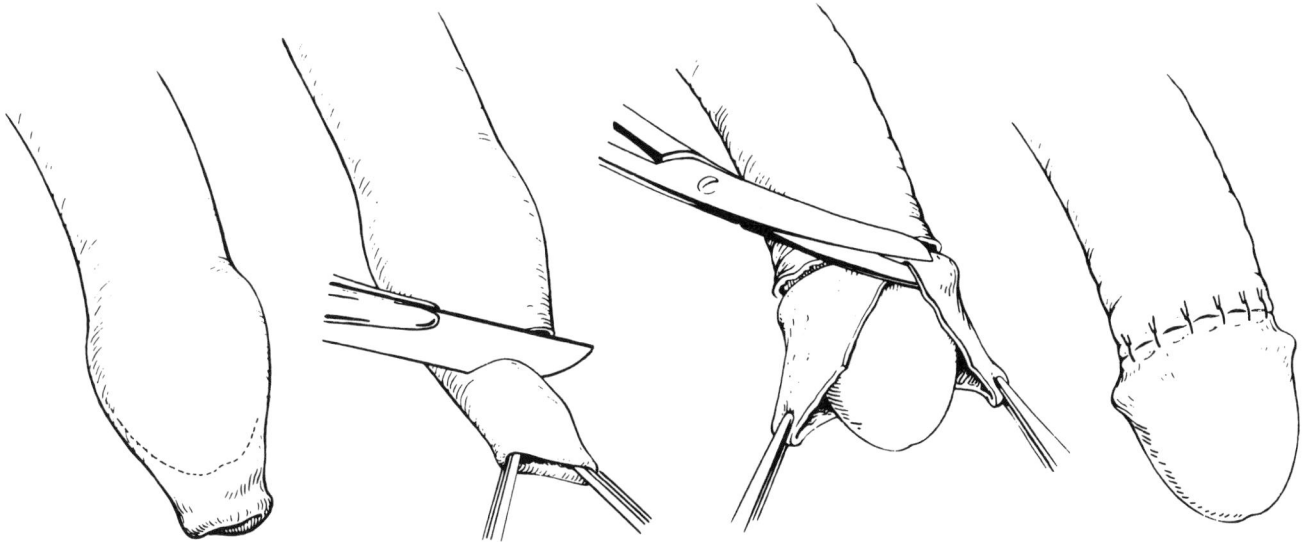

Foreskin          Foreskin grasped and incised          Foreskin being removed          Circumcision completed

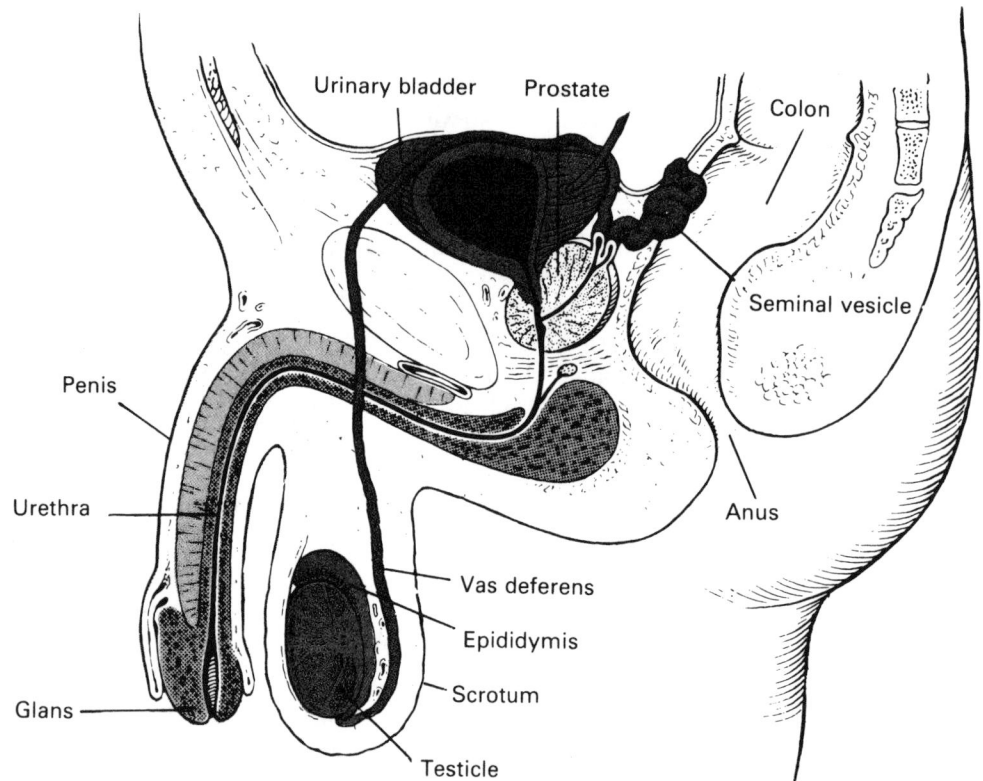

**The Male Organs.** *This diagram shows the penis, prostate, seminal vesicles, epididymis, and testicles. Sperm are manufactured in the testicles and are transmitted along the tube called the vas deferens and up into the seminal vesicles. The sperm are stored there and are emitted throught the channel of the penis (urethra). Sperm is mixed with fluid secreted by the prostate gland before it is ejaculated.*

**How long a hospital stay is necessary when circumcising an older child or adult?**

One to two days.

**Are there any harmful effects from circumcision?**

No.

## TUMORS OF THE PENIS

**Are malignant tumors of the penis common?**

No, and as stated previously, they seldom occur in circumcised males.

**Where is cancer of the penis usually located?**

Near the head of the penis, where it has the appearance of a protruding mass or a deep hard ulcer.

**In what age group is cancer of the penis most likely to occur?**

In middle and old age. It rarely occurs in youth.

**How is the diagnosis of cancer of the penis made?**

By taking a biopsy from the growth and submitting it to microscopic examination.

**With what other condition can a cancer of the penis be confused?**

One must distinguish a cancer from a venereal lesion such as a chancre.

**Is cancer of the penis related to sexual activity?**

No.

**What is the treatment for cancer of the penis?**

The best form of treatment is ampu-

tation of part or all of the penis, along with removal of the lymph glands in the groin that drain the penis.

**If the penis is amputated, how does urination take place?**

A small stump of penis is left to permit this function to continue.

**Can cancer of the penis be transmitted by sexual intercourse?**

No.

## THE SCROTUM AND TESTICLES

**What is the scrotum, or scrotal sac?**

A semi-elastic muscular sac covered by skin, located beneath the penis. It is divided into two compartments, each of which contains a testicle, an epididymis, and a spermatic cord.

### What is the composition and function of the testicle?

It is composed of a large number of tiny tubules known as the seminiferous tubules. It is here that sperm are produced. The testicle also contains cells that produce the male sex hormone, testosterone. The function of the testicle is to manufacture sperm and to allow them to be transported along the spermatic cord to the seminal vesicles. From the vesicles, the sperm are ejaculated during intercourse.

## INJURIES TO THE TESTICLE

### What is the treatment for an injury to the testicle?

The great majority of injuries, although extremely painful, are not serious and will heal by themselves. If the testicle is badly crushed or ruptured, it must be removed surgically.

### Can an injury to a testicle lead to sterility?

Severe damage to one testicle may cause it to lose its ability to transmit sperm, but if the other testicle remains normal, sterility will not result.

### Are injuries to both testicles very common?

No. Nature has a way of protecting these structures so that injury to both testicles is unusual.

## TUMORS OF THE TESTICLE

### What is the incidence of tumors of the testicle?

Malignant tumors of the testicle constitute about 5 percent of all malignant growths seen in males.

### Do tumors of the testicle occur more frequently in abnormally developed testicles and in undescended testicles?

Yes.

### When are tumors of the testicle most likely to occur?

In the third and fourth decades of life.

### Are all tumors of the testicle malignant?

No, but malignant growths are much more frequent than benign growths.

### How can one tell if a tumor of the testicle is present?

By the appearance of a slow, painless enlargement of the structure.

### What causes tumors of the testicle?

The cause is unknown.

### What is the treatment for these tumors?

Surgical removal should be carried out just as soon as the diagnosis is made. A radical procedure is performed if the growth is malignant.

This will also involve the removal of lymph glands in the abdomen.

### Is x-ray treatment of value in treating tumors of the testicle?

Yes. After surgery has been performed, x-ray treatment is often employed, especially in treating tumors known as *seminomas*.

### Is treatment with chemicals valuable for tumors of the testicles?

Yes. Recently it has been discovered that certain combinations of chemicals are extremely effective in destroying some malignant tumors of the testicle. They are also of great value in destroying metastases (spread of the tumor from its original site to another part of the body).

## UNDESCENDED TESTICLE

### What is an undescended testicle?

During the development of the embryo, the testicles are located in the abdomen. As the embryo grows, the testicles descend into the groin, and by the time the child is born, the testicles have reached the scrotal sac. Failure of such descent or incomplete descent is called undescended testicle (cryptorchidism). This may occur on one or both sides.

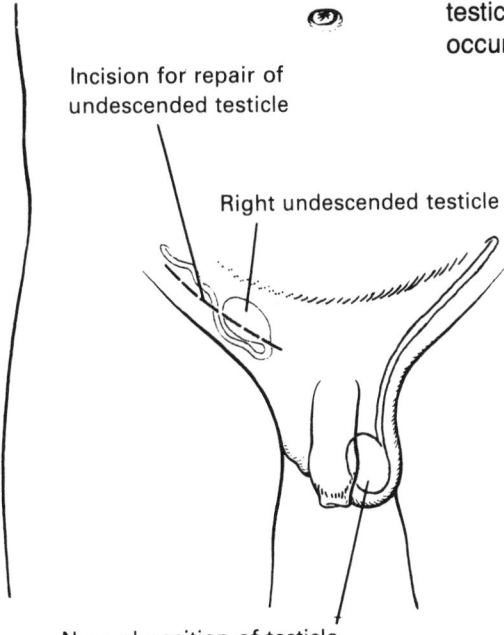

Incision for repair of undescended testicle

Right undescended testicle

Normal position of testicle

*Undescended Testicle. A right undescended testicle and a left testicle in normal position within the scrotal sac are seen in this diagram. The right testicle has not descended into the scrotum but remains high up within the inguinal canal. This is a birth deformity, which often requires surgical correction. In many cases of undescended testicles at birth, the testicles descend into the scrotum by themselves by the time the child is a year old.*

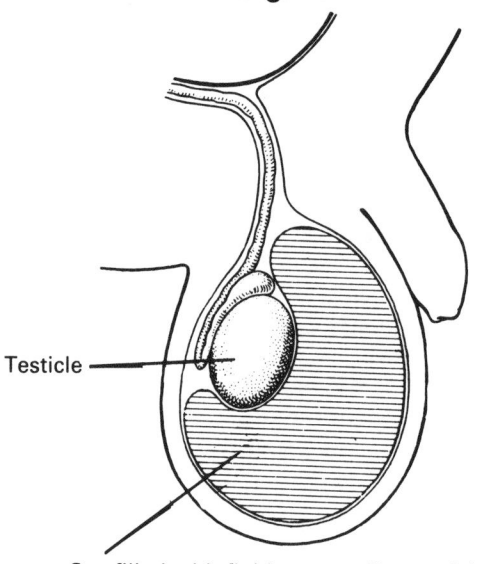

Testicle ———

Sac filled with fluid surrounding testicle

*Hydrocele. This is a rather common condition in which the sac surrounding the testicle is filled with fluid. Many infants born with a hydrocele may require no treatment, as the fluid will absorb before the child is a year of age. However, when the hydrocele persists, surgery for its removal should be performed. The testicle is rarely damaged by the presence of a hydrocele.*

**If there is an undescended testicle at birth, does it mean that the testicle will remain undescended?**

Not necessarily. A certain number of testicles will descend during the first year of life or during adolescence.

**What medical treatment can be given to encourage a testicle to descend into the scrotal sac?**

Hormone injections will sometimes cause the testicle to grow and to descend into the scrotal sac. This type of treatment should be tried when the child is young and before instituting surgery.

**Are undescended testicles often associated with the presence of a hernia?**

Yes.

**What is the best time to operate upon a child with an undescended testicle?**

Between five to seven years of age, although some surgeons feel the child is ready for this procedure beforehand.

**Must surgery be performed on all children with undescended testicles?**

Not if the testicle descends following a series of hormone injections.

**Are operations for an undescended testicle serious?**

No. They are no more serious than a hernia operation.

**How long a hospital stay is necessary for this procedure?**

About five to seven days.

**What operation is carried out for an undescended testicle?**

There are many methods of performing this procedure (orchidopexy). An incision three to five inches long is made in the groin, and the testicle and cord are delivered into the wound. The cord is lengthened by cutting away all the extra fibrous tissue and adhesions that may be surrounding it. The testicle is then brought down into the scrotal sac where it is anchored in place with sutures.

**Will undescended testicles function normally when brought down into normal position?**

Not always, since some of these glands are extremely small and underdeveloped. However, even if they fail to produce potent sperm, they will continue to secrete the important male sex hormone and thus maintain the male characteristics of the individual.

**Are the results of operations for undescended testicles good?**

Yes. The great majority of testicles can be brought down into the scrotal sac.

## HYDROCELE

**What is a hydrocele?**

It is a collection of clear fluid within a membranous sac surrounding the testicle. It may also occur in the spermatic cord.

**What is the cause of hydrocele?**

The cause is unknown.

**Does the presence of a hydrocele endanger the testicle?**

No.

**What is the treatment for hydrocele?**

In small infants, hydroceles have a tendency to disappear by themselves. If they occur in older children or in adults, surgery is indicated.

**What is the surgical treatment for hydrocele?**

Through a small incision in the groin, the hydrocele sac is excised completely, or part of it is removed and the remainder turned inside out and sutured behind the testicle.

**Are operations for hydrocele serious?**

No. They are considered to be minor surgical procedures.

**What are the results of surgery for hydrocele?**

Cure of the condition in almost all cases.

**Is there a nonsurgical treatment for hydrocele?**

Yes. The fluid within the hydrocele sac may be withdrawn through a needle and a solution may be injected to cause the walls of the sac to become sclerosed. This form of treatment is not as efficient as surgery and may occasionally result in infection.

### Do hernias and hydroceles often occur together?

Yes, and when this does happen, both conditions should be corrected surgically.

## TORSION (TWIST) OF THE TESTICLE

### What is torsion of the testicle?

For some unexplained reason in boys and young men, the spermatic cord and testicle may suddenly undergo a twist. This may be due to an excessively long cord, a developmental defect, or an injury.

### What are the symptoms of torsion of the testicle?

There is sudden pain, marked tenderness, and swelling in the region of the testicle and along the cord. If the scrotum is lifted up, there is increased pain. This differentiates this condition from epididymitis. Nausea and vomiting may ensue. When the twist takes place, the blood supply to the testicle is shut off. Unless the condition is remedied promptly, the testicle may become gangrenous.

### What is the treatment for torsion of the testicle?

Prompt surgery, with untwisting of the cord. In order to save the testicle, surgery should be performed within six to eight hours after onset. If, at operation, the testicle is found to be gangrenous and beyond salvage, it must be removed.

### Is torsion of the testicle a serious condition?

It is serious in that it may lead to loss of one testicle, but not serious insofar as danger to life is concerned.

Hospitalization for about a week is necessary.

## INFECTION OF THE EPIDIDYMIS (Epididymitis)

### What is the epididymis?

It is a structure immediately adjacent and connected to the testicle. It is made up of innumerable tubules containing the sperm that have been manufactured by the testicle.

### Are infections of the epididymis common?

Yes. In years gone by, when gonorrheal infection was so poorly controlled, many infections of this structure were seen. Today, however, antibiotic therapy has reduced the incidence of infection within the epididymis.

### What are some of the causes other than gonorrhea for infections of the epididymis?

It is sometimes encountered after an operation upon the prostate gland, or it may follow a cystoscopic examination. It frequently follows vigorous prostatic massage, which forces infected material from the prostate down the connecting duct to the epididymis.

### How can one prevent infections of the epididymis?

In operations, the best way to prevent it is to tie off and cut the vas deferens (the tube connecting the epididymis with the seminal vesicles) before carrying out surgery upon the prostate. In medical conditions such as prostatitis, massage should be carried out very gently, and the patient should void after treatment.

### What are the harmful effects of epididymitis?

In addition to being a very painful condition with swelling, fever, and

extreme tenderness of the testicle, epididymitis is often followed by sterility if it involves both sides.

### What is the treatment for acute epididymitis?

Treatment consists of bed rest, liberal fluid intake, the application of ice to the affected side, and the administration of antibiotics.

### How long does the acute phase of epididymitis last?

About five to seven days, but the swelling may not subside for several months.

### Is surgery ever necessary for epididymitis?

Yes, when an abscess has formed. This will require drainage.

### Does acute epididymitis ever become chronic?

Yes. There are cases in which the infection subsides only partially and flares up from time to time.

### What is the treatment for chronic or recurring epididymitis?

The surgical removal of the epididymis.

### Is epididymitis ever caused by tuberculosis?

Yes, occasionally.

## VARICOCELE

### What is a varicocele?

A varicocele is a varicose involvement of those veins that accompany the spermatic cord.

### What causes a varicocele?

It is thought to be a birth deformity. In 90 percent of cases, it occurs on the left side.

### How is a diagnosis of varicocele made?

When the physician examines the

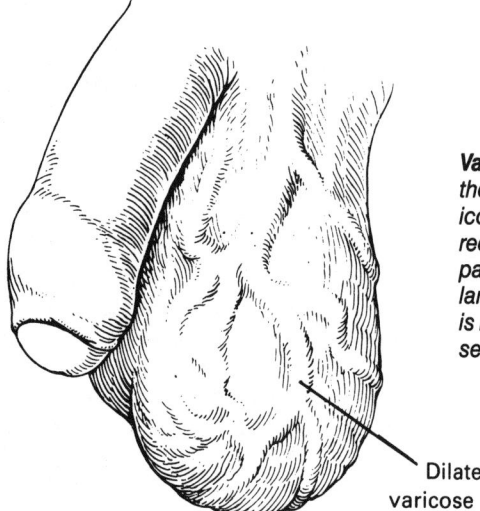

Dilated
varicose veins

*Varicocele. This is a condition in which the veins coming from the testicle are varicosed. In most instances, this condition requires no treatment. However, if there is pain in the area, or if the varicocele is very large, surgical removal of the varicosities is indicated. This type of operation is not serious, and results are uniformly good.*

scrotum, it will feel to him like a "bag of worms."

### What symptoms are caused by varicocele?

Usually none, although there may be a dragging sensation and a feeling of vague discomfort at the side of the scrotum.

### What is the treatment for varicocele?

Most varicoceles require no treatment. If they attain a very large size, then surgery is performed, with the removal of some of the veins.

### Are operations for varicocele serious?

No. They are carried out preferably through an incision in the groin. It may also be done through an incision in the scrotum, but this is more likely to shrink the testicle.

### Is there any medical treatment for varicocele?

Yes. A well-fitting scrotal support may be worn.

### Is fertility affected by varicocele?

Yes. Varicoceles are associated with male infertility in many instances. The infertility may be overcome in more than 50 percent of the cases by surgically tying off the varicocele.

# CHAPTER 43

# MEDICATIONS AND DRUGS

*(See also Chapter 4 on Adrenal Glands; Chapter 7 on Allergy; Chapter 26 on First Aid; Chapter 31 on Immunizations and Vaccinations; Chapter 34 on Infectious and Virus Diseases; Chapter 55 on Pituitary Gland)*

**Is it safe for a patient to medicate himself without a doctor's advice?**

It is absurd to assume that in every indisposition one should call the doctor before taking a simple medication such as a laxative or an aspirin. However, intelligent people will realize that the physician should be consulted whenever unusual symptoms develop. In such situations, it is dangerous for people to medicate themselves. In certain instances in which a patient is already under medication, has a chronic disease, or is pregnant, even the more common drugs should not be taken without the advice of the physician.

**If a physician has once recommended a medication, is it safe for the patient to take it again at a later date for what he considers to be a similar condition?**

This should be done only upon the instructions of the physician. If there is any doubt at all, a brief telephone call may serve to avert a serious mistake.

**Is it safe for someone to give a relative or friend a medication recommended for himself?**

No. This has been the cause of many serious mistakes. Lay people are not in a position to make an accurate diagnosis of another person's illness.

**How can one tell if a drug or medicine is still effective or whether it has lost its potency?**

Call the pharmacist or physician if in doubt. Many prescriptions have labels, which give an expiration date; look for this on the bottle. Any change in color or consistency of the preparation should be considered suspicious either of loss of efficacy or of a major change in its composition.

**Why is it that certain drugs can be bought directly across the counter while for others it is necessary to have a doctor's prescription?**

Over-the-counter sale of drugs is regulated by federal, state, and local health authorities. The decision on these drugs is generally based on their possible toxic action as well as on the nature of the illness for which the drug is intended.

**What controls are exercised by the government over the manufacture and sale of drugs?**

The federal government sees to it through its various agencies that all medicines and drugs released for public consumption are properly manufactured, contain accurate information on their labels, and are based upon research that shows evidence that they are efficient and safe for the illness for which they are prescribed.

**How reliable are the various advertisements one sees and hears over radio, television, and in the newspapers about drugs and medicines?**

It is safe to say that most manufacturers are a bit overenthusiastic concerning the value of their product. Some advertisements are cleverly misleading while still adhering to the letter of the law. On the whole, however, in America, one must say that advertisements maintain a rather high standard of accuracy. If they fail to live up to the law, the federal

agency concerned is quick to prosecute.

**How can one best safeguard against taking the wrong medicine or drug?**

Whenever in doubt about a medication, call your pharmacist or family doctor on the telephone.

**Should one ever take a drug or medicine when the label has come off or is difficult to read?**

No. It is much safer to throw away the medicine than to take it without being certain of what it is. A safe rule is to always read every label twice before taking medication.

**What medicines and drugs should be kept in the home medicine cabinet?**

Unless one lives in a very rural district, it is not wise to keep too many medications at home. First-aid materials, a mild antiseptic, aspirin, Tylenol, and a few other similar medications are all that should be kept in the home.

**What medicines and drugs are particularly dangerous to have around the house?**

All medications and drugs are particularly dangerous to small children who may overdose themselves. Even a laxative can be dangerous if taken in large quantities by a small child. All medications should be kept well out of reach of small children, especially insecticides, lyes, and chemicals of any type, including alcoholic beverages. In any event, people should always request "child-proof" bottles, which children cannot open.

**What makes a drug habit-forming?**

a. The inherent character of the drug.
b. The personality of the individual who takes the drug.
c. Any drug that relieves discomfort and produces a pleasant state of

mind or body is potentially habit-forming.

## Is there a difference between a habit-forming drug and a drug to which one has become addicted?

Yes. Drug addiction produces a physical and mental dependency upon the substance. Withdrawal of such a drug produces extremely intense physical, physiological, and emotional disturbance. Withdrawal of a habit-forming drug may cause mild psychological and emotional distress but rarely causes any physical symptomatology.

## Is it common for people to develop resistance or immunity to various medicines after taking them for a prolonged period of time?

This tendency definitely exists with certain drugs. For instance, certain bacteria will develop resistance to penicillin and other antibiotics. Also, increased tolerance or resistance to the effect of certain pain-relieving drugs or narcotics or sleeping pills sometimes occurs. However, most medications continue to exercise their therapeutic properties when used properly over prolonged periods of time.

## Is it true that the less medication a person takes, the better?

Yes. Medication should be taken only when necessary, and the doctor's orders should be followed closely. It is just as bad to take too little medication when it is indicated as it is to take too much.

## Can true drug addiction ever be cured?

Yes, though it is admittedly a most trying and difficult procedure.

## Are there satisfactory measures to cure and control overdoses of medications and drugs?

There is a method of treating overdoses of all medications and drugs. The most important point to remember is not to delay one moment in getting medical help. Also, it is important to try to induce vomiting as soon as possible.

## Why is it that so many physicians refuse to renew a prescription but will insist upon a return visit?

a. To check on the progress of the patient and the effect of the medication.
b. To make certain there are no new complications.
c. To reaffirm or alter a questionable diagnosis.
d. To alter dosage or to change the medication.
e. Certain medications are effective for only short periods and should not be taken for prolonged periods of time.

## Should pregnant women be especially careful about the medicines or drugs they take?

Yes, the less medication they take, the better. Some medications may have harmful effects upon the developing unborn child. They should never take medicines without first consulting their doctor.

## Is it harmful, at any time, to take a medication for too long a period?

Yes. Certain medications, while effective and harmless for short periods of time, will cause toxic symptoms if taken for too long a period. Consult your physician.

## ANTIBIOTIC DRUGS

### What are the antibiotics?

Antibiotics are chemical substances produced synthetically or by living microorganisms such as bacteria or fungi. They are used medically to combat disease produced by bacteria.

### How effective are the antibiotics?

Millions of lives have been saved since the antibiotics have been dis-covered. Pneumonia, streptococcal, staphylococcal, gonococcal, syphilitic, and other infections have been cured by the judicious use of the antibiotics.

### Are the antibiotics effective against virus infections?

Unfortunately, antibiotics do not seem to affect viruses. However, drugs to combat viruses are soon to be released for general use.

### Does one tend to develop resistance to the antibiotics?

The patient does not develop resistance to the antibiotics, but unfortunately many bacteria do develop resistance. Antibiotics should therefore be used wisely and sparingly.

### Are antibiotics helpful in the treatment of tumors or cancer?

At the present time, there are no known cures from the use of the antibiotics in the treatment of tumors or cancer.

### Is allergy to the antibiotics common?

Yes. However, a patient may be allergic to one antibiotic and not to others. Thus, allergic patients can be treated successfully with one or another of these drugs.

### Is it safe for someone to medicate himself with the antibiotics?

No! Antibiotics should be taken only upon a doctor's prescription, because self-medication may lead to unnecessary development of allergies to the antibiotics or to the development of resistance of certain organisms within the body to the antibiotics.

### Are harmful effects ever seen from an allergy to, or overdose of, antibiotics?

Occasionally. The allergic reactions may be most severe and may show themselves by skin rashes, bleeding tendencies, and hives. Antibiotics may cause serious damage to the kidneys, the bone marrow, the nervous system, or to the gastrointestinal tract. As in all other potent medications, their usage should be outlined and controlled under a physician's direction.

**Should prescriptions always be obtained before taking antibiotics?**

Yes.

**Are antibiotics effective against the common cold or influenza?**

No, but they are effective in preventing some of the complications of these infections.

# SULFA DRUGS
## (Sulfonamides)

**What are the sulfa drugs?**

A specific class of chemical substances, synthetically manufactured, which are effective in the treatment of a wide variety of bacterial and viral diseases. They are often used interchangeably or in conjunction with the antibiotics.

**How effective are the sulfa drugs in the treatment of infection?**

They represent a great weapon in the treatment of certain infections, especially those involving the urinary tract. Here, they are sometimes more effective than the antibiotic drugs.

**Do patients ever develop immunity or resistance to the sulfa drugs?**

Here again, the patients themselves do not develop a resistance or immunity to sulfa drugs, but certain bacteria do become resistant. Reactions of an unfavorable nature are quite uncommon when using the more modern sulfa drugs.

**Is it safe to medicate oneself with the sulfa drugs?**

No. These medications are powerful

and should be taken only upon a doctor's prescription.

**Is it necessary to drink large quantities of fluids when taking the sulfa drugs?**

Yes, as this will prevent crystals from precipitating in the kidneys and in the urine. However, recent improvements in the structure of the sulfa drugs have minimized this complication.

**Do the sulfa drugs ever adversely affect the blood-forming structures?**

This is now a rare occurrence. However, if taken over a prolonged period of time, it is wise to have a routine blood count taken. Also, it is wise to have the urine examined to note the appearance of crystals or blood cells.

**Are antibiotics more effective than the sulfa drugs in combating most infections?**

Yes, except for certain infections involving the urinary or gastrointestinal tracts.

**Are the antibiotics safer to take than the sulfa drugs?**

No.

# PAIN-RELIEVING DRUGS
## (Analgesics)

**What are the common analgesic medications?**

The most commonly used analgesic are salicylates, that is, aspirin and related medications. Other medications, including Darvon, Talwin, and Tylenol, have also come into wide use as pain relievers.

**How effective sre the analgesics in relieving pain?**

Aspirin and similar medications are usually very effective means for relieving pain. They are relatively mild in action and are of great use-

fulness. However, they are relatively ineffective against the more serious causes of pain, such as kidney colic, ulcer pain, etc.

**Is it safe to medicate oneself with the analgesics?**

Prescriptions are not usually required for the purchase of most mild analgesic medications. Some self-medication is permissible, provided it is done intelligently. In other words, their usage for temporary minor aches and pains is permissible. However, they should not be used for conditions that are severe and that continue over a prolonged period of time.

**Is there any harm in taking analgesics over a period of many weeks or months?**

Any condition that requires an analgesic to be taken for weeks or months warrants examination by a physician.

**For what common conditions are the analgesics usually prescribed?**

Minor muscle aches and pains, neuralgias, functional headaches, arthritis, menstrual cramps, and other conditions not requiring narcotics for relief.

**Is aspirin habit-forming?**

No.

**Does one develop an allergy or an immunity to the analgesic medications?**

Allergy to analgesics does occur and is frequently seen. However, these medications are quite remarkable in that long-term, frequent use is not commonly associated with loss of efficacy of the drug.

**Is it important to take the correct dosage of aspirin or other analgesic drugs?**

Definitely, yes. Incorrect dosage may be dangerous if too high or ineffectual if too low. Dosage will always vary according to the age and weight of the patient.

### Are analgesics such as aspirin ever dangerous to take?

Yes, when a patient is markedly allergic to them. Fatalities have been known to occur from taking just one aspirin tablet. Also, if a patient has an ulcer of the stomach or duodenum, aspirin may cause the ulcer to bleed. Therefore, patients with ulcers should use aspirin very sparingly. Analgesics are also dangerous if given in overdoses, especially to children.

### If a person is sensitive to one pain-relieving drug, is he likely to be sensitive to all of them?

Fortunately, no.

## BARBITURATES

### What are barbiturates?

They are medications that are commonly prescribed to allay nervous tension or for the purpose of inducing sleep.

### How effective are the barbiturates in inducing sleep and relieving nervous tension?

Although there is great variability in the susceptibility to barbiturates, generally speaking they are effective in relieving nervous tension and in inducing sleep. It must be mentioned, however, that the underlying cause for the nervous tension and lack of sleep cannot be helped by taking barbiturates.

### Should one medicate himself with barbiturates, or should he take these drugs only upon a doctor's prescription?

Most emphatically, barbiturates should only be taken under doctor's, as they are potentially harmful drugs.

### Is it safe to take barbiturates over a long period of time?

No, unless the physician permit this practice

### Are the barbiturates habit-forming?

Yes. In certain people, they may even cause addiction.

### Does one develop a resistance or immunity to barbiturates after taking them for a period of many months?

Yes. To achieve the same effect from barbiturates, users tend to require larger and larger dosages.

### What harm can result from an overdose of barbiturates?

Marked overdose of these medications may cause coma or death.

### For what conditions are the barbiturates commonly prescribed?

Nervous tension, irritability, convulsive states such as epilepsy, motion sickness, insomnia, overstimulated states, high blood pressure, etc.

### Are there drugs other than barbiturates that are effective for sedation?

Yes. Chloral hydrate and some of the newer nonbarbiturate drugs have been found to be effective. Tranquilizers are now being used extensively as sedatives instead of barbiturates.

### Are there instances when the above-named drugs are preferable to the barbiturates?

This will depend upon the individual patient's response and the particular preference of the prescribing physician.

## TRANQUILIZERS

### What are the tranquilizer medications?

These are chemicals that tend to allay tension and anxiety. They also depress brain function.

### Is it safe to medicate oneself with tranquilizing drugs?

Definitely not. People who feel they need a tranquilizer need medical at-tention first. The decision to prescribe these drugs should come from the physician and should not originate with the patient.

### Can one buy the tranquilizer drugs across the counter, or should a doctor's prescription be obtained?

According to law, these drugs should be prescribed by a physician. However, in many areas, this regulation is not strictly observed.

### Do people frequently develop tolerance to tranquilizers?

Yes. Tolerance develops with repeated use of tranquilizers. As a result, the patient requires ever-increasing doses to obtain the desired effect.

### How effective are the tranquilizers in calming the nerves?

They are effective in varying degrees. At best, they only give temporary relief from anxiety and tension.

### Is there any harm in taking tranquilizers regularly for a period of months or years?

Yes, as larger and larger doses are usually required, and addiction may result. In any event, these drugs should only be prescribed by a physician who should know when to discontinue their use.

### Can an overdose of tranquilizing drugs be dangerous?

Yes. Serious toxic reactions, and even deaths, have been reported from overdoses of tranquilizers.

### Are tranquilizers frequently prescribed?

They are the most widely prescribed drugs in the world. Therefore, physician supervision of their use is essential!

### Are tranquilizers a good substitute for narcotics, barbiturates, or analgesics?

Tranquilizers should not be considered in the nature of a "substitute" for any of these other types of drugs, although there is often an over-lap in their areas of usage.

## NARCOTICS

**For what purpose are the narcotics prescribed?**
They are the most potent pain killers and are prescribed only in situations where pain is intolerable or excruciating.

**Can narcotic drugs be obtained directly, or is it necessary to have a doctor's prescription?**
A doctor's prescription is mandatory.

**What advantages do the narcotics have over the pain-relieving drugs?**
Narcotics are many, many times more potent than the analgesic drugs.

**Should narcotics ever be used in place of the barbiturates or tranquilizers in order to produce sleep or relieve nervous tension?**
No! Narcotics should never be used in the treatment of insomnia or nervous tension.

**How can one tell if he is becoming addicted to a narcotic?**
The patient will experience an intense emotional craving for the narcotic as well as extremely unpleasant physical symptoms if the drug is not taken.

**Does one ever develop immunity or resistance to the effects of narcotics?**
One does not become truly resistant to narcotics, but frequent usage may lead to the necessity of ever-increasing dosages in order to produce the same effect.

**How quickly does one become addicted to some of the more powerful narcotics?**
It usually takes at least several weeks of repeated use to induce addiction. However, extremely susceptible people have been known to become addicted after only a few doses of a drug.

**Is there a cure for narcotic addiction?**
Yes, but it usually requires a great deal of effort and perseverance.

## LAXATIVES *(Purgatives)*

**Is it safe to take laxatives?**
In most cases, it is quite safe to take laxatives to relieve occasional or chronic constipation. This does not mean that frequent and repeated use is admissible.

**When should one *not* take laxatives?**
a. When there is acute abdominal pain.
b. When there has been progressively increasing constipation that appears to respond less and less to laxatives.
c. When there are symptoms such as chest pain, headache, or other signs not related to the bowel.
d. When there is evidence of bleeding from the intestinal tract, such as bloody stools or black stools.

**When should one consult his physician concerning the taking of laxatives?**
a. In all of the above instances or in any other situation where there is doubt as to the propriety of taking a laxative.
b. When one finds that he cannot get along without the repeated use of laxatives.

**Do laxatives tend to be habit forming?**
Definitely, yes.

**Do laxatives tend to lose their effectiveness if taken over a period of months or years?**
Yes.

**Can permanent damage be done to the bowels by prolonged usage of laxatives?**
Yes. The bowels may lose some of their ability to function naturally. In other instances, the frequent taking of laxatives may irritate the lining of the bowel and lead to certain types of colitis.

**How can one break the laxative habit?**
This is most difficult, and will require gradual weaning from the use of laxatives and a substitution of new habits. Foods plentiful in bulk and roughage should be taken. Most important of all, the individual must establish a fixed daily routine for bowel movements. It is important to consult your physician to make sure that no underlying disease is the cause for the chronic constipation.

**Are there any adequate substitutes for laxatives?**
Yes. There are several preparations that are not true laxatives but that form bulk and moisture in the intestinal tract.

**Can overdose of laxatives ever be dangerous?**
Yes. Certain of the ingredients in some of the laxatives can cause serious toxic reaction.

## WEIGHT-REDUCING DRUGS

**What are some of the common weight-reducing drugs?**
There are no true weight-reducing drugs but merely drugs that tend to make the patient lose his appetite. The most commonly used drugs are in the amphetamine group.

**Is it safe to take weight-reducing drugs without a doctor's prescription?**
No. Do not take another person's prescription simply because it works

for him; it may cause serious injury to *you*.

### Are the bulk-forming drugs safe to take in order to reduce appetite?

There are certain medications that form large bulk within the stomach and tend to make the patient lose his appetite. However, these drugs are not without danger and should only be taken when prescribed by a physician, as they sometimes cause intestinal disorders.

### Can weight-reducing drugs be taken over a prolonged period of time if the patient *is* supervised by a physician?

Yes.

### Is there a tendency for the effectiveness of the weight-reducing drugs to wear off if the drug has been taken over a prolonged period of time?

Yes.

### Are there any safe weight-reducing drugs which will permit the patient to eat a normal, full diet?

No. Unless the calorie intake is decreased, the patient will not lose weight.

## HORMONES

### What are hormones?

Hormones are chemicals secreted by the endocrine glands into the bloodstream, which affect the body mechanism as a whole.

### What are the common hormones within the body?

a. Pituitary hormones, secreted by the pituitary gland.
b. Thyroid hormones, secreted by the thyroid gland.
c. Parathyroid substance, secreted by the parathyroid gland.
d. Adrenal hormones, including cortisone and adrenalin, secreted by the adrenal gland.
e. Ovarian hormones, secreted by the ovaries.
f. Testicular hormones, secreted by the testicles.
g. Insulin, secreted by the pancreas.

### Can hormones be manufactured artificially so that they can replace a deficiency in one's own body?

Many, but not all, hormones can now be synthesized chemically.

### Should hormones ever be taken by a patient without a doctor's prescription?

No. Great harm may be done by improper usage of these powerful substances.

### How effective are the hormones in treating glandular deficiencies?

This varies markedly with the condition for which they are being used. Suffice it to say that there are numerous conditions, both glandular and nonglandular, in which hormones have great therapeutic value.

### What harm can result from taking hormones over a prolonged period of time without proper supervision?

If taken without proper supervision, hormones can cause severe imbalance in the chemistry of the body and may lead to serious illness and disorders. Hormones should only be taken under adequate supervision of a physician, who will make frequent tests to see if proper dosages are being given.

### Can the indiscriminate taking of hormones lead to cancer development in an organ?

To date there is no conclusive proof that an overdose of hormones can produce cancer, but it is conceded that certain hormones may well speed the growth and spread of latent malignancy. Thus, if a cancerous tendency exists, hormones must be given very cautiously.

### Do people ever develop allergies to hormones?

Yes; this occasionally takes place.

### Why is it that some hormones can be given in tablet form while others must be injected?

Some hormones are either destroyed by the digestive juices or are not properly absorbed in the intestinal tract. Such hormones must therefore be given by injection.

### Are hormones of value in the treatment of glandular insufficiency?

Yes. Certain hormones, such as thyroid, ovarian, testicular, etc., are of great value if properly utilized in the treatment of inactivity of the endocrine glands.

### What is cortisone?

This is a substance naturally produced by the adrenal glands. It belongs to the family of substances known as steroids.

### What is ACTH?

This is an abbreviation for the term adrenocorticotropic hormone. It is one of the substances normally secreted by the pituitary gland. Its function is to stimulate the adrenal gland to produce cortisone and cortisonelike chemicals.

### What conditions are ACTH and cortisone used to treat?

In recent years it has been discovered that both ACTH and cortisone are very effective in relieving a wide variety of diseases of inflammatory, allergic, or unknown origin. Some of the most common uses have been in various types of arthritis, rheumatic fever, allergies, sensitivities, lupus, nephrosis, etc.

### Are ACTH and cortisone curative when used for the above conditions?

No. They merely alleviate the conditions, but it is felt that they may forestall physical damage due to the active process of certain diseases for which they are used.

### Are ACTH and cortisone used in all cases of arthritis?

No. They are to be used only in severe cases of certain types of arthritis or in those that fail to respond to other forms of medication.

### Is cortisone now preferred over ACTH in the treatment of arthritis?

Yes.

### Can cortisone be harmful if given in excess quantity?

Yes.

### Should cortisone be given only under the supervision of a physician?

Yes! Improper and unsupervised use may cause serious damage.

### Does the effect of these drugs continue after they have been stopped?

Unfortunately, most of the beneficial effects of these drugs are completely lost after they have been discontinued.

### How is ACTH given?

ACTH is only effective when given by injection.

### How is cortisone given?

Cortisone and some of the related drugs are effective when given either by mouth or by injection.

## STIMULATING DRUGS

### What is a stimulating drug?

One that acts upon the higher nervous system to eliminate a sense of physical or emotional fatigue. They are also used to counteract depression, drowsiness, and other lethargic states.

### What are the more commonly used stimulating drugs?

Benzedrine, Dexedrine, ephedrine, and caffeine.

### For what purposes are stimulating drugs used?

a. To counteract mild depression.
b. To counteract certain neurological abnormalities.

### Do stimulating drugs tend to lose their usefulness if they are taken over a prolonged period of time?

Usually not.

### Can one develop an addiction or habituation to the taking of stimulating drugs?

Yes.

### Are stimulating drugs dangerous to take by oneself?

Most of these medications are potent chemicals and should be taken only upon a doctor's prescription.

### Is it harmful to take an overdose of the stimulating drugs?

Definitely, yes.

### Is caffeine a stimulant?

Yes.

### Can the caffeine in coffee cause insomnia?

In those people who are sensitive to its use, insomnia can definitely be caused by a cup or two of coffee in the evening.

### Does tea contain caffeine?

Yes. A cup of tea has approximately the same amount of caffeine as a cup of coffee.

### Does cocoa contain caffeine?

Only in insignificant quantities.

### Is alcohol a true stimulant?

No. On the contrary, alcohol is a depressant.

## PSYCHEDELIC OR HALLUCINATORY DRUGS

### What are hallucinatory drugs?

These are chemicals that when taken by mouth, by injection, or by inhalation, will cause changes in mental processes. Characteristic of these changes are hallucinations that deprive an individual of an appreciation of reality or cause him to interpret fantasy situations as real.

### What are the purposes of the hallucinatory drugs?

In actuality, they serve no useful purpose at the present time other than to give people a false sense of elation and to permit them a brief period of escape from the hardships of their reality existence. It is not true that there is an expanded intellect as a result of taking these drugs.

### What are some of the hallucinatory drugs?

The ones used most widely today are LSD and STP.

### What are some of the specific effects of these drugs?

Both LSD and STP may create a false sense of clairvoyance and often permit the user to think he has insights that he actually does not possess. Thus a person may be led to believe, during the period he is under the influence of these substances, that he can solve perplexing reality problems, or that he is powerful enough to overcome great physical and emotional obstacles that confront him.

### Are there harmful effects from LSD and STP?

Yes. It has been shown that rational thinking is often completely destroyed during the time that an individual is under the influence of these substances. Furthermore, many people have suffered permanent brain damage and damage to their chromosomes and genes from their use.

### Are there any beneficial effects from taking psychedelic drugs?

Not when taken by those in good

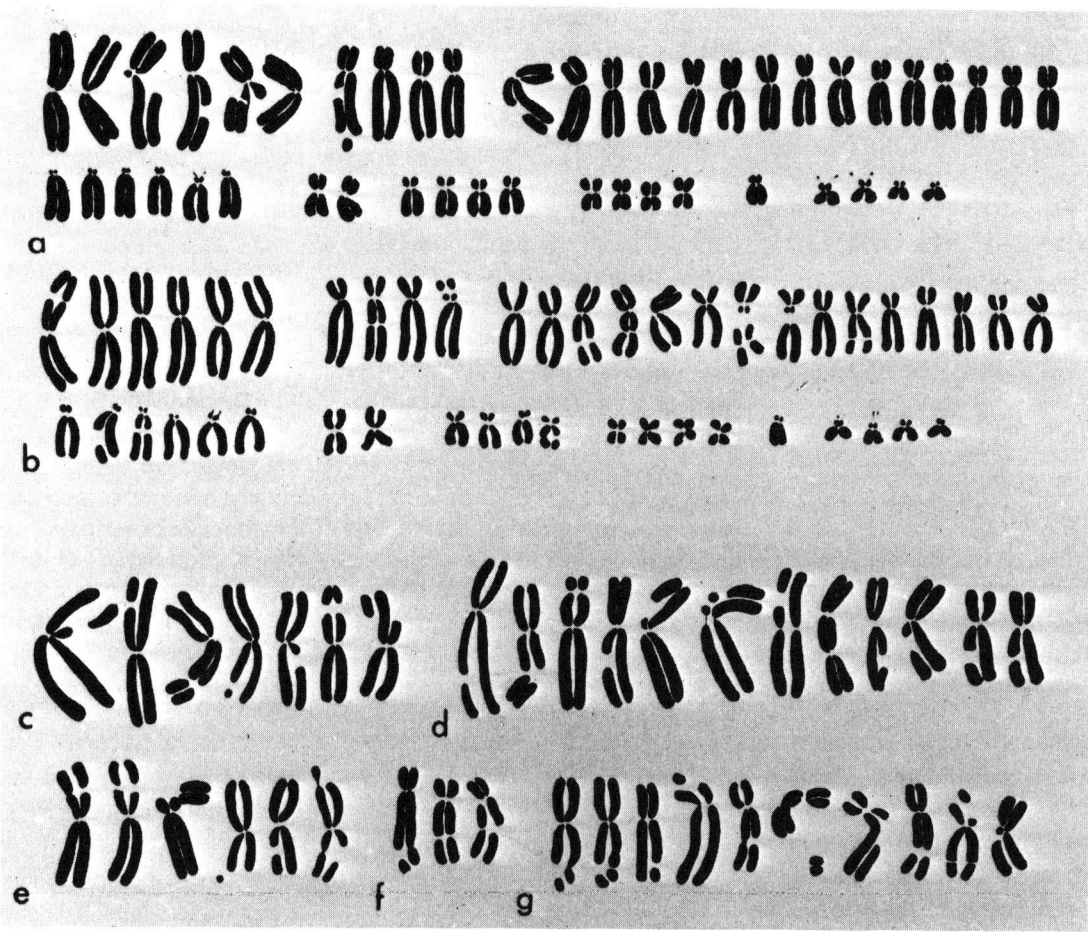

**Permanent Damage from Psychedelic Drugs.** In this karyotype, or chart of chromosomes, some of the chromosomes show breaks. This genetic damage can result from the use of psychedelic drugs.

health. However, some physicians do prescribe them to ease the anxiety and stress of those suffering from terminal illness.

## VENEREAL DISEASE DRUGS
*(See Chapter 77 on Venereal Disease)*

## VITAMINS
*(See Chapter 78 on Vitamins)*

# SUGGESTED DRUGS AND SUPPLIES FOR THE HOME

## Medical Supplies

Adhesive bandages, 1 box

Adhesive tape, 1 roll of 1 inch, 1 roll of 2 inch

Alcohol, 1 bottle of rubbing (70 percent alcohol, to be used as a skin antiseptic instead of iodine, etc.)

Applicators, 1 dozen with cotton tips

Bandages, 1 roll of 1-inch-wide gauze, 1 roll of 2-inch-wide gauze, 1 roll of 3-inch-wide (Ace semielastic)

Bedpan

Bell (so patient may summon aid if necessary)

Cotton, 1 large roll of sterile

Douche bag and attachments

Electric pad

Enamel basin (for preparing wet dressing; for bathing patient; etc.)

Enema bag and attachments

Flashlight

Gauze pads, 1 dozen sterile (paper wrapped) 2 X 2", 1 dozen sterile (paper wrapped) 4 X 4"

Glass drinking tube

Hydrogen peroxide, 1 bottle (for use as a skin antiseptic)

Icebag

Rubber pad (to go under sheets or to be used when wet dressings are being applied)

Rubber tubing, 2-foot length (for possible use as a tourniquet)

Scissors, 1 pair (preferably bandage scissors)

Steam inhalator and electrical attachments

Thermometers, 1 mouth, 1 rectal

Tweezers, 1 pair (for splinter removal)

Urinal

Vaseline, 1 tube or bottle of sterile

## Medicines*

Aspirin tablets, 1 bottle of 5 grains

Bicarbonate of soda, 1 box of powdered

Bicarbonate of soda tablets, 1 bottle of 10 grains

Boric acid, 1 box of powdered

Collyrium eyewash with eyecup, 1 bottle

Epsom salt, 1 box of powdered

Milk of magnesia, 1 bottle

Paregoric, 1 ounce bottle

Salt tablets, 1 bottle of 5 grains

Sodium perborate powder, 1 container (for mouthwash)

Talcum powder, 1 container of any bland type

Tincture of benzoin, 1 bottle

Witch hazel, 1 bottle

## Precautions

1. Every medication and bottle must be clearly labeled.

2. If label is not easily read, throw medication away.

3. All medications, no matter how mild, must be kept out of children's reach!

4. Read every label **twice** before giving medication.

5. Any poison or special medication should be under lock and key. Do **not** keep such a medication in your regular medicine cabinet where the whole family may get to it.

6. When in doubt as to the freshness of a medicine, throw it away.

7. Do **not** ever take a medication in the dark.

8. **Never** apply a hot/wet dressing unless it has been tested for intensity of heat by the patient himself. It is better too cool than too hot.

9. Do **not** go to sleep with an electric pad turned on.

10. Do **not** keep an icebag in place more than a half hour at a time.

*Please note that powerful medications such as strong sleeping tablets, narcotics, strong anticeptics such as iodine, and other special medications are **purposely** omitted from this list. Such drugs should be kept apart from the family medicine chest.

# CHAPTER 44

# MENTAL HEALTH AND DISEASE

*(See also Chapter 3 on Adolescence; Chapter 5 on Aging; Chapter 17 on Child Behavior; Chapter 35 on Inherited and Congenital Conditions; Chapter 45 on Nervous Diseases)*

## What is psychiatry?

Psychiatry is a branch of medicine devoted to the study, prevention, and treatment of disorders of the emotions, behavior, and the mind and is practiced by physicians who have completed several years of special training in the field. Some of the disorders treated by these doctors are associated with structural or chemical changes and are known as organic disorders. Others are the result of poor environmental adjustment and are known as functional disorders. Today there is evidence that many major mental illnesses, such as schizophrenia, may be both organic and functional in origin.

## What is psychology?

The biological science concerned with the study and evaluation of mental and emotional function.

## What is a psychologist?

A specially trained individual, usually not a physician, who has a Master's or Ph.D. degree in psychology. A psychologist may elect to teach, perform psychological testing, or engage in clinical practice that should be restricted to therapy of minor mental disorders.

## How common is mental illness?

Recent studies in the Western world place the incidence of mental disorders at approximately 15 percent of the population. The advances of the past thirty years have made it possible to obtain remission in the majority of patients who undergo appropriate psychotherapy.

## What are emotions?

They are the feelings of the human experience. The most common emotions are fear, love, hate, and anger. Anxiety is the fear of an unknown entity.

## What are neuroses?

They consist of a large number of functional disorders. Neuroses are commonly caused by internal conflicts, sometimes unrecognized or unconscious, which are manifested by anxiety, depression, phobias, or compulsions. These symptoms often control the personality of the people who suffer from them. Neurotic people are frequently described as being "high strung."

## What is the appropriate treatment for neuroses?

Psychotherapy aimed at resolving the patient's personal conflicts. Such therapy may be conducted by various mental health professionals, including psychiatrists, psychologists, and social workers. Newly developed drugs known as tranquilizers, given only under rigid medical supervision, may be helpful in relieving neurotic symptoms.

## What is neurasthenia?

Neurotic conflicts often manifest themselves by excessive fatigue in response to a slight exertion. There may be undue concern about the symptoms along with loss of appetite and consequent weight loss. Neurasthenic patients may also experience tension headaches, dizziness, insomnia, inability to concentrate, and depression. It is very im-portant for the psychiatrist to distinguish these patients from those suffering from a masked depression.

## What is meant by the term "nervous breakdown"?

This is a term used by lay people to refer to emotional or mental disorders.

## Can one have a "nervous breakdown" or become "insane" from overwork?

No, but bad work conditions can be a source of stress, and stress may precipitate an acute emotional crisis.

## Can a great disappointment or tragedy in one's life cause a nervous breakdown?

Losses and disappointments cause a form of depression known as grief or reactive depression, but they seldom lead to mental illness.

## What are psychoses?

These are major emotional and mental disorders that impair the person's ability to function at work, within his family, and in his social life. Psychoses are often associated with disorganized feelings, asocial behavior, an inability to concentrate, to think clearly, or to remember. Sometimes, the patient may experience hallucinations, the most common being those involving sight and hearing.

## Do neuroses often turn into psychoses?

There appears to be little or no relationship between the psychotic experience and neuroses.

## What is anxiety neurosis?

This is a form of emotional disorder characterized by excessive anxiety. Patients are irritable, apprehensive, tense, and many times overreact to routine life situations. Their sleep may be impaired. The sufferer from anxiety neurosis may also display physical manifestations such as trembling, rapid pulse, palpitation of the heart, excessive sweating, dizziness, and headaches. Gastrointestinal symptoms such as nausea, vomiting, or diarrhea may be present. While symptoms may occur in relation to obvious circumstances, often the attacks occur without an obvious cause. Along with physical symptoms, the anxiety neurotic has a severe sense of dread.

### What is insanity?

This term is important only for its legal significance. It implies that a person, as a result of his mental disability, may not be responsible for his actions. Psychiatrists who assist the legal profession usually determine whether a person is so impaired that he is incapable of distinguishing between right and wrong. Many patients who suffer from severe mental disorders may not be legally insane and therefore can be held responsible for their actions.

### What symptoms should alert a person to the need for psychiatric help?

a. Frequent or persistent depression.
b. Recurring anxiety and unfounded fears.
c. Irritability and uncontrolled temper.
d. Persistent fatigue.
e. Inability to carry on sustained work.
f. Frequent conflicts with one's associates.
g. Loss of appetite and progressive weight loss.
h. Frequent bouts of illness with no clear physical cause.

### Will seeing a psychiatrist help to prevent mental disorders?

In many instances, yes.

### Can one safely marry into a family in which a member is "insane"?

In general, one can say, yes. However, if several members of the family have experienced mental disturbances, there should be cause for

concern. Most disorders of a reactive type, and those that are related to a demonstrable organic cause, should not be regarded as deterrents to a marriage.

### What role does heredity play in mental disease?

Studies indicate that heredity plays some role in the transmission of major functional mental disorders. However, there is increased evidence that while a predisposition may exist, one would have to be exposed to serious environmental stresses in order to develop a full-blown disorder.

### What part does sex play in determining mental health?

Usually, sexual problems are the result, rather than the cause, of mental disorder. It should be stated that healthy sexual practices enhance the mental health of the individual.

### Does abuse in sexual practices cause disturbances in emotional health?

No.

### Does a lack of sex cause a disturbance in mental health?

In general, restricted sexual practices do not cause mental disturbances. In fact, celibacy is practiced by a great many people without apparent emotional trouble. Reactive problems arise in individuals whose sexual life, previously satisfactory, is impaired by life's events.

### How serious is the incidence of suicide?

Suicide represents a major problem in our society. The degree of emotional and mental impairment is not necessarily connected with suicidal intention, threats, and gestures. However, as a rule, people who talk about it and who have tried it constitute a serious risk. The expression of suicidal intention should always be taken seriously and treated by an expert professional.

### What is a compulsion neurosis?

Compulsions and obsessions are common neurotic symptoms. They are characterized by repetitive thoughts or actions that the patient is unable to control or overcome. A common compulsion is the repeated washing of one's hands when they are clean or excessive concern over cleanliness of one's body or home.

### What is the significance of an abnormal attachment to a parent, as in the case of a "mama's boy"?

People who show abnormal dependency on adults usually have not been able to mature emotionally into independence. They also may find it very difficult to adjust to common life situations.

### What is meant by the Oedipus complex?

An unconscious attachment of a son to his mother (the term originated in Greek mythology) usually associated with jealousy and fear of the father. An unresolved Oedipus complex may result in feelings of guilt and serious emotional conflict.

### What is meant by castration complex?

In psychoanalytic theory, it may be related to an unresolved Oedipal situation. It is manifested by anxiety about sex based upon a deep-seated fear of castration or inadequacy of the sexual organs.

### What are phobias?

Phobias are manifestations of neuroses and are based upon unreasonable fear of common objects or life situations. The most common phobias are claustrophobia (fear of closed-in spaces, such as elevators, tunnels, etc.) and agoraphobia (fear of open spaces).

### What is hypnotism?

Hypnotism is an altered sense of consciousness, which places the patient in a highly suggestible state.

Hypnotism often removes a patient's normal inhibitions. When performed by an experienced therapist, hypnotism can be of value in removing certain neurotic symptoms, or it may help in gathering information that the patient finds difficult to transmit when in a conscious state.

### Should hypnotism be performed by other than a trained mental health professional?

No. Hypnotic practices outside of medical therapy are highly objectionable as they may precipitate serious psychiatric disorder in a suggestible and susceptible individual.

### Is the use of tranquilizers helpful or dangerous for the emotionally ill person?

Tranquilizers, when used under strict medical supervision, can be very beneficial. However, it may be dangerous to continue them indefinitely because of the problems of addiction and tolerance. Powerful tranquilizing medications can also be used to commit suicide, and this risk must always be kept in mind when they are prescribed for emotionally ill patients.

### Is sleep necessary to mental health?

Recent studies indicate that sleep is essential to sustain mental health. Many psychiatric disorders have a tendency to impair the ability to sleep. Although it may be necessary to take sleeping pills during the acute phase of an illness, these medications should be discontinued as soon as possible.

### Is inability to sleep (insomnia) a serious symptom?

Persistent insomnia should be sufficient cause to seek psychiatric help.

### What is hysteria?

Suggestible patients often develop symptoms that have no basis in anatomical or medical fact. This reaction, frequently assuming a dramatic form, may involve the temporary loss of function of an arm or a leg or the senses of sight or hearing. The treatment for hysteria lies in solving the patient's underlying psychological conflict.

### What are psychosomatic symptoms and diseases?

These are a group of diseases of a physical character that are related primarily to emotional factors. Most common are some forms of high blood pressure, peptic ulcer, and colitis. This category also includes some of the so-called allergic conditions such as asthma, eczema, hives, and various conditions in which itching is a prominent symptom. Some physicians think that overactivity of the thyroid gland and some forms of diabetes may be psychosomatic in origin. Many headaches, including migraine, and certain forms of arthritis have been included in this category. The treatment of psychosomatic illnesses requires a combination of medical and psychological treatment.

### Are emotional symptoms imaginary?

No, they are *real* symptoms. This misconception may stem from the impression that if a symptom has no physical cause it is imaginary.

### Should a depressed person consult a psychiatrist?

Depression is a universal experience and very often does not require special psychiatric care. Should the symptoms persist, the person should consult a psychiatrist. He may discover and treat the underlying cause whether it is related to the patient's environment or to his makeup.

### When is psychiatric hospitalization indicated?

Serious acute psychiatric symptoms are best treated in a hospital. They may require only a short stay, often in a psychiatric unit of a general hospital. The average length of stay is about two weeks. If recovery is not complete within that period of time, intensive office psychotherapy or long-term psychiatric hospitalization may be indicated.

### How frequently is long-term psychiatric hospitalization advocated?

This form of residential treatment is very uncommon today because of recent advances in therapy and management. Most mental disorders are controlled before they achieve a chronic form. However, custodial and institutional care may be necessary for some patients suffering from organic mental symptoms or for those who exhibit violent or dangerous behavior.

### What is psychotherapy?

Treatment of emotional, behavioral, or mental illness by a qualified therapist. It can be of several varieties, depending upon the theories used by a particular therapist.

a. *Supportive therapy* is related to the specific problem at hand and may be carried out by intelligent, sympathetic people such as relatives, close friends, a member of the clergy, a family physician, etc.

b. *Uncovering therapy* is aimed at deeper and more persistent problems and is carried out by trained and highly experienced psychiatrists.

### What is the main aim of psychotherapy?

To bring to the patient's awareness the psychological conflicts that are bothering him. As a result of this newly gained knowledge, the symptoms decrease or disappear.

### What is cognitive psychotherapy?

A technique that helps people understand themselves better, adjust to their difficulties, and become more efficient in dealing with their problems and with the people with whom they have contact. The objective also includes the development of better values and standards.

### What is psychoanalysis?

It is a specialized form and technique of psychotherapy. Psychoanalysis is aimed at allowing the patient to become aware of the unconscious traits that underlie his personality and his difficulties. By this technique one hopes to eliminate the symptoms and improve the patient's reactions. Analysis operates solely through the patient, the therapist usually assuming a passive role. Dreams and free associations are used as a way to reach the unconscious.

### What is group therapy?

A method of psychiatric treatment in which a number of people meet under the leadership of a therapist and are treated together as one group.

### What are the objectives of group therapy?

Essentially the same as for individual therapy. Group therapy is particularly indicated when a person has difficulty in dealing with others. The group situation improves this function. It also helps by making available to the patient the experience of others so that he does not feel alone in his illness. Another advantage of group therapy is that it is less expensive than individual therapy.

### What are the disadvantages of group therapy?

The patient may find it difficult to express extremely personal problems. Also, he may feel that the attention of the psychotherapist is not exclusively aimed at his problems.

### How long does it take for psychotherapy to work?

Results depend upon many factors. After the patient and therapist have established a goal, the duration of the relationship is usually related to the severity of the disorder and frequency of treatment. Following completion of successful psychotherapy, many patients remain in contact with their therapist for follow-up care. This period may extend from a few months to two years or more.

### Is psychotherapy expensive?

Psychotherapy is considered by many to be expensive, but when one considers the amount of time that must be expended to get a result, it is not actually expensive. A major operative procedure, costing a large sum of money, lasts but a few hours. Psychotherapy, costing less, may require hundreds of hours of intensive treatment.

### Is there any surgical treatment for mental disease?

In the past, the surgical destruction of small areas of brain tissue (lobotomy) was advocated for certain types of mental illness. This operation has been abandoned because of the new advances in psychiatry.

### What are the different forms of psychoses?

The major psychoses include:
a. Schizophrenia.
b. Manic-depressive disorders.
c. Psychotic depression.
d. Paranoid disorders.
e. Depressions of the middle-aged.
f. Senile psychoses.
g. Arteriosclerotic psychoses.
h. Paresis (syphilitic psychosis).
i. Psychosis due to head injuries.
j. Psychosis due to brain tumors.

### What is depression?

Depression is a mental disorder manifested by a lowering of mood and spirits and a gloomy outlook. It is often associated with anxiety, tension, and agitation. The patient complains of lack of energy, lack of interest in things, inability to perform his usual activities, and a wish to remain isolated. These feelings are often associated with inability to sleep, loss of appetite, and weight loss. Under severe conditions, suicide becomes a distinct possibility.

### What are the different forms of depression?

Some depressions are manifestations of a neurosis and may arise as a response to circumstances. These are known as *reactive depressions*. In other cases, depression may be part of a change in the patient's biochemical makeup, such as the psychotic depressions of the manic-depressive disorders.

### What is involutional melancholia?

Until recently, the depression of middle age was thought to be a distinct entity, occurring in a person who was compulsive and fastidious and who was undergoing the hormonal changes of the fifth decade of life. Today this condition is not considered to be a specific illness.

### What is the treatment for depression?

a. Safeguard the patient who has expressed suicidal thoughts. This is best accomplished through short-term psychiatric hospitalization.
b. The administration of antidepressant medications, which act chemically upon the brain, such as lithium.
c. If the above two methods fail to achieve a favorable result, *electroshock therapy* may be indicated.
d. Psychotherapy should follow any one of the above forms of treatment.

### What is electroshock therapy?

Electroshock therapy is a form of physical treatment in which a small amount of electrical current is applied to the brain for a fraction of a second. The shock leads to a brief period of unconsciousness, following which there may be mild, temporary confusion, which will clear within three to five weeks. Shock therapy results in remission of symptoms in the great majority of cases.

## In what other conditions might electroshock therapy prove beneficial?

Severe forms of anxiety neurosis, manic states, and some forms of schizophrenia, especially the catatonic and acute types.

## Where can electroshock therapy be given?

In a psychiatrist's office, in an ambulatory clinic setting, or in a hospital.

## What are the manic-depressive disorders?

They are states in which the patient has wide swings in mood, going from a high manic phase to a low depressed phase or vice versa. During the manic phase, there is incessant restlessness, continuous talking, exhilarated mood with euphoria, and sleeplessness. The depressed phase has symptoms akin to those of any depression, as described above. Symptoms of the manic-depressive disorder vary markedly in degree and in duration.

## What is the outlook for a manic-depressive disorder?

The patient will recover from the episode and remain well for a shorter or longer period of time. Those whose symptoms recur within months are known as *rapid-cycling* patients, while those who go years between episodes are known as *slow-cycling* patients. Between episodes of the illness, patients show no outward manifestation of psychiatric disorder.

## What medication should people take who have had a manic-depressive disorder?

Lithium. If taken indefinitely under the supervision of a psychiatrist, it may prevent future relapses.

## Will most patients who have had an episode of a manic-depressive disorder have a recurrence?

Not if they take appropriate medications continually.

## Should a person on lithium still seek psychiatric therapy?

Yes. Such treatment will allow him to recognize the nature of his illness and will help to forestall a recurrence.

## Does pregnancy or having a baby cause mental disease?

Having a baby, by itself, is no specific cause for mental disorder. The stress of the pregnancy and of the delivery may, however, act as a nonspecific stimulus in triggering an emotional reaction that might have been latent.

## What is a postpartum psychosis?

In rare instances following confinement, a woman may develop an acute psychotic episode that may resemble schizophrenia, a manic state, or a depression. Today many psychiatrists think that such psychoses are not specific to the period following childbirth but are merely triggered by it.

## What is schizophrenia?

Schizophrenia is a mental disorder manifested by disturbances in thinking, impaired relation to reality associated with ideas of persecution, and auditory (hearing) hallucination. In its natural history, this psychosis usually first affects people of high school age. It recurs intermittently during one's life, especially during periods of emotional stress. Schizophrenia, which was previously known as dementia praecox, is of unknown origin, although there is strong evidence that it may be related to a derangement in the chemical makeup of one's brain.

## What is the treatment for schizophrenia?

Schizophrenia is treated today mainly by psychotherapy and by drug therapy. The condition may require repeated short-term hospitalization. The outlook for this condition has improved by involving the family in what is known as "family therapy." If one can discover the stresses that trigger the psychotic episodes, the schizophrenic individual can be helped through the avoidance of those stresses.

## What is the outlook for schizophrenia?

Schizophrenia is a chronic illness manifested by relapses and recurrences. Drug maintenance therapy and patient cooperation, however, may result in control of the symptoms over prolonged periods of time.

## What are paranoid reactions?

These are mental disorders in which the patient experiences ideas of persecution or grandeur. These false beliefs, known as delusions, lead the patient to the thought that people are out to harm him. His reality is distorted to prove these delusions. This disorder is often referred to by laymen as "persecution complex." Many serious psychiatric disorders are associated with paranoid delusions.

## What is the outlook for the paranoid patient?

In most instances, the symptoms persist and become chronic. For these people the outlook is poor, and they tend to retain their disturbed mental state. In a smaller number of cases, the condition is temporary, especially when it is associated with a toxic, physical disorder that is transient.

## Is there any specific treatment for the average patient with paranoia?

No.

## What does I.Q. mean?

The letters stand for Intelligence Quotient. This is a numerical figure arrived at by a ratio of *mental age,* as obtained by intelligence tests, to *actual age* of the person. The average Intelligence Quotient lies between 90 and 110. Mental deficiency lies below this level.

## What is meant by the term mental deficiency?

Mental deficiency—also known as developmental disability, mental retardation, or feeble-mindedness—implies a defect in understanding or comprehension, and a handicap in learning ability. The different degrees of impairment are known as idiot, imbecile, moron, or mentally retarded. The disorder, essentially organic in nature, may be related to injuries to the nervous system that occurred before birth, at birth, or after birth. Thus, associated signs of injury to the brain such as paralysis, abnormal movements, and occasionally cerebral palsy may be noted. The head may appear to be unusually small or unusually large, often because of increased accumulation of excess fluid within the head.

## What is Down's syndrome?

Also known as mongolism, this is a type of mental deficiency in which the child has oriental features. It has been clearly established on the basis of research that Down's syndrome is a genetic disorder related to a defect in the chromosomes and affected by heredity. Children with Down's syndrome are moderately retarded, usually passive and pleasant, and, to a limited extent, teachable. Some children with Down's syndrome may die young as a result of an overwhelming infection or a disorder of metabolism.

## What is idiocy?

This is the lowest form of mental development, easily recognizable early in life. The mental age never develops beyond two years. The I.Q. is below twenty-five. Physical deformities may be present, and convulsions are frequent. The idiot may never learn to speak. He can do very little for himself and requires constant supervision. Idiots occur about once in every thirty-five hundred births.

## What are imbeciles?

In this form of mental deficiency, the I.Q. falls between twenty-five and fifty. Speech is limited, learning is poor, but imbeciles can be taught simple tasks. Mental age ranges from two to seven years. Imbeciles occur about once in every fifteen hundred births.

## Do idiots and imbeciles require institutionalization?

In the past, it was thought that these children were cared for best in a specialized institution, but recently they have been considered for placement within willing families or in small, residential homes. This has led to a betterment in their life adjustment. In considering the placement of such a child in an institution, parents should give primary consideration to the welfare of the child.

## What is a moron?

This term is applied to the group whose I.Q. ranges from fifty to seventy. Again there is delayed development. These children look like any others, and there is no gross anatomical malformation. Usually the impairment is detected in school because they are unable to keep up with their schoolwork.

## Into what category do children with an I.Q. of seventy to ninety fall?

This level is considered to be mild retardation. These children can fit into society and lead a useful life, providing they receive adequate training and preparation.

## Is mental deficiency inherited?

Most mental deficiency is accidental. It occurs as a result of trouble at birth or follows acquired illness. There are, however, a few cases in which mental deficiency is inherited. A study of the unborn child's chromosomes in the mother's uterus allows the physician to diagnose some of the hereditary mental deficiency conditions.

## What is an idiot savant?

An individual of low mental development who may disclose a remarkable talent in one direction such as memory or mathematical calculation.

## What are the most common causes of mental deficiency?

a. Hereditary disorder.
b. A mother's illness during pregnancy such as German measles, the use of drugs, or excessive alcohol.
c. Difficulties arising from the delivery or from complications of pregnancy and delivery.
d. Injury of or infection in the brain during infancy or early childhood.
e. Inborn metabolic disorders as the result of abnormal chemical substances that have accumulated in the blood. One form is known as *phenylketonuria* or PKU. (See Chapter 35, on Inherited and Congenital Conditions.) This abnormal substance can be discovered by urinary tests, and the condition can be corrected by suitable diet. In these cases, brain damage can be prevented.

## Is there any treatment for mental deficiency?

Management is directed toward the full utilization of the child's resources. It is known that children with milder degrees of mental deficiency may be suitably trained to carry on useful work in society.

## Can mental deficiency be prevented?

No, but much can be done to diminish its incidence:

a. By following the instructions of one's obstetrician religiously. This will include the avoidance of excess smoking, eliminating the use of drugs, imbibing only small amounts of alcohol, eating a nourishing diet, and getting sufficient sleep during pregnancy.

b. By obtaining genetic counseling before pregnancy if there is a familial history of mental deficiency.

## STRESS

### What is the concept of stress?

The human body has within it certain innate mechanisms that allow it to protect itself from outside stresses. These stresses may be physical, such as excess heat or cold, or emotional, such as impending danger. The reaction of the body to the stress is called "adaptation." Adaptation is a complex mechanism involving the nervous system and the glandular (endocrine) system. These adaptation patterns vary, depending upon the nature of the stress and the basic character of the individual. In general, adaptational response to physical stress is physical; the adaptational response to an emotional stress is both psychological and physical. These latter responses may be expressed as an emotional pattern—anger, fear, disgust, etc.

### What are some physical stress reactions?

One of the most important is the reaction to a sudden or severe injury. The body may react to such an injury by a generalized response known as shock, a state in which the blood content of the body is redistributed to those organs that need it the most. However, like many adaptational mechanisms, if the shock is permitted to persist too long, it may lose its ability to act as a protective mechanism and may lead to death.

Another common physical adaptational reaction to a physical stress is allergy. The allergic response, whether in the form of hay fever, asthma, or hives, is the body's defense against a foreign substance (i.e., a pollen). However, when the protective response is too extreme (as in bronchial asthma), the reaction may be more serious than the stress that originally produced it.

### What are some emotional stress reactions?

Just as a physical stress (pollen) can provoke a physical reaction (asthma), so can a psychological stress (impending danger) provoke a psychological reaction (fear). The adaptational reaction of fear is biologically designed to better prepare the person for the danger. Thus, when confronted with danger, the adrenal glands pour forth certain secretions that better enable the body to withstand the stress. However, the psychological elements of fear may become so overwhelming as to completely incapacitate the individual, while the physical elements, if they persist long enough, may actually cause physical illness. Some physicians call these physical illnesses, which result from psychological stresses, psychosomatic diseases.

### What role does the stress mechanism play in health?

Certain of the stress reactions are essential for health. For example, the allergic reaction so troublesome to hay fever sufferers is the same mechanism as the one by which we develop immunity to certain diseases, either through actual exposure (you can have measles only once) or by inoculation (polio vaccine). Similarly, in any physical illness, the production of certain hormones by the adrenal gland is the means the body uses to fight disease, just as the doctor may fight disease when he prescribes drugs or medications.

### What part does the stress mechanism play in physical disease?

It is thought that impaired adaptational responses, whether overactive or underactive, may result in actual physical disease. Allergy, as mentioned above, may be an example of a physical adaptational response that has gone askew. High blood pressure, on the other hand, is considered by many to be the result of an emotional adaptational response becoming overactive. When a person becomes excited, his pressure rises and he becomes more affected. However, if excitement persists too long, his high blood pressure becomes fixed and he becomes physically ill.

On the other hand, the adaptational organs in certain illnesses react as though they were exhausted. For example, the adrenal glands may excrete an insufficient amount of hormone (cortisone). Under such circumstances, the body may react defectively, and diseases such as arthritis or colitis may result. The administration of the adrenal hormone (cortisone) will help the patient return to normal.

### Is the stress reaction a helpful or harmful one in maintaining health?

This will depend upon the severity of the stress and the intensity of the adaptational reaction. Basically, the stress reaction is beneficial since it is the biological system of self-protection. However, if the adaptational system becomes either overactive or exhaustive, it may produce actual physical or mental disease.

### What are the "so-called" adaptation diseases"?

They are those brought about through constant exposure to chronic stress.

**What is the relation of the stress mechanisms to the so-called "psychosomatic disorders"?**
Psychosomatic disorders are considered by many physicians to be the physical results of prolonged emotional tension. Such diseases as high blood pressure, peptic ulcer, and overactivity of the thyroid gland fall into this category. Other diseases such as arthritis, colitis, and allergies, are considered to be the effect of underactivity of the adaptational system through exhaustion.

**What role is stress supposed to play in the aging process?**
It is thought by many investigators that aging is in some measure the result of frequent and continued insult that the body suffers over a prolonged period of time. Hardening of the arteries, for example, may result from prolonged high blood pressure, which may be an adaptational response. The endocrine glands, especially, tend to become exhausted by frequent stresses and strains of life, and their underactivity tends to accelerate the aging process. It would appear that to prolong life, one should avoid excessive stresses of any type.

# CHAPTER 45

# NERVOUS DISEASES

## (The Brain, Spinal Cord, and Nerves)

*(See also Chapter 35 on Inherited and Congenital Conditions; Chapter 46 on Neurosurgery; Chapter 53 on Physical Therapy and Rehabilitation; Chapter 77 on Venereal Disease)*

**What is the structure of the nervous system?**

It is made up of the following:

a. The central nervous system, which includes the brain and spinal cord.

b. The peripheral nervous system, which is composed of nerves that leave the spinal cord and go to muscles (motor nerves) and nerves that carry sensation from the limbs and body (sensory nerves) to the spinal cord.

c. The autonomic (sympathetic) nervous system, composed of nerves that regulate the bowels, bladder, blood vessels, and functions of the body, such as sweating, heart rate, blood pressure, etc.

**What are the cranial nerves?**

These are twelve pairs of nerves that extend from the brain through various openings in the skull and supply various structures in the face, head, and in certain, organs.

**What are the organs supplied by the various cranial nerves?**

a. Cranial nerve I (olfactory) is concerned with the sense of smell. Damage to this nerve may result in loss of taste as well as smell, since recognition of flavor is an olfactory function.

b. Cranial nerve II (optic) is connected with the eyes and has to do with vision.

c. Cranial nerves III, IV, and VI control the movements of the eyes.

d. Cranial nerve V (trigeminal) has to do with sensation in the face and the eye and controls the muscles that take part in chewing.

e. Cranial nerve VII (facial) controls the muscles of the face, eyelids, and forehead and carries taste from the anterior two-thirds of the tongue.

f. Cranial nerve VIII (acoustic and vestibular) has to do with hearing and the sense of balance.

g. Cranial nerve IX (glossopharyngeal) carries sensation from the throat, taste from the posterior third of the tongue, and is involved in the act of swallowing.

h. Cranial nerve X (vagus) goes to the heart, stomach, and intestinal tract. It is also concerned with swallowing and speech. Paralysis on one side results in hoarseness; paralysis on both sides results in the loss of voice.

i. Cranial nerve XI (spinal accessory) controls certain muscles in the neck and shoulders.

j. Cranial nerve XII (hypoglossal) controls the tongue.

**What are the spinal nerve roots?**

The spinal cord has pairs of nerves, called roots, emerging at regular intervals from both sides of the cord. On each side there is a posterior branch for sensation and an anterior one for motor control. These roots combine to form the peripheral nerves, which are then distributed outside the spinal column to various organs and structures. These nerves control all the muscles and glands and also carry sensation from all over the body.

**Generally speaking, how does the nervous system function?**

The nervous system is composed of nerve cells and supporting tissue centered in the brain and spinal cord, with widespread extensions all through the body. Its function is the transmission and coordination of stimuli and their integration into the phenomena that make up mental activity and behavior. Impulses conveying sensory impressions such as touch, taste, hearing, sight, and smell are carried to the brain along pathways called afferent nerves. Glandular secretion and muscular activity, on the other hand, are achieved by impulses that originate in the central nervous system and travel in an outward direction along pathways called efferent nerves. The orderliness that characterizes normal human activity is rendered possible only because of the high degree of organization of the nervous system. This fact becomes apparent when a part of this elaborate system is disturbed by a disease process.

## NEURITIS *(Neuropathy)*

**What is neuritis?**

Neuritis is a term used to denote damage to a nerve regardless of the cause. Most authorities prefer the term *neuropathy*, unless the damage is of an infectious origin.

**What are the causes of neuropathy (neuritis)?**

a. An accident causing direct injury to a nerve.

b. Pressure upon a nerve due to a poorly healing fracture, from bone fragments of the fracture, from scar tissue, or from a tumor that is growing and pressing upon the nerve.

c. Pressure upon a nerve as it exits from the spinal column, as in arthritis or in the case of a herniated disk.

d. There can be many causes of neuropathy of a diffuse type. It may be part of a deficiency disease, such as one encounters with lack of vitamins (as in beriberi); it may be seen with chronic alcoholism or in cases of advanced diabetes. Various toxic agents, such as lead, may affect the peripheral nerves and produce neuropathy. Finally, various generalized infections of the body can affect the peripheral nerves.

## What is polyneuritis?

A term used to designate a condition in which many of the peripheral nerves are involved.

## What are some of the symptoms of neuropathy?

a. Tingling, described as pins and needles, and numbness in the hands and feet or in the region supplied by the nerve.
b. Muscular weakness and wasting of the muscles in the involved area.
c. Absent or reduced muscle reflexes in the area supplied by the involved nerves.
d. Loss of sensation in the affected part.
e. Pain, although this is not necessarily a constant finding in neuritis.

## What is brachial neuropathy?

It is a term applied to a painful nerve affliction of an arm. It may be caused by a herniated disk in the neck region, osteoarthritis compressing a nerve root, cervical rib (a congenital anomaly), or it may follow fracture of a lower cervical vertebra, the shoulder, or the upper arm.

## What is sciatica?

This is a general term used when pain radiates down the back of the thigh and leg. It is frequently caused by a herniated disk, osteoarthritis, or a narrow vertebral canal. It may also occur as a result of injury or diabetes.

## What is a herniated intervertebral disk?

See Chapter 46, on Neurosurgery.

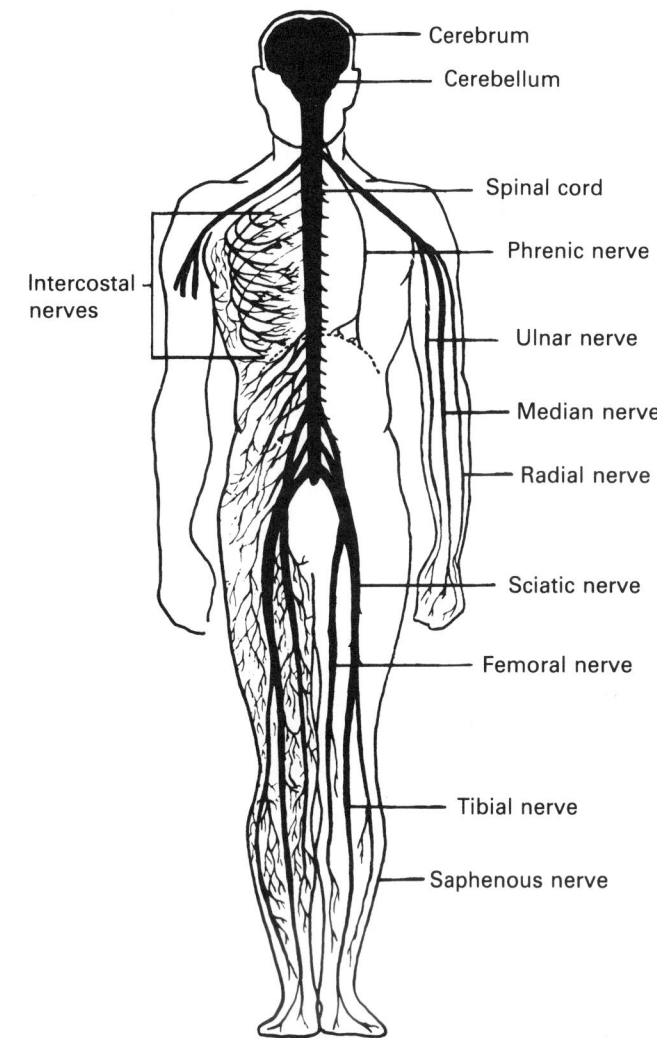

**The Nervous System.** *This diagram shows the brain and its nerve attachments. Every part of the body is supplied by nerves, and all of these nerves connect with the brain. Some nerves carry impulses toward the brain: these are called afferent nerves. Other nerves carry impulses away from the brain: these are called efferent nerves. Nerve tissue shows very little tendency to regenerate once it has been destroyed; thus we see relatively little recovery in people who have been paralyzed for more than several months.*

## What is trigeminal neuralgia (tic douloureux)?

It is a disorder of the fifth cranial nerve, the trigeminal, which supplies the face. This is a very painful condition characterized by episodes of sudden excruciating pain in the face coming in paroxysms and lasting for a short time. The attacks may be brought on by chewing, talking, exposure to cold, or by touching a sensitive point on the face or the mouth. These paroxysms of pain have a ten-dency to recur over a period of time varying from weeks to months. Effective relief of pain may be obtained in some patients with Dilantin or Tegretol. Should medication fail to relieve pain, other procedures may become necessary to perform. Destruction of the nerve can frequently be accomplished through the use of radio-frequency current administered through a needle placed in the region from which the nerve originates at the base of the skull. In the exceptional case, it may become necessary to sever the nerve surgically in order to produce lasting relief of pain. This procedure, however, leaves the patient with a permanently numb face. (See Chapter 46, on Neurosurgery.)

### What is meant by "shingles"?

This disease is also called herpes zoster. It is an inflammation of one of the posterior roots of the spinal cord. It is characterized by severe, persistent burning pain and a skin eruption of small blisters along the course of the nerve.

### What causes shingles?

It is believed to be caused by a virus, closely related to the one producing chickenpox.

### What is the course of shingles?

The pain may be very severe and may last from a few to many weeks or months. In most cases, it subsides by itself.

### What is the treatment for shingles?

There is no known specific treatment to cure this disease. Pain-relieving medications may be required. The great majority of patients get well by themselves.

### What is Bell's palsy (facial paralysis)?

It is an inflammation of the facial nerve resulting in paralysis of half of the face. The face and mouth sag on the affected side, and the eye fails to close completely. It may occur at any age and affect either sex.

### What is the cause of facial paralysis?

The cause is not known, but many people attribute it to having been exposed to a draft over a prolonged period of time.

### What is the course of facial paralysis?

It usually lasts for two to three months and then has a tendency to clear up by itself.

### Is complete recovery from facial paralysis usually the ultimate outcome?

Most cases make a near-complete recovery, but a small proportion of people are left with some permanent weakness of the involved side of the face.

### What is the treatment for facial paralysis?

Since the eye fails to close completely, it should be protected by wearing glasses that enclose the entire eye or by placing a shield over the eye. Electrical stimulation is often applied to the weak facial muscles. The value of this form of therapy is questionable. Steroids (cortisone, etc.) given from the outset may protect the nerve from permanent damage.

## CEREBRAL PALSY

### What is cerebral palsy?

This is not a single disease but a group of neurological disorders affecting children and beginning at birth. Children with cerebral palsy have difficulty in walking and may have many involuntary movements of the limbs and muscles of the face. It often affects speech and makes it blurred and difficult to understand. There may be no mental impairment, or mental impairment may, in some cases, be severe. The muscular condition is characterized by a stiffness or spasticity of the limbs, resulting in an awkward or stiff-legged gait.

### What causes cerebral palsy?

It is thought that a difficult labor, an excessively prolonged labor, or lack of oxygen to the unborn infant during labor may be the cause of certain cases. Some cases are due to actual injury to the brain during delivery. Others are due to a disorder within the germ cells that is passed on to the infant; that is, in some there is a hereditary basis. Some cases are thought to be the result of illness in the mother during the first twelve weeks of pregnancy. Also, certain cases are thought to be due to cycts of the brain with which the child is born.

### Is there any effective medical treatment for cerebral palsy?

Yes. Children with cerebral palsy can be greatly benefited by persistent and prolonged education and other physical measures aimed toward rehabilitation and better control of muscles.

### Is there any effective surgical treatment for cerebral palsy?

Yes. There are a large number of operative procedures performed upon the muscles, tendons, and bones that can be very helpful in aiding the locomotion of a patient with cerebral palsy. Some of these operations relieve muscle spasm; others relieve the contractures of jonts that are so characteristic of this disease. Through modern reconstructive and rehabilitative surgery, many children with cerebral palsy who were formerly unable to walk can now get about in fairly satisfactory fashion. Also, it has recently been discovered that certain nerve pathways in the base of the brain may be responsible for some of the spastic conditions associated with cerebral palsy, and certain neurological surgical procedures are being developed to sever these pathways and thus relieve some of the spasm associated with this condition.

### Should children with cerebral palsy be sent to special schools if possible?

Yes. The rehabilitation methods being used today are a striking advance over former years. Excellent results are now being obtained by special educators in this particular field of rehabilitation.

**Does cerebral palsy get worse as the child grows older, and does it result in premature death?**

No. The children tend to improve as they reach adulthood, and many of these people lead normal, healthy lives.

## HYDROCEPHALUS
*(See Chapter 46 on Neurosurgery)*

## BRAIN TUMORS

**Are brain tumors common?**

Yes. The brain is a frequent site of tumor formation.

**What symptoms do brain tumors cause?**

a. Persistent and recurring headaches.
b. Progressiver weakness of an arm or leg or perhaps more than one limb at a time.
c. Disturbances in sensation, such as numbness.
d. Impairment of vision, such as double vision or loss of sight in one eye.
e. Dizziness or vertigo.
f. Convulsions.
g. Sudden episodes of headache and vomiting.

**Are most headaches indicative of a brain tumor?**

Absolutely not. Headaches alone, unaccompanied by some of the other symptoms listed above, are rarely caused by brain tumors.

**How are brain tumors diagnosed?**

A careful examination is first performed by either a neurologist or neurosurgeon, who will then obtain x rays of the skull and a CAT scan. This latter test is extremely sensitive and can usually detect a tumor undetectable by any other means.

These studies can be performed without hospitalization.

**Are brain tumors ever curable?**

Yes, some forms are. (See Chapter 46, on Neurosurgery.)

## ENCEPHALITIS

**What is encephalitis?**

An acute inflammation of the brain.

**What are some of the symptoms of encephalitis?**

Headache, fever, vomiting, paralysis, delirium, convulsions, stupor, and in some cases, coma.

**What causes encephalitis?**

Any one of a number of viruses. It may also occur as a complication of measles, whooping cough, or mumps. Infrequently it may occur with severe infections such as pneumonia and typhoid fever, or as a toxic reaction accompanying any disease with prolonged high fever.

**Is encephalitis ever seen in an epidemic form?**

Yes, most often during war periods and in war camps. It is also seen in localized areas involving a town or city.

**What is the treatment of encephalitis?**

Unfortunately, there is no specific treatment.

**What is the outcome of encephalitis?**

The majority of patients will recover completely. However, when the disease exists in epidemic form, there may be a considerable initial mortality. There may also be partial recovery in some patients who will be left with serious mental deficiencies.

**Is encephalitis sometimes called "sleeping sickness"?**

Yes.

**Does encephalitis ever lead to the development of symptoms years after the acute attack?**

Yes. Certain people who have recovered from encephalitis may develop tremors, palsies, and various other disorders later on.

## MENINGITIS

**What is meningitis?**

An infection of the coverings of the brain and spinal cord.

**What are the symptoms of meningitis?**

The rather abrupt onset of fever, severe headache, stiff neck, and, often, coma. On tapping the spine, inflammation may be discovered in the spinal fluid, and examination of the spinal fluid under the microscope will reveal inflammatory cells or even the germ that has caused the meningitis.

**What are the various causes of meningitis?**

Some are caused by infection with pus-forming bacteria; others may be due to an infection spreading from the middle ear or the sinuses. Other types of acute meningitis are caused by viruses. There are still other types of meningitis occurring with tuberculosis and syphilis.

**How is the diagnosis of meningitis made definitely?**

By tapping the spine and analyzing the spinal fluid.

**What is the treatment for meningitis?**

This would depend completely upon the causative agent. Those types caused by the pus-forming bacteria can be successfully treated with the antibiotics or with the sulfa drugs. Most of the types caused by viruses must be treated symptomatically.

Special treatment is now available

for meningitis caused by tuberculosis or syphilis.

## Can meningitis be cured?

Yes. The great majority of cases can now be cured by the newer drugs that are available.

## SYPHILIS OF THE NERVOUS SYSTEM

### How does syphilis affect the nervous system?

In former years, syphilis was a common cause of diseases of the nervous system. Modern treatment of syphilis has been so successful that this is a rare disease today. One variety, still seen occasionally, is syphilitic meningitis.

### What is pareses (general paralysis)?

This was a disease encountered much more frequently years ago when syphilis involved the brain itself. It resulted chiefly in a mental disorder.

### What is locomotor ataxia (tabes)?

This is a disease in which syphilis mainly affects the spinal cord and leads to a staggering gait.

### Can syphilis of the nervous system be treated effectively today?

Yes. The antibiotics are very effective in treating this disease if it is diagnosed during its earlier stages.

## CEREBROVASCULAR ACCIDENTS ("Strokes")

### What are cerebrovascular accidents?

These are commonly called strokes, or aopolexy. These conditions are the result of a more or less abrupt interruption of the blood supply to some area of the brain.

### What happens when a person has a stroke?

The patient develops one of the following conditions:

a. The closure of a blood vessel in the brain due to a clot (thrombosis).
b. A blood clot from elsewhere in the body is carried to a blood vessel in the brain, thus blocking the vessel.
c. One of the blood vessels in the brain ruptures, causing hemmorhage.

### What is a cerebral thrombosis?

A form of stroke in which the artery, which is the seat of arteriosclerosis, becomes progressively narrower through thickening of its wall. Eventually, complete closure of the vessel takes place and blood flow is interrupted. The area of brain normally supplied by that blood vessel will degenerate and die. Usually, paralysis of one or more limbs is found on the opposite side of the brain (hemiplegia). Loss of speech will also occur if the thrombosis is on the dominant hemisphere, which is usually the left side of the brain in a right-handed person and the right side of the brain in a left-handed person.

### Are the symptoms of cerebral thrombosis ever caused by narrowing and hardening (arteriosclerosis) of the carotid arteries in the neck?

Yes. The carotid arteries, which carry blood to the front half of the brain, are most frequently involved. For symptoms to develop, the carotid artery would have to be approximately 80 percent narrowed.

### What is a "small" stroke?

This refers to an interruption in the flow of blood to an area of the brain resulting from a condition that lasts from a few minutes to twenty-four hours and is followed by recovery. Such an episode is too short to cause much permanent brain dam-

age and is referred to as a transient ischemic attack. If, however, the condition lasts longer than twenty-four hours, a small amount of brain tissue may die. This dead area of the brain is called an infarct.

### What is ischemia?

Decreased or interrupted flow of blood through an artery.

### Can several transient ischemic attacks occur without producing any permanent brain damage?

Yes.

### Is it possible to predict the outcome following a "small" stroke?

No. It is impossible to determine initially if the episode will be transient or will become permanent. It has been estimated that nearly 75 percent of patients with a complete stroke have a history of transient ischemic attacks. In other words, a warning of a potential catastrophe occurs in most cases.

### What, if anything, can be done to prevent such a catastrophe from occurring?

See Chapter 46, on Neurosurgery.

### What is cerebral embolism?

A condition in which an artery of the brain becomes blocked by a blood clot originating from some distant site.

### What symptoms develop from a cerebral embolus?

If the embolus is small, a transient ischemic attack with full recovery usually takes place. If the clot occludes a larger blood vessel, there may be loss of consciousness and complete paralysis, usually on one side of the body. If the dominant side of the brain is involved, there will be loss of speech (aphasia).

### Can anything be done for such a patient?

See Chapter 46, on Neurosurgery.

## What causes cerebral hemorrhage?

This occurs when a blood vessel within the brain ruptures. Stroke is most common in people with high blood pressure or in a disease where bleeding takes place. If a large blood vessel is involved, the patient may die rather quickly. If the blood vessel is small, a small area of the brain may be damaged, and the patient often makes a good recovery.

## Can a hemorrhage in the brain be treated surgically?

See Chapter 46, on Neurosurgery.

## Are there other forms of cerebral hemorrhage?

Yes. Bleeding into the subarachnoid space surrounding the brain may occur.

## What is the subarachnoid space?

This is a narrow space between the brain and its outside covering, the dura mater. It contains cerebrospinal fluid and blood vessels carrying blood to and from the brain.

## What is the cause of bleeding into the subarachnoid space?

This results most frequently from rupture of an aneurysm. Less often it is caused by a malformation of an artery or vein of the brain.

## What is an aneurysm?

An aneurysm is a saclike dilatation of a blood vessel. Aneurysms are generally located along the major blood vessels at the base of the brain. Symptoms are produced by sudden rupture of the sac, resulting in bleeding. Severe headache, drowsiness, and loss of consciousness usually ensue. Sometimes the headache will be of short duration without loss of consciousness.

## Aside from bleeding, what other symptoms can be produced by an aneurysm?

Pressure on the optic nerve may result in blindness; pressure on other parts of the brain may lead to epileptic seizures.

## What is an arteriovenous malformation?

An arteriovenous malformation is a cluster of abnormally large blood vessels that may be located on the surface of the brain or within the brain substance. Symptoms may be produced by rupture of a blood vessel, resulting in headache and drowsiness similar to an aneurysm.

## Are aneurysms treatable?

See Chapter 46, on Neurosurgery.

## Are arteriovenous malformations amenable to surgery?

See Chapter 46, on Neurosurgery.

# EPILEPSY (Convulsive Seizures)

## What is epilepsy?

A disorder characterized by convulsions, seizures, or spells, in which there is temporary loss of consciousness or memory. Since there are many causes for these seizures, the epilepsy may only be a symptom. Neurologists, therefore, prefer to use the term "convulsive state" rather than epilepsy.

## Are there different types of epileptic seizures?

Yes.
a. Grand mal. Characterized by a generalized convulsion.
b. Petit mal. Meaning a "small attack," in which the patient has a brief lapse of contact with his surroundings, after which he resumes his usual activities.
c. Psychomotor seizures. These may be associated with purposeful movements, incoherent speech, smacking of the lips, and amnesia.
d. Jacksonian seizures. These are caused by local areas of irritation

of the brain. They usually begin with a jerking of the face or hand and a gradual spread to involve adjacent parts of the body. Consciousness will generally not be lost as long as the seizure remains confined to half of the body. This type of seizure is most commonly associated with lesions such as brain tumors or a scar in brain tissue.

## What are the common symptoms of the major epileptic convulsions?

a. Loss of consciousness.
b. Shaking convulsions, in which the arms and legs undergo strong repetitive to-and-fro movements for a short period of time.
c. Biting of the tongue and frothing at the mouth.
d. The patient may soil or wet himself.

## What are the causes of epilepsy?

a. It may be caused by any condition or disease affecting the brain, such as a tumor, scar, blood vessel disease, injury, or infection.
b. It may be caused by a birth injury.
c. There may be hereditary epilepsy.
d. There are a great number of patients with epilepsy in whom the cause is unknown.

## What is the usual age at which epilepsy has its onset?

It begins most often at puberty, but may even appear earlier on in childhood.

## Does epilepsy affect both sexes equally?

Yes.

## Are people with epilepsy mentally retarded or below average in mentality?

Not necessarily. Many of them are normal or even above average in intelligence.

## Can epilepsy be controlled?

Yes. The great majority of cases can

be controlled so that seizures are reduced to a minimum. There are excellent medications on the market that reduce or eliminate convulsions.

### Can epilepsy be cured?

Not really. The frequency of seizures can be markedly lessened when a specific cause for seizures can be found and treated, i.e., removal of a brain tumor. Even then, however, the patient will generally require anticonvulsive medication for the control of seizure activity despite successful removal of the tumor.

### What is the first-aid treatment for a patient who is having a convulsion?

Guard him from injury. If he is on the floor, let him remain there. Put a pillow under his head. If possible, bring the tongue forward to prevent it from being swallowed. Place a spoon between his teeth to prevent tongue-biting.

### How frequently is epilepsy encountered?

Statistics show that about 1 percent of people have epilepsy.

### Is epilepsy inherited?

From 10 to 25 percent of patients give a history of epilepsy in some other member of the family. However, it is important to note that there is only a one in ten chance that a child in a family in which there is epilepsy will develop the condition. If only one parent has epilepsy, the chance of a child developing epilepsy is one in forty.

### Is epilepsy a bar to marriage?

No.

### Should an epileptic have children?

If there is an evident cause for the epilepsy, heredity will play no part, and the patient can have children without any hesitation. If there is a family history of epilepsy on one side only, the chances of having epilep-

tic children are very slight. Where there is a positive family history on both sides, serious consideration should be given to not having children.

### Does a child who has a convulsion associated with high fever or some childhood disease have epilepsy?

No. Usually, this is a different kind of condition, having no association with true epilepsy. Sometimes, however, convulsions during fever in early childhood are followed by epilepsy later on.

### Should epileptics be permitted to live a normal life and to engage in a gainful occupation?

Yes. They can be taught how to keep medicated so that their chances of having a seizure are minimal. They should not engage in such occupations as will be dangerous should a seizure occur.

### What are the precautions an epileptic should take?

a. He should not drive an automobile unless he is sure that his attacks are well controlled with medication.

b. He should abstain from drinking alcohol.

c. He should not swim alone.

d. Total fluid intake should be limited to approximately three or four glasses per day.

e. He should take medications as prescribed and should *never* stop without consulting his doctor.

f. An adequate supply of medication should always be on hand.

g. Unnecessary stress and emotional strain should be avoided.

h. Every individual who is subject to seizures should carry a card with him stating that he is subject to convulsive attacks. Such a card will be most helpful to first-aiders or others who are present when a seizure takes place. The card should give precise instructions on how to handle the seizure.

## FAINTING

### What is fainting?

Fainting, or syncope, is a brief, temporary loss of consciousness resulting from a transient reduction in the circulation of blood to the brain.

### What are some of the causes of fainting?

a. Emotional upset.

b. Too sudden a fall in blood sugar (hypoglycemia.)

c. An overdose of insulin in a diabetic patient.

d. Certain heart conditions.

e. Extreme pain.

f. Cerebral arteriosclerosis, or hardening of the arteries to the brain, causing decrease in the caliber of the artery. This narrowing of the blood vessel may occur in the carotid arteries in the neck.

### Do patients ever die in a faint?

This is extremely rare, as most patients who faint regain consciousness by themselves.

### What should be done for a patient who has fainted?

See that he lies flat and that his head is at a level with or below the level of the rest of his body. Loosen the patient's collar so that he can breathe easily.

## COMA

### What is coma?

It is a state of unconsciousness from which the patient cannot be aroused.

### What are some of the more common causes of coma?

There are many:

a. A toxic agent, such as excessive alcohol or excessive consumption of sleeping pills.

b. Severe brain injury.

c. Severe infection, such as meningitis or encephalitis.

d. Brain tumor or a stroke due to cerebral thrombosis, embolus, or hemorrhage.
e. A complication of diabetes due to excessively high blood sugar.
f. Overdoses of insulin, resulting in too low blood sugar.
g. Uremia, with failure of kidney function.

### What is the treatment of coma?

To ascertain the cause and to treat it. Hence, diagnosis is the most important initial step. Patients who are in coma should be hospitalized immediately so that the various tests can be instituted that will determine the cause.

## HEADACHE

### What is the significance of headache?

Headaches are among the most common of symptoms and frequently constitute the most difficult problem confronting both physician and patient. Headache is a symptom, not a disease. As such, headache may occur from a wide variety of disorders. It may be associated with disease involving some of the sense organs, such as the eyes, nose and sinuses, or ears. It may be due to disease of structures within the head, involving the brain. Most often, however, it results from fatigue, tension, or anxiety. Another frequent cause of headache is a general disturbance of bodily function, such as a systemic disease associated with fever.

### Are headaches ever caused by allergies?

Yes.

### Should a patient with frequent headaches consult his physician?

Yes.

### What is migraine?

It is a common condition character-ized by paroxysmal headache, occurring in bouts, often affecting only one side of the head and frequently preceded by visual disturbances. Between attacks, the patient feels perfectly well.

### What is the cause of migraine?

The cause is unknown, but it frequently affects several members of a family.

### Is emotional tension ever a cause of migraine?

Yes, frequently.

### Can migraine ever be cured?

An individual attack may be stopped with medication, but there is no treatment that can guarantee a true cure.

### Will a competent neurologist be able to distinguish between a headache caused by a serious nerve or brain disease and one that is caused by a less serious condition?

Yes. The neurologist has many methods for distinguishing the various causes of headache.

## VERTIGO

### What is vertigo?

It is a symptom in which there is a sense of rotation of one's surroundings and a sense of loss of balance in space. The patient is unable to maintain his equilibrium during an episode of vertigo.

### What is the significance of vertigo?

It indicates a disturbance in the apparatus that controls the sense of equilibrium. This apparatus includes the structures in the inner ear and the nerves that connect the inner ear with the brain. It also includes the blood vessels that supply the inner ear and the nerves in the area.

## MÉNIÈRE'S DISEASE

### What is Ménière's disease?

An illness characterized by sudden paroxysms of vertigo, nausea, and vomiting, in which the patient lies down and is unable to move because of loss of equilibrium. Usually the paroxysm is of short duration, lasting anywhere from minutes to hours. It subsides gradually, and the patient is then well for long intervals. During the acute disturbance, there may be noises in one ear, such as buzzing, hissing, or whistling. After a number of such attacks there may be decreased hearing in that ear. The cause for this disease is not definitely known but has been attributed to increased fluid or edema in the inner ear.

### What is the treatment for Ménière's disease?

In the acute phase, there must be complete rest. Sedatives and other medications may be helpful. Fluid intake should be limited, and salt should be eliminated from the diet. Diuretics are given to reduce the water content of the body. In rare instances, cutting the vestibular portion of the eighth nerve may be necessary.

## MUSCULAR DYSTROPHY

### What is muscular dystrophy?

Muscular dystrophy is an inherited muscular disorder usually affecting several members of one family. It often begins in childhood and is evidenced by various muscles becoming weak with progressive weakening of the hips, thighs, back, shoulders, and arms. Such patients have trouble in walking, rising from the prone position, and in elevating their arms. Ultimately, the muscles will waste away, although there may be a transitory phase of the disease in which some muscles appear enlarged.

**What is the outlook for a patient with muscular dystrophy?**

The condition is likely to progress slowly and become worse over a period of years. Although the condition may seem to be arrested for a time, there is ultimate progression to a fatal outcome.

## MULTIPLE SCLEROSIS
### (Disseminated Sclerosis)

**What is multiple sclerosis?**

A disease of the central nervous system resulting in what is called demyelination, or loss of the myelin sheaths, which cover the nerve fibers. This occurs usually in small patches and is characterized clinically by the rapid development of symptoms that persist for a varying period of time and then recede. A period of freedom from symptoms is called a remission. Later, additional episodes occur that also tend to remit. The average case displays a series of intermittent and remittent illnesses affecting various parts of the nervous system. In most people the disorder is progressive, although the rate of progress varies markedly in different cases. Common symptoms are:

a. Temporary loss of vision in one or the other eye.
b. Temporary weakness of limbs, awkwardness, and clumsiness of movement (termed ataxia).
c. Stiffness of the limbs (spasticity).
d. Bladder trouble resulting in loss of urine or difficulty in voiding, etc.

**What is the cause of multiple sclerosis?**

The cause is unknown.

**What is the outlook for a patient with multiple sclerosis?**

This is a progressive disease, which ultimately leaves the patient bedridden. It may take many years to reach such a state, and some fortunate people may live out an almost normal life span without becoming too greatly incapacitated.

**Is there any effective treatment for multiple sclerosis?**

At this time there is no specific cure. Many forms of treatment have been helpful, but none is consistently successful. Many of the symptoms can be alleviated, and it must be remembered that the natural history of this disease includes long periods of spontaneous improvement.

## PARKINSONISM
### (Shaking Palsy)

**What is Parkinsonism?**

A disease of the brain characterized by muscular rigidity and tremor. The rigidity is of a particular kind that slows up all movements and produces an expressionless face, The tremor, or shaking, is rhythmic, slow, and is present even when the patient is resting. It may affect one or both sides of the body. This disorder affects middle-aged and elderly people and is generally progressive, though often very slowly so. Ultimately, patients tend to become helpless. The condition is also known as paralysis agitans, although actual paralysis does not occur.

**What is the cause of Parkinsonism?**

Most varieties are due to hardening of the cerebral arteries or are the result of brain damage caused by a previous illness such as encephalitis. Others are caused by degeneration of certain parts of the brain.

**Is there any affective medical treatment for Parkinsonism?**

Yes. A number of medications are available that are effective. Also, psychotherapy may be of benefit by helping patients with this disease to keep physically and socially active and by helping them adjust to, and accept, their illness.

**Can surgery ever be helpful in Parkinsonism?**

Yes. (See Chapter 46, on Neurosurgery.)

## FRACTURED SKULL
*(See Chapter 46 on Neurosurgery)*

## CEREBRAL CONCUSSION
*(See Chapter 46 on Neurosurgery)*

## LUMBAR PUNCTURE
### Spinal Tap

**What is a lumbar puncture, and why is it performed?**

It is a procedure in which the physician taps the spinal canal to obtain a sample of the cerebrospinal fluid. This fluid bathes the brain and the central nervous system. By this procedure, it is possible to measure directly the intracranial pressure and thereby detect any increase in pressure, such as occurs with tumors of the brain. The constituents of this fluid are altered in different ways by different diseases of the central nervous system. This procedure is often of great significance and yields information of the greatest importance to the doctor in diagnosing and managing the patient's illness. Thus, with infections of the nervous system, examination of the cerebrospinal fluid helps to determine the nature of the infecting organism. It is also important in attempting to establish a diagnosis of a ruptured cerebral aneurysm as it may reveal leakage of blood, a warning symptom.

## PNEUMO-ENCEPHALOGRAPHY

**What is pneumoencephalography?**

This is a special form of x ray of the

brain and contents of the skull. In this procedure, air is injected into the space around the brain and spinal cord by way of a spinal puncture. The air finds its way into the ventricles (normal cavities) of the brain, and since it is transported to the x rays, it may disclose any distortion or enlargement of these cavities. Encephalography often reveals the presence and location of a brain tumor. However, this test is rarely performed because of the availability of the CAT scan.

## BRAIN SCAN

### What is a brain scan?

It is a test given after the intravenous injection of a radioactive substance, in which the brain scanned to note how the radioactive substance is deposited in the brain tissue. Variations from the normal pattern of deposit will accurately portray the presence of a brain tumor or cyst.

## THE CAT SCAN

*(See also Chapter 79 on X ray)*

### What is a CAT scan?

It is an x-ray technique wherein many computerized pictures of tiny sections of an organ are taken. Study of CAT scans of the brain often reveals the presence of even the smallest tumors or abnormalities.

### Are there other names for the CAT scan?

Yes. The technique is known as computerized axial tomography.

### Is a CAT scan the same as a CT scan?

Yes.

### Can CAT scans of the brain outline tumors or cysts that are too small to be seen by any other diagnostic tool?

Yes.

## ELECTRO-ENCEPHALOGRAPHY

### What is electroencephalography?

A procedure that records the electrical activity going on in the brain. By a process of considerable magnification, this activity is recorded as brain waves on a strip of paper. The normal pattern of these waves is quite characteristic, but it is often modified by disease. Thus, epilepsy causes typical changes in the brain waves. Tumors, strokes, and injuries may also alter the pattern in a special way. For convenience, the procedure is referred to by the abbreviation of EEG.

### Is electroencephalography a helpful and accurate diagnostic aid in brain disease?

EEG has extreme limitations as a diagnostic tool. However, it often serves a useful function in following the course of epileptic patients.

### Has the EEG been replaced as a diagnostic aid in brain disease by the CAT scan?

Yes, in most instances.

### What is one of the main uses of the EEG today?

The procedure is used most frequently to determine brain death. The absence of brain waves shows brain death.

### What is angiography of the brain?

It is a method by which a liquid that is opaque to x rays is injected into the circulation, usually through a vessel in the neck, arm, or leg. During this procedure, x rays of the brain are taken that reveal its circulation. Alterations from normal patterns often signify the presence of brain tumors or cysts. (See Chapter 79, on X ray.)

# CHAPTER 46

# NEURO-SURGERY

*(Brain, Spinal Cord, and Nerve Surgery)*

*(See also Chapter 44 on Mental Health and Disease; Chapter 45 on Nervous Disease; Chapter 55 on Pituitary Gland)*

## What is the scope of neurosurgery?

Neurosurgery is that branch of medicine dealing with the surgical treatment of diseases of the nervous system, including the brain, spinal cord, and peripheral nerves. Injuries, infections, tumors, various congenital abnormalities, ruptured disks, certain painful states, and intracranial hemorrhage are among the conditions that can be helped by the neurosurgeon.

## Generally speaking, how does the nervous system function?

The nervous system is composed of nerve cells and supporting tissue centered in the brain and spinal cord, with widespread extensions all through the body. Its function is the transmission and coordination of stimuli and their integration into the phenomena that make up mental activity. Impulses conveying sensory impressions such as touch, taste, hearing, sight, and smell, are carried to the brain along pathways called afferent nerves. Glandular secretion and muscular activity, on the other hand, are achieved by impulses that originate in the central nervous system and travel in an outward direction along pathways called efferent

nerves. The orderliness that characterizes normal human activity is rendered possible only because of the high degree of organization of the nervous system. This fact becomes apparent when a part of this elaborate system is disturbed by a disease process.

The nervous system is divided anatomically into two components, a central and a peripheral. The brain and spinal cord make up the central portion; the peripheral part is composed of all the nerves that establish communication with the rest of the body. The peripheral component consists of twelve pairs of cranial nerves, which arise from the brain and leave through openings in the bones of the skull, thirty-one pairs of spinal nerves, which emerge through openings in the vertebral column, and a complex network of nerves called the autonomic or sympathetic system. The function of the autonomic system is to transmit nervous impulses to the intestinal tract, bladder, heart, glands, and blood vessels.

## What is the appearance of the brain?

The brain is a soft, grayish white structure, hemispherical in shape, with innumerable folds. It is nourished by many blood vessels that permeate its substance. It is continuous with the spinal cord, which emerges through an opening in the base of the skull. Both the brain and spinal cord are covered by membranes (the dura, arachnoid, and pia) and by a liquid called cerebrospinal fluid. Within the brain itself are a number of communicating cavities also containing cerebrospinal fluid.

## How does one gain surgical access to the brain?

The operation for exposing the brain is called a craniotomy. As a general rule, craniotomy is performed under general anesthesia, though at times

local anesthesia is preferable. In preparation for surgery, the entire head is shaved and the scalp cleansed thoroughly with soap and water. A skin antiseptic is then applied, and all but the area to be operated upon is covered with sterile drapes. The scalp is incised, usually in a semicircular manner, and a number of holes are drilled in the underlying skull. The holes are connected by means of a wire saw or air drill bone cutter, thereby freeing a block of bone that is detached from the remainder of the skull. Directly underneath the bone are the membranes overlying the brain. These are incised, thus exposing the brain. Progress in surgical technique, mainly through use of the operating microscope, has made it possible to gain access to almost any part of the brain with reasonable safety!

## What is the appearance and function of the spinal cord?

The spinal cord is an elongated, cylindrically shaped structure, which measures approximately eighteen inches in length and occupies the canal within the vertebral column. It consists of bundles of nerves, and its function is to act primarily as a conducting mechanism. Sensory impulses travel toward the brain, while impulses concerned with muscular contraction and movement descend in the opposite direction. Connections with various organs and structures are established by means of spinal nerves that are attached to the cord throughout its length.

## How is the spinal cord exposed?

An incision is made in the center of the back, and the muscles overlying the spinal column are spread apart. Parts of the arches of the exposed vertebrae are then removed, thereby bringing into view the spinal cord enclosed within its membranes. This operation is known as a laminectomy.

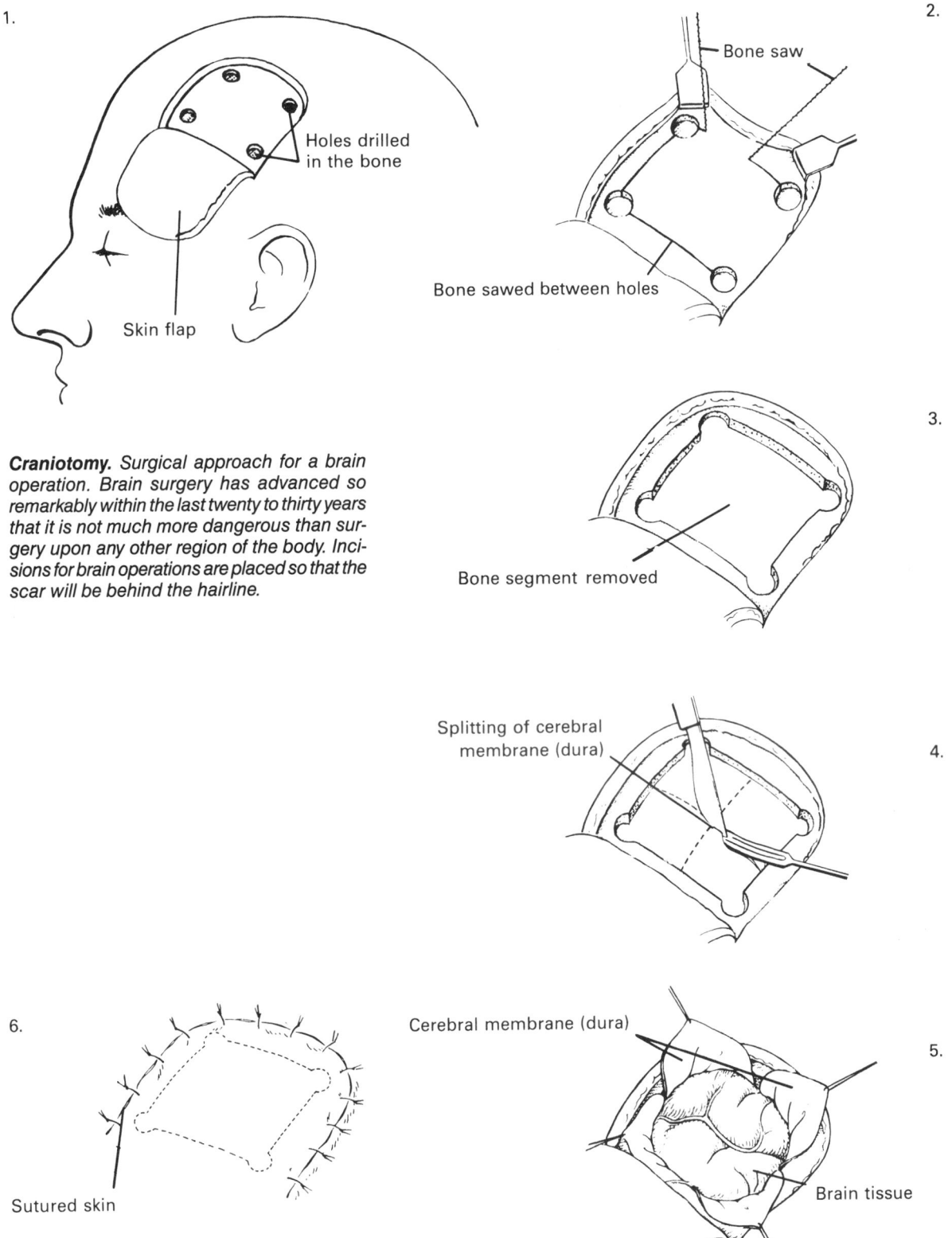

1.

Holes drilled in the bone

Skin flap

2.

Bone saw

Bone sawed between holes

3.

Bone segment removed

4.

Splitting of cerebral membrane (dura)

5.

Cerebral membrane (dura)

Brain tissue

6.

Sutured skin

**Craniotomy.** *Surgical approach for a brain operation. Brain surgery has advanced so remarkably within the last twenty to thirty years that it is not much more dangerous than surgery upon any other region of the body. Incisions for brain operations are placed so that the scar will be behind the hairline.*

## SKULL AND BRAIN INJURIES
### (Lacerations, Concussion, Fracture)

### Are all head injuries serious?

No, on the contrary, head injuries vary in seriousness from the relatively minor laceration of the scalp to the severe bruising of the brain associated with profound unconsciousness. Fortunately, the skull affords considerable protection to the underlying brain substance. Many head injuries damage only the relatively unimportant superficial tissues. Those of a more severe nature may fracture the skull and cause serious brain damage, such as a laceration or contusion.

### Is a laceration of the scalp serious?

Scalp lacerations frequently look more serious than they really are because of their great tendency to bleed. The bleeding usually stops by itself or after pressure has been applied. Surgical repair of the wound is necessary in cases of extensive laceration. The hair around the wound is shaved and the laceration cleansed before it is sutured. Careful inspection of the wound is necessary to be certain that the injury has not involved the skull or underlying brain.

### What is the significance of loss of consciousness following a head injury?

It signifies that an injury to the intracranial contents has taken place! X rays should always be taken in such cases because of the possibility of a skull fracture. Patients who have lost consciousness, if only for a few seconds, should be observed carefully for a day or two for evidence of hemorrhage within the skull.

### What is meant by a concussion?

Concussion is a term applied to a head injury that has resulted in loss of consciousness for a brief period.

### What is the treatment for a concussion?

No specific treatment is required in uncomplicated cases, as spontaneous recovery is the rule. The patient should, however, be watched for the development of increasing drowsiness and weakness of the limbs on one side of the body. Such symptoms are usually caused by bleeding within the skull.

### Is a fractured skull a serious injury?

Yes. Skull fractures result from a severe blow or fall upon the head. However, it must be emphasized that it is not the extent of the fracture that determines the seriousness of the injury but the amount of damage to the underlying brain. In other words, a small fracture accompanied by widespread brain damage may be much more dangerous than an extensive skull fracture that has caused little brain damage.

### Is the patient's state of consciousness an important factor in regard to the severity of the injury as well as the ultimate outcome?

Yes. The depth and duration of coma or stupor vary in proportion to the severity of the injury.

### What is the proper first-aid treatment for a head injury with loss of consciousness?

a. Place the patient on his side or in a semiprone position. This will lessen the danger of aspiration of secretions.
b. Hemorrhage from a scalp wound should be controlled by pressure with a sterile dressing or clean handkerchief.
c. Transport the patient on a stretcher; avoid bending his head or trunk.
d. Be sure the patient's airway remains unobstructed.

### Is there any specific treatment for injury to the brain?

No. There is no specific treatment for brain injuries as such. Fortunately, most patients recover spontaneously. Good nursing care is essential. Comatose patients must be turned frequently to avoid pressure sores. Soiled bed linen must be changed promptly. Urinary incontinence may require insertion of a catheter in the bladder or may be dealt with by other methods. The importance of maintaining a clear airway so as to avoid interference with respiration cannot be overemphasized. It may be necessary at times to introduce a tube through an incision in the windpipe (tracheotomy) in order to facilitate respiration. The danger of aspiration resulting from vomiting and the accumulation of secretions requires the frequent use of mechanical suction. Maintenance of nutrition in a comatose patient usually necessitates the administration of fluids intravenously for a few days after which a tube is inserted into the stomach for purposes of feeding.

### Is it necessary to operate on all cases of head injury?

No.

### What are the indications for surgery?

a. An open wound (i.e., compound fracture).
b. The presence of indriven or depressed fragments of bone, which may irritate the brain (depressed skull fracture).
c. Intracranial hemorrhage developing as a complication.
d. A persistent leak of cerebrospinal fluid through the nose.

### Is the occurrence of bleeding within the skull following a head injury a serious complication?

Yes. Signs of increasing pressure within the skull will develop.

### What is the prognosis of increased intracranial pressure?

This depends in large part on the

Fragments of bone driven into brain tissue

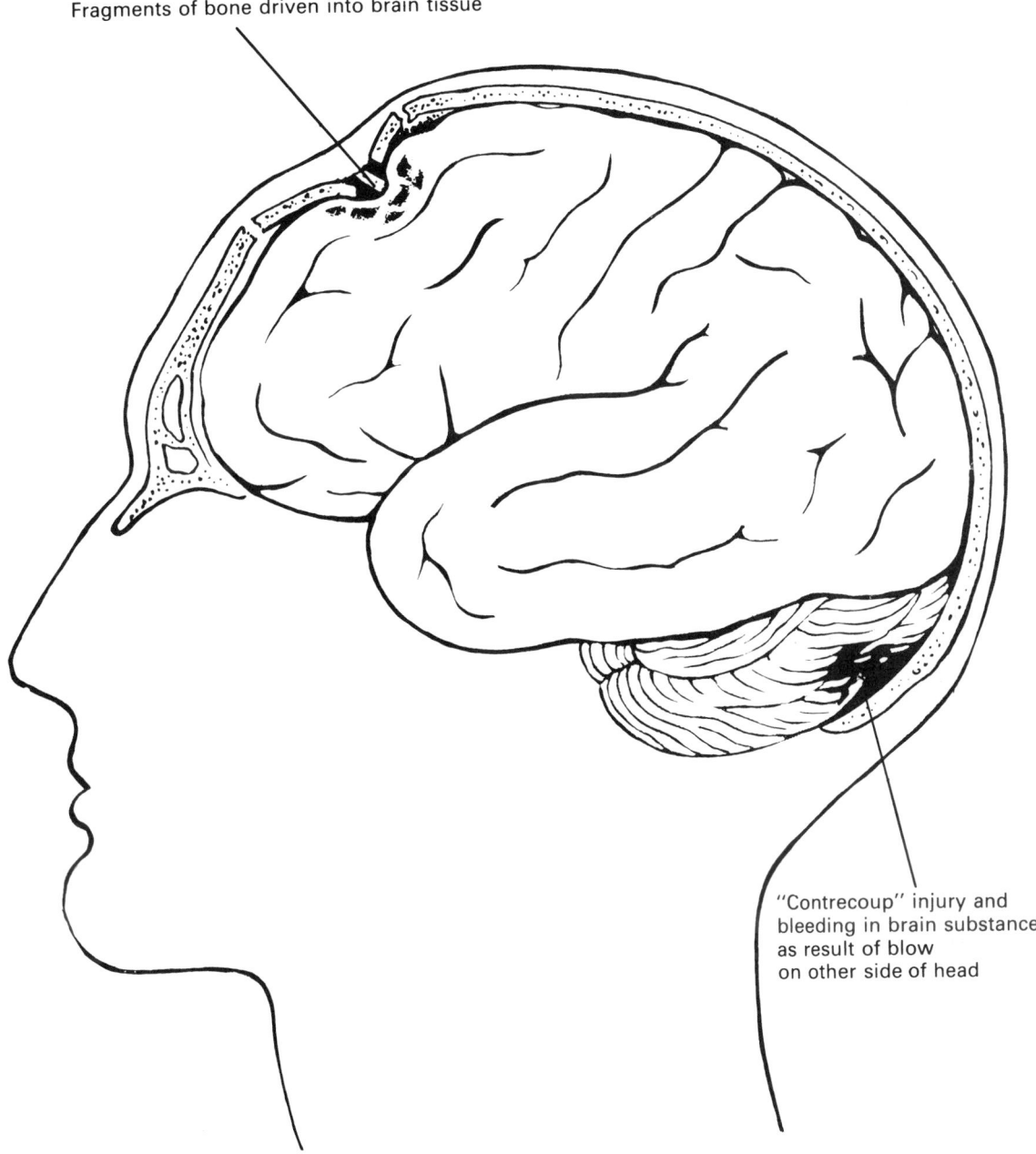

"Contrecoup" injury and bleeding in brain substance as result of blow on other side of head

***Depressed Skull Fracture.*** *This diagram shows a depressed skull fracture with some of the bone fragments being driven in toward the brain substance. This is a serious condition demanding surgery to relieve the pressure that such bone fragments might create upon the brain and to minimize the possibility of the patient developing epilepsy at a later date due to scarring. Often a severe blow on one side of the skull will produce a hemorrhage or laceration of brain substance on the opposite side of the skull. Such a condition is called a "contrecoup" injury.*

cause of the bleeding. Bleeding may be extradural, subdural, or intracerebral—only the latter is within the brain itself.

An extradural hemorrhage results from a tear of the middle cerebral artery. If recognized early and treated surgically, recovery occurs in most cases. A subdural hemorrhage may follow head trauma and is associated with a much higher morbidity and mortality even when handled promptly. An intracerebral hemorrhage is even more dangerous, as it is within brain substance.

## Is surgery necessary in all cases of increased intracranial pressure?

No. Increased intracranial pressure may be caused by cerebral edema (brain swelling). This is best treated with medication.

## How does intracranial hemorrhage following injury manifest itself, and what can be done about it?

Evidence of hemorrhage within the skull may appear within a matter of hours after an injury or may be delayed for weeks or even months. Seemingly slight injuries may be followed by intracranial bleeding; thus a careful lookout for this complication must be maintained. Intracranial bleeding occurring soon after an accident constitutes a surgical emergency. It is manifested by increasing drowsiness and weakness of the limbs on one side of the body.

Prompt recognition of the condition and operation to stop the bleeding and remove the blood clots are imperative to avoid a fatal outcome. Even the suspicion of hemorrhage is sufficient to warrant an immediate exploratory operation. This is a relatively minor operative procedure, performed under local Novocain anesthesia. A small incision is made in the scalp in front of and above the ear, and a hole is drilled in the skull. Should the exploration fail to disclose the presence of a hemorrhage, no harm will have been done. On the other hand, failure to operate when a clot is present will cost the patient his life!

The symptoms of hemorrhage that appear at a late stage, weeks or months after an injury, consist of headache, drowsiness, and mental confusion. This type of bleeding presents a much less urgent problem, although treatment is similar to that for the more acute variety. Blood clots may be evacuated through a small opening in the skull, although at times a more extensive surgical procedure is necessary.

## Does intracranial bleeding ever occur during early life?

Yes. Intracranial hemorrhage (subdural hematoma, or clot overlying the brain) resulting from injury is sometimes encountered during infancy. The trauma may have occurred inadvertently at the time the baby was born. Early diagnosis and surgical treatment are essential to prevent permanent brain damage.

## Is physical or mental disability a common sequel of head injury?

Considering the frequency with which head injuries occur, the incidence of serious aftereffects is remarkably small. In most cases recovery is complete. At times, however, symptoms such as headache, dizziness, irritability, etc., persist following an injury (posttraumatic or postconcussion syndrome). These do not, as a rule, indicate any serious underlying disorder or complication. It must be realized that there is a strong emotional component to every physical injury, and this is particularly true when the accident has involved the head. Psychological disturbances and emotional instability after skull and brain injuries can often be minimized by careful explanation of the exact nature of the injury. Above all, it is important to assure such patients that their ability to return to a completely normal life need not be impaired when they have recovered fully from the physical effects of the accident.

## SURGICAL INFECTIONS OF THE SKULL AND BRAIN

## Do all types of infection of the skull or brain require surgical treatment?

No. Surgery is not indicated in cases in which the infection is widespread (encephalitis, meningitis) and in which there is no localized collection of pus to drain.

## How does the brain or its coverings become infected?

Sinusitis and, less often, injury are the most common causes of infection of the bones of the skull (osteomyelitis). An abscess within the brain occurs as a result of the spread of an infection from an adjacent structure, such as the sinuses or ears, or from a distant part of the body, usually the lung. It may also be caused by a penetrating wound of the skull or by a compound skull fracture.

## Is osteomyelitis of the skull serious?

Yes. Unless it is adequately treated, there is danger of the spread of infection to the brain. This type of infection is encountered less often than in the days before the advent of chemotherapy and antibiotics.

## What does the surgical treatment of osteomyelitis entail?

Removal of the diseased bone and provision for drainage of pus. Antibiotics are administered concurrently.

## How serious is a brain abscess?

Brain abscess is a very serious condition, despite the fact that its incidence has diminished markedly and the outlook for successful treatment has improved considerably as a result of the introduction of antibiotics. It is treated by surgical excision or drainage.

## TUMORS OF THE BRAIN

## How common are tumors of the brain?

The brain is a frequent site of tumor formation.

## Are there different kinds of brain tumors?

Yes. The term intracranial tumor is used to denote any one of several types of growths that may be present within the skull. A tumor may originate from the skull, from the membranes or nerves external to the brain, or from the brain itself. Still another source of origin is the pituitary gland at the base of the skull. Finally, cancerous growths arising elsewhere in the body may spread by means of the bloodstream to involve the brain secondarily.

### What determines the outlook in a particular case of brain tumor?

The nature of the growth and its location. Tumors arising from the coverings of the brain (meningiomas) and the nerves of the brain (neurofibromas), when surgically accessible, may be completely removed and the patient cured. As these tumors represent 20 percent of all growths within the skull, it is obvious that many patients can look forward to complete recovery.

Approximately 50 percent of brain tumors develop within the brain substance itself (gliomas). With few exceptions, these tumors are not sufficiently well localized to be removed completely. Their rate of growth varies, being exceedingly rapid in the more malignant varieties. Some may grow slowly over a period of years, while others may go on to a rapid termination within a much shorter time. Even when complete cure cannot be accomplished, many people with this type of brain tumor can be helped by surgery. However, a brain tumor incompletely removed eventually recurs, and the ultimate outlook depends upon its rate of growth. The growth of some of these tumors is retarded by x-ray treatment, which is therefore often carried out after surgery. Chemotherapy may also be helpful.

### What are the chances of surviving an operation for a brain tumor?

Since the introduction of the operating microscope, many nonmalignant tumors in locations heretofore considered to be inaccessible can be successfully removed. The operative mortality has been reduced to 2 to 8 percent.

### What are the most common symptoms of brain tumors?

Headache, vomiting, disturbances of vision, and various specific symptoms, depending on the location of the tumor, such as paralysis or convulsions.

### What causes brain tumors?

The cause is unknown.

### Are brain tumors hereditary?

No.

### Can the exact location of a brain tumor be determined before operation?

In most instances, yes.

### How is the location of a brain tumor determined?

The CAT (computerized axial tomography) scan, a new x-ray device, can usually locate a tumor in the earliest stage of development. The CAT study pinpoints the tumor's location for the surgeon. Notwithstanding this fact, an angiogram is also performed. This entails injecting a material into an artery for the purpose of outlining the blood vessels of the brain so that they can be seen on x ray. By noting any displacement from their normal position, the location of a tumor is confirmed. In addition, by knowing the location of these blood vessels, they can often be spared during the course of the tumor removal.

### Is it possible to determine before operation whether a brain tumor is benign or malignant?

Not in all cases, though at times one can be reasonably certain.

### What kind of anesthesia is used for brain surgery?

General anesthesia, through a tube placed into the trachea (windpipe).

### Where are the incisions made in cases of brain surgery?

Over any part of the scalp, depending on the location of the underlying condition.

### Is the scar resulting from brain surgery disfiguring?

No. Insofar as possible, the incisions are made within the hairline, and the eventual scar is inconspicuous.

### Are blood transfusions administered during ihe course of brain operations?

Yes, very often.

### How long do brain operations take to perform?

The time element varies depending on the nature of the condition requiring surgery and the procedure to be performed. Some operations can be completed within two to three hours; others, done under the operating microscope, may require eight to twelve hours.

### Can patients safely withstand this type of surgery for many hours?

Yes. Improved anesthetic techniques and supportive measures make it possible for lengthy operations to be performed safely.

### How soon after a major brain operation can the surgeon tell if the patient will survive?

Usually within a few days.

### Are special nurses necessary after brain operations?

Yes, for several days.

### How long a hospital stay is necessary after a major brain operation?

Two to three weeks.

### Must one take special care of the wound area after a brain operation has been performed?

Not usually. The only cases that require special attention are those in which the piece of bone removed at operation has not been replaced.

## Do brain tumors, once removed, tend to recur?

Only if incompletely removed.

## Can a patient who has had a brain tumor successfully removed live a normal life?

Yes.

## Do brain tumors occur in children?

Yes. Brain tumors during childhood are not at all uncommon. Certain types of tumors are especially prevalent in children, and they tend to occur predominantly in certain locations within the brain. Both benign and malignant varieties are encountered. Their treatment is similar to that of tumors in adults, and the results obtained are comparable. Children withstand brain surgery as well as adults.

## Are cobalt or high voltage x-ray treatments, rather than surgery, ever recommended for brain tumors?

Yes. Cobalt or x-ray treatment is used when a spreading tumor involves the speech area of the brain.

## If vision is lost because of a brain condition, does it ever return?

If vision is lost as a result of increased pressure within the skull, the outlook for recovery is not good. In cases in which vision is damaged, surgery may prevent further impairment or result in improvement. Loss of vision due to direct pressure of the tumor on the optic nerves may be helped considerably through surgery.

## If hearing is lost because of a brain tumor, is it ever regained after surgical removal?

A brain tumor causing loss of hearing usually arises from the auditory nerve, and hearing will not return despite the removal of the tumor.

## Can a patient who has lost the power to speak be taught to speak again after removal of a brain tumor?

Yes. Very often this is possible with intensive effort and training in cases in which brain tissue has not been destroyed.

## Can patients regain the use of their limbs following removal of a brain tumor?

Yes, in many cases. Complete recovery, however, does not always take place.

## Is a patient's mentality usually affected by a brain operation?

As a rule, no. The patient's mental reaction is primarily determined by the nature and location of the disease from which he is suffering.

## Will the removal of a brain tumor result in a cessation of convulsions?

The frequency of the convulsions may be diminished, but they are not always eliminated completely. Hence the administration of anticonvulsant medication should be continued following operation. Even in cases in which convulsions did not occur preoperatively, the use of anticonvulsant medication postoperatively is advisable as a precautionary measure.

# STROKE/INTRACRANIAL HEMORRHAGE

## What is meant by cerebral hemorrhage?

Bleeding occurring within the substance of the brain or on its surface.

## What are the common causes of cerebral hemorrhage?

a. Hardening of the arteries (arteriosclerosis) and high blood pressure are the most common causes of hemorrhage within the brain. This type of hemorrhage usually occurs after the age of forty.

b. Bleeding may also take place in younger individuals as a result of rupture of a malformed blood vessel. Most often, the malformation is a saclike dilatation of a blood vessel (aneurysm). Occasionally it consists of a cluster of abnormally large blood vessels (angioma).

c. Injury to the brain may also cause intracranial hemorrhage.

## Is a cerebral hemorrhage synonymous with a stroke?

Not entirely. The term "stroke" includes several conditions, one of which is cerebral hemorrhage.

## Is cerebral hemorrhage serious?

Yes, regardless of cause.

## Is surgery ever indicated for a cerebral hemorrhage?

Yes, when the patient develops signs of increased intracranial pressure (pressure within the skull), such as gradually deepening coma. It is possible to remove a blood clot from most regions of the brain through a small opening in the skull.

## What is the role of surgery in the treatment of malformation of the intracranial blood vessels?

Because these deformed vessels often rupture and cause intracranial bleeding, they constitute a threat to life. Obviously, it would be desirable to discover them and, wherever possible, to institute treatment *before* they cause hemorrhage. Unfortunately, evidence of hemorrhage is often the first indication of their presence. The use of radiopaque substances in order to outline the blood vessels of the brain (arteriography) is especially useful in cases in which an abnormality of the blood vessels is suspected. Various methods of surgical treatment have been devised, but unfortunately, such operations, when feasible, frequently entail considerable hazard.

# OTHER BRAIN OPERATIONS

### Can aneurysms of blood vessels within the skull be helped through surgery?

Yes, once their exact location has been pinpointed. Then with the aid of the operating microscope, it is often possible to remove them. This operation requires great skill and delicacy.

### Can arteriovenous malformations be removed surgically?

Yes, in some instances.

### Is surgery ever performed to remove a cerebral embolus?

Yes, in cases in which a major blood vessel is blocked by the clot and the exact location can be determined before surgery. In some cases, the blood vessel is opened and the clot is removed. In other cases, the clotted, obstructed portion of the blood vessel is bypassed.

### What is a bypass procedure?

The operation is called a superficial temporalcortical anastomosis. It involves suturing an artery from outside the brain to a blood vessel on the surface of the brain, thus bringing blood to an area of the brain that has been deprived of its blood supply. Such operations are performed with utilization of the operating microscope.

### Is surgery ever performed for a small stroke?

Yes. This condition is characterized by transient paralysis, periods of unconsciousness, loss of sensation in parts of the body, etc., and is thought to be caused by an abnormality of the carotid artery in the neck. In these cases, the carotid artery is found to be narrowed by arteriosclerosis and its inner lining containing calcified plaques. To overcome the condition, the carotid artery is opened, and its diseased inner lining is scraped out. The procedure is known as an endarterectomy. (See Chapter 13, on Blood Vessel Surgery.)

### How dangerous is a carotid endarterectomy?

There is a 2 to 3 percent chance that the patient will develop a stroke during the operative procedure.

### Can plaques in the carotid artery always be removed surgically?

No. The narrowing of the vessel and the plaques may be located at the base of the skull where they cannot be reached surgically. In such cases, an arterial bypass operation is performed.

### What is meant by trigeminal neuralgia (tic douloureux, trifacial neuralgia)?

Trigeminal neuralgia is a disease occurring mostly in middle-aged and elderly people, characterized by severe, recurrent paroxysmal pain in the face. Its cause is unknown.

### What is the surgical treatment for trigeminal neuralgia?

Today the nerve-cutting operations have been largely abandoned and replaced with newer procedures. One such procedure involves displacement of an abnormal blood vessel that presses against the trigeminal nerve at its point of origin, while another involves the application of radio-frequency current to the nerve. These operations largely do away with the annoying numbness created by the nerve-cutting procedures.

### How effective is the new procedure for relief of trigeminal neuralgia?

It works in about 75 percent of cases.

### Is surgery ever indicated in the treatment of epilepsy?

Yes, though relatively infrequently. Epilepsy may occur in the absence of any demonstrable cause (idiopathic) or may result from the presence of some structural abnormality in the brain, such as a tumor, abscess, blood vessel malformation, or scar. It is essential to differentiate the idiopathic cases from those due to a known organic disease. The cause of idiopathic epilepsy is unknown and treatment is designed exclusively for the purpose of controlling the seizures. Medication is employed in the management of this type of case.

An entirely different problem is presented by the patient whose seizures are not idiopathic in nature. Control of the seizures must still be achieved, but, in addition, the underlying condition must also be treated. It is this type of case that may require surgical treatment. Thus an operation is indicated if the basic condition is a tumor, abscess, or depressed fracture. Surgery may be advisable in cases of epilepsy due to scar formation if the seizures cannot be effectively controlled by medication. Certain patients with uncontrollable psychomotor epilepsy, characterized by the performance of some sort of automatic activity during a period of amnesia, may also be benefited by surgery.

### What is the role of surgery in the treatment of mental disease?

The operation originally devised for the treatment of mental disease (lobotomy) has been abandoned. In fact, at the present time the role of surgery in the treatment of psychiatric illness is not altogether clear.

### Is surgery of value in the treatment of Parkinsonism (shaking palsy)?

There is no longer any reasonable doubt that selected cases of Parkinsonism may be appreciably benefited by surgical treatment. While best results are achieved in patients with unilateral (one-sided) involvement, there are apparently no absolute contraindications to surgery, including old age. The operation is not wholly devoid of risk, but the proportion of untoward effects is relatively small. This type of surgery requires special training and equipment and should be performed only at a suitable neurosurgical center. The operation is usually done under local anesthesia. In addition to the tremor (palsy), other types of involuntary movements may be helped by surgical treatment.

### What is meant by hydrocephalus?

Hydrocephalus is a disorder of infants in which the head enlarges abnormally because of an excessive amount of cerebrospinal fluid within the brain. Interference with the circulation or absorption of cerebrospinal fluid is responsible for an excessive accumulation. The size of the head may reach enormous proportions.

### What is the treatment for hydrocephalus?

While spontaneous arrest may occur, cases of progressive hydrocephalus should be treated surgically in the hope of avoiding or minimizing damage to the brain. Various types of surgical procedures have been performed in the past. The operation currently favored involves diverting the cerebrospinal fluid from the cavities of the brain into the abdomen, utilizing a polyethylene tube and a one-way valve to prevent back flow. The procedure is called a ventriculoperitoneal shunt. An occasional revision of the shunt may be-

come necessary to lengthen the tubing to accommodate the growth of the child or to replace a blocked tube.

## SPINAL CORD BIRTH DEFORMITIES
### (Congenital Malformations, Developmental Anomalies)

### What are the common malformations involving the spinal cord?

Incomplete closure of some part of the vertebral canal is a fairly common developmental deformity and usually causes no symptoms (spina bifida occulta). It may, however, be associated with a protrusion or herniation of the membranes covering the spinal cord. Such a protrusion may contain cerebrospinal fluid only (meningocele), or it may contain nerve elements and even part of the spinal cord itself (meningomyelocele).

### How does a meningocele or meningomyelocele manifest itself?

Infants with these conditions are born with a noticeable lump on the back. Inclusion of nerve structures in the malformation usually is accompanied by varying degrees of paralysis of the lower limbs, the bowel, and the urinary bladder.

### Can a child be born with more than one malformation?

Yes. Hydrocephalus often occurs or

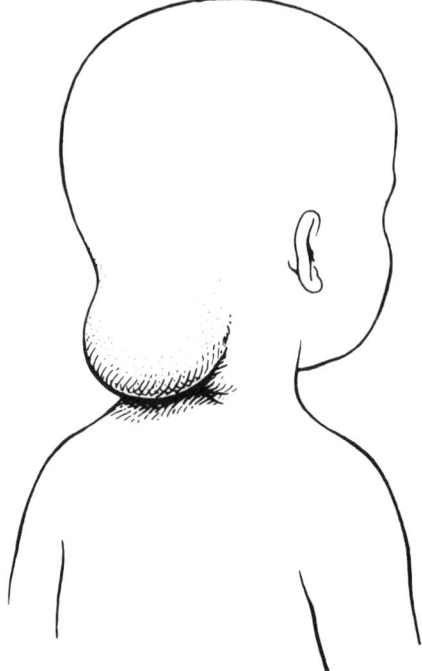

*Meningocele. The lump on the back of this child's neck is a meningocele. It contains cerebrospinal fluid and some nerve elements. Paralysis often results from this malformation.*

develops in association with a meningocele.

### Can anything be done to remedy a developmental defect (meningocele, meningomyelocele)?

Nothing can be done to correct an existing paralysis. Operation is performed solely for the purpose of repairing the deformity. Occasionally, in cases in which the sac is very thin and threatens to rupture, surgery may be required soon after birth.

## TUMORS OF THE SPINAL CORD

### What are the usual symptoms resulting from a tumor of the spinal cord?

Backache, together with weakness and numbness of the limbs, and disturbances referable to the bladder and bowels.

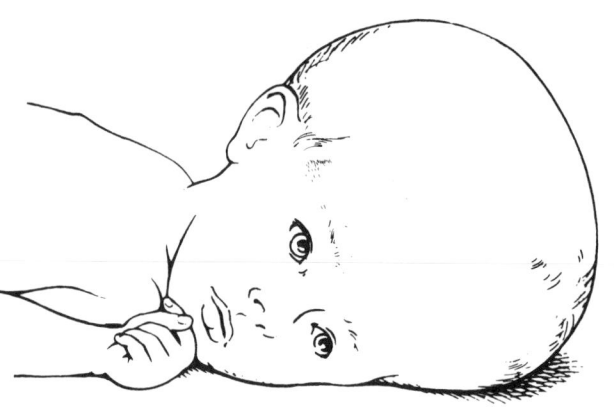

*Hydrocephalus. This drawing shows the abnormally large head of an infant with hydrocephalus. The swelling is caused by an excess of cerebrospinal fluid within the brain.*

**Are there different kinds of tumors of the spinal cord?**

Yes. The spinal cord may be affected by tumors compressing it from without or growing within its substance. About 50 percent of these tumors originate from the membranes overlying the cord or from a spinal nerve.

**How is the diagnosis of a spinal cord tumor established?**

The presence of a spinal cord tumor may be suspected on the basis of the history and examination of the patient. Spinal puncture usually reveals an obstruction to the free flow of cerebrospinal fluid. Examination of the spinal fluid often provides useful information. The diagnosis may be further confirmed by introducing a radiopaque substance into the cerebrospinal fluid and subjecting the patient to fluoroscopy. This procedure is called myelography. Normally, the radiopaque substance flows freely when the patient is tilted in either direction. A tumor will act as an obstruction to the flow of the radiopaque substance, thus verifying the diagnosis and providing evidence of its exact location.

**What are the results of surgery in the treatment of spinal cord tumors?**

Tumors originating from the membranes overlying the spinal cord or from a spinal nerve can usually be totally removed and the patient cured or greatly improved. Some tumors growing within the substance of the spinal cord can be removed when the microscope is used. When total removal cannot be accomplished, x-ray therapy may halt tumor growth. Not infrequently, a cancer that has originated in some other part of the body spreads to involve the spinal cord. The outlook in such cases is especially poor, though x-ray treatment and, occasionally, surgery may prove temporarily beneficial.

**Can paralysis caused by a spinal cord tumor be relieved by surgery?**

Yes. In the vast majority of cases, when the tumor is not malignant, it can be removed completely and the patient cured or improved without fear of recurrence of the tumor.

**Are operations upon the spinal cord dangerous?**

No more so than a major operation elsewhere.

**What kind of anesthesia is used when operating upon the spinal cord?**

General anesthesia, as a rule, administered through a tube in the trachea (windpipe).

## RUPTURED INTERVERTEBRAL DISKS (Herniated Slipped Disks)

**What is a ruptured disk?**

The space between two adjacent vertebrae is called an intervertebral disk and is composed of an outer rim of firm fibrocartilage and an inner, softer portion. When, as the result of an injury, the inner portion presses against a nerve root, the patient experiences radiating pain. This sequence may occur anywhere along the course of the spinal column and may cause pain and symptoms at the affected level. The most common site is at the lumbar level, producing pain in the low back, thigh, and calf. This condition is sometimes referred to as a slipped disk.

**How is the diagnosis of a ruptured disk established?**

The diagnosis may be strongly suspected on the basis of the history of the patient and a physical examination. Plain x rays of the spine may or may not provide additional useful information. Myelography (x rays outlining the spinal canal) usually resolves all doubt as to diagnosis. A CAT scan may also reveal the presence of a herniated disk.

**What is the treatment of a ruptured disk?**

Conservative measures such as bed rest, traction, nerve blocks, local heat, medications to relieve spasm, and physical therapy, are worth a trial in the treatment of this condition. Should pain and disability persist after a reasonable period of conservative treatment or should there be recurrent attacks, operation is indicated.

**Are disk operations dangerous?**

No.

**Is it necessary to fuse the spine after a disk operation?**

Only in a very small proportion of cases.

**How long a hospital stay is required for a disk operation?**

About seven to ten days.

**How successful are operations for ruptured disk?**

About 85 percent of patients are completely or considerably relieved of pain. This presupposes that patients have been carefully selected for surgery and truly have a herniated disk.

**Do ruptured disks ever recur?**

They may, though infrequently.

**Does the removal of a ruptured disk ever result in paralysis?**

No.

**Does removal of a ruptured disk affect one's sex life?**

No.

## SPINAL CORD INJURIES

**What are the common causes of spinal cord injury?**

Injuries of the spinal cord usually occur in association with fractures or dislocations of the spinal column. Falls, automobile and driving accidents, and gunshot wounds are the most frequent causes. The spinal cord may escape injury at the time a spinal fracture is incurred, but careless transportation of the patient from the scene of the accident may result in damage to the spinal cord.

### How does a spinal cord injury manifest itself?

The manifestations of spinal cord injury include varying degrees of paralysis, loss of sensation, and inability to control the bladder and bowels.

### What is the outlook for recovery following spinal cord injury?

In cases in which there is a complete paralysis and loss of all forms of sensation, the outlook for recovery is very poor. The retention of some degree of spinal cord function, no matter how slight, renders the outlook infinitely better than when all function is lost. If evidence of complete interruption of the spinal cord persists for more than a few days, it is unlikely that any improvement will occur. Regeneration of divided fibers does not occur in the spinal cord.

### Is surgery of value in the treatment of spinal cord injury?

In most cases of spinal cord injury, operation is useless. There are occasional exceptions, but, as a rule, all that can be accomplished is to institute orthopedic measures to treat the spinal fracture or dislocation. Reduction of the fracture so as to achieve stability and normal alignment of the bones may require operative treatment.

### Is there any hope for the patient who remains paralyzed?

The management of the patient who remains paralyzed is a complex problem beyond the scope of this discussion. Suffice it to say, after prolonged training it is possible to rehabilitate many of these unfortunate paraplegics so that they can lead a reasonably normal and useful life.

## SURGERY FOR INTRACTABLE PAIN

### Are operations on the spinal cord performed for the relief of pain?

Yes. The neurosurgeon is often called upon to relieve pain that fails to respond to medication. Such pain is usually caused by advanced cancer. The location of the pathways within the spinal cord conducting pain being known, it is possible to cut them and afford the patient relief. This type of operation is known as a cordotomy. It is also possible to cut the nerves (as they enter the spinal cord) that supply a particular region of the body. By depriving that area of all sensation, pain is eliminated. This procedure is called a rhizotomy.

Another neurosurgical procedure is called medial longitudinal myelotomy, which is used primarily to control pelvic pain. This is a procedure that is used more frequently in Europe than in the United States. The operation involves making a longitudinal cut into the lower portion of the spinal cord. The only fiber tracts that are cut are those that carry pain. There is risk, however, that bladder and bowel function may be disturbed. Hence it is best performed in patients who already have these functions impaired.

### Does an operation upon the spinal cord for the relief of pain (cordotomy) result in paralysis?

As a rule, no. However, complications such as varying degrees of weakness (paralysis) and/or impairment of bladder control can occur.

## PERIPHERAL NERVES

### What is a peripheral nerve?

One that conveys impulses between the spinal cord and some other part of the body. It may transmit impulses concerned with muscular contraction as well as stimuli conveying sensory impressions.

### How do nerve injuries occur?

They may occur as a result of blunt

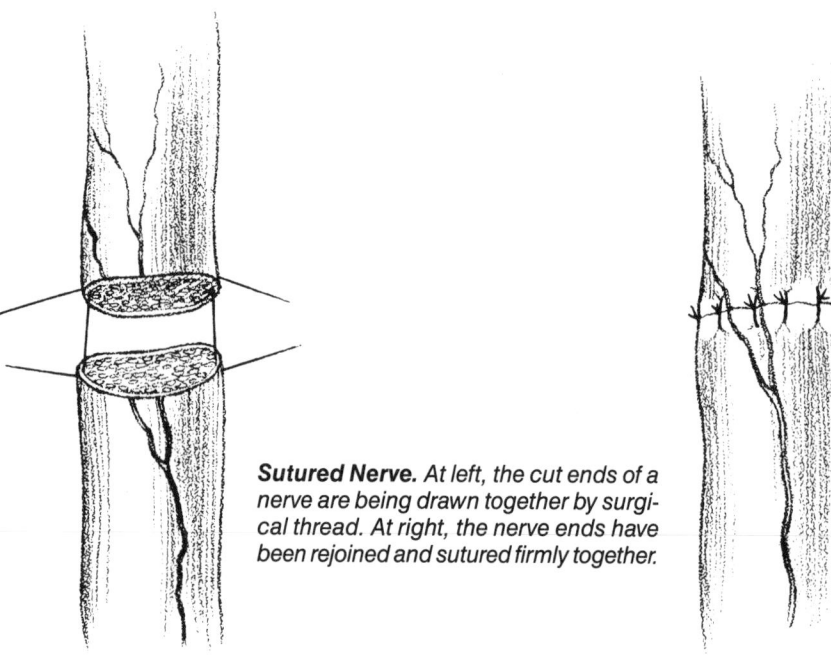

*Sutured Nerve. At left, the cut ends of a nerve are being drawn together by surgical thread. At right, the nerve ends have been rejoined and sutured firmly together.*

trauma, punctures, lacerations, incisions, or penetrating (gunshot or stab) wounds.

## Where do peripheral nerve injuries occur most commonly?

In the limbs.

## What are the symptoms of peripheral nerve injury?

Paralysis of the muscles and loss of sensation over a specific area supplied by that particular nerve.

## What is the role of surgery in the treatment of peripheral nerve injuries?

Nerves are capable of regrowth and resumption of function provided the cut ends are accurately united. This is precisely what the surgeon seeks to accomplish at operation. A good result is not always achieved following surgery. However, with the advent of the operating microscope, small nerves can be sutured with much greater accuracy.

## Is surgery necessary in all types of nerve injury?

No; only in cases in which a nerve has been severed.

## Can tumors arise from peripheral nerves?

Yes. Fortunately, such tumors are usually benign and can be removed completely.

# CHAPTER 47

# THE NEWBORN CHILD

*(See also Chapter 33 on Infant Feeding and Bowel Function; Chapter 35 on Inherited and Congenital Conditions; Chapter 57 on Pregnancy and Childbirth)*

## How can it be determined that a newborn child is normal?

This is usually the first question asked of a pediatrician. It can be answered only after a thorough examination of the newborn baby. This should always be done within the first few days of life. Many of the little abnormalities found within the first few days will disappear spontaneously and should cause no concern.

## Do newborn babies ever display slight difficulty in breathing?

Yes. At birth there may be an excessive collection of mucus in the baby's throat. The nursery nurse will suction this out and thus improve the baby's breathing.

## Why does a newborn baby's head sometimes have a peculiar shape?

The elongated or irregular shape of the baby's head is caused by "molding," which takes place during the birth of the baby. The head will usually return to its normal shape in one to three weeks, although it may take longer in some instances.

## Is there a chance of injuring the "soft spot" fontanelle) on the baby's head?

No. This area is rarely injured, and ordinary washing and touching will not hurt it.

## May a newborn child's head be washed?

Yes.

## Why do some newborns have an egg-shaped swelling on the head?

This may occur because of bleeding beneath the skin of the scalp as a result of pressure during passage down the birth canal. It does not extend into the skull, does not involve the brain, and will be slowly absorbed, leaving no aftereffects.

## Is it significant if a baby is born with very little hair?

No. Many babies are born with very little hair; others will lose some of the hair they do have. Baby hair may fall out, but new hair will grow in later. There may even be some fine, downy hair on the body or forehead. This, too, will disappear in a short time.

## What special care is needed for the baby's scalp?

Wash the scalp with soap and water two or three times a week. Use baby oil at other times. This prevents the formation of scalp crusts or "cradle cap." If cradle cap forms, it can be washed thoroughly and combed out with a fine comb. In some instances your doctor will give you a salve to be applied to the scalp to prevent the reformation of this crust.

## What care should be given to the baby's eyes, ears, and mouth?

It is not necessary to wash the baby's eyes and ears or to cleanse the nose or mouth. Nature has provided fluids and secretions for cleansing them without any outside assistance. If any wax accumulates on the outside of the ears, it may be washed away gently, but do not poke into the ear canals.

## Does anything need to be done about a short membrane (frenum) under the baby's tongue?

In most instances nothing needs to be done, particularly if the baby can protrude the tongue adequately. This so-called "tongue-tie" does not affect speech or produce any lisp. The old practice of clipping this membrane is no longer followed, except when it is very thick, very short, or actually affects the ability of the baby to protrude the tongue beyond the lip margins.

## Why do some babies have a slightly yellow color (jaundice)?

Many babies will develop this light yellow skin color about the third to fifth day of life. This is normal, and nothing needs to be done about it. It will disappear spontaneously in about seven to ten days. This is called physiologic jaundice. If jaundice appears earlier or is more intense or increases instead of disappearing, it will require the attention of your doctor for diagnosis and treatment.

## What are the many small red spots on the baby's skin, seen during the first few days of life?

These are a reaction to the amniotic fluid, which surrounded the baby in the womb. They will disappear in a few days.

## Why does the newborn infant's skin peel?

After having been in a fluid environment for nine months, some infants' skin will peel. The skin is very sensitive at this stage and may react to rubbing, washing, warmth, or irritation of clothing. The reaction may cause some redness or peeling of the skin.

## What is the meaning of small pus pimples on the abdomen or in the groin?

This is the result of a skin infection called impetigo of the newborn. It will clear readily with antibiotic ointments or washing with an antiseptic soap. In some cases antibiotics may also be used internally.

### What is the meaning of a bluish spot at the base of the spine?

This spot has no significance and will disappear in time, perhaps within a year. Similar spots may be present over the buttocks. No treatment is necessary.

### Why do babies lose weight during the first few days of life?

All mothers seem to be concerned about this early loss of weight, yet it occurs with every newborn baby. In breast-fed infants it occurs because the milk does not appear in the mother's breast until the third or fourth day after delivery. In bottle-fed babies, it occurs because of the very small amounts of formula fed to the baby.

### What is the reason for the eyedrops given to newborn babies?

Practically all communities require that some antiseptic be instilled into a baby's eyes as soon as it is born to prevent the possible spread of any infection from the mother's vagina. In some states, silver nitrate is used. In other places it is permissible to use a few drops of penicillin solution or some other antibiotic. Such drops will prevent a gonorrheal eye infec-

tion if the mother is affected with this disease.

### What is the meaning of the marks over the baby's eyes?

Some babies are born with small pressure marks on the eyelids, on the forehead, and over the back of the neck. These have no significance and will usually disappear in a few weeks, though occasionally they may last several months.

### Will the color of the baby's eyes change?

The color of the eyes at birth will not be the final color. It usually takes up to six months for the final color to be established.

### When does a newborn learn to focus his eyes?

At about two to three months of age.

### Is it natural for a newborn's eyes to appear crossed?

Yes. Not all newborns can make their eyes synchronize perfectly during the first year of life. Do not conclude that the baby's eyes are crossed until such a condition persists beyond the age of one to one and a half years.

### Why do some babies have small blood spots in their eyes?

These spots are caused by tiny

hemorrhages in the conjunctiva, or covering, of the eyeball and will disappear without leaving any aftereffects.

### Does the puffiness of the baby's eyes have any significance?

No. This, too, is temporary.

### Why does the baby have some discharge from the eyes on the second or third day?

The discharge is usually caused by the drops that were instilled at birth. It will disappear within a few days.

### Why are the baby's breasts swollen?

Most babies, boys and girls alike, have some swelling of the breasts at birth or soon thereafter. This is caused by a hormone that was circulating through both the mother's and baby's bloodstreams. It is the hormone that induces the production of milk in the mother's breasts.

### What treatment is necessary for swollen breasts?

None, unless the breasts become red, inflamed, and tender. The swelling and any milk secretion will subside without treatment.

### Why do some babies have small white spots on their noses?

These are due to collections of skin

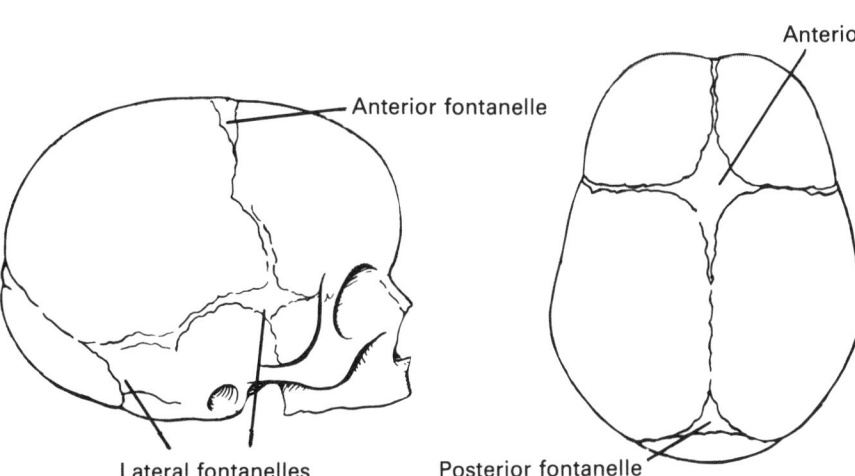

*Fontanelles of the Skull of the Newborn. The spaces between the skull bones are covered by taut connective membranes. The posterior fontanelle closes itself shortly after birth; the anterior (large) fontanelle closes at eight to fifteen months. Contrary to popular belief, injuries to these areas are very rare.*

Anterior fontanelle

Anterior fontanelle

Lateral fontanelles

Posterior fontanelle

oil, which have not been able to escape from the oil glands. Usually the surface film will come off in the washing, and the white oil collections will disappear.

### Is it necessary to circumcise a male infant?

Circumcision is practiced by some people as a religious ritual. Nowadays, it is advised by most physicians for all babies in order to safeguard cleanliness in the area of the penis. Also, the incidence of cancer of the penis is practically nil if circumcision has been carried out in infancy. However, circumcision is not medically essential. (See diagram in Chapter 42, on The Male Organs.)

### When can a circumcision be done?

In cases where it is done as a ritual procedure, the circumcision is usually done on the eighth day of life. It may, however, be done safely on the third or fourth day of life. In some hospitals, the obstetrician will perform circumcision as soon as the baby is born. It is essential that the baby's bleeding time be determined prior to circumcision in order to uncover any abnormal bleeding tendency and to avoid possible postoperative hemorrhage.

### What care should be given after circumcision?

The bandages may be removed in two to three days. Little care other than cleansing is required.

### Does the rectal area need any special handling?

No. Just wash gently with soap and water, as any other part of the body.

### Does the vaginal area need any special handling?

No. Just the ordinary cleansing, preferably with a motion going from the vaginal area backward toward the rectal area.

### Will a hernia result if the umbilical cord was tied off long?

The umbilical cord is usually tied off about one to two inches from the baby's body. This entire area will dry up and fall off in about a week, leaving a moist area of healing. This, in turn, will dry and heal a few days later. The length of the tied cord will not influence development of a hernia.

### What care should be given after the cord has fallen off?

The area should be cleansed with a little alcohol, applied on a cotton applicator, twice a day until it is completely healed. This will take about a week or ten days. If there is a little bleeding, don't be disturbed by it. Occasionally, a small area of "proud flesh" may be found remaining at the navel. This can be cauterized by the baby's physician and will then heal promptly.

### Is an abdominal binder or belly-band necessary?

No. These do not help in the healing of the cord, nor do they prevent a rupture or hernia from forming. Only a dry, clean gauze dressing needs to be applied to the area while it is healing.

### What is the significance of swelling of the scrotum?

In most cases it is caused by an accumulation of fluid. This condition is called a hydrocele. The majority of hydroceles in newborns disappear by themselves within a year after birth. However, it is important for the physician to examine all swellings in the scrotum to make sure that a hernia (rupture) is not present.

### Can crying cause a hernia in a baby boy?

No. Hernia is a developmental defect present at birth.

### Why do some newborn babies' legs appear bowed?

This is due to the position in which the legs were crossed in the uterus. This bowing will disappear in time without treatment.

### How soon may the baby have a sponge bath?

As soon as the baby is taken home from the hospital.

### How soon may the baby have a tub bath?

As soon as the umbilical area has healed completely. In the case of a male baby who has been circumcised, it is wise to wait until the circumcision area is healed too. This will usually take about seven to ten days.

### At what temperature should the baby's room be kept?

Seventy to 72°F. during the day; 65° to 70°F. at night. A room that is too warm is just as harmful as one that is too cold. Always be sure there is some air entering the room, and avoid the use of kerosene or gas stoves in the room for heating purposes.

### When may the baby be taken out of doors?

As soon as the mother is able, providing the weather is good. Start with a quarter hour the first day, a half hour the second day, and so on. Don't take the baby out if the weather is very cold (below 40°F.), windy, or damp. Be sure the baby is adequately protected from the direct glare of the sun.

### When should visitors be permitted to see the new baby?

It is best to keep all visitors away from the newborn for the first week or two. Certainly, anyone with a cold or sore throat should be kept away. After this period, healthy people may be allowed to see and hold the baby.

**Does a baby have to be taken out of doors every day?**

No. Fresh air from an open window is just as healthful. Avoid going out in bad weather just as one would do for oneself.

**Can a newborn baby be given a pacifier if he cries excessively?**

Yes. If it is found to satisfy him, it does no harm.

**May pictures of the newborn baby be taken with a flashbulb?**

Yes. The flashbulb will not in any way affect the baby's eyes.

**May brothers or sisters visit a newborn baby?**

Yes. Many hospitals allow sibling visits. It is reassuring to them that their mother is well, and exciting to see the new arrival.

## PREMATURE BABIES

**What is meant by a premature baby?**

Ordinarily, any baby born before term (nine months) is considered premature. Because we are not sure of the exact length of pregnancy in all cases, all babies who weigh less than five and a half pounds are considered premature and are treated accordingly.

**Do premature babies tend to have more defects than other newborns?**

Yes. However, the great majority are structurally normal.

**What special care is required for premature babies?**

Most premature babies are best cared for in a hospital where special facilities are available. They may require an incubator or a heated crib. Special formulas must be made, and feedings are often given by tube or dropper.

**When can a premature baby leave the hospital?**

If the baby is thriving, he may be taken home when he weighs about five pounds.

**What are the chances for survival of a premature baby?**

The smaller and less mature the baby, the less are his chances of survival. However, many more babies are being saved today than ever before. A baby over four or four and a half pounds has an excellent chance if there are no defects in his heart, brain, or lungs. Babies between four and five pounds have a 90 percent or better chance of survival. Those between three and four pounds have better than a 50 percent chance, but those below three pounds have a considerably poorer chance.

**Does a baby under two pounds have any chance?**

Occasionally such a baby may survive, but it has only a 5 percent chance.

**Does the length of the pregnancy have anything to do with survival rate?**

Yes. The longer the pregnancy, the better the chances of the baby's survival.

**If a baby is carried to full term but weighs very little, will he have a better chance than a premature baby of equal weight?**

Yes.

**Is it true that seven-month babies have a better chance than eight-month babies?**

No. This is a common misconception.

**Is oxygen supplied to every premature baby?**

No. It is supplied only when necessary for the respiration of the premature baby and then only in a special

concentration and only for a few days. It has been found that excessive use of oxygen may be harmful to the baby's eyes.

**How long does the baby stay in an incubator?**

As long as it needs the added oxygen or warmth.

**Are the cribs heated for premature babies?**

Some of the open-air cribs are heated and used when the baby is removed from the incubator.

**Can a premature baby be transported from home to hospital or from hospital to hospital?**

Yes. There are special ambulances that have portable incubators. These supply heat and oxygen to the baby while he is being transported.

**Can any hospital care for a premature infant?**

The larger prematures can be treated in any hospital, but the smaller ones require the special facilities that are present in what are called "Premature Centers."

**Is the premature baby fed right after birth?**

No. Usually a wait of a day or longer is advised.

**Can a premature baby suck from a nipple?**

The larger prematures can, but not the smaller ones.

**How are the smaller premature infants fed?**

A polyethylene tube is inserted through the nose into the baby's gullet and then down into the stomach. Small amounts of formula are then "fed" into the stomach by way of this tube.

**Can the feeding tube stay in the stomach for several days?**

Yes.

**How long is the tube kept in place?**
Until the baby can suck from a nipple. This may take several days or weeks.

**Is this tube harmful or painful if kept in for prolonged periods?**
No.

**What amounts are fed the baby?**
At the start, as little as half a teaspoon (2cc.) at a time. Such feedings may be given every hour or two. The amounts are increased very slowly, depending upon the baby's tolerance and weight gain.

**Does the premature baby require any special dietary supplements?**
Yes. Vitamins may be given earlier, and iron drops may be added to the milk because the premature baby has not been able to store a supply of vitamins and iron that he would have normally received from his mother during the last month or two of uterine development. Also, small amounts of calcium are sometimes added to the baby's diet.

**What other treatments are given to premature babies?**
Some babies require additional fluid by vein or under the skin if they cannot absorb sufficient quantities through the stomach tube.

**Is there a tendency for a premature baby to be anemic?**
Yes, and he may remain so for several weeks or months.

**Are transfusions ever required by premature babies?**
Rarely. However, if the hemoglobin is very low, it may be necessary to give a blood transfusion. Most prematures will respond satisfactorily to iron supplements in the diet.

**Are prematures given routine baths and similar care?**
It is usually advisable not to handle them too much, although the skin must be watched very carefully.

**Are premature babies ever given antibiotics?**
Yes. In some hospitals, antibiotics are given routinely to prevent secondary infections, to which such babies may be prone.

**Is any special care given to the eyes or ears of the premature baby?**
Usually not. Their eyes should be examined about once a week to determine any evidence of disturbance.

**Does prematurity affect the baby's heart or lungs?**
Not ordinarily, although premature babies are more susceptible to a rare lung condition known as hyaline membrane disease.

**Will prematurity affect the baby's later mental development?**
If there are no organic brain defects at birth, the premature baby, with good care, should develop normally after he has been discharged from the hospital. In some cases he may be a little slower in his early development, but he will catch up by completion of the first year of life.

# CHAPTER 48

# THE NOSE AND SINUSES

*(See also Chapter 7 on Allergy; Chapter 39 on Lips, Jaws, Mouth, Teeth, and Tongue; Chapter 56 on Plastic Surgery; Chapter 71 on Throat; Chapter 75 on Upper Respiratory Disease; Chapter 79 on X ray)*

### What is the structure of the nose?

The nose is made up of bone and cartilage and contains two cavities that are separated by a septum. The nose acts as a natural airway for respiration; it acts as an air conditioner by filtering, moistening, and warming the air that is breathed; and it functions as the organ of smell. Also, the hairs within the nose prevent dust from gaining access to the throat, and a mucus that lines the membranes of the nose further settles out dust and bacteria, thus protecting against infection.

## FRACTURED NOSE

### Is fracture of the nose a frequent occurrence?

Yes. It is the most common facial fracture because of the exposed position of the structure and because the nasal bones are thin and delicate.

### Is bleeding from the nose always indicative of the presence of a fracture?

No. There are a considerable number of injuries accompanied by bleeding in which the nasal bones are intact.

### Does bleeding from the nose always take place with a fracture?

No.

### Should x rays be taken to determine nasal fracture?

The diagnosis of a recent nasal fracture is made by clinical examination. It is advisable to take x rays, however, as they will show more specifically where the fracture is located. These x rays are very hard to evaluate and can be easily misread. X rays are usually not necessary after a fracture has been set, as one can determine by observation whether the nose has been restored to a normal appearance.

### How soon after a nasal fracture occurs should it be treated?

As soon as possible, preferably within a few hours, for at this time manipulation of the fragments and setting of the fracture can be accomplished easily. If this is not possible, the fracture must be set within two weeks of the injury. After two weeks have elapsed, the bones have usually healed to a degree, making it extremely difficult to bring them back into proper alignment. Usually, one must wait six months before repairing a nasal fracture that had not been set within two weeks of the time of the injury.

### What methods are used to set a fractured nose?

a. External manipulation by the hand of the surgeon.
b. Insertion of special instruments into the nasal cavity to push out depressed bony fragments.
c. Open surgery in complicated cases and in neglected cases.

### Is it necessary to use anesthesia to set a nasal fracture?

Almost all cases can be set under local anesthesia. In children, a general agent may be used.

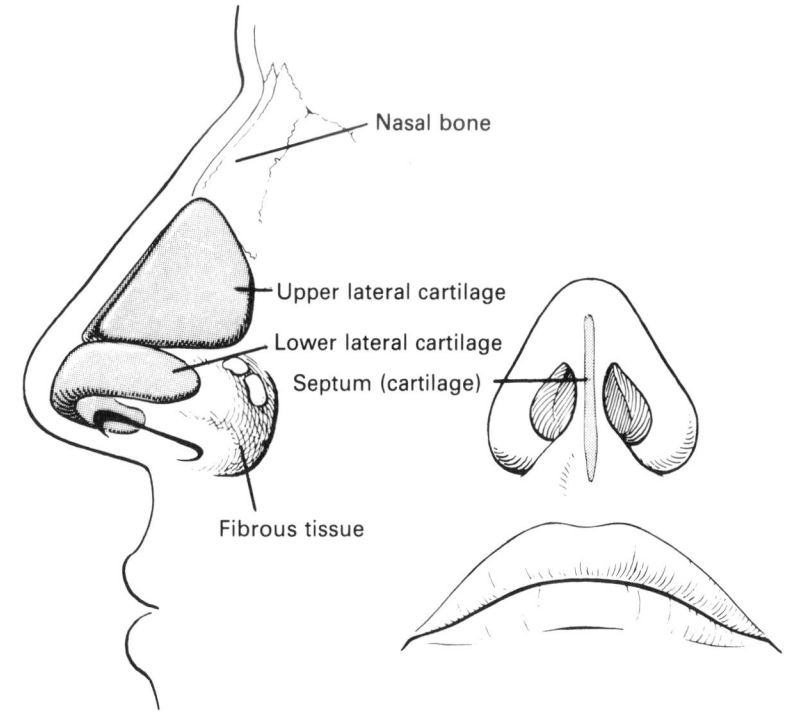

Nasal bone

Upper lateral cartilage

Lower lateral cartilage

Septum (cartilage)

Fibrous tissue

***Anatomy of the Nose.*** *This diagram shows the normal anatomy of the nose. The bones in the nose are quite fragile, and fracture occurs frequently. Fortunately, the nose can be restored to its normal shape without too much difficulty.*

**Is hospitalization necessary for a fracture of the nose?**

Only if there is an extensive or compound fracture, or if general anesthesia is necessary. Also, when there are accompanying injuries that require hospitalization.

**How long does it take a fracture of the nose to heal?**

Nasal fractures heal rapidly because of the rich blood supply in the area. Bone healing usually takes place within two to three weeks. The bones are healed solidly within six weeks, by which time full physical activity may be resumed.

**How long does the swelling of the nose persist after a fracture?**

Slight swelling usually persists for six months to a year, but the greatest part will subside within two to three weeks.

**Is a fracture of the nose usually followed by a permanent deformity?**

No. However, there may be some thickening at the site of the fracture. In children under twelve to fourteen years of age, severe fractures can disturb the growth centers of the nose and lead to delayed deformities of the nose.

**Are antibiotics used following the setting of a nasal fracture?**

No, unless the nasal bones have been exposed (compound fracture) or an infection already exists in the area of nasal fracture.

**What can be done to correct a poor result after the setting of a fracture of the nose?**

Plastic surgery can be performed to restore the nose to normal appearance.

**How long should one wait before advising plastic surgery to restore the appearance of a broken nose that has healed poorly?**

At least six months should pass from

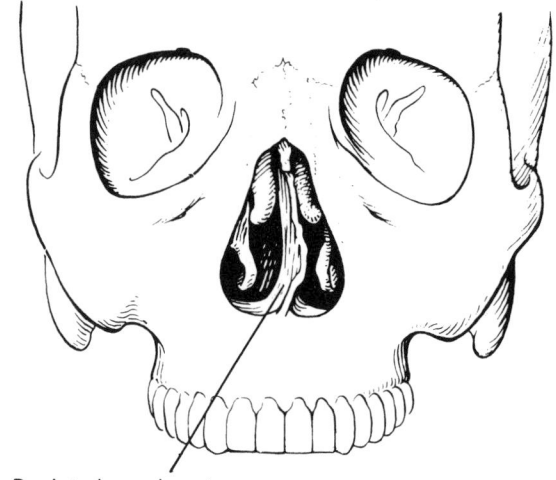

Deviated nasal septum

***Deviated Nasal Septum.** This is a common condition affecting the nose. It may occur as a result of injury, or it may be present from birth. A markedly deviated septum interferes with normal breathing and should be corrected surgically.*

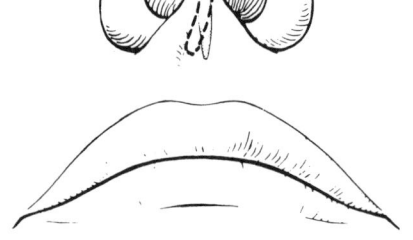

Distortion of nose caused by deviated septum

the time of the original injury. This is advisable because there may be persistent swelling for that length of time, and the degree of deformity cannot be accurately determined until all swelling has subsided.

**Will the proper setting of a fractured nose guarantee that there will be no permanent deformity?**

Unfortunately, no. Even if a fracture is set perfectly, the healing process may cause overgrowth of bone with resultant deformity. Also, injury to the septum may cause septal deviations, which can result in the nose having a twisted appearance.

## DEVIATED SEPTUM

**What is a deviated nasal septum?**

The nasal septum is the partition in the nose that divides it into two

chambers. It is composed of cartilage and bone. When this partition is crooked and not in the midline, it is called a deviated, or deflected, septum. Most people have a slight septal deviation.

**What causes a septum to become deviated?**

Many cases are due to faulty development. However, injuries to the nose, such as dislocation or fracture, can cause the formation of this defect.

**Does the presence of a deviated septum cause symptoms?**

Usually not. Many people have markedly deflected septums without nasal blockage. When there are symptoms, they take the form of blockage of the free and easy passage of air through one nostril, and/or headaches.

### How can a deviated septum that causes nasal blockage be corrected?

This is corrected by performing an operation known as submucous resection of the nasal septum. One must make sure that the nasal blockage is not caused by enlarged turbinates. If this is the situation, the turbinates, not the septum, must be treated.

### Is a submucous resection a dangerous operation?

No. The operation is performed through an intranasal incision. The membranes on either side of the bony and cartilaginous septum are elevated, and spurs, ridges, and deformed sections of the bones and cartilage are cut away. The operation is performed under local anesthesia.

### At what age should submucous resection be carried out?

As this is an elective operation, it should not be done until the nasal bones have developed full growth, usually when the patient is about sixteen years of age or older.

### How successful are operations for deviated septum?

In well-selected cases, the results are exceptionally good, although it is not always possible to straighten a crooked nose perfectly.

### Are there any complications to this operation?

Very rarely there may be bleeding when the nasal packing is removed. This can be readily controlled by the surgeon.

### How soon after an operation for a deviated septum can one return to work?

Usually within ten to twelve days.

### How long a period of hospitalization is necessary?

Two to four days.

### Is a submucous resection operation ever performed at the same time as a plastic operation to improve the appearance of the nose?

Yes. The two procedures are often combined and done at the same time.

### Are the results of a plastic operation upon the nose affected by the presence of a deviated septum?

No. However, when a plastic surgeon notes the presence of a deviated septum, he may repair it at the same time.

## NASAL POLYPS

### What are nasal polyps?

They are grapelike masses of swollen tissue that protrude from the sinuses and the internal side walls of the nose.

### What are thought to be the causes of nasal polyps?

They are thought to be due to an allergy.

### What symptoms are caused by nasal polyps?

If the polyps are small and few in number, there may be no symptoms. Frequently they will be large enough to obstruct the airway and cause difficulty in breathing. Occasionally, polyps will be so large as to extrude from the nostrils.

### What is the treatment for nasal polyps?

When polyps are obstructive, they should be removed surgically. However, the basic treatment should be directed toward determining the cause of the condition and toward preventing recurrence of the polyps.

### What operation is performed for the removal of the polyps?

A polypectomy is usually performed under local anesthesia in the surgeon's office or in the hospital. The polyps are grasped with a wire snare and removed as close to their attachment as possible.

### Does this operation keep one from work for a long time?

No. Most patients may return to work the day following surgery.

## NASAL SINUSES

### What are the nasal sinuses, and where are they located?

The sinuses are mucous membrane-lined air spaces and are located within the bones of the face and skull. They communicate through small openings with the nasal cavity. The frontal sinuses are located within the bone just above and behind the eyebrows; the maxillary sinuses are located within the bones of the cheeks beneath the eyes; the ethmoid sinuses are located near the side of the nose and inner aspect of the eyes and extend backward into the skull; the sphenoid sinus is located deep in the skull above the level of the throat.

### What is the function of the sinuses?

These air-lined spaces lighten the weight of the head and contribute toward the resonance of the voice.

### Is inflammation of the sinuses (sinusitis) a common condition?

Sinusitis is one of the most common conditions encountered in the entire field of medicine. It consists of an inflammation of the mucous membrane lining of one or more of the sinuses. When all the sinuses are involved, the condition is called pansinusitis.

### What causes sinusitis?

It is usually secondary to an infection in the nasal cavity, although the maxillary sinus may become infected as a result of an extension from a tooth infection in the upper jaw. Swimming, diving, and injuries or fractures of the bones overlying the sinuses may also block the sinus openings, and allergies with nasal polyp formation may also predispose to sinusitis.

### Are sinus infections more likely to occur in certain climates?

Yes. Those who live in damp, muggy climates or in areas in which there are marked fluctuations in temperature are more prone to develop sinus infections. Also, those who constantly breathe polluted air show a greater tendency toward sinusitis. People who live in dry, warm, equable climates show the lowest incidence of sinus infection.

### What are the symptoms of sinusitis?

They vary according to the sinus involved. The most common symptoms are:
a. Tenderness over the infected sinus.
b. A nasal quality to the voice.
c. Nasal obstruction, with discharge from the nose or down the back of the nose.
d. Severe headache, which is worse on lowering the head.
e. Elevated temperature.

### How is the diagnosis of sinusitis made?

Sinusitis is usually suspected when a cold has persisted for more than a week. The presence of pain or tenderness over the affected sinus, headache, and the symptoms enumerated above will tend to establish the diagnosis. It can be confirmed by transillumination of the sinus with a strong light in a dark room and by taking x rays.

### What is the treatment for sinusitis?

Most cases will respond well to medical treatment. This should consist of bed rest, steam inhalations, warm compresses to the affected sinus area, nose drops to lessen the congestion of the nasal mucous membranes, and the use of antibiotic and antihistaminic drugs. If the fever is high, medicines such as aspirin should be used. If the pain is severe, pain-relieving drugs such as codeine may be used. Further medical treatment in the physician's office will consist of nasal packs and various methods of removing the nasal discharge by the use of suction. Cultures of the sinus discharge are frequently taken to determine the exact germ involved and to test the sensitivity of these bacteria to the various antibiotic drugs.

### Which sinuses are most prone to develop inflammation?

The maxillary, frontal, and ethmoid sinuses.

### What cases of sinusitis require surgery?

Those that fail, after a prolonged period of time, to respond to the above-mentioned medical management.

### What operations are carried out for sinusitis?

The aim of all operations for sinusitis is to obtain adequate drainage and, in some cases, to remove diseased mucous membranes and bone. Most of these operations are done under local anesthesia, but some may require general anesthesia.

### What operations are usually performed upon the maxillary sinus?

a. Simple puncture of the sinus through the nose, with irrigation and suction.
b. The cutting of a large window in the side wall of the nose into the sinus to promote drainage.
c. A radical sinusotomy, in which the mucous membrane lining the sinus is lifted away from the underlying bone and scraped out. In this operation, the incision is made inside the mouth beneath the upper lip.

### What operations are performed on the frontal sinus?

Formerly, the frontal sinus was irrigated through the nose, but this is rarely done today. If surgery is necessary, an incision is made in the skin below the inner portion of the eyebrow, and a small hole is cut in the bony floor of the frontal sinus. If the infection has involved the surrounding bone, it may become necessary to do a radical frontal sinusotomy. In this event, a larger incision is made, and the entire bony floor of the frontal sinus is removed. Although frontal sinus operations are serious, the results are usually good, and the majority of patients recover completely.

### What operations are performed on the ethmoid sinuses?

These sinuses can usually be approached and scraped out through the nose. If the infection is severe or has involved the sphenoid sinus or has broken through to involve the tissues about the eyes, it may be necessary to do an external ethmoidectomy. In this event, the incision is simply a prolongation downward of the same type of incision that is made for a frontal sinus infection.

### What operations are used for inflammation of the sphenoid sinus?

Under local anesthesia, this sinus can be probed and irrigated through the nose. As a severe sphenoid infection may lead to brain infection or blindness, it is sometimes necessary to do a radical operation in conjunction with a complete ethmoidectomy.

### How effective is sinus surgery?

The great majority of cases are improved through surgery.

### How long a hospital stay is necessary after major sinus surgery?

Usually about seven days.

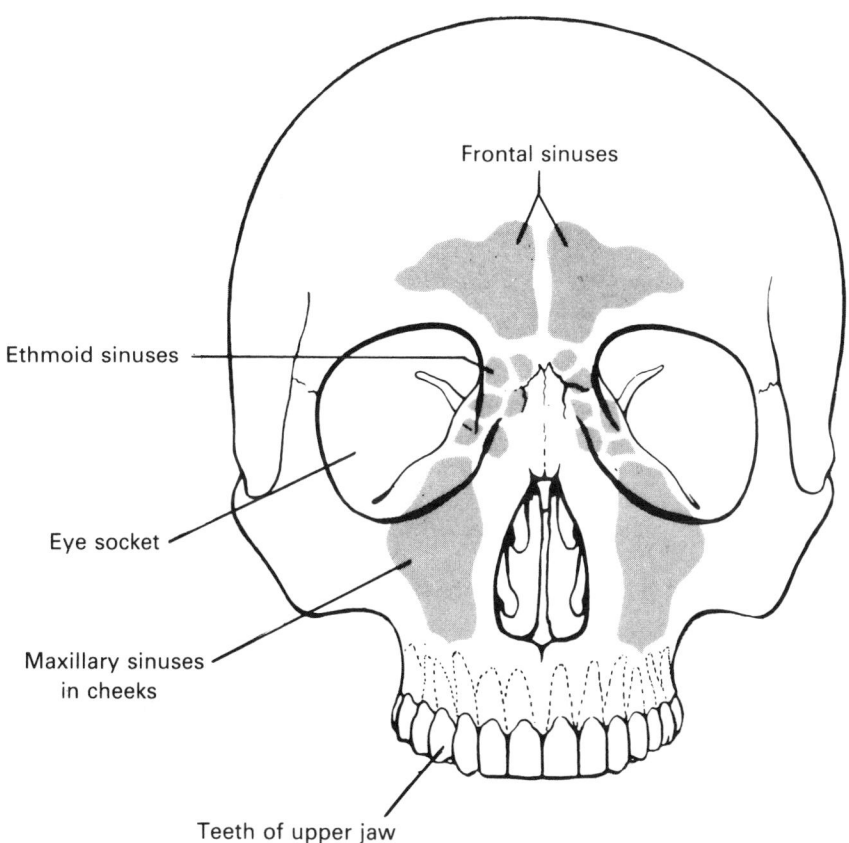

Frontal sinuses

Ethmoid sinuses

Eye socket

Maxillary sinuses
in cheeks

Teeth of upper jaw

*Diagram of the Nasal Sinuses.* Sinuses are air spaces within the bones of the skull whose main purposes are to lighten the skull and to give resonance to the voice. The sinuses are a frequent site of infection, and, unfortunately, these infections tend to be chronic.

**Does sinusitis ever recur after surgery?**

Yes, but in a small minority of cases.

**How does one treat recurrent sinusitis?**

It is treated as a new infection and is handled in the same way as an original infection.

## TUMORS OF THE NOSE AND SINUSES

### Are tumors of the nose and sinuses common?

The benign tumors are rather common. Among these, one would include nasal polyps, warts, and hemangiomas (small blood vessel tumors). Fortunately, malignant tumors are not very common in this area.

**What is the treatment for benign tumors of the nose or sinuses?**

Most of these can be removed readily under local anesthesia in the surgeon's office.

**What is the treatment for malignant tumors of the nose and sinuses?**

Cancer of the nose or sinuses is treated by wide surgical removal of the growth and surrounding tissues. Extensive plastic surgery is usually performed at a later date, after the physician is reasonably sure that all of the cancer was completely removed.

**How successful is surgery for tumors of the nose and sinuses?**

Surgery for benign tumors is uniformly successful. The success of surgery for cancer depends upon the time at which the surgery is performed and upon the degree of malignancy. If the surgery has been done before the cancer has spread to distant tissues, the expectation of cure is good. Modern surgical techniques may include the lifesaving measures in which large sections of the nose, face, cheek, the roof of the mouth, or the floor of the orbit are removed.

**Can cosmetic reconstruction be carried out after radical surgery upon the nose and sinuses?**

Yes. Modern advances in technique in plastic surgery can effect remarkable restoration toward normal appearance.

## NOSEBLEEDS

**What causes nosebleeds?**

In many cases, there is no apparent cause. However, there may be local or general causes or a combination of both:

a. Injury to the nose or the base of the skull with or without fracture.
b. Foreign body in the nose.
c. Operations upon the nose.
d. Violent coughing, sneezing, or nose blowing.
e. Nose picking.
f. Ulcerations caused by diseases such as syphilis and tuberculosis.
g. Benign or malignant tumors within the nose or sinuses.
h. Varicose veins of the mucous membranes of the nose.
i. An acute inflammation of the mucous membrane lining of the nose as occurs in allergy, sinusitis, or the common cold.

**What are some of the general causes of nosebleeds?**

a. High blood pressure.
b. Blood disorders such as hemophilia, pernicious anemia, purpura, scurvy, leukemia, and jaundice.
c. Atmospheric changes such as mountain climbing, diving, or descending to great depths within the sea.
d. Excessive dry heat such as is found in homes and buildings heated during the winter months.

**How can one distinguish between a nosebleed caused by a local condition and one caused by a general condition?**

If the bleeding arises from one nostril only, the cause is more likely to be local. Also, thorough nasal examination will reveal a bleeding point or other local cause.

**How can nosebleeds be controlled?**

There are really two types of nosebleeds. Over 90 percent occur in the anterior part of the nose, arising from the septum or more rarely from the anterior ethmoid area. The point of bleeding can usually be found and controlled by cauterization under local anesthesia. This can be done by chemicals such as silver nitrate or by electric coagulation.

**What should be done as a first-aid measure for nosebleed?**

Since the vast majority occur in the anterior part of the nasal septum, they can be simply controlled by continuous pressure applied to the side of the nose from which the bleeding arises. It is well to put a small piece of cotton in the nose, possibly moistened with some nose drop if available. Pressure against this piece of cotton should be maintained for at least ten minutes. The person should be sitting up with his head tilted forward to prevent blood from trickling down his throat; also, because bleeding from a vein will decrease if the head is higher than the heart.

**What can be done for bleeding arising from the posterior part of the nose?**

This type cannot be self-treated. People with this condition must be hospitalized, as it is usually necessary to pack the posterior part of the nose through the mouth.

**How long is the nasal packing left in place?**

The posterior packing is left in place for about a week. Anterior packing should be removed gradually, starting generally about the fourth day.

**What is the treatment for nosebleeds that arise from a general condition?**

Expert medical advice must be obtained, and treatment of the underlying disease must be instituted.

## PLASTIC SURGERY OF THE NOSE (*Rhinoplasty*)

**Can all nasal deformities be corrected through plastic surgery?**

Almost every deformity can be corrected to a certain degree.

**What are the common types of nasal deformity?**

a. A twisted nose.
b. Deformities of the tip of the nose or nostrils.
c. Depression of the bridge and ridge of the nose, called "saddle-nose."
d. Hump nose or hook nose.

**Is there a standard appearance for the nose?**

No. Each plastic operation upon the nose should be individualized for each patient. Different peoples and races have different standards of beauty or acceptability.

**What is meant by the expression "a perfect nose"?**

In the absolute sense, there is no such thing as a perfect nose. The best one can say is that a nose should fit the face.

**What are some of the important factors in determining the results of plastic surgery upon the nose?**

a. The age of the patient. The best results are obtained in those from sixteen to thirty years of age.
b. The skin. The quality of the skin, including its thickness, thinness, and tendency toward oiliness.
c. The extent of the deformity. The greater the deformity, the more difficult it is to get a perfect result.
d. The type of deformity. Certain

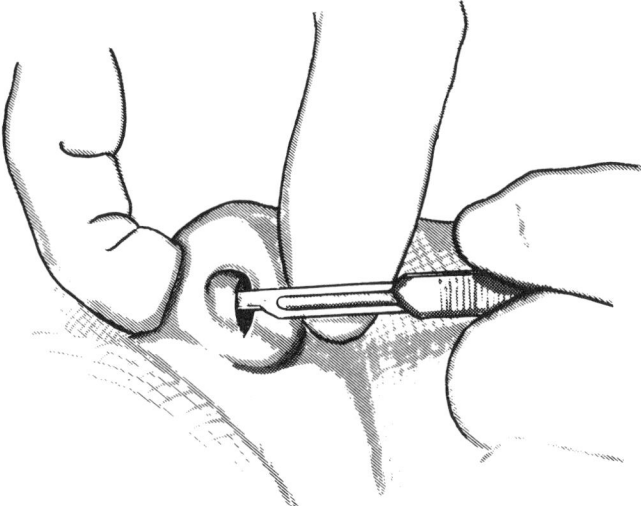

Incision within the nostril
for deviated septum
or plastic operation

***Plastic Surgery upon the Nose.*** *The incisions for plastic operations upon the nose are made within the nostril so that no scar will be visible after the operation is completed. Considerable swelling follows most nasal plastic operations, and it may take several weeks or months for it to subside completely.*

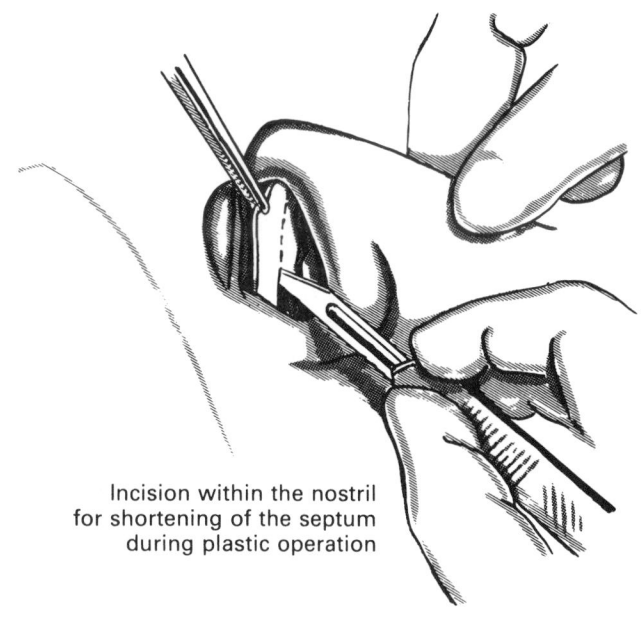

Incision within the nostril
for shortening of the septum
during plastic operation

types of deformity are much harder to cure than others, especially severely twisted noses.

e. The mental stability of the patient. The results are poorer among neurotic patients who have a tendency to worry about insignificant defects.

**Are the results good when an operation is performed upon a child rather than upon an adult?**

The surgeon should wait until the nose is fully formed; this does not take place until the child has attained at least age sixteen. There are exceptions, however, when a

rhinoplasty can be performed on a younger child (twelve to fifteen).

**What operation is performed for a plastic procedure on the nose?**

All the incisions are made within the nose, and the skin of the nose is loosened or undermined to free it from the bone and cartilage, which make up the framework of the nose. The frame work of the nose is then cut and shaped according to a plan laid out before the operation. The skin then falls back upon the reshaped frame work and is sutured into position. A dressing is placed on the outside of the nose to help maintain the new position of the bone and cartilage. Packing is normally not used. As time passes, the skin will attach itself to the newly shaped bony and cartilaginous framework of the nose.

**Are any scars visible after plastic operations upon the nose?**

No, because incisions are made within the nasal cavity. If the nostrils are made smaller, external incisions are used, but they are well hidden.

**Is it possible for the patient to select the type of nose he desires?**

Only to a certain degree. The surgeon must first overcome the defects of the nose and then he will try to create a result pleasing to his patient. The patient must understand clearly before surgery that an exact prediction cannot be made as to the specific appearance of the nose after surgery.

**Can the patient obtain a good approximate idea of what his nose will look like after surgery?**

Yes. An approximation can be foretold.

**What materials are used to build up a nose?**

The best substance, or graft, is a piece of bone or cartilage taken from the patient himself. Bone, when

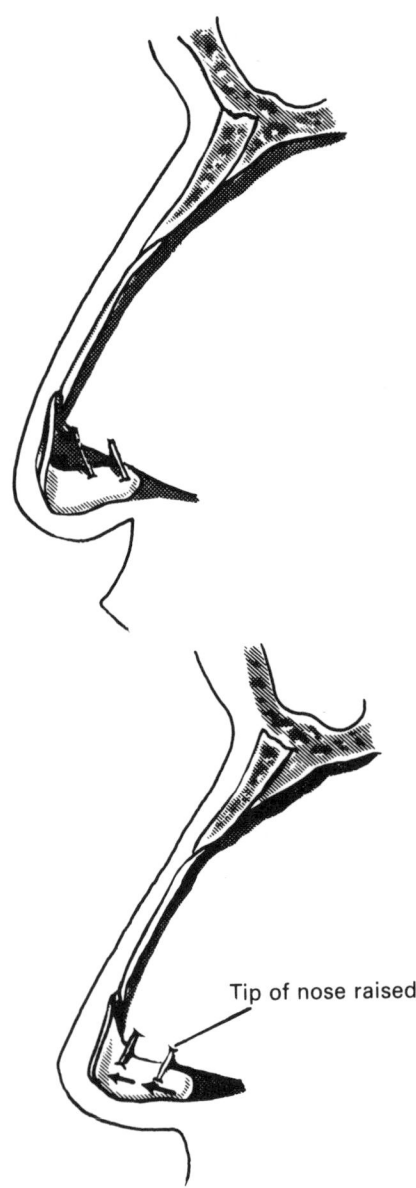

Tip of nose raised

*Plastic Surgery Upon the Nose. Plastic operations on the nose are usually performed under local anesthesia and require but a short hospital stay. Although marked improvement follows almost all plastic operations upon the nose, the patient should understand that the exact shape the nose will take cannot always be predicted.*

used, is taken from the hip or shinbone. Cartilage, which is more commonly used than bone, may be taken from the nasal septum, the ear, or from a rib cartilage.

### How long does a plastic operation upon the nose take to perform?

Approximately one hour.

### What anesthesia is used?

Local anesthesia, fortified by sedation.

### Are plastic operations upon the nose painful procedures?

No.

### How long a hospital stay is necessary?

Two to four days.

### Is it common for the eyes to be discolored or swollen after this operation?

Yes. This will begin to subside in approximately forty-eight hours but may not completely disappear for a week or two.

### When are the dressings and packings removed from the nose after a plastic operation?

External dressings are removed anywhere from twenty-four hours to seven days after surgery. Nasal packings, if used, are removed twenty-four to forty-eight hours postoperatively.

### Does a plastic operation upon the nose affect the sense of smell?

No.

### How long after a plastic operation on the nose can one breathe normally?

The nose may feel "stuffy" for up to two weeks.

### After a nose has healed completely following a plastic operation, must special care be exercised not to injure it?

No. A healed nose following plastic surgery is just as strong as any other nose.

### Do noses that have undergone plastic surgery tend to sag and change shape months or years later?

No. They will heal in the position that is present immediately following the surgical procedure.

### May swelling of the nose persist even for several months after plastic surgery?

Yes. It may take several months or even a year for the nose to attain its absolute permanent shape and for all of the swelling to disappear.

### How soon after a plastic operation on the nose can one return to work and to social functions?

In approximately two weeks, even though some swelling may remain. Contact sports and physical activity can begin six weeks after surgery.

### Is it possible to repeat a plastic operation if the result of the first operation is unsatisfactory?

Yes; but it is best to wait at least six months before repeating the surgery so that stabilization of healing has had an opportunity to develop.

### How successful are plastic operations upon the nose?

The overall improvement is almost always good, and the general degree of satisfaction is high. When results are poor, they can often be remedied by reoperation.

# CHAPTER 49

# THE PANCREAS

*(See also Chapter 19 on Diabetes Mellitus; Chapter 27 on Gall Bladder and Bile Ducts; Chapter 66 on Small and Large Intestines; Chapter 70 on Stomach and Duodenum)*

## Where is the pancreas, and what are its functions?

The pancreas is a flat yellowish gland that stretches across the upper abdomen for a distance of approximately five inches. It lies on the posterior abdominal wall between the lowermost extent of the stomach and the upper margin of the transverse colon. Its head is attached to, and is surrounded by, the curve of the duodenum. The pancreas has two main functions:

a. To manufacture various enzymes (chemical substances) that help to digest the food in the intestinal tract.

b. To manufacture and secrete into the blood stream the hormone known as insulin, which regulates the rate at which sugar is utilized by the body.

## How do pancreatic secretions reach the intestines?

Through long ducts or tubes that course the entire width of the pancreas and empty into the duodenum.

## What are the most common diseases of the pancreas?

a. Pancreatitis.
  1. The acute type.
  2. The chronic, or recurring, type.
b. Abscess of the pancreas.
c. Diabetes.

d. Hyperinsulinism, or overproduction of the hormone that causes sugar to be burned by the body.
e. Cysts of the pancreas.
f. Benign tumors of the pancreas.
g. Cancer of the pancreas.

## How does an upset in the pancreas become evident?

There may be upper abdominal pain, with nausea and vomiting, particularly after eating large meals. Failure to produce sufficient insulin will become evident by the development of diabetes.

## PANCREATITIS (Inflammation of the Pancreas)

## What causes acute inflammation of the pancreas (pancreatitis)?

In some instances it is thought to be caused by infected bile backing up into the pancreatic ducts; in other instances it is caused by bacteria that invade the pancreas directly through its blood supply. It is not unusual for pancreatitis to have its onset shortly after one has eaten large quantities of food or imbibed excessive amounts of alcohol. Gallstones are frequently associated with pancreatitis.

## Is pancreatitis a serious disease?

Yes, especially in its acute form, which can be accompanied by severe hemorrhage, overwhelming toxemia, and death. However serious it is, the great majority of those affected will recover.

## What are the symptoms and signs of acute pancreatitis?

a. Elevation of temperature.
b. Pain, tenderness, and distention in the upper abdomen.
c. Nausea and vomiting.
d. An increase in the quantity of amylase and lipase (chemical enzymes) circulating in the blood.
e. Signs of shock in severe cases,

secondary to hemorrhage and toxemia.

## What are the symptoms of chronic or recurring pancreatitis?

When it recurs, it usually takes the form of an acute episode. Chronic indigestion, a bloated feeling, and vague abdominal pains are seen in the chronic form of the disease. In some cases, it is associated with diabetes.

## What is the treatment for acute pancreatitis?

a. No food by mouth is given; fluids and glucose (sugar) are given through the veins.
b. Antibiotics are sometimes given to control bacterial infection within the gland.

## Is a patient with acute pancreatitis often subjected to surgery?

Yes. Surgery is often recommended because the exact diagnosis has not been established, and it is necessary to rule out other upper abdominal emergencies for which surgery is mandatory. Surgery is also performed for the complications of pancreatitis such as abscess or cyst formation.

## What operative procedures are carried out when operating upon pancreatitis?

The fluid that is secreted into the abdominal cavity in cases of pancreatitis is drained. If the gall bladder or bile ducts are found to contain stones, and if it is thought that this is a contributing factor in the causation of the pancreatitis, the stones are removed and the gall bladder or bile ducts are drained with rubber tubes.

## Does disease within the gall bladder or biliary system often incite pancreatitis?

Approximately half the cases of pancreatitis are associated with gallstones, and many physicians feel that this is one of the main factors

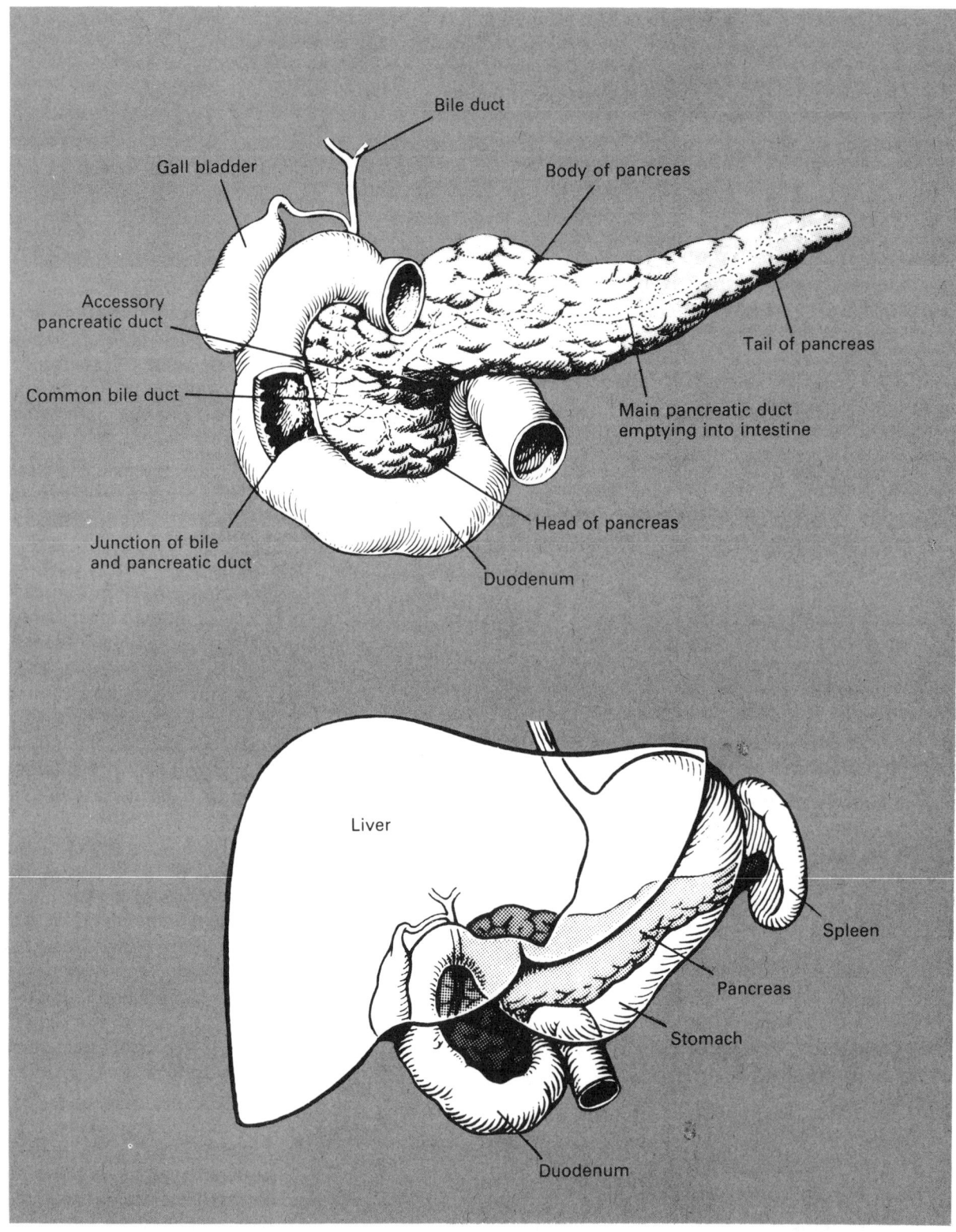

**Anatomy of the Pancreas.** *This diagram shows the location and the relations of the pancreatic gland within the upper portion of the abdomen. The pancreas is important in that it secretes enzymes that help digest food. It is also the organ that manufactures insulin, the hormone that controls the metabolism of sugar. Failure of the insulin-producing cells within the pancreas results in diabetes.*

leading to the development of pancreatitis.

**Is alcoholism frequently associated with pancreatitis?**

Yes, in perhaps 50 to 70 percent of cases.

**Does pancreatitis have a tendency to recur?**

Yes, unless the underlying condition, such as gall bladder disease, is corrected.

**How can pancreatitis best be prevented?**

By eating a bland, low-fat diet, by not overeating, and by restricting alcohol intake. Also, any disease within the gall bladder or bile ducts must be eradicated.

**Is pancreatitis usually associated with diabetes?**

Usually not. It is remarkable that thise cells that manufacture insulin do not appear to be involved very often when pancreatitis occurs. It is only in the very severe case that diabetes may ensue.

## ABSCESS OF THE PANCREAS

**When is an abscess of the pancreas most apt to develop?**

Following an attack of acute pancreatitis.

**Does this occur frequently?**

No. It is found usually only after very severe cases in which the pancreatitis has caused destruction of a portion of the gland.

**How is a diagnosis of pancreatic abscess made?**

By studying the history of a previous episode of pancreatitis and by noting pain and tenderness in the upper abdomen, along with temperature elevation. These symptoms come on several days or weeks after an attack of pancreatitis has appeared to subside. A sonogram may demonstrate the presence of an abscess, as may a CAT scan. (See Chapter 79, on X ray.)

**What is the treatment for an abscess within the pancreas?**

a. Administration of antibiotic drugs.
b. Surgical drainage of the abscess.

**What are the chances for recovery following surgery for a pancreatic abscess?**

The great majority of patients will get well, but the wound may drain pus for quite some time.

## DIABETES MELLITUS
*(See Chapter 19 on Diabetes)*

## HYPERINSULINISM
*(Hypoglycemia)*

**What is hyperinsulinism?**

It is a condition in which the insulin-producing cells (the cells of the islets of Langerhans) manufacture and secrete an excessive amount of insulin into the bloodstream.

**What causes hyperinsulinism?**

Some cases are caused by a tumor (adenoma) or multiple tumors within the pancreas involving an overgrowth of those cells that manufacture insulin. Other cases are caused by an upset in metabolism of the gland, with resultant secretion of abnormally large quantities of insulin into the bloodstream.

**What are the symptoms of hyperinsulinism?**

Abrupt episodes of intense hunger, trembling of the hands, black spots before the eyes, mental confusion, fainting, and, in severe cases, convulsions with loss of consciousness. Examination of the blood at the time of these attacks will show an extremely low level of circulating sugar. In some patients, ulcers of the duodenum may develop.

**What type of person is most likely to be affected by hyperinsulinism?**

Young adults are more prone than older people to develop hyperinsulinism.

**Is hyperinsulinism always accompanied by a tumor of the pancreas?**

No. There are many cases in which examination of the pancreas will reveal no abnormality. Microscopic examination of a portion of the pancreas, however, may sometimes show overgrowth of the insulin-producing cells without true tumor formation.

**How large are adenomas of the pancreas?**

They are small lesions measuring no more than a half to one inch in diameter. They cannot be felt on abdominal examination, but they may appear on sonography (see Chapter 67, on Sonography) or on a CAT scan (see Chapter 79, on x ray).

**What is the treatment for hyperinsulinism?**

At first, medical management is attempted. This will consist largely of giving low quantities of sugar in the diet so as not to excite or overstimulate insulin production. If this form of treatment is unsuccessful, then an exploratory abdominal operation is carried out for the presence of a tumor (pancreatic adenoma) or tumors.

**What form of surgery is carried out for hyperinsulinism when no tumor of the pancreas is discovered at operation?**

Some surgeons feel that a portion—such as a half or two-thirds—of the pancreas should be removed. Others feel that this is not beneficial and carries with it too great a risk.

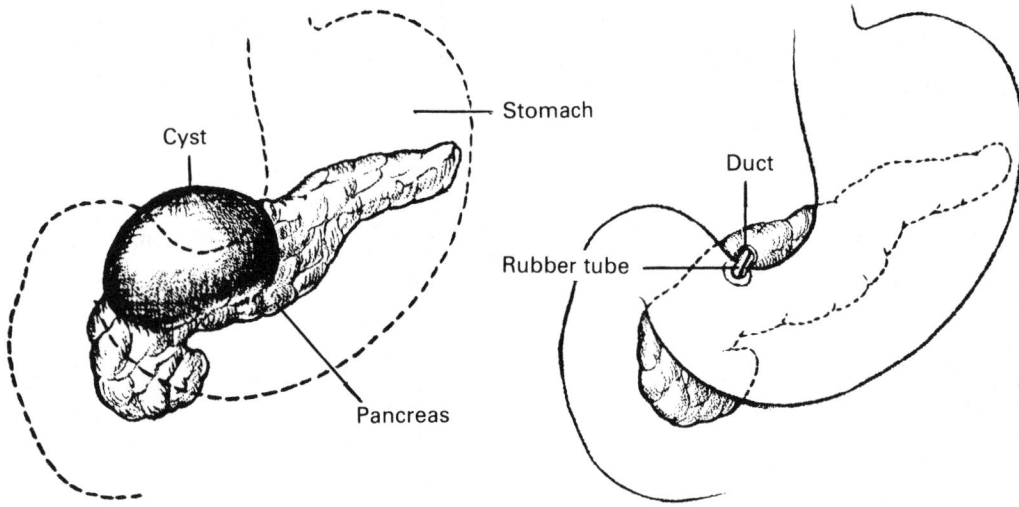

Cyst

Stomach

Duct

Rubber tube

Pancreas

*Cyst of the Pancreas. In the drawing at left, a cyst of the pancreas is shown. The dotted outline of the stomach is superimposed. Below, a rubber tube has been inserted from the duct of the pancreas into the stomach. This will drain the cyst of its fluid in a few weeks, and it will collapse.*

**If a benign adenoma of the pancreas is found, can it be removed surgically?**

Yes. This is not a dangerous procedure, and the patient is usually cured of his hyperinsulinism.

**Does recovery from hyperinsulinism take place?**

Yes, in the great majority of cases. However, it is important to carry out a thorough examination of the patient to make sure that some other endocrine gland, such as the pituitary, thyroid, or adrenal, is not responsible for the upset in pancreatic function.

**What is the Zollinger-Ellison syndrome?**

This is a condition in which there are severe ulcers of the stomach or duodenum caused by a special kind of tumor of the pancreas.

**What is the treatment for the Zollinger-Ellison syndrome?**

If an isolated tumor of the pancreas is located, this should be removed. Unfortunately, the condition is not always associated with a discernible tumor, and in these instances it may be necessary to remove the entire stomach in order to prevent new ulcers from forming.

## CYSTS OF THE PANCREAS

**What are cysts of the pancreas, and how often do they occur?**

It is thought that blockage of one of the pancreatic ducts may cause cysts to form, or that they are the end result of an episode of pancreatitis. When cysts do occur (they are an uncommon lesion), they may vary in size from that of a grape to a watermelon.

**Are cysts of the pancreas dangerous?**

No. The small ones may be ignored. It is only the large ones that require attention when they press upon and interfere with the function of neighboring organs.

**How is the diagnosis of a cyst of the pancreas arrived at?**

The larger cysts can be felt by the examining physician as a painless, rounded swelling in the upper abdomen. Others may be diagnosed by taking a sonogram or CAT scan.

**What surgery is advocated for a cyst of the pancreas?**

The cyst is removed, or if this is not technically feasible because of its size, attachments, or location, it is merely drained of its fluid contents.

Several rubber drains are inserted into the cyst cavity and are left in place for several weeks until the cyst collapses and fills in by itself. In some cases, the wall of the cyst is stitched to the stomach or small intestine and its contents permitted to drain internally. This method often leads to a rapid cure.

**Are there any permanent aftereffects from cysts of the pancreas?**

No. Digestion and pancreatic function usually return to normal within several weeks to a few months.

## BENIGN TUMORS OF THE PANCREAS

**What is the most common benign tumor of the pancreas?**

A growth involving those cells that manufacture insulin. (See the section on Hyperinsulinism in this chapter.)

**Do these benign tumors ever develop into cancer?**

Yes. This is one of the main reasons why surgery should be undertaken when a pancreatic tumor is suspected.

## CANCER OF THE PANCREAS

**Is cancer of the pancreas encountered very often?**

Unfortunately, it is one of the most common of all abdominal cancers and carries with it the lowest rate of permanent cure.

**What causes cancer of the pancreas?**

The cause is not known.

**Where are most cancers of the pancreas located?**

The majority are located in the head of the pancreas, adjoining the duodenum. Most benign tumors of this organ are located farther to the left side in the body or tail of the pancreas.

**What are symptoms of cancer of the pancreas?**

Pain in the upper abdomen, usually radiating to the back. Also, because the cancer is usually located in the head of the pancreas, its growth creates pressure on the bile ducts, and this will result in obstruction and the slow onset of jaundice. The patient experiences loss of appetite, weight loss, and progressive weakness. Jaundice may not be noted if the growth involves the body or tail of the pancreas.

**What are the chances for cure in cancer of the pancreas?**

Not very great, although operations have been evolved in which the entire pancreas and the surrounding duodenum can be removed. Unfortunately, even with these extensive procedures, it is not often that the cancer can be eradicated completely.

**Will the patient develop diabetes after removal of the pancreas?**

Yes. However, other organs in the body tend to take over the metabolism of sugar, and the patient often does not die from diabetes.

**What is the life expectancy after a diagnosis of cancer of the pancreas has been made?**

Approximately six to eighteen months. It must be remembered, though, that a considerable number of cases have been reported in which permanent cure has followed removal of the entire gland.

**Can one anticipate greater progress in the diagnosis and treatment of cancer of the pancreas?**

Yes. The use of the CAT scan has been successful in discovering pancreatic cancers when they are extremely small and give no symptoms. Thus, surgery will be much more successful in curing this disease.

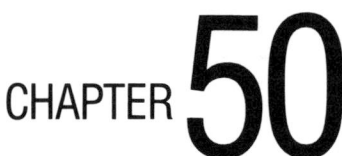

CHAPTER **50**

# PARASITES AND PARASITIC DISEASES

*(See also Chapter 34 on Infectious and Virus Diseases; Chapter 38 on Laboratory (Pathology) Tests and Procedures)*

### What is an animal parasite?

One that lives at the expense of its host.

### Are there organisms other than animal that are parasitic?

Yes. Parasites include bacteria, viruses, and fungi, as well as animals. However, in the medical sense, parasitology (the study of parasites) is generally restricted to the animal parasites of man.

### How do parasites gain entry to the human body?

Through contaminated food or drink, by direct contact with the skin or mucous membranes, or through infected blood-sucking insects. A certain type of dysentery can be transmitted through sexual contact, especially in homosexual practices.

### What are common parasites that gain entry to the body by means of contaminated food or drink?

These include intestinal protozoa *(Entamoeba histolytica* and *Balantidium cofi),* roundworms *(Ascaris lumbricoides* and *Enterobius vermicularis),* tapeworms such as the fish tapeworm *(Diphyllobothrium latum)* or the beef tapeworm *(Taenia solium),* etc.

### What are examples of parasites that gain entrance through the skin or mucous membranes?

Hookworms and the itch mite.

### What is the most common parasite to be transmitted by an infected blood-sucking insect?

The malarial parasite, which is transmitted by an infected mosquito.

### Once parasites gain access to the body, can they multiply there?

Not all animal parasites multiply in the body. This is particularly true of infestations with worms. However, the malarial parasites and amebae, among others, multiply within the body.

### Is anyone actually immune to parasitic infestation?

No.

### How can parasitic disease be avoided?

The practice of good sanitary habits, having a pure water supply, avoidance of contact with infected material, and control of carriers of infection (mosquitoes, lice, etc.) are some of the best means of avoiding infection. Some of these involve measures of public health that may be worldwide in scope, such as the control of mosquitoes, ticks, etc.

### Is it possible to harbor more than one parasite at a time?

Yes. Multiple infestation is very common.

### Are there any areas of the world where parasitic diseases are more prevalent than others?

Yes. People living in the tropics or semitropics have a relatively high incidence of parasitic infestation. Those areas where sanitation is poorly handled also have a high incidence of parasitism. Food habits are also important. Scandinavians who commonly eat or sample raw fish have higher infestation rates

from the fish tapeworm than people who are careful to cook this food thoroughly before eating.

### How is a diagnosis of parasitic disease made?

The only certain way is by identifying the organism in body excrement (stool or urine), body fluids, or tissues. At times, skin testing and other laboratory tests may be helpful in arriving at a precise diagnosis.

### Are there any specific blood changes in parasitic disease?

No, although an increase in the number of certain circulating white blood cells (eosinophils) may be suggestive. In malaria or certain other parasitic diseases, the parasite may be identified microscopically by examining a blood smear. In such cases, an absolute diagnosis can be made.

### Is there any effective treatment to cure parasitic diseases?

In most instances, specific treatment *is* available, and the infestation can be eradicated. The treatment, however, varies with each particular parasite.

## AMEBIASIS

### What is amebiasis?

This is an infestation from a one-celled animal parasite called an ameba. There are several types of amebae that are disease producing, the most important of which is called *Entamoeba histolytica.* It generally causes an intestinal disease known as amebic colitis, or dysentery. The parasite may at times invade other organs of the body, including the liver and brain.

### Where is amebiasis found?

It is found throughout the world, but most commonly in the tropics and semitropics. It should be noted that there was quite an outbreak in

Chicago some years ago. With the vast increase in world travel, no country is immune to this type of infection.

**How is amebiasis transmifted?**

From person to person through ingestion of contaminated food or drink.

**What are the symptoms of amebic colitis (dysentery)?**

Recurrent attacks of diarrhea, abdominal pain, tenderness, and loss of weight.

**How is the diagnosis made?**

By demonstrating the parasite in the feces or tissues of the patient. Blood tests, too, may help in confirming the diagnosis.

**Is amebiasis a serious disease?**

Yes. Not only can debility be great, but severe infection may cause death. Complications are not uncommon in untreated cases.

**Are the chances for recovery favorable in amebic dysentery?**

Yes. There are several drugs that cure the great majority of cases. These include metronidazole, tetracycline, Diodoquin, etc. Treatment must be intensive and should be supervised by an expert in the field.

**Are there other protozoan parasites of the intestine?**

Yes, the whipworm *(Trichuris)* may invade the large intestine.

## TRICHOMONAS VAGINITIS

**What is *Trichomonas vaginitis*?**

This is an infestation of the human vagina with the parasite *Trichomonas vaginalis*. It can cause an inflammatory condition associated with a heavy vaginal discharge. Since the parasite is sometimes found in the male urethra, the infec-

tion'can be readily passed from male to female.

**Is *Trichomonas* infection serious?**

No. It is not a serious disease, but it sometimes proves difficult to eradicate completely. Recently, new fungicides taken orally have proved most effective in overcoming these infestations.

## LEISHMANIASIS

**What is leishmaniasis?**

It is a group of diseases caused by certain protozoan parasites called leishmania. These include kala azar, espundia, and oriental sore. These are serious diseases seen in tropical countries. Sometimes they are seen in the United States in returned military personnel who have served in infected areas. Kala azar has a very high mortality rate in untreated persons. Espundia and oriental sore are diseases in which the skin is principally affected. The outlook for these conditions is much better than in kala azar, and treatment is usually curative.

## AFRICAN SLEEPING SICKNESS

**What is African sleeping sickness?**

This is a parasitic disease caused by a protozoan called *Trypanosoma*. There are at least two different types known. The disease is transmitted by biting flies (tsetse flies). The disease is extremely serious, and unless treated, death occurs in most cases.

## SCHISTOSOMIASIS

**What is schistosomiasis?**

Schistosomiasis is a rather common parasitic disease caused by a blood fluke harbored by infected snails. People who bathe in fresh water con-

taining the snails are infected by the flukes, which penetrate the skin and gain access to the bloodstream. There they grow and invade many organs, causing anemia, intestinal upsets, and general debility. The disease is prevalent in Puerto Rico and other Caribbean countries.

## CHAGAS' DISEASE

**What is Chagas' disease?**

This is a disease caused by a *Trypanosoma*, which is limited to the Western Hemisphere, notably to Brazil. It is transmitted by the bite of a triatomid bug. The disease is a serious one and is attended with a high mortality rate.

## MALARIA

**What are the various types of malaria?**

There are at least three different types, each caused by a different malarial parasite. These include tertian malaria caused by *Plasmodium vivax*, quartan malaria caused by *Plasmodium malariae*, and estivo-autumnal malaria caused by *Plasmodium falciparum*.

**How is malaria transmined to humans?**

By inoculation through the bite of an infected *Anopheles* mosquito.

**Where do the malaria parasites live in humans?**

In the red blood cells, which they destroy.

**How are the different types of malarial parasites distinguished?**

By their specific appearance in the blood and by the difference in clinical picture and symptoms that each produces.

**How common is malaria?**

It is still one of the most prevalent diseases in the world, especially in tropical and underdeveloped countries. The World Health Organization is working hard to bring the disease under control.

### Where is malaria found?

It is undoubtedly one of the most important diseases of the warm climates of the world. However, it is found as far north as southern Sweden. Many servicemen returned from Viet Nam with malaria.

### Are any people immune to malaria?

All native races where malaria is common have a considerable resistance to the disease, but this may be the result of repeated infections causing a buildup of relative resistance. In all probability, there is little or no natural immunity to malaria.

### What are the symptoms of malaria?

Episodes of shaking chills and fever in severe paroxysms, usually spaced at regular intervals.

### What is the outlook for untreated malaria?

Untreated malaria is rarely fatal except in the estivo-autumnal type, where the outlook is always grave.

### What is the treatment for malaria?

There are a number of drugs that are very effective against the malarial parasites. These include chloroquine, quinine, and Plasmochin.

### Can these drugs be used successfully to suppress or prevent the development of malaria?

Yes.

### Should an individual known to have had malaria ever be used as a blood donor?

No. Such an individual might be a carrier of parasites, and the disease could thereby be transmitted to the recipient of the blood transfusion.

## WORM DISEASES

### What are roundworms?

Roundworms are animals that vary in size from forms barely visible to the naked eye to those that are as large around as a lead pencil and almost a foot in length. They look something like an ordinary earthworm.

### What are some of the roundworms that infest man?

These include *Trichinella spiralis* (trichinosis); *Ascaris lumbricoides* (common roundworm of hogs and man); *Necator americanus* (North American hookworm); *Ancylostoma duodenale* (Old World hookworm); etc.

### How is trichinosis acquired?

The parasites normally form cysts in the muscles of hogs. When pork that is incompletely cooked is eaten by man, the parasites are released in the body and make their way into the muscles of man.

### Is trichinosis a common disease?

Yes. It has been estimated that almost twenty-eight million persons throughout the world are infested, three-fourths of which live in North America.

### Is trichinosis a serious disease?

Although trichinosis is rarely fatal, a serious infection can cause death.

### Can trichinosis be treated successfully?

Once the parasites enter the muscles, there is no specific treatment.

### Can trichinosis be prevented?

Yes, by thoroughly cooking pork and pork products before eating.

### Where does the human whipworm reside?

The whipworm *(Trichuris trichiura)* normally resides in the cecum and appendix of man.

### How is whipworm infection acquired?

By eating the eggs of the whipworm, which reside in soil contaminated by feces.

### How is the diagnosis of whipworm infection made?

By finding the eggs in the human stool.

### Can whipworms cause diarrhea?

Yes. They can cause chronic diarrhea.

### Can whipworms cause appendicitis?

Occasionally, the worms may provoke an attack of acute appendicitis, but this is not held to be one of the truly frequent causes.

### How can infection be prevented?

Sanitary disposal of feces and thorough washing of the hands before meals are effective preventive measures.

### What is the treatment for whipworm infestation?

The drug metronidazole is effective treatment.

### How do hookworms get into the human body?

Free-living larval forms can penetrate the intact skin. They generally gain access through the skin between the toes of individuals who walk bare foot in soil contaminated with human feces.

### Is hookworm infection a serious disease?

Yes. The disease is seen in the southern states, where it causes severe anemia, malnutrition, and diarrhea. "Potbelly" is a common finding in children infected with hookworm.

### What is "ground itch"?

This is the first lesion produced by hookworms as they gain access to the body through the skin.

**Where do the adult hookworms reside?**

In the intestinal canal.

**How is the diagnosis of hookworm made?**

By finding the eggs in the human stool.

**How can hookworm disease be prevented?**

As in most roundworm diseases, it is important to dispose of human feces carefully. Also, in infected areas, it is most important to wear shoes at all times!

**Where does the human pinworm, or seatworm, normally reside?**

In the cecum, appendix, and large intestine.

**Why are they called seatworms?**

Because they tend to migrate about the anus, especially at night, and cause severe itching in that region of the body.

**What types of individuals are most commonly infected with pinworms?**

Children.

**Do pinworms ever infect an entire family?**

Yes. This is common.

**How does one get a pinworm infection?**

By eating the eggs of pinworms. Scratching the infected skin about the anal area may result in eggs being picked up by the fingernails. If the hands and nails are then not cleaned frequently and thoroughly, infection can be spread to others, or reinfection of the same individual can occur when the fingers are placed in the mouth.

**How is a diagnosis of pinworm infection made?**

By finding the eggs in the feces or perianal skin.

**Do pinworms ever cause other diseases?**

Yes. They are an occasional cause of acute appendicitis. Also, the severe itching they induce may result in nervousness, irritability, and emotional instability.

**How can pinworm infection be prevented?**

a. Scrupulous attention to personal hygiene is important.
b. The nails must be cut short.
c. Toilet seats must be thoroughly scrubbed.
d. Individuals known to be infected should be treated. Also, they must discontinue scratching themselves about the anal region.

**Is the common roundworm of man (Ascaris) the same as the one found in the intestine of hogs?**

Apparently not. Although the two worms look exactly alike, infection from hog to man, or vice versa, does not occur.

**Is Ascaris infection very serious?**

Usually not. Prompt treatment is curative.

**What is filariasis?**

This is a serious debilitating infection seen in the tropics, which is caused by a tiny worm (wuchereria bancrofti). The worms block the lymph channels of the limbs, resulting in tremendous enlargement of structures. The condition is also known as elephantiasis.

**Is filariasis ever seen in this country?**

Yes, but only in people who have returned from areas of the world where the disease is normally found.

**What is a fluke worm?**

This is a flatworm that has no true body cavity like the roundworms. The fluke worms generally have suckers, by means of which they attach themselves to the human body.

**What fluke worms are parasitic in man?**

The blood flukes or schistosomes, the Chinese liver fluke, the oriental lung fluke, and many others.

**Where are the fluke worms found?**

They are worldwide in distribution but are mainly found in the warmer climates.

**What are the common tapeworms infesting man?**

a. The pork tapeworm (Taenia solium).
b. The beef tapeworm (Taenia saginata).
c. The fish tapeworm (Diphyllobothrium latum).
d. The dog tapeworm (Echinococcusgranulosus).

**Why are these worms "tapeworms"?**

Because they consist of a series of flat segments attached to a head (scolex) and because they resemble an elongated flat tape measure.

**Where do tapeworms commonly reside?**

In the intestine, where they anchor themselves by means of their scolex (head).

**How is tapeworm infection usually acquired?**

By eating foods that contain the larvae of the worms. Thus the fish tapeworm is acquired by eating infected fish that has been improperly cooked, etc.

**How can tapeworm infection be prevented?**

Proper cooking of fish, pork, or beef will kill the worms they harbor. This will prevent infection from these parasites when the food is eaten. In respect to other tapeworms such as the dog tapeworm, care must be taken not to come in contact with the feces of these animals. Sanitary disposal of human and animal excretions is an important consideration.

## How long do tapeworms measure?

They vary in length from a fraction of an inch to over twenty feet for the beef tapeworm.

## How is the diagnosis of tapeworm infection made?

When the adult worm inhabits the intestinal canal, the diagnosis is made by finding the eggs or segments of the worm in the feces.

## Why is it necessary to recover the head or scolex of the worm in order to cure a tapeworm infection?

The worm grows from the head down. Unless the head is removed from the body, the worm will continue to live and grow.

## How does one find the head?

In treated cases, the stool specimens are collected and carefully strained and examined for the presence of the scolex.

## What is an echinococcus cyst?

This is the larval form of the tapeworm of dogs, *Echinococcus granulosus*. The adult worm is commonly infective of dogs. Man acts as the intermediate host. Commonly, sheep, cattle, and hogs are the reservoir hosts, but many cases of human infection are known.

## Is an *Echinococcus* infection serious in man?

Yes. The larvae invade the liver, lungs, and sometimes the brain, and may give rise to serious symptoms.

## What is the treatment for an *Echinococcus* infection in man?

It is generally surgical and will involve the removal of the cyst from the infected organ. This may be serious and dangerous if the brain, lung, or liver is involved.

# CHAPTER 51

# THE PARATHYROID GLANDS

*(See also Chapter 37 on Kidneys and Ureters; Chapter 72 on Thyroid Gland)*

### Where are the parathyroid glands, and what is their function?

They are four small pea-sized structures located behind, and attached to, the thyroid gland in the neck. They are sometimes embedded within thyroid substance and are not easily located even when surgical dissection is carried out. The parathyroid glands secrete a hormone (parathormone) that is responsible for the maintenance of balance in calcium and phosphorous metabolism.

### Do tumors of the parathyroid glands occur very often?

Yes. They are a rather common occurrence. Fortunately, these tumors are seldom malignant.

### What happens when there is overproduction of parathyroid hormone (hyperparathyroidism)?

This results in an increase in the amount of calcium circulating in the bloodstream and in the excretion of an abnormally large amount of calcium in the urine.

### What harm results from overactivity of the parathyroid glands?

a. It can lead to the formation of stones in the kidneys and subsequent impairment of kidney function.

b. Such overactivity can cause calcium to be withdrawn from the bones.

### How is the diagnosis of parathyroid overactivity made?

By performing a blood chemical examination and finding a high level of calcium and parathormone. Also, by noting characteristic changes in bony structure, as seen on x-ray examination. All patients who have kidney stones should be checked for the possible presence of parathyroid disease.

### What are the dangers of demineralization of calcium from the bones?

The bones become weakened, brittle, form cysts, and fracture easily.

### Does overactivity of the parathyroid glands lead to marked bone deformity?

Yes. This condition, known as osteitis fibrosa cystica, is often associated with grotesque deformities of the bones.

### What is the most common cause of overactivity of the parathyroid glands?

A tumor in one or more of the glands.

### Does hyperparathyroidism lead to the formation of kidney stones?

Yes, in a large number of instances.

### What is the treatment for hyperparathyroidism?

Surgical removal of the gland in which a tumor is present.

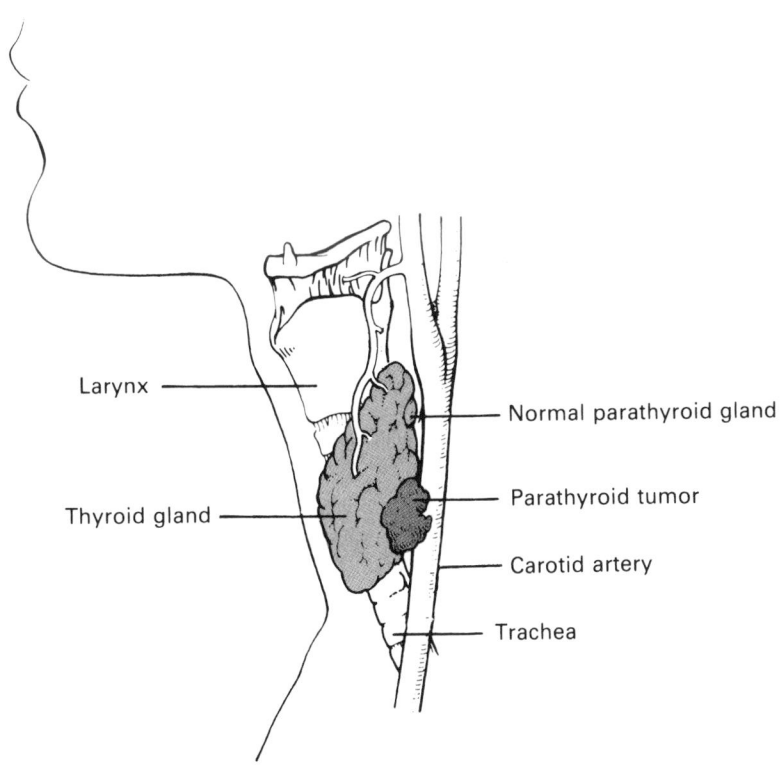

***Anatomy of the Parathyroid Glands.*** *This diagram shows the parathyroid glands as they are located behind the thyroid of the neck. One of these glands is pictured as normal in size; the larger one illustrates tumor formation. Parathyroid tumors, by stimulating excessive secretion of the parathyroid hormone, cause cyst formation and bone deformities. Surgical removal of a parathyroid tumor can be carried out successfully and will result in a cure.*

**Is removal of a parathyroid tumor a dangerous operative procedure?**

No. It is no more serious than an ordinary thyroid operation, and recovery can be anticipated without great disability or discomfort.

**What type of incision is made in operating upon the parathyroid glands, and where on the body is the incision made?**

The same type of collar incision across the lower neck as is made in performing a thyroid operation.

**Are these scars disfiguring?**

No. They usually heal as a thin white line.

**Will the bone cysts heal and the bone deformities disappear after removal of a parathyroid tumor?**

There is a remarkable improvement after this procedure in that the cysts fill in and calcium returns to the bone substance. However, all deformities do not disappear if they have been present for a long time or have been very extensive.

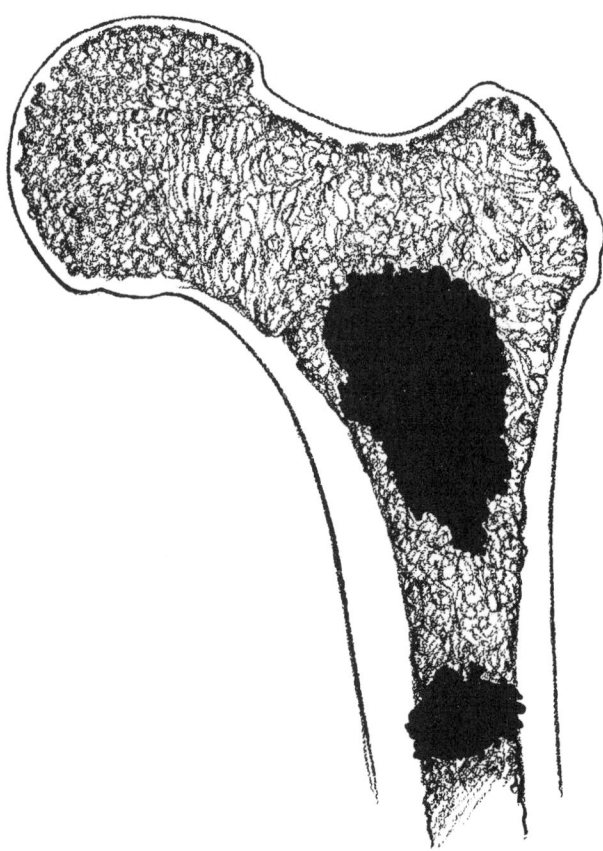

**Bone Cysts.** *In cases of overactivity of the parathyroid glands, the bones are deprived of calcium and become subject to cysts and tumors, as shown here.*

**Is the cause for the hyperparathyroidism always found upon operation?**

Not in all cases. Occasionally, despite all indications that a tumor is present, none is found in the neck. This may be due to the fact that a parathyroid gland has developed in an abnormal position in the neck, or even in the chest cavity. In such cases, to produce a cure, one must find the gland and remove it.

**What symptoms are caused by underactivity of the parathyroid glands (hypoparathyroidism)?**

a. Sudden spasms and cramps in various muscles.
b. In severe cases, tetany, with characteristic involuntary contractions of the muscles or convulsions, takes place.

**How is the diagnosis of underactivity of the parathyroids made?**

a. By examining the blood and finding an abnormally low calcium level.
b. By tests that demonstrate excess muscle irritability.
c. By noting the occurrence of characteristic cramps of the muscles and tendons of the hands and feet and by the onset of convulsive seizures.

**What is the treatment for underactivity of the parathyroid glands?**

a. Large doses of Vitamin D taken regularly.
b. Large supplementary intake of calcium in the form of tablets.

**Will this treatment cure underactivity of the parathyroids?**

A cure will not result, but patients with this condition can be maintained in reasonably good health indefinitely by adequate doses of the above medications.

**Is there any surgical treatment for underactivity of the parathyroids?**

Attempts have been made to graft these glands from animals and humans, but most of these procedures have resulted in failure.

**Is parathyroid function ever disturbed as a result of an operation upon the thyroid gland?**

Yes. In complicated cases, usually those with recurrent goiter, the parathyroids are sometimes injured or inadvertently removed along with the goiter.

**What happens when the parathyroid glands have all been removed?**

Symptoms of underactivity (hypoparathyroidism), such as muscle cramps and tetany (convulsions), may develop.

**Must all four of the parathyroids be removed before symptoms of underactivity develop?**

Yes.

**How soon after surgery upon the parathyroid glands can one do the following:**

Get out of bed:
   Twenty-four to forty-eight hours.
Leave the hospital:
   Five to seven days.
Bathe:
   Five to seven days.
Return to normal activity:
   Four weeks.

# CHAPTER 52
# PERITONITIS

*(See also Chapter 9 on Appendicitis; Chapter 43 on Medications and Drugs; Chapter 66 on Small and Large Intestines)*

## What is peritonitis?

Peritonitis is an inflammation of the peritoneal (abdominal) cavity, usually caused by bacteria resulting in pus formation. It can also be caused by chemical irritation secondary to an inflammation of the pancreas, the rupture of an ulcer, or from spillage of bile.

## What is the peritoneal cavity?

It is the free space within the abdomen surrounding the various organs such as the stomach, intestines, gall bladder, appendix, liver, spleen, etc.

## What are the most common causes for peritonitis?

a. Rupture of an abdominal organ, such as the appendix, small or large bowel, the gall bladder, etc.
b. Spread of infection from an inflamed organ such as the Fallopian tube or ovary.
c. A wound of the abdominal wall that has extended into the peritoneal cavity, such as a gunshot or stab wound.

## What are some of the symptoms and signs of peritonitis?

a. Pain in the abdomen.
b. Tenderness on pressure over the abdominal organs.
c. Loss of appetite, along with nausea and vomiting.
d. Distention of the intestines.
e. Temperature elevation.
f. Characteristic x-ray findings.

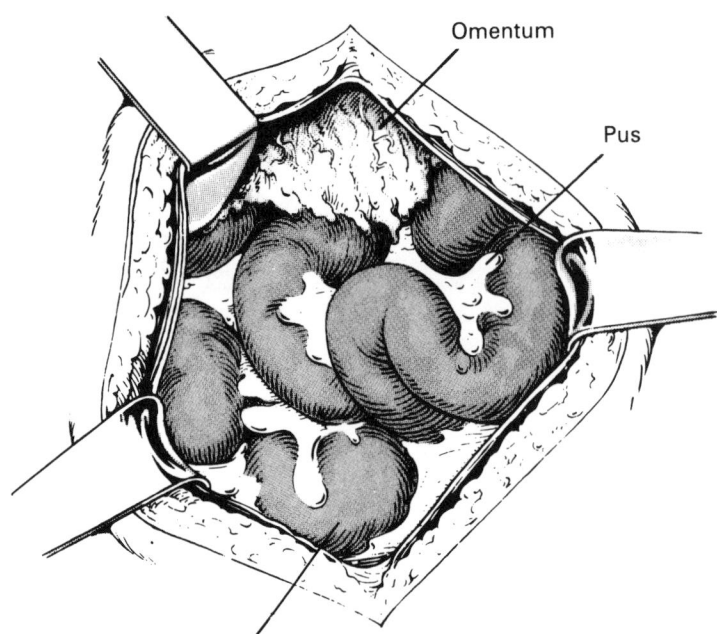

**Peritonitis.** *This diagram shows peritonitis, a condition in which pus is present between the coils of intestine. Peritonitis is a most serious condition and requires surgery in order to eliminate the cause for the discharge of pus into the abdominal cavity.*

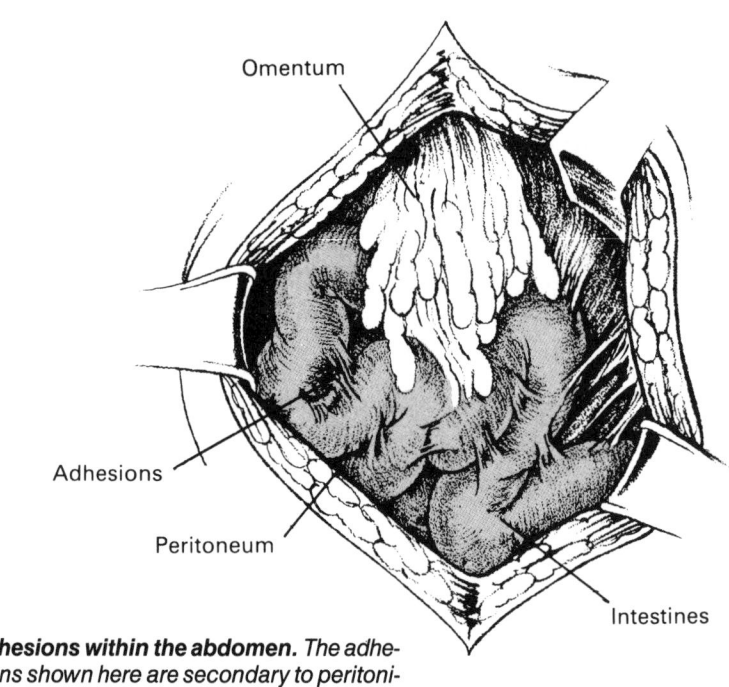

**Adhesions within the abdomen.** *The adhesions shown here are secondary to peritonitis, and they must be surgically removed to prevent intestinal obstruction.*

**Is peritonitis a serious condition?**

Yes, as it results in severe toxemia. Untreated cases often lead to death because of overwhelming bacterial infection.

**What are the methods of treating peritonitis?**

a. Prompt surgery to remove the underlying cause, such as an acutely inflamed appendix or gall bladder.
b. Removal of pus from the peritoneal cavity by suction and the insertion of rubber drains that exit on the abdominal wall. This is to conduct to the exterior any new pus that may form.
c. If peritonitis is due to the rupture of an organ such as the stomach, duodenum, or intestine, immediate surgery should be performed to repair the holes in these structures.
d. The giving of massive doses of antibiotic drugs.
e. During the acute phases of peritonitis, a tube is inserted through the nose into the intestinal tract to keep it free from distention, and the patient is fed intravenously.

**How can peritonitis be prevented?**

a. By early attention to abdominal pain, with prompt treatment of the underlying condition. Appendicitis or acute gall bladder disease, if treated without delay, will not be complicated by rupture and consequent peritonitis.
b. Do not give laxatives to people with acute abdominal pain! Many an appendix has ruptured as the result of injudicious giving of a laxative.
c. Gonorrhea in the female should be treated early and strenuously. This will prevent the infection from spreading from the vagina into the uterus, Fallopian tubes, and out into the peritoneal cavity.

**What are the chances for recovery from peritonitis?**

With the institution of prompt and adequate surgery and the administration of large doses of antibiotics, the chances for recovery are excellent, provided the underlying cause of the peritonitis has been eradicated.

**How long does it take for recovery from peritonitis to take place?**

This will vary according to the cause of the peritonitis, the type of bacteria involved, the length of time it was in existence before active treatment was begun, and how far it has spread throughout the peritoneal cavity. Early cases of peritonitis may subside within a week; others of long standing may require several weeks for the patient to recover.

**Are there any permanent aftereffects of peritonitis?**

Recovery is usually complete, but in some instances extensive adhesions may form. These can lead to the development of intestinal obstruction weeks, months, or even years after the peritonitis has subsided.

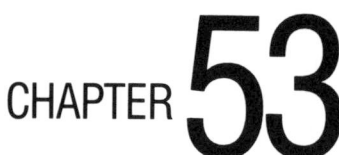

CHAPTER 53

# PHYSICAL THERAPY AND REHABILI-TATION

*(See also Chapter 5 on Aging; Chapter 10 on Arthritis; Chapter 14 on Bones, Muscles, Tendons, and Joints; Chapter 46 on Neurosurgery)*

## What are physical therapy and rehabilitation?

Physical therapy is that branch of medicine that aims toward full restoration of strength and function to sick or injured structures and toward maximizing disabled abilities. Physical therapy employs exercise, light, heat, electricity, manipulation, water, and other mechanical agents in order to restore activity to an injured part of the body.

Rehabilitation employs physical therapy in conjunction with attempts at psychological and social services and vocational retraining for handicapped people. Rehabilitation is directed not only toward the permanently handicapped but also toward the temporarily injured or ill patient.

## What methods does physical therapy employ?

a. Heat therapy.
 1. Baking lamps.
 2. Infrared rays.
 3. Hot compresses.
 4. Diathermy.
 5. Paraffin baths.
 6. Steam baths.
 7. Ultraviolet rays.
 8. Natural sunlight.

b. Hydrotherapy.
 1. Whirlpool baths.
 2. Swimming tanks and pools.
 3. Tub baths.
c. Electrical stimulation.
 1. Galvanic current.
 2. Faradic current.
d. Massage.
e. Exercises.
 1. Passive exercises. These are muscular movements carried out by the physical therapist, not by the patient himself. Passive exercise is most applicable to those who have been paralyzed and cannot move by themselves.
 2. Active exercises. These are taught by the physical therapist but carried out by the patient.
f. Manipulation. This is carried out by physical therapists, nurses, or the physician in charge of the case in order to restore motion to a stiff or "frozen" joint. Some of these procedures can be performed without anesthesia; others require anesthesia to overcome pain and spasm.
g. The application and teaching of proper use of braces, plaster casts, artificial appliances and limbs, crutches, canes, walking aids, supports, and ambulation retraining.

## HEAT THERAPY

### In general, how does heat help an injured part?

It has two main beneficial effects:
a. It increases the blood supply to the injured area, thus permitting nature to better heal the injury.
b. It relaxes spasm of blood vessels and muscles, thus promoting normal healing processes.

### Are there different forms of heat therapy?

Yes. There are several types with varying degrees of penetrative powers.

### What are some of the instruments used for heat treatments?

a. An ordinary baking lamp. This does not have great penetrative powers but will help to a certain degree in improving circulation and in relaxing spasm.
b. Infrared machines. Infrared rays have some penetrative power but do not go deep into the tissues.
c. Diathermy machines, both long-wave and short-wave. These have considerable penetrative power and send heat waves into the substances of muscles, tendons, bones, and other deep-lying tissues.
d. Conductive heat. This is a type of heat in which there is direct conduction from the heat source into the body tissues. Hydrotherapy, hot baths, moist or wet dressings, and other procedures fall into this category.

### Is it safe to employ heat treatments without medical supervision?

No. Whenever heat therapy is used, it should be prescribed by a physician. Severe burns can result from the improper use of heat, whether it is merely in the form of a hot-water bottle or whether it is short-wave diathermy. Furthermore, the patient is not in a position to know whether heat is the proper form of therapy or whether it will actually be harmful in certain conditions. A physical therapist can instruct one in the proper use of various types of heat treatments.

### What types of illness or injury are aided by heat therapy?

These are so numerous that it would be impossible to enumerate all of them. A few of them are:
a. Arthritis of certain types.
b. Bursitis, during some of its stages.
c. Muscle sprains or inflammation.
d. Muscle spasm.
e. Still joints, tendons, and muscles, following prolonged immobilization such as after fractures.

How often do heat treatments have to be given to be effective?

They should be given almost daily to have their best effect.

## ULTRAVIOLET (UV) LIGHT THERAPY

### How is light used in the treatment of patients?

Ultraviolet light rays are used quite extensively in the treatment of certain skin diseases.

### Should ultraviolet light rays be used without a doctor's supervision?

No. This is a dangerous procedure, as severe burns and damage to tissues may result from their improper use.

### Do the ultraviolet lamps sold in drugstores deliver many ultraviolet rays?

These are usually inferior instruments and do not deliver the type and quantity of rays required for adequate therapy. However, they are not without danger, as burns to the eyes, skin, and other structures can result from their overuse.

## HYDROTHERAPY

### What is hydrotherapy?

It is a form of physical therapy utilizing water.

### What are the benefits of hydrotherapy?

Swimming tanks, whirlpool baths, hot sprays, and hot tub baths are all excellent for relaxing spasm and increasing the blood supply to various areas of the body.

### Is hydrotherapy valuable as an aftertreatment for paralysis?

Yes. Swimming relaxes muscles and allows those that have poor function to be used more effectively.

### Will whirlpool bath treatments aid a fractured part in returning to normal function more quickly?

Yes. Such treatments tend to relax spasm and allow for more active motion in stiff muscles, joints, and tendons.

### Are whirlpool baths beneficial in treating sprains, strains, lumbago, etc.?

Yes.

## ELECTRICAL STIMULATION

### Is electricity used very often as a form of treatment in cases of neuritis or paralysis?

No. Electrical stimulation will not cause a damaged or paralyzed nerve to return to normal.

### What are the most frequently used types of electrical stimulation?

Galvanic and faradic current. These can be applied by a specially devised machine.

### Will the giving of electrical treatments cause a facial paralysis to heal more quickly?

Probably not. This condition is a self-limited one, and the rate of recovery of the nerve will not depend to a very great extent upon electrical stimulation.

### How is electrical stimulation used as a form of treatment?

By stimulating a muscle to contract during the period that its nerve is not functioning properly, it is often possible to keep the muscle in better tone.

### Is the application of electrical stimulation helpful in making the diagnosis of disease?

Yes. It is extremely helpful in distinguishing the cause of the nerve paralysis or muscle degeneration.

## MASSAGE

### Is it safe for a patient to have himself massaged without a doctor's prescription?

No. Much harm can come from improper massage, as muscles and joints can be damaged by too strenuous and overzealous a masseur.

### What information should be given to the physiotherapist before massage is undertaken?

It should be stated whether the massage is to be deep or light, whether it is to be carried out to stimulate or to quiet down muscles, tendons, and joints.

### When is it bad to use massage?

a. When it is used to bring about weight reduction. Massage by itself does not lead to weight loss.
b. Where there is a lump or mass present. This may be a tumor, and massage can do it great harm.

### What are the beneficial effects of properly administered massage?

a. It tends to relax muscles.
b. It tends to increase motion of joints, muscles, and tendons.
c. It tends to increase the blood supply to the area.

## EXERCISE

### Are exercises valuable in the treatment of bone, muscle, joint, and other diseases?

Most definitely, yes. Properly prescribed exercises can do a tremendous amount of good for conditions involving the muscles, bones, joints, tendons, and nerves.

### Are there specific exercises that aid specific conditions such as a slipped disk, lumbago, whiplash, wry neck, and illnesses such as cerebral palsy and muscular dystrophy?

Yes. Expert medical attention by orthopedic and rehabilitation specialists will often result in great improvement in the above conditions.

## Can anyone prescribe exercise, or should one go to a specialist in the field?

This has become a highly specialized field, and the various types of apparatus and exercises to be used should be prescribed by an expert in this field of medicine.

## Is it necessary for exercises to be conducted frequently and under controlled conditions?

Yes. Most failures in physical exercises are the result of an improperly prescribed program or infrequent exercise periods.

## REHABILITATION

### What are the goals of rehabilitation?

a. To restore the patient to as near normal a physical condition as possible.
b. To improve the patient's emotional and psychological state so that he makes full use of his capabilities and adjusts to his disability.
c. To improve the patient's social adjustment so that he may resume his place within his family and community.
d. To enable the patient to assume an active vocational or educational status.

### Have rehabilitation methods improved within the last fifteen to twenty years?

The advancement in this field has been one of the most remarkable in all of medicine. No longer do we think in terms of people being "crippled." Rehabilitation methods have enabled the vast majority of handicapped people to be useful, productive, self-sustaining members of society.

## For what patients are rehabilitation methods most valuable?

a. For the patient with a disabling birth deformity.
b. For the paralyzed patient.
c. For the patient with an amputation.
d. For the patient with incapacitating diseases of the nerves, muscles, bones, or joints.
e. For the patient who has partially recovered from a long and debilitating illness but who has not yet been able to resume normal physical, emotional, or social activity.

## What percentage of those who have had prolonged illness require some form of rehabilitation?

It is estimated that 50 percent of all long-term hospitalized medical patients and 50 percent of all orthopedic patients need some type of rehabilitation service after their discharge from the hospital.

## During what phase of illness is rehabilitation most needed?

During the convalescent period. It is extremely important that people who have recovered from serious illness be encouraged to return to normal activity as quickly as possible. There is a tendency for many of the chronically ill to "adjust" to their illnesses and to display a lack of interest in resuming full activity.

## Is there a tendency for people to accept their status as an invalid?

Yes. It is sometimes observed that people who have been cared for as total invalids for prolonged lengths of time have a tendency to accept their situation. Rehabilitation measures must therefore counteract this natural tendency, and people must be encouraged to function independently and return to normal living, if this is possible.

## Where can one find information

concerning rehabilitation services?

There are a great many excellent voluntary organizations that specialize in giving information concerning rehabilitation and in leading one to an agency that will render such services.

## PHYSICAL THERAPY AND REHABILITATION FOR OLDER PEOPLE

### Is rehabilitation for older people worthwhile?

Yes. Great advances have been made in recent years toward reeducation and rehabilitation of older people who have been handicapped as a result of injury or disease. Specialists in physical medicine have discovered ways of increasing the physical capacity of handicapped older people and of restoring any of their lost abilities.

### What are some of the general areas in which rehabilitation is most helpful?

a. People who have been partially paralyzed by a stroke can often be taught to walk again and to get the most use possible out of their paralyzed limbs.
b. Those who have lost their ability to speak can, in some instances, benefit greatly from speech therapy. Others who are unable to have their speech restored are taught methods of expressing themselves so that they can be understood by people who come in contact with them.
c. Those who are deformed or crippled by arthritis are taught exercises to limber their stiff joints, to preserve those joints that are unaffected, and to get the maximum use out of their hands and feet.
d. People with permanent joint, bone, nerve, or muscle infirmities are supplied with appliances to

support their bodies, to maintain as near-normal posture as possible, and to get the most use possible out of partially damaged structures.

e. Special ways to walk, to get up and down curbs or stairs, to sit and stand, have been devised for people who are disabled.

f. People who have undergone amputation of a limb are taught how to use artificial limbs and appliances.

g. Great advances have been made in rehabilitating patients paralyzed due to injury to the spinal cord.

h. Those afflicted with Parkinson's disease are given special treatment and training for rigid muscles; they are given speech therapy and occupational training that will help them work with their tremor and palsy.

i. Occupational retraining is given to fit in with existing deformities.

j. Psychotherapy is given to aid those who are depressed and to better adjust the handicapped person to the world in which he lives.

**Can people who have been invalids for many years ever be helped through rehabilitation techniques?**

Yes. Some who have not used their arms or walked for years can be taught how to do so again. Of course, the sooner the rehabilitation is started after an injury, the better the final results will be.

**Should older people who need rehabilitation go to physicians who specialize in rehabilitation?**

Yes. Rehabilitation techniques are highly specialized, and only doctors who confine their practice to this field will be able to give expert care. These doctors are called physiatrists.

**How soon after a stroke can rehabilitation measures be started?**

Within a day or two. One of the first procedures is to control the patient's position in bed so that unnecessary contractures will not set in. Also, exercises of a passive type will be instituted so that muscles and joints do not become stiff. As soon as the patient has regained consciousness, he will be shown how to assist himself.

**How are psychological factors used in aiding rehabilitation?**

Seeing others improve as a result of treatment has an uplifting effect on patients who are depressed by their misfortune. Group therapy and classroom techniques may prove especially beneficial. Also, patients will often form stimulating new relationships with others who have similar needs.

**Is it safe for people in their sixties, seventies, or eighties to take physical therapy treatments such as ultraviolet rays, heat treatments, baths, or diathermy?**

Yes, but physical therapy should be under the supervision of a specialist in this field of medicine. There are real dangers in permitting older patients to treat themselves without medical supervision. Older patients require special care because they are more sensitive to the effects of physical therapy.

**Can heat treatments improve the deep circulation in the legs of older people?**

Not measurably. Most older people with impaired circulation have hardening of the arteries, and no amount of physical therapy will alter the underlying condition. Surgical methods of treatment offer much more hope in this regard for severely impaired patients.

**What specific precautions should older people take in the use of heat?**

a. Temperature should be carefully regulated so that burns do not result from excessive heat.

b. Electric pads, heating or baking lamps, or hot-water bottles should be applied only on the order of and under the supervision of a nurse or other qualified attendant. They should be removed immediately if the skin becomes mottled or turns red.

c. Heat should not be applied when the patient is about to go to sleep, and it should be removed as soon as a patient dozes off.

d. Heat should not be applied to a patient who has just received a narcotic or sedative. The medication may dull his sensibilities to such an extent that he will be unaware of the heat's intensity.

e. Cold applications should not be left in place for more than a half hour at a time. Damage to circulation or frostbite may result.

**Is it safe for older people to take hot cabinet baths or Turkish baths?**

Healthy, active older people can tolerate these baths well, but it is unwise to "sweat out" someone who is ill or underweight. The loss of large quantities of body fluids and salt can be dangerous.

**Are whirlpool baths, hot tub baths, and swimming tanks safe for older people?**

Yes, but the temperature of the water must be watched carefully so as not to cause a burn. Also, if older people have a tendency to faint or are unable to communicate easily, they must be watched very carefully while they are in the water.

**Is it ever possible to train handicapped people to use other muscles when paralysis has damaged those that are ordinarily used?**

Yes. This process is one of the great techniques of those who specialize in the fields of rehabilitation. Many people who were totally bedridden have been taught to walk again through use of old muscles for new functions.

# CHAPTER 54

# PILONIDAL CYST

*(See also Chapter 60 on Rectum and Anus)*

## What is a pilonidal cyst?

It is an irregularly shaped cyst located in the lower back just above and between the cheeks of the buttocks.

## What is the cause of these cysts?

It is thought that they are caused either by a defect in the development of the embryo or by ingrown hairs that become encysted.

## How frequent are pilonidal cysts?

Almost 5 percent of all people have pilonidal cysts.

## Do these cysts tend to be inherited or to run in families?

No.

## How is it that these cysts rarely evoke any symptoms until early adult life?

Hair grows within these cysts, and this may take a long time. Eventually, however, it is common for infection to take place within the cyst, and then pus will form and the patient will become aware of a pain in the region.

## How can one know if he has a pilonidal cyst?

By the formation of a lump between the buttocks, by a yellowish discharge that appears from time to time on the underwear, and often by pain, tenderness, and abscess formation in the region.

## How does the physician make the diagnosis of a pilonidal cyst?

There are one or more small openings in the skin that lead into the cyst. From these openings, one often sees hair protrude, and when infected, pus exudes through these openings.

## What are the harmful effects of a pilonidal cyst if not treated?

a. The cyst may become markedly enlarged and may tunnel in several directions for a distance of several inches.
b. There may be a chronic discharge and discomfort in the region.
c. An abscess may form, which will cause extreme pain and high temperature.
d. In rare instances, these cysts may turn into malignant growths.

## Is there any way to prevent the development of a pilonidal cyst?

No.

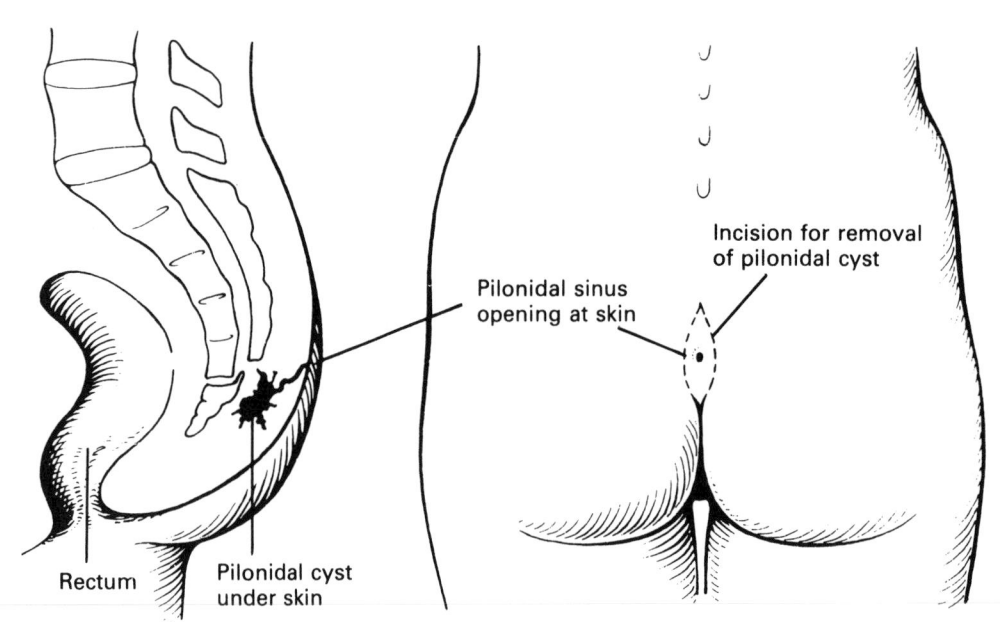

Pilonidal sinus opening at skin

Incision for removal of pilonidal cyst

Rectum

Pilonidal cyst under skin

***Pilonidal Cyst and Incision for Its Removal.*** *This diagram shows the location of a pilonidal cyst and outlines the incision made to remove the cyst. Pilonidal cysts are encountered frequently in young adults and are thought by most investigators to be birth deformities. Other more recent investigators feel that they are caused by ingrown hairs.*

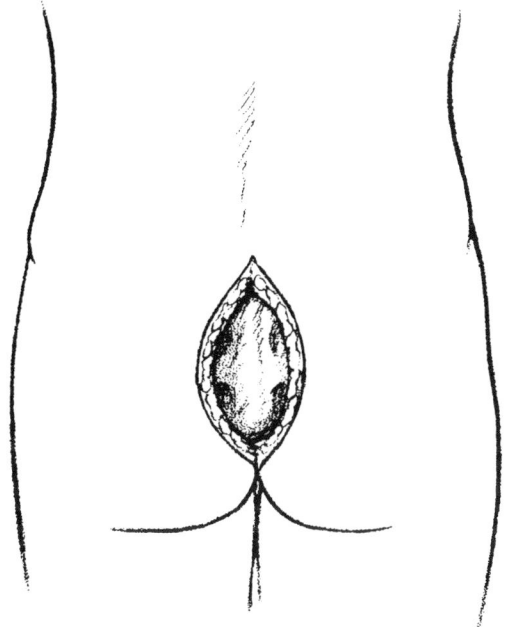

*Removal of Pilonidal Cyst. The hole, left after the removal of the cyst, contains packing. The hole will gradually close by itself, and the packing will be removed.*

### What is the treatment for a pilonidal cyst?

Surgical removal.

### How is the surgical treatment carried out?

By wide excision of the skin, subcutaneous tissue, and the entire cyst-bearing area extending down to the tissue overlying the sacral bone. Most surgeons pack these wounds wide open and permit them to fill in gradually from the bottom. A few surgeons close the skin tightly after removing the cyst, but this method is followed by recurrence in a large percentage of cases.

### Are operations for pilonidal cysts serious?

No. They are considered to be minor operative procedures.

### What type of anesthesia is used?

Epidural, spinal, or, in rare instances, a local anesthetic such as Novocain is given.

### Are there any special preoperative measures that are necessary?

No.

### Is there a great deal of postoperative discomfort?

Yes. A moderate amount of pain will be felt in the operative area. Also, there may be some discomfort because of the inability to move the bowels for a few days after the removal of a pilonidal cyst.

### Will bowel function eventually return to normal after this operation?

Yes, within a few days.

### How soon after the removal of a pilonidal cyst can the patient get out of bed?

The day following surgery.

### How long a hospital stay is usually necessary?

Approximately four days.

### Are these wounds often packed and left open?

Yes.

### Does the packing have to be removed?

Yes. Usually within four to six days.

### Is it painful when the packing is removed?

Yes.

### What special postoperative routines are advised after the removal of a pilonidal cyst?

Tub baths, frequent changes of the dressings, visits to the surgeon's office every few days, and the maintenance of cleanliness in the area.

### How long does it take these wounds to heal?

Anywhere from four weeks to four months, unless they have been closed tightly at surgery. The latter type of case may have complete healing within two weeks, but the chances of recurrence are much greater.

### Does one have to remain out of work throughout the entire time the wound is healing?

No. Many patients can return to work within two to three weeks after this operation. However, they will have to make frequent visits to their surgeon's office for change of dressing.

### Is there a tendency for these pilonidal cysts, once removed, to recur?

Yes, in approximately 2 to 5 percent of all cases.

### For how long must one be wary of recurrence after an apparently successful operation?

Recurrences have been noted as long as one to two years after surgery.

### What is the treatment for recurrence?

Reoperation, making sure to leave the wound wide open so that it fills in solidly from the bottom.

### How soon after a pilonidal operation can one do the following:

Bathe:
    Four to seven days.
Walk out in the street:
    Five to seven days.
Drive a car:
    Two to three weeks.
Return to work:
    Three weeks.
Resume sexual relations:
    Three to four weeks.
Resume all normal activities:
    As soon as the wound has healed completely.

# CHAPTER 55
# THE PITUITARY GLAND

*(See also Chapter 4 on Adrenal Glands; Chapter 46 on Neurosurgery; Chapter 72 on Thyroid Gland)*

## What is the pituitary gland, and where is it located?

The pituitary is a small, nut-sized structure measuring about a half inch in diameter. It is located at the base of the skull within a hollowed out area of bone known as the sella turcica.

The pituitary is divided into two parts, an anterior and a posterior portion, each of which contains different types of cells and secretes different types of hormones into the bloodstream. The posterior lobe is connected with that part of the brain known as the hypothalamus, which produces the hormones that are stored in the posterior portion of the pituitary gland.

## What is an endocrine gland?

It is a gland that secretes a hormone into the bloodstream. The hormone has a specific effect upon another organ of the body.

## What is a hormone?

A chemical substance that is produced by an endocrine gland and is transmitted through the bloodstream to a target organ located in another part of the body.

## What hormones are secreted by the pituitary gland, and what are their functions?

a. The anterior portion of the pituitary secretes several hormones that in-fluence the activity of other endocrine glands, such as the thyroid, the adrenals, the ovaries, and the testicles. Sometimes the pituitary stimulates these glands to greater activity, at other times it inhibits their activity. Secretions from the anterior portion also control growth mechanisms.

b. The posterior pituitary contains hormones that regulate the excretion and retention of water from the kidneys. It also produces a hormone known as oxytocin, which stimulates contraction of the uterus.

## Do endocrine glands such as the adrenals, thyroid, etc., ever influence the activity of the anterior pituitary?

Yes, as an example, when the adrenal secretion reaches the desired level, it will act to inhibit the pituitary from producing more of its secretion.

## Is the pituitary gland referred to as the "master gland"?

Yes, because it appears to control the function of all the other endocrine glands within the body.

## Does the pituitary gland often undergo tumor formation?

Yes, especially the anterior portion of the gland. The posterior portion is rarely, if ever, the site of tumor growth.

## How common are pituitary tumors?

They account for 10 percent of all growths within the brain and skull.

## What are the most frequently encountered types of pituitary tumors?

Adenomas are seen most often. The majority are benign, but occasionally they become malignant.

## What are the various types of pituitary adenomas?

a. The chromophobe adenoma, making up approximately 75 per-cent of all pituitary tumors. This tumor does not secrete a hormone.
b. Prolactin adenomas.
c. Growth hormone adenomas.
d. Corticotropin-secreting adenomas.

## What symptoms and signs result from a pituitary tumor of the chromophobe type?

a. Headache.
b. Disturbances in vision due to pressure of the tumor upon the optic nerves of the eyes. There may be loss of wide vision, with vision restricted to objects that lie straight ahead.
c. If the tumor grows large, it may compress and interfere with the secretion of hormones by the gland.
d. Loss of menstruation is a not uncommon symptom in the female.
e. Loss of libido "sexual desire" is not uncommon in the male.
f. As these tumors grow, they tend to compress the bones of the sella turcica, which surround the pituitary. On x ray, changes in the bones of the sella turcica can be seen.

## What symptoms occur with prolactin-secreting adenomas of the pituitary?

An excessive production and secretion of prolactin in the female may cause cessation of menstruation and the secretion of milk from the nipples.

## How does one diagnose a prolactin-secreting tumor?

a. By noting a high level of the hormone prolactin on examination of the blood.
b. By the findings of absent menstruation and the secretion of milk from the breasts.

## What are the symptoms and signs of growth hormone tumors of the pituitary gland?

a. If the tumor appears before pu-

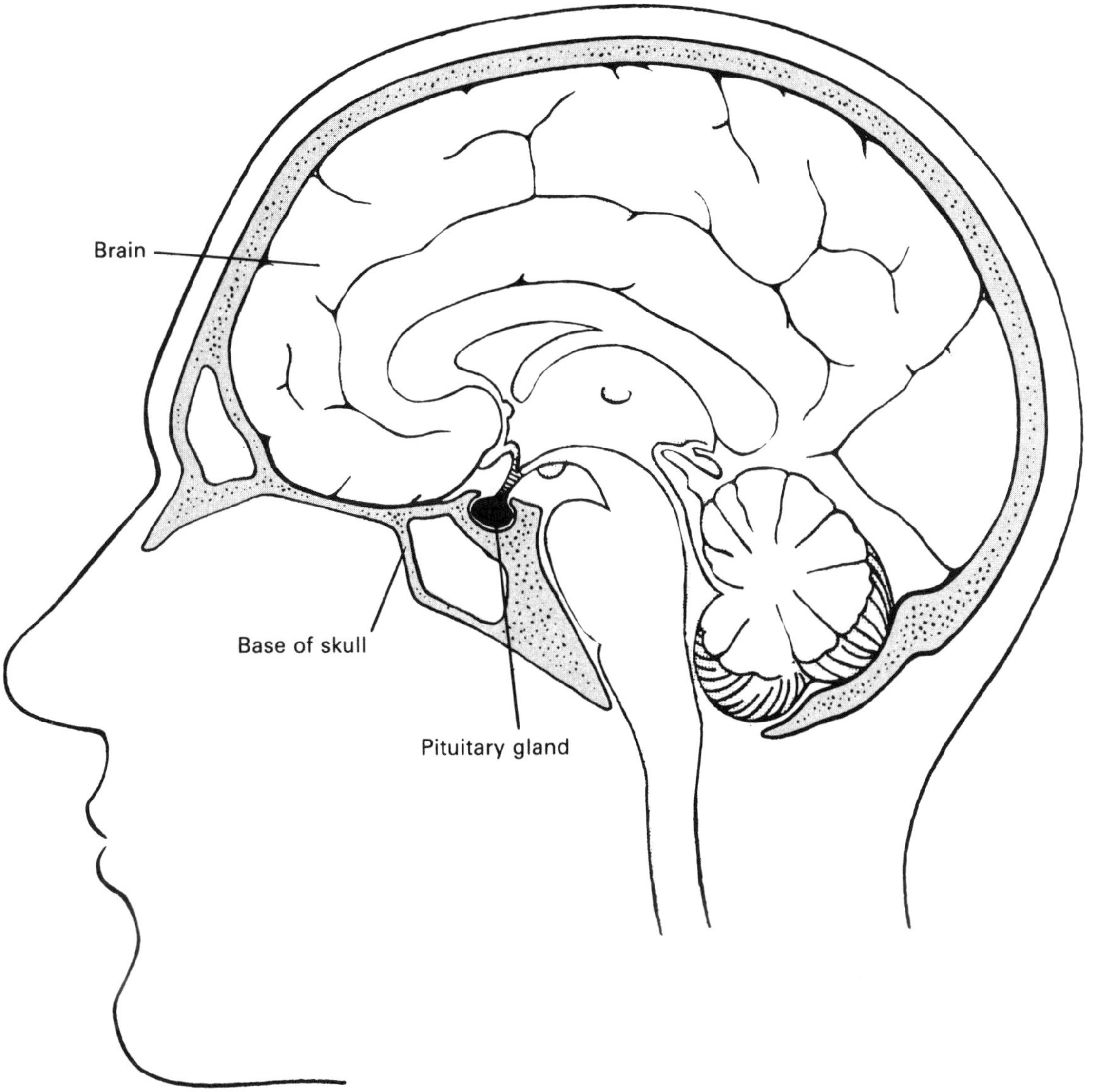

**Brain**

**Base of skull**

**Pituitary gland**

**Anatomy of the Pituitary Gland.** *This diagram shows the pituitary gland as it nestles within the bony structure of the skull. A tumor within the pituitary gland will press upon the optic nerves that supply the eyes, and this may lead to impairment of vision.*

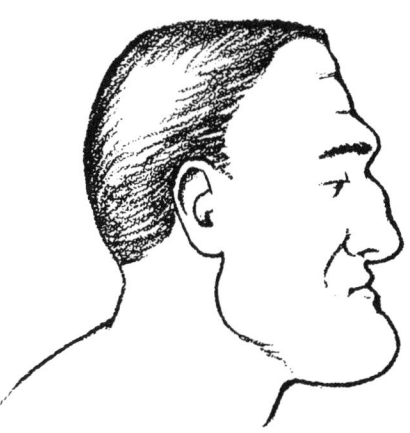

berty, the child may grow to be a giant. This type of tumor is responsible for most adults who attain seven and a half to eight feet in height.

b. If the tumor becomes active during adulthood, a condition known as acromegaly will appear. This is characterized by bony overgrowth of the face, hands, and feet, muscle weakness, diabetes, high blood pressure, and premature hardening of the arteries, unless the tumor is treated adequately.

## What symptoms and signs are caused by corticotropin-secreting tumors of the pituitary?

Cushing's syndrome results from this tumor. The condition is characterized by:

a. Marked weight gain.

b. Marked elevation of blood pressure.
c. A "moon-shaped" appearance of the face.
d. A hump that develops in the lower neck and upper back.
e. Bluish red streaks on the abdomen.

## Is Cushing's syndrome more common in women than men?

Yes. It is three times more common in women.

## What is the treatment for pituitary tumors?

They are best treated through surgery, although some tumors can be effectively treated by radiation "x-ray" therapy.

## Through what type of incision is the pituitary gland reached?

a. Most often an incision is made above the gums of the upper jaw through the nasal cavities and the sphenoid sinus to the floor of the bony cavity that surrounds the gland (the sella turcica).
b. If the pituitary tumor is very large, it may be necessary to approach it through an incision into the skull, namely, a craniotomy.
c. In rare instances, both an incision above the gums and a craniotomy are necessary in order to remove the entire tumor.

## Is the whole gland always removed when a pituitary tumor is present?

Not necessarily. Sometimes, only the tumor is removed.

## If the entire pituitary gland has been removed, will this affect hormone secretions?

Yes. It may be necessary to administer these hormones either through pills or by injections.

## Is x-ray therapy ever combined with surgery in the treatment of pituitary tumors?

Yes, if postoperative studies reveal that the gland is still secreting an excess of hormones.

## If x-ray therapy is effective in removing pituitary tumors, why is it not utilized more often?

Because the radiation frequently results in severe hormonal defects that require lifelong hormone substitution therapy. Also, it takes much longer to destroy a pituitary tumor by x-ray radiation than by surgery.

## Are medications ever used in treating pituitary tumors?

Yes. Some of the growth hormone tumors and some of the prolactin-secreting tumors can be controlled through medications. However, they cannot reduce the size of the tumors.

## Do children ever develop tumors of the pituitary gland?

Yes. The so-called craniopharyngioma occurs in children and results in underactivity of the pituitary gland.

## How is a craniopharyngioma diagnosed?

a. By noting signs of underactivity of the gland, especially prior to puberty.
b. By characteristic x-ray findings of the sella turcica and the area above it.

## What are the chances for recovery from an operation upon the pituitary gland?

About 95 percent.

## How long a hospital stay is necessary?

Usually about ten days.

## How long do these operative procedures take to perform?

Two to three hours.

## Do tumors of the pituitary gland ever recur?

Yes. A small percentage of tumors do recur, in which event x-ray therapy or reoperation is indicated.

## Do tumors of the pituitary often spread to other parts of the body?

No.

## Is the pituitary gland ever operated on to slow down the growth of breast cancer?

Yes. It has been found that total removal of the pituitary gland will cause a remission of cancerous growth in certain cases where cancer of the breast has spread to other parts of the body.

## What is diabetes insipidus?

It is a disorder caused by an inadequate production of the antidiuretic hormone by the posterior portion of the pituitary gland.

## What are the symptoms of diabetes insipidus?

a. Tremendous, excessive thirst.
b. An excretion by the kidneys of tremendous amounts of water.

## Can diabetes insipidus be treated effectively?

Yes. There are available potent extracts of the posterior pituitary gland that can be given to the patient by injection or as a snuff. However, the condition is not curable, and the patient must continue to receive these hormones for the rest of his life. Recently, new chemical drugs have been used to further alleviate this condition.

## Is there any relationship between diabetes insipidus and so-called "sugar diabetes"?

No.

## Are diseases of the pituitary gland preventable?

No.

## Are there conditions other than diabetes insipidus that may influence the function of the posterior portion of the pituitary gland?

Yes. Its function may be affected by

disease processes involving the brain, such as strokes, head injuries, infections, hydrocephalus, or brain tumors.

**Can a normal child who appears to be small in stature be made to grow taller by the giving of pituitary hormones?**

Probably, yes. Recent work utilizing purified extracts of the growth hormone from the human pituitary gland would so indicate. However, at the present time, such material is not generally available.

**Is there any effective way to stimulate growth in a child who appears to be undersized?**

One must determine the cause of the growth retardation. If it is found to be due to underactivity of the thyroid gland, the administration of thyroid hormone will stimulate the child to grow. If the growth retardation is due to inadequate nutrition and intake of vitamins, the restoration of an adequate diet and vitamin and mineral intake will also cause the child's growth to spurt. And finally, as mentioned above, if the condition is due to insufficient pituitary gland activity, growth hormone might be administered. Again, it is necessary to emphasize the fact that the pure growth hormone has only recently been isolated and is not available for general use.

**Is there any safe and effective way of stopping a child from growing too tall?**

No.

**Are there any disease states that result from underactivity of the pituitary gland (hypopituitarism)?**

Yes. If underactivity occurs in childhood, growth will be retarded markedly. Children so affected will remain small but well proportioned. They retain a childlike appearance throughout life. This condition is responsible for dwarfism.

If underactivity of the pituitary commences during adulthood, growth cannot be stunted. However, such a situation will lead to a depression in the function of all the other endocrine glands, such as the thyroid, the adrenals, the ovaries, and the testicles.

**Is pituitary dwarfism inherited?**

No. If pituitary dwarfs marry and have children, they usually have normal-sized children.

**What are some of the other symptoms of hypopituitarism?**

Weakness, general apathy, loss of energy, and, in some cases, mental disturbance. The skin takes on a wrinkled appearance as seen in old age. There may be lowering of the blood sugar and loss of appetite and weight.

**What is the treatment for underactivity of the anterior pituitary?**

If the condition is due to a tumor of the pituitary, then x-ray therapy or surgery may be helpful. Medical treatment will consist of replacement of the deficient hormones by injection or oral medication.

**Can the serious effects of underactivity of the anterior pituitary be counteracted by treatment?**

To a major extent, yes.

CHAPTER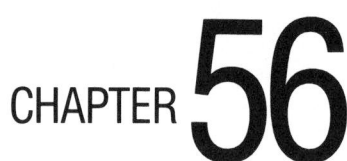

# PLASTIC SURGERY

*(For specific surgery, see chapters on the organs involved, such as Chapter 15 on Breasts; Chapter 48 on Nose and Sinuses)*

## What is plastic and reconstructive surgery?

A branch of surgery devoted to restoration, repair, and correction of malformations of tissues. It concerns not only return to normal appearance but also the restoration of function. The field has several subdivisions, including:

a. Cosmetic surgery.
b. Hand surgery.
c. Management of congenital defects.
d. Management of burns, wounds, and other acquired defects.
e. Head and neck cancer surgery, including reconstructive surgery following the various cancer operations.

## What is the difference between cosmetic and reconstructive plastic surgery?

Cosmetic surgery deals with improving or restoring the appearance of tissues or organs, such as the nose, face, eyes, or breasts. The reconstructive phase of plastic surgery deals with the restoration of both appearance *and* function.

## What parts of the body and what conditions are most commonly operated upon by the plastic surgeon?

While it is commonly thought that the plastic surgeon is limited to operations upon the face and neck, this is not the case. The well-trained plastic surgeon deals with a great many disorders that are located in other parts of the body. Here is a partial list of those conditions in which plastic surgery frequently plays a role:

a. Deformities of the nose (rhinoplasty).
b. Aging of the face (meloplasty, rhytidoplasty).
c. Aging of the eyelids (blepharoplasty).
d. Lop or bat-ear deformities (otoplasty).
e. Unsightly scars anywhere on the body.
f. Receding or protruding chins.
g. Cleft lip or cleft palate deformities.
h. Breast surgery, including making the breast larger (augmentation mammoplasty), making the breast smaller (reduction mammoplasty), or elevating the breast to a more youthful position (dermal mastopexy).
i. Reconstruction of the breast following cancer surgery.
j. Body sculpturing surgery, including surgery on the abdomen (abdominal lipectomy), the thighs, buttocks, arms, and other areas of the body.
k. The management of burns from the early stages through to the reconstructive phase, involving reconstruction of the eyelids, nose, face, hands, release of contractures, and cosmetic improvement of burned areas.
l. The use of skin grafts, composite grafts, pedicle flaps, and free flaps (flaps completely removed from the nerve and blood supply) to reconstruct deformities of the body.
m. Replantation surgery, involving the use of microsurgical techniques to replace amputated portions of the body including fingers, hands, feet and legs, the nose, ears, and the lips.
n. Deformities of the male or female genitals.
o. The removal of skin blemishes, skin cancers, and other tumors of the body.

## Should one go to a plastic surgeon to have plastic surgery performed?

When plastic surgery is indicated, a Board-certified plastic surgeon should be consulted. Your county medical society will have a list of those physicians who are qualified.

## Is special training necessary for a physician to become a plastic surgeon?

Yes. Most plastic surgeons are first trained in general surgery for a period of four to six years. They then undergo training in plastic surgery for an additional two to three years.

## Are the results of cosmetic surgery permanent?

In those conditions in which cosmetic surgery is directed to the improvement of form, such as in operations upon the nose, ears, abdomen, or breasts, the results are permanent. In those cases in which cosmetic surgery is directed to the problems of aging, the results last a significant amount of time but they are not permanent. Specifically, cosmetic surgery is successful in removing wrinkles for a period of time but the natural aging process cannot be halted, and therefore wrinkles will eventually reappear. Using modern techniques, it is now possible to perform an eyelid operation that will last successfully for eight to ten years. New techniques in the facelift, specifically the use of platysmal muscle flaps in the neck, have made it possible to achieve results that will last anywhere from seven to ten years. Of course, results may vary considerably from patient to patient.

## Should plastic surgery be performed upon children, or is it wiser to wait until they have attained maturity?

Plastic surgery can be performed

with great success on children. There are, however, time factors that must be kept in mind. With respect to deformities of the nose, it is generally wise to wait until the child is fifteen or sixteen years of age until the nose is fully developed. To operate at a younger age invites the possibility of creating a nasal deformity that will appear at a later date. Deformities of the ears can be operated upon when the child is approximately five years of age. At this time the ears have attained 85 to 90 percent of their normal adult size. This is fortunate because it is wise to operate upon the child before he begins school where he may suffer the criticism of his classmates. In regard to scars and skin growths, it is generally best to wait until the child is older before operating. The skin of young children is highly elastic and surgery at a very early age may lead to wide and unattractive scars.

**Can the plastic surgeon always predict the outcome of the operation he is going to perform?**

This can be done with reasonable certainty in many instances, although the exact appearance can never be predicted. Much of the final result will depend upon the inherent healing properties of the specific patient. As everyone knows, individuals heal differently and age differently depending upon their genetic background, their nutrition, and their general body type.

**In performing reconstructive surgery, what tissues of the body can be used?**

a. Skin is often used in reconstruction, taken as a thin split-thickness graft or as a full-thickness graft.
b. Grafts of cartilage, bone, fat, muscle, nerve, or blood vessel are frequently employed.
c. Composite grafts, which consist of more than one type of tissue, such as skin and muscle, skin and cartilage, muscle and bone, skin and fat, etc.

d. Flaps, which are segments of tissue usually involving more than one element, such as skin and fat, skin and muscle, etc., which are elevated from the surface of the body but are left attached to their blood and nerve supply. They are later transferred from one part of the body (the donor area) to the recipient area where the flap is needed. If the flap must travel a large distance, it will be detached from one part of the body and allowed to grow in at another part. Often, however, a flap is simply rotated or transposed directly from one site to another. For example, in reconstructing the face after a cancer operation, one may take a flap from the neck and move it up to the area where it is needed. The site from which the flap has been taken is then closed, using surrounding tissue to fill in the defect.
e. Free flaps, the utilization of which represents a new concept, which has literally revolutionized the field. Using microsurgical techniques, segments of tissue can be removed from one part of the patient's body along with their arteries, veins, and nerves. In the new location, the arteries, veins, and nerves of the donor tissue are reattached to the arteries, veins, and nerves in the recipient area. This method of grafting involves just one procedure, thus obviating the many-stage procedures formerly necessary with pedicle grafts and flaps. Also, it permits tissues to be transplanted from distant parts of the patient's body.

**Can a plastic surgeon always tell in advance how skin will heal and whether the scars will be smooth or ugly?**

This is not always possible. There are certain broad categories of skin types that tend to heal better than other types. The plastic surgeon must evaluate each patient individually and plan his operation specifically for him, keeping in mind his

body type, his skin tone, and his genetic and ethnic background.

**Can tissues be transferred from one individual to another?**

This is generally not done in reconstructive surgery, although in the treatment of burns, skin from other human beings, cadavers, or even animals can be used. Also, cartilage or bone from animals can sometimes be used in humans. As an example, cartilage from a cow is occasionally used in the reconstruction of the nose or chin.

**How do skin grafts work?**

a. Split-thickness grafts. These grafts are composed of only part of the full thickness of the skin, excluding the deepest portions of the hair follicles and sweat glands. The skin at the donor site regrows from cells in the remaining hair follicles and sweat glands. The split-thickness graft is then placed over and sewn in position at the recipient site. The recipient site must be clean, as a graft will not "take" in an infected area. Thin split-thickness grafts will derive new blood supply from the recipient site within thirty-six to forty-eight hours and will be well fixed by seven to ten days after grafting. The thicker the skin graft, the longer it will take to obtain new blood supply and to become well fixed. Thin split-thickness grafts may take months before they are able to produce oils to keep them soft and pliable. Therefore, they must be protected and lubricated regularly.
b. Full-thickness grafts. These grafts include all layers of the skin but do not include the underlying fatty subcutaneous tissues. Obviously, if a full thickness of skin is taken, the donor site will not grow new skin and must be closed either by suturing or by placing a split-thickness graft over it.
c. Pinch grafts. Small bits of skin, less than a half inch in diameter,

are occasionally placed in ulcerated areas.

## For what conditions are skin grafts advocated?

a. Ulcerated areas that fail to heal naturally.

b. Areas that have been destroyed by radiation.

c. Burn areas.

d. Areas that are devoid of skin because of an injury.

e. Areas where skin had to be removed during the course of a surgical procedure.

f. Areas involved in skin cancer or malignant moles (melanomas).

g. Areas in which there are marked contractures, such as in the neck, the joints, or fingers.

h. Congenital birth deformities in which normal skin is lacking.

## What are flaps?

These are grafts composed of skin and underlying tissues, including subcutaneous tissue and sometimes muscles, nerves, blood vessels, etc. One portion of the flap remains attached to its original site while the rest is transplanted to the recipient site. At a later date, when blood supply has been established at the recipient site, the flap is detached from its origin and is swung around to cover the entire recipient area.

## Is a pedicle graft a form of flap?

Yes, but it contains only skin and subcutaneous tissues.

## When are flaps used?

a. In cases where function or form will be greatly handicapped by the presence of a skin graft. Also, in cases where resiliency, stretchability, and contours are very important. (In breast reconstruction, flaps are often employed.)

b. In patients who have large defects resulting from extensive cancer operations or from severe accidents.

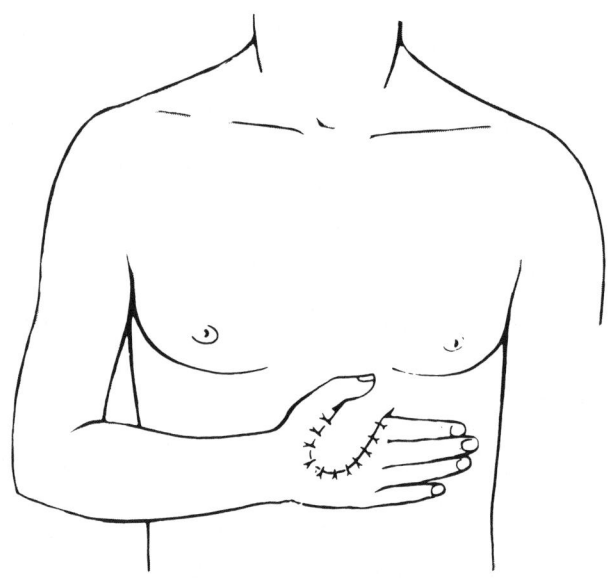

Pedicle graft taken from skin of body and grafted onto back of hand

**Skin Grafts.** *Together these diagrams show a pinch graft, wherein just a small segment of skin is lifted out from one part of the body and placed over a raw area elsewhere; a split-thickness graft, which takes a segment of the upper layers of the skin; a full-thickness graft, which removes all the layers of the skin; and a pedicle graft, in which a segment of skin is partially detached from one area and attached to another part of the body.*

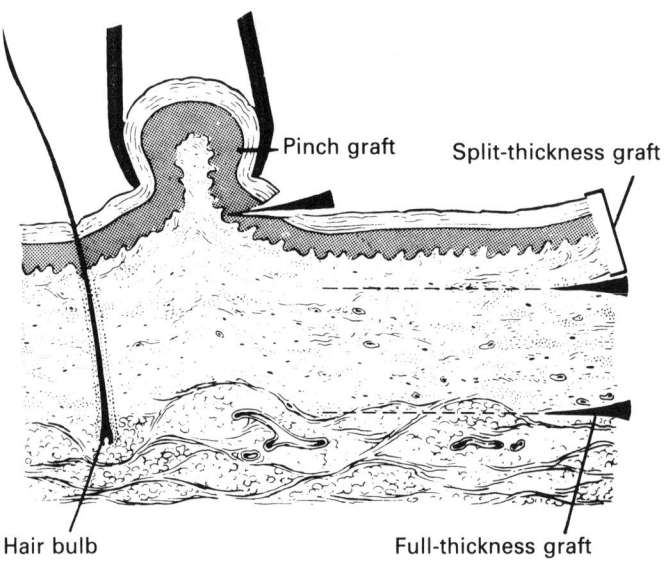

## What are the advantages of flaps over ordinary skin grafts?

A flap has the advantage not only of replacing skin but also muscle, cartilage, blood vessels, bone, etc.

## What is a free flap?

It is one that is transferred microsurgically, thus permitting blood vessels, nerves, tendons, and other tissues to be transplanted. Their use has opened a whole new era in reconstruction. (See Chapter 61, on Replantation Surgery.)

## What is a mesh graft?

It is a graft containing multiple perforations, which allows the skin to expand so that it can cover many times the area it would cover without the perforation. In some cases, a mesh graft can cover three, six, or nine times the area a nonperforated graft can cover.

**How is a mesh graft obtained?**

By a special instrument known as a mesh grafter.

**Where are mesh grafts best used?**

a. In burn cases in which large areas are devoid of skin and where many donor sites have already been utilized.

b. At sites where there may be some residual infection, a mesh graft has a better chance of taking than a nonperforated graft.

c. In diabetic patients who naturally have slow healing processes.

**Do mesh grafts heal with good cosmetic result?**

Usually, no. For this reason they are seldom employed on exposed parts of the body. Moreover, they often have a rough surface.

**What principles should be followed in obtaining skin grafts?**

a. Donor skin must be taken from an uninfected, clean area.

b. The donor site should be an unexposed part of the body.

c. Whenever possible, the donor site and the recipient site should be of the same, or nearly the same, color.

d. The recipient site must be uninfected and must have a good blood supply.

e. The skin graft must be well fixed to the recipient site. If it is not well fixed, it will shift so that new blood vessels will be unable to grow into it.

f. The graft must remain fixed for several days by pressure dressings and by keeping the recipient area immobile.

**Will grafted skin be of the same color as surrounding skin?**

Usually it is a lighter color, lacking natural pigment. The area of a split-thickness graft may also heal with a raised scar.

**Are thicker split-thickness grafts preferable to thin ones?**

Yes, because they give a better cosmetic appearance and shrink less than thin ones.

**Will hair regrow at sites where a split-thickness graft has been used?**

No, because the hair follicles have been left behind at the donor site.

**Where are the full-thickness grafts most desirable?**

a. Over weight-bearing areas such as the soles of the feet.

b. Over areas that will be subject to pressure, such as the palms of the hands.

c. In reconstructing cosmetically im-

portant areas such as the eyelids, the nose, the ears, and visible parts of the face.

**How does one know when a graft has taken?**

The graft will appear warm to the touch, and its color will be a light purplish red. Grafts that have not taken turn a dark bluish black, are wrinkled in appearance, and appear much like a scab.

**Is grafted skin usually the same quality as the normal skin?**

No, but the thicker the graft, the more it approximates normal-looking skin.

**How long does it take grafted skin to acquire the properties of surrounding normal skin?**

It will be several months before grafted skin develops all the characteristics of normal skin, and in many instances, it never does.

**Can a donor site be used again?**

Yes, if a split-thickness graft has been taken from it. However, several weeks must pass before another graft can be taken. Also, eventually, scarring intensifies, rendering the donor site unusable.

**Is it important to prevent grafted skin from becoming sunburned?**

Yes. Grafted skin lacks pigment and is therefore extremely sensitive to the rays of the sun.

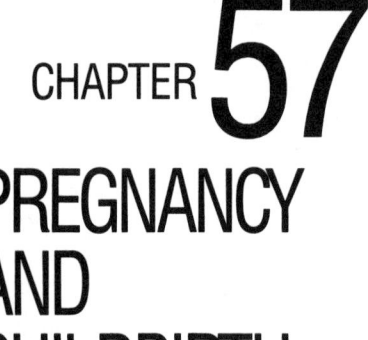

# CHAPTER 57

# PREGNANCY AND CHILDBIRTH

*(See also Chapter 11 on Birth Control; Chapter 25 on Female Organs; Chapter 69 on Sterility, Fertility, and Male Potency)*

## THE PRENATAL PERIOD

### Are classes of instruction for prospective parents available?

In nearly every community in the country, classes are made available for both prospective mothers and fathers. In these classes, the anatomy, physiology, and complications of pregnancy are discussed. Such classes are extremely useful and will help to relieve the fears that some young people have about the experience of becoming parents. It is just as important for the prospective father to attend these classes as for the mother. In most communities, classes are also available to the parents for instruction in natural childbirth.

### What are the symptoms of pregnancy?

a. The most consistent symptom is a missed menstrual period.
b. Enlargement of the breasts and tenderness of the nipples occurring within the first few weeks of pregnancy.
c. Increased frequency of urination within the first few weeks of pregnancy.
d. Nausea and vomiting, known as "morning sickness." This symptom may begin during the second month of pregnancy. Actually, the symptoms are not limited to the morning but may occur at any time.
e. In later pregnancy, abdominal enlargement becomes apparent.
f. Movements of the baby, known as "feeling life," start between the fourth and fifth month of pregnancy.

### Do these symptoms always indicate pregnancy?

No. Some of these symptoms may be found with other conditions. However, when these symptoms are correlated with specific physical findings, the diagnosis of pregnancy is easily made.

### How soon after the onset of pregnancy can the obstetrician make a positive diagnosis?

At approximately the time of the second missed menstrual period, that is, after four to six weeks of pregnancy. Of course, the diagnosis could be made with a high degree of accuracy by taking a pregnancy test some two to three weeks after the first missed menstrual period.

### What are the characteristic physical signs of pregnancy?

a. Enlargement and softening of the uterus.
b. Bluish discoloration and softening of the cervix.
c. Brownish discoloration of the area around the nipples.
d. After the ninth or tenth week, the fetal heartbeat can be detected with a special stethoscope.
e. A sonogram will detect the presence of a pregnancy as early as six to eight weeks after conception. This procedure, however, is not done routinely.

### Is a missed menstrual period always indicative of pregnancy?

No! A hormone imbalance, a debilitating disease, or severe emotional upset may occasionally cause a woman to miss a menstrual period.

### Does menstruation occur during pregnancy?

No. Menstruation is a term applied to regular bleeding from a nonpregnant uterus.

### Is vaginal bleeding always considered to be abnormal when the uterus is pregnant?

No. Slight bleeding is not uncommon during the first three months of pregnancy.

### Is it necessary to take a careful medical history of a pregnant woman?

Yes. This is very important, and such a history should include a complete family and personal history. Such familial conditions as diabetes, tuberculosis, twins, etc., are important to know as soon as a woman becomes pregnant. Also, the history of previous surgery or previous serious medical illness, such as a cardiac condition, a kidney condition, or allergic disease, is extremely important to note.

### Why is it so important to take a careful medical history?

Because the presence of one of the above conditions may influence the obstetrician to alter his management of the pregnancy and its subsequent delivery.

### What are some other important medical conditions that should be known about a pregnant woman?

a. Previous pelvic infection.
b. A history of infertility.
c. The woman's correct age, as well as her husband's age.
d. Previous obstetrical history.

### What kind of physical examination should be conducted upon a pregnant woman?

A complete physical examination, including thorough investigation of the heart, lungs, breasts, abdomen, and pelvis. The patient's blood pressure and weight should be checked at each prenatal visit. The importance of these findings will become apparent when toxemias of pregnancy are discussed.

### Must all pregnant women be examined internally?

Yes! There is no substitute for a thorough internal examination. Abnormalities of the uterus, tubes, ovaries, or bony pelvis can be detected most readily by a pelvic examination.

### Is there a danger of miscarriage following an internal examination?

Certainly not!

### What laboratory tests should be performed?

a. A complete blood count.
b. A complete urine analysis.
c. An examination of the blood for syphilis.
d. An examination of the blood to determine the Rh type.
e. A blood sugar test or a glucose tolerance test if diabetes is suspected or if there is a family history of diabetes.
f. Blood chemical analysis, especially if kidney disease or liver disease is suspected.

### Can the obstetrician tell during an early examination if a Cesarean section will be necessary?

No.

### How does the obstetrician determine when the baby is to be born?

The most common method is to count 280 days from the beginning of the last regular menstrual period.

### How accurate can the obstetrician be in determining the date of the baby's birth?

The obstetrician's prediction will usually be accurate within a two-week range from the date of the child's birth.

### Is there any such thing as a normal pregnancy diet?

Yes. The diet should be a balanced one with approximately fifteen hundred to two thousand calories. The diet should be high in proteins, minerals, and vitamins, with a moderate amount of carbohydrates and a minimum of fats, salt, and spices.

### What specific items are important to include in pregnancy diets?

Milk, eggs, cheese, meat, poultry, green vegetables, garden vegetables, and fruits.

### How much weight should the average pregnant woman gain?

About fifteen to thirty-five pounds, depending upon the woman's size, the baby's size, and the amount of water the particular patient retains in her tissues.

### Does the mother's weight influence the size of the baby?

No.

### Should vitamins be taken during pregnancy?

In a well-balanced, controlled diet, extra vitamin intake is not necessary. However, because of the eating habits of most people today, it is perhaps best to take supplementary vitamins to counteract any possible deficiency.

### Should a pregnant woman have an extra intake of calcium?

Yes. Calcium is included in the prenatal vitamin and mineral capsule the obstetrician will prescribe.

### Should iron be taken during pregnancy?

Yes, when some degree of anemia exists. Some investigators believe that the routine use of iron through-out pregnancy will prevent the onset of anemia.

### Is anemia a common occurrence during normal pregnancy?

Yes.

### Should salt intake be limited during pregnancy?

Only if the patient has an elevated blood pressure.

### Is it safe for a pregnant woman to drink alcoholic beverages?

An occasional cocktail, highball, glass of beer or wine is not harmful. Excessive intake of alcohol, however, may be harmful to both the baby and the mother.

### Is smoking permitted during pregnancy?

Yes, but in moderation. Heavy smoking during pregnancy may be harmful both to the baby and the mother.

### What restrictions on physical activity should be imposed upon pregnant women?

The normal pregnant woman may engage in all of the usual physical activities as long as she is able to do so without discomfort. As pregnancy progresses, her ability to do so may decrease. Very strenuous or excessive physical activity should be curtailed at all times.

### Are miscarriages frequently caused by strenuous physical activity?

No.

### Is bending, stretching, or raising the arms harmful to the pregnancy?

Absolutely not!

### What is the best clothing to wear during pregnancy?

a. A good brassiere is essential to support the enlarging breasts.
b. A firm girdle will give the patient a

feeling of support and relieve some of the lower abdominal or lower back or thigh discomfort that sometimes accompanies the later months of pregnancy.

c. Low or medium heels should be worn. This is particularly important as there is a tendency to slip and fall during the later months of pregnancy—and high heels are conducive to such accidents.

d. A garter belt should be used to support stockings. *Elastic garters around the legs or thighs should never be worn!*

e. Elastic stockings may be worn if there is a tendency to develop varicose veins.

**Why are elastic garters not to be worn?**

Because they may produce varicose veins.

**Is bathing permitted during normal pregnancy?**

In the early months of pregnancy, tub baths or showers are permitted. In the later months, showers are preferable over tub baths, as stepping into and out of a tub may lead to falls.

**Is ocean bathing or pool bathing permitted during pregnancy?**

Yes. Care should be taken to stay away from rough water and to avoid too strenuous activity, such as diving.

**What special care should be given to the breasts during pregnancy?**

a. A good supporting brassiere is essential.

b. If the nipples are inverted, an attempt to bring them out should be made. This is done by grasping the nipple gently and pulling with a slight rotating movement in an outward direction.

c. Where there is a discharge from the nipples, cotton or gauze pads should be used as a protective measure.

d. Nipples should be washed regularly with a mild soap.

**Are pregnant women permitted to travel in an automobile, train, or plane?**

Yes, except when there is the threat of miscarriage, as evidenced by vaginal bleeding or abdominal cramps.

**Is miscarriage ever caused by a bumpy automobile, train, or plane trip?**

No. This is a common misconception with no scientific substantiation.

**Should pregnant women drive automobiles?**

Yes.

**Is sexual intercourse permitted during pregnancy?**

Yes, until the end of the eighth month. However, if there has been any vaginal bleeding, intercourse should be avoided.

**How often should a pregnant woman visit her obstetrician?**

Throughout the first six months, a visit every four weeks is indicated. During the seventh and eighth months, the patient should visit the doctor every two to three weeks and then once a week for the last four weeks. Women should not hesitate to phone or visit their obstetrician at any time should a question arise!

**Why are regular, periodic visits important during pregnancy?**

To spot the onset of complications at the earliest possible time and to prevent them in some instances. Weighing the patient, taking her blood pressure, examining the urine, listening to the baby's heartbeat, judging the growth and development of the baby, etc., are helpful ways of making sure that everything is going well. Also, a regular visit will offer an opportunity to answer the mother's questions, to reassure her, and to allay any unfounded fears.

**At what stage of pregnancy does the abdomen become visibly enlarged?**

Usually after the third month. At the fifth month, the top of the uterus is at the level of the navel. At the eighth month, the top of the uterus reaches the bottom of the breastbone. In the ninth month, the baby settles in the pelvis, and the abdomen looks slightly smaller again.

**Should the pregnant woman take extra rest periods?**

Yes, as pregnant women may become easily fatigued.

**How soon after the onset of pregnancy does the mother "feel life"?**

Fetal movements, or "quickening," are first noticed about the fifth month after the last menstrual period. At first these are just faint, fluttering movements, but later, actual marked movements are felt almost continually.

**Can the baby's movements be felt every day?**

Not necessarily. Nor are they felt all day long. In many instances, only occasional movements are felt once or twice during the course of a day.

**What is "lightening"?**

When the baby's head drops into the pelvis, the woman experiences a lighter feeling in the upper abdomen. In first babies, this occurs about three weeks before labor begins in 80 percent of cases.

**Can a mother tell when lightening takes place?**

Yes, sometimes. There is a feeling of more breathing space, and the mother notes a lowering of the height of the abdomen. She may also feel increased pressure within the pelvis and greater difficulty when walking.

**Can the obstetrician determine beforehand if labor will be easy or difficult?**

No. The kind of labor the mother will have is an unknown factor. The obstetrician can tell only if the pelvis is adequate or inadequate. He can also tell whether the baby is in the right position or if there is a pelvic abnormality. However, a good strong labor can overcome most difficulties. Even a large baby can come through the average pelvis without harming the mother or damaging itself.

**When does the obstetrician usually take pelvic measurements?**

Pelvic measurement is performed during the first visit. This is done by vaginal and rectal examination.

**What information does the obstetrician obtain from such an examination?**

a. The general size of the various planes of the pelvis, such as the inlet, the mid-pelvis, and the outlet.
b. The configuration or bony type of pelvis.
c. Any abnormalities in the soft tissues or bones in the region.

**Is the cause for morning sickness known?**

No, although it is thought to be associated with the large amount of female hormones that are produced during early pregnancy. Also, emotional upset seems to play a role in the condition.

**What is the treatment for the nausea and vomiting of pregnancy (morning sickness)?**

a. In the presence of repeated attacks of nausea and vomiting, frequent small feedings and plenty of fluids are advised.
b. Safe preparations, including antispasmodics, antacids, vitamins, motion sickness tablets, etc., have been given to treat this condition.

c. Severe cases that fail to respond to ordinary measures may have to be hospitalized and treated with intravenous feedings to restore fluid and mineral balance. Some of these women have an underlying psychological problem and may require treatment by a psychiatrist to tide them over this difficult period.

**Do nausea and vomiting have any effect upon the developing embryo?**

No.

**Is it common for pregnant women to have excess production of saliva?**

Yes. This is a frequent complaint, often replacing nausea and vomiting.

**Is special care of the teeth necessary during pregnancy?**

Yes. Proper oral hygiene must be exercised. A sufficient amount of calcium must be included in the diet. This is usually obtained by the drinking of milk and by taking a prenatal tablet containing calcium.

**Should women receive dental treatment during pregnancy?**

Yes. Dental care can be carried out throughout all of pregnancy without the fear of precipitating a miscarriage. However, it is best not to take a general anesthetic without the consent of the obstetrician.

**How is constipation treated during pregnancy?**

By eating those foods that tend toward regularity. Fresh and stewed fruits, bran cereals, and buttermilk should be included in the diet. If these measures are unsuccessful, mild laxatives may be used. Mineral oil is to be avoided since it may interfere with digestive processes.

**Are hemorrhoids a frequent complication of normal pregnancy?**

Yes, particularly in the later months.

They are caused by the pressure of the baby upon the large veins in the pelvis.

**What is the treatment for hemorrhoids during pregnancy?**

a. Rectal suppositories to relieve pain.
b. Medications to soften the stool.
c. The application of witch hazel or ice packs to the anal region if pain is severe.
d. The application of anesthetic ointments in the presence of severe pain.
e. When a large hemorrhoid has clotted and produces severe pain, it may be necessary for a small incision to be made in order to evacuate the blood clot.
f. In rare instances, it is necessary to operate and remove the hemorrhoids, especially if there is repeated or continuous bleeding or protrusion of large hemorrhoids through the anal outlet.

**What causes frequency of urination during pregnancy?**

a. Pressure of the enlarging fetus upon the dome of the bladder.
b. Infection of the bladder (cystitis).

**What is the treatment for frequency of urination?**

a. If frequency is due to pressure of the baby, the mother can do very little about it.
b. When the frequency is due to infection, active treatment is carried out by giving sulfa drugs or antibiotics.

**Are varicose veins of the legs very common during pregnancy?**

Yes. These are due to back pressure upon the pelvic veins by the enlarging uterus.

**What is the treatment for varicose veins during pregnancy?**

a. Any constricting garters must be immediately removed.

b. An elastic bandage encircling the entire leg or elastic stockings should be used to give even support to the veins of the extremity.

**Is surgery advocated for varicose veins during pregnancy?**

No.

**Do varicose veins ever disappear after delivery?**

Many of them will disappear or become much smaller. Each subsequent pregnancy may cause an aggravation, both in the symptoms and in the size of the varicosities.

**Is it natural for women to have a vaginal discharge during pregnancy?**

Yes. Some slight increase in vaginal secretion is entirely normal. However, an erosion of the cervix or a fungus infection of the vagina may cause discharge associated with an itch in the region of the vulva. Such conditions are usually treated during pregnancy.

**Are douches used to treat vaginal infections during pregnancy?**

No. They are not used because of the danger of extending the infection into the uterine cavity.

**What causes backaches during pregnancy?**

The most common cause is the change in posture that is adopted to compensate for the enlarging abdomen. In other words, the patient attempts to change her center of gravity.

**What is the treatment for backache?**

The use of a firm girdle or support will tend to relieve most backaches. However, some discomfort may be noted despite all measures.

**What causes leg cramps during pregnancy?**

A change in posture, which places a new kind of tension upon leg muscles.

**How are leg cramps treated?**

a. Immediate relief can often be obtained by standing on tiptoe and bending the knees or by pressing the toes against the end of the bed or against a wall.
b. If cramps are due to insufficient calcium, calcium and antacid tablets will frequently control them.

**What causes swelling of the feet, ankles, or other parts of the body during pregnancy?**

a. Pressure on pelvic veins. This is usually noticeable after standing for several hours and is relieved by rest in bed. Such swelling has no clinical significance.
b. Varicose veins. Such swelling is treated by the use of elastic bandages or stockings.
c. In some patients with elevated blood pressure (toxemia), swelling may appear in the lower limbs and also in the fingers, the face, the back, or abdominal wall.

**What causes the heartburn so frequently noted during pregnancy?**

It is usually caused by excess stomach acidity and is seen most commonly in the later months of pregnancy. It is associated with belching and a sour taste in the later months of pregnancy.

**What is the treatment for heartburn in pregnancy?**

The simplest remedy is to take small sips of milk. If this is unsuccessful, antacid powders or similar preparations should be taken. (Antacids containing bicarbonate of soda should be avoided.)

**What is the cause of dizzy spells during pregnancy?**

In early pregnancy, particularly in hot or humid weather, dizziness or fainting spells are rather common and are not considered serious. In the later months of pregnancy, if they are associated with other symptoms, such as tissue swelling, spots before the eyes, or nausea and vomiting, they may be an evidence of elevation of blood pressure.

**Is it particularly important for pregnant women to avoid taking patent medicines?**

Yes. No medication should be taken by a pregnant woman unless precisely prescribed by the obstetrician. It has been found lately that deformities of the embryo can be caused by taking drugs that will interfere with the normal development of the embryo. The best rule to follow is when in doubt, do *not* take the medication. This is particularly true during the first twelve weeks of pregnancy.

**Can the fetus be affected by emotional instability of the mother or by strife in the mother's surroundings?**

A new science is developing known as *fetology*. This branch of medicine is now studying the effects of the environment upon the developing embryo, and it has been discovered that the child might very well be influenced by upheavals in its mother's surroundings. For instance, it has been noted that the fetus's pulse rises precipitously when there is screaming, yelling, or loud noises or when the mother is emotionally upset. Moreover, an emotionally unstable mother may neglect her diet, may smoke or drink too much, or may in other ways fail to provide her embryo with the best environment in which to develop.

# LABOR
## (Delivery and Confinement)

**What is the usual normal mechanism of delivery?**

The most normal mechanism is one in which the baby's head comes first.

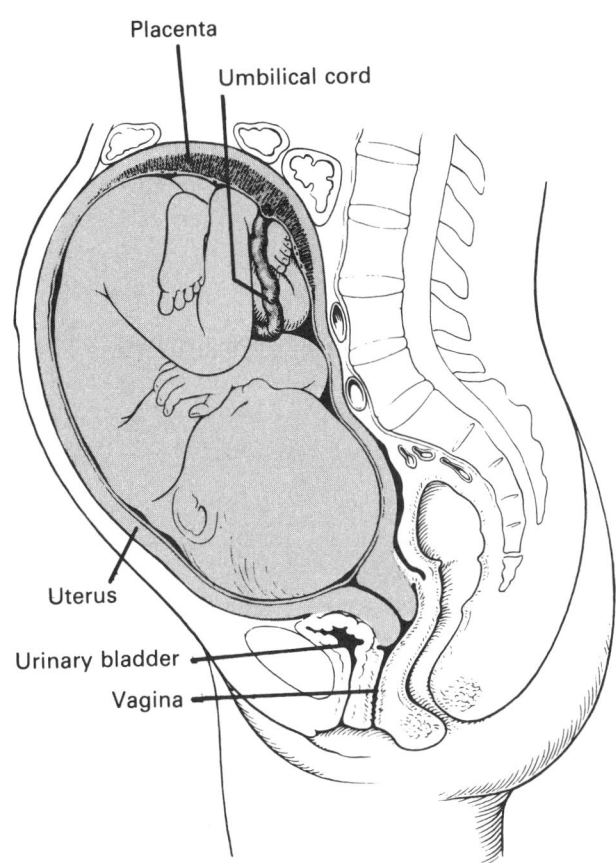

Placenta

Umbilical cord

Uterus

Urinary bladder

Vagina

*Head Presentation During Labor. This is the most common of all positions. During labor, the head molds so that it conforms to the contour of the inner aspect of the mother's pelvic bones. This makes passage through the birth canal easier.*

This is called vertex (head) presentation, and the head is termed the leading, or presenting, part.

### Can the obstetrician determine what part of the baby is going to come first?

Yes, by examining the abdomen or by an ultrasound test known as sonography. (See Chapter 67, on Sonography; Chapter 79, on X ray.)

### What parts other than the head sometimes present themselves just before or at the onset of labor?

The buttocks or legs may come first. This is called breech presentation. Occasionally, a baby's arm or shoulder will be the presenting part. Such a situation will complicate delivery. Sometimes the baby's head, instead

of being bent toward its chest, is extended or bent backward. This then becomes a face, or brow, presentation. This, too, constitutes a complication of delivery.

### What causes abnormal presentation?

In many instances, the cause is unknown. In other cases, it is caused by:
a. Abnormal shape of the mother's pelvis.
b. Tumors, such as a fibroid of the uterus.
c. Placenta previa, in which the afterbirth is implanted beneath the level of the baby's head.
d. Abnormalities of the baby itself.
e. Looping or twisting of the cord around the body of the fetus.

### What is done when the baby is found to be in an abnormal position?

The treatment for abnormal position depends upon many factors, such as:
a. The number of pregnancies the woman has already had.
b. The type of abnormality encountered.
c. The presence or absence of active labor at the time of discovery of the abnormal position.
d. The stage of labor present when the abnormal position is encountered.
e. The presence or absence of ruptured membranes.
f. The size of the baby.
g. The general condition of the mother.

All of these factors will influence the obstetrician in deciding what course to take. Some abnormal positions spontaneously convert to normal as labor progresses; others can be assisted by the obstetrician to return to normal presentation. Some babies may be delivered without complication even with the abnormal presentation. Finally, in certain instances, the obstetrician may resort to Cesarean section to carry out delivery.

### How can a woman tell when labor is beginning?

Labor begins any one of three ways:
a. Abdominal pains or contractions.
b. Rupture of the bag of waters.
c. Staining from the vagina.

### How are these signs identified?

Contractions or pains are identified by a feeling of tightness in the abdomen, with discomfort in the back radiating around to the front, or pain high in the abdomen radiating down toward the pelvis. There may also be a tight feeling in the thighs. In early labor, contractions are irregular and last for only a few seconds.

After a few hours, the contractions come closer together, last longer, and are more painful. If the bag of waters breaks, there may be just a little trickle of fluid or a big gush may ensue. If the bag of waters breaks before contractions have begun, the contractions will usually follow within twenty-four hours. When staining occurs, contractions usually follow within twenty-four to forty-eight hours.

## What are the various stages of labor?

a. The first stage is calculated from the onset until complete dilatation (opening) of the cervix or mouth of the womb.

b. The second stage begins at the time of complete dilatation of the cervix and ends with delivery of the baby.

c. The third stage begins with the delivery of the baby and ends with the delivery of the placenta, or afterbirth.

## How long does normal labor last?

In first babies, the average duration of the first stage of labor is approximately eighteen hours. After the first baby, the average duration of the first stage is less than eight hours.

In first babies, the second stage of labor lasts about an hour. After the first baby, the second stage is usually less than an hour.

The third stage of labor usually lasts only a few minutes but occasionally continues as long as an hour. The modern obstetrical trend is to cut the third stage of labor as short as possible by removing the afterbirth quickly.

## What is meant by "false labor pains"?

In the later months of pregnancy, the muscles of the uterus are extremely irritable and may undergo frequent contractions. These contractions resemble labor only in that there is a sense of tightening. False labor pains have no effect on dilating the cervix or pushing the baby downward.

## Is it ever necessary to treat false labor pains?

Yes. Sedatives are sometimes given to lessen the awareness of these annoying contractions.

## When should the patient starting labor go to the hospital?

This is a variable factor and depends upon each obstetrician's method of management. Some of the important considerations are:

a. The farther the patient lives from the hospital, the sooner she should depart for it.

b. If it is the first baby, it will probably be longer in coming, and the patient can take more time before departing for the hospital.

c. Patients with known abnormalities or complications of pregnancy should be hospitalized earlier than others.

## At what stage of labor is hospitalization mandatory?

With the first baby, when good strong contractions occur every five minutes for one full hour. With subsequent pregnancies, depending on the distance from the hospital, when contractions are occurring every ten to fifteen minutes.

## Is it always better to go to the hospital early?

Not necessarily. In normal pregnancy, it is better for the patient to stay at home until labor is well established. If there have been previous pregnancies and there is a history of rapid labor, it is perhaps better to leave for the hospital earlier than usual.

# INDUCED LABOR

## What is meant by "labor by appointment" or "induced labor"?

This is a method of initiating labor artificially. It is done in some cases because of a medical condition such as

high blood pressure, diabetes, etc. When properly carried out in suitable cases, it can be accomplished without harm to baby or mother.

## What are the advantages of induced labor?

a. The mother comes to the hospital in the morning after a good night's sleep. She can fast before coming to the hospital so that her stomach is empty prior to delivery.

b. She can make arrangements before she leaves for the hospital to have her other children taken care of.

c. Her husband can arrange his affairs so that he is at the hospital during labor.

d. The doctor can schedule the labor at a time when he is free of office hours or other duties that might keep him from attendance.

e. The hospital staff is alert and fully staffed during the daytime hours when labor is being induced.

f. All hospital activities, such as those that take place in the blood transfusion department, the x-ray department, the laboratories, the operating rooms, the delivery rooms, etc., are fully staffed and ready to carry out any necessary procedure during the day hours.

## How is labor induced?

a. By artificially breaking the water bag with a sterile instrument. This is a painless procedure and requires no anesthetic.

b. By the use of pituitary extract injections to stimulate contractions of the uterus.

## Can all patients be delivered by induced labor?

No! Certain conditions must be present before induced labor is advised. These are:

a. The patient must be at, or near, the regular time for delivery (not sooner than thirty-eight weeks after the onset of pregnancy).

b. The baby should be in a normal

position of presentation, with the head down in the pelvis.

c. The cervix should be soft, thinned out, and slightly open.

If the above conditions are met, there are virtually no dangers to either mother or baby from induction of labor.

## NATURAL (PREPARED) CHILDBIRTH

### What is natural childbirth?

This term refers to the method of management in which special care is taken to prepare the patient psychologically for pregnancy, including the prenatal period, labor, and the postpartum period (the period following delivery).

### What is prepared childbirth?

This is another name for natural childbirth.

### What are the aims of natural childbirth?

To banish unwarranted fears, thus preventing tension and, in this way, reducing pain to a minimum. The vicious cycle of fear/tension/pain is difficult to break once it has been established. If natural childbirth can do away with the element of fear, the vicious cycle is abolished.

### How does natural childbirth work?

It is accomplished by a course of instruction in the mechanism of pregnancy and by establishing a closer relationship between the patient and obstetrician. Also, the patient develops a familiarity with the hospital area and personnel so that the eventual labor and delivery will not take place in a strange atmosphere.

### Must one take a formal course in natural childbirth?

Not necessarily, but most large communities do have such courses. They include visits to the hospital, lectures by hospital physicians and nurses, instructions in breathing exercises, and, in some instances, specific instructions as to what should be done when labor approaches.

### Should the husband participate in natural childbirth?

Yes, so that he can be an emotional aid to his wife during times of expectant stress. In hospitals where natural childbirth is practiced, husbands remain in the labor and delivery rooms with their wives.

### Does natural childbirth mean delivery without sedatives or anesthesia?

Not at all! The patient is always aware of the fact that sedatives are available if she or her obstetrician thinks they are necessary. Anesthesia is also available if needed. However, the patient who practices natural childbirth and is emotionally prepared for labor will require a minimum of both sedatives and anesthesia. The patient should feel no shame or disgrace if she needs assistance from these agents. Natural childbirth is not an endurance contest!

### What are the advantages of natural childbirth?

a. A better understanding of the role to be played in pregnancy.
b. A more relaxed, emotionally stable attitude throughout pregnancy.
c. Less discomfort, as a result of understanding and relaxation.
d. A sense of well-being and active participation in the most natural of all human phenomena.

### Are there any advantages to the baby in natural childbirth?

Yes. The baby is often more alert at birth, breathing and crying takes place spontaneously and is not delayed, and there is more chance for a spontaneous delivery because of the ability of the mother to assist during the second stage of labor.

### What are the disadvantages of natural childbirth?

The only disadvantage arises in the patient who is emotionally unsuited for the experience. Such patients may build up more tension than normal by hiding their fears, and thus they will defeat the primary aim of natural childbirth.

### What happens when the patient reaches the hospital in labor?

In most institutions, after registering at the desk, the patient is accompanied by an aide to the labor floor. She is then admitted to a labor room, undressed, and given a gown or short jacket to wear. If she is in active labor, she is examined immediately by her own obstetrician, if he is present, or by one of the hospital residents or interns. This examination determines the stage of labor she is in. The pubic region is then shaved, and frequently an enema is given.

### Is the obstetrician always notified immediately upon admission of a patient to the hospital?

Yes. The obstetrician is always contacted by the intern or resident as soon as the exact stage of labor has been determined.

### Will hospital personnel delay the delivery of the child if the patient's obstetrician is not available?

No. This is not good practice and is rarely done. All well-qualified hospitals have intern and resident staffs that are sufficiently well trained to perform a delivery if it takes place prior to the arrival of the patient's private obstetrician.

### How often does a delivery take place before the obstetrician gets to the hospital?

Today this is a rare occurrence because patients are instructed explicitly on when to leave for the hospital. Also, transportation facilities are such today that the obstetrician can get to the hospital without too great a delay.

## What other tests are performed upon the patient following hospitalization?

The blood pressure is taken, a sample of urine is examined, and the baby's heartbeat is listened to and recorded. A blood count is taken, and the patient is given a physical examination of the heart and lungs by the house physician. A history is taken either by the house physician or supplied to the hospital records by the obstetrician from his office charts.

## How is the progress of labor determined?

a. By vaginal examinations. This tells the extent of dilation of the cervix and the position of the presenting part of the baby.
b. Also the progress of labor is monitored with an apparatus attached to the mother's abdomen. This gives a continuous recording of the fetal heartbeat and the contractions of the uterus.

## Who performs examinations upon the patient during labor?

Examinations are performed by the obstetrician, the house physician, and in some smaller institutions by obstetrical nurses who are experts in the field.

## Should the obstetrician be in attendance throughout all of labor?

With first babies, this is not necessary, and in most recognized hospitals throughout the country, the obstetrician is expected to visit his patient only periodically. During the first stage of labor, the patient is observed by the house physicians and nursing staff. If labor is rapid and progressing quickly, the obstetrician will naturally remain within easy reach of the labor floor. With second or subsequent babies, because of the shorter labor, most obstetricians remain on the labor floor or in the hospital throughout the entire course of labor.

## How is severe pain relieved during labor?

a. By giving narcotic drugs.
b. By epidural anesthesia. This involves an injection of an anesthetic agent outside the spinal canal.

## What types of anesthesia are used in delivery?

a. Local injection with Novocain of the skin of the perineum. This will allow the obstetrician to enlarge the opening with a surgical incision (episiotomy).
b. Pudendal block, the use of Novocain injected into a group of nerves in the perineum. This anesthetizes the area of the vagina so that an episiotomy can be performed painlessly.
c. Epidural block or spinal anesthesia. These methods utilize Novocain or similar drugs that are injected into openings in the vertebral column in order to produce anesthesia in the region of the vagina and outlet.
d. Inhalation anesthesia. This will include such gases as nitrous oxide, cyclopropane, Fluothane, or ether, in conjunction with the administration of oxygen.

## What determines the type of anesthesia that will be used?

Each type of anesthesia has its advantages and disadvantages, and every institution has anesthesiologists with special preferences. There are innumerable considerations in determining which anesthesia shall be used for an individual patient. Where there are expert anesthesiologists available, the decision should be left to them. The obstetrician will always confer with the anesthesiologists and state his preference for his patient.

The condition of the unborn child is as important a factor in determining anesthesia as the condition of the mother. For instance, premature babies do not tolerate inhalation anesthesias very well. In such a case, the mother may be delivered by a local block anesthesia or may be permitted to have a spontaneous delivery without any anesthesia at all.

## How is the condition of the baby checked during labor?

a. By continuous monitoring of the baby's heartbeat. Irregularities in the baby's heartbeat are an indication that something is wrong.
b. The appearance of meconium (the contents of the child's bowel) in the vagina is an indication of fetal distress. This finding is correlated with the heartbeat, and together they form a picture of fetal difficulty.

## What is the treatment for fetal distress?

The rapid delivery of the baby.

## What does the obstetrician do when the head is stretching the vaginal opening?

He enlarges the opening by making an incision along the edge of the vagina. This is called an episiotomy. The head, shoulders, and the rest of the body will then emerge. Such an eventuality is called a spontaneous delivery. Occasionally, pressure applied by an assistant who presses gently on the top of the uterus will hasten the delivery. If the baby does not exit from the vagina after this stage is reached, forceps may be employed. (See the section on Forceps Delivery in this chapter.)

## What is the advantage of an episiotomy?

It prevents tearing of the vagina or perineum near or through the rectum.

## When is an episiotomy performed?

Just before expected delivery, after

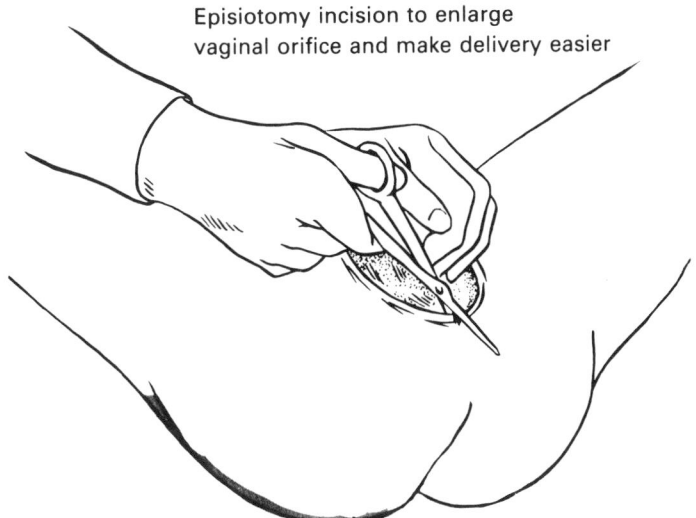

Episiotomy incision to enlarge vaginal orifice and make delivery easier

*Episiotomy and Delivery of the Afterbirth. In order to prevent tearing as the head comes through the opening of the vagina, it is common practice for the obstetrician to make a surgical incision (episiotomy) to allow more room for the child to emerge. This incision is repaired immediately after delivery. The afterbirth is delivered by gentle pressure by the obstetrician over the uterus. This usually occurs within a few minutes after the baby is born.*

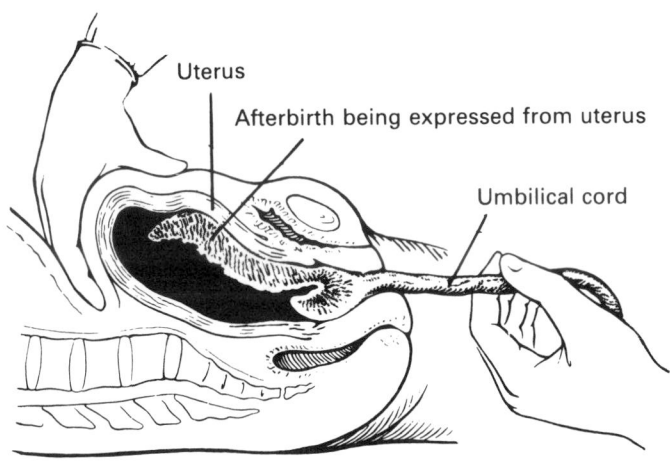

Uterus

Afterbirth being expressed from uterus

Umbilical cord

the skin has been anesthetized, and the baby's head is pressing on the outlet.

### When is the incision of an episiotomy repaired?

Immediately after delivery of the baby, while the patient is still under anesthesia.

### How long does it take an episiotomy incision to heal?

It heals in a matter of a few weeks.

### Do stitches have to be removed from an episiotomy wound?

No, as absorbable sutures are used.

### Is an episiotomy performed in most deliveries?

Yes.

### How is the afterbirth (placenta) removed?

By gentle pressure on the uterus and gentle pulling on the cord. If any difficulty arises, it should be removed

manually by the obstetrician, who inserts his hand into the uterus, separates the afterbirth carefully from the lining of the uterus, and removes it.

### How is the baby separated from the umbilical cord?

At birth, the baby is placed on the mother's abdomen or on an adjoining table. The umbilical cord is then clamped or tied about an inch from the baby's abdomen and is cut across with a scissors.

## FORCEPS DELIVERY

### What are forceps?

In obstetrics, forceps are instruments used to help deliver the baby's head.

### When are forceps used?

a. When the second stage of labor has been prolonged and the mother has been unable to push the baby out.
b. When the mother is tired and can no longer assist in the labor.
c. When the baby's head is not in the proper position to be delivered and must be rotated by the forceps.
d. When, because of one factor or another, the baby's head has not come completely through the pelvis to reach the opening of the vagina.
e. When signs of fetal distress appear and it is urgent to deliver the baby quickly rather than wait for natural processes to take their course.

### Are forceps dangerous to the baby?

When used properly by a qualified obstetrician at the proper time and for a correct indication, forceps are not at all dangerous and cause no injury to the baby. As a matter of fact, they are helpful to the baby because their application will aid earlier delivery and thus cut down on the period of time the child's head will be subject to the pressure of the birth canal.

## Are forceps dangerous to the mother?

No.

## Are there different types of forceps?

Yes. There are many types used for different purposes. Some are used to rotate the baby's head, some are used for traction on the head, others are used to exert traction in various directions to effect delivery of the head. Still others are used to deliver the head when the baby is in a breech position.

# BREECH DELIVERY

## What is a breech delivery?

One in which the baby's buttocks or feet are delivered first.

## Is breech delivery an abnormal situation?

In a certain sense this is an abnormal situation, but in the hands of a competent obstetrician, breech delivery can be carried out with safety to both mother and child.

## How often does breech delivery take place?

In approximately 3 percent of all deliveries.

## What causes breech presentation?

a. An abnormal pelvis.
b. Birth deformities of the uterus.
c. Fibroid tumors of the uterus.
d. Abnormalities of the fetus.
e. A placenta that is placed abnormally low within the vagina.
f. Multiple pregnancy.
g. An excessively large amount of fluid surrounding the baby.

## If the first baby is a breech, will all other pregnancies be breech?

Not necessarily.

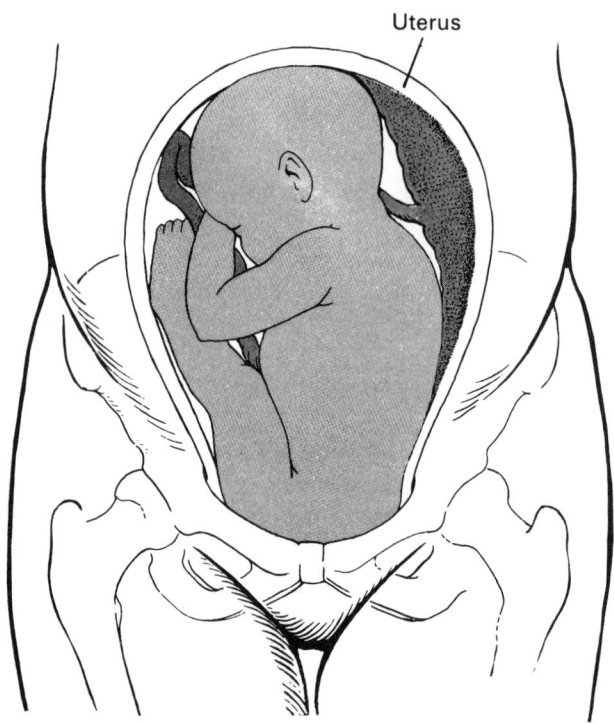

*Breech Presentation. This is less common than the head position, but most breech babies are delivered without too much difficulty. An infant presenting in this position will have less time for the head to mold to conform to the pelvic bones. Therefore, children in breech position with large heads are sometimes delivered by Cesarean section.*

## At what stage during pregnancy does the baby assume a breech position?

This may not take place until actual labor has been established. It is not at all uncommon for the baby to change its position from day to day or even from hour to hour until the very terminal stages of pregnancy. Most breeches, however, are found at about the eighth month of pregnancy.

## How is the breech position diagnosed?

a. By examination of the abdomen and noting that the head is in the upper part of the uterus.
b. By sonograms (ultrasound examination).
c. By vaginal examination during labor.

## How is breech position treated?

This is usually decided after the on-

set of labor. In first babies, the size and shape of the mother's pelvis must be accurately gauged since the large diameter of the baby's head will not be shaped or molded during a breech labor. Therefore such determinations must be made accurately before labor has progressed too far. If labor is good, and the pelvis is adequate in size, and the baby is not unduly large, labor is allowed to progress naturally. If labor is poor, or the pelvis is inadequate in size, or the baby is suspected of being large, a Cesarean section is indicated. Cesareans are performed more frequently for breeches occurring during the first pregnancy, no matter what the size of the baby.

## If a breech is found, should the patient go into the hospital at an earlier stage of her labor?

Yes, as the determination as to management must be made at an earlier stage of labor.

## PROLAPSED CORD

### What is a prolapsed cord?

It is a condition in which the umbilical cord drops down below the presenting part (the head or the breech) and comes through the cervix into the vagina. It may be only a partial prolapse, with the cord lying alongside the head, or a complete one in which the cord escapes through the cervix into the vagina all by itself.

### How often does prolapsed cord occur?

In about one out of two hundred cases.

### When is prolapsed cord seen most often?

After the membranes have ruptured in cases in which the baby is in an abnormal position or the head has not dropped down far enough into the pelvis.

### Is there danger to the baby from a prolapsed cord?

Yes, since the circulation through the cord will be interfered with by compression between the bony parts of the baby and the mother. Such an interruption of circulation may cause the baby to die.

### How is the diagnosis of prolapsed cord made?

a. By signs of fetal distress, such as slowing or irregularity of the heartbeat or presence of meconium in the vagina.
b. By the presence of the cord in the vagina or protruding from the vagina.

### What is the treatment for prolapsed cord?

Immediate Cesarean section.

### What emergency measures should be carried out if the cord prolapses while the patient is still at home?

The patient should be brought immediately to the hospital.

### Is there any way to anticipate or prevent prolapse of the cord?

No.

## MULTIPLE BIRTHS
### (Twins, Triplets, and Quadruplets)

### How often do twins occur naturally?

About once in eighty cases. If fertility pills (Clomid) have been given, the rate is higher.

### How often do triplets occur naturally?

About once in eight thousand cases. If a fertility medication (Pergonal) has been given, the incidence is greater.

### How often do quadruplets occur naturally?

About once in every 700,000 cases. Here, too, if Pergonal has been given, the incidence is greater.

### What is meant by identical twins?

These are twins who have developed from one egg. These twins usually look exactly alike.

### What are dissimilar (fraternal) twins?

They are those that have developed from two separate eggs. These twins may be of different sexes and do not look any more alike than two brothers or two sisters or a sister and brother.

### What causes twin births?

a. Identical twins result from the complete splitting of one egg after it has been fertilized.
b. Dissimilar (fraternal) twins result from the release of two eggs from the ovaries and the fertilization of each egg by a separate sperm.

### Is the tendency toward multiple births inherited?

Yes.

### Can multiple births occur when there is no family background of such births?

Yes.

### Is it possible to cause a woman to develop multiple births?

Within recent times it has been discovered that the giving of certain hormone medications to a woman prior to conception may stimulate her to develop multiple births. There are on record many cases of multiple births that have occurred in women who have taken these hormones.

### When can twins or multiple births be diagnosed?

With the use of sonograms, multiple births can be diagnosed as early as the tenth week of pregnancy.

### How does the obstetrical management of multiple births differ from that of single births?

The obstetrician will observe the patient more closely for signs of toxemia and for possible premature labor. A patient with twins or multiple births is usually admitted to the hospital at an earlier stage in labor.

### How is labor of multiple births managed?

The presentation of the first baby is determined and the patient is managed accordingly. Most babies will deliver head first. The second most common situation is one in which one baby delivers head first and the other by breech presentation. Sonograms are used to determine the position of each baby.

## INERTIA LABOR

### What is inertia labor?

It is a condition characterized by poor contractions of the uterus. Inertia labor may be primary, that is, the contractions may be poor from the very start; or it may be secondary,

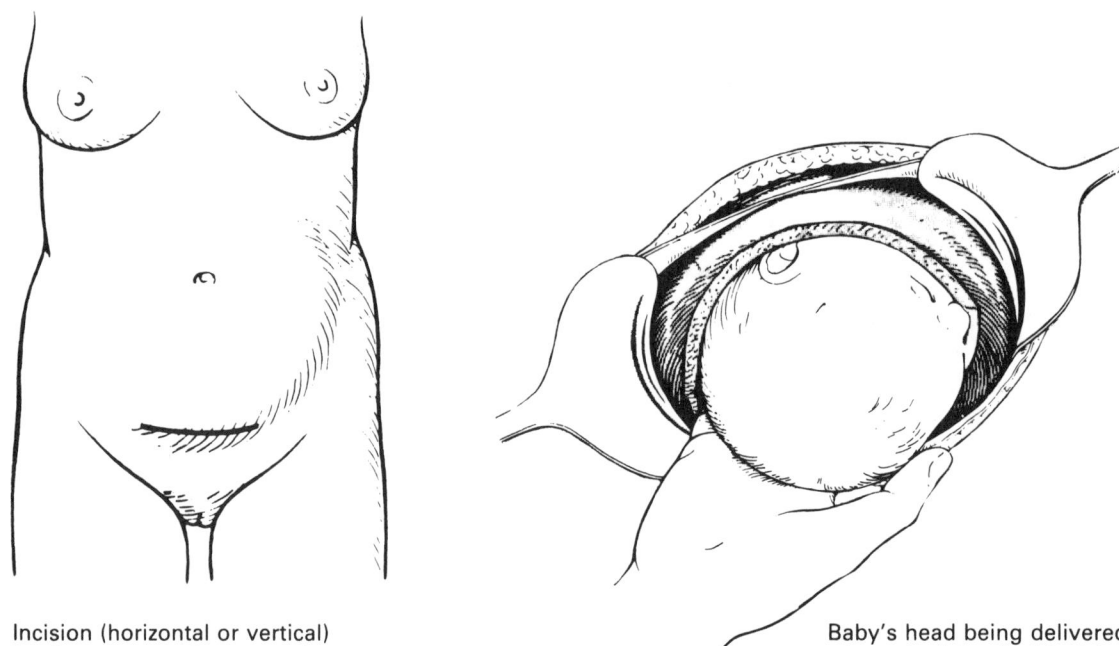

Incision (horizontal or vertical)
for Cesarean section operation

Baby's head being delivered
through abdominal incision

*Cesarean Section. This diagram shows how a child is delivered through Cesarean section. An operative incision is made in the abdominal wall, the uterus is opened, and the child is withdrawn therefrom. The afterbirth is then removed from the uterus, the uterine wall is sutured, and the abdominal wall is closed in the same manner as after any abdominal operation. Cesarean section is a safe operative procedure.*

that is, after a prolonged period of good labor, the contractions become weak and ineffective.

### What are the causes of inertia labor?

Primary inertia may develop in an overdistended uterus, such as one containing a very large baby or twins, or it may develop in those uteri that have too much fluid. Tension and fear may also play a role in the causation of primary inertia.

Secondary inertia is caused by prolonged labor. This situation arises when the mother's pelvis is not adequate for the size of the baby's head or when some abnormal presentation exists. In other cases, it is caused by failure of the cervix to dilate.

### What is the treatment for inertia labor?

Assuming that the presentation is normal, the pelvis is adequate, and the baby's head has entered the mother's pelvis, inertia is treated primarily with medication to stimulate the uterus to contract regularly and more forcefully. If some abnormality is present, such as abnormal position of the baby, this may involve performing a Cesarean section.

## CESAREAN SECTION

### What is a Cesarean section?

It is an operation devised to deliver a baby surgically by an incision in the abdomen and then into the uterus.

### Is Cesarean section a major operation?

Yes.

### How often are Cesarean sections performed?

In about 20 percent of all deliveries in the United States.

### Is Cesarean section a safe procedure?

Yes. It is virtually as safe as delivery through the vagina when performed by a competent obstetrician.

### What are the indications for Cesarean section?

a. Disproportion, where the baby's head is too large or the mother's bony pelvis is too small to allow delivery from below.

b Fetal distress, which refers to situations in which the life of the unborn child is endangered.

c. Prolonged or ineffective labor that fails to respond to the usual methods of stimulation and where normal vaginal delivery seems improbable in a reasonable time.

d. Placenta previa, when the afterbirth (placenta) lies in front of or below the baby's head. This is fraught with danger to the mother and baby because of the danger of hemorrhage.

e. Abruptio placenta, when the placenta separates from the uterus before the delivery of the baby has taken place and where bleeding is too brisk to permit waiting for delivery from below.

f. Abnormal presentation, such as one in which the baby is coming down with an arm or a shoulder first and delivery from below is almost impossible without great danger.

g. Prolapsed cord, where the umbilical cord comes out through the vagina before delivery and delivery is not thought to be imminent.

h. Breech presentation in first pregnancies, where the obstetrician fears some disproportion between the baby's head and the pelvis.

i. Preeclampsia or eclampsia, where elevated blood pressure and other symptoms make delivery urgent as a lifesaving measure.

j. Previous surgery, such as:
   1. Previous Cesarean section.
   2. Removal of fibroid tumors from the uterus.
   3. Previous plastic operations upon the vagina, where delivery from below may lead to rupture of the cervix or vaginal structures.

k. A fibroid of the uterus or an ovarian cyst or other tumor that obstructs the pelvis and prevents the normal passage of the baby through the birth canal.

### When was Cesarean section first performed?

It is thought that it was first performed in the sixteenth century A.D. The name has evolved from the tale that Julius Caesar was delivered by this method, but there is no historical substantiation for this legend.

### Are all of the above indications for Cesarean sections absolute?

No. It must be understood that there are many variable factors that will help the obstetrician make his decision.

### When will the obstetrician know whether a Cesarean section will be necessary?

This varies considerably. He may know on his first examination of the patient during the early days of pregnancy, or he may not know until after labor has been in progress for several hours.

### What types of anesthesia are used for Cesarean section?

a. General anesthesia.
b. Spinal or epidural block.
c. Caudal.
d. Local anesthesia, in rare instances.

The type of anesthesia will be determined by the mother's condition and the preference of the obstetrician, the patient, and the anesthesiologist.

### Where is the incision made by Cesarean section?

In the lower abdomen, either by a longitudinal or transverse incision.

### How is the baby delivered in Cesarean section?

After the abdominal wall has been opened and the wall of the uterus has been incised, the surgeon's hand is inserted into the uterus, and the baby is gently lifted out. The cord is tied off in the usual manner, and the surgeon again inserts his hand and separates the afterbirth from the uterine wall. The incision in the uterus is then sutured with two layers of stitches and the abdomen is closed.

### How long does it take to perform a Cesarean section?

Anywhere from forty-five to sixty minutes.

### How many Cesarean sections is it safe for a woman to have?

In the absence of complications, a woman may be allowed to have as many Cesarean sections as she wishes.

### Is it true that most women who have had one Cesarean section will be delivered by the same method in future pregnancies?

As a general rule this is true.

### Is Cesarean section a painful operation?

Not particularly.

### When does the patient get out of bed after Cesarean section?

The day following surgery.

### Are special nurses necessary?

They are not essential but are helpful for the first few days.

### How long after Cesarean section will vaginal bleeding continue?

For two to three weeks, followed by the usual discharge that ensues after any pregnancy.

### Does Cesarean section interfere with subsequent menstruation?

No.

### How long after Cesarean section will the first menstrual period appear?

In about six weeks.

### Can a baby be breast-fed after Cesarean section?

Yes.

### Can a patient who has once had a Cesarean section ever be delivered from below in subsequent pregnancies?

Yes. However, such a patient must be watched very closely from the very onset of labor, and the operating room must be alerted at all times to perform an emergency Cesarean section should a complication arise.

### How long a hospital stay is necessary after Cesarean section?

About eight to ten days.

### Does Cesarean section interfere with future pregnancies?

No.

**How soon after Cesarean section can a woman safely become pregnant again?**

As soon as she wishes.

**How soon after Cesarean section can one do the following:**

Shower:
  One week.
Bathe:
  Four weeks.
Douche:
  Six weeks.
Drive an automobile:
  Five to six weeks.
Resume sexual relations:
  Six to eight weeks.
Resume all normal activities:
  Eight to ten weeks.

## POSTPARTUM HEMORRHAGE
*(Hemorrhage Following Delivery)*

**What is meant by postpartum hemorrhage?**

Loss of excessive blood following removal or delivery of the afterbirth (placenta).

**What causes postpartum hemorrhage?**

a. Failure of the uterus to contract following prolonged labor, overdistention of the uterus due to a large baby, or overdistention of the uterus due to excessive fluid within its cavity.
b. Retained placental tissue, which allows bleeding to take place behind it.
c. A laceration of the vagina, cervix, or uterus that has occurred during labor.

**Is postpartum hemorrhage dangerous?**

The real danger exists in failure to recognize its presence or severity. A great deal of the danger has been overcome by modern methods of recognition and treatment and by the availability of blood for transfusion.

**When is postpartum hemorrhage most likely to occur?**

Either within the first few hours after delivery or, in delayed hemorrhage, several days after delivery.

**What is the treatment for postpartum hemorrhage?**

a. If the patient is at home, she should be hospitalized immediately.
b. If she is in the hospital, blood is given to replace the loss if necessary.
c. The cause must be established and appropriate corrective measures instituted promptly.

**What specific measures are carried out to eradicate the cause of hemorrhage?**

a. If it has taken place as a result of failure of the uterus to contract, medications are given to bring about contraction.
b. If a laceration of the vagina, cervix, or uterus is present, it must be sutured surgically.
c. If the hemorrhage has been caused by retained placental tissue, this must be removed.

## THE POSTPARTUM PERIOD
*(After Delivery)*

**When is the patient allowed out of bed after delivery?**

Usually within the first twelve hours.

**How soon after delivery can the patient eat and drink?**

Fluids may be taken within the first four hours. Full diet is resumed within the first twelve hours. If a prolonged inhalation anesthesia has been given, fluid and food intake may be delayed.

**Is it common to require a catheterization after delivery?**

Yes. Difficulty in passing urine soon after delivery is not at all uncommon.

**How soon after delivery does the average patient have a bowel movement?**

Usually on the third day. A laxative is given on the second day. If there is no result by the third day, an enema may be administered.

**When do the breasts become engorged and tender after delivery?**

By the third or fourth day.

**If the mother does not breast-feed the child, how are the breasts treated?**

a. A good, firm support is worn.
b. An ice bag is applied if the breasts are painful.
c. Pain-relieving medicines and sedatives are given if necessary.

**If the mother decides to breast-feed her child, how soon will the milk start to come in?**

By the second or, at the latest, third or fourth day.

**How are the breasts treated when the mother stops breast-feeding?**

a. By applying a firm brassiere.
b. By giving pain-relieving medications.

**What is the treatment for tender nipples?**

If they become too tender, a specially designed nipple shield will permit the mother to nurse without experiencing pain. Also, a special medicated cream for the nipple can be applied.

**Can a mother continue to breast-feed if the nipples bleed, crack, or become inflamed?**

Yes, if she wears a specially designed nipple shield and uses the special cream.

**How are breast infections treated?**

a. By the giving of antibiotics.
b. By warm compresses to the breast.
c. If a localized abscess has formed, it must be incised and drained surgically.

**Do hemorrhoids ever develop after delivery?**

Yes. They are a common complication and should be treated by the taking of lubricants to soften the stool and by the application of warm compresses or witch hazel to the area. Anesthetic ointments applied to the anal area may also help to relieve pain.

**Are the stitches in the vaginal region painful after delivery?**

Yes. Some pain and tenderness is present for a few days. This pain is frequently alleviated by warm compresses and by the giving of mild sedatives.

**What is the average length of hospital stay after delivery?**

This varies. Some obstetricians discharge patients as early as the third or fourth day; others hold their patients for five or six days.

**How soon can one go out of doors after delivery?**

Usually, about a week after leaving the hospital.

**How soon after delivery can one return to all normal activity?**

In approximately four weeks.

**How long does vaginal staining continue after delivery?**

The vaginal discharge is called the lochia; it usually continues for several weeks after delivery. It is not uncommon to have a vaginal discharge until the first menstrual period.

**How soon after delivery does the first menstrual period occur?**

Usually within six weeks, but it may vary from five to eight weeks or longer.

**How soon after delivery may one shower?**

Within a day or two after returning home.

**How soon after delivery may one bathe?**

Not until four weeks after delivery.

**How soon after delivery may one douche?**

After the obstetrician performs the routine six-week postpartum examination.

**How soon after delivery may sexual relations be resumed?**

After six weeks. It should be remembered that the first few attempts may be accompanied by pain or discomfort, but this will resolve itself within a short time.

**How soon after delivery may one do housework?**

This varies markedly, but most women begin to resume their normal household duties within two to three weeks after delivery.

**Should the patient stay in bed after leaving the hospital?**

No, but she should get into the habit of having a daily rest period for the first few weeks.

**Is a special diet necessary after normal delivery?**

No. A well-balanced diet is all that is necessary.

**How soon do the female organs return to normal after delivery?**

The uterus returns to normal by the sixth week. The breasts also return to normal size within approximately six weeks. The abdominal muscles seem to take longer to return to normal and may be lax and weak for several months after delivery. This condition can be helped greatly by exercise.

**Is special treatment of the cervix necessary after delivery?**

The cervix should be inspected after the first or second menstrual period following delivery. If it is then found to require treatment, it will be carried out by the obstetrician.

**How soon after delivery is it safe to have another baby?**

From a purely physical point of view, it is safe to become pregnant as soon as the effects of delivery have worn off, that is, within two months. However, the burden of caring for a newborn and the added household duties often make it advisable to space children more widely.

**Are women who have recently had babies more susceptible to infections?**

Yes; for some incompletely understood reason, women who have just given birth to a child are particularly prone to develop infections. They should avoid contact with people who have upper respiratory infections, and they must protect their nipples, as breast abscess is a common postpartum infection.

**Are women easily fatigued, and do they tend to be depressed following childbirth?**

This often does occur and is a natural phenomenon.

## COMPLICATIONS OF PREGNANCY

**What are the danger signs that might indicate the onset of a complication of pregnancy?**

a. Increased swelling of the feet and ankles.

*(continued)*

b. Sudden marked increase in weight.

c. Disturbances in vision, such as disturbing "spots before the eyes" or double vision.

d. Severe, persistent headaches.

e. Severe abdominal pain, especially in the upper abdomen.

f. Repeated vomiting.

g. Abdominal cramps, with or without bleeding from the vagina.

h. Vaginal bleeding at any time after the onset of pregnancy.

i. A marked decrease in the output of urine.

j. Repeated episodes of fainting.

k. Failure to feel the baby moving for more than one day, if this occurs after the sixth month of pregnancy.

## Heart Disease in Pregnancy

**Should a patient with heart trouble allow herself to become pregnant?**

This will depend upon the type of heart disease, the presence or history of episodes of heart failure, and the ability of the patient to carry on normal activity without excessive fatigue.

**Can most cardiac patients go through pregnancy?**

Yes. Contrary to common belief, even damaged hearts are able to tolerate pregnancy.

**What type of cardiac patient will have the most difficulty in carrying through a pregnancy?**

A patient who has had episodes of heart failure or one who has been unable to carry out ordinary physical activity during nonpregnant periods.

**Is the heart patient managed differently during pregnancy?**

Yes. Such a patient should be observed by both the obstetrician and the cardiologist. She is seen more frequently than the average pregnant woman, and she is advised to rest more. If there are any signs of heart failure, the patient is hospitalized immediately.

**Is delivery by Cesarean section always necessary for cardiac patients?**

No. Cardiac disease in itself is not an indication for Cesarean section, although the cardiac patient is often better served by Cesarean section as she will not have to undergo the stress of labor.

**Can surgery for rheumatic heart disease help a pregnant woman?**

Yes. In many cases where indications for heart surgery exist and the symptoms are on the increase, surgery becomes mandatory. This surgery can be performed as late as the sixth month of pregnancy. Most women will tolerate the procedure well and will be benefited considerably.

**Can cardiac patients have more than one baby?**

Yes, providing there is no evidence of heart failure and the patient is supported by the watchful care of both obstetrician and cardiologist.

## Pyelonephritis in Pregnancy

**What is pyelonephritis?**

It is an infection of the kidney frequently seen during pregnancy.

**What causes pyelonephritis during pregnancy?**

Pyelonephritis is a bacterial infection arising from the bowel, the bladder, or some other source. During pregnancy, there is an abnormal amount of pressure on the ureters that causes them to become partially obstructed and to interfere with free drainage of urine from the kidney. This situation predisposes toward the development of infection.

**Is pyelonephritis serious during pregnancy?**

Not usually. Treatment today with antibiotics makes the disease easily controllable. However, if untreated, there is danger of permanent kidney damage.

**Does pyelonephritis in the mother affect the child?**

No.

**At what stage of pregnancy is a woman most likely to develop pyelonephritis?**

During the later months, when pressure upon the ureters is greatest.

**What are the symptoms of pyelonephritis?**

Urinary frequency, burning on urination, pain in the region of the kidneys or down along the course of the ureters. There may also be chills, fever, nausea, and vomiting.

**What is the treatment for pyelonephritis?**

a. Large increase in the intake of fluids.

b. The giving of sulfa preparations or antibiotics.

**How long does pyelonephritis usually last?**

Approximately three to four days.

## Diabetes in Pregnancy

**Does the finding of sugar in the urine during pregnancy always indicate diabetes?**

Not necessarily. Lactose is often present in the urine of pregnant women during the later months of pregnancy, and this will give a positive test for sugar in the urine. Lactose in the urine does not represent diabetes.

**How is diabetes diagnosed during pregnancy?**

a. By the presence of glucose in the urine.

b. By tests showing an elevation of the sugar level in the blood.

c. By a blood test known as a glucose tolerance test.

### Are all of these tests performed during every pregnancy?

No. Routine urine examinations are done for glucose. If a positive sugar test is found or if there is a family history of diabetes, then further investigation is carried out.

### Are there certain types of women who should be scrutinized with particular care for the development of diabetes?

Yes; women who have had previous obstetrical difficulty such as miscarriage, stillbirth, or toxemia, or women who have had large babies weighing more than nine pounds at birth. Also, patients who give a family history of diabetes should be investigated with special thoroughness.

### Is special treatment carried out for the potential diabetic?

Yes. She is more closely watched for signs of toxemia or other complications of pregnancy.

### Are known diabetics a particular problem during pregnancy?

Yes. They must be followed by both the obstetrician and the medical specialist throughout the entire pregnancy. Control of the diabetic status is more difficult to maintain because of the presence and demands of the growing fetus.

### Must diabetics always be delivered by Cesarean section?

No.

### What effect does pregnancy have on diabetes?

Pregnancy interferes with the ready control of diabetes, and therefore the diet and the insulin dosage must be altered frequently to meet changing situations. It is not uncommon for these patients to require periods of hospitalization at various stages of pregnancy in order to regulate their diabetes.

### What effect does diabetes have on pregnancy?

a. There is a higher-than-normal incidence of miscarriage.
b. Diabetic women tend to have excessively large babies with difficult delivery. Because of this, there is often a high percentage of disproportion between the size of the baby's head and the mother's pelvis.
c. There is a higher incidence of toxemia of pregnancy, with increased dangers to both mother and child.
d. There is a higher-than-usual incidence of fetal death during the last months of pregnancy in a severe diabetic.

## Toxemia of Pregnancy

### What is toxemia?

It is a disease peculiar to pregnancy characterized by high blood pressure, damage to the blood vessels, the liver, and especially to kidney function. As a matter of fact, all body processes are disturbed in a woman suffering from toxemia of pregnancy.

### How often does toxemia of pregnancy occur?

It is thought to occur in about 10 percent of all pregnancies, but in the great majority of these instances the toxemia is mild.

### What causes toxemia?

The cause is unknown.

### What are the various types of toxemia?

a. Toxemia that is peculiar to pregnancy, such as preeclampsia and eclampsia.
b. Toxic states that are not peculiar to pregnancy, such as high blood pressure, kidney disease, and disease of the blood vessels.

### What type of patient is most likely to develop preeclampsia or eclampsia?

Those who have had previous high blood pressure, kidney disease, or liver disease. However, many patients with no history of previous illness may develop toxemia during pregnancy.

### Do patients with twins have a particularly high incidence of toxemia?

Yes.

### Do diabetic women have a special tendency toward the development of toxemia?

Yes.

## Preeclampsia

### What are the symptoms of preeclampsia?

There may be no symptoms in mild cases, but in the more severe form, during the last three months of pregnancy, the following may be present:
a. Nausea and vomiting.
b. Headaches.
c. Diminished output of urine.
d. Spots before the eyes or double vision.

### What are the signs of preeclampsia?

a. Swelling or edema of the face, hands, and most commonly of the ankles and legs.
b. Albumin in the urine.
c. Elevated blood pressure.
d. Unusual and marked gain in weight.
e. Abnormal blood chemistries.

### Is there any way to prevent preeclampsia?

The greatest part of prenatal care today is directed toward prevention of toxemia and early detection of the disease when it does appear. Routine examination of blood pressure, urine, weight, swellings, etc., are all done to detect early signs of toxemia. With early detection, preventive measures may be carried out.

## Who is most likely to develop pre-eclampsia?

The young woman who is having her first baby, the diabetic, the overweight patient, and the woman who is having multiple births.

## What is the treatment for preeclampsia?

The following measures are advocated:

a. Table salt and sodium are limited markedly.

b. Mild sedatives are given, and the patient is kept quiet in a darkened room.

c. Hospitalization is advised if the patient fails to respond to the above measures.

d. Termination of pregnancy is advocated if hospital treatment is ineffectual.

e. Early delivery of the baby.

## What methods are used to terminate pregnancy in preeclampsia?

a. If a short labor seems probable, induction and delivery from below is indicated.

b. If a relatively short labor is not anticipated or if induction fails, a Cesarean section is advised. This latter situation occurs if the woman is having her first child.

## What are the harmful effects of preeclampsia?

During pregnancy, there is danger to the baby and the mother for the following reasons:

a. Premature separation of the placenta with resulting hemorrhage is quite common in preeclampsia.

b. The disease may progress to true eclampsia with dangerous convulsive seizures.

c. Permanent kidney damage may

result unless treatment is carried out conscientiously.

d. Infant mortality is much higher than normal in preeclamptic women.

## What are the chances of full recovery from preeclampsia?

Treatment, as outlined above, will keep most cases of preeclampsia under control until the baby is delivered. After delivery of the baby, almost all patients recover quickly with a return to normal kidney function and normal blood pressure within a few days. A small number of patients may take several weeks to regain normalcy.

## Does preeclampsia usually clear up by itself without treatment?

No!

## Does preeclampsia tend to recur during subsequent pregnancies?

Yes. There is a tendency toward recurrence.

## Are there ever any serious aftereffects of preeclampsia?

Yes, when there has been underlying disease of the kidneys or blood vessels before the pregnancy. In such cases, the elevated blood pressure, the impaired kidney function, and the damage to the blood vessels are further aggravated by the preeclampsia.

## Are any precautions necessary after the woman with preeclampsia has delivered?

If kidney function, liver function, blood pressure, etc., have returned to normal, then no aftercare is necessary. It is important, however, that these patients be checked periodically by their physicians.

## Can a woman who has had preeclampsia permit herself to become pregnant again?

Before advising another pregnancy,

one must weigh carefully the severity of the disease, the response to treatment, the presence of underlying permanent disease, and the number of babies the woman has had thus far. The mere history of one episode of preeclampsia is not a contraindication to subsequent pregnancy.

## Eclampsia

### What is eclampsia?

Eclampsia represents the end result of a preeclamptic state. In rare instances, it comes on spontaneously without evidence of preeclampsia.

### How often does eclampsia occur?

In one out of eight hundred cases.

### What is the cause of eclampsia?

The cause is unknown.

### When does eclampsia occur?

Usually in the last few months of pregnancy. The most common time is just before the onset of labor, but it may sometimes occur during labor or in the first twenty-four hours after delivery.

### Is eclampsia serious?

Yes. There is much increased risk to mother and baby when eclampsia exists.

### What are the signs of eclampsia?

a. Convulsions.

b. Decreased or absent urinary output.

c. Extremely high blood pressure.

d. Large quantities of albumin in the urine.

e. Coma.

f. Marked changes in blood chemistry.

### How is eclampsia treated?

a. By immediate hospitalization.

b. By giving sedatives to control the convulsions.

c. By giving fluids intravenously.

d. By stimulating urinary output.

e. By the use of drugs to bring down the blood pressure.

f. By emptying the uterus as soon as the convulsions have been controlled for a period of twelve to eighteen hours. If induction is possible, delivery from below is carried out. If this is not feasible, then Cesarean section is undertaken.

### What are the chances of recovery from eclampsia?

If recognized early and treated properly, the chances for complete recovery are good. If unrecognized or untreated, the results may end in maternal and fetal fatality. This is an important reason why women should make frequent visits to the obstetrician *during* pregnancy.

### Are there any permanent aftereffects of eclampsia?

If the eclampsia was treated early and effectively, there may be no permanent aftereffects at all, providing that there was no preexisting condition such as kidney or blood vessel disease.

## Placenta Previa

### What is placenta previa?

It is the presence of the placenta in the lower part of the uterus, below or in front of the presenting part of the baby. In this condition, the placenta encroaches upon the opening of the cervix into the vagina.

### What causes placenta previa?

The exact cause is not known.

### What types of placenta previa exist?

a. Partial placenta previa, in which only part of the internal opening of the cervix is covered by the placenta.

b. Complete placenta previa, in which the entire opening of the cervical canal is covered by the placenta.

### How often does placenta previa occur?

Approximately one in eight hundred cases.

### What is the anatomy of placenta previa?

The placenta (afterbirth) is implanted at the edge of the internal orifice of the cervix instead of higher up on the wall of the uterus. As the lower part of the uterus thins out during delivery and prepares for labor, the internal opening enlarges. This causes a separation of the placenta from the wall of the cervix with resultant bleeding.

### Can placenta previa be prevented?

No.

### What are the signs of placenta previa?

The most important sign, and actually the only sign, is painless bleeding during the later months of pregnancy. This may vary from just a trickle of blood to a gush of heavy bleeding. The bleeding may stop immediately or may continue until it endangers the life of the patient.

### What are the harmful effects of placenta previa?

a. There is danger of severe hemorrhage.

b. Placenta previa usually requires early termination of the pregnancy. This may result in premature infants, with all the disadvantages of prematurity.

### How is the diagnosis of placenta previa made?

By taking a sonogram (ultrasound examination), which will show the location of the placenta.

### Is hospitalization absolutely necessary in all cases of placenta previa?

Yes.

### What is the most frequent time for placenta previa to occur?

During the last two or three months of pregnancy.

### What is the treatment for placenta previa?

a. Bed rest to permit the pregnancy to approach full term.

b. With a partial placenta previa, delivery from below is often possible.

c. With a complete placenta previa, Cesarean section is indicated.

### What are the chances of recovery from placenta previa?

With conscientious treatment in the hospital, almost all patients will recover.

### Are there any aftereffects of placenta previa following the delivery?

No, unless the mother is markedly anemic from blood loss.

### Is it safe for a woman who has had a placenta previa to have another pregnancy?

Yes.

### Does placenta previa tend to recur in subsequent pregnancies?

No.

## Abruptio Placenta

### What is abruptio placenta?

It is the premature separation of a normally placed placenta from the uterine wall.

### When does abruptio placenta usually occur?

When the blood pressure is markedly elevated.

### What causes abruptio placenta?

The exact cause is not known, but there is a close relationship between abruptio placenta and the various types of toxemias of pregnancy. It is thought that with elevated blood pressure, as in toxemia, the placenta is forced off the wall of the uterus.

### How often does abruptio placenta occur?

About one in five hundred cases.

### What types of abruptio placenta are there?

a. Partial separation of the placenta.
b. Complete separation of the placenta.

### What takes place after the placenta separates from the uterine wall?

There is bleeding between the uterine wall and the placenta, and this may spread and cause further separation of the placenta.

### Is there any way to prevent abruptio placenta?

Only by good prenatal care and the early treatment of any toxemia that may exist.

### What are the signs of abruptio placenta?

Some, or most, of the following signs may be in evidence:
a. Pain or tenderness when touching the area over the uterus during the last days of pregnancy.

b. The finding of an abnormally rigid or hard uterus on abdominal examination.
c. Nausea and vomiting.
d. Signs of toxemia, including elevated blood pressure.
e. Fainting, with a weak pulse and other signs of blood loss.

### Is there always external bleeding with abruptio placenta?

No. The bleeding may be concealed and may remain contained within the uterus.

### What are the results of abruptio placenta?

a. An extremely high fetal mortality.
b. The blood-clotting mechanism of the mother may be disturbed so that dangerous hemorrhage may result.

### What is the treatment for abruptio placenta?

Treatment is first directed toward combating any shock that is present. Blood replacement in the form of transfusions must be given immediately if indicated. Pregnancy must be terminated either by induced labor or by the performance of a Cesarean section. If the clotting mechanism of the blood has been disturbed, this must be corrected by the giving of

substances such as fibrinogen. If the wall of the uterus has been badly damaged by the hemorrhage, a hysterectomy may have to be performed following the Cesarean section.

### What are the chances of the mother's recovery from abruptio placenta?

If the diagnosis can be made early and the proper treatment is carried out promptly, recovery takes place in the vast majority of cases.

### What are the chances for a live baby in abruptio placenta?

This will depend upon the degree of separation of the placenta, the amount of bleeding that has taken place, the state of maternal shock when the separation occurs, and the speed at which treatment has been carried out.

### Are there any aftereffects of abruptio placenta if treatment has been carried out promptly and adequately?

No.

### Is there a tendency for abruptio placenta to recur with subsequent pregnancies?

No.

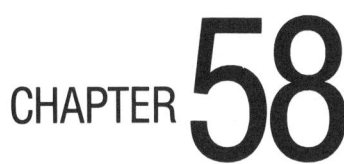

CHAPTER **58**

# PREOPERATIVE AND POST-OPERATIVE ROUTINES

*(See also Chapter 8 on Anesthesia; Chapter 26 on First Aid in Emergencies; Chapter 36 on Intensive Care Unit (ICU))*

## INFORMED CONSENT

### What is meant by informed consent?

Every adult patient who is in possession of his mental faculties must sign permission for surgery or any invasive procedure to be performed upon him. Before signing such consent, the patient must be given a complete description of what the physician or surgeon intends to do and what the outcome will probably be.

### What is an invasive procedure?

Any maneuver that involves entering the body with an instrument. Cardiac catheterization, colonoscopy, needle biopsy of the liver, etc., fall into this category.

### Must informed consent be written?

Yes. Most hospitals have a consent form, which the patient will be asked to read. After reading it, the patient signs in the presence of a witness, who also signs.

### Can a spouse sign a consent form for his mate?

Not if the mate is of sound mind and is an adult.

### Will the informed consent tell of the possible complications of a particular procedure?

There is a space for the intern or resident physician to fill in the details of possible complications for a particular procedure. Thus, the form may say that there is a certain chance of infection, that there is a certain percentage of cases wherein the procedure will fail to do what it set out to do, etc.

### Can a parent sign informed consent for a minor?

Yes.

### Must an informed consent form be signed if the patient is unconscious or if an emergency situation makes him incapable of signing?

No. In such cases, operations may proceed without consent. However, under such circumstances, a member of the family who accompanies the patient may sign for him, or a member of the family may be reached by telephone.

### Should a patient be asked to sign a consent form after he has already received sedative or narcotic medications?

No, unless it is an emergency procedure.

## PREOPERATIVE MEASURES

### Can the patient, by proper preoperative preparation, improve his chances for a smooth operative and postoperative course?

Yes. There are many things a patient can do to make the surgeon's task easier and his own discomfort less.

### What can the patient do to help himself before entering the hospital?

a. Smoking. It is much better for the patient to smoke as little as possible for a few days before he is to be operated upon. This will lead to a smoother anesthesia, with less chance for postoperative complications such as coughing, inflammation of the trachea, lung congestion, etc.

b. Alcohol. It is wise not to drink heavily for a few days before contemplated surgery. Excessive drinking may have harmful effects upon the liver, and it is important that liver function not be impaired when major surgery is being performed.

c. Sleep. Patients should have at least eight hours' sleep for a few nights before major surgery. A rested body will respond better to the trauma of surgery.

d. If there are loose teeth, they should be pulled prior to hospital admission, and if the planned operation is an elective one, infected gums should be treated, and decayed teeth should be taken care of.

### What are some of the routine procedures that will be carried out in the hospital?

a. Bowel function. As the bowels may not move for several days after an operation, an enema is given the night before most surgical procedures. This is not carried out where there is an acute inflammation within the intestinal tract or abdomen.

b. Food intake. It is always best to operate upon a patient whose stomach is empty. Fasting for ten to twelve hours before surgery is a routine procedure.

c. Sedatives. To insure a good night's rest before surgery, adequate doses of sleeping pills are usually prescribed.

d. Narcotics. In order to have the patient in a calm, semiconscious state, an injection of Demerol, morphine, or a similar drug is given one or two hours before the patient goes to the operating room.

*(continued)*

e. Preparation of the wound area. It is customary to shave a very wide area around an operative site. This is done to insure surgical sterility. Thus the entire abdomen is shaved for an abdominal operation, and an entire limb may be shaved for surgery upon an arm or leg.

f. Teeth. Before the patient goes to the operating room, all false teeth or dentures are removed so that they are not dislodged during the giving of anesthesia. It is always wise to inform the anesthesiologist if you have a loose tooth in your mouth so that this may be attended to before the operation.

g. Intravenous injections. If a patient is dehydrated or if he is in need of special medications such as vitamins, proteins, sugars, or antibiotic drugs, these may be given prior to surgery.

h. Blood transfusions. Surgeons find that their patients react much better to major operative procedures when there is no anemia. Therefore, people who have lost marked amounts of blood or who are exceptionally anemic may be given blood by transfusion before surgery.

i. Stomach tubes. For certain kinds of abdominal operations, particularly those upon the gastrointestinal tract, it is advisable to have the stomach completely empty. A tube is therefore inserted through the nose into the stomach and attached to a suction apparatus. This may be done the night before surgery or early the morning of surgery. These tubes are often left in place throughout the operative procedure and for a few days thereafter.

j. Catheterization. Patients will be much more comfortable postoperatively if their bladder is empty. In order to insure this, a tube (catheter) is sometimes inserted into the bladder before the patient goes to the operating room; the tube may be left in place during the operative procedure and for some time thereafter.

k. Wearing apparel. No matter how minor the operative procedure and no matter how limited the area to be subjected to surgery, it is general practice to remove all clothing before a patient goes to the operating room. He will then be dressed in a cap and a short gown and will have something to cover his legs. This is done because the patient's clothes are not surgically clean and therefore should not be worn in an operating room.

## POSTOPERATIVE MEASURES

### What are the usual measures carried out immediately after an operation?

a. Recovery rooms. All hospitals have recovery rooms staffed by personnel specifically trained in the care of the postoperative patient. In such rooms are all the various types of apparatus necessary to combat any possible postoperative complication. It is customary for patients not to return directly to the preoperative room, but to remain in the recovery room anywhere from a few hours to as long as a full twenty-four hours.

b. ICU. Extremely sick postoperative patients are usually sent to the Intensive Care Unit. (See Chapter 36, on ICU.)

c. Position in bed. Patients are usually placed flat in bed on returning from the operating room. It is customary for children to be placed lying face down on their abdomen and for adults to lie flat on their back. If the patient's blood pressure has dropped as a result of the surgery, it is sometimes customary to raise the foot of the bed above the level of the patient's head. This allows more blood to flow to the head and helps to raise blood pressure. In operations upon the neck or chest, the patient is often placed in a semisitting position immediately after operation.

After full reaction and recovery from the anesthesia, the patient is urged to change his position frequently and to move his limbs about in bed. This stimulates circulation, thus reducing any tendency toward the development of blood clots in the veins of the extremities.

d. Airways. The patient may have a tube extending into his trachea from the anesthesia, which is left in place until he regains consciousness, or the anesthesiologist will often place an airway into the patient's mouth that extends into the back of the throat. The airway will prevent the patient from swallowing his tongue or developing an obstruction to the free passage of air from the outside into his lungs. It will stay in place until he regains consciousness and, depending upon respiratory function, may sometimes stay there for additional hours or days.

e. Ambulation. Modern surgery advocates that the patient get out of bed as soon as he possibly can after surgery. This practice, called early ambulation, has been found to minimize lung complications and circulatory disturbances. Many patients can get out of bed the same day as major surgery; others can be gotten up and walking within one to two days after surgery. There are, however, a small number of patients who must remain in bed for a week or longer after an operation.

f. Stomach tubes. Distention of the stomach after an operation is a common occurrence, which can cause great distress and discomfort. To avoid this, a tube is passed through the nose into the stomach and allowed to remain there for a day or two. To make sure the stomach remains deflated, this tube is sometimes attached to a suction apparatus.

g. Food and fluid intake. Most patients are extremely thirsty after operation, particularly when fluids have been withheld preoperatively. Small amounts of water or tea may be taken within a few hours after surgery if patients have not been operated upon for a condition within the stomach or intestinal tract. (Such patients are usually forbidden to drink or eat for two to three days and are fed by intravenous fluids.) When the latter situation is not applicable, patients may have small amounts of a soft bland diet the day following surgery and may return to a regular diet within three or four days.

h. Catheterization. Difficulty in urinating for a day or two after surgery is a common occurrence. This is particularly true when spinal anesthesia has been used or after an operation involving the lower abdomen, the female organs, or the rectum. In order to avoid the uncomfortable feeling of a distended bladder that cannot be emptied, it is routine procedure to pass a tube into the bladder at regular intervals. In certain cases, the catheter may be left in place for a few days. The ability to urinate always returns, but repeated catheterization may be necessary for several days.

i. Narcotics. Since all people have varying degrees of pain following surgery, it is customary for narcotics to be prescribed. Pain-relieving narcotics or sedatives are given, if necessary, every few hours for the first day or two after surgery. The patient should be cautioned not to seek these medications unnecessarily, as they may retard the rate of recovery. However, there should be no fear of drug addiction, because this does not occur within the short space of time it takes a patient to convalesce.

j. Antibiotics. Whenever there is a chance that infection may retard operative recovery, the surgeon will order antibiotic drugs to be given either by injection or by mouth. It is very important for the patient to inform his surgeon if he is sensitive or allergic to any of the antibiotic drugs. Fortunately, the large number of antibiotic drugs available makes it possible to find one to which the patient is not sensitive or allergic.

k. Blood transfusions. Every major operation is associated with a certain amount of blood loss. If this amount is sizable, the surgeon will order a transfusion to replace the loss. It should not be concluded merely because blood is being given that the patient's condition is precarious.

l. Enemas. Bowels often do not function satisfactorily for the first four, five, or six days after abdominal surgery. Failure to have a bowel movement should be no cause for alarm. Enemas are often prescribed on the third, fourth, or fifth day to remedy this situation.

m. Wound dressings. Dressings of operative wounds vary according to the type of procedure that has been performed. Wounds with drains may be dressed every day or every other day after surgery. Clean, tightly closed wounds may not be dressed until the sixth, seventh, or eighth day, when the sutures or clips are to be removed. Most dressings are not painful, but if pain is to be associated with the dressing, the surgeon will often prescribe a sedative or narcotic.

n. Suture or clip removal. As mentioned above, sutures or clips may be removed on the sixth, seventh, or eighth day after surgery. There is very little pain and discomfort associated with the removal of clips or sutures.

o. Blood tests. Following major surgery, it is essential that the patient's blood chemistries be carefully monitored. Chemical imbalance interferes greatly with recovery from surgery. Thus blood will be drawn frequently and sent to the laboratory for various analyses.

p. Hospital discharge. Within recent years it has been found that recovery from surgery is accelerated by early discharge from the hospital. It is up to the surgeon, not the patient, to determine when discharge shall take place.

# CHAPTER 59

# THE PROSTATE GLAND

*(See also Chapter 37 on Kidneys and Ureters; Chapter 42 on Male Organs; Chapter 76 on Urinary Bladder and Urethra)*

## Where is the prostate gland, and what is its function?

The prostate is a part of the male genital apparatus, located near, and surrounding, the outlet of the urinary bladder. It is the size of a horse chestnut, and its main function is to secrete a liquid that comprises the bulk of the seminal fluid.

## What are the principal diseases affecting the prostate gland?

a. Infections (prostatitis).
b. Enlargement of the gland associated with the aging process (benign hypertrophy).
c. Cancer.

## How is the prostate examined?

a. Because of its proximity to the rectum, the examining physician can obtain much information about the gland by inserting his finger into the patient's rectum.
b. Additional information can be obtained by examination through a cystoscope.

## What is the usual route by which infection reaches the prostate gland?

a. By direct extension from the outside, up the urethra.
b. Less often, by bacteria being brought to the gland through the bloodstream.

## What bacteria are most likely to infect the prostate?

The gonorrhea germ; also other bacteria, such as staphylococcus, streptococcus, or colon bacillus.

## What are the symptoms of infection in the prostate?

Fever, pain in the lower part of the back, frequency of urination, pain upon voiding, infected and bloody urine.

## What is the treatment for prostatic infections?

a. Bed rest.
b. Administration of the appropriate antibiotic drug.
c. Liberal intake of fluids.
d. Avoidance of alcoholic beverages and spicy foods.
e. Administration of sedatives to relieve tension and pain.
f. Avoidance of sexual intercourse.
g. In chronic cases, repeated gentle massage of the gland.
h. Hot sitz baths.

## Is surgery often necessary in the treatment of prostate infections?

Usually not, except when an abscess has formed.

## What is chronic prostatitis?

A low-grade, persistent inflammation that manifests itself by low back pain, urinary disturbance, sexual disturbance, and sometimes a morning discharge from the penis.

## What is the treatment for chronic infections of the prostate?

a. The use of antibiotics.
b. Periodic gentle massage of the prostate by insertion of the finger into the rectum.
c. Hot baths.

## Are most infections of the prostate curable?

Yes, although there is a tendency for the more stubborn and chronic infections to recur from time to time.

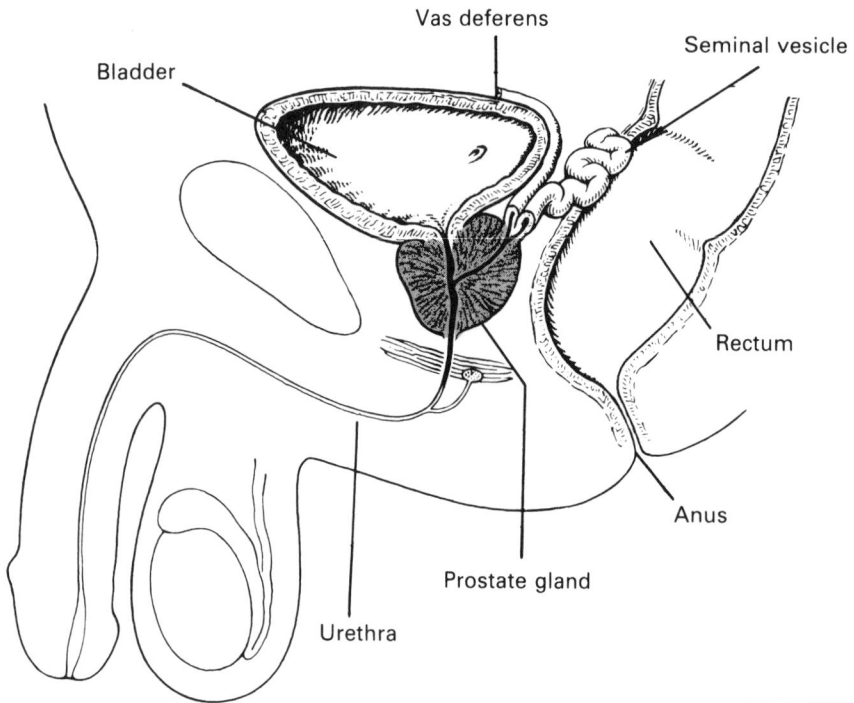

**The Prostate Gland.** *This diagram shows the location of the gland as it surrounds the outlet of the urinary bladder. The prostate gland, for some unknown reason, tends to enlarge as a man ages. The function of the prostate is to secrete the fluid in which the sperm are carried.*

# BENIGN ENLARGEMENT OF THE PROSTATE
## (Prostatism)

### What is benign enlargement of the prostate?

A condition in which portions of the gland slowly enlarge over a period of years. Malignancy does not occur in this type of enlargement.

### Is it natural for all men to have enlargement of the prostate when they grow older?

Yes. Beginning at forty to forty-five years of age, almost all men have a slowly enlarging prostate.

### Will all men develop symptoms from prostatic enlargement?

No. Most men go through life without having difficulty. It must be remembered that enlargement of the prostate accompanies normal aging processes.

### How can one tell if the enlargement of his prostate requires medical attention?

There will be interference with normal urination.

### Why does enlargement of the prostate interfere with urination?

An enlarging prostate compresses the outlet of the bladder.

### What may be the eventual outcome of prostatic enlargement?

It may cause a sudden inability to urinate. This condition is known as acute urinary retention.

### Is there any relationship between the amount of sexual activity and enlargement of the prostate?

No.

### Do all men with enlargement of the prostate have to undergo surgery?

No. Only one in four men has any symptoms at all. Of those who do have symptoms, only one in four requires surgery.

### Is there any satisfactory medical treatment for enlargement of the prostate?

Treatment with hormones, advocated by some physicians, does not help this condition! Massage of the gland may help at times to relieve symptoms partially, but will not actually reduce the size of the gland. If there is an infection associated with the enlargement, its control may relieve symptoms.

### What are the most common symptoms of enlargement of the prostate?

a. Frequency of urination during the day.
b. The need to void several times during the night (nocturia).
c. Hesitancy in starting the flow of urine.
d. Diminution in the size and force of the urinary stream.
e. Dribbling before and after urination.
f. Burning on urination.
g. Eventual inability to void (acute urinary retention).
h. Bleeding on urination.

### What is the effect of enlargement of the prostate upon the bladder and kidneys?

Since the main function of the bladder is to expel urine, it is obvious that an obstruction such as enlargement of the prostate will force the bladder to work harder to discharge the urine. As a result, the wall of the bladder becomes thickened, more muscular, and heavier. Eventually, the bladder fails to empty itself completely with each voiding. This residual urine increases in amount and ultimately creates abnormal back pressure up the ureters toward the kidneys. Along with the dilatation of the ureters there is some impairment of kidney function, and the general health of the patient suffers. Permitted to progress untreated, such a condition may lead to complete kidney failure, with resultant uremia and death.

### What harm does incomplete emptying of the bladder do to the patient?

It results in stagnation of the urine, with consequent infection. The infection usually spreads up the ureter to the kidney as well. Ultimately, from stagnation of the urine over a period of years, stones may form in the bladder. The increased work and pressure on the bladder wall may cause local "blowouts," known as diverticula. These are saclike protrusions from the wall of the bladder; they may contain stagnant urine, or stones may develop within them. Incomplete emptying of the bladder may cause day and night frequency of urination.

### What operations are carried out for enlargement of the prostate?

a. Suprapubic prostatectomy. This is an operation in which an incision is made in the midline of the lower abdomen, and the bladder is opened. The prostate gland is removed through the open bladder in either one or two stages. A rubber tube is then placed in the bladder for a period of days. When the tube is removed, the normal urinary stream flows through the urethra as it did preoperatively.
b. Retropubic prostatectomy. This is a surgical procedure in which the incision is made in the lower abdomen directly over the prostate, and the prostate is removed without opening the urinary bladder.
c. Perineal prostatectomy. This is an operation in which an incision is made in the perineum (the space below the testicles and in front of the rectum). The prostate is removed through this incision.
d. Transurethral resection of the

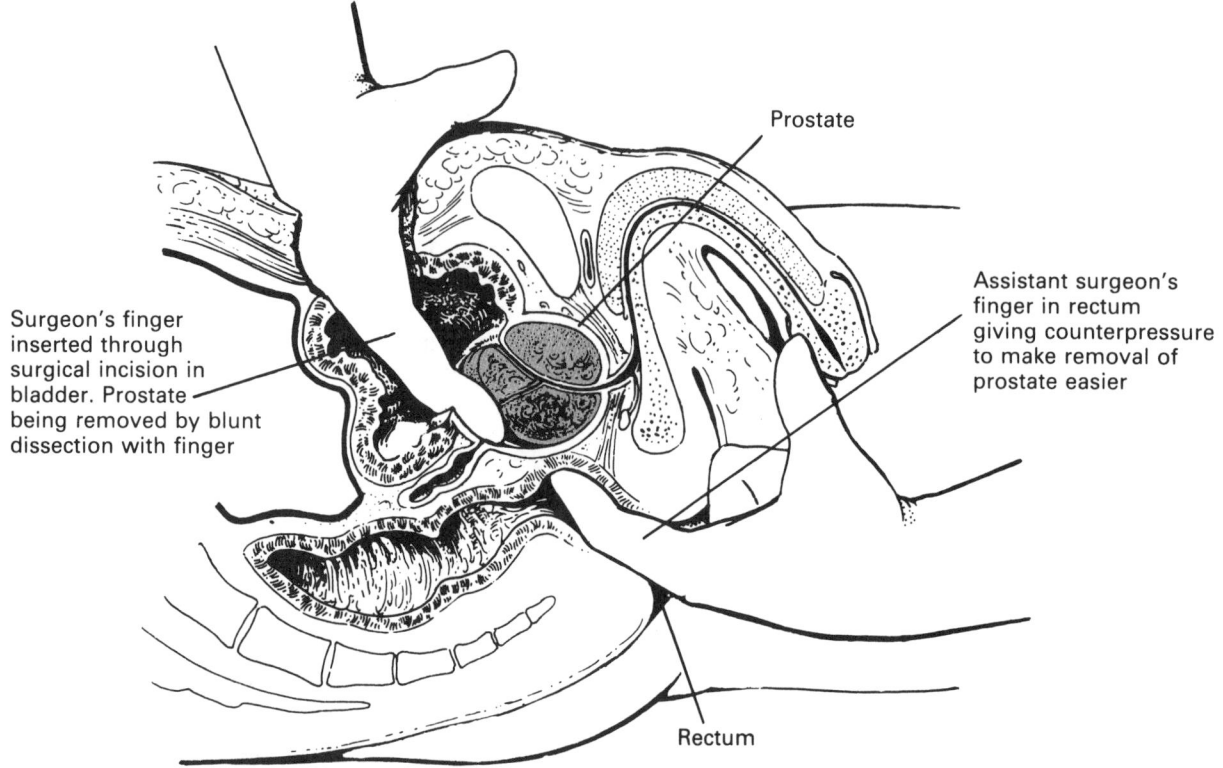

**Prostate**

**Assistant surgeon's finger in rectum giving counterpressure to make removal of prostate easier**

**Surgeon's finger inserted through surgical incision in bladder. Prostate being removed by blunt dissection with finger**

**Rectum**

*Removal of the Prostate Gland through the Open Bladder. This demonstrates how the enlarged portion of the gland that surrounds the bladder neck is removed.*

prostate. This is a procedure in which part of the obstructing portion of the prostate is burned away with a cutting loop that is passed through a cystoscope. No external incision is made for this procedure.

### What will determine which procedure is chosen?

a. The size of the prostate gland.
b. The presence or absence of stones or infection in the bladder.
c. The presence or absence of bladder diverticula.
d. The status of kidney function.
e. The general health of the patient.

### Is any one procedure preferable for removal of the prostate?

No. Each procedure has its definite indications, depending upon the particular findings in any given case.

### What is meant by a "two-stage" prostate operation?

In some instances—because of poor general health or impaired kidney function, infection, stones, or associated diseases such as heart trouble or high blood pressure—it is too risky to remove the gland directly. In these cases, a period of preliminary urinary drainage is required; when this is carried out, it is called a first-stage (cystotomy) prostate operation. In this operation, the bladder is opened surgically and is allowed to drain onto the abdominal wall. After a suitable interval of time, when kidney function has returned to normal, infection has subsided, and any bladder stones that are present have been removed, the prostate is then excised by the surgeon, who inserts his finger into the bladder and shells out the gland.

This procedure is the second stage of the operation.

### Is the entire prostate gland removed when performing a prostatectomy?

In actuality, no. A rim of normal gland tissue is usually left behind.

### Are operations upon the prostate serious?

Yes, but with our present-day knowledge and with the use of better surgical techniques and the aid of antibiotics, the vast majority of patients undergoing prostatic surgery can look toward a safe and satisfactory recovery.

### What is a cystostomy?

It is the first stage of a two-stage prostate operation in which a rubber tube is placed into the bladder through an abdominal incision.

**Is it ever necessary to operate upon the prostate gland as an emergency procedure?**

Yes, if acute obstruction to the passage of urine develops secondary to an enlarged prostate.

**How long is the period between the two stages of this operation?**

This may vary from a week to an indefinite period of time, depending upon the improvement in the general condition of the patient.

**Does the prostate ever enlarge again and cause urinary obstruction after it has once been removed?**

Not if a thorough removal has been carried out. Occasionally, after a transurethral resection through a cystoscope, prostatic tissue may grow and cause some obstruction.

## CANCER OF THE PROSTATE

**How common is cancer of the prostate?**

It is generally agreed that somewhere between 10 and 20 percent of all men past fifty years of age will develop cancer of the prostate, and it becomes increasingly more common with age, so that among those who live into the nineties, almost all will have prostate tissue that may be termed malignant. The activity is low, and these men usually succumb to some other more active disease.

**At what age is cancer of the prostate most apt to occur?**

In the sixties, seventies, and eighties.

**What are the symptoms of cancer of the prostate?**

Unfortunately, early cancer of the prostate produces few, if any, symptoms. It is only when the disease has become advanced that it makes itself known. The only way to detect early cancer of the prostate is to examine the gland at regular intervals. For this reason, it is important that men over fifty years of age have a yearly examination of the prostate gland.

**How is a positive diagnosis of cancer of the prostate made?**

a. Cancer of the prostate feels much firmer and more irregular on rectal examination than benign enlargement.

b. It is distinguished from benign enlargement by taking a biopsy of the gland, usually by way of a biopsy needle inserted through the rectum, and submitting it to microscopic examination.

**Do all cases of cancer of the prostate cause symptoms?**

No. It has been found that in many individuals, the tumor may lie dormant for an indefinite period, never causing symptoms or spreading to other parts of the body.

**Is there any medical treatment for cancer of the prostate?**

Yes. Some relief may be obtained by giving large doses of female sex hormones. In some cases, the growth of the tumor is retarded by the suppression of male hormone secretion, which results from the administration of the female sex hormone.

**Does simple benign enlargement of the prostate ever become cancerous?**

Such a transition is extremely rare. Most cancers start as cancers.

**For how long can the female sex hormones be effective in retarding the progress of cancer of the prostate?**

Although this form of treatment is not curative, it may suppress a cancerous growth and prolong life for many years.

**Is x-ray therapy helpful in treatment of cancer of the prostate?**

Yes. An x-ray machine known as the *linear accelerator* has proved to be very effective in the control of this disease.

**Are there any radioactive substances that are helpful in the treatment of cancer of the prostate?**

Yes. The injection of radioactive iodine directly into the gland appears to give promising results. This method of treatment is still in its early stages of development.

**What is the surgical treatment for cancer of the prostate?**

a. In early cases, the treatment is removal of the entire gland (radical prostatectomy).

b. In more advanced cases, removal of the testicles is also performed.

c. Surgical removal of the adrenal glands or the pituitary gland has been reported as retarding the rate of growth and extension of far advanced cancers of the prostate. These, however, are drastic procedures used only as a last resort.

**Will operations for removal of the prostate cause impotence?**

Ordinary prostatectomy does not cause impotence. However, a radical operation for removal of the prostate gland usually does cause impotence. Since many of the patients are in the twilight years of their active sex life, this is often not a matter of major concern.

**Will operations upon the prostate gland result in inability to control urination (incontinence)?**

Temporary loss of control can follow surgery upon the prostate. However, this will clear up within several weeks to several months in the great majority of cases.

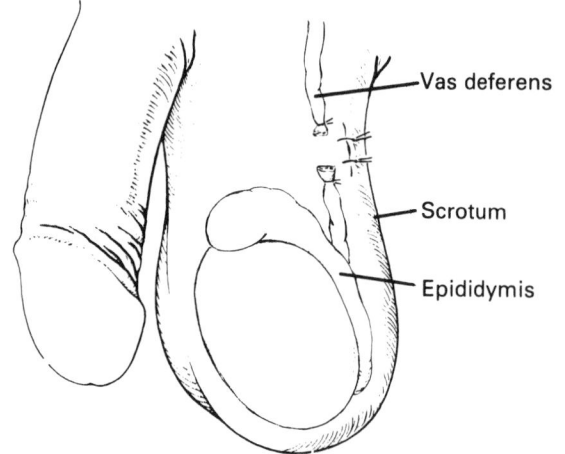

*Vasectomy.* This drawing shows a vas deferens that has been cut and the ends tied off. The small incision in the scrotum is closed with two stitches. The operation, done to prevent inflammation of the epididymis in prostate surgery, also creates sterility, as sperm from the testicle can no longer be carried through the vas to the seminal vesicles.

**Does loss of urinary control occur after ordinary prostatectomy for benign enlargement?**

Very rarely, and then for a few weeks only.

**How long a hospital stay is necessary for prostate operations?**

For one-stage prostate operations, twelve to fourteen days. For two-stage operations, three to four weeks.

**Are special nurses advisable after operations upon the prostate?**

Yes, for a period of three to four days.

**Are blood transfusions employed in operations upon the prostate?**

Yes, although hemorrhage following these operations is much less likely to occur today than in former years.

**How long a period of convales-** **cence is necessary after an operation upon the prostate?**

Four to five weeks.

**Does enlargement of the prostate ever recur after removal?**

Once in a very great while, regrowth of gland tissue may take place. This is treated by reoperation, with removal of more of the gland.

**Do stones ever form in the prostate gland?**

Yes, this is not an uncommon finding, particularly in glands that have been infected over a period of years.

**What is the treatment for stones in the prostate?**

They are operated upon only when accompanied by symptoms such as those caused by enlargement of the prostate.

**What type of anesthesia is used for a prostate operation?**

This will depend upon the general condition of the patient. Continous epidural anesthesia (see Chapter 8, on Anesthesia) is the anesthesia of choice, although spinal or general anesthesia may be used.

**How does urine leave the body after a prostate operation?**

If a suprapubic prostatectomy has been performed, a tube is placed from the bladder to an incision in the abdominal wall. When a retropubic prostatectomy is done, or when a transurethral resection is done, a rubber catheter is placed in the urethra temporarily to drain the urine.

**What is the usual interval of time before the resumption of normal voiding?**

Following suprapubic prostatectomy, approximately nine days; after retropubic prostatectomy, approximately one week; after transurethral resection, approximately five to seven days.

**Is it common practice to tie off the vas deferens (vasectomy), leading from the testicle when performing a prostatectomy?**

Yes, this is done as a preliminary measure to prevent inflammation of the epididymis, a structure adjacent to the testicle. However, those who undergo transurethral prostatectomy often do not require the procedure.

CHAPTER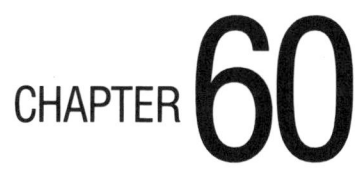

# THE RECTUM AND ANUS

*(See also Chapter 66 on Small and Large Intestines)*

### What is the anus?

The last inch or one and a half inches of the intestinal tract.

### What is the rectum?

That portion of the bowel extending up from the anus for a distance of six to eight inches.

### Is rectal or anal disease common?

Nearly a third of all adults at one time or another suffer from some local disease of the anus or rectum, such as hemorrhoids, fissures, or fistulas.

### Is it necessary for the maintenance of good health to have a bowel movement every day?

No. Bowel habits vary widely among normal people.

### Is it normal to have one or two movements daily?

Yes, for some people.

### Can a person lead a normal life if he moves his bowels only every other day or every third day?

Yes, providing he has a regular pattern of bowel function.

### Does the type of food that one eats affect bowel function?

Yes.

### What foods are best avoided when one has acute rectal or anal disease?

a. Highly seasoned spicy foods.
b. Alcoholic beverages.

### What determines regularity of bowel movement?

a. The formation of good habits in early childhood.
b. The eating of a well-rounded diet containing plenty of fresh fruits and fresh vegetables.
c. A good general state of health.

### Will good bowel habits in childhood usually lead to good habits when one is older?

Definitely, yes.

### Is it harmful to take a lubricant such as mineral oil over a prolonged period of time?

No, if it is really necessary for normal function. However, it should not be taken at the same time of day as vitamin-rich foods, as it may interfere with vitamin absorption.

### Should a person take a laxative when he has abdominal pain?

Never! This practice can be dangerous—particularly if the cause of the pain is appendicitis or some other inflammatory process in the intestinal tract.

### Is a change in one's bowel habits significant of disease?

Yes. Very often it means that there is trouble. Recurrent diarrhea or constipation should lead one to have a thorough medical survey of his intestinal tract.

### What abnormalities in bowel function should cause one to seek medical advice?

a. Episodes of diarrhea.
b. Episodes of constipation.
c. Change in the appearance or caliber of the stools.
d. Blood in the stool.
e. Black-colored stool.
f. Mucus in the stool.

### Are there any laxatives that are better than others?

The milder the laxative, the better.

Lubricants or stewed fruits are preferred for the relief of constipation.

### When is it permissible to take laxatives?

Occasionally, when there is a period of constipation in a patient who ordinarily has normal bowel function.

### When is it permissible to take lubricants?

When there is a tendency toward chronic constipation in an older person.

### When should enemas be taken for constipation?

Only when the patient is otherwise in good health and has no other symptoms referable to the intestinal tract.

### Is there any adequate treatment for chronic constipation?

Yes. Eat plenty of fresh fruit and vegetables and develop regular habits. Also, the taking of lubricants or bulk-forming medications may prove helpful.

### Is there a tendency for constipation to become more prevalent as one grows older?

Yes. The abdominal muscles (important in aiding bowel evacuation) tend to weaken.

### How does one treat constipation in children?

a. Train the child toward regular bowel habits.
b. Give the child a well-rounded full diet.
c. If necessary, give the child lubricants to aid him until he develops regularity.

### What is the best treatment for constipation in adults or older people?

a. Make sure there is no underlying disease of the large bowel, rectum, or anus.
b. Improve dietary habits.
c. Establish regular bowel habits.

*(continued)*

d. Use bulk-forming medications or, if necessary, lubricants.

## Of what significance is blood in the stool?

It may be caused by:

a. Excess straining at stool when constipated.
b. Hemorrhoids or some other anal condition.
c. An acute colitis associated with diarrhea.
d. A chronic colitis.
e. A benign tumor, such as a polyp.
f. A malignant tumor of the rectum or bowel.

## What is the significance of a black stool?

It is caused by bleeding high in the intestinal tract, as from an ulcer. Certain iron medications when taken orally, can also cause black stools.

## What is the significance of mucus in the stool?

Mucus does not necessarily signify a disease process, as many people, especially women in middle life, have mucus in the stool when no real disease exists. However, it should be checked by a physician.

## Is it harmful for one to strain at the stool for prolonged periods of time?

Yes. This can lead to hemorrhoid (pile) formation.

## Are colonic irrigations helpful in curing disease?

No. Years ago certain colon conditions were treated by this method, but now it has been proved that they are of little, if any, benefit.

## Is it true that people who do not have a regular bowel movement are likely to become sluggish, have headaches, and feel weak?

They may develop such symptoms because of the psychological effect upon them. However, there is no sound physical reason why constipation for a day or two should cause these reactions.

## HEMORRHOIDS (Piles)

### What are hemorrhoids?

They are varicose dilatations of the veins, which drain the rectum and anus.

### What causes hemorrhoids?

It is felt that these veins break down and their valves become incompetent because of the strain placed upon them by irregular living habits. Chronic constipation, irregularity of bowel evacuation, and prolonged sojourns on the toilet are thought to be conducive toward hemorrhoid formation. Pregnancy, because of the pressure of the baby's head in the pelvis, also leads toward hemorrhoid formation.

### How common are hemorrhoids?

This is the most common condition in the anal region and affects almost 25 percent of the population at one time or another.

### How can one tell if he has hemorrhoids?

There are one or more swellings or bulges about the anus that become more pronounced on bowel evacuation. There is also a sense of fullness in the anal region, more pronounced on bowel evacuation. Hemorrhoids are frequently painful and may be accompanied by considerable rectal bleeding.

### Is there any way to prevent getting hemorrhoids?

Yes, to a certain extent. Regular bowel evacuation, the eating of a good diet with sufficient roughage, and the avoidance of straining at stool will diminish the chances of getting hemorrhoids.

## How can a positive diagnosis of hemorrhoids be made?

Your physician will be able to tell by a rectal examination whether hemorrhoids are present.

## What are the various forms of treatment for hemorrhoids?

a. Medical treatment, which includes the taking of lubricants to ensure a regular stool and the use of medicated suppositories inserted into the rectum.
b. The injection treatment if the hemorrhoids are of the internal type.
c. Surgical removal of the hemorrhoids.
d. Banding hemorrhoids by placing rubber bands around them. This procedure can be effective for internal hemorrhoids only.

## Do all types of hemorrhoids respond to the injection treatment?

No. Only the internal type can sometimes be successfully treated by this method.

## What can happen if hemorrhoids are not treated?

a. They may bleed severely and cause a marked anemia with all of its serious consequences.
b. The hemorrhoids may become thrombosed (clotted), producing extreme pain in the region.
c. The hemorrhoids may prolapse (drop out of the rectum and not go back in again).
d. Hemorrhoids may become strangulated and gangrenous.
e. Hemorrhoids may become ulcerated and infected.

## Does neglect of hemorrhoids ever lead to the formation of cancer of the rectum?

No, but the abrupt development of hemorrhoids is occasionally secondary to the development of a tumor in the large bowel.

**What determines whether or not surgery is recommended for hemorrhoids?**

Many hemorrhoids cause no symptoms whatever and require no treatment. Those that cause symptoms and do not respond to adequate medical management must be operated upon.

**Will the surgeon perform other tests before performing hemorrhoidectomy?**

Yes. The surgeon will perform a sigmoidoscopy to make sure there is no disease high up in the rectum above the hemorrhoids. He may also recommend a barium enema x-ray examination of the large bowel.

**Can sigmoidoscopy reveal the presence of a cancer in the rectum or lower bowel?**

Yes. That is the main value of performing this examination.

**How and where is the sigmoidoscopy performed?**

It is done in the surgeon's office by the passage of a sigmoidoscope into the rectal canal. A sigmoidoscope is an instrument about ten inches long that allows direct visualization of the entire rectum and the lower portion of the large bowel (the sigmoid).

**Is sigmoidoscopy a painful examination?**

No. Only slight discomfort accompanies sigmoidoscopy.

**Is there any other test recommended when a patient has hemorrhoids and the physician thinks disease in the large bowel may also be present?**

Yes. A colonoscopic examination is advised. This entails the passage of a long, flexible instrument through the rectum and into the large bowel. Through the colonoscope, disease of the large bowel may be visualized as far as several feet from the anus. (See Chapter 22, on Endoscopy.)

**Are hemorrhoids sometimes an indication that other disease exists in the lower intestinal tract?**

Yes. That is the reason sigmoidoscopy, colonoscopy, and x rays are advocated before the decision is made to remove the hemorrhoids.

**Is hospitalization necessary when hemorrhoids are to be removed?**

Yes. The hospital stay will last anywhere from four to five days.

**Is hemorrhoidectomy a serious operation?**

No. The risks are negligible.

**What are the chances for full cure following the removal of hemorrhoids?**

Well over 95 percent.

**Is there a tendency for hemorrhoids to recur?**

Yes, but the number of such instances is small.

**Is hemorrhoidectomy followed by much pain?**

Yes, for the first week or two after the operation.

**What is done when the hemorrhoids are removed?**

The varicosed veins are dissected out from the surrounding tissues and are ligated and cut away.

**What anesthesia is used?**

Caudal anesthesia, a low spinal anesthesia, or general anesthesia is usually given. Occasionally, local anesthesia is employed.

**How long does it take to perform a hemorrhoid operation?**

Approximately fifteen to twenty minutes.

**Are any special preoperative measures necessary before hemorrhoidectomy?**

No, except to see that the bowel is empty before operation.

**What special diet is necessary after hemorrhoidectomy?**

The avoidance of highly seasoned foods and alcoholic beverages.

**How soon after a hemorrhoid operation will bowel function return to normal?**

It may take several weeks before bowel function returns completely to normal.

**What special postoperative measures are usually advised?**

A lubricant, such as mineral oil, is taken twice a day, and the patient is told to sit in a tub of warm water two or three times a day. Frequent postoperative visits to the surgeon will be necessary.

**Is it common to have bleeding at the stool following a hemorrhoid operation?**

Yes. This may continue for a few days to a few weeks after operation.

**How soon after a hemorrhoid operation can one do the following:**

Bathe:
  Three to four days.
Walk out on the street:
  Four to five days.
Walk up and down stairs:
  One to two days.
Perform household duties:
  Seven days.
Drive a car:
  Two weeks.
Resume sexual relations:
  Three to four weeks.
Return to work:
  Two to three weeks.
Resume all physical activities:
  Four to six weeks.

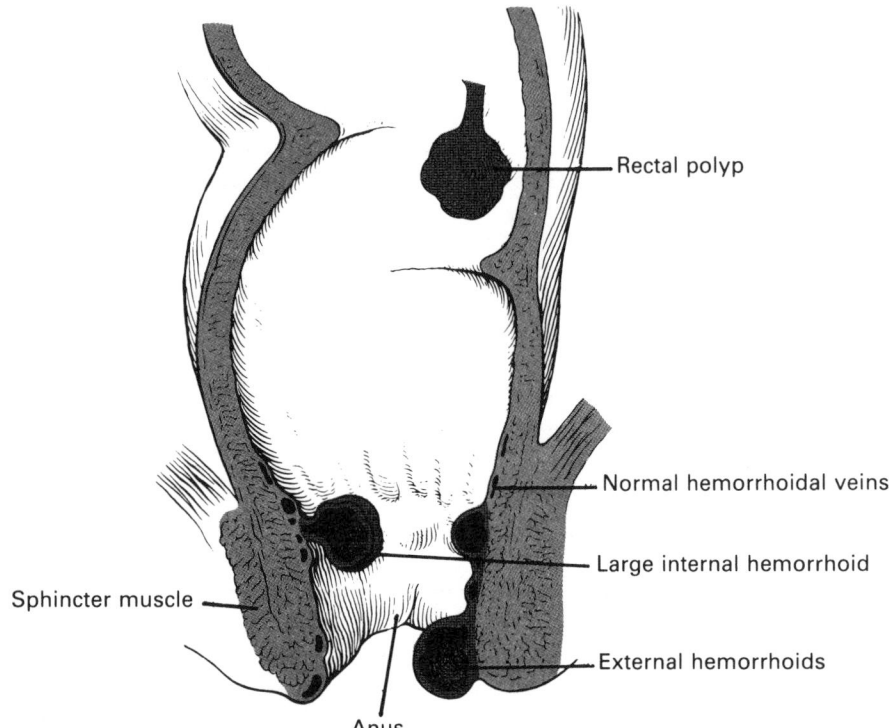

Rectal polyp

Normal hemorrhoidal veins

Large internal hemorrhoid

Sphincter muscle

External hemorrhoids

Anus

*Rectal Polyps and Hemorrhoids. Rectal polyps are benign tumors found within the rectum. They are thought to be the forerunners of cancer, and for this reason they should be removed surgically. Hemorrhoids are varicose veins within the rectum. When they bleed and cause pain, they should be removed surgically.*

**Should one return for regular checkups after a hemorrhoid operation?**

Yes, about every six months.

## POLYPS OF THE RECTUM AND ANUS

### What are polyps?

Polyps are wartlike growths of the anal or rectal mucous membrane, which may vary in size from that of a small pea to that of a golf ball or even larger.

### Where are polyps found?

Polyps can be found anywhere in the large bowel, from the anal orifice upward.

### What causes polyps?

Polyps are growths, like other tumors. The exact cause is unknown.

### How common are polyps?

They are the most common tumor within the intestinal tract.

### Who is most likely to develop polyps?

Polyps are seen in all age groups, but tend to make their appearance more often during the fourth, fifth, and sixth decades of life.

### Do polyps tend to run in families or to be inherited?

Only the multiple polyps of the large bowel. This is a distinct disease. It is called multiple polyposis, and should be distinguished from the isolated, individual polyp so often found in the rectum or about the anal region.

### How can one tell if he has a polyp?

Polyps near the anal region sometimes extrude on bowel evacuation and can be felt. But the most com-

mon symptom is painless bleeding from the rectum on bowel evacuation in a patient who has no other anal or rectal disease.

### How does the surgeon make the diagnosis of rectal polyps?

Polyps can often be seen by direct visualization through an anoscope or sigmoidoscope.

### What harm can polyps do if untreated?

Some polyps will undergo cancerous changes if not removed. Simple removal of polyps can prevent this from happening!

### What is the treatment for polyps?

Polyps of the anus and rectum should be removed. If small enough, this can be carried out in the surgeon's office. If the polyps are large or high up in the bowel, they must be removed in the hospital.

### What operative procedure is performed?

Through an anoscope or sigmoidoscope, a snare is placed around the polyp and the base of the polyp is burned with an electric needle. Thus, through the rectal canal, the polyp is withdrawn along with the tightened snare. Polyps high in the large bowel can frequently be removed through a colonoscope. (See Chapter 22, on Endoscopy.)

### How can one tell if a polyp is becoming malignant?

The excised polyp is sent to the laboratory and a microscopic examination is carried out.

### How soon will the laboratory report be available?

Within two to four days.

### What is done if the polyp has proved to be malignant?

An abdominal operation is performed for the removal of that segment of involved bowel.

### How long a period of hospitalization is necessary?

For the ordinary polyp, a one-day stay is all that is required.

### Are any special preparations necessary before performing polyp removal?

No; just the ordinary cleansing of the bowel.

### What special postoperative measures are advised after polyp removal?

A lubricant such as mineral oil should be used, and the patient should follow a bland diet.

### Do polyps tend to recur?

Once removed, a polyp rarely recurs unless there are malignant changes within it. However, people who have formed one polyp may develop others.

### Can a polyp be removed through the rectum if it is high up in the colon?

Yes, in some cases. An instrument known as a colonoscope can be inserted far up into the bowel, and a polyp may be removed through it.

### How soon after a procedure of this kind can one return to normal activity?

Usually within two to three days.

### Will bleeding continue for a few days after polyp removal?

This sometimes occurs and should not occasion alarm.

## FISSURE IN ANO

### What is a fissure in ano?

It is an ulceration or split in the mucous membrane of the anus.

### What causes a fissure?

Chronic constipation, with overstretching of the mucous membrane at the anal outlet. The cracked sur-face becomes infected and an ulcer forms. The ulcer tends to remain, as it is kept open by the stretching at bowel evacuation.

### What are the symptoms of fissure in ano?

Pain on moving the bowels, accompanied by a slight amount of bleeding.

### What is the treatment for fissure in ano?

Medical treatment may result in healing in many cases if carried out early. It will consist of taking lubricants such as mineral oil and the placing of medicated suppositories into the rectal canal. Those patients who fail to respond to medical management must be operated upon.

### What kind of operation is performed for fissure in ano?

The fissure is removed with a small elliptical incision, and the underlying sphincter muscle is cut so as to relax the anus for a period of time.

### Are the hospital procedures and the preoperative and postoperative measures the same for fissure in ano as for hemorrhoid operations?

Yes. (See the section on Hemorrhoids in this chapter for the answers to these questions.)

### How long does it take for fissures to heal following surgery?

Three to four weeks.

### Do fissures in ano ever recur?

Yes, but only in rare instances.

### Does the sphincter muscle heal, and will bowel function return to normal after an operation for a fissure?

Yes. Healing takes place within a few weeks, and bowel function will return to normal.

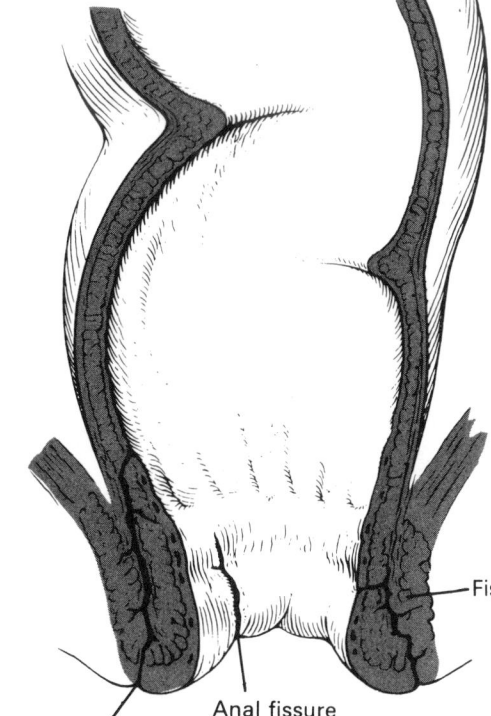

*Fissure in Ano and Fistula in Ano. This diagram shows two very common conditions about the anus and rectum. A fissure is much like a split lip, since it is caused by a crack in the mucous membrane lining the anus. As the anus dilates during a bowel movement, the mucous membrane splits, preventing the fissure from healing. A fistula is a tunnel, or tract, leading from the inside of the anus or rectum to the outside surface of the skin. It tends to become chronically infected, and in order to obtain a cure, it must be removed surgically.*

Fistula

Anal fissure

Fistula on skin surface

## ABSCESSES AND INFECTIONS ABOUT THE ANUS
### (Perirectal and Perianal Abscess)

**Are abscesses in the area about the anus and rectum very common?**

Yes.

**What causes these abscesses?**

It is thought that the infection originates in the lining wall of the anus or rectum and tunnels its way out toward the skin.

**What is the treatment for these abscesses?**

These abscesses should be incised very early in their course and drained widely.

**Do these abscesses always heal completely?**

No. Some of them will open and close for several weeks or months, eventually resulting in fistula formation. (See the section on Fistula in Ano in this chapter.)

**Is hospitalization necessary to open these abscesses?**

Only the large, extensive abscesses that are accompanied by great pain and high temperature must be opened, under anesthesia, in a hospital. The less severe ones can be opened under local anesthesia in a surgeon's office.

## FISTULA IN ANO

**What is a fistula in ano?**

An abnormal communication between the mucous membrane lining of the rectum or anus and the skin surface near the anal opening. A fistula is therefore a tunnel, or tract.

**How common is fistula in ano?**

Fistulas comprise approximately one-fourth of all conditions about the anus or rectum.

**What causes fistulas?**

They represent the end result of an infection that has originated in the rectal or anal wall and that has tunneled its way out to the skin surface.

**Are fistulas ever caused by tuberculosis?**

A very small percentage of fistulas are associated with tuberculosis of the lungs, However, today this is an extremely rare occurrence.

**What are the symptoms of fistula in ano?**

The patient usually gives a history of a painful boil or abscess alongside the rectum that opened and discharged pus at some time previously. The abscess closed and opened alternately over a period of several weeks or months, leaving a small discharge but causing relatively little pain.

**What happens if a fistula in ano is not treated?**

The fistulous tract tends to spread and tunnel about the rectum and may reach the surface at several points alongside the rectum or anus. Also, the sphincter muscle controlling the outlet may be damaged by an untreated fistula.

**What is the treatment for fistula?**

All fistulas that fail to heal over a period of several weeks should be operated upon.

**What kind of operation is performed?**

The fistulous tract is removed or laid open widely. This usually includes cutting the sphincter muscle, as in the operation for a fissure in ano.

**Are the hospital procedures and the preoperative and postoperative measures for fistula in ano similar to those for fissure in ano and hemorrhoids?**

Yes. (See the section on Hemor-rhoids in this chapter for the answers to these questions.)

**What are the chances for cure of a fistula after surgery?**

Excellent. Only rarely will a fistula recur. Occasionally, a large extensive chronic fistula will recur and reoperation will become necessary to effect a permanent cure.

**Does bowel function return to normal after a fistula operation?**

Yes, within a few weeks.

**How long do fistulas take to heal?**

This is a more extensive operation than a fissure operation, and the tissues may take from six to ten weeks to heal fully.

## PRURITUS ANI
### (Itching Anus)

**What is pruritus ani?**

It is a chronic itching of the skin around the anus.

**What causes pruritus ani?**

a. The skin in this area is moist, highly sensitive, and is soiled repeatedly by feces.
b. This skin area is often allergic to irritating soaps, clothing, etc.
c. Associated anal conditions, such as hemorrhoids, fissures, colitis, etc., may cause irritation and set up an itching/scratching pattern.
d. Highly neurotic or disturbed people tend to develop pruritus ani much more frequently than others.

**What are the symptoms of pruritus ani?**

a. Uncontrollable itching, worse during hot weather and at night.
b. Irritation and burning of the skin around the anus.

**What is the treatment for pruritus ani?**

There have been innumerable treatments carried out, but none has proved completely effective in all cases. If an allergy is present, it must be discovered and treated. If any associated anal condition is present, it must be eliminated. The anus must be kept clean and dry. Soaps must be used infrequently and cautiously. There are many salves that can bring considerable relief when used properly, especially ointments containing cortisone and itch-relieving ingredients.

### Can excessive use of soap and water be harmful in pruritus?

Yes. Soap and water may irritate rather than benefit the condition.

### How long can pruritus last?

It tends to be chronic, and many people have it for years.

### Does recovery ever take place spontaneously?

Yes. Often the condition disappears by itself.

### Is psychotherapy ever valuable in the treatment of pruritus ani?

Yes, if the patient is an emotionally disturbed person.

## PROLAPSE OF THE RECTUM

### What is prolapse of the rectum?

It is an extrusion of the mucous membrane lining of the rectum through the anal opening.

### When does prolapse occur most often?

When straining at the stool.

### Who is most likely to have this condition?

Young children and older people.

### What causes prolapse?

Excessive straining at the stool, sometimes associated with diarrhea or constipation, in a person with a weak musculature.

### What is the treatment for prolapse of the rectum?

Some cases require no treatment other than improved bowel habits and the eradication of the associated diarrhea or constipation. Others may require some form of surgical bolstering of the muscle supports of the anal canal and excision of redundant mucous membrane.

### What kind of operation is performed?

For the minor type of prolapse, an operation around the rectum is performed. For the major types, an abdominal operation is carried out, with shortening of the rectum and a reconstruction of the musculature that holds the rectum in place.

### Are operations for prolapse more often necessary for older people than for children?

Yes.

### Are operations for prolapse successful?

Yes, but there are many failures in advanced cases in older patients.

## CANCER OF THE RECTUM AND ANUS

### Is cancer of the rectum or anus a common condition?

Yes. It is one of the most frequently encountered malignant growths in the entire body.

### What causes cancer of the rectum?

The cause is unknown, but it is a medical fact that many cancers in this region originate from the benign polyps described above.

### Is cancer of the rectum preventable?

To a certain extent, insofar as periodic rectal examinations and sigmoidoscopic examinations may uncover a benign condition that might

have resulted in cancerous degeneration if it had not been removed.

### How is the diagnosis of cancer of the rectum made?

a. By examination with the physician's finger, which is inserted into the rectal canal.
b. By taking a piece of the tumor tissue and submitting it to microscopic examination. (This is a simple office procedure.)

### What symptoms are caused by cancer of the rectum?

a. The outstanding symptom is blood in the stool.
b. There may also be a change in bowel habits.

### At what period in life is cancer of the rectum seen most often?

It may come on at any time, but is most usual in middle and later life.

### What is the surgical treatment for cancer of the rectum?

There are three main methods:
a. Removal of the entire rectum and approximately two to three feet of bowel. An artificial opening for the passage of stool (colostomy) is fashioned on the abdominal wall.
b. In some cases, when the cancer is high up in the rectum, it is possible to remove the cancer-bearing portion of the rectum and to reestablish bowel continuity. In such an instance, a colostomy is unnecessary.
c. In localized, superficial rectal cancers it is occasionally advisable merely to burn out the tumor through an instrument inserted through the anus. This operation is advocated more often for older patients and those who might not, because of poor general health, be able to withstand a more extensive surgical procedure.

### What are the above operations called?

a. An abdominoperineal resection.

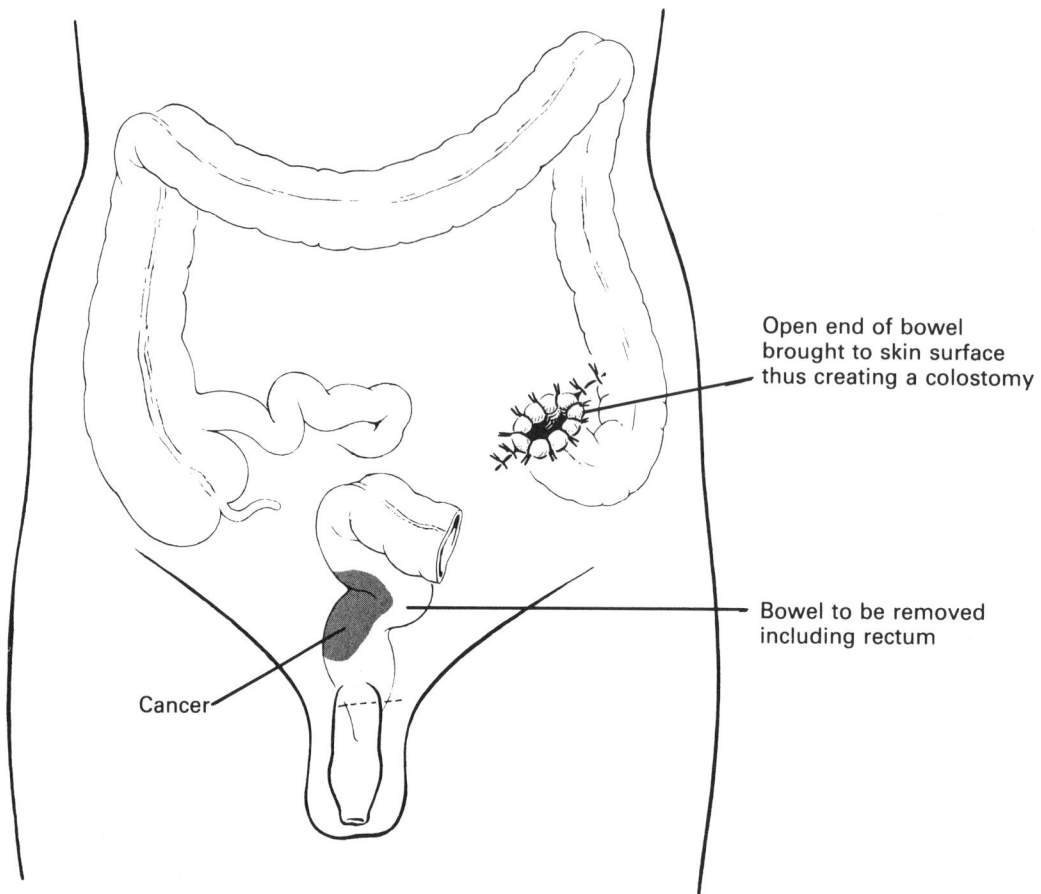

Open end of bowel brought to skin surface thus creating a colostomy

Bowel to be removed including rectum

Cancer

**Removal of the Rectum and Part of the Colon for Cancer.** *This diagram illustrates what is done for the cure of cancer of the rectum. This operation results in a cure in the majority of cases, provided the cancer has been discovered and operated upon before it has spread to other structures.*

b. An anterior resection.
c. Fulguration of the tumor.

### Are the results the same for all three procedures?

Most surgeons seem to think that the best chances for cure result from the abdominoperineal resection or the anterior resection.

### Is surgery for cancer of the rectum dangerous?

Today surgical recovery takes place in well over 95 percent of cases. However it is a major procedure that takes two to three hours to perform and necessitates hospitalization for several weeks.

### Is cancer of the rectum ever curable?

Definitely, yes! More than half the cases can be cured if seen at a stage before the tumor has spread to other parts of the body.

### Can a patient lead a full, normal existence with the rectum removed?

Yes. There are many thousands of people who engage in all activities despite the fact that they have no rectum. They learn to care for their colostomy in such a manner that the bowel is emptied at a set time each day, permitting them full activity. Various bags are applied over the colostomy opening that seal in any feces or odor while the patient is away from home.

# CHAPTER 61

# REPLANTATION SURGERY

*(See also Chapter 14 on Bones, Muscles, Tendons, and Joints)*

### What is meant by replantation?

Reattachment of an amputated part with restoration of its blood flow and the repair of severed structures such as bones, muscles, tendons, and nerves.

### Can replantation surgery save severed parts in the majority of cases?

No, because the special circumstances required for successful replantation are not present in most instances.

### What must be done in cases of amputation if replantation is to be made possible?

a. The amputated part should be wrapped in a clean, moistened handkerchief, towel, or bandage. It should then be put in a sealed plastic bag.
b. The plastic bag is immersed in ice or cold water. This will permit the amputated part to survive longer.
c. The patient should be transported

*immediately* to the emergency room of a nearby hospital. (The larger the hospital, the more apt it will be to have surgeons who are trained in replantation, and the more apt the hospital will be to have essential equipment for this type of surgery.)

### How soon after amputation must replantation be carried out?

Within a few hours at the most. The amputated part will not survive if a longer interval occurs.

### Is replantation of an amputated part ideally carried out by a team of surgeons?

Yes. The most successful results are obtained when orthopedists (bone

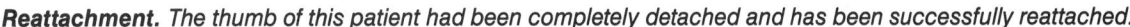

*Reattachment. The thumb of this patient had been completely detached and has been successfully reattached.*

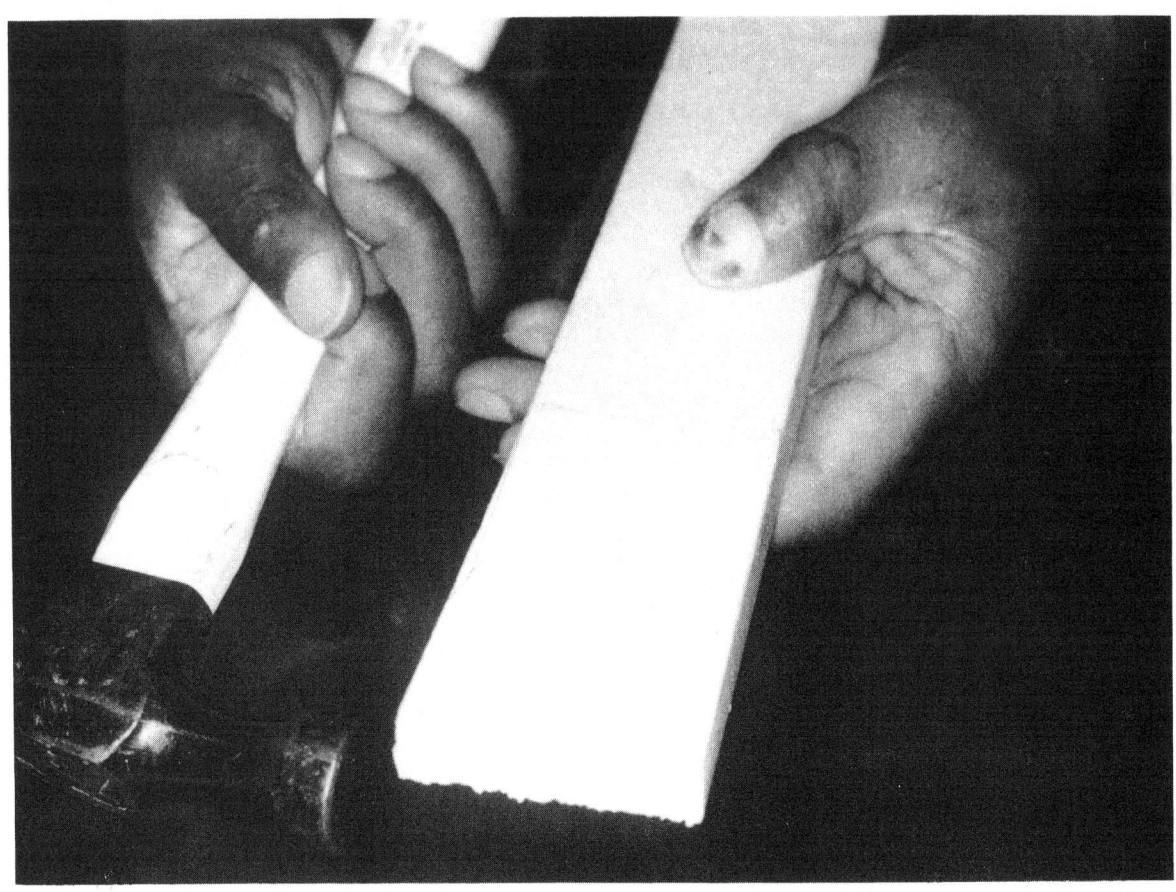

surgeons), vascular surgeons (blood vessel surgeons), neurosurgeons, and plastic surgeons all work together.

### What recent advances have made replantation more successful?

a. The working together of a team of surgeons.
b. The development of microsurgery, permitting extremely small blood vessels and nerves to be reunited (anastomosed) accurately.
c. The judicious use of heparin to keep blood from clotting in the amputated part.
d. Better methods of preservation of the amputated part until reattachment surgery can be performed.
e. The use of antibiotics to prevent infection.

### Under favorable circumstances, what are some of the parts of the body that might be reattached?

a. Fingers.
b. Hands.
c. Arms.
d. Legs.
e. Ears.
f. Noses.
g. Scalps.

### Should every amputated part be replanted?

No. Each injury requires careful evaluation. Some parts are too severely damaged to be replaced. If it appears feasible that some useful function may be restored, then replantation should be considered.

### Is surgery with microscopic techniques used in most cases of replantation?

Yes, because it enlarges the view of small structures, enabling the surgeon to carry out more accurate stitching together of severed parts.

### Is it frequently necessary to cut away crushed and dead tissue before attempting replantation?

Yes. This is essential. Crushed parts will not mend, and function will not be regained.

### Will the cutting away of damaged tissues sometimes lead to a deformed finger, hand, arm, or leg?

Yes, but this is a small price to pay if function can be restored. A shortened finger, hand, or limb is preferable to an absent one.

### How long may it take to perform a replantation procedure?

A finger may take only two to three hours; major replantation of a hand, arm, leg, etc., may take anywhere from eighteen to twenty hours to perform.

### Does replantation surgery frequently require several operations?

Yes. Further operations upon the bones, blood vessels, tendons, and nerves may be necessary over a period of weeks or months.

### What is successful replantation?

Survival of the replaced part is not true success. Success means a return of useful function.

### Does function return immediately after surgery?

No. Many months of postoperative therapy are necessary to regain movement, feeling, and strength in a reattached part.

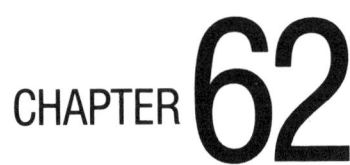

# CHAPTER 62

# RHEUMATIC FEVER

*(See also Chapter 10 on Arthritis; Chapter 14 on Bones, Muscles, Tendons, and Joints; Chapter 29 on Heart; Chapter 45 on Nervous Diseases)*

### What is rheumatic fever?

Rheumatic fever is a specific disease thought to be bacterial in origin and characterized by attacks of fever that last anywhere from several weeks to several months and that tend to recur over a period of many years. In addition, there may be inflammatory heart, joints, skin, lungs, and nerves.

The disease is seen most frequently between the ages of five and fifteen, but may occur at any age.

### Is rheumatic fever a common disease?

Not anymore, because of the widespread use of the antibiotics when someone has tonsillitis or a streptococcus infection of the throat.

### What is the cause of rheumatic fever?

Rheumatic fever often has its onset a few weeks after a sore throat, tonsillitis, ear infection, or other infections caused by the streptococcus. However, it is felt that a peculiar kind of individual susceptibility is necessary for this relationship to develop.

### Is heredity a factor in the susceptibility to rheumatic fever?

Rheumatic fever has definitely been noted to be more prevalent in certain families than in others. However, it is not known whether this is caused by a hereditary predisposition or because the environment and living habits are predisposing.

### Can an individual have rheumatic heart disease without a known previous history of rheumatic fever?

Yes. In most cases, a careful inquiry into the individual's history will uncover significant data to indicate a previous episode of rheumatic fever. However, there are many instances where careful investigation does not bring to light a past episode of rheumatic fever. The characteristic heart symptoms and signs will, nevertheless, permit a diagnosis of rheumatic heart disease to be made, even without such a history.

### How does rheumatic fever affect the joints?

In the acute illness, all degrees of joint involvement may occur. These vary from vague discomfort in the extremities to severe pain in one or more joints, with swelling, redness, heat, and extreme tenderness on touch or motion. Commonly affected are the joints of the knees, ankles, elbows, and wrists. However, any other joint may be affected.

A characteristic of rheumatic fever is the "migratory" nature of the joint involvement; that is, the inflammation may settle in one joint and subsequently subside, only to crop up in another joint.

### Does rheumatic fever cause permanent joint damage or crippling?

No. Once the acute illness subsides, the joints revert to a perfectly normal condition, without residual damage. Even repeated attacks of rheumatic fever do not permanently damage the joints.

### What organs may be permanently injured by an attack of rheumatic fever?

While it is true that during the active stage of this disease many organs may be involved, almost all except the heart escape serious permanent damage.

### How does rheumatic fever affect the heart?

During the acute stage, rheumatic fever may set up areas of inflammation:
a. Within the heart muscle itself, causing myocarditis.
b. On the inner lining of the heart and on the heart valves, causing endocarditis.
c. On the outer lining of the heart, causing pericarditis.

### What is the effect of rheumatic fever upon the heart during the active and acute stage?

The patient may have any degree of heart involvement. It may be so mild as to be undetectable clinically. It may be so severe as to be rapidly fatal. Fortunately, fatalities in the initial attack of acute rheumatic fever are rare and are becoming even more rare with newer methods of detection and treatment.

### What are the later effects of rheumatic fever upon the heart?

The most important medical feature of rheumatic fever is the effect it has upon the heart valves. This usually becomes manifest a number of years after the acute attack even when the patient has recovered completely and, for all practical purposes, appears and feels perfectly normal. However, the initial inflammatory lesion in the valves of the heart may lead to extensive scar tissue formation. As a result of this process, the valves become distorted, damaged, and incapable of performing their duties adequately. The greater the number of attacks of acute rheumatic fever, the more extensively the heart valves are damaged.

### How can one tell if he has rheumatic valvular damage?

By complete examination, supplemented, if necessary, by other procedures, such as electrocardiography and x-ray studies of the heart.

### What is the significance of valvular damage?

a. As previously described, the heart valves are situated between the various chambers and exits of the heart. Their function is to keep the blood circulating in one direction and to enable the work of the heart to be utilized in the most efficient manner by the circulatory system. Depending upon the manner in which the valves are injured and distorted, they may either cause greater resistance to the natural forward flow of blood or they may permit backward leakage of blood from one chamber to the preceding chamber. Both abnormal processes may occur in the same damaged valve.

Because of the defective valves, the heart must work harder to accomplish its work. Eventually, the chambers of the heart become dilated, the heart muscle becomes strained, and the entire organ becomes less and less capable of performing the job required of it. (See Chapter 29, on The Heart.)

b. Injured heart valves are particularly prone to superimposed bacterial infection. The occurrence of this complication results in a bacterial endocarditis, a most serious disease, which, until recently, was associated with an extremely high mortality.

c. Patients with rheumatic valvular disease are also prone to form blood clots on the inner lining of the heart. These may, in time, break loose and be carried by the circulation to various parts of the body, where they will cut off the circulation to vital organs and cause profound tissue damage (embolism).

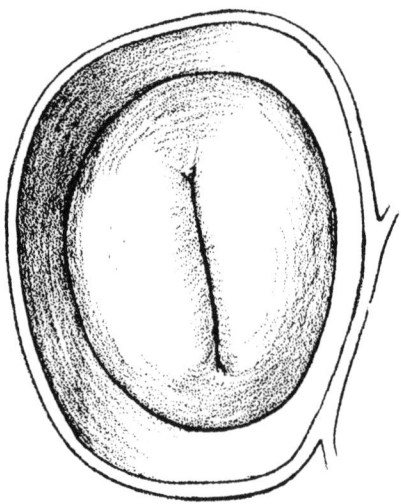

**Normal Mitral Valve.** *This strong, tightly closed mitral valve lies between the atrium and ventricle, the two chambers on the left side of the heart.*

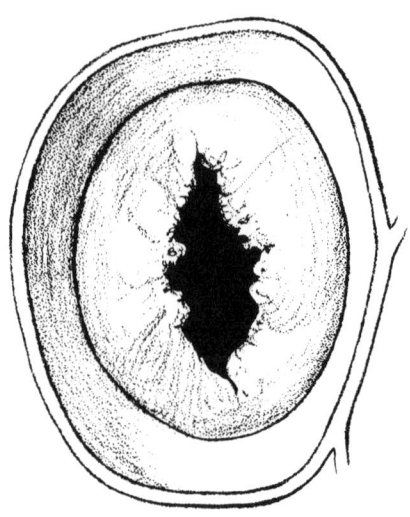

**Damaged Mitral Valve.** *This mitral valve, weakened and distorted by rheumatic fever, is subject to infection and will cause the heart to work harder.*

d. Patients with rheumatic valvular disease may develop disorders in the rhythmicity of the heart contractions, such as fibrillation. This will sharply curtail the efficiency of the heart and may lead to heart failure.

### Does one attack of rheumatic fever inevitably lead to heart damage?

Not always.

### Can damaged heart valves be helped?

Yes. If the damage is extensive, surgery is often indicated. The destroyed valves are replaced with efficient artificial valves.

### What signs warn of the possible presence of rheumatic fever?

a. Unexplained fever.
b. Unexplained joint or muscle pains.
c. The appearance of nodules over bony prominences such as the elbows, back of the hand, feet, kneecaps, skull, spine, and other areas. (The skin can usually be moved over rheumatic nodules.)
d. Peculiar and unexplained skin rashes.
e. Chorea (St. Vitus' dance).
f. Recurrent spontaneous nosebleeds.
g. Recurrent abdominal pains.
h. Shortness of breath on exertion.
i. Pain in the heart region.

### What is the likelihood of recurrence of rheumatic fever?

Prior to present day treatment, the incidence of recurrence was approximately 75 percent when the first attack occurred during early childhood. If the first attack occurred in an older individual, the possibility of recurrence is much less, and recurrence is found rarely among those whose initial attack takes place in adulthood.

### How long does an attack of chorea last?

An attack usually lasts from several weeks to several months. It usually terminates in complete recovery.

### Is rheumatic fever contagious?

No.

**What is the treatment of acute rheumatic fever?**

a. Bed rest for as long as the attack lasts. This may be for several weeks.

b. Antibiotic drugs, given regularly for an extended period of time.

c. Aspirin in sufficient doses to relieve fever and inflamed joints.

d. Cortisone and/or related drugs, depending upon the severity of the condition and the individual preferences of the attending physician.

**Can recurrent attacks of rheumatic fever be prevented?**

Experience over the past few years has shown that recurrent attacks of this disease may be reduced or eliminated by repeated dosages of penicillin, sulfonamides, and other antibiotics to susceptible individuals while they are well.

**Is the extraction of teeth of benefit to a patient with rheumatic fever?**

Usually not, unless the teeth are infected.

**Is tonsillectomy of any value in the treatment of rheumatic fever?**

Usually not. Tonsillectomy is advised only when there is definite evidence of disease within the tonsils, not as a routine procedure for the sake of helping in the treatment of rheumatic fever.

**What special precautions are necessary for a patient with rheumatic fever who is undergoing dental treatment?**

The patient should receive antibiotics and be carefully supervised by his physician. These precautions are carried out to prevent bacteria from lodging on the heart valves.

CHAPTER **63**

# THE SALIVARY GLANDS

*(See also Chapter 18 on Contagious Diseases; Chapter 39 on Lips, Jaws, Mouth, Teeth, and Tongue)*

## Where are the salivary glands, and what is their function?

The salivary glands are:

a. The parotid glands, located in front of and a little below each ear.

b. The submaxillary glands, located just about an inch in front of and below the angle of the lower jaws.

c. The sublingual glands, which lie in the floor of the mouth under the tongue. These glands manufacture and secrete saliva, which reaches the mouth through ducts (tubes) leading from the glands to the oral cavity.

## Are the salivary glands often involved in inflammatory processes or infections?

The parotid glands are involved considerably more often than the other glands, particularly when mumps—a virus infection—is present. In the days before the liberal use of the antibiotic drugs, pus-forming infections of the parotid gland were seen some-times as a complication of major surgery or in debilitated patients. Such a condition, acute parotitis, is now a rarity.

## Do abscesses or infections ever involve the submaxillary glands?

Occasionally, especially when a stone has blocked the submaxillary duct leading into the mouth. Marked swelling, pain, tenderness, and infection may take place if the duct remains obstructed. These symptoms are aggravated by chewing or eating.

## How can one tell if there is a stone blocking the submaxillary duct?

In some instances, the stone can be felt by placing the examining finger within the mouth along the duct. X-

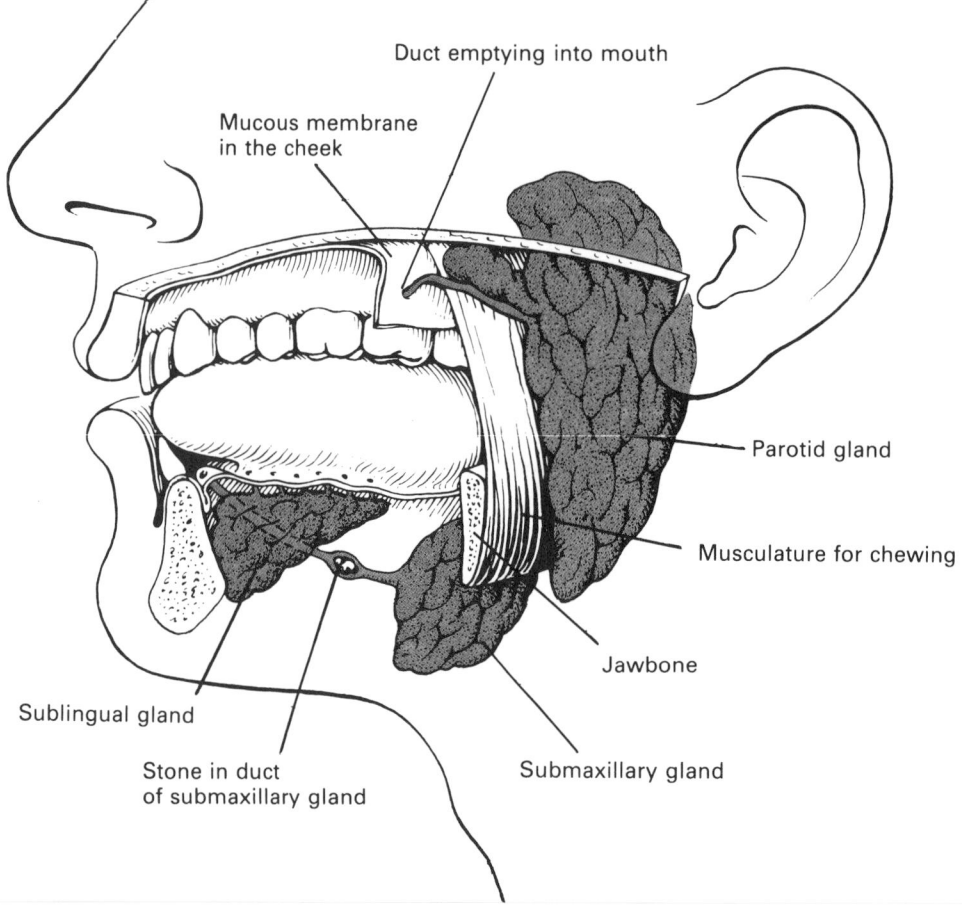

Duct emptying into mouth

Mucous membrane in the cheek

Parotid gland

Musculature for chewing

Jawbone

Submaxillary gland

Sublingual gland

Stone in duct of submaxillary gland

*Anatomy of the Salivary Glands. This diagram not only shows the anatomical relations of the salivary glands, but shows a stone in the submaxillary gland below the angles of the jaw. Such stones often cause marked pain and swelling. The stones can be removed by making an incision into the duct.*

ray examination will demonstrate the stone's presence on occasion. In the remainder of cases, the diagnosis must be made by the clinical history and symptoms.

### What is done about a stone in one of the salivary ducts?

It should be removed surgically under local anesthesia by making an incision into the duct and lifting out the stone.

### Do stones, once removed, have a tendency to recur?

Occasionally.

### If an abscess has formed in the submaxillary gland, what treatment is recommended?

Simple incision and drainage of the abscess if it has spread beyond the confines of the gland, or removal of the entire gland if the abscess is localized to the gland itself.

### Where is the incision made for the removal of the submaxillary gland?

Beneath the chin and off to the side of the midline. An incision approximately two to three inches long is necessary for the removal of the gland.

### Is it ever necessary to remove the parotid gland?

Yes, but only when a tumor has formed, not for abscess formation.

### What is the treatment for an abscess within the parotid gland?

Incision and drainage, usually in the hospital under general anesthesia.

## SALIVARY GLAND TUMORS

### Are tumors of the salivary glands common?

Yes, particularly the so-called "mixed tumors," which involve the parotid gland.

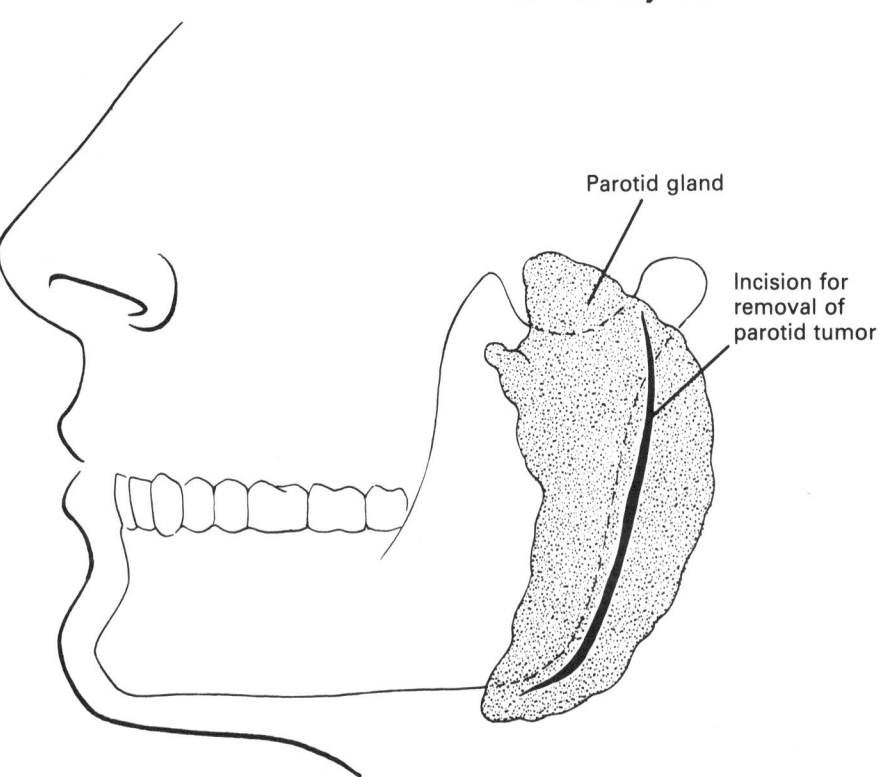

*Incision for Operation upon the Parotid Gland. The parotid gland is often the site of tumor formation, and such tumors should be removed. Most cases of parotid tumor can be cured, since these growths are not usually of a high degree of malignancy. While performing the surgery, great care must be exercised not to injure the facial nerve that courses through the gland.*

### Are tumors of the parotid gland usually malignant?

No. Most parotid tumors are benign, but the gland often does become involved in a cancerous growth.

### Do parotid tumors tend to recur once they are removed?

Yes, about one in five may recur even if they are benign.

### How can one tell if a salivary tumor is benign or malignant?

The benign tumors grow slowly and are usually surrounded by a capsule. Many of them are freely movable beneath the skin. Malignant tumors of the salivary glands grow rapidly and become adherent to the skin and surrounding tissues. Of course, following removal, microscopic examination will result in a conclusive diagnosis.

### Does the removal of one of the salivary glands interfere with digestion or adequate production of saliva?

No.

### Are operations upon these glands dangerous?

No, but operations for the removal of parotid tumors are long and tedious to perform. Great care must be exercised to avoid injury to the nerve filaments of the facial nerve that course through the parotid gland. Injury to this nerve will result in a certain amount of facial paralysis.

### What anesthesia is used for operations upon the salivary glands?

General anesthesia for the major surgical procedures; local anesthesia for minor operations.

**Where is the incision made for operations on the parotid gland?**

In front of the ear and down along the angle of the jaw on to the neck.

**Are the operative scars disfiguring following surgery on the parotid or submaxillary glands?**

No. Fine thin lines are usually obtained several months later when these wounds have healed completely.

**Is it always possible to avoid injury to the facial nerve when operating to remove a tumor of the parotid gland?**

No. It is sometimes necessary to disturb or even cut a branch of the nerve when removing an extensive growth of the parotid gland. However, this is not a frequent occurrence, and when it does happen, it is excusable on the grounds that the most important consideration is the total removal of the offending tumor.

**What happens if the facial nerve is injured during the removal of a parotid tumor?**

The face becomes partially paralyzed and distorted with a drooping and twisting of one side of the mouth. In rare cases, a branch of the nerve to the eyelid may be injured, and this will interfere with the patient's ability to close his eye completely.

**If the facial nerve has been injured, is the face deformity permanent?**

More or less, although the deformity tends to become less prominent as time passes.

**Can these nerves be repaired successfully once they have been cut?**

They are very small in diameter, some being no wider than ordinary sewing thread. It is therefore most difficult to find their ends and sew them together again. Recently, by means of ingenious muscle and nerve transfers, it has become possible to restore the face to near-normal appearance. To accomplish this, the services of an expert plastic surgeon are required.

**Do the wounds from these operative procedures have a tendency to drain?**

Yes. They may drain saliva onto the skin for many days or weeks postoperatively. However, the drainage will eventually subside and the wounds will heal completely.

**How soon after the salivary glands are operated upon can one resume eating?**

Fluids are taken for the first few days after surgery; then a normal diet may be resumed.

**How long a hospital stay is necessary following surgery upon these glands?**

Most patients can leave the hospital within four to five days after surgery.

**If a parotid tumor recurs, is it possible to get a cure by reoperation?**

Yes. A more extensive removal of parotid tissue will bring about a cure in the great majority of cases.

**What is the treatment for a tumor of the submaxillary or sublingual glands?**

Complete removal of the gland.

**Are operations for tumors of the submaxillary or sublingual glands successful?**

Yes, unless the procedure has been carried out for a rapidly growing cancer of these structures. Such malignant involvement is, fortunately, a rare occurrence.

# CHAPTER 64

# SEX AND HUMAN SEXUALITY

*(See also Chapter 3 on Adolescence; Chapter 17 on Child Behavior; Capter 25 on Female Organs; Chapter 42 on Male Organs; Chapter 44 on Mental Health and Disease; Chapter 77 on Venereal Disease)*

**What determines the sex of a child?**

The type of male sperm that fertilizes the egg. Usually, about half of the male sperm contain the Y-sex chromosome and the other half contain the X-sex chromosome. If a sperm containing the Y-sex chromosome fertilizes the egg, the child will be a boy; if a sperm containing the X-sex chromosome fertilizes the egg, the child will be a girl.

**Does the female's egg have anything to do with the determination of sex?**

No.

**How is it that some women give birth to a majority of boys while others have a majority of girls?**

This occurs because some men's sperm do not have an equal number of X and Y chromosomes. Thus, a man whose sperm contain a preponderance of X-sex chromosomes is more likely to produce girls, and vice versa.

**Can a man's sperm be examined to note distribution of X-sex chromosomes versus Y-sex chromosomes?**

Yes. This is done microscopically.

**Can sex be predicted before birth?**

Yes, by a test known as *amniocentesis*. This test involves the insertion of a long, thin needle through the abdominal wall into the pregnant uterus. Some of the fluid surrounding the fetus is withdrawn through the needle and is examined microscopically. Within the fluid there are always superficial skin cells that the growing fetus has shed. These cells are examined microscopically for the presence of chromatin bodies. If these bodies are seen, the fetus is female. Male cells do not contain these chromatin bodies.

**Is amniocentesis a safe procedure?**

Yes, when done properly, it in no way interferes with the pregnancy.

**Is there such a thing as changing a person's sex?**

Yes, but only to a certain extent. A male undergoing a trans-sex operation can have his penis and testicles removed, and through plastic surgery can have an artificial vagina constructed. He can then grow breasts by continually taking female sex hormones.

Similarly, a woman can have her breast tissue, uterus, tubes, ovaries, and vagina excised surgically. However, the construction of a functioning penis is not feasible. The taking of male sex hormones may cause hair to grow on her face and her voice to deepen.

**Is it ever possible for a transformed male to impregnate a female?**

No.

**Is it ever possible for a transformed female to become pregnant?**

No.

**How soon after conception can it be determined whether a woman is carrying a male or female embryo?**

By about the fourth month of pregnancy.

**What is a hermaphrodite?**

A person born with development of sex organs bearing some of the characteristics of both male and female. It is often necessary to perform an operation to remove a piece of glandular tissue and submit it to microscopic examination to determine whether it is of ovarian or testicular origin. There are also certain examinations of blood cells and skin that help indicate whether the person is predominantly male or female.

**What is a pseudohermaphrodite?**

A person who possesses the sex gland (ovary or testicle) of one sex, but whose secondary sex organ (penis or vagina) has been modified by excesses or deficiencies of certain hormones.

**When does sexual interest first manifest itself?**

Very early during the life of the child. During the first years of life, children discover that their genital area is a source of pleasure. Frequently, they engage in manual stimulation of their genitals. This is considered a normal phenomenon. Parents should not punish or threaten their child because of this activity.

**At what age should children be told about sex?**

There is no specific age, but when they ask questions, they should be answered honestly and without signs of embarrassment. It is unwise to avoid their questions, and it is equally unwise to give them more information than they seek, or to give them incorrect information.

**Is there value in sexual education?**

Yes. Most schools provide it today, and it constitutes a very important part of a child's learning process. Accurate information, well dispensed, can do much to prevent sexual problems in adolescent and adult life.

**What should be the parent's attitude toward the child who masturbates?**

It is perhaps wisest for the parent to ignore this practice. Care should be taken not to be threatening or punitive so as not to create neurotic guilt feelings that could affect the child's sexual attitudes in the future.

**Is masturbation an indication of emotional or mental disturbance, or does it lead to such disturbances?**

No. The old belief that masturbation could cause neurotic or mental illness is false. However, a sense of guilt about masturbating may create emotional anxieties.

**Is sexual contact essential for normal living?**

No. It is a common belief that sexual intercourse is a necessary component of normal adult living. Some people live happy, fruitful lives in a completely celibate state. However, in many cases, lack of sexual contact is part of, or the result of, an emotional disturbance.

**Can physical or mental harm result from a lack of sexual contact?**

Many maladjusted people erroneously attribute their unhappiness to lack of sex contacts, when in fact the lack of sexual contact may be the product of the maladjustment.

**What part do the hormones play in one's sexual desires?**

Hormones, along with the psychological attitude, play a significant role in conditioning an individual toward sexual experiences; that is, hormones stimulate desire.

**Is it true that the early development of sexual attitudes determines to a great extent the subsequent patterns of adult sexual behavior?**

Definitely, yes!

**Physiologically, what is the age of maximum sexual activity for the male and the female?**

According to some investigators, the teen years constitute the period of greatest activity for males, whereas the late thirties and early forties are the years of greatest sexual urge in females.

**Do men normally have a greater sexual desire than women?**

No.

**Does a person's desire for sex vary from time to time, or does a person who is uninterested tend to remain uninterested throughout life?**

Sexual desire may vary greatly from time to time.

**Does the removal of the uterus, tubes, or ovaries alter a woman's sexual desire or ability?**

No.

**What is nymphomania?**

A neurotic form of behavior in women in which there is excessive sexual desire and activity without actual gratification.

**What is the significance of the erotic dream?**

It is a normal phenomenon, occurring most often in adolescence and early adulthood.

**Should someone with a serious heart condition limit sexual activity?**

Yes, as it may place too great a physical strain on the heart. People who have had recent attacks of coronary thrombosis should consult their physician before resuming sexual relations.

**What is meant by the term "oversexed"?**

This is a neurotic form of behavior in certain women or men and is often typified by those who have relations indiscriminately and excessively without accompanying feelings of love or affection. (The word "oversexed" is not a medical or psychiatric term.)

**What diseases can be transmitted through sexual contact?**

See Chapter 77, on Venereal Disease.

**What is meant by the term "undersexed"?**

There are many people whose interests in life include little desire for physical relations. The term "undersexed" is therefore a purely relative term, of little meaning.

**What are the most common sexual disorders?**

In the man, premature ejaculation and impotence; in the woman, frigidity and painful intercourse.

**What are the most common causes of sexual malfunction?**

a. Deep-seated psychological problems.
b. Physical problems such as diabetes, neurological disorders, arteriosclerosis, etc.
c. Structural malformations of the genitals, especially those present since birth.
d. Surgical removal of the penis or testicles in the male or of the vagina in the female because of disease.

**What is frigidity?**

Lack of sexual desire and inability to attain an orgasm in a woman.

**What causes frigidity?**

It is almost always an emotional phenomenon that has its origin in neurotic attitudes toward sex. Many of these attitudes begin in early childhood, and as one matures, they lie deep in the individual's unconscious memories, where they continue to exert an important influence upon sexual behavior and reactions.

**Does frigidity have any influence on one's ability to bear children?**

None whatever. It is a common misconception that women must attain climax in order to conceive.

**Is there a satisfactory treatment for frigidity?**

Psychotherapy may be helpful, but the therapy must be intensive and prolonged. Sex therapists, too, may be helpful in treating frigidity.

**What is impotence?**

The inability of the male to achieve a satisfactory erection and thereby initiate intercourse.

**Is impotence caused by physical or mental disturbance?**

In many cases, it is caused by an emotional or mental disturbance. However, physical causes due to impaired blood supply to the penis as the result of arteriosclerosis are also major causes of impotence.

**At what age in life do men usually become impotent?**

This varies markedly. Many men are potent and fertile in their seventies and eighties. If they have diabetes or premature arteriosclerosis, they may become impotent in their forties or fifties.

**What is the treatment for impotence?**

In many cases, psychotherapy and/or sex therapy is indicated. Impotence due to arteriosclerosis can often be treated successfully through surgical methods. (See Chapter 69, on Sterility, Fertility, and Male Potency.)

**Is the use of hormones successful in the treatment of impotence?**

Usually not, unless the patient is quite advanced in age or unless there is a definite hormone deficiency.

**What is the difference between impotence and sterility in men?**

Impotence is the inability to have sexual relations. Sterility means the inability to fertilize an egg. Some men may be potent but sterile; others may be fertile but impotent.

**What is premature ejaculation?**

It is the experience of rapid orgasm, either before or soon after insertion of the penis into the vagina. Premature ejaculation interferes with successful sex relations and is often accompanied by a sense of failure in the male and a feeling of lack of fulfillment in the female.

**Is premature ejaculation a form of impotence?**

Not really, since the male who ejaculates prematurely is perfectly capable of an erection.

**Can premature ejaculations be overcome?**

Yes. Physicians, psychiatrists, and sex therapists are successful in curing most men who have this problem. Patience on the part of both mates is essential in eradicating premature ejaculation.

**What causes homosexuality?**

It is generally conceded to be a condition arising from emotional problems and attitudes within the home during early childhood. The development of homosexuality hinges upon the relationship of the child to the parents and to brothers and sisters, Some investigators believe homosexuality is related to hormonal or hereditary factors.

**How early in life can one detect a homosexual tendency?**

It can sometimes be detected during early adolescence.

**What should be done if homosexual tendencies appear in an adolescent or young adult?**

The individual should be referred to a competent psychiatrist who will decide if treatment is indicated or contraindicated.

**Can homosexuality be reversed?**

If an individual wants to become heterosexual, it is possible in some instances through psychiatric guidance.

**Can a heterosexual person be persuaded to become homosexual?**

Only if the tendency has existed in a latent form. Also, if circumstances are such as to deprive the individual of heterosexual outlets for prolonged periods of time.

**Is homosexuality on the increase today?**

It is not thought to be. However, homosexual individuals hide their attitudes much less today than heretofore. Thus the public gets the impression that homosexuality is on the increase.

**Is it wise to seek medical advice on sex matters before marriage?**

Yes. All couples should consult with their family doctor before marrying. Many young people harbor erroneous information and ideas about sex, which cause unfounded fears and which interfere, at times, with healthy marital adjustment.

**Can a doctor tell, on physical examination, whether a young couple will be physically suited to one another?**

It is exceedingly rare that two people are anatomically or physically "unsuited" to one another. Almost all incompatibility is psychological in origin, not physical!

**Can prolonged sexual inhibitions and sexual misinformation during youth and early adulthood be harmful to a mature sexual relationship?**

Yes. Children and adolescents should be as well informed on sex matters as they should be about any other important phase of living. Failure to educate them properly in sex matters may lead to sexual maladjustment in adult life.

## Where can one obtain reliable information on sexual subjects?

Most family physicians are well equipped to answer questions relating to sex. Also, one may write to the American Medical Association Information Service, in Chicago.

## Is the first sex act always very painful for a woman?

No. There may be some pain, but a tender attitude on the part of the man and proper instruction may avoid a great deal of pain.

## Do virgins always bleed upon first contact?

No. This is a common misconception.

## What is the most common cause of sexual incompatibility?

Psychological disturbance in either or both of the partners.

## Can sexual incompatibility be treated effectively?

Yes, by psychotherapy and/or sex therapists.

## Is simultaneous climax necessary for a well adjusted sexual relationship?

No, but it is desirable. Many couples can learn, over a period of time, to attain this state.

## Does the failure of a woman to reach climax indicate that she does not love her mate?

No.

## Is it natural for men to reach a climax more rapidly than women?

Yes, usually.

## Can excessive sexual relations be harmful to general health?

It depends on one's definition of "ex-

cessive." Harm may arise when one or both parties is maladjusted. If both are happy and content, there is no such thing as "too much love."

## Is it psychologically or physically harmful for people to have incomplete sexual relations?

Not if both parties are satisfied through such relations. It may be harmful if one of the parties is left sexually unsatisfied.

## Is there a normal frequency of sexual relations?

No.

## Is there a normal pattern of sexual behavior?

There is no definite pattern. Whatever gives the two people the most happiness is appropriate and normal for them. This involves wide variations in sexual practices and frequency of lovemaking.

## Can sexual relations be consummated during menstruation without harmful effects?

Yes. However, it is often considered unpleasant.

## Is it possible to become pregnant without actually having intercourse?

This occurs only in exceedingly rare instances. When it does take place, sperm must of necessity be deposited in large numbers in and around the vaginal orifice. (Of course, it does *not* take place from kissing or from bathing in the same tub that a man has recently used.)

## What is dyspareunia?

Painful intercourse.

## Is painful intercourse a physical or psychological condition?

It is usually psychological, but sometimes may have physical components if the female has an inflammation or abscess or mechanical pelvic abnormality.

## Is there any effective treatment for dyspareunia?

Yes. Psychotherapy and/or sex therapy if the condition is emotional in origin; medical treatment of the physical condition if physical factors are present.

## What constitutes sexual abnormality in a sexual relationship?

This is most difficult to answer. What is considered perverse in one society is considered normal in another society. The primary gauge should be the happiness of the couple and their mutual agreement on sex practices. Most physicians agree that if a couple is happy in their life together, their practices fall within that broad, but poorly defined, classification of "normal." Sadism and masochism that are abhorrent to one member of the couple constitute sexual abnormality.

## What are common causes for lack of sexual fulfillment?

a. An inability on the part of the couple to discuss sexual matters openly and candidly. One or the other, or both, may not reveal how they actually feel about the sex relationship.

b. A fear of failure in the performance of the sex act. The male, the female, or both, may feel sexually inadequate.

c. Hidden resentments and feelings of anger may interfere with sexual response and destroy erotic pleasure.

d. A failure to vary the sex act.

e. Performance of sexual relations in an inappropriate place where interruption may take place unexpectedly.

f. Lack of cleanliness and hygiene by either, or both, parties.

## What is the remedy for the common sexual malfunctions?

Sex therapy today is based upon the knowledge that some disorders are emotional in origin while others are caused by physical factors. Before treatment is begun, a thorough investigation is carried out by both medical and psychological questioning and examination. Once the causes have been determined, effective therapy can be implemented.

### What is the duration of sexual activity?

Contrary to popular belief, sexuality begins early in life and continues, in varying degrees, throughout all of life. Some people have an intense interest in sex from early childhood through old age; others have little interest throughout their entire lives.

### Does middle age have a significant impact on sexual activity?

There may be some decrease in sexual activity associated with a decreased secretion of hormones. However, such physical factors need not alter sexual activity. Psychological factors play a more important role. (In this connection, one notes many widows and widowers who were sexually inactive during the later years of their former marriages become extremely active sexually when they embark upon a new relationship.)

### What are some of the more common reasons for decreased sexual desire?

a. Severe physical illness.
b. Depression, stress, anxiety, and fatigue.
c. Fear of being sexually incompetent.
d. Any condition in which pain may interfere with the pursuit of erotic matters, such as severe back pain, bursitis, etc.

### What effect does alcohol have on sexual relations?

Alcohol in small or moderate quantities may heighten sexual desire and relax tensions. However, in large quantities, alcohol is a depressant and depresses the nerves that control the sex centers in the brain. Inebriated people are much less likely to enjoy normal sex relations.

### What is the effect of drugs on sex?

Some drugs, such as narcotics and those given to lower high blood pressure, diminish sexual desire (libido). Other drugs, not often prescribed, may intensify sexual urges.

### Does increased sexual desire improve sexual fulfillment?

Usually it does. One is much more apt to reach climax when the mate is sexually attractive.

# CHAPTER 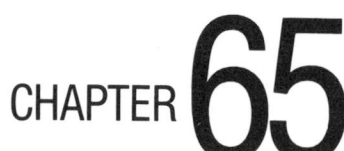65

# SKIN AND SUB-CUTANEOUS TISSUES

*(See also Chapter 2 on Abscesses and Bacterial Infections; Chapter 7 on Allergy; Chapter 16 on Cancer; Chapter 18 on Contagious Diseases; Chapter 26 on First Aid; Chapter 50 on Parasites and Parasitic Disease; Chapter 77 on Venereal Disease)*

**Does diet influence complexion?**

Yes. Certain foods may aggravate existing skin conditions. However, this does not always apply. People can be guided best by their own experience and by medical advice.

**Are cosmetics harmful to the skin?**

When used judiciously on a normal skin they are not harmful and, in fact, may even be helpful. However, in certain skin conditions, cosmetics can do harm, particularly when they produce plugging of the skin pores or when people are allergic to certain cosmetics.

**Does massage help skin tone?**

Not actually. As a matter of fact, after a plastic operation upon the face, massage can be harmful.

**Are skin creams ever beneficial?**

Yes, in certain skin conditions characterized by dryness. However, skin creams should be prescribed by a physician, as there are ingredients in some of the commercial products that may be harmful to certain skins. Vaseline is as effective as any of the more expensive commercial products.

**Are the "hormone" creams ever beneficial to the skin?**

In some instances. However, these medications should be used only on a doctor's prescription.

**Is suntanning beneficial to one's skin and health?**

Not particularly. As a matter of fact, more harm than good comes from overexposure to the sun.

**What harm can come from overexposure to the sun?**

An actual burn may result. Also, certain tendencies toward development of skin tumors may be aggravated by repeated overexposure to the rays of the sun. Then, too, there are skin diseases that can result directly from sun sensitivity. Blonds, redheads, blue-eyed, fair-skinned people particularly should avoid overexposure to the sun.

**Are sunscreens protective against the harmful effects of the sun's rays?**

Definitely, yes. These can be prescribed by a dermatologist or bought in a drugstore.

**What can be done to prevent skin wrinkles?**

Nothing. Wrinkles can be treated by plastic surgery in certain cases, but the benefit is usually of a temporary nature.

**Are the commercial products safe and useful in the treatment of cracking skin and chapped hands?**

Yes; some are quite efficient.

**Can one prevent the formation of brown spots that appear on the face as one grows older?**

No, but avoiding the sun will diminish their intensity. The public erroneously considers brown spots to be associated with liver conditions.

**Is there any relationship between the condition of the hair, fingernails, and skin?**

Yes. The nails and hair are actually part of the skin in the general sense of the term.

**Are clay packs and mud baths beneficial to the skin?**

Psychologically, they give many people a feeling of improved skin and well-being. Otherwise, they are of no benefit.

**Is the careful use of ultraviolet rays beneficial to people without skin difficulties?**

Only insofar as being suntanned gives them a sense of improved health. Actually, there is no physical benefit, and care must be exercised not to produce a severe burn!

**Are skin conditions ever caused by a lack of vitamins in the diet?**

Occasionally. Consult your physician for a general checkup, and he will tell you if vitamins need be taken.

**Is there any specific treatment for excessively large pores in the skin of the face?**

No, except that the face should be kept clean so that the pores are less noticeable.

## ACNE

**What is acne?**

A condition characterized by the appearance of blackheads and pimples on the face and frequently the chest and back. It occurs most often in adolescents and young adults.

**Is it normal for adolescents to have a mild degree of acne?**

Yes.

**What causes acne?**

To the best of our knowledge, the condition represents a disturbance in glandular function in the skin due to changes in certain hormone secretions.

### Does acne always require treatment?

Yes. If the pimples and blackheads are numerous and the patient is physically and psychologically disturbed by their presence, treatment is very important. Treatment will diminish and prevent the occurrence of scarring.

### Is acne curable?

Proper management can, in the great majority of cases, produce either a marked improvement or complete cure.

### Is it dangerous to squeeze blackheads?

Yes, if done improperly. Your physician should give instructions as to the exact method of carrying out this procedure.

### Is it important for the patient with acne to wash his face frequently with soap and water?

Yes. The regular use of a proper cleansing agent three to four times a day is very helpful. However, some skins are extremely sensitive, and care must be exercised not to cause irritation.

### Is sunlight helpful for acne?

Yes. The condition improves considerably during those months in which exposure to sun is increased.

### Are ultraviolet treatments beneficial?

Yes. Such treatments should be carried out under a doctor's supervision.

### Are x-ray treatments beneficial in the treatment of acne?

Modern treatment methods such as antibiotics and the newer local preparations are much safer and more effective than x-ray treatments for this condition. Moreover, x-ray therapy is used very sparingly because of the possible harmful effects it may have if overexposure results.

### Does acne leave scars on the skin?

In many cases, when treated properly, little scarring remains. However in some patients, scarring may be a very serious problem, particularly because of the bad psychological effect upon the patient.

### What is the treatment for acne scars?

In the last few years, a technique of *skin planing* (dermabrasion) has been developed. This consists of grinding away the superficial layers of the skin down to the bottom of the scar. When the skin heals, either the scar is gone or the pitting of the skin is diminished, so that the general appearance is considerably improved.

### How is skin planing carried out?

With an abrasion machine, which revolves and scrapes off the superficial layers of skin.

### Is skin planing a painful procedure?

No, because the skin is anesthetized with a local anesthetic while the planing is being performed.

## IMPETIGO

### What is impetigo?

Impetigo is a contagious infection of the skin, which occurs most often in children, but may also occur in adults.

### Is it very contagious?

Yes.

### What does impetigo look like?

It begins ·as a blister that rapidly changes to a crust. The spots are seen, as a rule, on the exposed parts of the body, such as the face and hands.

### How is impetigo treated?

With oral antibiotic drugs and with the local applications of antibiotic ointments.

### Are these ointments effective in curing impetigo?

Yes. Cure will result within a few days.

### What precautions should be taken to avoid spread of impetigo to other members of the family?

Each individual should use his own disposable towel, his own eating utensils, and should sleep in a bed by himself.

## ATHLETE'S FOOT

### What is athlete's foot?

A fungus infection of the skin of the feet.

### What is a fungus?

A fungus is a very small, microscopic type of plant cell, which may grow on the skin and, under certain conditions, may produce an infection.

### Is athlete's foot a common condition?

Yes. It is one of the most frequently encountered of all skin conditions.

### Is athlete's foot contagious?

Yes, but not highly so.

### How can athlete's foot be prevented?

By keeping the feet clean, cool, and dry. This means changing shoes and socks daily. Dry the skin between the toes thoroughly after bathing. Make sure soap between the toes is thoroughly rinsed out before completing the bath. Finally, use a foot powder.

### Why do some people have repeated attacks of athlete's foot?

This is usually due to poor foot hygiene. However, there may be a focus of infection in one of the toenails. Unless such a focus is cleared up, recurrences (particularly during warm weather) may be anticipated.

### Does athlete's foot ever spread to other parts of the body, such as the hands or groin?

Yes.

### What is the treatment for athlete's foot?

There are several highly effective fungicidal preparations that will control athlete's foot. Some fungus infections can be cured by internal medication, which, of course, should be given only under the doctor's supervision.

## ECZEMA

### What is eczema?

This is a general term used to describe an itching, oozing inflammation of the skin.

### What part of the body is most often affected?

The hands, arms, and other parts of the body may also become involved. In children, the face is the most common site.

### What is housewife's eczema?

This is an irritation of the hands, usually due to the excessive or careless use of detergents and other chemicals used in the routine of housework. The condition is more prevalent in cold weather.

### Do the majority of women develop eczema from detergents?

No. Most women have a skin that is resistant to the irritative effects of the common detergents.

### What precautions should one take to avoid housewife's eczema?

a. If the hands are known to be sensitive, it is a good idea to use rubber gloves with a cotton lining while doing work involving contact with these chemicals.
b. Do not wear gloves for more than fifteen minutes at a time.
c. Avoid the use of excessive hot water while wearing gloves.
d. Turn the gloves inside out every two or three days to allow them to dry thoroughly.

### Is the use of protective creams important or helpful in the prevention and management of this condition?

Yes, but it is advisable that the creams be prescribed by a physician. No two skins are exactly alike, and certain creams that may be helpful for one person, may be harmful for another.

## BATHING AND THE SKIN

### How often should people bathe?

People with dry skin will find that excessive bathing may irritate their skin and cause unnecessary itching during cold weather. Such people should rarely bathe more than once or twice a week. However, if one's occupation involves exposure to excessive dirt, more frequent bathing will, of course, be necessary.

### What can those with sensitive skins do to cut down on skin irritation resulting from bathing?

Superfatted soaps and bath oils can be used, which may prove very helpful. Also, such people should not use scrubbing brushes on their bodies.

### How can those who must restrict their bathing to once or twice a week keep their bodies clean?

Simple water baths, without soaping, may be taken more frequently.

### Is the skin less sensitive to bathing during warm weather?

Yes.

## PERSPIRATION AND BODY ODORS

### What causes excessive sweating?

This is usually a manifestation of an unstable circulation or a nervous overactivity of the sweat glands in the skin. It is very common in adolescents and young adults.

### Does excessive sweating require treatment?

As a rule, no. However, if the skin shows signs of being irritated or damaged by the excessive sweating, then certain preparations may be used to offset it.

### Are the patented advertised deodorants helpful in stopping perspiration and perspiration odors?

Yes, but people with sensitive skins must guard against irritation from these preparations.

### What causes body odors?

Failure to bathe, especially under the arms and in the groin. Also, certain bacteria acting on sweat form substances that are odoriferous. Some detergents contain a chemical that destroys these bacteria and thus does away with the offensive odor. Perfumes merely disguise body odors.

## COLD SORES (Herpes Simplex)

### What is herpes simplex?

It is a viral infection of the skin and certain areas of mucous membranes.

### Are cold sores caused by the herpes virus?

Yes. The sores usually occur on the lips of the face.

### What causes herpes of the lips?

Some people seem to get cold sores whenever the face is overheated.

This may occur following exposure to wind or sun, during the course of other infections with fever, or in association with a menstrual period.

### Can one prevent cold sores?

To a great extent, yes, especially when it is caused by excessive exposure to wind or sun.

### Is there a relationship between herpes simplex and cancer?

Some investigators feel that cancer of the cervix may be related to an initial herpes infection.

### Do men ever get herpes simplex of the penis?

Yes, and this may be transmitted by intercourse to the cervix.

### Do herpes infections tend to recur?

Yes, and some physicians believe that some people are herpes virus carriers and harbor the virus for years at a time.

### Is there any way to immunize or get rid of a persistent herpes virus infection?

Very encouraging results have been obtained recently with a substance known as acyclovin. However, this work is in its experimental stage.

## SHINGLES (Herpes Zoster)

### What is shingles?

A virus infection of the skin, which appears along the course of one of the nerves—most often around the chest. The patient with shingles is usually found to have had chickenpox in childhood.

### Is this condition very painful?

Yes. Several days after the onset of pain, a rash appears along the line of the nerve. It is the combination of the pain and the appearance of a typical rash that makes the diagnosis apparent.

### How long does shingles usually last?

The rash usually lasts two to four weeks. However, the pain may last longer—for several weeks or months.

### Is shingles contagious?

No.

### Is this condition serious?

Not as a rule. However, in some cases, the pain may last for several weeks or months after the rash has gone and may get very severe.

### What is the treatment for shingles?

There is no specific treatment for this condition. Relief of pain with appropriate drugs is the most important measure to be taken.

### Does shingles eventually disappear by itself?

Yes.

## RINGWORM

### What is ringworm?

A fungus infection of the skin due to a small microscopic plant.

### Are there different types of ringworm?

Yes. When ringworm involves the scalp it is known as tinea capitis; when it involves the feet it is known as athlete's foot; when it occurs on the body it is known as tinea corporis; in the groin it is known as tinea cruris.

### Is ringworm contagious?

Yes, to a certain extent. It is not as communicable as some of the contagious diseases, such as measles, chickenpox, etc. However, in a family where one person has ringworm, certain simple precautions like the use of one's own towels, slippers, etc., is advisable.

### Is there an ointment that will cure all types of ringworm?

No. The treatment of ringworm depends entirely upon the particular type as well as the individual in whom it occurs.

### Can ringworm be cured?

Yes. Medication given by mouth, especially in scalp ringworm, has been able to shorten the treatment considerably. This, however, must be done under the doctor's supervision.

### How is scalp ringworm recognized?

As a rule, it occurs only in children. Small spots on the scalp where the hair has fallen out or broken off should arouse one's suspicions. There is a special lamp (Wood's light) that causes infested hairs to light up or "fluoresce," thus helping to establish the diagnosis.

### Is ringworm a very serious condition?

No, inasmuch as it does not endanger life, but every attempt should be made to clear it up and to prevent recurrences.

## THE HAIR

### Is there any satisfactory treatment for baldness?

Baldness may be of several different types. A proper diagnosis as to the type of baldness is important, as certain types cannot be helped. Your physician can advise you if you have the kind of condition that will respond to treatment. Don't waste money on advertised patent medicines or so-called "cures"!

### Is baldness inherited?

Not directly, but one does inherit a tendency toward becoming bald.

### Does scalp massage help baldness?

No.

**Do the medicines so widely advertised to the public actually help in growing hair on bald heads?**

No.

**What is alopecia?**

Alopecia is a technical term used to describe loss of hair.

**Are there different types of alopecia?**

Yes. One type, alopecia areata, is a patchy loss of hair that is unrelated to the usual types of baldness. This type usually responds to treatment, but it may recur.

**How does one treat the ordinary type of baldness occurring in young men?**

Examination of the scalp is the first important step. If there is any disease of the scalp itself, correction of such a condition may often prevent the further loss of hair.

**Does the appearance of premature gray hair or premature baldness have any significance as to general health?**

None whatever. It is often a family trait and has nothing to do with premature aging or length of life.

**Does cutting or shaving the hair make it grow heavier?**

No. This is a common misconception.

**How often should the hair be shampooed?**

This varies with the individual. Some people require frequent shampooing, two or three times weekly. Others, because of the structure of their hair, would do well to shampoo it no more than once every two weeks.

**Can anything be done for excessive growth of hair on a young woman's face or body?**

Yes. It can be removed by electrolysis. In some cases, excessive growth of hair is due to a disordered functioning of one of the endocrine glands. For this reason, it is important before embarking upon treatment to investigate the patient's general health.

**How is excessive growth of hair on a normal person treated?**

Depilitories, if used carefully, may be helpful. However, the most effective method of removing excessive hair is by electrolysis.

**What is electrolysis?**

A procedure whereby a small needle is introduced into the hair follicle and an electric current is passed through the needle, thus destroying the root of the hair. The hair is then removed by the operator. If done accurately, electrolysis will result in permanent removal.

**Is electrolysis dangerous?**

Not if performed properly upon skins that can tolerate it.

**Does one have to see a physician for electrolysis?**

No. There are many competent electrologists who can remove hair properly.

**Is it safe to treat hairy moles by electrolysis?**

No. A physician's advice is essential before electrolysis is used on moles.

**Is it dangerous to dye the hair?**

When the preliminary patch test has been satisfactorily completed to make certain that there is no allergy or sensitivity to the chemicals used, and when the dyeing is done by trained, skilled operators, then it is harmless.

## SEBORRHEIC DERMATITIS AND DANDRUFF

**What is seborrheic dermatitis?**

A skin condition that causes dandruff when it involves the scalp.

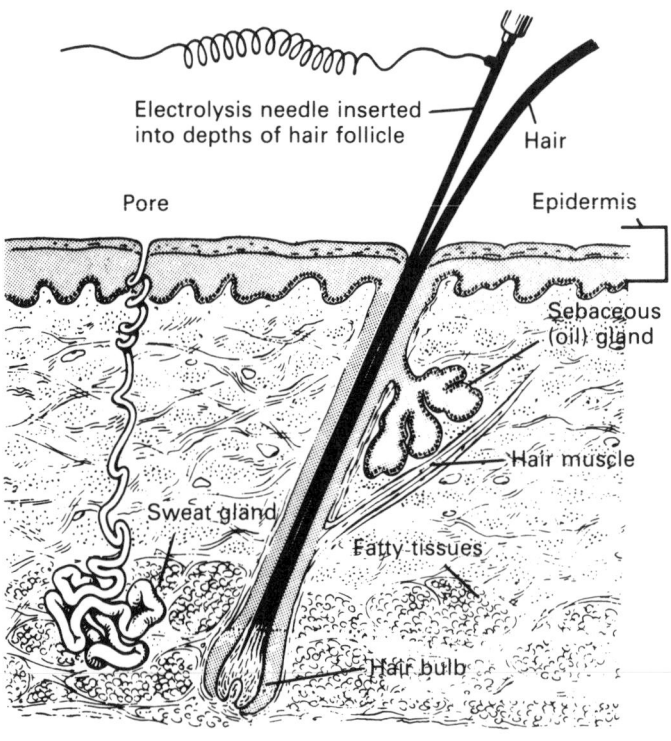

Electrolysis needle inserted into depths of hair follicle

Hair

Pore

Epidermis

Sebaceous (oil) gland

Hair muscle

Sweat gland

Fatty tissues

Hair bulb

*Technique for Electrolysis (Hair Removal). The needle electrode is placed deep into the hair follicle and an electric current is passed through it to destroy the hair and the hair follicle so that regrowth will not take place.*

## What is dandruff?

Dandruff is a term used to describe the appearance of flakes and scales in the scalp. It is due, as a rule, to a disordered functioning of fat glands that nourish the hair.

## Is dandruff contagious?

No.

## Is there any effective treatment for dandruff?

Yes. Your physician can prescribe certain preparations that will either cure or control this condition.

# CHILBLAIN

## What is chilblain?

Chilblain is an itching and painful burning and redness of the fingers, toes, nose, or ears associated with prolonged exposure to cold, damp weather.

## Is chilblain essentially the same as frostbite?

No, but the condition is caused by exposure to bad weather for prolonged periods of time.

## Is it necessary to seek medical advice for chilblain?

Yes, as chronic chilblain is associated with disturbances in the circulation in the skin.

# KELOID

## What is a keloid?

A reaction of the skin following a laceration, abrasion, or wound, in which there is excessive scar formation. Instead of a flat, thin white line of healing, there is marked thickening, elevation, and redness of the healed scar.

## What causes keloid scar formation?

The cause is unknown. Some peo-ple have a type of skin that heals in this manner.

## What is the treatment for keloids?

The most successful treatment is injecting cortisone into the area of the lesion before and after surgical removal. Also, good results have been obtained by giving x-ray treatments to the area after removal of the keloid.

## When is a patient most likely to get a good result from the removal of a keloid?

The longer the interval between the development of a keloid and its surgical removal, the better the result. It is not wise to remove a keloid until it has been present for at least two years.

## Is there any way of knowing in advance whether one will develop keloids following an operation?

No, unless previous operations have been followed by such scars, or if they have appeared following injuries or other conditions.

# SCABIES

## What is scabies?

A skin condition due to a mite, a small parasite or insect.

## How does one recognize scabies?

An itching and eruption develops between the fingers, on the wrist, around the breast, on the buttocks and genitals. The itch is worse at night.

## Does scabies often affect children?

Yes. It is one of the most common conditions of the skin affecting children. It is usually caught from a schoolmate or playmate.

## Does scabies often affect more than one member of the family?

Yes.

## Is scabies contagious?

Yes.

## Is scabies curable?

Yes. There are medications that bring about prompt cure.

# LICE

## What types of lice affect humans?

a. Head lice.
b. Body lice.
c. Genital lice.

## How can one recognize head lice?

There are small nits that are seen clinging to the hairs themselves. These nits look like dandruff. However, when one tries to remove them, it becomes apparent that they are tightly adherent to the hair and will not come away like dandruff.

## Are there other ways of diagnosing head lice?

Yes. In many cases, in addition to the nits, lice can be seen moving around the scalp and among the hairs.

## Is the treatment of head lice difficult?

No. Today there are several preparations that make treatment very simple. Shaving the head is no longer necessary, nor does one have to soak the scalp with some of the old-fashioned, foul-smelling preparations that were popular many years ago.

## How can one recognize the presence of body lice?

There are scratch marks on the backs of people who have body lice.

## Where do body lice live?

Usually in the seams of dirty clothing or underwear, not actually in the skin.

## What is the treatment for body lice?

Sterilization of all garments and frequent bathing.

### What are "crabs"?

A form of louse infestation that involves the hair around the genitals.

### What is the treatment for crabs?

There are several ointments, which, when applied properly, bring about prompt cure.

### Is this condition contagious?

Yes. It is contracted by either wearing clothing worn by one already infected with the disease, by sexual contact, or by sleeping in the same bed with an individual who is infected.

### Must the hair be shaved in treating crabs?

No.

## PSORIASIS

### What is psoriasis?

A chronic skin disease characterized by reddish silvery patches and plaques appearing anywhere on the body but having a predilection for the elbows, knees, and scalp.

### Can psoriasis be inherited?

There is some evidence that certain families show a higher frequency of this disease than others.

### Can psoriasis be cured?

Treatment may be effective in causing the spots to disappear, but they have a tendency to recur from time to time.

### Is psoriasis contagious?

No.

### Is psoriasis a common skin condition?

Yes. It is one of the most prevalent.

### Is there a standard form of treatment for psoriasis?

No. Treatment varies with the individual case, and many different methods may be used over a period of months or years.

### Does psoriasis tend to get better by itself as one grows older?

No.

### Does psoriasis ever shorten or endanger life?

No.

## LUPUS

### What is lupus?

Lupus is a term used to designate certain skin diseases that are seen on the face but often involve other parts of the body. Lupus is sometimes associated with involvement of the internal organs.

### Are there different forms of lupus?

Yes. One type, called lupus vulgaris, is a form of skin tuberculosis.

### What is lupus erythematosus?

A disease usually occurring on the central part of the face in what is called the "butterfly area" extending across the nose to both cheeks.

### Is sun exposure dangerous in lupus erythematosus?

Yes. It may aggravate the condition considerably.

### Is lupus erythematosus serious?

Yes. Some forms of this condition remain localized in the face and can be treated effectively by certain medications. Other forms are associated with involvement of other parts of the body and are so serious that they may not respond to treatment.

### Is lupus erythematosus ever fatal?

In rare instances. However, newer forms of treatment, particularly with the cortisone group of medications, have been very effective in controlling it.

## PITYRIASIS ROSEA

### What is pityriasis rosea?

A relatively common skin disease occurring, as a rule, in the spring and autumn of the year.

### How can pityriasis rosea be recognized?

It begins with a reddish patch on the chest, back, arms, or legs. This patch may look similar to ringworm and is called the "mother" or "herald" patch. Within a few weeks after its appearance, a rash suddenly appears on the entire body and may be accompanied by fever, itching, and a feeling of malaise.

### Is pityriasis rosea contagious?

No.

### What is the treatment for pityriasis rosea?

There is no treatment other than medication to relieve itching.

### Does pityriasis tend to clear up by itself even if untreated?

Yes. It will disappear in approximately six weeks.

## VITILIGO

### What is vitiligo?

Loss of pigment in the skin in patchy areas. These areas do not tan and are therefore more apparent in the summer on exposed areas of the body.

### What causes vitiligo?

The cause is unknown.

### Is there any treatment for vitiligo?

There are new drugs that are sometimes effective, but these are not without danger, and careful medical supervision is necessary while taking them.

## POISON IVY

### Is poison ivy a skin allergy?

Yes. It is due to hypersensitivity to a substance present on the leaves of the poison ivy plant.

**Is the skin ever allergic to plants other than poison ivy?**

Yes. Certain people may be allergic to other plants such as primrose, sumac, poison oak, etc.

**Is poison ivy contagious?**

No.

**Can poison ivy be prevented?**

There is as yet no injection or medication that will prevent attacks of poison ivy with any degree of certainty.

**How can one avoid getting poison ivy?**

By learning to recognize the plant and avoiding it.

**Is it necessary to have direct contact with the poison ivy plant to contract it?**

Yes. It is not gotten merely by being in the vicinity of the plant, although the smoke of burning ivy leaves can cause the condition.

**What is the best treatment for poison ivy?**

There are many simple "anti-itch" preparations, which have a soothing effect. The new cortisone drugs are effective in shortening the course of the disease, but they must be used under careful medical supervision.

**How long does poison ivy last?**

It may last from one to six weeks.

**Does one attack of poison ivy give any immunity against future attacks?**

No.

## SURGICAL CONDITIONS OF THE SKIN AND SUBCUTANEOUS TISSUES

**How frequently do people develop tumors or cysts of the skin or tissues directly beneath the skin (subcutaneous tissues)?**

Very few people go throughout life without developing a tumor or cyst of the skin or subcutaneous tissues.

**What are the common conditions of the skin or subcutaneous tissues that may require surgery?**

a. Sebaceous cysts. These cysts, or sacs, may form when the pores of sebaceous glands become plugged and the secretions accumulate and cannot gain exit.

b. Moles (nevi). Almost all people have moles somewhere upon their bodies. They may be nonpigmented, brownish, or blue-black in color. They may be extremely small or may grow to large size. Some people are born with these moles, but most moles develop in childhood or later in life.

c. Warts (verrucae). These, too, occur in most people at one time or another during their lives.

d. Blood vessel tumors of the skin (hemangiomas). These may occur at any time from birth to old age and are recognized as red spots on the skin. They vary in size from that of a pinhead to several inches in diameter. They may be flat or raised. In children, many of these lesions disappear by two and a half years of age. The flat lesions, known as "port-wine" nevi, do not disappear, and treatment of them is not very effective.

e. Fibrous tumors (fibromas). These appear as hard lumps in the skin or beneath the skin and are usually the size of a cherry pit.

f. Fatty tumors (lipomas). These occur directly beneath the skin in the fatty tissues. They may vary in size from that of a pea to that of a grapefruit or even a watermelon.

g. Ganglions. These are thin-walled cysts of the tendons or joints and are most commonly seen on the back of the wrists of children and young adults.

h. Cancers of the skin (epitheliomas). These are found most often upon exposed portions of the body in people in middle or older age. Epitheliomas are very common but do not tend to spread or kill the patient. They are curable.

**Do all sebaceous cysts, warts, moles, blood vessel tumors, fibromas, lipomas, etc., have to be removed surgically?**

No. They should be operated upon when they show increase in size, when they are in an area subject to repeated irritation, when they become infected, when they become painful, or when they bleed repeatedly.

**Where are procedures for removal of these tumors and cysts usually carried out?**

Small sebaceous cysts and warts are often removed in the surgeon's office. Moles, blood vessel tumors, ganglions, fibrous or fatty tumors, and cancers are removed in the hospital.

**What anesthesia is used for the removal of these lesions?**

Most can be removed with use of local Novocain anesthesia.

**Is it necessary to remain in the hospital after these operations?**

Often it is permissible to go home the same day as the operation. If a large tumor has been removed or if the surgery has been extensive, it may be advisable to stay for two to three days.

## SEBACEOUS CYSTS

**Are sebaceous cysts known by any other name?**

Yes. They are also called wens or dermal cysts.

**What are the common sites for sebaceous cysts?**

They may appear anywhere on the body, but are more commonly seen on the scalp, face, and back.

**If a sebaceous cyst gives no pain, must it be removed?**

Yes, if it begins to enlarge. These cysts have a great tendency to become infected if left in place over a prolonged period of time.

**Are sebaceous cysts dangerous?**

No.

**Can a sebaceous cyst be removed when it is infected?**

Usually not. At this stage, it can only be opened surgically and the pus drained out. Removal is performed at a later date, when all of the infection has subsided.

## MOLES

**Are moles (nevi) dangerous?**

The great majority are not dangerous.

**How does one know whether a mole is malignant or likely to become malignant?**

A mole, or birthmark, that suddenly begins to increase in size or change in color, or one that bleeds or is irritated by clothing, should be examined carefully to see if it is potentially malignant. Most of these moles prove to be benign, but early removal may be instrumental in preventing them from developing into cancer at some future date.

**Will the surgeon or dermatologist know which mole should be removed and which can be safely let alone?**

Yes.

**What is the proper treatment for a mole that has suddenly undergone changes?**

Wide surgical removal including normal skin and subcutaneous tissue around the mole. If a mole happens to be large, it may be necessary to put a skin graft in its place to cover

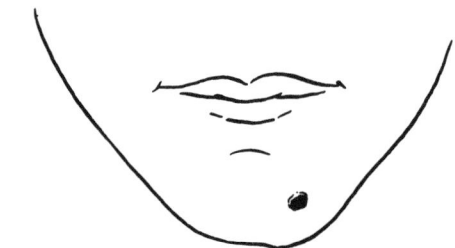

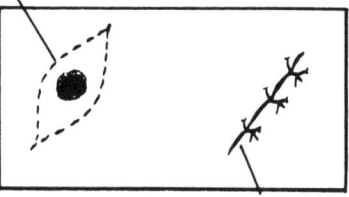

*Excision of a Mole. Most deeply pigmented moles should be treated by surgical removal rather than by electric needle fulguration. Certain moles, especially the bluish black type, have a tendency to undergo malignant changes. For this reason, any mole that starts to grow or change color should be removed.*

Elliptical incision in skin surrounding mole

Sutured skin

the skin defect remaining from its removal.

**Is it wise to cauterize brown or blue-black moles with an electric needle?**

No. Surgical removal is the best treatment.

## WARTS

**What causes warts?**

Warts are thought to be caused by a filtrable virus.

**Do warts ever come from handling frogs?**

No. This is a common misconception.

**Must all warts be removed?**

No. Sometimes the removal of one large wart will result in the others disappearing by themselves.

**Is there any effective way to prevent warts from forming?**

No, except that existing warts should not be picked at or irritated, as this may lead to the formation of others.

**Do warts disappear when untreated?**

Yes, in some people.

**What are the standard treatments for most warts?**

If they are to be removed at all, the most frequent way to do it is with an electric needle. Other warts are removed with surgical excision.

**Do all of these methods prove successful in curing warts?**

Yes, but some recur even when removal is thought to be thorough.

**If a wart is properly removed, is there a tendency for it to re-form?**

No, but new ones may develop elsewhere in the body.

**Do warts on the soles of the feet (plantar warts) produce many symptoms?**

Yes. They may be very painful and should be removed.

## BLOOD VESSEL TUMORS

**What is the significance of a blood vessel tumor of the skin (hemangioma)?**

The smaller tumors have no significance at all. Larger ones should be surgically removed or destroyed with an electric needle or by freezing with carbon dioxide snow.

**Do blood vessel tumors often turn into cancer?**

No. This is an exceedingly rare occurrence.

**Do blood vessel tumors tend to bleed?**

If they are located superficially in the skin and if they happen to be injured, active bleeding may take place.

**What is the treatment for bleeding from a blood vessel tumor?**

Direct, firm pressure over the bleeding point until a physician can treat it.

## FIBROUS TUMORS (Fibromas)

**Where are fibrous tumors (fibromas) most frequently located?**

In the skin of the arms or legs, but they may occur anywhere on the body.

**What is the treatment for fibromas?**

If they grow or if they cause pain, they should be removed by surgical excision.

**Do fibromas tend to form cancer?**

No. This is exceedingly rare.

**Do fibromas tend to recur once they have been removed?**

No.

## FATTY TUMORS (Lipomas)

**Are fatty tumors (lipomas) very common?**

Lipomas are about the most common of all benign tumors occurring in the human body.

**Where are lipomas usually located?**

They occur anywhere in the body within the subcutaneous tissues or between muscle bundles.

**Are lipomas painful?**

Usually not.

**Do lipomas tend to turn into malignant tumors?**

This occurs extremely rarely and is characterized by sudden, rapid growth of the tumor.

**When should a lipoma be removed?**

When it shows evidence of growth, when it is irritated or subject to injury because of its location, or when it becomes painful or unsightly.

## GANGLIONS

**What is a ganglion?**

A cyst of a tendon or a joint, most commonly appearing about the wrist area. Ganglions are also seen on other parts of the body, particularly on the fingers and feet.

**What is the treatment for a ganglion?**

Surgical removal, if it tends to grow or to become painful.

**Is it wise to break a ganglion by hitting the wrist with a book or other object?**

No. This is bad treatment and may be followed by recurrence.

**Do ganglions ever recur once they have been removed?**

Yes, in about 10 percent of the cases.

**What is the treatment for a ganglion that recurs?**

Surgical removal a second time.

## SKIN CANCER

**Is cancer of the skin curable?**

Practically every cancer of the skin, if treated early enough, is completely curable.

**What are some of the early signs of skin cancer?**

It is rarely possible for a patient to make a diagnosis himself. However, a good principle to follow is that a person should consult his physician whenever he has a localized sore that fails to heal within a month's time.

**What is the treatment for skin cancer?**

a. It can be removed with a surgical excision, including surrounding healthy skin and underlying subcutaneous tissue.
b. Certain skin cancers can be burned away with an electric needle.
c. Other skin cancers can be obliterated by x-ray radiation or other radioactive substances.

**Where does skin cancer occur most frequently?**

On the exposed surfaces of the body, around the nose and eyes, or on the back of the hands.

**Is the cause for skin cancers known?**

In certain instances, the cause can be attributed to repeated or constant irritation. Some skin cancers can be caused by the irritation of petroleum or petroleum products, phosphorus, or other substances that have repeated contact with the skin of the hands over a period of many years. It has been noted that those who have been repeatedly overexposed to sunlight during the course of their lives are more prone to the development of skin cancer.

CHAPTER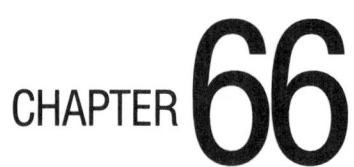

# THE SMALL AND LARGE INTESTINES

*(See also Chapter 16 on Cancer; Chapter 49 on Pancreas; Chapter 60 on Rectum and Anus; Chapter 70 on Stomach and Duodenum)*

## What is the small intestine?

It is that part of the intestinal tract extending from the duodenum (immediately beyond the stomach) to the junction with the large intestine at the ileocecal valve located in the lower right part of the abdomen.

## How long is the small intestine?

If its coils were straightened out, it would extend for approximately twenty feet.

## What is the main function of the small intestine?

By secretion of certain chemicals, called enzymes, it breaks down various foods into their basic components, thus permitting their absorption through its mucous membrane. The food elements enter into the lymph and bloodstream and travel to the liver, where they are further altered for eventual use by the tissues of the body.

## In what form are foods absorbed through the wall of the small intestine?

As carbohydrates (sugars), fats, and proteins. Also, chemical components of foods such as potassium, sodium, chlorides, calcium, iron phosphorus, etc., are absorbed through the small intestinal lining.

## Is water absorbed through the small intestinal lining?

Yes.

## Is the small intestine essential to life?

Yes, since it is the main area from which foods and chemicals are absorbed. However, at least half of it can be removed when necessary in cases of disease, and the remaining portion will be capable of sustaining normal nutrition and digestion.

## What is the large intestine?

It is that portion of the intestinal tract arising at its junction with the small intestine at the ileocecal valve, located in the lower right portion of the abdomen and ending with the anal orifice.

## Are there other names for the large intestine?

Yes. It is referred to as the colon or large bowel.

## How long is the large intestine?

Approximately five to seven feet.

## What is the main function of the large intestine?

Contrary to common belief, a large proportion of the stool is made up of bacteria, not of food waste or leftover undigested food particles. It is the function of the large bowel to absorb the water from this fecal stream that has come to it from the small intestine and to propel it forward toward eventual evacuation through the anal opening.

## Does the large intestine play a major role in the digestion and absorption of food?

No. Its main function is water absorption, although certain essential chemicals are absorbed by the first portion of the large bowel.

## Is the large intestine essential to life?

No. In cases of advanced ulcerative colitis, it is sometimes necessary to remove the entire large intestine, including the rectum and anus. This state is compatible with active living.

## What takes over the function of the large intestine when it is removed?

The terminal few feet of the small intestine. The end of the small intestine is brought out onto the abdominal wall and serves in place of an anal opening. This is called an ileostomy.

## CHRONIC CONSTIPATION

### What is constipation?

Difficulty in having a bowel movement or irregularity and infrequence of bowel movements.

### What are the most common types of constipation?

a. Functional constipation, caused by poor bowel habits, improper eating habits, irritable colon, spastic colitis, or emotional disturbances.
b. Organic constipation, caused by paralytic or mechanical obstruction to the passage of stool. Such things as adhesions, tumors of the bowel, stricture of the anus or rectum, or inflammatory conditions may produce organic constipation.

### Is there a certain type of person who is more apt to develop constipation?

Yes. Neurotic, highly strung people may develop spasm of the bowel with consequent constipation. Also, the indolent, slovenly type of person, whose habits are irregular, may develop chronic constipation.

### Is it necessary to have a bowel movement every day?

No. Many people normally move their bowels only every second or third day.

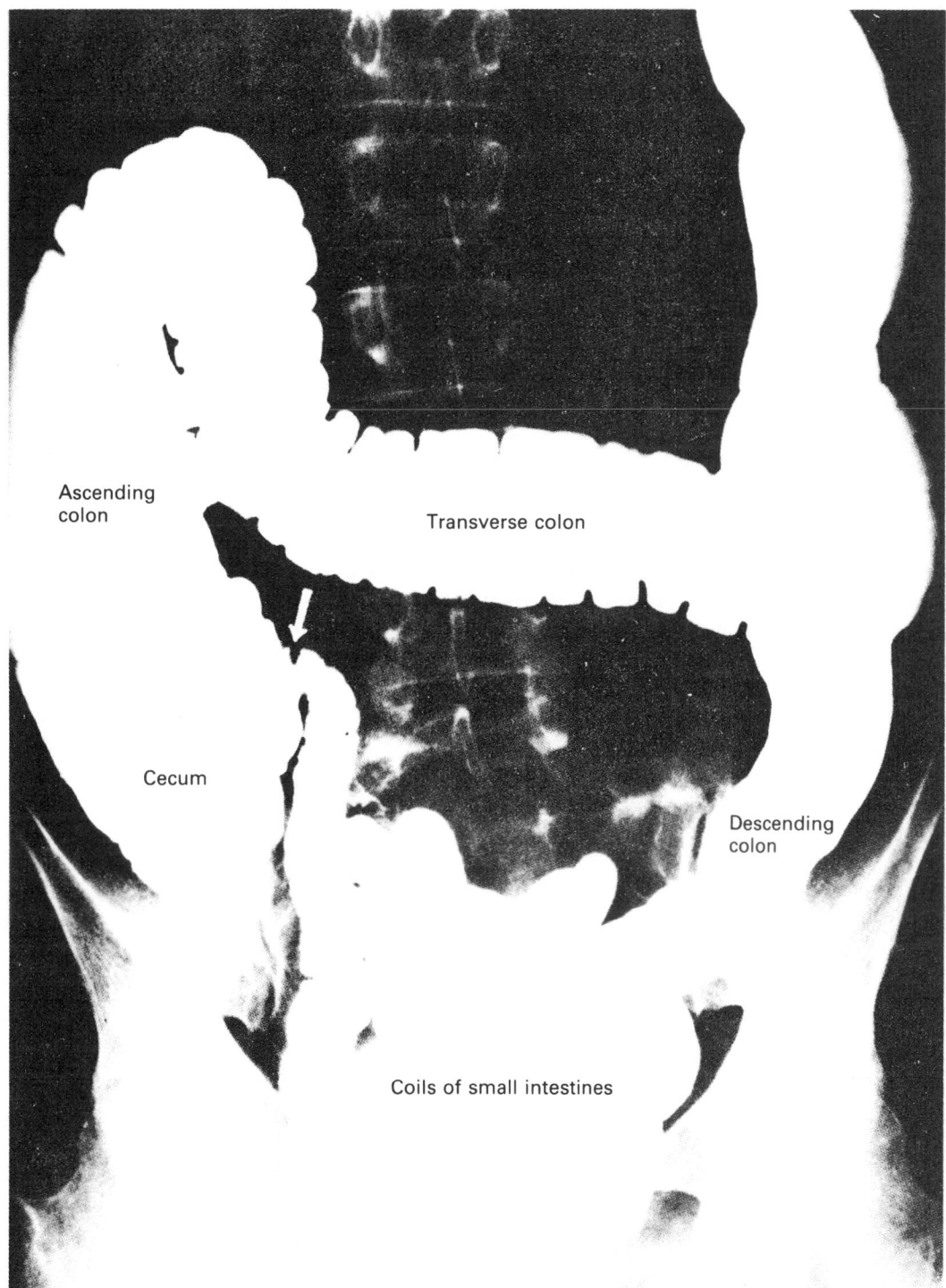

**X ray of Small and Large Intestine.** *The small intestine can be seen emptying into the large intestine (arrow). The ascending colon travels up the right side of the abdomen, the transverse crosses the abdomen, and the descending colon goes down the left side of the abdomen toward the rectum.*

### Does failure to move the bowels for a day or two cause symptoms such as headache, loginess, etc.?

If these symptoms are produced, they are usually of emotional origin, for there are no real physiological ill effects from constipation of such brief duration.

### Is it harmful to take enemas frequently?

Yes, as they may disrupt the normal rhythmic action of the bowels. Also, too frequent enemas, or improperly administered enemas, may injure the lining membrane of the large intestine.

### Is it harmful to take lubricants, such as mineral oil, for long periods of time to relieve constipation?

No, if it is really necessary. Mineral oil is not a laxative and serves merely to lubricate the stool and thus aid bowel evacuation. Mineral oil does not significantly interfere with the absorption of vitamins from the intestinal tract, especially when it is taken just before going to bed at night.

### What is the treatment for chronic constipation?

a. For functional constipation, the patient must be told to discontinue the use of laxatives, enemas, irrigations, etc. He must be placed on a good diet and made to develop regular habits. Psychotherapy is necessary so that the patient stops relating physical complaints to his bowel function.

b. Organic constipation must be treated actively to remove, through either surgical or medical methods, the disease causing the obstruction and constipation.

### What is autointoxication?

There is no such thing. People erroneously think that symptoms such as headaches, dizziness, dullness, etc., are due to constipation. This is rarely true.

### Is constipation curable on a permanent basis?

Yes, if one adheres permanently to the advice of the physician.

### Should a patient with chronic constipation be examined rectally?

Yes. It is always a good idea to rule out the possibility of an organic cause for the constipation.

### Should a patient with chronic constipation submit to x-ray examination of his intestinal tract?

Yes, particularly if there is a change in the character of the stool or if blood is noticed.

### Are colonic irrigations helpful in treating chronic constipation?

Usually not. They should be taken only upon a physician's advice.

## DIARRHEA

### What is diarrhea?

The passage of frequent, loose, unformed stools.

### What are common causes of diarrhea?

a. The simplest cause is gastroenteritis, caused by eating spoiled or infected foods or a food to which one may be allergic.

b. Other common causes include the diarrheal diseases, such as dysentery, ulcerative colitis, regional ileitis, diverticulitis, etc.

c. Some of the infectious diseases, such as typhoid fever and cholera, will cause severe diarrhea.

d. The taking of large doses of laxatives or purgatives will cause temporary diarrhea.

e. Diarrhea is often encountered as a functional disturbance among nervous, highly strung, neurotic people.

### Is there a certain type of person who is more apt to develop diarrhea?

Yes. The nervous, highly sensitive individual seems to be more prone to develop diarrhea as a reaction to an upsetting or tension-creating situation.

### When should one consult his physician because of diarrhea?

a. When it continues unabated for more than a few days.

b. When it is accompanied by other symptoms, such as high fever, aches and pains, and a general feeling of being ill.

c. When there is blood in the stool.

### How can one distinguish between functional diarrhea and that caused by serious disease within the bowel?

Functional diarrhea subsides spontaneously within a few days. Diarrhea caused by serious disease may continue for weeks, may be associated with generalized symptoms elsewhere in the body, and may be accompanied by blood in the stool. In addition, stool examination by a competent laboratory may reveal a germ or parasite that is causing the diarrhea.

### Should examination of the rectum be performed on people who have prolonged diarrhea?

By all means—a digital, sigmoidoscopic, and possibly a colonoscopic examination should be carried out.

### What is the treatment for diarrhea?

This depends entirely upon the cause. Most diarrheas due to eating spoiled or infected food subside spontaneously. Other diarrheas demand the specific treatment required to kill the particular causative agent.

### Should x rays of the intestinal tract

be performed on those who have prolonged diarrhea?

Yes, if other means of investigation fail to reveal the cause.

**Is it important to have the stools examined in determining the cause for prolonged diarrhea?**

Yes. A thorough search for parasites, eggs of parasites, and bacteria must be made.

**Are medications that bind the bowels helpful in the treatment of prolonged diarrhea?**

No. They merely delay treatment.

**Are laxatives ever given to end diarrhea?**

Not usually. Certainly, they should not be given unless advised by the physician.

**Will the taking of antibiotic drugs ever cause diarrhea?**

Yes! Many of the -mycin group of antibiotics will cause a serious and prolonged diarrhea. This condition is called pseudomembranous enterocolitis and is one of the main reasons why people should take antibiotics only upon the explicit recommendation of their physician.

**How do antibiotics sometimes cause diarrhea?**

By destroying certain necessary bacteria that should normally grow within the intestinal tract. When these bacteria are destroyed, others that are not sensitive to the particular antibiotic being given (usually staphylococci germs) grow in large numbers and produce an irritation of the mucous membrane lining of the bowel.

## GASTROENTERITIS
*(See Chapter 70 on Stomach and Duodenum)*

**What is gastroenteritis?**

An acute inflammation of the lining of the small intestine and the stomach.

**What causes acute gastroenteritis?**

There are several causes:
a. A virus, as in intestinal grippe.
b. Allergy to certain foods or drink.
c. Eating spoiled foods.
d. Food poisoning.
e. Taking certain medications that produce overactivity of the small intestine.
f. Taking poisons.
g. Overindulgence in alcohol.
h. A true inflammation caused by a germ, such as typhoid fever, dysentery, or cholera, etc.

**What are the symptoms of acute gastroenteritis?**

Gastroenteritis usually begins suddenly with loss of appetite and nausea, followed by abdominal cramps, vomiting, and diarrhea. This is followed by excessive weakness and a feeling of prostration. Fever is present if gastroenteritis is of infectious origin. The abdomen becomes distended and tender, usually in the midabdominal region or in the lower abdomen over the region of the small intestine.

**How long does acute gastroenteritis usually last?**

Two to three days.

**How can one distinguish between acute gastroenteritis and other conditions?**

By carefully noting the history of the signs and symptoms and by noting the absence of other more serious signs, such as muscle spasm and rigidity of the abdominal wall.

**Does one have to be operated upon for acute gastroenteritis?**

No, but differential diagnosis between this condition and other conditions that do require surgery, such as appendicitis or rupture of the bowel, etc., must be made.

**What is the treatment for acute gastroenteritis?**

a. Absolute bed rest.
b. Abstinence from food for twenty-four to forty-eight hours.
c. Sedatives to calm the patient.
d. Medications to diminish bowel activity.

**Does recovery from gastroenteritis usually take place?**

Yes, unless the enteritis is caused by an overwhelming dose of a true poison or severe food poisoning caused by a specific organism, the botulinus germ.

## REGIONAL ILEITIS

**What is regional ileitis?**

An inflammatory disease affecting the lower portion of the small intestine.

**What causes regional ileitis?**

The cause is unknown, although it is thought to be caused by a germ or viruses that have not yet been isolated.

**Are there any other names for this condition?**

Yes. It is also called terminal ileitis or regional enteritis.

**Is regional ileitis a common condition?**

Yes. It is most often seen in adolescence and in people in their thirties and forties.

**How is the diagnosis of regional ileitis made?**

It is usually established by characteristic x-ray findings.

**What are the signs and symptoms of this disease?**

It may have its onset with acute at-

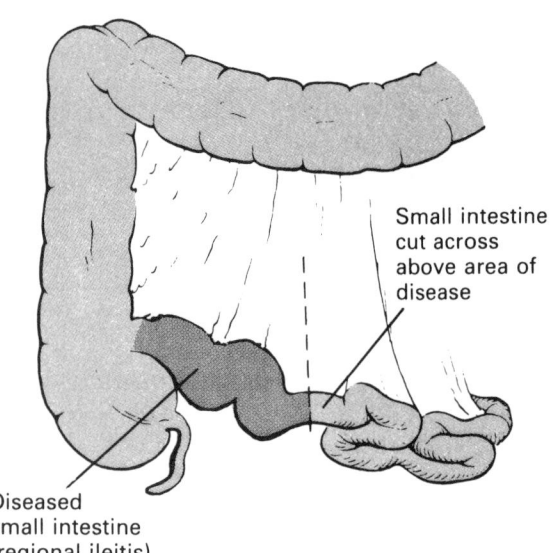

Small intestine cut across above area of disease

Diseased small intestine (regional ileitis)

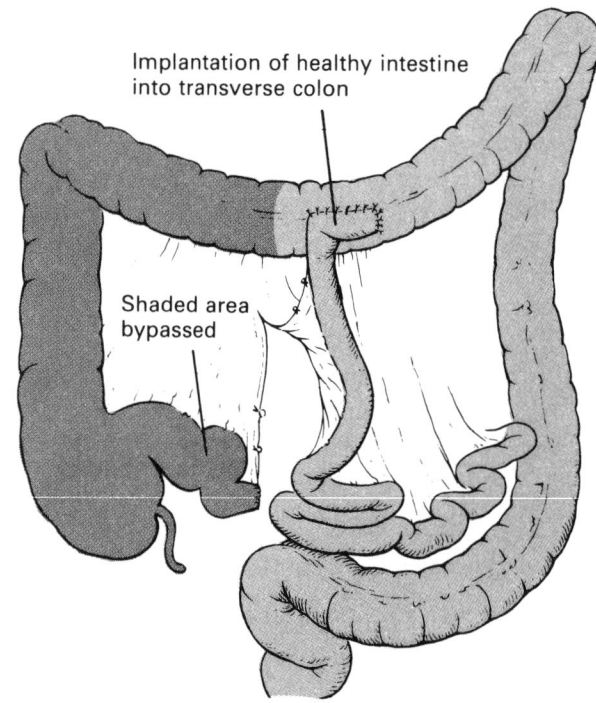

Implantation of healthy intestine into transverse colon

Shaded area bypassed

*Operation for Regional Ileitis.* This diagram shows how the small intestine is cut across above the diseased area, and the healthy small bowel is sutured to the transverse colon, thus short-circuiting the inflamed portion.

just a few days and disappear, never to return again.

b. In the more severe form, there are repeated attacks of fever, abdominal cramps, and loose stools. Eventually, there may be abscess formation within the bowel and small intestinal obstruction.

### What is the treatment for regional ileitis?

a. In the milder cases, bed rest, a bland diet excluding spices and alcohol, and the administration of antibiotic drugs. Emphasis is laid upon avoidance of excessive work and emotional strain. Some of the newer steroid (cortisone) drugs have been found to give remarkable relief in acute cases.

b. When the disease is far advanced, surgical treatment is necessary. This may involve removing the inflamed portion of the small bowel and joining normal bowel above it to the transverse colon (ileotransverse colostomy). In certain cases, the inflamed bowel is not removed, but the normal small intestine above the inflammation is joined to the large bowel, thus bypassing the inflamed bowel. The inflammation subsides in the great majority of cases, because the fecal stream does not course over the inflamed intestine.

### What is the outlook for recovery in a patient with regional ileitis?
Excellent.

### Is there any way to prevent regional ileitis?
Unfortunately, since the cause of this condition is not known, recommendations to avoid it cannot be given.

### Is there a type of individual who is more prone to develop regional ileitis?
It is thought that the overworked, fatigued, highly strung individual is more likely to develop this condition.

tacks of lower or midabdominal cramps, several loose stools per day, loss of appetite, and a mild fever. The condition often subsides after a few days but recurs at intervals over a period of weeks. Eventually, the inflammation of the small bowel may cause obstruction to the passage of stool. There will then be marked abdominal distention, nausea, vomiting, and inability to move the bowels.

### What is the course of this disease?

a. In the mild form, an attack may last

However, well-adjusted people also may develop regional ileitis.

**Does regional ileitis, once subsided, have a tendency to recur?**
Yes, in a small number of cases.

**Can one lead a normal life after part of the small bowel has been removed or bypassed?**
Yes. There are some twenty feet of small intestine, and less than half are necessary for the maintenance of normal intestinal function.

**Does regional ileitis tend to run in families or to be inherited?**
No.

**Should special diet be followed after an episode of regional ileitis?**
Yes. A bland diet should be followed for a period of months or even years.

## MECKEL'S DIVERTICULUM

**What is a Meckel's diverticulum?**
It is an outpouching, or fingerlike projection of the small intestinal wall, occurring within the terminal twelve inches or so of the small intestine. It is present from birth and represents a defect in development.

**Is this a common condition?**
No. It is rare.

**What is the significance of Meckel's diverticulum?**
It sometimes becomes inflamed, in much the same way as an appendix becomes inflamed.

**How can a diagnosis of an inflamed Meckel's diverticulum be made?**
The patient, usually a child, will have abdominal pain, tenderness in the midabdominal region, slight fever, and a bloody diarrhea.

**What is the treatment for this condition?**
When the diagnosis has been made,

surgery should be performed promptly, as the inflamed or infected diverticulum may hemorrhage or rupture. Surgery will involve the removal of the diverticulum, a procedure quite similar to the removal of the appendix.

**Is this a serious operation?**
It is a major operation, but complete recovery is the usual outcome.

**How long will it take before recovery from an operation for Meckel's diverticulum?**
Approximately the same postoperative course ensues as that following appendectomy.

## INTUSSUSCEPTION

**What is intussusception?**
It is a condition in which one part of the bowel telescopes through another part.

**What causes intussusception?**
Usually, an inflammation or tumor interferes with normal bowel contraction. The normal intestine above the region of inflammation or tumor continues to contract with force greater than the intestine below, thus producing a telescoping of the bowel above into the bowel below.

**What is the most frequent site for intussusception?**
The small intestine telescopes through into the large intestine at the point where they join, that is, in the lower right portion of the abdomen.

**Who is most likely to develop this condition?**
Most cases occur in children in their second, third, or fourth year of life.

**How is the diagnosis of intussusception made?**
By noting the presence of abdominal pain, the feeling of a mass (lump) in

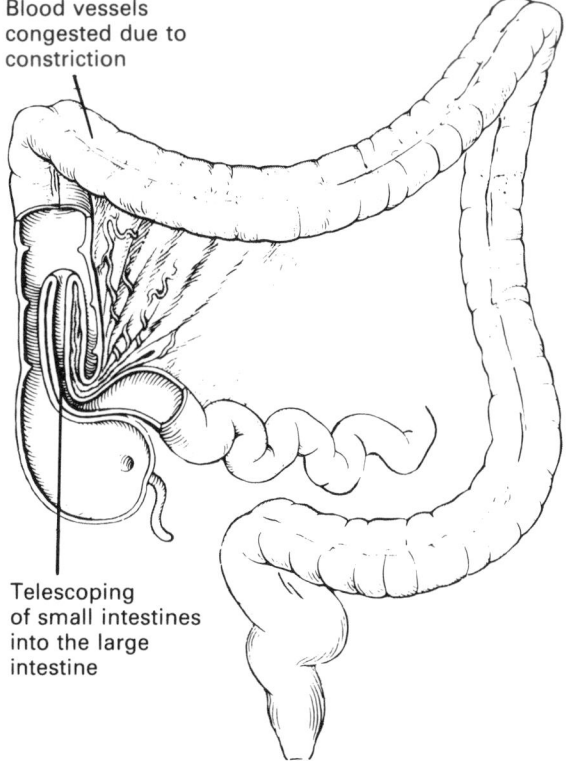

Blood vessels congested due to constriction

Telescoping of small intestines into the large intestine

*Intussusception of the Small Bowel. Intussusception is a condition in which one portion of bowel telescopes into another. In this diagram the small bowel intussuscepts into the large intestine. This condition occurs most often in children and demands surgery within a few hours in order to avoid gangrene of the bowel.*

the lower right portion of the abdomen, and by characteristic x-ray findings. Bloody diarrhea is also a frequent occurrence in this condition.

### What is the treatment for intussusception?

a. In most cases an abdominal operation is performed, and that portion of the bowel that is telescoped is gently pulled out into its normal position.

b. In certain cases the condition can be relieved medically by instilling under pressure a barium mixture into the rectum. This must be done by one who is completely familiar with the technique. Under fluoroscopic viewing the barium is permitted to fill the large intestine and is allowed to exert pressure upon the telescoped small bowel until it retracts into a normal position.

### Is the medical treatment successful in most cases of intussusception?

At the present time, only a small percentage of cases can be relieved by this technique, and it is still necessary to operate upon the majority of those children who have this condition.

### Once the telescoped bowel has been withdrawn, does it tend to telescope again?

Once this condition has been corrected surgically, it is highly unlikely that it will occur again.

### What are the chances for recovery from intussusception?

Excellent, providing the diagnosis has been made within the first day or two.

### What are the dangers of intussusception?

The bowel that is telescoped may become gangrenous because of strangulation of its blood supply. This may result in peritonitis and death, if undiscovered.

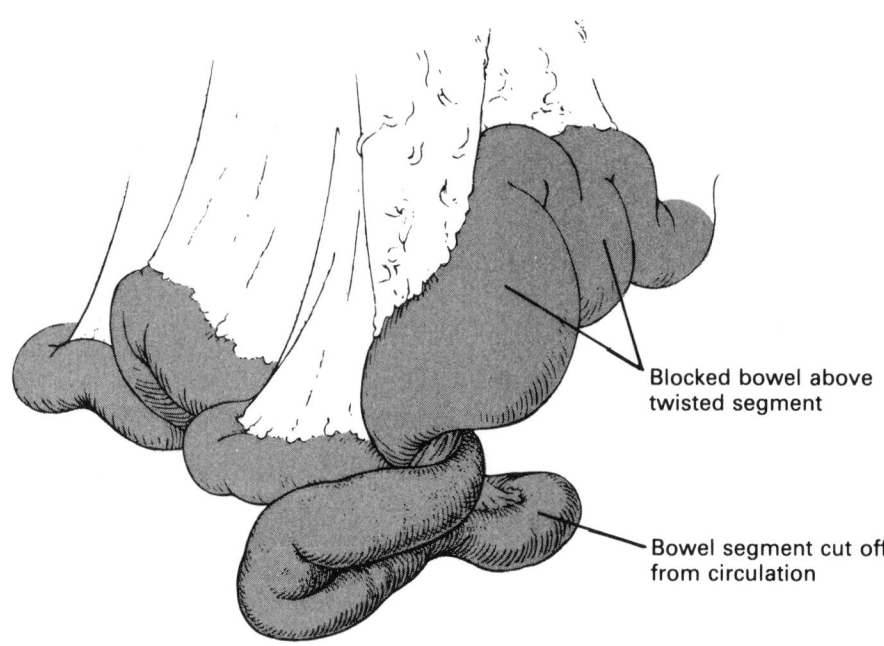

*Volvulus. In volvulus, the bowel undergoes a twist, which may cut off its circulation and lead to gangrene. Treatment is surgical and involves straightening out the bowel and removing the cause for the twist.*

Blocked bowel above twisted segment

Bowel segment cut off from circulation

## VOLVULUS

### What is volvulus?

It is a rotation, or twist, of a segment of small or large bowel upon its stalk (mesentery). Such a twist may cut off the blood supply to this segment of the bowel and thus produce gangrene.

### Where is volvulus most likely to take place?

In the large bowel, most often in the sigmoid colon in the lower left side of the abdomen.

### What causes volvulus?

It is frequently caused by a tumor of the large bowel or by adhesions secondary to a previous inflammation or operation. In some cases it is attributed to an abnormally long mesentery (stalk).

### Who is most likely to develop volvulus?

It is seen more often in elderly people or those who have lost large amounts of weight.

### What are the symptoms of volvulus?

Acute abdominal pain, nausea and vomiting, obstruction of the intestine, fever, tenderness of the abdomen, and characteristic x-ray findings.

### What is the treatment for volvulus?

Prompt surgery in which the twisted bowel is untwisted and any cause for the abnormal rotation, such as adhesions or a tumor, is removed.

### Once a twisted bowel has been untwisted, is it likely to recur?

Not if the cause for the volvulus has been removed.

### Will recovery take place?

Yes, in the majority of cases, if the diagnosis is made soon enough. In cases where the diagnosis is made late, gangrene may have set in and peritonitis may already have developed. If this has occurred, the chances for recovery are markedly diminished.

# DIVERTICULITIS AND DIVERTICULOSIS

### What is diverticulosis?

A condition in which there are pouches of mucous membrane that poke through the muscle wall of the large bowel.

### What is the cause of diverticulosis?

It is thought that there is a weakness in the bowel wall at various points where blood vessels pierce it.

### What is the difference between diverticulitis and diverticulosis?

Diverticulitis is a disease in which there is an inflammation of one or more of these pouches or protrusions.

### Is diverticulosis a common condition?

Yes. It is thought that approximately one in ten people have such diverticula. The great majority, however, have no symptoms secondary to this condition.

### If the majority of people with diverticulosis have no symptoms, how is the existence of the condition discovered?

It is usually discovered by characteristic x-ray findings that are seen when a routine gastrointestinal x-ray series is taken.

### What are the chances of developing diverticulitis if one has diverticulosis?

The great majority of those people who have diverticulosis never have any symptoms whatsoever. Only about 10 percent develop inflammation or diverticulitis.

### If one has diverticulosis, is there any way to avoid getting diverticulitis?

No. Although various types of diet have been prescribed, they are not significantly influential in determining whether an episode of diverticulitis will ensue.

### What diets are prescribed for diverticulosis?

Two diametrically opposed diets. One advocates an extremely high roughage component; the other a very low roughage component. Both advocate the developing of regular bowel habits and the avoidance of markedly spicy foods. (See Chapter 20, on Diet.)

### What is the treatment for diverticulitis?

In the mild cases, medical treatment is all that is required. This will include:

a. Bed rest.
b. Bland diet.
c. Intensive antibiotic treatment.

### Can most cases of diverticulitis be brought under control with medical management?

Yes. Only one in ten of those people suffering from an initial attack of diverticulitis require surgery.

### When is surgery necessary for diverticulitis?

a. When there have been recurring attacks.
b. When the diverticula threaten to rupture, or actually do rupture, causing peritonitis.
c. When the inflammation is so bad that it forms localized abscesses or fistulas that extend from the bowel into adjacent organs such as the bladder.
d. When there is repeated massive hemorrhage from the diverticula.

### What operations are indicated in the treatment of diverticulitis?

a. If the inflamed diverticula have

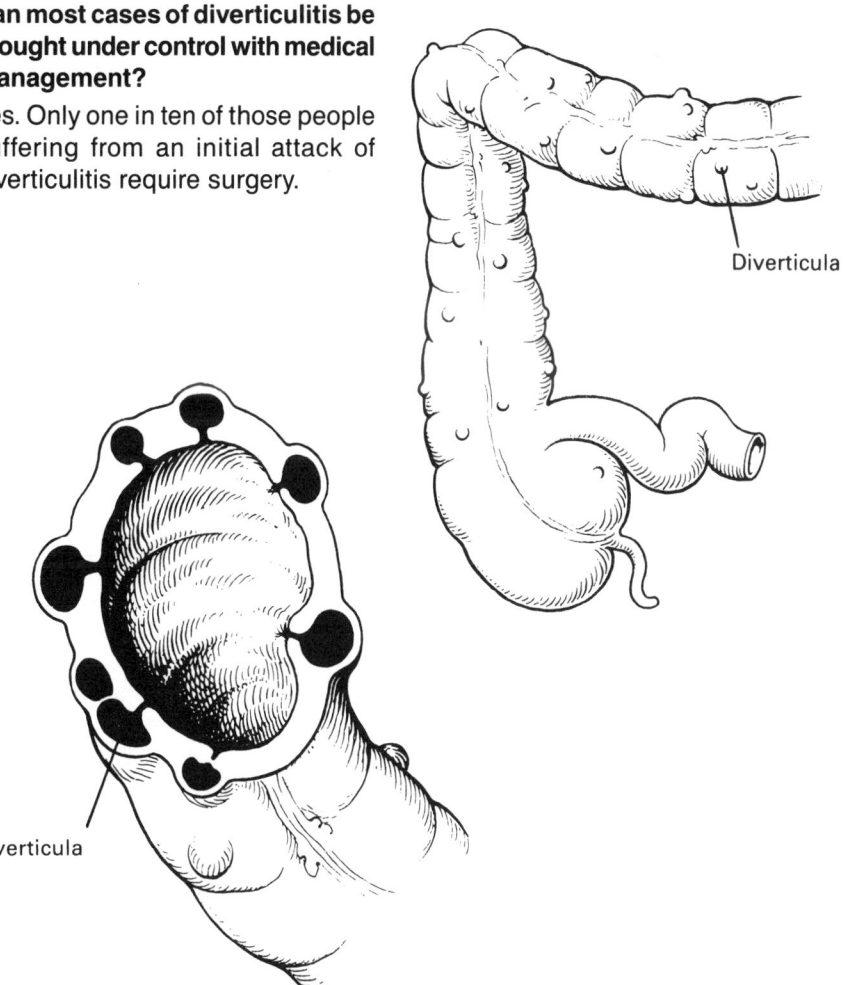

Diverticula

Diverticula

*Diverticulosis. This is a condition in which there are many small outpouchings or blisters on the wall of the large bowel. These blisters cause no harm unless they become inflamed (diverticulitis), or unless one of them ruptures, causing peritonitis.*

ruptured and formed abscesses, the abscesses must be drained. In such cases, it may be necessary to perform a colostomy (an opening from the bowel onto the abdominal wall) in order to divert the fecal stream from the diseased area.

b. The ideal treatment for an area of localized diverticulitis is to remove the diseased portion of bowel and to join the healthy bowel above to healthy bowel below.

### Are operations for diverticulitis dangerous?

They are serious operations, but recovery is the general rule.

### Does diverticulitis often recur after surgery?

Only if diseased loops of bowel have been left behind.

### How long a period of hospitalization is necessary for diverticulitis?

If one waits for the acute inflammation to subside without surgery, three or more weeks of hospitalization may be necessary. If surgery is performed, the patient may be ready to leave the hospital within two to three weeks.

### Is it often necessary to perform several operations in order to cure this condition?

Yes. The first operation may consist merely of drainage of the abscess secondary to a ruptured diverticulitis and performing a colostomy to divert the feces; the second stage may be carried out to remove the diseased segment of bowel; and a third-stage operation may be required to close the opening in the bowel and restore the normal course of the fecal stream.

### Are operations for diverticulitis always done in stages?

No. Whenever possible, the surgeon will attempt to remove the diseased bowel and restore continuity all in one operation. Unfortunately, this is not always possible.

### Can the patient return to a normal existence after an attack of diverticulitis?

Yes, except that he must be careful about his diet and his bowel function.

## COLITIS

### What is colitis?

Colitis is classified as functional or organic. Functional colitis includes the so-called "spastic colitis" and "mucous colitis." These are not instances of true inflammatory colitis but represent merely an irritable colon. Organic colitis is caused by true disease processes that are very serious indeed. Ulcerative colitis, amebic colitis, typhoid fever colitis, etc., fall into this category.

## SPASTIC (MUCOUS) COLITIS

### What is spastic, or mucous, colitis?

It is a condition in which the large bowel contracts violently and goes into spasm on the slightest provocation. Such bowel often secretes large quantities of mucus, which appear in the stool. Spastic and mucous colitis are also called *irritable colon*.

### What causes mucous, or spastic, colitis?

Functional disorders that are thought to be caused by emotional instability and as a reaction to undue stress.

### Who is most prone to develop colitis?

Young women and men who have deep-seated, unsolved emotional problems.

### What are the symptoms of mucous, or spastic, colitis?

a. Abdominal discomfort, flatulence, and vague crampy pains.

b. Irregular bowel habits, with alternating diarrhea and constipation.

c. Passage of a large amount of mucus in the stool.

### How does one make a diagnosis of spastic, or mucous, colitis?

It is very important to rule out more serious conditions, such as ulcerative colitis or a tumor of the bowel. This can be done by taking careful note of the symptoms, by examining the bowel through a sigmoidoscope or colonoscope, and by x-ray examination.

### What is the treatment for irritable colon (spastic, or mucous, colitis)?

a. It is important to treat the patient psychologically, and in certain cases, psychiatric help should be obtained.

b. It is important to discontinue the use of laxatives or enemas, as this will interfere with return to normal bowel function.

c. The patient must be instructed to develop regular eating habits and regular bowel habits. He must avoid highly seasoned food and alcohol in large quantities.

### Do people get well from spastic, or mucous, colitis?

Yes, but they tend to have recurrences under mental stress, when they have gone off their diet, or when they return to the use of laxatives or enemas.

### Is spastic, or mucous, colitis a dangerous condition?

No. People with these conditions can lead active normal lives despite their irritable colons.

### Does mucous colitis, or spastic colitis, lead to the formation of cancer?

No.

### Are the antispasmodic or tranquilizing medications helpful in the treatment of this condition?

Yes. These drugs often relieve the

spasm and permit the patient to develop regular bowel habits. The new tranquilizing drugs have also proved somewhat helpful in relieving emotional stress.

## CHRONIC ULCERATIVE COLITIS

### What is chronic ulcerative colitis?
A very serious inflammatory disease of the large bowel. It is accompanied by bouts of fever, anemia, bloody diarrhea, weakness, and a characteristic set of generalized symptoms, including joint aches and pains.

### What causes ulcerative colitis?
The cause is not definitely known, but many investigators feel that the disease is bacterial in origin. Emotionally disturbed people in their twenties or thirties are more prone to develop this condition than emotionally stable and older individuals.

### What are the symptoms of this condition?
Ulcerative colitis often has its onset in early youth or adulthood, with continuing diarrhea, abdominal cramps, and the appearance of blood and mucus in the stools. There may be as many as fifteen to twenty or even thirty movements a day. If this keeps up, the patient becomes markedly dehydrated, and develops high fever and a profound anemia.

### What is the usual course of ulcerative colitis?
The condition may continue for several weeks and then subside, only to appear again at a later date within the next few months or years.

### How is the diagnosis of ulcerative colitis made?
a. By noting the characteristic symptoms.
b. By examining the large bowel through the sigmoidoscope or colonoscope and noting the characteristic signs of inflammation and ulceration.
c. By noting characteristic x-ray findings.

### What is the treatment for ulcerative colitis?
a. In mild cases, medical management is advised. This includes a bland diet, antibiotic drugs, and the prescribing of cortisone or a similar medication. The majority of early cases subside under this regime.
b. In advanced or recurrent cases, surgery is often necessary. This may involve the removal of the entire large bowel. When this procedure is carried out, the small bowel (ileum) is brought out onto the abdomen in the form of a permanent ileostomy.

### What are the chances for recovery from a severe case of ulcerative colitis?
The chances are excellent, provided surgery is performed at an appropriate time on those patients who do not respond to medical treatment after a thorough trial.

### When the entire large bowel has been removed, will the patient always have an ileostomy opening on his abdomen?
Yes, but the great majority of patients learn to manage their ileostomy effectively.

### Is it ever possible to save the rectum when operating upon a case of ulcerative colitis?
In a small number of cases of ulcerative colitis, the rectum is not involved in the disease process and can be preserved. In some cases, although they are unfortunately not very many, the small bowel (ileum) can be stitched directly to the rectum at the time of the initial surgical procedure. In other cases, an ileostomy is performed at the initial procedure and the patient is permitted to make an operative recovery.

Then, some months or years later, if it is discovered that the rectum is completely free of the disease process, the ileostomy can be taken down and the ileum can be stitched to the rectum. It must be emphasized that this procedure cannot be performed on the great majority of those who must undergo surgery for ulcerative colitis.

### Will the patient with an ileostomy be able to lead a full life?
Yes. There are literally thousands of people with permanent ileostomies who go to business and perform all the functions that normal people perform.

### Is psychotherapy helpful in treating ulcerative colitis?
Yes, but only when the patient is seen early in the course of the disease.

### Is there any way to prevent ulcerative colitis?
No, but if prompt and early treatment is carried out, a great deal can be done to prevent the disease from getting worse.

### What may happen if surgery is not performed upon a patient with severe chronic ulcerative colitis?
a. Eventually, death may ensue from an acute attack that involves fever, dehydration, and uncontrollable diarrhea.
b. Cancer of the bowel will develop in a large percentage of those patients who have an active ulcerative colitis for more than ten years.

## COLITIS DUE TO BACTERIA OR PARASITES

### What types of colitis are caused by bacteria or parasites?
Dysentery may be caused either by bacteria (bacillary dysentery) or by an amebic parasite (amebic dysentery).

### How is dysentery contracted?

By drinking water or eating foods infected with the specific germs or parasites that cause the disease.

### Is there any way to prevent dysentery?

Yes, by avoiding improperly prepared foods when visiting foreign countries and by avoiding inferior restaurants where hygienic supervision of the employees is inadequate.

### Is there any effective treatment for dysentery?

Yes. Cure can be brought about by the administration of specific medications, provided they are given early in the course of the disease.

### Is dysentery a common form of colitis?

It is seen much more often within recent years because of increased travel to tropical countries. Also, members of the armed services who have been on overseas duty have contracted dysentery and have brought it back to this country.

### Can people recover completely from amebic or bacillary dysentery?

Yes, when treated early and intensively. If permitted to go untreated, there is a tendency toward the development of chronic dysentery and serious complications, including the formation of amebic abscesses within the liver or other organs.

### Is there a tendency for dysentery to recur?

If inadequately eradicated, recurrent attacks do take place.

## INTESTINAL OBSTRUCTION

### What is acute intestinal obstruction?

It is one of the most serious of all surgical conditions within the abdomen.

Intestinal obstruction is caused by an interference with the progressive advance of intestinal contents through the intestinal canal.

### What are the most common conditions that produce intestinal obstruction?

a. A tumor either inside or outside the bowel that presses upon and blocks the passageway.
b. Adhesions causing constriction of the bowel.
c. A twist of the large bowel, as in volvulus.
d. A loop of bowel becoming caught and obstructed within a hernia sac (strangulated hernia).

### What are the symptoms of intestinal obstruction?

a. Distention of the abdomen.
b. Inability to move the bowels and complete inability to pass gas.
c. Repeated episodes of vomiting.
d. Colicky abdominal pains.
e. Typical x-ray findings showing obstruction.

### Is intestinal obstruction always complete?

No. Partial obstruction takes place first. This will be evidenced by increasing constipation and abdominal distention over a period of several days.

### What happens when intestinal obstruction is not relieved?

The abdomen becomes greatly distended and vomiting becomes progressive until eventually the patient may vomit feces. Chemical balance is upset because of loss of intestinal juices, and death may result from overwhelming toxemia. In other instances, an overdistended bowel may rupture, causing a rapidly fatal peritonitis.

### Does intestinal obstruction ever disappear without surgery?

Yes, occasionally, if it is caused by a twist, kink, the telescoping of one

segment of bowel in another, or by an inflammation of the lining of the bowel. These conditions sometimes subside spontaneously, thus relieving the obstruction.

### What is the treatment for partial intestinal obstruction?

A tube is inserted through the nose and down through the stomach into the small intestine. By attaching this tube to a suction apparatus, the bowel is deflated and much of the fluid and gas is removed. To sustain the patient, fluids, sugar, and other necessary chemicals are given by intravenous injection.

### How is a definite diagnosis of intestinal obstruction made?

By noting the symptoms and by taking x rays. Intestinal obstruction of mechanical origin is suspected when one notes a scar on the abdomen from a previous operation. This may suggest that a loop of bowel is obstructed by a kink that has formed secondary to an adhesion.

### What type of operation is performed to cure intestinal obstruction?

If it is caused by an adhesion or kink, the obstructing tissue is severed with a scissors. If the obstruction is due to a tumor, that segment of the bowel must be removed.

### Is it ever necessary to perform more than one operation for acute intestinal obstruction?

Yes. The most important consideration is to relieve the obstruction as soon as possible. This often requires a preliminary colostomy, a procedure in which the bowel is brought out onto the abdominal wall, a small opening made into it, and feces permitted to drain from it.

### Is a permanent colostomy necessary following intestinal obstruction?

Usually not. After the obstruction has

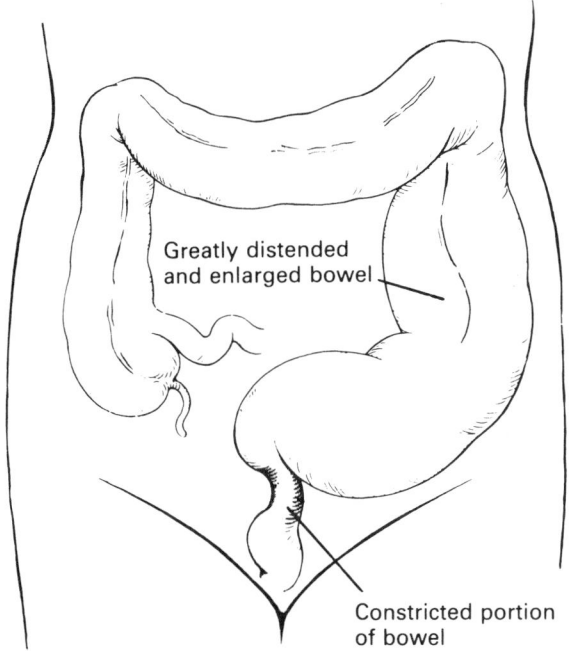

Greatly distended
and enlarged bowel

Constricted portion
of bowel

*Hirschsprung's Disease.* This is a condition present since birth, in which a constricted portion of the bowel prevents passage of stool in a normal fashion. As a result of this, the bowel above becomes markedly distended and enlarged. This disease can now be cured surgically by removing the constricted portion of bowel.

subsided, the surgeon will investigate the patient more thoroughly to discover the exact cause and the precise location of the obstruction. He will then reoperate, remove the underlying cause for the obstruction, and, at a subsequent date, close the colostomy and reestablish normal bowel continuity.

### What are the chances for recovery from complete intestinal obstruction?

The great majority operated upon within twenty-four to forty-eight hours after onset will recover. If the process has gone on for several days, many will die no matter what is done for them.

## HIRSCHSPRUNG'S DISEASE *(Megacolon)*

### What is megacolon or Hirschsprung's disease?

A condition, present since birth, in which the large bowel is tremendously enlarged and distended. A contracted portion, usually only a

few inches long, is found in the sigmoid part of the left colon and is thought to be the cause for the enlarged and distended bowel above.

### Why is a portion of the bowel constricted in megacolon?

It is thought that certain nerves, which give the bowel the ability to relax and dilate, are missing in this area of the bowel wall.

### In whom is megacolon seen?

In young children.

### What are the symptoms of megacolon?

a. Inability to move the bowels. Some children never have a normal bowel movement and can evacuate only when they receive an enema.
b. The abdomen in these children is tremendously distended due to the enlarged bowel.

### How is the diagnosis of megacolon made?

By noting the symptoms and by taking x rays that will reveal the characteristic picture of huge distention of

the bowel above an area of constriction.

### What is the treatment for Hirschsprung's disease?

The great majority of cases require surgery. The constricted segment of bowel is removed, and the bowel above is sutured to the rectum below.

### Is megacolon curable?

Yes, in almost all cases.

### Is this a dangerous operation?

No, but it is a very serious operation, as it involves removal of a segment of bowel.

### Is there a tendency for the condition to recur after surgery?

No. Almost all cases are cured permanently.

### Can a child lead a normal life after an operation for Hirschsprung's disease?

Yes. The physical and mental development following cure of this condition is astonishingly rapid.

## TUMORS OF THE SMALL AND LARGE INTESTINES

### Where are most tumors of the intestinal tract located?

The great majority occur in the large bowel. Small intestinal tumors are rare in comparison to large bowel tumors.

### What types of tumors exist in the intestinal tract?

a. The benign, noncancerous tumors, such as polyps or muscle tumors (myomas).
b. Cancer of the bowel or allied conditions such as lymphomas or sarcomas.

### Do the benign tumors of the bowel ever turn into cancer?

Yes. This is one of the main reasons

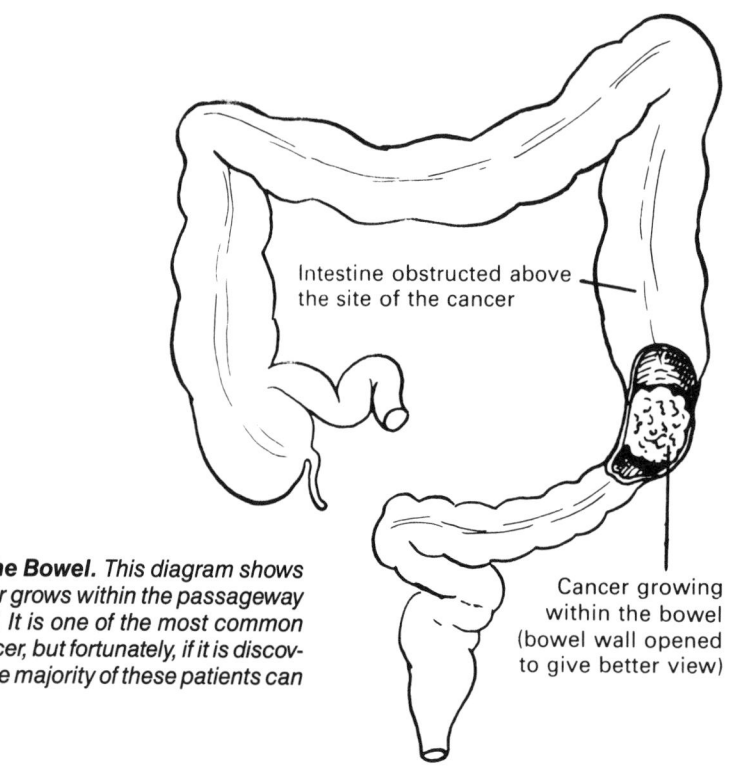

*Cancer of the Bowel. This diagram shows how a cancer grows within the passageway of the bowel. It is one of the most common forms of cancer, but fortunately, if it is discovered early, the majority of these patients can be saved.*

Intestine obstructed above the site of the cancer

Cancer growing within the bowel (bowel wall opened to give better view)

velopment of polyps and other precancerous lesions may run in families.

### How reliable are x rays in making a diagnosis of cancer of the bowel?

These tests are very accurate and will show a deformity of the lining of the bowel at the site of the tumor.

### What is the proper treatment for tumors of the bowel?

Surgery, as soon as a definite diagnosis is established.

### What kind of operations are performed for tumors of the bowel?

a. For the benign, noncancerous tumors, simple removal of the tumor at its base is all that is necessary.

why people with intestinal symptoms should consult their doctors promptly.

### How can one tell if he has a tumor within his bowel?

Bleeding from the rectum and a change in one's normal bowel habits are the two most reliable warning signs.

### Is there any way to prevent tumor formation?

No, but regular physical examinations, including a rectal examination and a sigmoidoscopic examination, are advisable whenever symptoms develop.

### What is a colonoscope?

It is a pliable, hollow, lighted instrument that enables the entire length of the large bowel to be visualized. Through it, polyps high up in the colon can be removed.

### How can one tell if he has a polyp?

Painless rectal bleeding is the most

characteristic sign. Larger polyps high in the large bowel may cause intermittent colicky pain or temporary episodes of obstruction.

### What is the treatment for polyps?

Those that are within ten inches of the anus can be removed through a sigmoidoscope, either in the surgeon's office or in a hospital. Those located higher up in the colon may be removed through a colonoscope or by opening the abdomen surgically.

### What is the incidence of cancer of the bowel?

It is one of the most common of all cancers!

### When is cancer of the bowel most likely to take place?

During the sixth and seventh decades of life.

### Does cancer of the bowel tend to run in families or to be inherited?

No, but a tendency toward the de-

*Tumor Removal. The tumor shown below will be removed along with the part of the intestine indicated between the dotted lines. The severed ends of the intestine are then sewn together.*

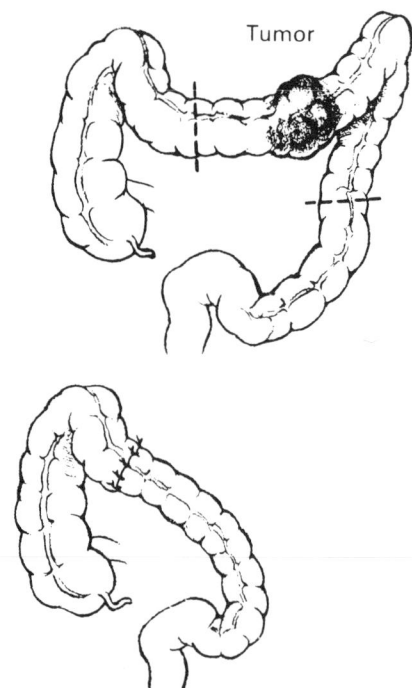

Tumor

b. Whenever possible, a malignant tumor, along with a generous portion of bowel above and below, is removed. The ends of normal bowel are then joined to one another above and below. If the passageway cannot be reestablished, an artificial opening (colostomy) is made on the abdominal wall. The surgeon's main goal is to remove the entire tumor even though this sometimes necessitates making a permanent artificial opening.

## Are operations for removal of bowel tumors serious?

Yes, but surgical recovery takes place in well over 95 percent of all cases.

## How often can a permanent cure be effected through surgery for cancer of the bowel?

The latest results show that more than 50 percent of all people will live for a period of five or more years after successful surgery for cancer of the bowel.

## Is there a tendency for growths within the bowel to recur?

The one that has been removed does not often recur, but in about 5 to 10 percent of cases, people will develop a tumor elsewhere within the bowel.

## How often should one go for a checkup after removal of a bowel tumor?

At least once every year, or at any time when new symptoms develop.

## How does the surgeon decide whether or not to make an artificial opening (colostomy)?

Whenever the bowel continuity can be reestablished, the surgeon will do so. However, he will never leave any tumor tissue behind if he can help it.

## Are all colostomies permanent?

No. Some are made merely to relieve the obstruction caused by a tumor of the bowel.

## When will a surgeon decide to close the colostomy?

When he knows that he can reestablish the normal passageway. This may take place several weeks or months after the original operation.

## Can one lead a normal life with a permanent colostomy?

Yes. The great majority of people learn how to control their colostomy so that it functions with almost the same kind of regularity as their normal rectum.

## Do people who have colostomies have an odor?

No. They learn how to keep their colostomies clean most of the time. Also, specially constructed bags are often placed over the opening to trap and destroy any odors.

## Can other people detect that a patient is wearing a colostomy bag or that he has a colostomy?

No. There are many thousands of people who enjoy all activities without discomfort to themselves or anyone around them.

## Can a patient live a normal life with a large portion of his bowel removed?

Digestion and nourishment can be normal even when the entire large bowel has been removed. Also, at least half of the small bowel can be removed and still permit normal nutrition.

## How can the surgeon distinguish between a benign tumor of the bowel and a malignant one?

The general appearance is impor-

tant, but tumors of the bowel are always subjected to microscopic examination. Such examination will reveal the exact nature of the growth.

## Can the examining surgeon always tell when a patient has a tumor of the bowel by examining the abdomen?

No. This is why it is so important to have x rays of the intestinal tract taken as a routine procedure whenever there are intestinal symptoms. Also, all people over forty-five years of age, whether they have symptoms or not, should undergo a gastrointestinal x-ray examination.

## Do tumors of the bowel ever take place in young people?

Yes. Occasional cases are seen in adults in their twenties or thirties.

## How long a hospital stay is necessary for surgery upon the large bowel?

These operations are among the most complicated of all surgery and may require several weeks of hospitalization. Very specialized preoperative and postoperative care is necessary, including preparation of the bowel with frequent cleansing enemas and the administration of antibiotic and chemotherapeutic drugs. These medications will prevent peritonitis from developing postoperatively.

## Is peritonitis a common complication of surgery upon the bowel?

It used to be years ago, but today, with the antibiotic drugs, the inside of the intestinal tract can be brought almost to a state of sterility. This permits the surgeon to operate in a clean field and relieves the fear of the development of postoperative peritonitis.

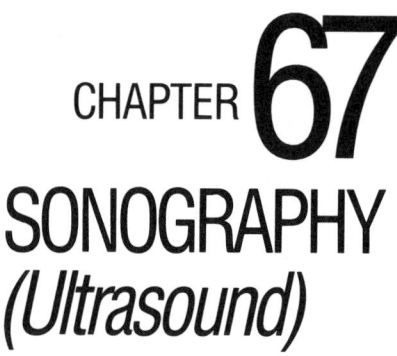

# CHAPTER 67

# SONOGRAPHY
# (Ultrasound)

## What is sonography?

Sonography is a diagnostic method based upon the reflection of ultrasonic waves that occur at the boundaries between different tissues within the body.

## Is ultrasonography the same as sonography?

Yes.

## How is sonography performed?

The patient lies on a table, and the ultrasound machine is placed over the part to be examined. There is a long arm of the sonograph, called a transducer, which is pressed against the skin and moved in various directions. Ultrasound waves are emitted from the transducer and enter the body. The waves bounce against internal structures and are reflected out and up through the transducer. The reflections are translated via a computer into actual images that can be seen on a viewing screen. Based upon these images, a diagnosis can be made. Polaroid photographs of the images are taken to serve as a permanent record of the sonographic findings.

## What creates the sonographic images?

The varying densities of the structures subjected to the ultrasound waves. This takes place in much the same way as x rays show light and dark shadows as they pass through structures of varying densities.

## Is sonography painful?

No. The test is completely noninvasive; no injections are given; nor is it necessary to swallow any medication prior to taking the test. However, large quantities of water should be drunk prior to having a sonogram of the pelvic organs, as it will lead to better images.

## Does the body react to the ultrasound waves that enter the body?

No.

## Is there any connection between the ultrasound waves and x rays, or x-ray radiation?

None whatsoever. The ultrasound waves are not x rays!

## Who interprets ultrasound examinations?

In most institutions, this is a function of the x-ray department. As a consequence, radiologists who are trained in interpreting variations in shadows usually interpret sonographic findings.

## Are there similarities in the appearance of sonographic pictures and those seen on x rays?

There is similarity in that both methods of investigation depend upon diagnosis of variations of shadows and outlines. However, the actual pictures do not look alike.

## Is sonography dangerous?

It is considered completely harmless.

## Is sonography valuable and safe for the evaluation of pregnancy?

Yes. It can do the following:
a. Tell the age of the pregnancy.
b. Tell whether the pregnancy is in the uterus or in the tube (ectopic pregnancy).
c. Tell whether the fetus is of normal size for the age of the pregnancy.

d. Tell the position of the fetus within the womb.
e. Tell whether the fetus is structurally normal, including whether its head is of normal size, whether all four limbs are present and normal, etc.
f. Tell the position of the placenta. This is very important in cases in which placenta previa is suspected. (See Chapter 57, on Pregnancy and Childbirth.)

## Can sonography tell the sex of the unborn child?

Occasionally, one can see the image of the male genitals on a sonogram. However, the child's sex is much more accurately foretold by performing amniocentesis.

## Has any harm ever come to a mother or baby through sonography?

No cases have been reported in which any harm has come either to mother or child through sonography.

## What are some of the major applications of sonography?

a. In denoting heart or lung abnormalities.
b. In noting tumors, cysts, or abscesses of the liver.
c. In diagnosing the presence of gallstones.
d. In spotting cysts, tumors, or other abnormalities of the pancreas.
e. In showing cysts, tumors, or malformations of the kidneys.
f. In diagnosing aneurysms or other abnormalities of the aorta.
g. In diagnosing enlarged lymph nodes (glands).
h. In spotting cysts or tumors within the abdominal cavity.
i. In diagnosing diseases of the pelvic organs such as cysts or tumors of the uterus, tubes, and ovaries.
j. In diagnosing various conditions in pregnancy as mentioned above.

## Is sonography helpful in diagnos-

**ing conditions within the skull or in conditions within bones?**

No. The ultrasound wave reflections are of no value in these conditions as they cannot penetrate the thick bones.

**Is sonography helpful in diagnos-**

**ing conditions within the stomach and intestinal tract?**

No.

**Will sonography replace the need for x rays?**

Most physicians think this will not occur. The two methods of investiga-

tion supplement and complement each other. However, in some instances such as gallstones, an x ray may become unnecessary if the condition is clearly demonstrated on sonography.

# CHAPTER 68
# THE SPLEEN

*See also Chapter 12 on Blood and Lymph Diseases; Chapter 73 on Transplantation Organs)*

## What is the spleen?

The spleen is a solid purple-colored gland, which is soft and elastic in consistency, located in the posterior portion of the abdomen on the upper left-hand side beneath the rib cage. It measures approximately five inches in length, three inches in width, and two inches in thickness.

## What is the function of the spleen?

It is a blood-lymph gland concerned with iron metabolism, blood cell storage, and the manufacture and destruction of blood cells. During development of the embryo, the spleen manufactures both red and white blood cells. After birth, this function is taken over by the bone marrow. During childhood, and to a lesser extent during adulthood, the spleen produces cells that help destroy bacteria and other inert particles that are brought to it by the bloodstream. It is also responsible for the destruction of old, worn-out red blood cells and for the storage of great quantities of blood, which it discharges into the bloodstream during times of strain or stress.

## What are some of the common diseases and disorders of the spleen?

a. Congenital hemolytic anemia (hemolytic jaundice). This condition is characterized by an enlarged spleen, anemia, and mild jaundice. It is thought to be the result of a defect in the structure of the red blood cells that makes them particularly susceptible to damage. Hemolytic anemia tends to run in families and makes its appearance during childhood.

b. Thrombocytopenic purpura. This is a common disease seen in young adults. It is diagnosed by the appearance of hemorrhagic areas in the skin, which appear like bruises, along with bleeding from the nose, gums, or vagina. This type of purpura is caused by a deficiency in blood platelets and by a prolongation of the bleeding time of the blood. (Platelets are necessary for normal blood clotting.)

c. Hypersplenism. This is a general classification for many disorders in which there is enlargement and overactivity of the spleen, as evidenced by excessive destruction of blood elements.

d. Tumors of the spleen. Benign tumors, cysts, or malignant tumors in the spleen are quite rare, but they do occur nevertheless.

e. Sickle cell anemia. This is an inherited anemia seen chiefly among black people. Diagnosis is made by noting that some of the red blood cells are sickle shaped.

f. Gaucher's disease. This is a chronic disease, running in families, accompanied by huge enlargement of the spleen. It is seen most often in young women.

g. Cooley's anemia, or Mediterranean anemia. This type is seen in childhood and manifests itself by a large hard spleen and by deformed red cells. There are also characteristic x-ray findings in the bones.

h. Rupture of the spleen. This is a common accident caused by a sudden, severe blow to the abdomen in the region of the spleen. Rupture of the spleen is accompanied by shock, evidences of hemorrhage, and tenderness in the upper left part of the abdomen.

## In what other conditions is the spleen found to be enlarged?

a. Leukemia.
b. Lymphoma.
c. Malaria.
d. Cirrhosis of the liver.
e. Thrombosis (clot) of the splenic vein.
f. Tuberculosis.
g. Infectious mononucleosis.
h. Bacterial endocarditis.
i. Certain virus infections.

## Does an enlarged or diseased spleen cause any symptoms?

If the enlargement is very great, it may cause pressure on other abdominal organs. Sometimes the spleen can grow to the size of a watermelon, and when this happens it produces a dragging, heavy sensation in the abdomen.

## How does an overactive spleen harm the patient?

It can result in excessive destruction of blood elements, with resultant anemia, insufficient white blood cells and blood platelets.

## How does one distinguish the various diseases of the spleen?

a. By a familial history of splenic diseases.
b. By the appearance of the blood on microscopic examination.
c. By other special blood tests.
d. By the appearance of the spleen on a radioactive scan.

## What are the harmful effects if diseases of the spleen are not treated?

a. Anemia may result in marked weakness, pallor, and shortness of breath.
b. Low white blood cell levels may result in serious infections.
c. Low blood platelet levels may lead to bleeding.

## Is there usually satisfactory medi-

**cal treatment for diseases of the spleen?**

No. It is often necessary to remove the spleen surgically to relieve some of the disorders affecting this organ. However, tuberculosis can sometimes be treated effectively with drugs, and malignancies can benefit from chemotherapy and radiation.

**Does an enlarged spleen always mean that surgery is necessary?**

No. Other factors, as determined by blood studies, are necessary to make this decision. Certain conditions, such as Hodgkin's disease,

leukemia, Gaucher's disease, and cirrhosis of the liver are seldom benefited by removal of the spleen.

**What conditions *are* benefited by removal of the spleen?**

a. Thrombocytopenic purpura.
b. Congenital and acquired hemolytic anemias.
c. Certain cases of hypersplenism.
d. Primary tumors of the spleen.
e. Rupture of the spleen.
f. Certain cases of malignant lymphoma (Hodgkin's disease).

**What conditions may occasionally**

**derive some benefit from removal of the spleen?**

a. Gaucher's disease.
b. Cooley's anemia.

**Does the size of the spleen determine the need for surgery?**

No. Some of the best results are obtained in cases in which the spleen is only slightly enlarged or not enlarged at all.

**When does removal of the spleen become an emergency procedure?**

When it has ruptured, surgery must be performed immediately as a

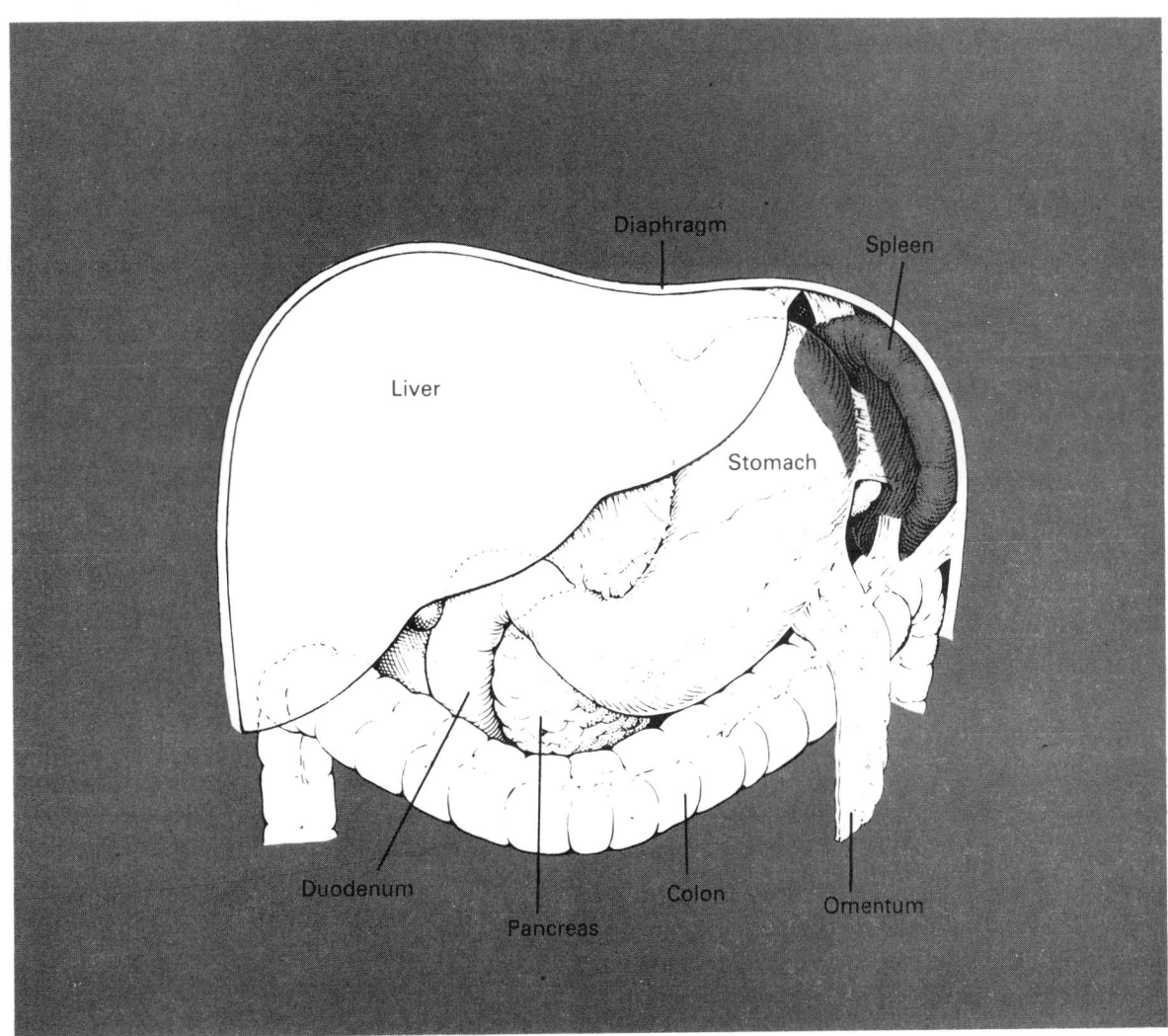

**Anatomical Relations of the Spleen.** *The spleen is an organ located in the upper left portion of the abdomen, beneath the ribs. During the life of the embryo, the spleen manufactures blood cells. After birth, it is concerned with the destruction of old, worn-out blood elements.*

lifesaving measure. Occasionally, the tear in the spleen can be sutured and the organ saved from removal.

### Is removal of the spleen a dangerous operation?

No. The mortality rate from this procedure is very low, except when performed upon patients who are in the terminal stages of their illness.

### When is it harmful to remove the spleen?

When its removal may lead to a lessening of the body's ability to fight off infection. This is especially important among small children.

### Will other structures within the body take over the functions of the spleen after it has been removed?

Yes. The bone marrow and certain cells called reticuloendothelial cells will perform some of the spleen's functions.

### Can people lead a normal life after removal of the spleen?

Yes, provided that the condition for which the spleen has been removed is alleviated. However, they must take special precautions to avoid infections, and when an infection does occur, they must be treated vigorously with antibiotic medication.

### Do diseases of the spleen often clear up by themselves, without treatment?

Yes, if the underlying cause for the splenic condition is cured, such as a bacterial or viral infection.

### What kind of anesthesia is used for operations to remove the spleen?

General inhalation anesthesia.

### What special preoperative preparations are necessary?

In certain cases, blood transfusions and vitamins will be given beforehand to fortify the patient. In other cases, it may be necessary to prepare the patient by giving him corti-sone or similar substances before, during, and for some time following surgery.

### How long does splenectomy (removal of the spleen) take to perform?

From three-quarters of an hour to two hours, depending upon the size of the organ and its adhesions to adjacent structures.

### Where is the incision made for removal of the spleen?

An incision five to eight inches long is made in the upper left portion of the abdomen.

### What special postoperative measures are necessary?

Blood studies must be carried out frequently to determine the progress of the patient. These studies may indicate what medications should be given. Blood transfusions, vitamins, and steroid medications such as cortisone are often administered postoperatively. In some instances, antibiotic medications are given for prolonged periods of time to ward off bacterial infections.

### How soon after splenectomy do bleeding tendencies disappear if the operation is successful?

This may take place immediately postoperatively, or within a few days.

### Are special nurses needed after operations upon the spleen?

Yes, for a few days.

### How soon after surgery can the patient get out of bed?

Within a day or two.

### Does the spleen ever grow back once it has been removed?

In performing a splenectomy, it is essential to determine the presence or absence of accessory spleens. The original spleen, once removed, will not grow back again, but accessory spleens may grow to a large size if not removed at the original operation.

### What are accessory spleens?

These are small structures, usually no larger than a nickel or a dime, which are identical in structure to the spleen and are located in the vicinity of the spleen. They are found in a small percentage of all normal people.

### Are there any permanent aftereffects of removal of the spleen?

Yes, but usually they do not interfere with the patient's leading a normal life.

### Is it safe to become pregnant after removal of the spleen?

Yes, unless the spleen has been removed in the hope of improving a condition that still persists in the body.

### How soon after removal of the spleen can one do the following:

Leave the hospital:
Ten to twelve days.
Bathe:
Ten to twelve days.
Walk out on the street:
Ten days.
Walk up and down stairs:
Ten days.
Perform household duties:
Six weeks.
Drive a car:
Six weeks.
Resume sexual relations:
Six weeks.
Return to work:
Eight weeks.
Resume all physical activities:
Eight to ten weeks.

### Should a patient be rechecked periodically after removal of the spleen?

Yes. It is especially important to have the blood examined every few weeks after the spleen has been removed.

Such studies will reveal whether the anemia has been alleviated and whether normal blood production and destruction have been resumed. Bone marrow studies will also be carried out to obtain further information on blood cell production. It is very important that children who have undergone splenectomy be safeguarded against infections as the chances of complicating blood poisoning are increased greatly.

### What is a splenic puncture?

It is a diagnostic procedure performed to make a specific diagnosis of a disease within the spleen.

### How is a splenic puncture carried out?

A long needle is inserted, under local anesthesia, through the lower left chest wall directly into the spleen. The needle is attached to a syringe and the plunger is pulled out, thus causing some of the splenic cells to pass up through the needle into the syringe. These cells are then sent to the pathology laboratory for microscopic examination.

### Is splenic puncture a dangerous procedure?

Not when carried out by one familiar with the technique.

### What is the special value of a diagnostic splenic puncture?

There are many cases of splenic disease in which blood examination and examination of the bone marrow will not reveal the exact diagnosis. In certain of these cases, a final conclusion can be determined only through examination of spleen tissue itself.

# CHAPTER 69

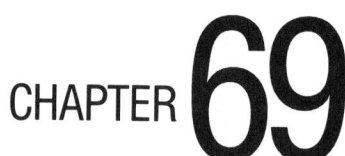

# STERILITY, FERTILITY, AND MALE POTENCY

*(See also Chapter 25 on Female Organs; Chapter 57 on Pregnancy and Childbirth; Chapter 64 on Sex)*

### What is sterility?

Sterility is the inability to reproduce. Since this definition connotes an absolute and irreversible state, it is more appropriate to use the term *infertility*. Infertility indicates a more temporary state that may, under certain circumstances, be reversed.

First-degree sterility relates to those couples who have failed to conceive after at least one year of effort. Second-degree sterility refers to those couples who have had one or more children and have then failed to conceive after repeated attempts over a prolonged period of time.

### How often does sterility occur among married couples?

Although there are no absolutely accurate statistics, it is estimated that approximately one out of every five marriages fails to produce a living offspring.

### How long does it take the average couple to conceive for the first time?

Pregnancy will usually take place within a year, providing the couple has intercourse two to three times weekly and refrains from using con-traceptive measures. The wife who conceives within the first month or two after trying is not the average woman. It is not at all unusual for normal young people to try for eight to ten months before being successful.

### Must a woman have an orgasm for conception to take place?

No! Climax plays no role whatsoever in conception.

### What factors are necessary for pregnancy to take place?

The woman must produce an egg from her ovaries; the Fallopian tubes must be open; healthy sperm must reach the egg while it is in the Fallopian tubes; there must be a place within the lining of the uterus for implantation of the fertilized egg; the woman must produce the proper hormones to nourish the fertilized, implanted egg.

## FEMALE STERILITY

### What are some of the common causes of sterility (infertility) in women?

a. Failure to ovulate or produce an egg. This can be the result of a congenital defect in the chromosomes, such as is seen in Turner's syndrome, or it can be due to an acquired abnormality in a female who is structurally normal.
b. Blocked Fallopian tubes, either due to infection or to a birth deformity in which the tubes are obstructed.
c. Glandular imbalance, particularly involving the pituitary gland, the thyroid, the adrenal glands, or the ovaries.
d. Failure of the sperm to pass through the cervix and up into the uterus. This may be caused by obstruction or infection at the cervix, the entrance to the womb.
e. Psychological factors, often elu-sive, vague, and difficult to evaluate. It has been known, however, that some sterile women will be able to conceive after a period of psychotherapy.
f. There is a large group of women who fail to conceive without any discernible cause. In view of the fact that scientists are learning more all the time about the nature of chromosomes, genes, and cellular structure, it is quite likely that this group will be understood more fully, and many additional reasons for sterility will be found.

### Must all of these factors be present to prevent conception?

Obviously, no. These factors may exist singly or in combination. It must be understood that infertility is a relative term and that minimal degrees of a number of factors can be as effective in causing sterility as one major factor.

### What is the "fertile period" of the month?

The middle of the menstrual cycle, when ovulation takes place. In a twenty-eight-day cycle, this is usually about twelve to sixteen days after the onset of the menstrual period.

### What is the "barren period" of the month?

Seven to nine days before the menstrual period, during the menstrual period, and the three to five days immediately following the menstrual period, depending upon the cycle and length of menstruation.

### During how many days of the month is conception possible?

Since healthy sperm must be deposited in the vagina within two days before ovulation and not longer than two days after ovulation, it is obvious that out of the entire cycle of twenty-eight days, fertilization of an egg can occur on only three to four of those days.

### Can one determine the "fertile period" and the "barren period" accurately?

In a woman who menstruates regularly, these periods can be determined with some accuracy by studying the basal body temperature charts from day to day.

### If a woman fails to ovulate, how is this fact recognized?

a. By taking a careful menstrual history and noting any irregularities.
b. By recording basal temperatures over a period of several months, a definite curve will develop which will show whether or not the patient is ovulating.

c. By taking a biopsy of the lining membrane of the uterus just before the expected date of menstruation, the gynecologist can tell whether ovulation is present or absent.
d. Vaginal smears can be studied microscopically to reveal whether ovulation has taken place.

### Can a woman be successfully treated if she fails to ovulate?

Yes. In the majority of cases, a glandular study will reveal the cause for failure to ovulate and will point the way toward the proper hormonal treatment. This will involve a careful study of the activity of the pituitary

gland, the thyroid gland, the adrenal glands, and the ovaries.

### What treatment is given a woman who fails to ovulate because of a glandular problem?

She is given a hormone called Clomid. This is very effective in causing ovulation.

### How is a biopsy of the lining of the uterus (endometrial biopsy) performed?

This is an office procedure performed on an examining table. A speculum is inserted into the vagina and the cervix is grasped with a clamp. A small metal instrument is

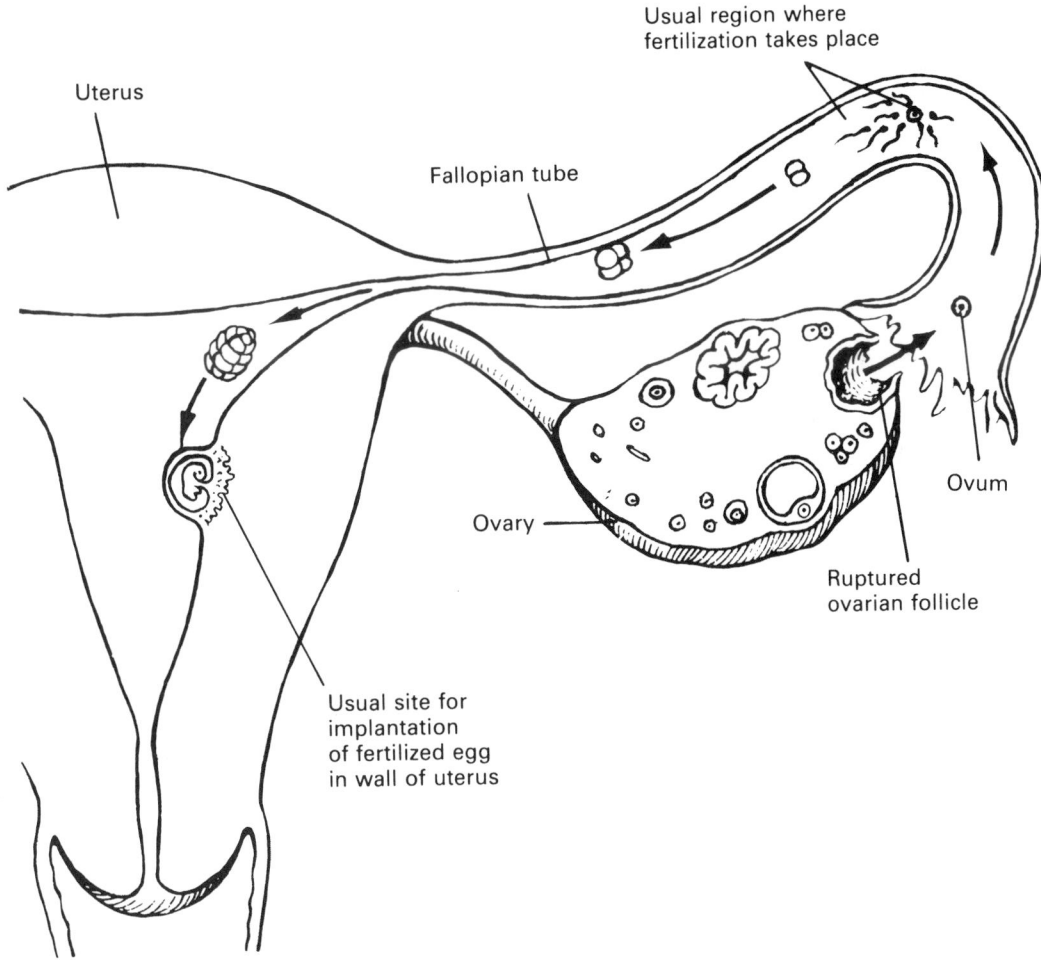

*Fertilization of an Egg by a Sperm.* This diagram demonstrates the route that sperm travel in order to reach the egg in the Fallopian tube. After fertilization has taken place in the tube, the egg descends to the uterus, where it implants in the uterine wall.

then inserted through the cervix into the uterus and the lining is scraped.

### Is the taking of an endometrial biopsy a painful procedure?

There is slight discomfort, but it takes only a few minutes to perform and has no unpleasant aftereffects.

### What precautions should be taken before doing an endometrial biopsy?

It is important to determine that the patient is not pregnant at the time the biopsy is taken. For this reason, abstinence is advised from the time of the previous menstrual period until the time the biopsy is taken. This is necessary because an early pregnancy would be disturbed by an endometrial biopsy.

### Will the patient bleed for two or three days after the taking of an endometrial biopsy?

Yes.

### What are the common causes of blocked Fallopian tubes?

a. Previous inflammation of the pelvic organs, most frequently caused by gonorrhea, tuberculosis, or some other germ.
b. Peritonitis, most often secondary to a ruptured appendix.
c. Spasm of the Fallopian tubes due to tension and emotional factors.
d. A fibroid in the upper portion of the uterus, which shuts off the entrance of the Fallopian tubes.
e. Endometriosis.

### How are blocked tubes diagnosed?

a. By performing the Rubin test. This involves the pumping of a gas (carbon dioxide) through the cervix into the uterine cavity and noting that the gas has entered the abdominal cavity.
b. By an x-ray examination involving the insertion of a radiopaque dye into the cervix to outline the uterine cavity and tubes (hysterogram).

### How is the Rubin test performed?

As an office procedure, the patient is instructed to report about five to seven days after a menstrual period. On the examining table, the cervix is exposed and grasped with a clamp. A thin tubular instrument is inserted into the cervical canal. One end of this tubular instrument is attached to a container of carbon dioxide and to a recording machine. By the proper use of the valves, carbon dioxide is administered and passed up into the uterus at known pressures. The only outlet for this gas is through the Fallopian tubes into the abdominal cavity. If the tubes are open, the gas escapes into the abdominal cavity and the pressure recorded on the machine falls. If the gas does not go into the abdominal cavity, the pressure on the machine is maintained or is elevated. By listening through the abdominal wall with a stethoscope, the escape of gas through the tubes can actually be heard.

### If the tubes are open, will the patient experience pain from the Rubin test?

Yes. The gas entering the abdominal cavity often produces pain in the shoulder region within five to ten minutes. This pain will subside in a short time and is not serious.

### Is there any danger to the Rubin test?

If proper precautions are taken, there is little chance of anything going wrong with this test. In occasional cases, an inflammatory disease within the Fallopian tubes may be aggravated by this procedure.

### Can a patient resume sexual relations following a Rubin test?

Not until two days after the test has been performed.

### How is a hysterogram performed?

This test is performed in essentially the same manner as the Rubin test, except that the radiopaque dye is in-serted through the cervix, and the results are obtained by taking an x-ray picture.

### What precautions should be taken before a hysterogram is performed?

It must be ascertained that no infection exists within the vagina, uterus, or tubes.

### Can blocked tubes ever be opened?

Yes, an operation known as tuboplasty is successful in reopening tubes in approximately 20 percent of cases, providing the lining of the tubes has not been damaged by previous infection. Occasionally, performance of the Rubin test itself, by expanding the tubes, will overcome the blockage.

### What can be done if the blocked tubes are due to spasm or emotional factors?

The giving of antispasmodic medications and the treatment of the patient's emotional problems will often result in the release of sperm and in the opening of the tubes.

### How does glandular or hormonal imbalance cause infertility?

By preventing ovulation or by failing to produce a proper atmosphere for the implantation of the fertilized egg in the wall of the uterus.

### Are there any specific tests to note the presence or absence of glandular imbalance?

Yes. Hormone studies can be carried out by specific tests upon the urine and blood. Also, chemical analyses may give a clue to the existence of glandular disturbance.

### Can glandular imbalance be overcome?

Yes, in some cases, by appropriate treatment with hormones. An endocrinologist can best handle this type of case.

**Does the cervix often block the passage of healthy sperm into the uterus?**

Yes. This occurs frequently when the cervix is infected or blocked by the presence of thick mucus.

**Are there any tests to determine the ability of the sperm to penetrate the cervix?**

Yes. The Huhner test is performed by examining the sperm after they have been deposited in the vagina. The patient comes to the office about two hours after intercourse, and samples from the vaginal canal and from the cervix are taken and are examined under a microscope. Where a normal sperm analysis exists, a comparison of the sperm in the vagina and in the cervix will give a clue as to the ability of the sperm to penetrate into the uterus.

**Should a woman remain in bed, lying on her back, for ten to fifteen minutes after intercourse if she desires to become pregnant?**

Yes, in order to give the sperm adequate time to penetrate the cervix.

**If the failure of the sperm to pass through the cervix is due to an infection of the cervix, can this situation be corrected?**

Yes, by cauterizing the cervix and by using antibiotics to get rid of the infection.

**Is conception ever interfered with by a vagina that is too acid?**

Yes. This is sometimes overcome by taking an alkaline douche with bicarbonate of soda before intercourse.

**Do fibroids of the uterus ever cause infertility?**

Yes, when the fibroids are located just beneath the lining of the uterus (submucous). Also, if the fibroids block the entrance to the Fallopian tubes, the sperm may not be able to reach the egg.

**Do cysts of the ovaries ever cause infertility?**

Yes, when the cyst is the type that results from, or causes an upset in, hormone production and balance. Pregnancy will often occur when such cysts are removed surgically.

**If infertility is thought to be due to emotional factors, how can it be treated?**

In many cases of this kind, psychotherapy has proven of great value and is often followed by conception.

**Is sterility in a woman often caused by the prolonged use of contraceptive jellies?**

No. It has never been proved that the use of these substances will interfere with conception, once they have been discontinued.

**Will the prolonged use of contraceptive pills interfere with subsequent ability to conceive?**

Usually not, but in an occasional case the prolonged use of the pill may be associated with decreased conceptive ability for a few months after stopping the medication.

**Can sterility result from "overindulgence" in intercourse?**

No, but men with low sperm counts should have intercourse no more than twice weekly.

**What is meant by artificial insemination?**

It is the introduction of live sperm, either the husband's or a donor's, in the vicinity of the cervix.

**When is artificial insemination employed?**

a. In cases where the Huhner test reveals that the husband's sperm (even though healthy) are not being deposited into the cervix, the sperm are collected and are deposited into the cervix by the gynecologist.

b. In cases in which the husband is sterile—that is, he possesses no live healthy sperm—and husband and wife consent, a sperm donor is employed.

**How is artificial insemination carried out?**

The patient reports to the office at an appointed time. She is placed on an examining table and a speculum is inserted into the vagina. Live sperm, taken either from the husband or from a donor, are injected with a syringe into the opening of the cervix. A small rubber cap that fits the cervix is then placed over the cervix to keep the sperm in contact with the cervix for a period of approximately a half hour.

**At what time of the month is artificial insemination carried out?**

When it has been determined by investigation that the patient is ovulating.

**How often is artificial insemination attempted?**

During one menstrual cycle, it should be done approximately three times. These should be just before, during, and after the ovulation date. This procedure should be repeated every month for four to six months.

**How often is artificial insemination successful?**

In a high proportion of cases, provided the female is physically normal.

**How is a sperm donor selected?**

The donor must be a healthy male who has been examined and found free of disease. A thorough history should be obtained to make sure that the donor's family is free from inherited physical or mental disease. (Such donors are usually recruited from college students, medical students, or interns.) The donor must remain anonymous to the couple! The couple must also remain anonymous to the donor! Complete accord must be reached, and consent must be given by husband, wife, and donor in writing, preferably in the presence of an attorney.

### What are the dangers involved in artificial insemination?

There are no physical dangers, but there may be some emotional injury to the husband when a donor is used. There may also be legal or religious entanglements, and these should be considered very carefully before artificial insemination is embarked upon.

## MALE STERILITY (Infertility)

### Is the male an important factor in sterility?

Yes. Any attempt to overcome infertility that does not have the complete cooperation of the male is worthless and should not be undertaken. *About 30 to 40 percent of all infertile marriages are due to failure of the male, not the female!* Complete studies of the husband must be carried out by the urologist in all cases of infertile marriages.

### What constitutes sterility in the male?

A sterile man is one who either has no sperm or has an insufficient number of normal, active sperm to make conception possible.

### What is the difference between sterility and infertility in the male?

Sterility implies an absolute impossibility of conception or fertilization. In the male, this would be a situation in which there are no sperm to ejaculate. On the other hand, infertility suggests that conception and fertilization are possible but not likely because of poor semen.

### What is a sperm count?

The ejaculate, which usually amounts to about a teaspoonful, normally contains upward of sixty million sperm per cubic centimeter. This count is obtained by microscopic examination of the ejaculate.

### Are there any other features of the ejaculate that are important to examine?

Yes. The motility of the sperm, as well as their anatomical appearance and characteristics (morphology), is important to note.

### What are the common causes of absence of sperm?

a. There are some developmental abnormalities in males that may cause them to be born without the ability to produce sperm. Such conditions have just recently been discovered through study of chromosomes and genes.

b. Old age is often accompanied by the loss of the ability of the testicle to produce sperm. This varies widely among individual men and may not have its onset in some until the eighth or ninth decades of life.

c. Orchitis, an inflammation of the testicle, may result in loss of sperm production. This is not uncommon following an attack of mumps in an adult. Other infections can also cause this form of male sterility.

d. Sperm may be absent because there is an interference with their migration from the testicle to the ejaculate. A previous infection, such as gonorrhea, may cause blockage of the passageway (the vas deferens) from the testicle to the seminal vesicle.

e. Of course, when the testicles are absent or are undescended (see Chapter 42, on Male Organs), no sperm will be produced.

### How can one tell whether the testicles are capable of producing sperm?

By careful examination of the semen. In some cases, if additional information is needed, a biopsy of the testicle is performed.

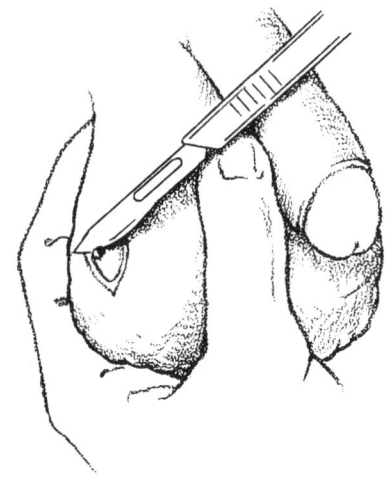

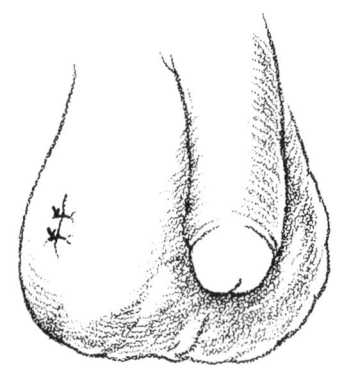

*Testicular Biopsy.* Through a small opening in the scrotum, a snip of testicular tissue is removed for biopsy in order to determine whether infertility has resulted from damage to the testicle. The incision in the scrotum is then sutured as shown in the bottom diagram.

### How is a biopsy of the testicle performed?

It is done in an operating room of a hospital under light general anesthesia. A small incision is made in the skin of the scrotum and through this a small piece of testicle is snipped away and is submitted for microscopic examination.

### What causes a low or reduced sperm count?

A natural reduction in the sperm content of the ejaculate follows frequent intercourse, a generalized debilitating disease, surgical operations, or any situation that temporarily weakens or depresses body activities. Low sperm counts of this type may be of a temporary nature. In other cases, however, men who are perfectly normal in all other respects may have low sperm counts.

### What are the most common causes of a reduced sperm count?

a. Glandular or endocrine disorders.
b. Inflammation of the testicles secondary to mumps, gonorrhea, tuberculosis, or other diseases.
c. Diseases of the testicles that result in their shrinkage (atrophy), such as interference with their circulation, etc.
d. Old age.
e. Elevated temperature of the scrotum over prolonged periods of time.
f. The presence of a varicocele.
g. Unknown causes.

### Can a sterile male be potent?

Yes. One thing has nothing to do with the other.

### Is treatment of sterility in the male ever successful?

Yes, in certain cases. When the problem is one of a low sperm count, various types of hormone treatments are available to raise the count. If a varicocele is present, surgery to correct the condition results in fertility in more than 50 percent of cases. Recently it has been found that prolonged lowering of the temperature of the testicles may produce marked increase in the sperm count and thus may overcome sterility.

### Is treatment for male sterility always successful?

No, and the results are often unpredictable. However, treatment should always be carried out because in a certain percentage of cases, pregnancy will result.

### Are there other methods for treating male sterility?

Yes. Any local disease should be eradicated. If there is an infection or a constriction of the urethra, this should be attended to. If there is an inflammation of the prostate gland, this must be corrected. If there is any disease within the scrotum, such as a hydrocele, this should be treated surgically. If impotence exists, it should receive treatment.

### How is it that parties to an infertile union, with no apparent abnormality on examination, will sometimes become divorced, remarried, and become fertile?

In some matings, despite the fact that each partner is found to be physically sound, there is a psychological or chemical barrier to conception. When such people remarry, subsequent circumstances may be such that these barriers no longer exist, and pregnancy results.

### At what age do most men become infertile?

This varies markedly. Some men remain fertile throughout their entire lives, even into the eighth and ninth decades of life. Some, due to congenital conditions, never become fertile at any time in their lives.

## POTENCY AND IMPOTENCE

### What is impotence?

The inability to consummate the sexual act.

### How common is impotence?

Impotence occurs many times during the life of the normal male. Such episodes are usually transient and pass spontaneously. True, continued impotence may be due to psychological disturbance, to long-standing diabetes, to arteriosclerosis of the vessels supplying the penis, or to the aging process.

### What percentage of cases of impotence is due to psychological disturbances?

It was thought until recently that im-

potence in approximately 90 percent of the cases was psychological in origin. However, it is now known that a much greater percentage is caused by organic diseases such as arteriosclerosis, diabetes, etc.

### Are potency and male sterility related?

No.

### What are some of the common causes of impotence?

a. Psychological disturbances.
b. Aging, resulting in poor blood supply to the penis.
c. Local disease of the genital organs.

### Can a man be potent yet sterile?

Yes. Many men are able to effect intercourse in a normal manner, but their semen contains no live sperm. Such men are potent but sterile.

### At what age do men usually become impotent?

If the man is healthy, both psychologically and physically, he may remain potent far into his seventies and eighties. Of course, if he is not attracted toward a particular female, he may become impotent at any age, even in his twenties or thirties.

### Will giving male hormones overcome impotence?

Only in the occasional cases in which the testicles are so damaged that they secrete no male sex hormones.

### Are premature ejaculations a sign of real impotence?

No. In such cases there is no inability to attain an erection. It is a psychological condition that can be overcome through proper advice and treatment by a psychiatrist or urologist.

### Will "overindulgence" in sex lead to premature impotence?

No. There is no proof that the sexual

activity of the male will have any organic effect upon the age at which he becomes impotent.

### What are some of the methods of treating impotence?

a. If the condition has been determined to be psychological in origin, then psychotherapy should be instituted.

b. If the condition is definitely shown to be of glandular origin (very rare), then hormones should be given.

c. If the impotence is due to arteriosclerosis of the vessels supplying the penis or to psychological problems that have not been solved despite intensive therapy, then one of two procedures may be carried out:

1. A plastic implant can be inserted surgically into the penis. One type affords the patient a permanent erection, sufficient to permit intercourse; the other type of implant is attached to a pump mechanism whereby the patient can force sufficient silicone into the penis so as to maintain an erection during the period of intercourse.

2. Operations have been devised to transfer an artery from the abdominal wall to the penis, thus increasing its blood supply sufficiently to permit intercourse.

### Is there a real male menopause?

It is commonly believed that there is a period in a man's life during which he has menopausal changes, but this may not be medically true. The age at which men become impotent, or at which they become infertile (sterile), varies widely. And the two conditions may be unrelated to each other. In other words, a man may lose his potency at an early age but may remain fertile far into his later years. Conversely, a man may be potent long after he has reached seventy or so years of age, but may have a very low or nonexistent sperm count,

### Are operations successful in overcoming impotence?

a. The use of plastic implants has proved highly successful in a large number of cases.

b. Operations to improve the blood supply to the penis are still in the experimental stage.

# CHAPTER 70

# THE STOMACH AND DUODENUM

*(See also Chapter 23 on Esophagus; Chapter 27 on Gall Bladder and Bile Ducts; Chapter 40 on Liver; Chapter 49 on Pancreas; Chapter 66 on Small and Large Intestines; Chapter 79 on X ray)*

## What is the stomach?

The stomach is a hollow, pouchlike structure lying beneath the diaphragm under the ribs on the left side of the abdomen. The empty stomach is a sac measuring about six to eight inches in length by three to four inches in width.

## What is the function of the stomach?

It is a common misconception that the stomach digests most of our foods. Its main function is to churn the food we have swallowed and to break it down into smaller particles. Its acid juice merely initiates digestion; the more important phases of digestion take place in the small intestine. Very little is absorbed directly through the stomach wall, except certain minerals, water, and alcohol.

## What are the most common conditions affecting the stomach?

a. Chronic dyspepsia (indigestion).
b. Hyperacidity (too much acid).
c. Acute gastritis.
d. Chronic gastritis.
e. Ulcer.
f. Pyloric stenosis (obstruction of the stomach outlet).
g. Upside-down stomach (diaphragmatic hernia).

h. Benign tumors.
i. Cancer.

## Where is the duodenum?

The duodenum is that segment of the small intestine extending for several inches immediately beyond the stomach. It is considered along with the stomach because conditions affecting the stomach so often affect the duodenum, too.

## What is the function of the duodenum?

The wall of the duodenum manufactures juices (enzymes) that help digest foods. It is also the portion of small intestine into which the bile is deposited and the segment where the pancreatic juices empty.

## What are the most common diseases of the duodenum?

a. Inflammation of the duodenum (duodenitis).
b. Duodenal ulcer.

## Do diseases of the stomach or duodenum tend to run in families or to be inherited?

No.

## What kind of person is most likely to develop trouble in the stomach or duodenum?

The energetic, nervous, neurotic type in the twenties, thirties, or forties. Men more commonly have stomach or duodenal trouble than women.

## Is there any method to minimize stomach trouble?

Yes. To lead a well-ordered, sensible, adjusted life and to eat a moderate, bland diet at regular meal times. Excessive smoking and drinking, too, react badly on the stomach in certain people.

## What are the most common symptoms of trouble in the stomach or duodenum?

a. Heartburn.

b. Belching.
c. Nausea.
d. Vomiting.
e. Pain high in the abdomen.
f. Loss of appetite.
g. Weight loss.

## How does the physician make a precise diagnosis of stomach or duodenal disease?

a. By taking a careful history of the exact symptoms.
b. By fluoroscopic and x-ray examination, with the swallowing of barium to visualize the lining of the stomach and duodenum.
c. By passing a tube and analyzing stomach and duodenal contents.
d. By looking directly at the stomach and duodenal linings through an *endoscope*, a flexible instrument with mirrors in it. The endoscope is passed through the mouth down into the stomach.

## Can the eating of improper foods and poor dietary habits lead to stomach and duodenal disease?

Yes, if continued over a prolonged period of time.

## Is it true that certain combinations of foods, such as ice cream and pickles, will cause stomach upsets?

Not necessarily. It depends upon individual tolerance to certain foods.

## Is it true that certain combinations of foods will cause "food poisoning"?

No. Food must be spoiled or infected to cause food poisoning.

## Can one eat normally when part of the stomach has been removed?

Yes, but the amount of food should be reduced somewhat and the frequency of feedings increased.

## Can one live a normal life if part of the stomach has been removed?

Yes. This occurs frequently when one has had a gastrectomy (removal of part of the stomach) for ulcer. (See the section on Peptic Ulcer in this chapter.)

**Is it true that emotional instability, overwork, or worry can cause stomach trouble?**

Definitely, yes. There is a marked psychic factor in conditions of the stomach and duodenum.

## INDIGESTION *(Dyspepsia)*

**What are the common symptoms of indigestion?**

A sense of fullness in the upper abdomen, heartburn, acid regurgitation of food, nausea, and vomiting.

**What is heartburn?**

A sensation of burning in the upper abdomen that ascends to the chest. Also, there is the taste of sour food in the back of the throat due to regurgitation of food from the stomach up into the esophagus.

**What causes indigestion?**

a. Excess secretion of stomach juices and acid.
b. Eating too much.
c. Eating too rapidly.
d. Eating improperly prepared foods.
e. Eating too highly seasoned foods.
f. Eating the wrong foods, such as those containing too much fat, grease, etc.
g. Eating infected or spoiled foods.
h. Drinking too much alcohol.

**What is the treatment for indigestion?**

a. Fasting for several hours, or even for an entire day.
b. Eating a light bland diet.
c. Taking one of the innumerable medications that will neutralize excess secretion of stomach juices and acidity.
d. The administration of one of the antispasmodic medications to cut down on excess contractions of the stomach and duodenum.

**Is it true that certain people are immune to the symptoms of indigestion and upset stomach?**

Certain people tend to have "stronger stomachs" than others. Nevertheless, if improper food intake occurs or if infected material is eaten, even the strongest stomach can react violently!

**Is it a good practice for someone to make himself vomit when his stomach feels upset?**

If this can be done without too much distress, it is often good treatment to empty the stomach when it is upset.

**Are the terms "acute gastritis," "upset stomach," and "acute indigestion" really used to describe the same condition?**

Yes, although some people erroneously associate the term "acute indigestion" with a heart attack.

**What are the symptoms of an upset stomach?**

Nausea, vomiting, cramps in the upper abdomen, loss of appetite. These occur usually within an hour or two after eating something that disagrees with the patient.

**How can one differentiate between an upset stomach and a more serious condition such as appendicitis, a gall bladder attack, or a heart attack?**

This is frequently difficult, and all people who have severe upper abdominal pain should contact their physician. Self-treatment is unwise if one has these symptoms.

**Is it safe to take a laxative for an upset stomach or acute indigestion?**

No, unless advised by your doctor.

**When should one call a doctor for abdominal pain?**

a. Whenever the pain is severe and the patient feels unable to tolerate it.

b. Whenever the pain persists for more than a few hours.

**Are there any particular foods that are more apt to cause indigestion than others?**

Yes; spoiled foods or foods that have been allowed to stand out in an open kitchen for several hours in hot weather (such as salads). Also, highly seasoned and greasy foods.

**Is it true that certain foods cannot be eaten with other foods because they are incompatible?**

No. This is a common misconception.

**Is the drinking of liquids at mealtime a bad habit?**

On the contrary, it aids digestion.

**Should one avoid heavy meals before going to sleep at night?**

Yes. It is best to permit all the organs of the body to rest during sleep.

**Should one eat more lightly in hot weather than in cold weather?**

Yes.

**Is it a poor idea to eat a heavy meal immediately before swimming?**

Yes, because the blood flow is diverted to the digestive tract instead of serving the muscular system, where it is most needed at such times. However, it has not been proved that eating before swimming will cause cramps and thus endanger the life of the swimmer.

**How great a part do the emotions play in indigestion?**

A very strong part. Every conceivable abdominal or intestinal symptom can be caused by emotional upset.

**Is it true that a person tends to have more stomach trouble as he grows older?**

Yes.

**Are there certain foods that must**

be avoided when drinking alcoholic beverages?

No. It is an erroneous notion that certain foods will cause violent upset if taken along with an alcoholic beverage. Of course, an upset stomach may follow drinking excessive quantities of alcohol no matter what food is taken along with it.

**Is it harmful to take iced drinks when one is overheated?**

No, except when large amounts are taken rapidly.

## STOMACH ACIDITY

**Does the normal stomach contain acid?**

Yes. Hydrochloric acid is secreted by the cells of the stomach in order to aid digestion.

**Will excess stomach acids cause symptoms?**

Yes. It is thought that excess acid is an important factor in the formation of an ulcer of the stomach or duodenum. Excess acid may also be associated with heartburn, inflammation of the stomach lining (gastritis), or inflammation of the duodenum (duodenitis).

**Will lack of acid in the stomach cause symptoms?**

Usually not, as the acid is not essential to normal digestion. On the other hand, in later life, a lack of acid is thought to make one slightly more prone to the development of a stomach tumor.

**Can one live normally without stomach acid?**

Yes. Approximately 10 percent of all people have low acid or absence of acid in the stomach.

**What causes lack of stomach acid?**

a. Most people with lack of acid (achlorhydria) are born with it.

b. As people grow older and get into the seventh and eighth decades of life, they tend to manufacture less acid.

**What are the symptoms of lack of acid?**

Usually there are none. Occasionally, a patient with low acid experiences some difficulty in digesting large quantities of meats.

**What causes excess stomach acidity?**

The exact cause is unknown. It is known that the emotionally disturbed, energetic, dynamic types tend to secrete more acid. Also, certain highly seasoned foods, tobacco, and alcohol will cause the stomach lining to secrete large quantities of hydrochloric acid.

**How does the physician test for acid in the stomach?**

a. By passing a tube through the nose or mouth into the stomach and analyzing the material that is withdrawn. This is "gastric analysis."

b. There is a urine test that gives a fairly accurate picture of stomach acidity.

**If a person has high stomach acidity, does this mean he will always have high acid?**

Not necessarily. The factors producing excess acidity, such as periods of emotional strain, may subside, and the acid content of the stomach may then return to normal.

**How effective are the commonly advertised antacid medications?**

Very effective to counteract excess acidity for a short period of time. However, they do not cure the condition; relief is only temporary.

**Is there any serious harm in taking antacid medications over a long period of time?**

No, but it is much wiser to seek medical aid to relieve the underlying cause of the excess acidity (hyperacidity).

**What is the best treatment for excess stomach acidity?**

a. Frequent bland feedings every two to three hours.

b. Abstinence from smoking, alcohol, and highly seasoned foods.

c. Taking of antacid medications and certain gastric inhibitory medicines such as Tagamet (cimetidine).

d. Attempting to live a more well-ordered, controlled emotional life.

**What is the best treatment for lack of acid in the stomach?**

Usually, no treatment is required. However, if symptoms do occur, appropriate amounts of dilute hydrochloric acid can be taken orally.

**What role does excess stomach acidity play in the cause of ulcers of the stomach or duodenum?**

It is thought that the greatest single contributory factor toward ulcer formation is chronic hyperacidity.

## ACUTE GASTRITIS AND GASTROENTERITIS

**What is acute gastritis?**

It is an inflammation of the lining of the stomach caused by bacteria, viruses, chemical irritants, or by eating spoiled foods.

**What are the symptoms of acute gastritis?**

Nausea, vomiting, upper abdominal cramps, fever, bleeding from the mucous membrane lining of the stomach.

**Is gastritis sometimes associated with a similar inflammation of the small intestine?**

Yes, and the condition is therefore referred to as gastroenteritis.

**Is ptomaine poisoning another name for acute gastritis or gastroenteritis?**

Yes, but this is no longer a term used by physicians.

**What is the treatment for acute gastritis or gastroenteritis?**

a. Bed rest.
b. Abstinence from food.
c. Moderate fluid intake when nausea subsides.
d. Antispasmodic and antacid drugs.
e. Drugs to quiet excess intestinal activity and to halt the diarrhea.

**How soon do people with acute gastritis or gastroenteritis get well?**

The condition usually subsides within one to three days. If it does not, examinations should be carried out to determine whether some more serious underlying disease exists.

**How does one distinguish between acute gastritis and acute gastroenteritis?**

The latter condition is accompanied by violent midabdominal and lower abdominal cramps with episodes of diarrhea. When only the stomach is involved, diarrhea is not present.

**Is it necessary to operate for acute gastritis?**

No. This is a medical condition that will clear up with medical management.

## CHRONIC GASTRITIS

**What is chronic gastritis?**

An inflammation of the lining of the stomach, which persists over a long period of time.

**What causes chronic gastritis?**

The cause is not definitely known, but it is thought that prolonged and excessive use of spices, alcohol, and other irritants may eventually lead to a chronic inflammation of the stomach lining.

**What are the symptoms of chronic gastritis?**

Upper abdominal discomfort and pain, heartburn, and a sense of fullness in the region. Also, loss of appetite, loss of weight, nausea, and vomiting. With certain types, there may be hemorrhage, with the vomiting of blood or the passage of a black stool.

**How does the physician make a diagnosis of chronic gastritis?**

From the history of symptoms plus characteristic x-ray findings and by inspecting the stomach lining through a gastroscope.

**What is the best way to prevent getting chronic gastritis?**

Avoid those substances that are thought to be predisposing toward the disease.

**What is the treatment for chronic gastritis?**

a. Stop smoking.
b. Refrain from alcoholic beverages.
c. Eat frequent, small, bland meals, with plenty of milk.
d. Refrain from eating spicy foods.
e. If the chronic gastritis is associated with excess stomach acidity, take appropriate antacid medications or possibly Tagamet.
f. If there is an absence of acid, then medications will be given along with liver extracts and vitamins.

**Does chronic gastritis ever clear up?**

Yes, some cases will, after adequate treatment for several months. Others do not clear up but can be kept under control.

**Is it ever necessary to operate for chronic gastritis?**

Only if there is repeated hemorrhage.

**Does chronic gastritis ever terminate in other diseases?**

Yes. It has been found that certain types of chronic gastritis (hypertrophic gastritis) seem to predispose toward ulcer formation, while other types (atrophic gastritis) predispose toward cancer of the stomach.

**How can one tell the progress of chronic gastritis?**

a. By noting the activity of the symptoms.
b. By a medical checkup every few months, with x rays of the stomach.
c. By direct examination of the stomach lining through a gastroscope.

**What is the difference between chronic hypertrophic gastritis and chronic atrophic gastritis?**

Hypertrophic gastritis gives many of the symptoms of ulcer, is associated with excess acid secretion, and may be accompanied by hemorrhage. Atrophic gastritis may be associated with loss of appetite, low or absent acid secretion, and anemia.

## INFLAMMATION OF THE DUODENUM (Duodenitis)

**What is duodenitis?**

An inflammation and irritability of the duodenum.

**What causes duodenitis?**

It is usually associated with excess acidity and with all the other factors that lead to the development of an ulcer.

**What are the symptoms of duodenitis?**

Very similar to those of ulcer. (See the section on Peptic Ulcer in this chapter.)

**How does the physician make a diagnosis of duodenitis?**

By noting the symptoms and by observing the characteristic findings of an irritable and spastic duodenum on x-ray examination and on direct examination through endoscopy.

**What is the treatment for duodenitis?**

The same as for peptic ulcer.

**Is it ever necessary to operate for duodenitis?**

No. This is strictly a medical condition.

**Will duodenitis clear up by itself, if untreated?**

It may, but it has a tendency to become chronic if not treated.

**How effective are present-day measures in relieving duodenitis?**

An ulcer regime will cause most cases to subside after a period of several weeks or months.

**Do people who have had duodenitis at one time tend to develop it again?**

Yes, if they are careless with their diet, drink to excess, and fail to observe medical instructions.

# PEPTIC ULCER (Ulcers of the Stomach, Duodenum, or Esophagus)

**What is meant by the term "peptic" ulcer?**

It is a general term used to describe an ulcer in the stomach, duodenum, or the lower end of the esophagus.

**What causes peptic ulcer?**

The exact cause is not known, but the common underlying factor in almost all cases is hyperacidity, or the secretion of excess acid by the stomach.

**What types of peptic ulcer are there?**

a. Duodenal ulcer is the most common form.
b. Stomach (gastric) ulcer is next in frequency.
c. Esophageal ulcer is the least frequently encountered ulcer.

**How common is an ulcer of the stomach or duodenum?**

About one in every ten adults is thought to have a duodenal ulcer at some time or other. About one in every hundred adults will have a gastric ulcer at some time or other.

**What type of person is most likely to develop peptic ulcer?**

The energetic, dynamic, highly emotional person who is beset by many frustrations but who works at a fast pace in a highly civilized society. Men get ulcers more often than women.

**Do ulcers of the stomach or duodenum tend to run in families or to be inherited?**

Not really, except that there is a tendency for children to develop along the same lines as their parents. Thus, neurotic parents with ulcers may have offspring who develop the same tendencies.

**Do ulcers tend to be multiple?**

Yes, frequently more than one ulcer is present at a time.

**What actually takes place when an ulcer of the stomach or duodenum is present?**

The lining mucous membrane is eaten away and eroded, leaving a raw, uncovered area in the wall of the stomach or duodenum. Ulcers may vary in size from that of a pinhead to that of a half-dollar.

**Is there any way to lessen the chances of getting an ulcer?**

a. Don't smoke.
b. Drink alcohol only in moderate amounts.
c. Eat bland foods.
d. Attempt to live within the bounds of one's ability and capacity.

**Is the size of an ulcer significant?**

Not necessarily. Small ulcers may bleed or rupture almost as easily as large ulcers. As a general rule, however, the larger and deeper the ulcer, the more difficult and the longer it takes to heal.

**How can one tell if he has an ulcer?**

The most characteristic symptoms are gnawing hunger pains in the upper abdomen occurring between meals. The pains are usually relieved for several hours by eating. Other symptoms include sour taste in the mouth, belching, and heartburn, relieved by the taking of antacid medications.

**What tests are performed to make a positive diagnosis of peptic ulcer?**

Most cases can be demonstrated by x-ray studies of the stomach and duodenum and by direct examination through a gastroscope.

**What are the harmful effects of peptic ulcer?**

In addition to the pain and continued discomfort that ulcer patients suffer, there are the following possible complications:

a. A gastric (stomach) ulcer, if untreated, may develop into cancer. This happens in about one in fifteen cases.
b. As ulcers become chronic, they may form scar tissue, which will obstruct the outlet of the stomach.
c. Ulcers may rupture and cause peritonitis.
d. Ulcers tend to cause severe hemorrhage. Death from loss of blood can occur during a bleeding episode.

**What is the treatment for peptic ulcer?**

More than 90 percent of all ulcers respond to medical treatment and require no surgery. Standard medical treatment for a patient suffering from a peptic ulcer consists of:

a. Special ulcer diet, with frequent feedings of milk and cream.
b. Abstinence from spicy foods, alcohol, etc.

*(continued)*

c. Antacid medications.

d. Special medications that act through the nervous system so as to cut down on the secretion of gastric juice and acid, such as Tagamet (cimetidine).

e. Stop smoking.

The remainder who do not respond to medical treatment should be operated upon if:

a. It is a gastric ulcer that shows no healing within a few weeks or months, as these ulcers have a tendency to become cancerous.

b. When pain and discomfort continue over the years despite conscientious attempts to bring about a cure through medical management.

c. When there is obstruction to the stomach outlet.

d. When the ulcer ruptures or threatens to rupture.

e. When there are repeated episodes of severe hemorrhage.

**Do ulcers, once healed through medical management, have a tendency to recur?**

Yes. As long as the stomach pours out an excess of acid, there is a danger of a new break occurring in its lining, with a resultant ulcer.

*At right and on opposite page:*
***Subtotal Gastrectomy for Ulcer.*** *These diagrams demonstrate the operative procedure frequently used for cure of a stomach or duodenal ulcer. The results from this operation are good, with cure of the ulcer resulting in more than 90 percent of cases.*

**What are the causes for recurrence of healed ulcers?**

Failure to maintain an ulcer dietary regime; continuation of smoking and drinking alcoholic beverages; the persistence of those situations in life that lead to emotional instability and stress.

**What actually takes place in the lining of the stomach when an ulcer heals?**

The lining membrane (mucosa) and a certain amount of scar tissue grow back over the raw, ulcerated surface.

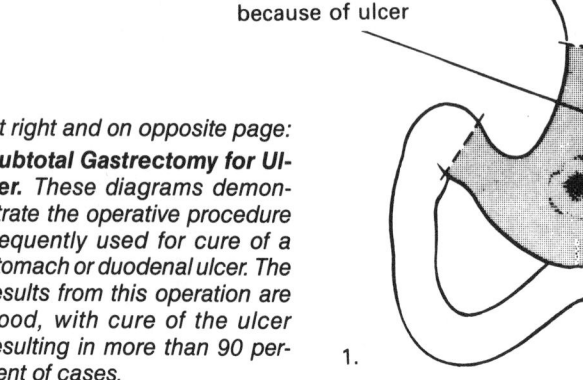

Shaded portion of stomach to be removed because of ulcer

1.

**Why is it more important to remove an ulcer of the stomach than an ulcer of the duodenum?**

Stomach ulcers may form cancer; duodenal ulcers do not.

**Are operations for peptic ulcer serious?**

Yes, but approximately ninety-nine out of a hundred will recover from the surgery.

**What operations are performed to cure peptic ulcer?**

There are several procedures, each of which has special indications, and each of which results in cure in well over 90 percent of cases.

1. For an ulcer located in the stomach (gastric ulcer), a subtotal gastrectomy is done. This involves the removal of approximately three-fourths of the stomach, and the remainder is joined to the small intestine. (See accompanying diagrams.)

2. For an ulcer in the duodenum (the most common form of peptic ulcer) one of the following operations is performed:

a. A vagotomy, in which the vagus nerves (which stimulate the stomach to secrete acid) are cut and approximately 50 percent of the stomach is removed.

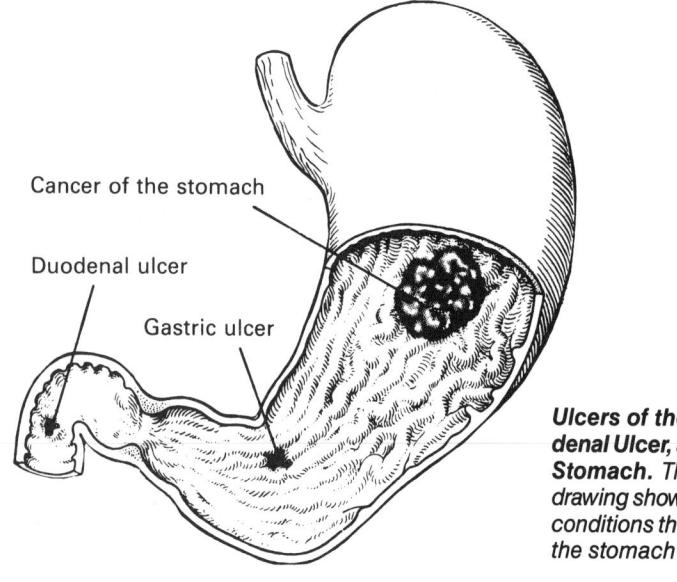

Cancer of the stomach

Duodenal ulcer

Gastric ulcer

***Ulcers of the Stomach, Duodenal Ulcer, and Cancer of the Stomach.*** *This is a composite drawing showing three separate conditions that sometime affect the stomach or duodenum.*

# SKIN AND SKIN DISEASES

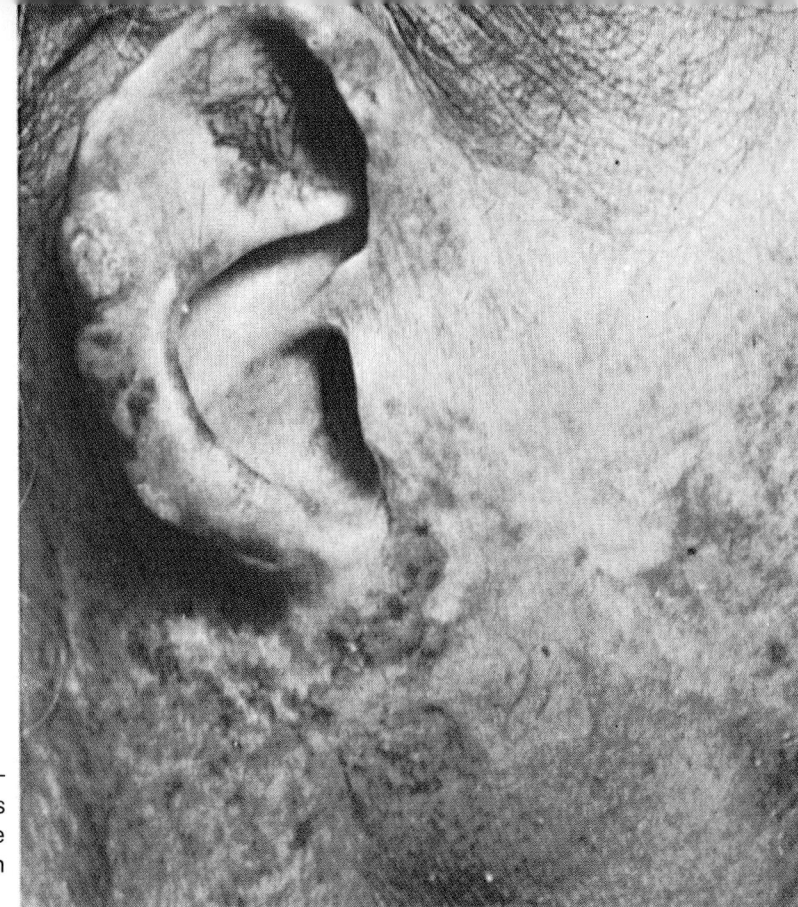

Tuberculosis of the skin (lupus vulgaris), a rare condition today, has extensively affected the skin of the ear of the patient in the photograph at right.

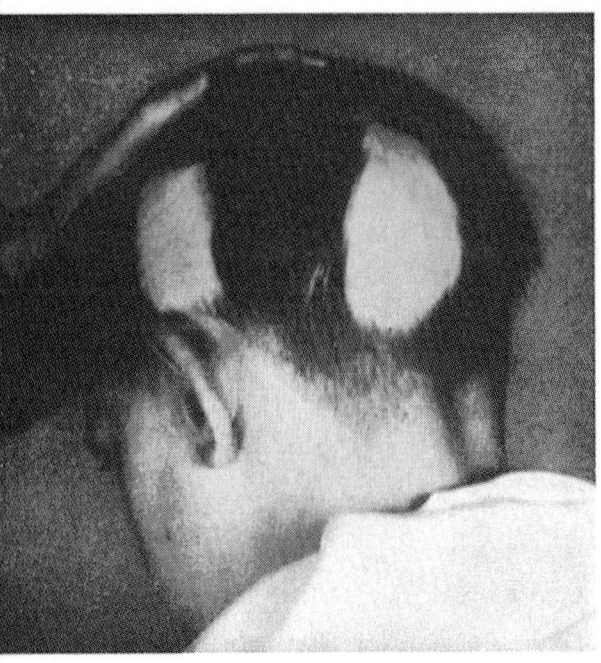

Alopecia areata, or loss of the hair in patches, is characterized by perfectly smooth, shiny bald areas (above). The condition comes on rather abruptly, lasts for several months, and then may disappear spontaneously.

Psoriasis (below) is a very common skin disease which tends to last off and on for many years. Characteristically, the rash appears on the knees and elbows, but may also affect the trunk. Fortunately, itching is not a marked feature in this condition, and some of the newer drugs are helpful in causing a remission or disappearance of the rash for lengthy periods.

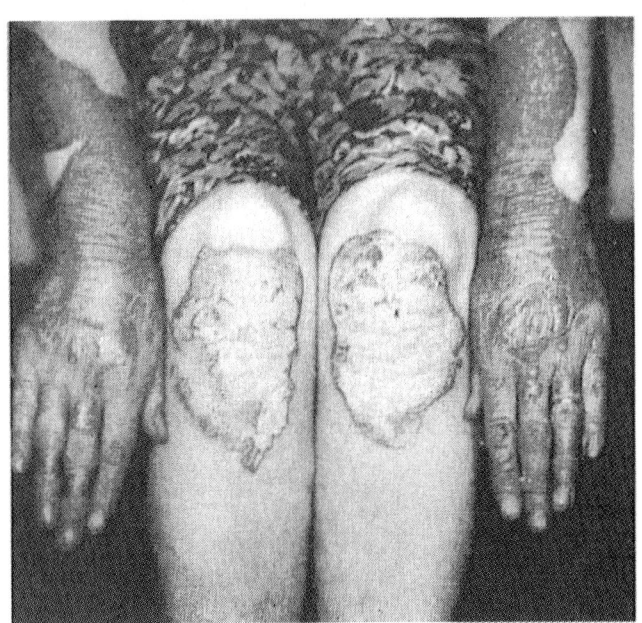

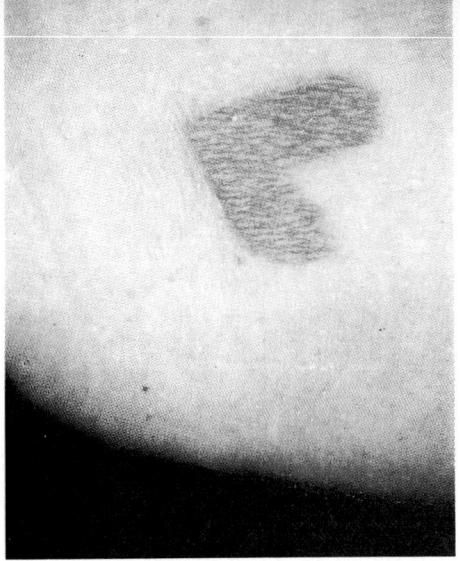
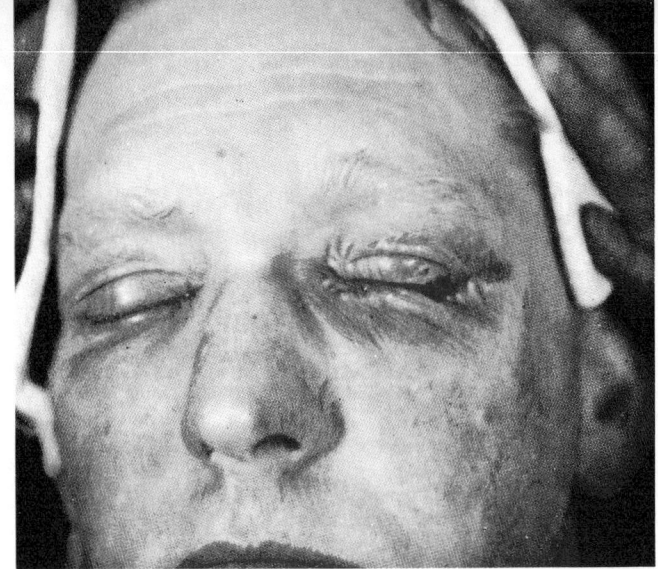

The contact eczema reaction illustrated above, left, is due to sensitivity to lipstick that was applied, as a test, to the skin of the arm. The reaction illustrated above, right, is due to sensitivity to an eye lotion. If the offending substance is withdrawn, most contact eczema disappears spontaneously within a few days.

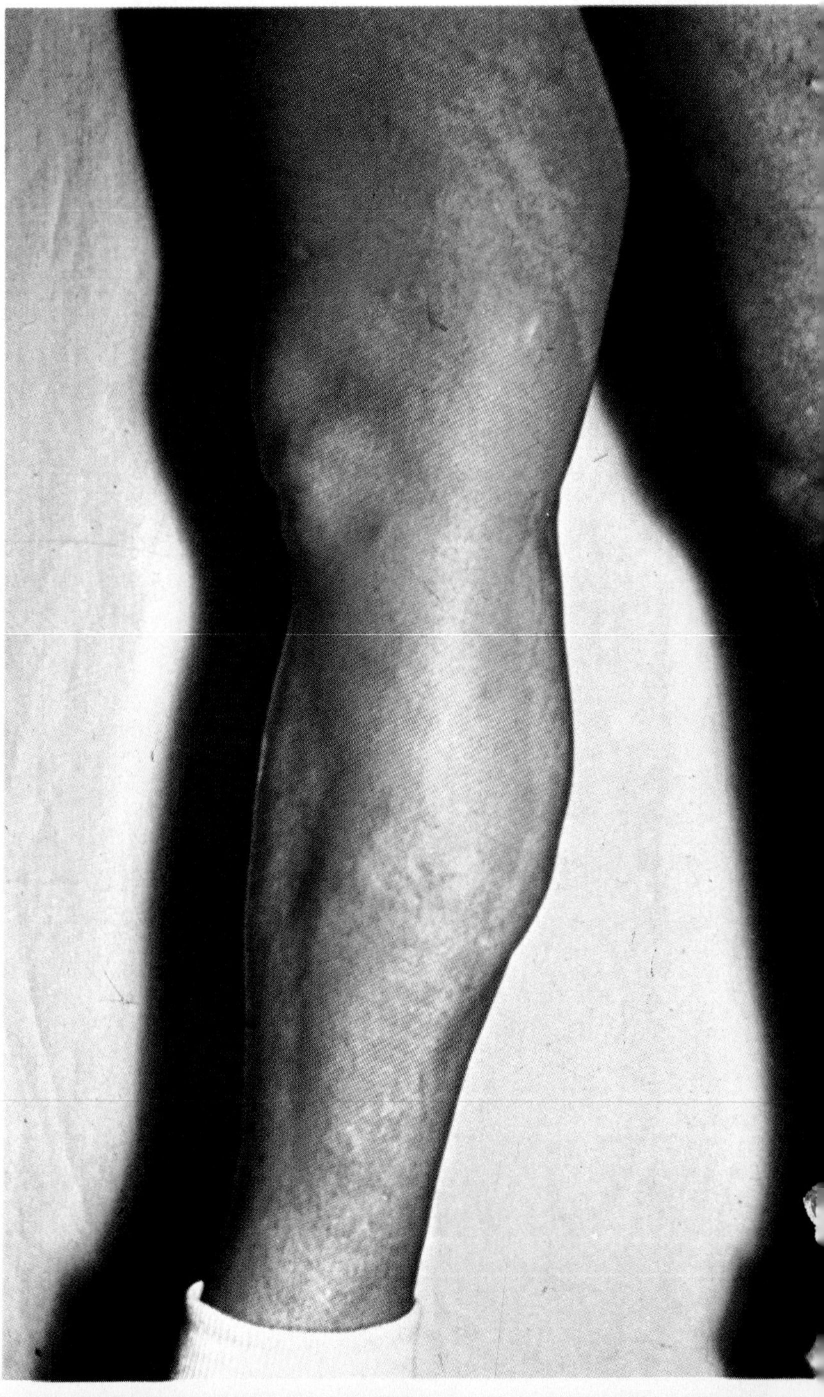

Urticaria, or hives, is a condition characterized by intensely itching wheals. Occasionally a giant hive, like the one at right, may be several inches in diameter.

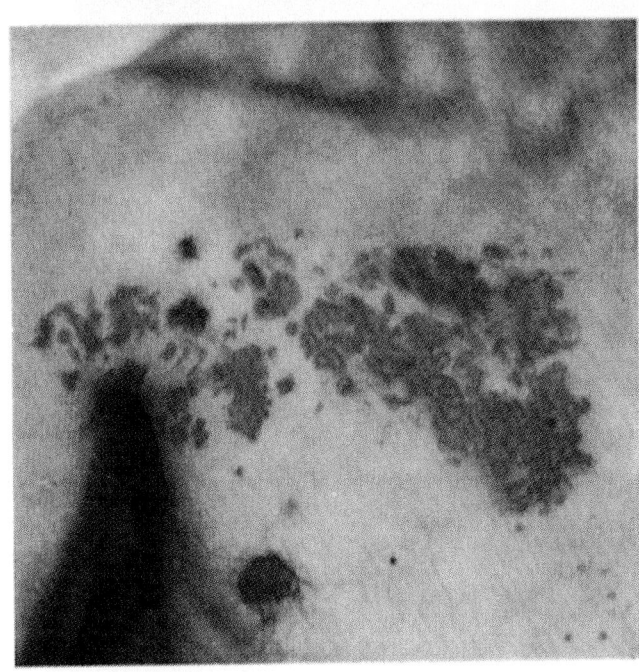

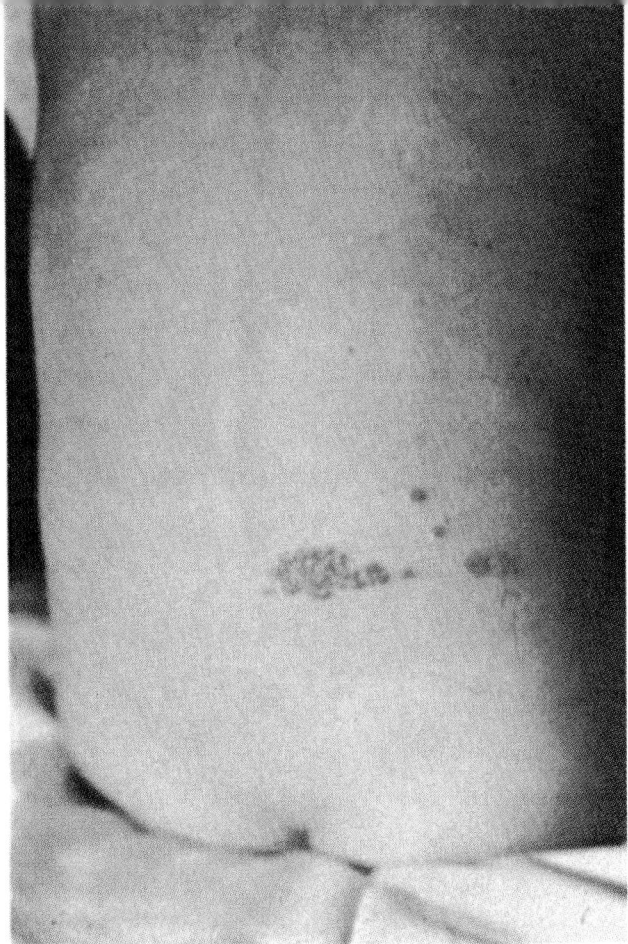

Herpes zoster, or shingles, illustrated here by three typical cases, is a skin eruption thought to be due to a virus infection of a nerve. The lesions are usually distributed along the course of a nerve on the chest or abdomen and may cause sufficient pain and discomfort in the early, pre-eruptive stages to be mistaken for a more serious disease.

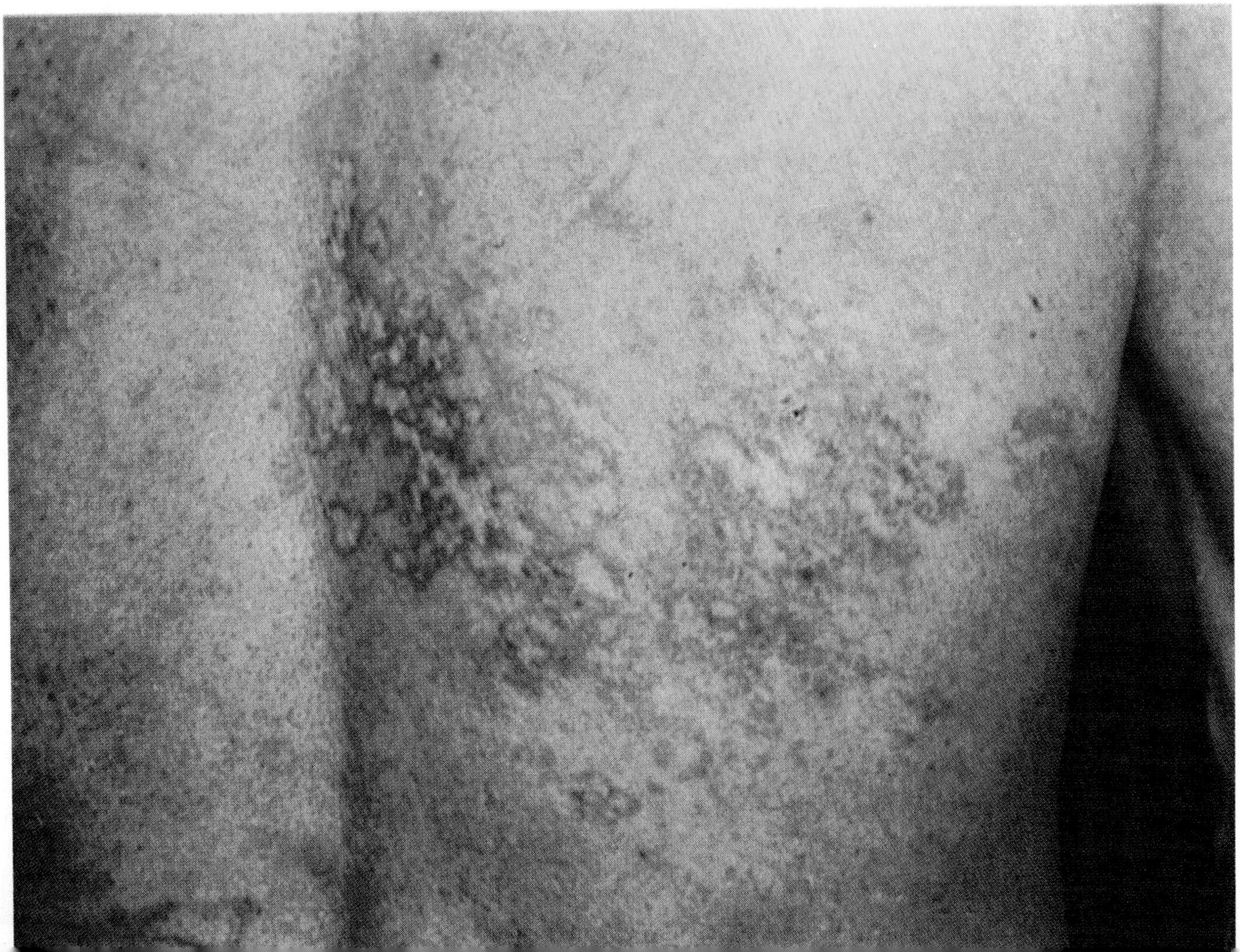

The characteristic impetigo lesion, which occurs most frequently on the face, has superficial crusts that often separate and leave a raw base. The condition is very contagious and sometimes causes epidemics in infant nurseries. Fortunately, impetigo can be cured rather quickly with the application of antibiotic ointments.

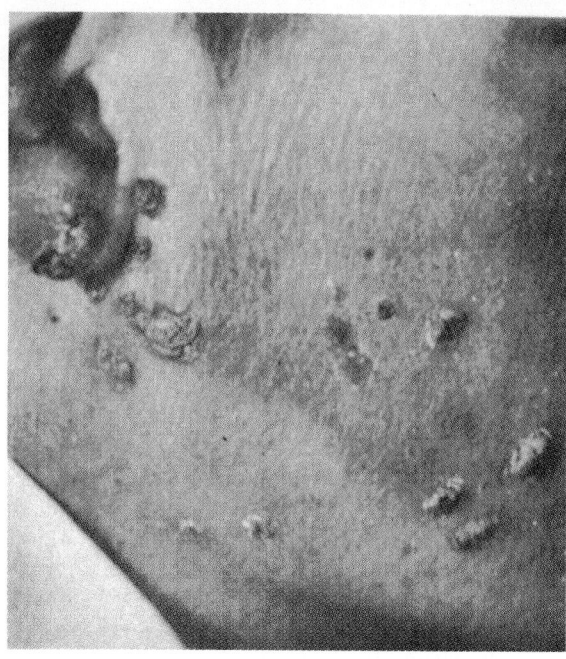

A carbuncle is a large, deep-seated inflammation of the skin which discharges pus from multiple points. Each one of the compartments of the underlying abscess must be drained in order to ensure a cure.

The photograph below illustrates a pustular blister of the skin, an infection usually caused by a staphylococcus.

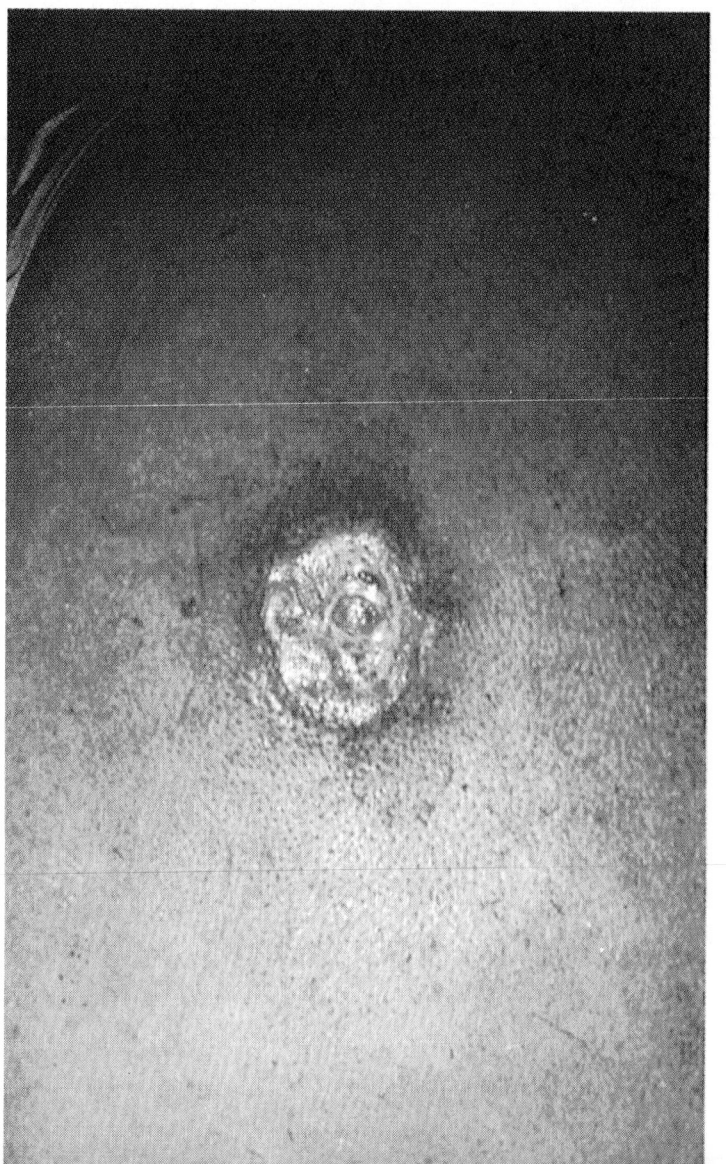

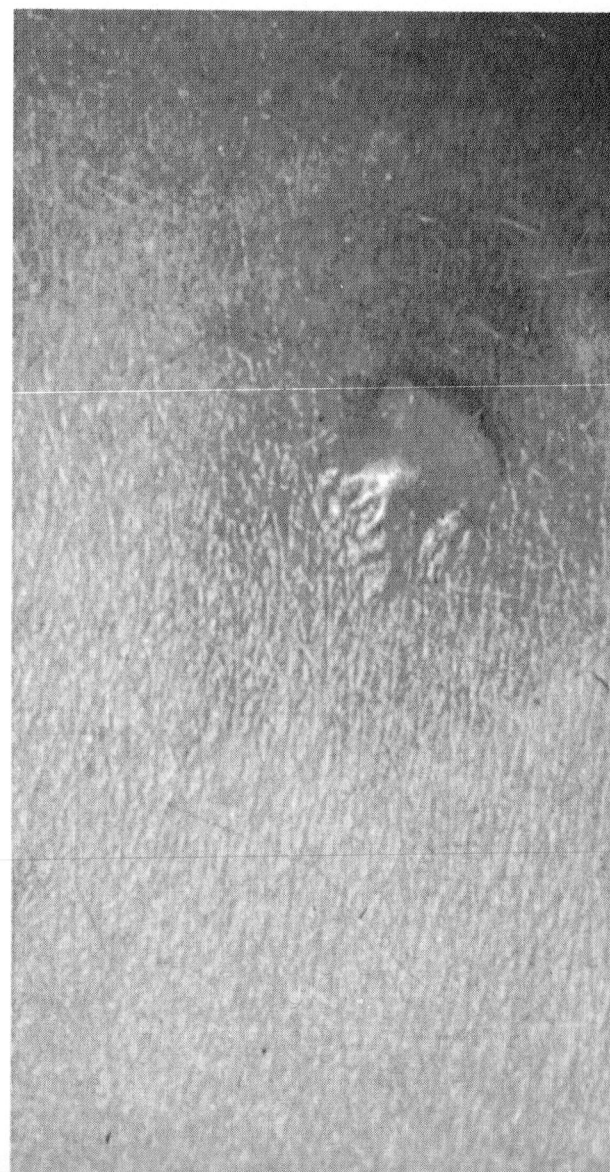

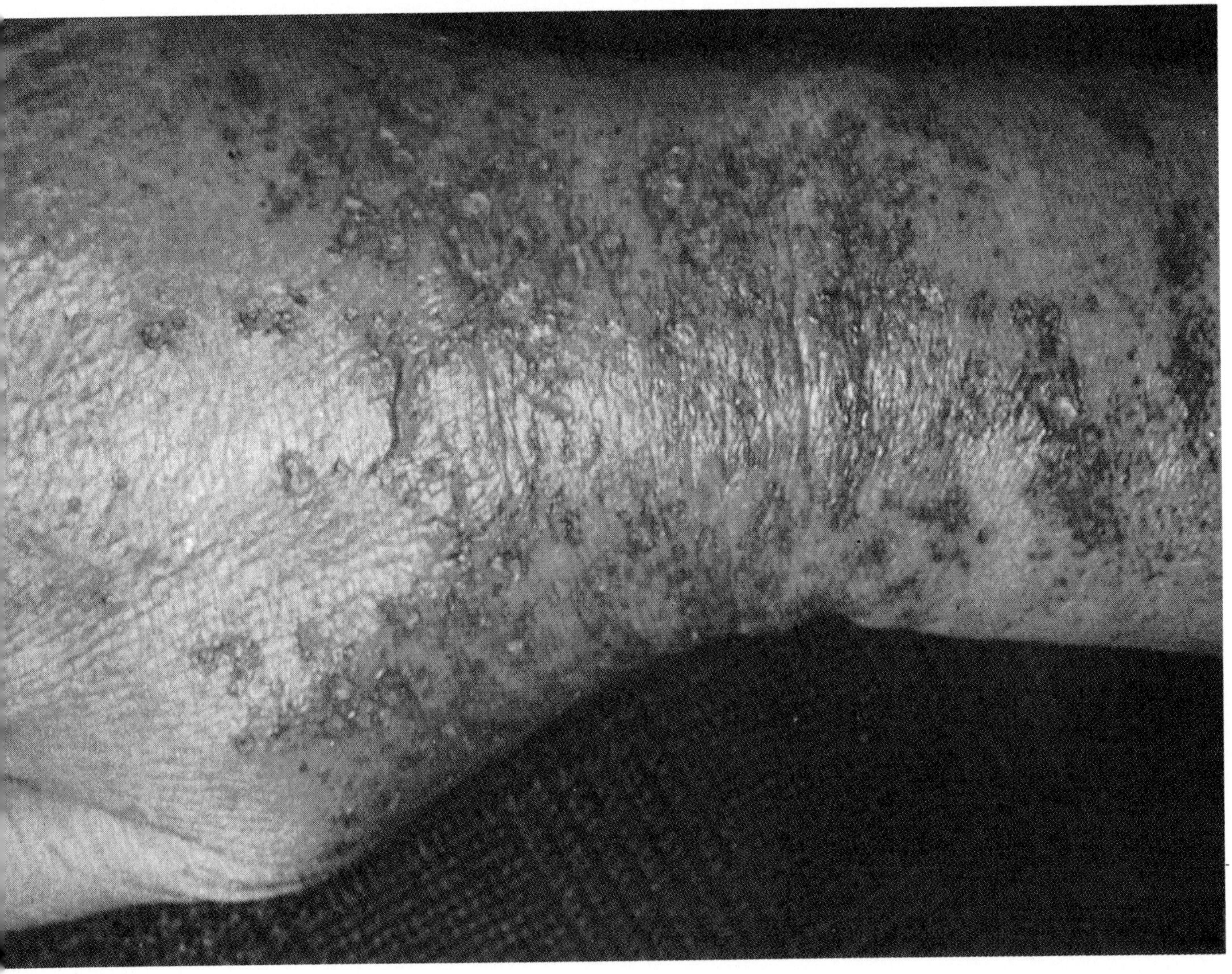

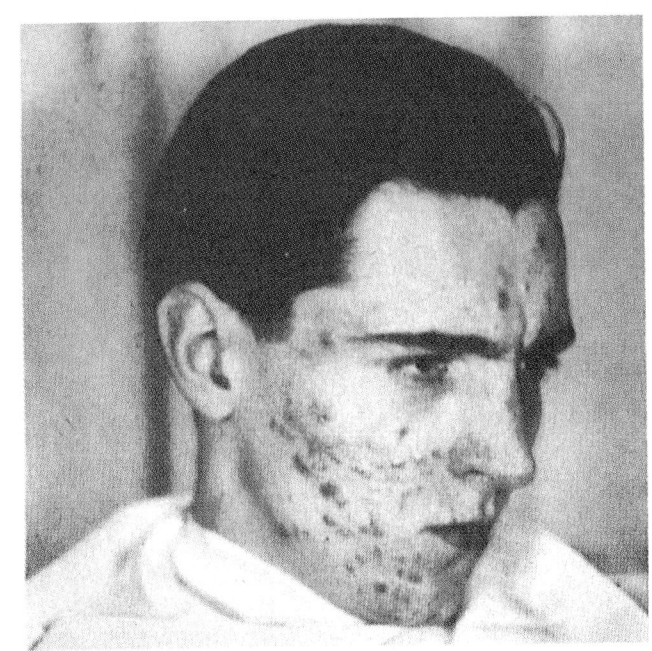

Pyoderma is a bacterial infection of the skin, which is sometimes encountered in persons who have severe, debilitating disease located elsewhere in the body.

Acne, with its characteristic lesions consisting of small abscesses, may be the most common skin disorder. It occurs very frequently in adolescents and young adults. The offending bacteria is usually the staphylococcus.

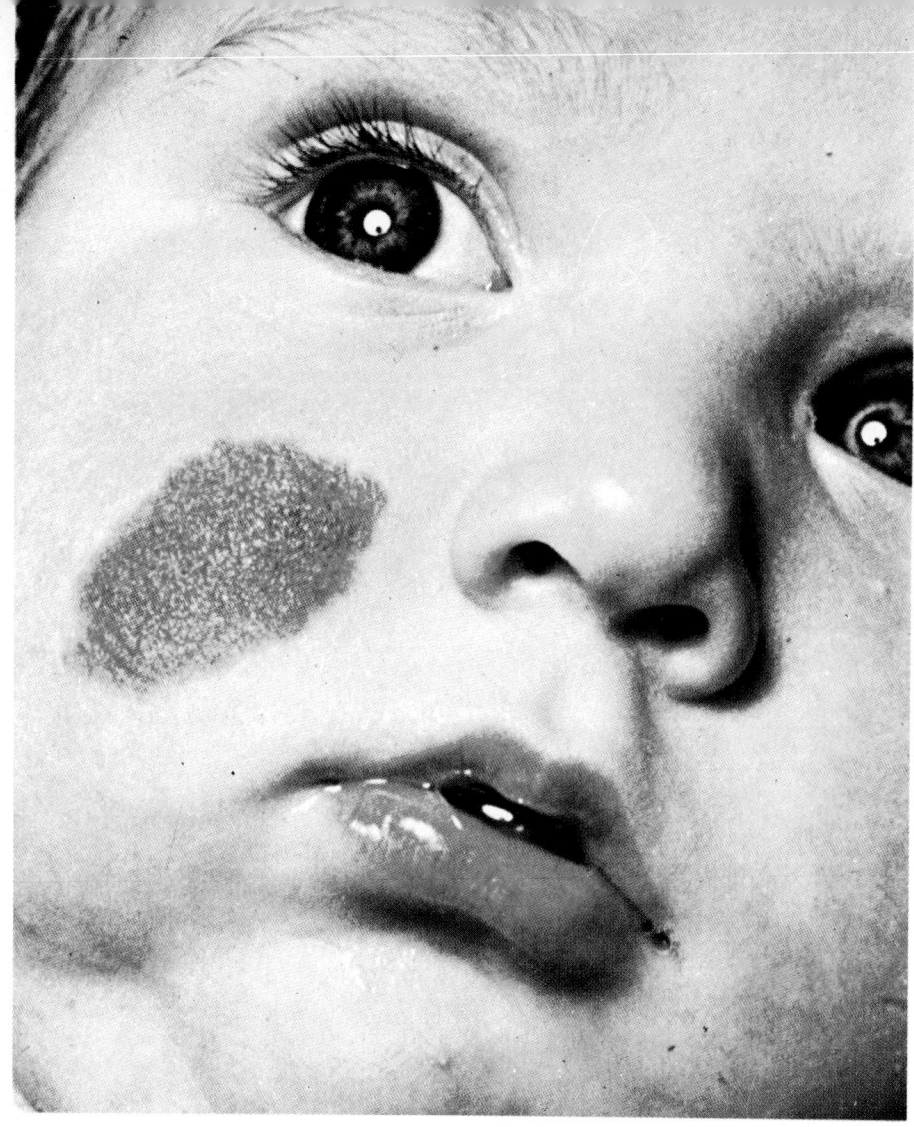

Children are often born with moles that enlarge as the child grows older. Moles that are markedly disfiguring should be removed surgically.

Some moles, or nevi, are darkly colored. Others, like the one in the photograph below, are almost colorless.

Verrucous moles have a warty appearance and may contain areas of dark pigmentation along with areas devoid of pigment.

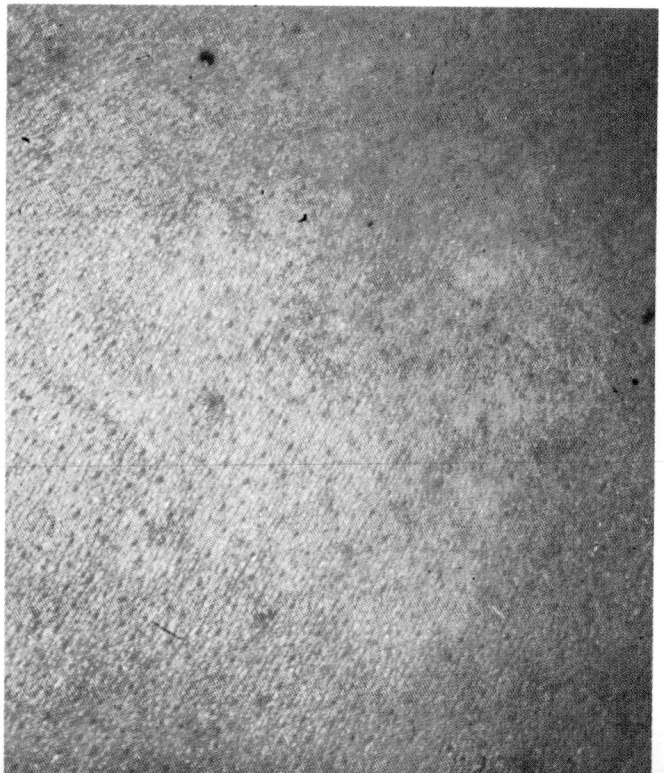

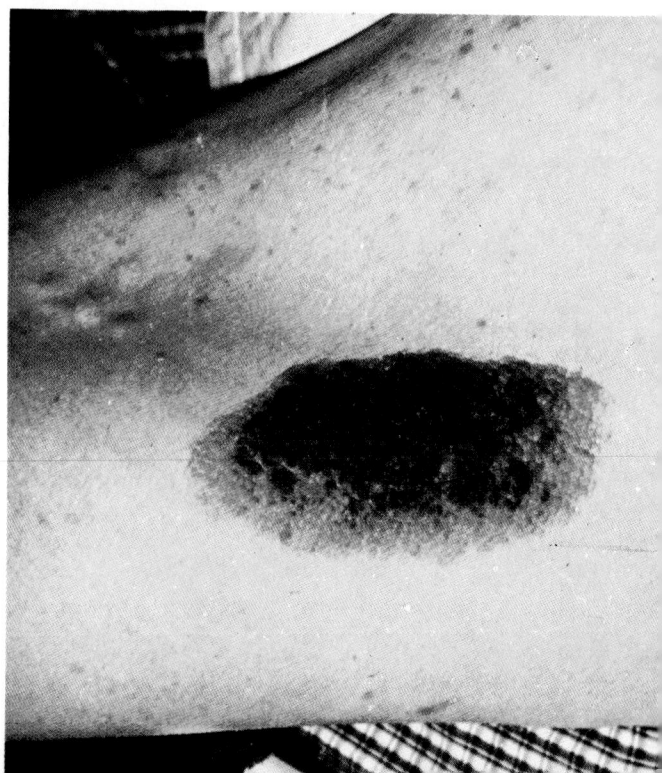

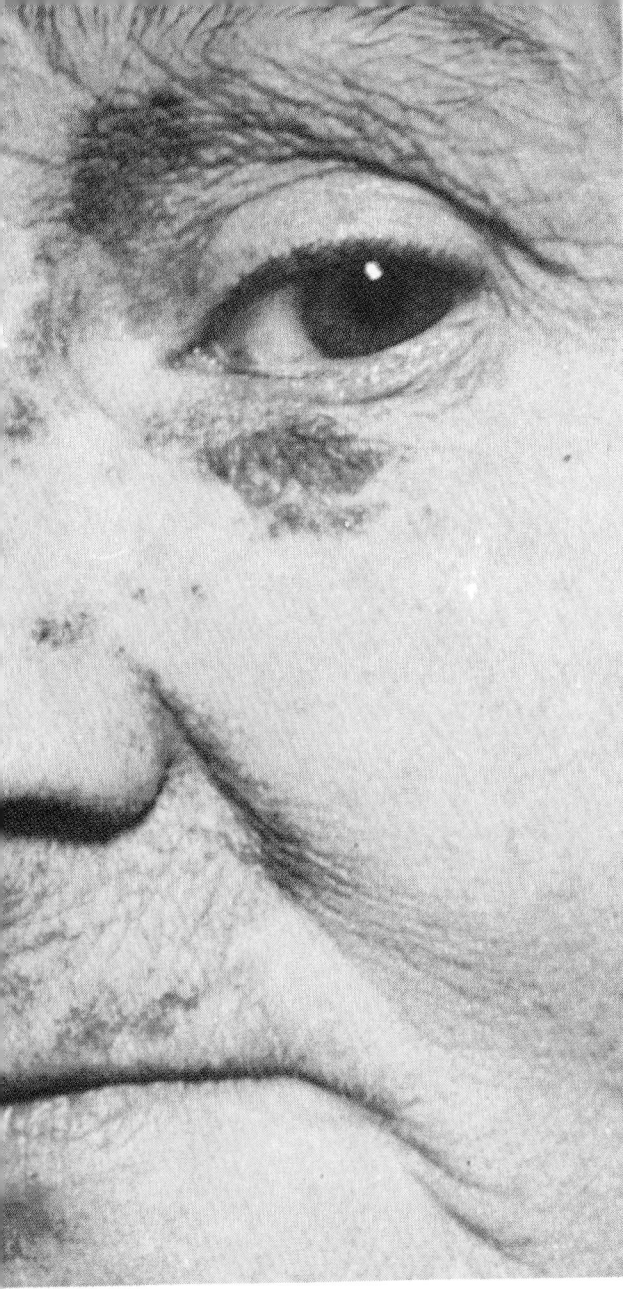

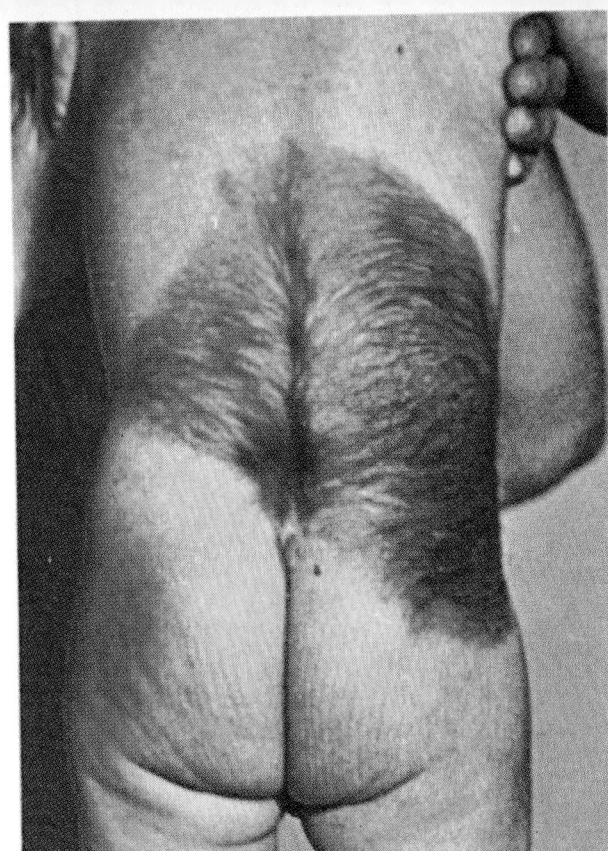

Hairy moles, such as this one which covers a huge area of the lower back and buttocks, are not uncommon.

Some moles, such as the telangiectatic nevus shown in the photograph at the left, look very much like blood vessel tumors or "wine stains."

Plastic surgery, including skin grafts, may be required after the removal of a mole from the face.

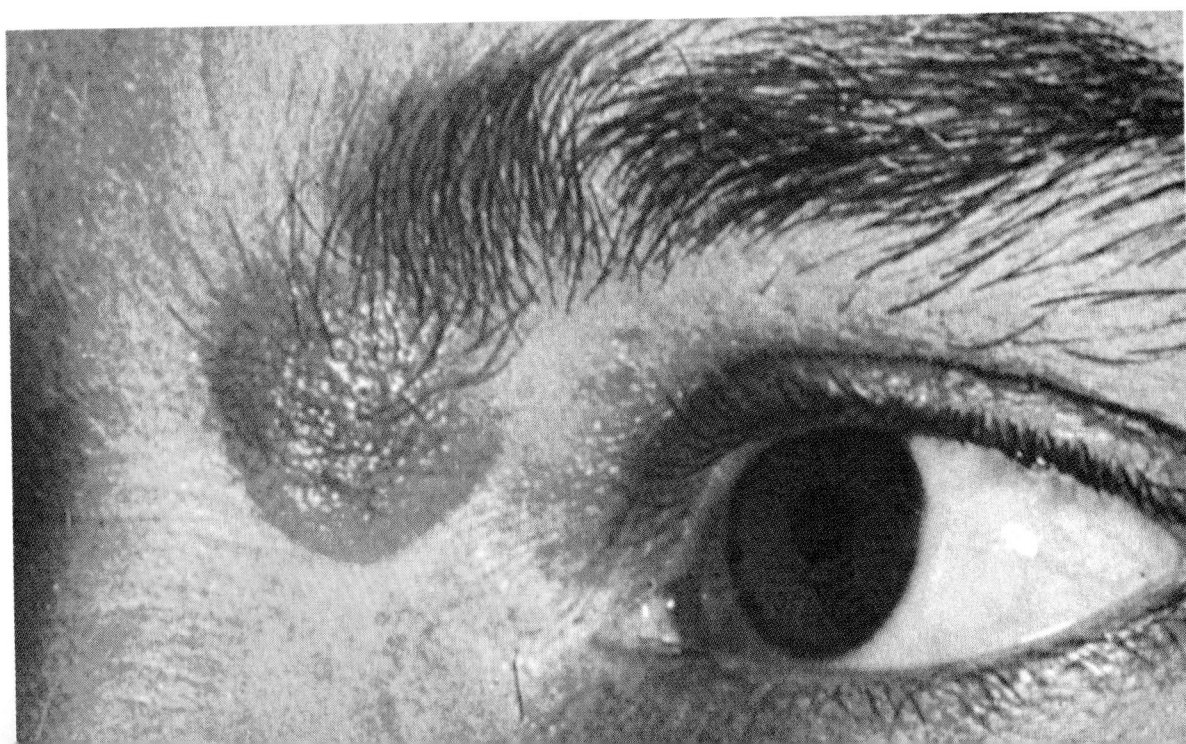

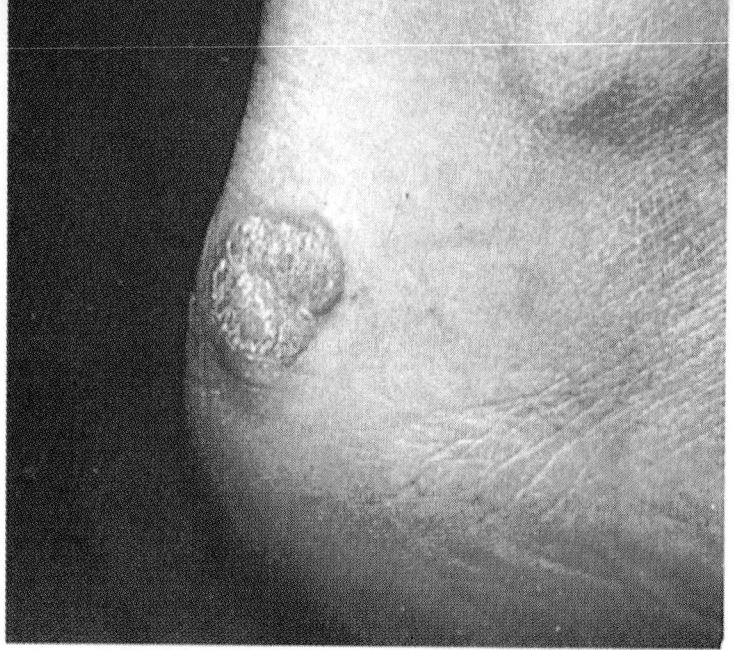

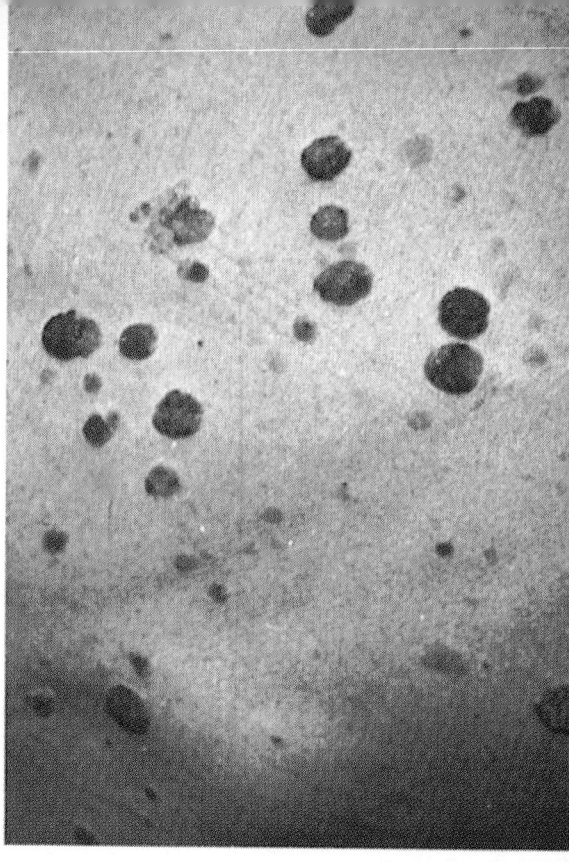

The common wart, which nearly everyone develops at some time in life, is thought to be caused by a virus. Many warts disappear spontaneously; others require treatment.

Seborrheic warts (at right) are sometimes deeply pigmented and mole-like in appearance.

As one ages, brown spots that resemble moles often develop on the body. Such lesions, illustrated below, are known as senile keratoses.

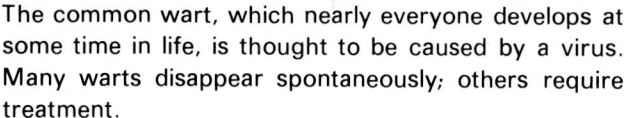

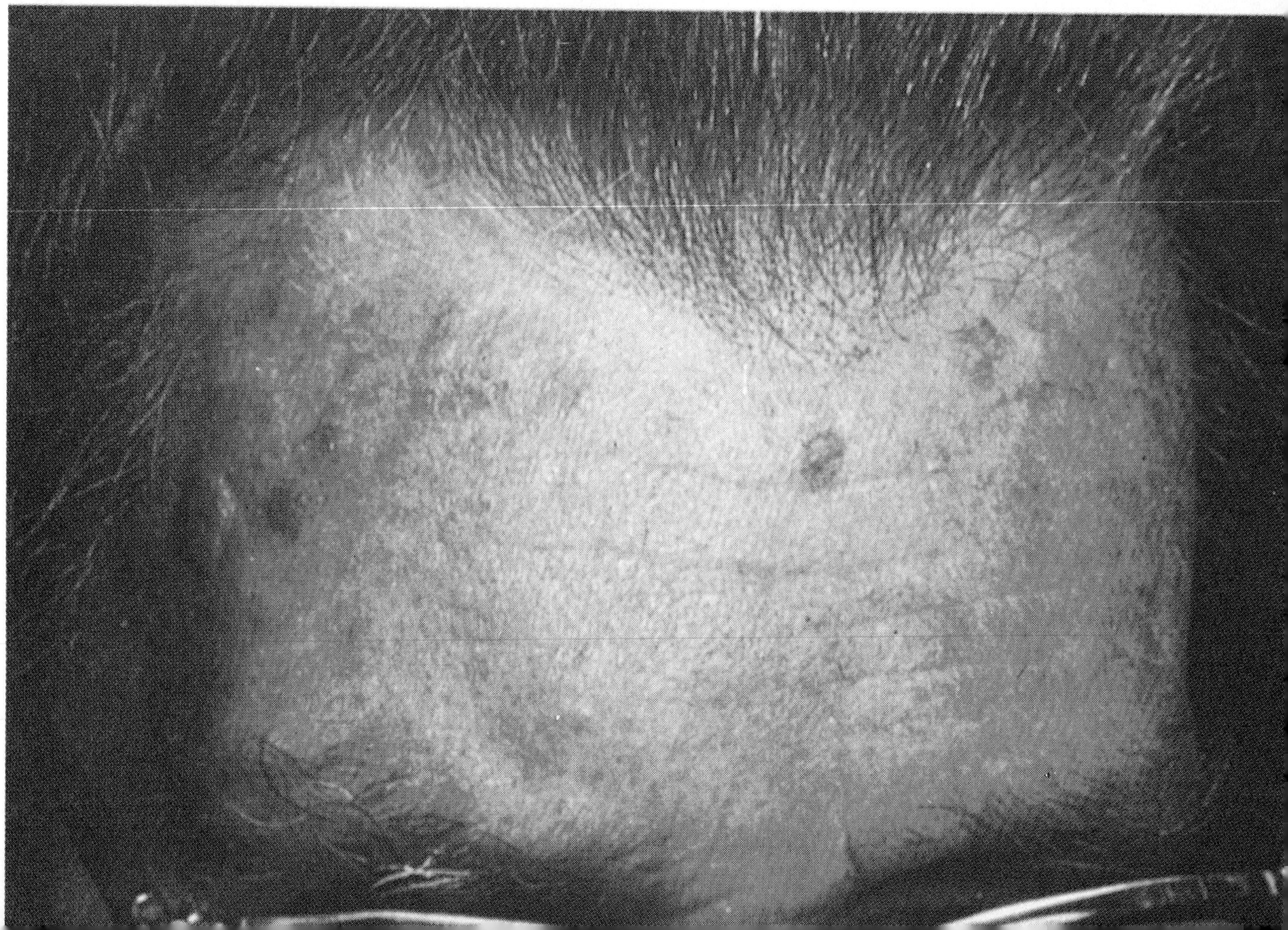

As one ages, the tiny capillaries in the skin may become very fragile and sometimes rupture, creating the reddish coloration of the skin illustrated in the photograph at right.

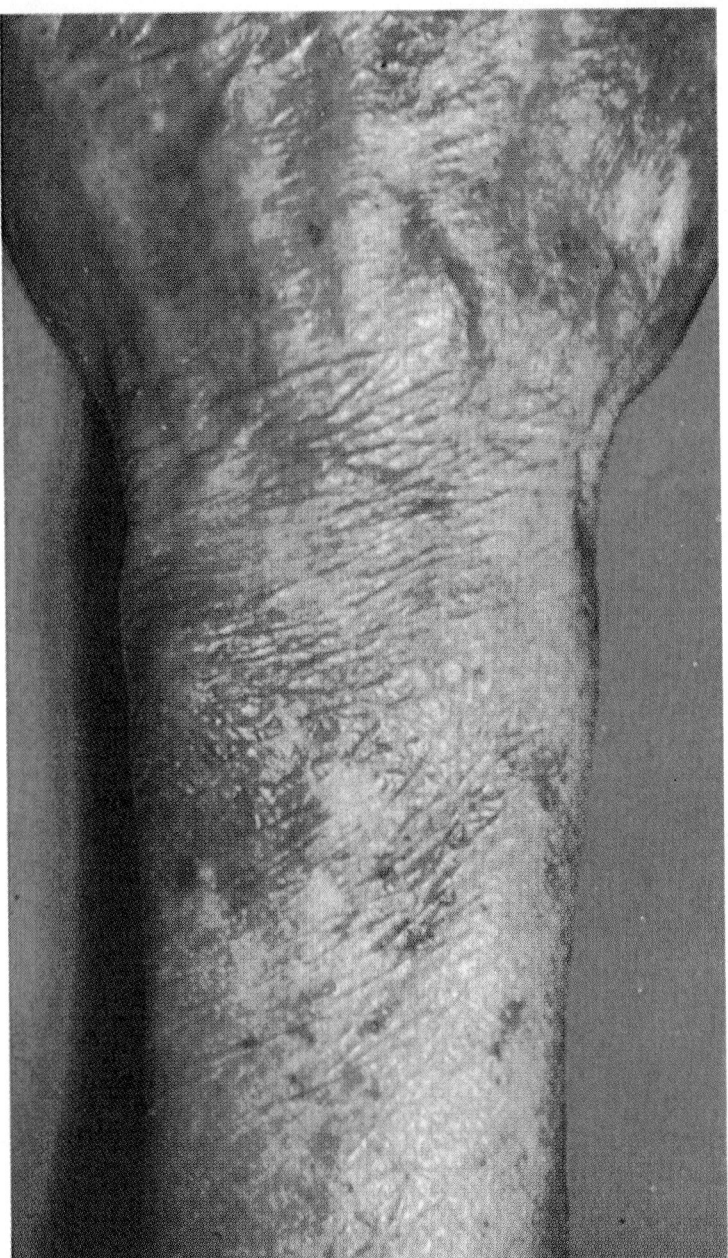

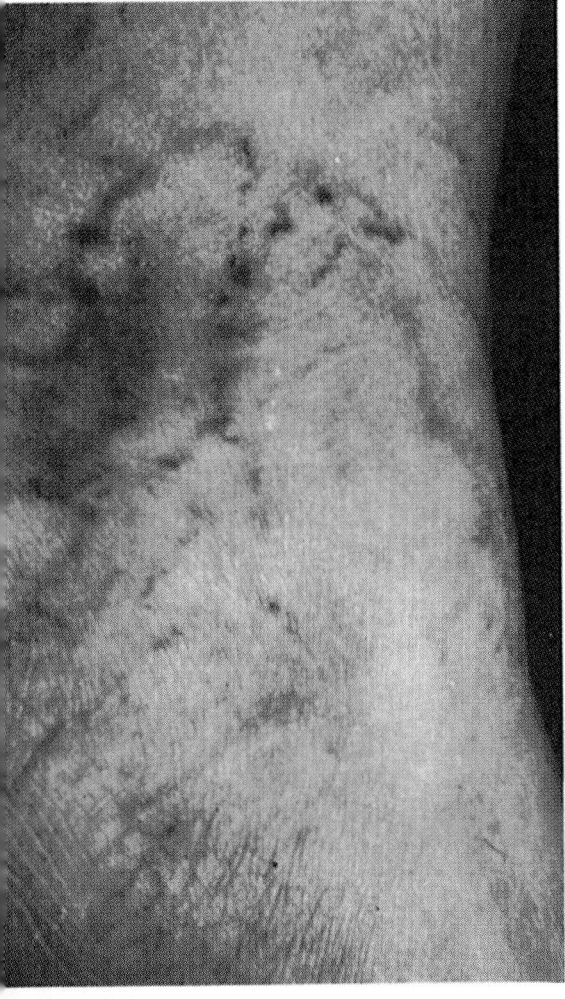

Varicose veins (*above*) affect mainly the blood vessels in the lower limbs. Such varicosities are associated with a breakdown of the valves of the veins and poor drainage of blood from the legs up toward the heart.

A keloid, or overgrown scar, is illustrated at right. The cause of keloids is unknown, and their removal is sometimes followed by the formation of an even larger keloid.

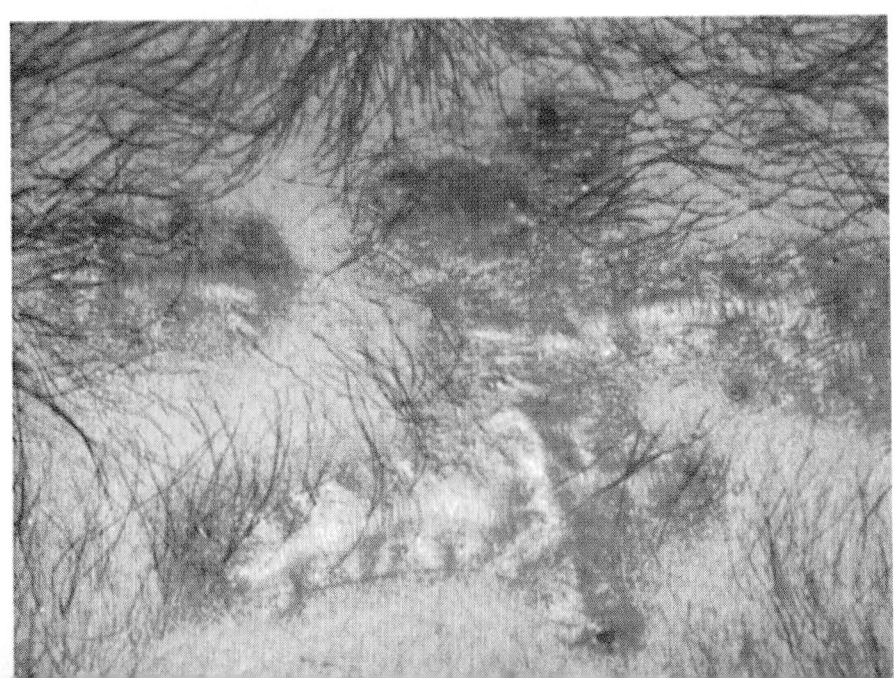

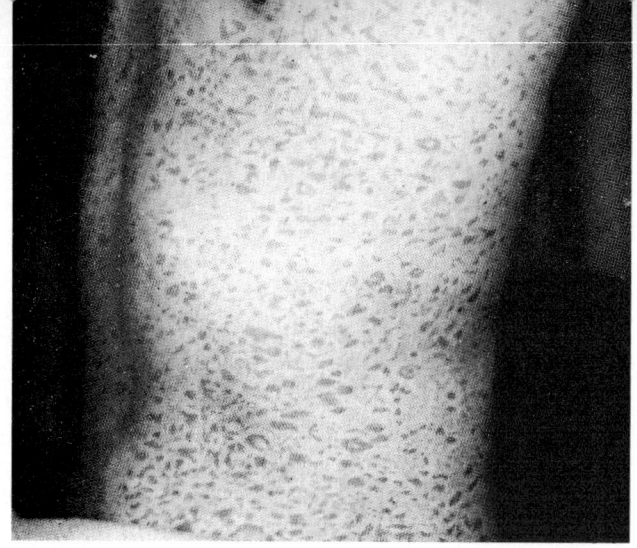

Pityriasis rosea is a common skin eruption affecting the trunk, the upper arms, and the thighs, which lasts for four to six weeks and then disappears. The cause is unknown, but some people believe that it may be a systemic disease, because it is often accompanied by fever and a feeling of malaise.

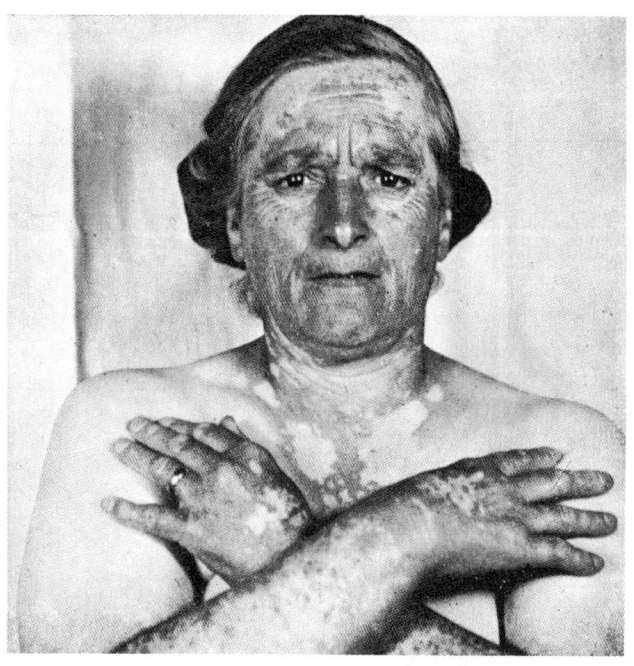

Vitiligo is a condition that is characterized by spotty loss of pigment in the skin while skin texture remains perfectly normal. Women with vitiligo upon exposed surfaces often use cosmetics to make the skin tones appear to blend naturally.

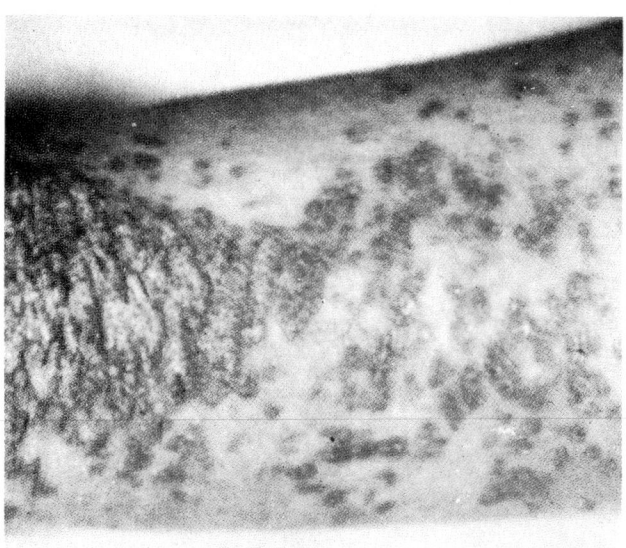

Lichen planus is a disease that often affects the skin on the limbs and is characterized by discrete, reddish, plaquelike areas. Sometimes, milky white spots on the lining of the mouth also occur.

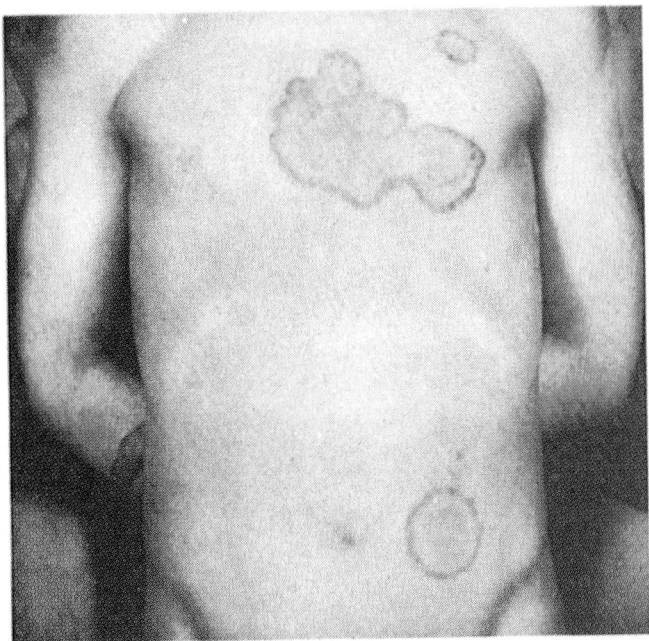

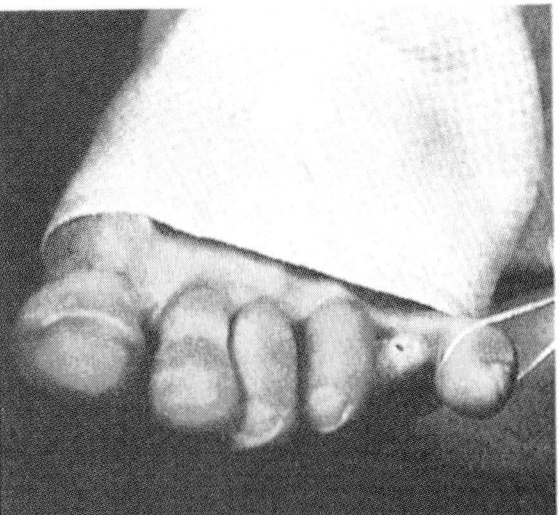

Ringworm, a skin disorder caused by a fungus, can affect any part of the body. When the feet are affected, the condition is known as "athlete's foot"; there are many preparations which are effective in the treatment of this condition, but it has a tendency to recur.

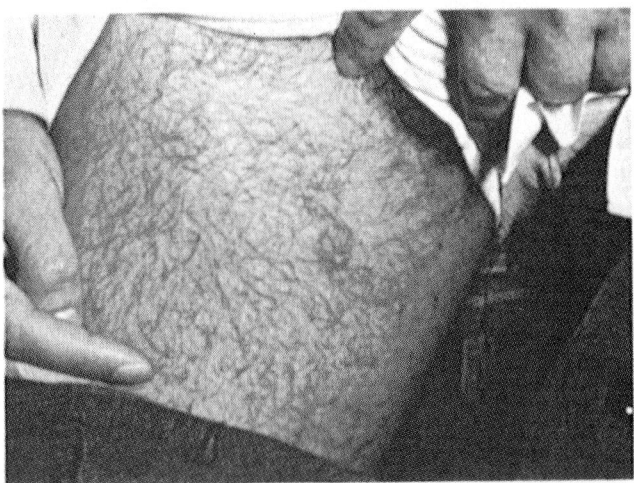

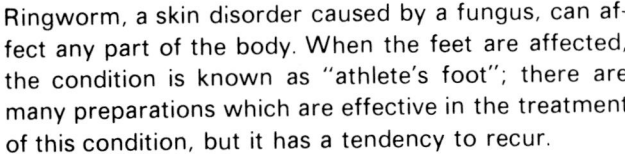

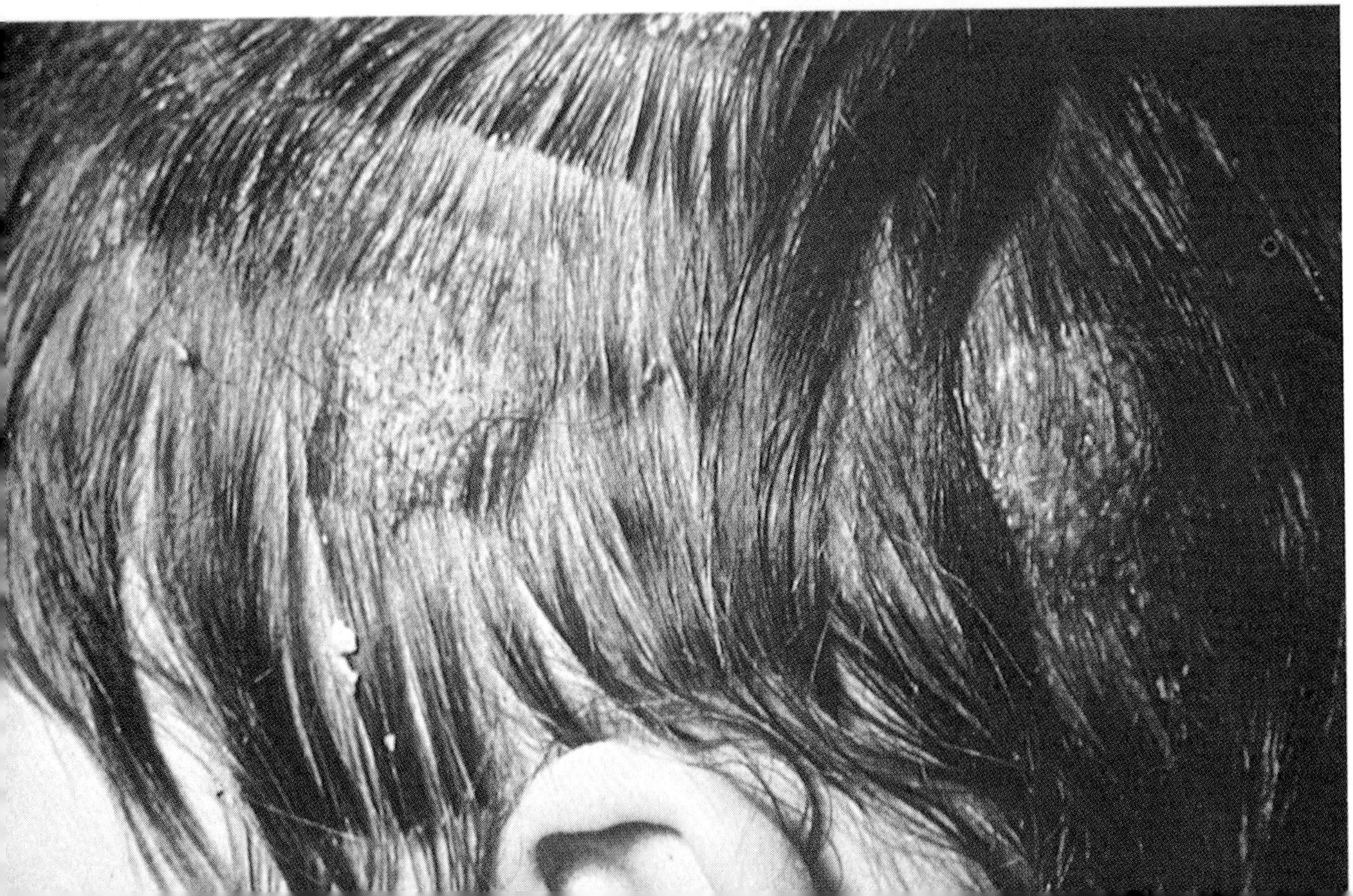

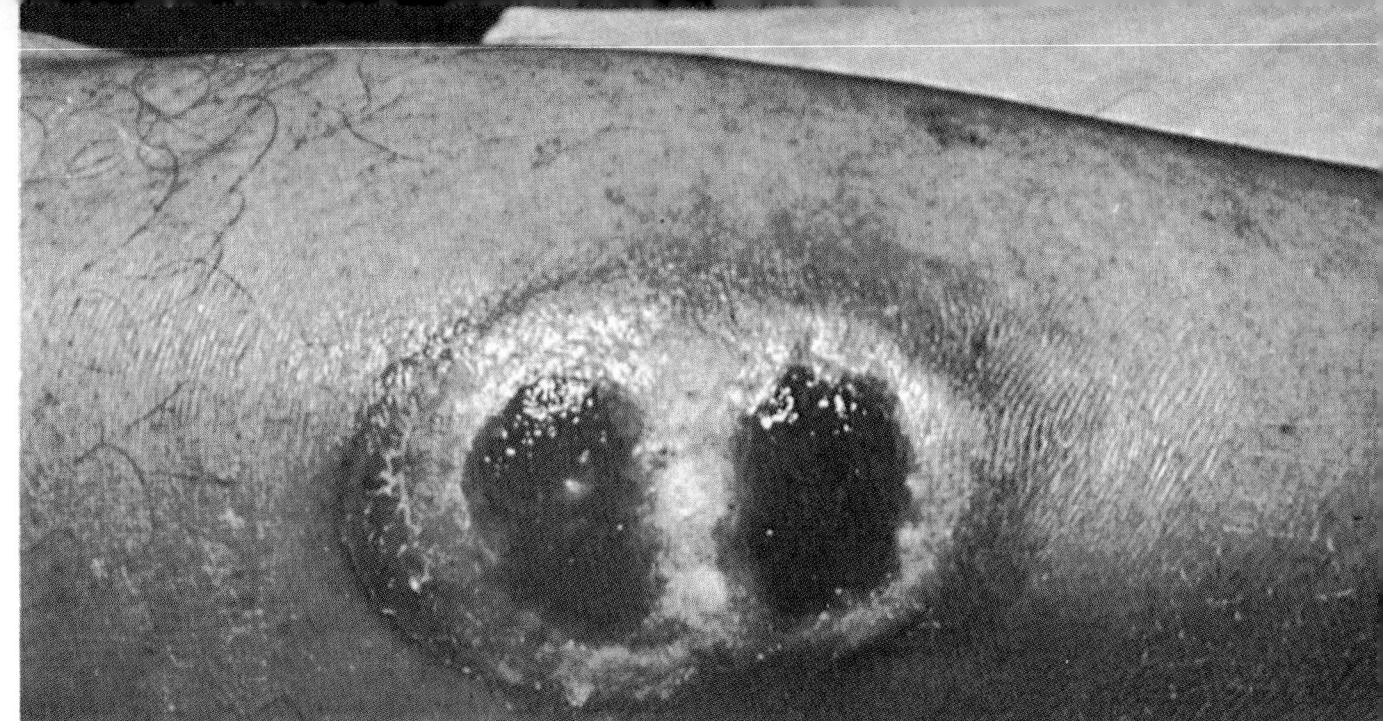

Skin cancer can occur anywhere on the body, but is seen most often on areas exposed to prolonged irritation or to intense sunlight. The cancer illustrated above, however, is located on an area of skin that is normally covered.

A cancer of the skin of the nose, known as a "rodent ulcer" (*left*), is a common form of cancer.

Basal cell cancer, illustrated below, is the most common form of skin cancer. It can nearly always be cured by surgical removal or by x-ray treatment.

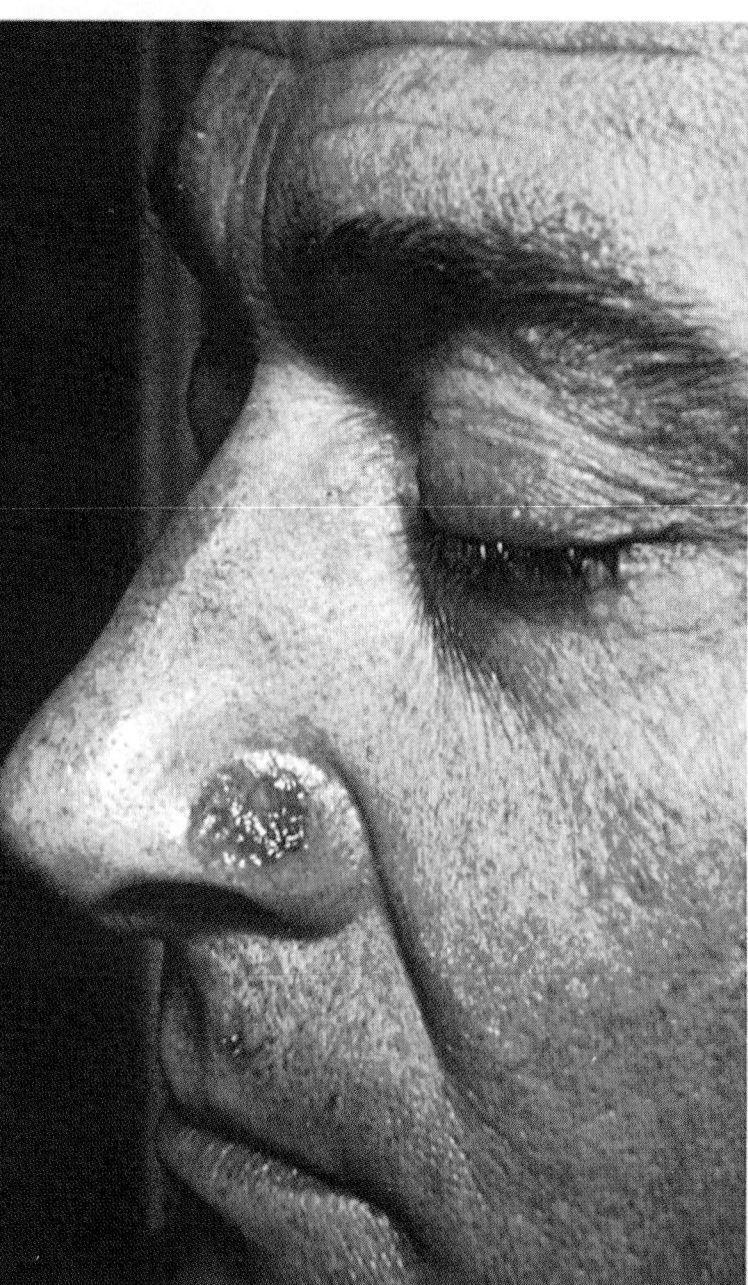

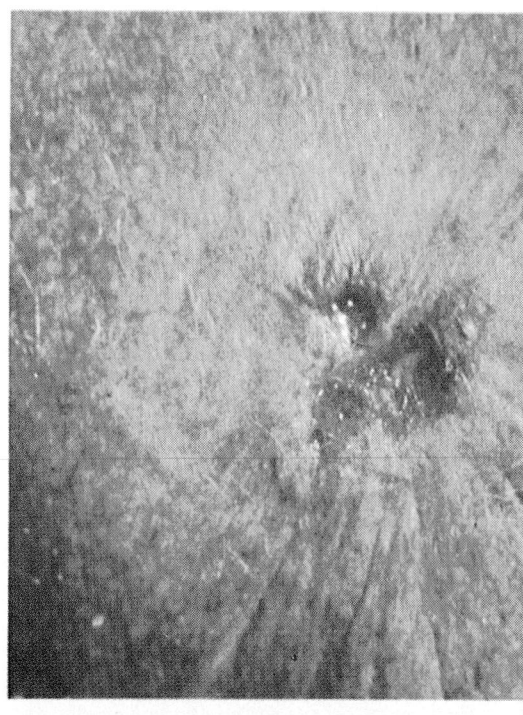

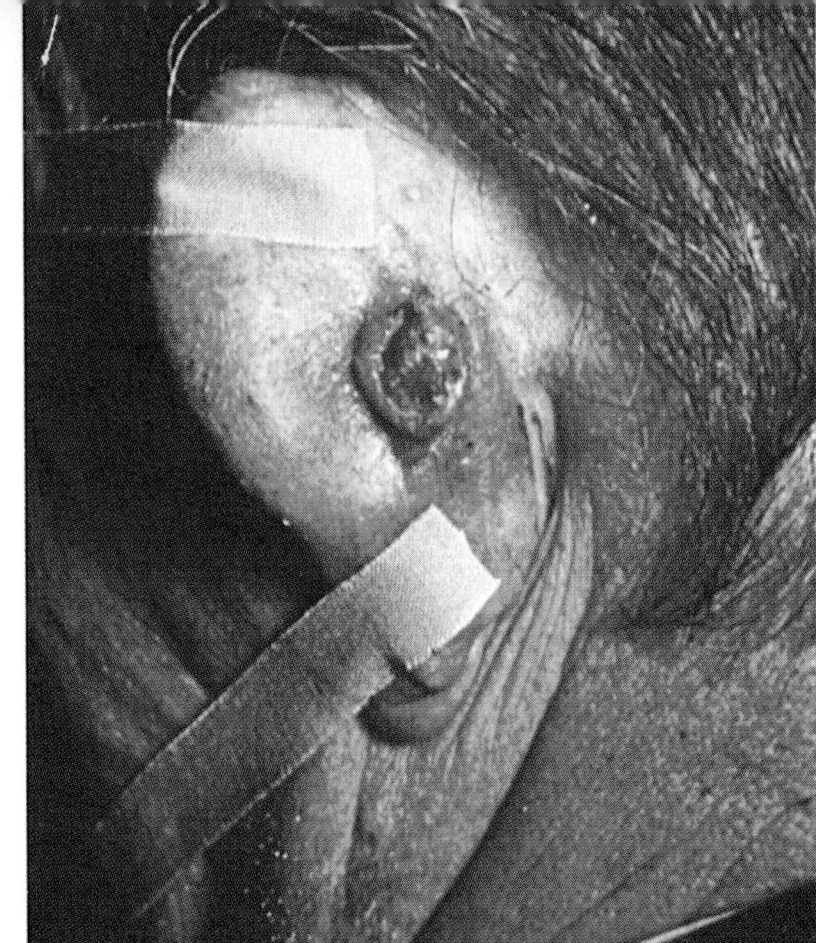

The ear is also a common location for skin cancer. This lesion is located on the back of the ear, but the most frequent site is the upper tip of the ear.

A melanoma is a malignant mole which must be removed surgically to prevent spread.

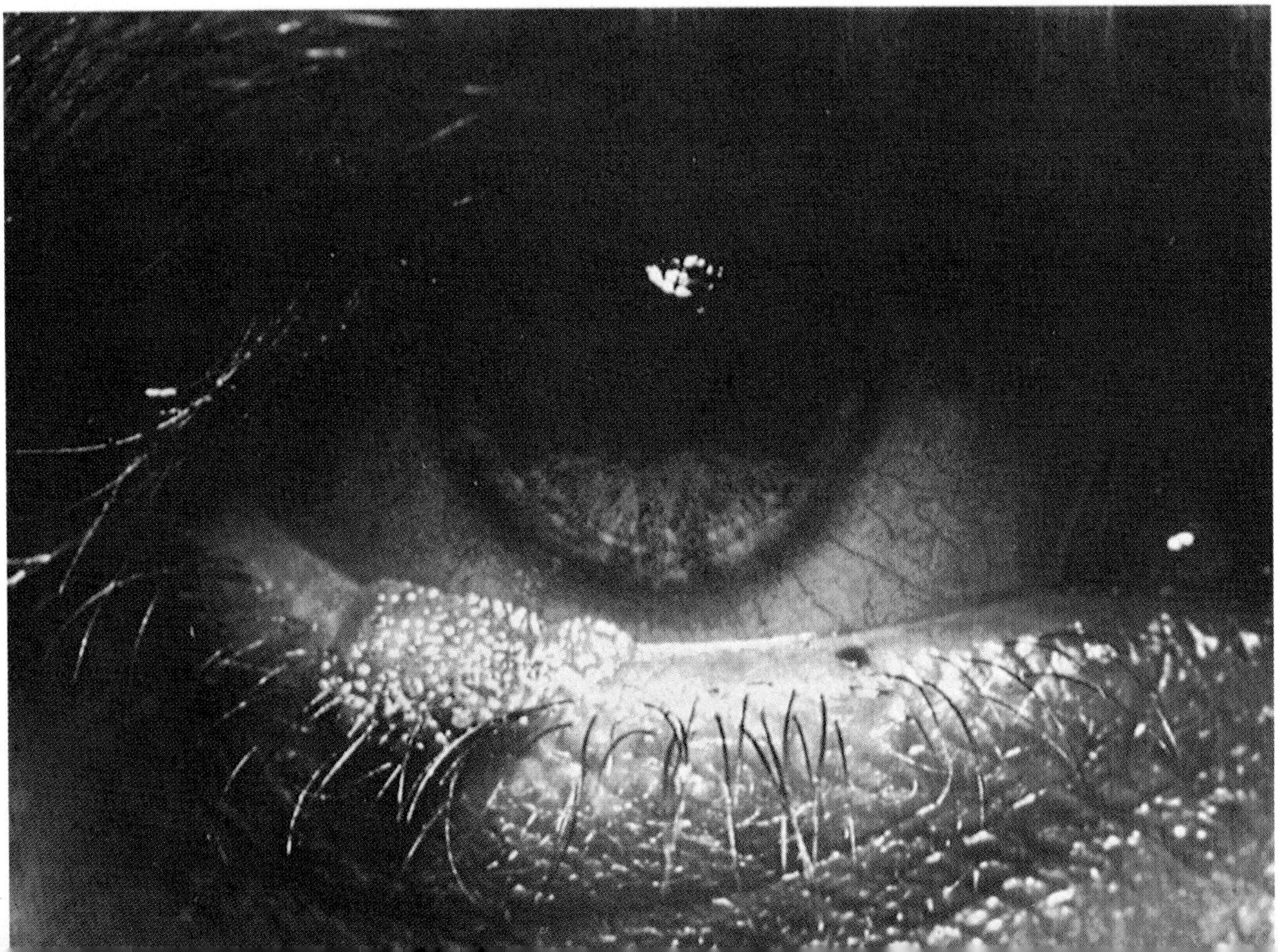

## STOMACH ULCERS

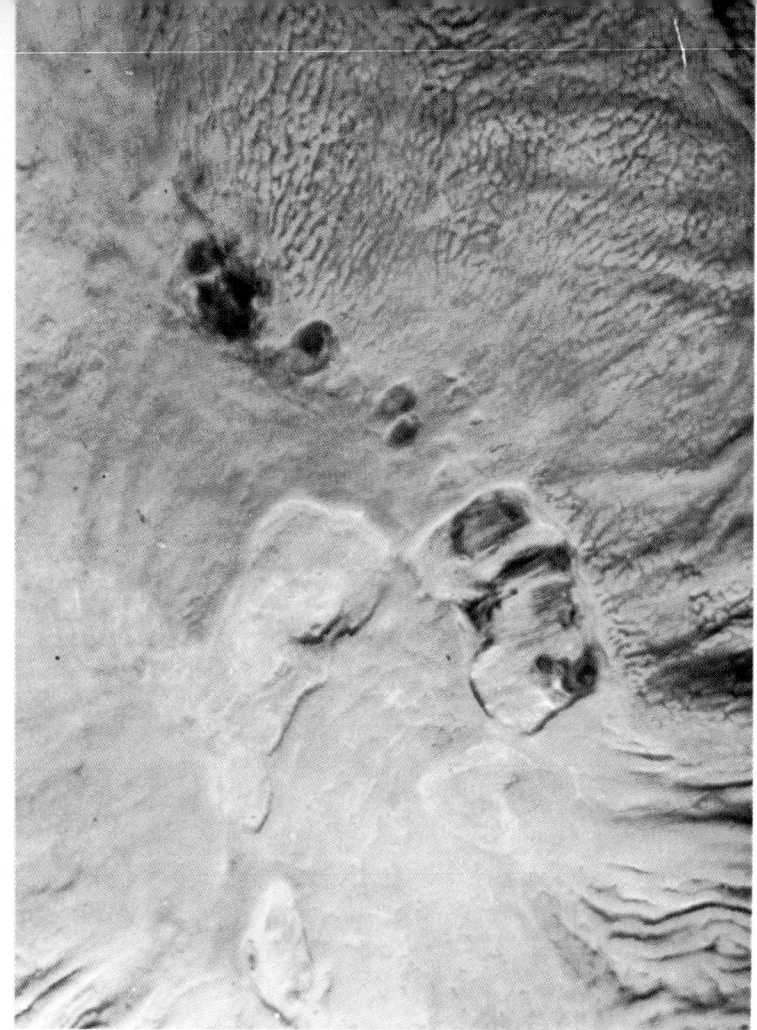

Ulcers of the stomach are often multiple. The bluish discoloration at the base of some of the ulcerations in the photograph at the left is caused by clotted blood.

One of the dangers of peptic ulcers is their tendency to rupture like the perforated stomach ulcer below.

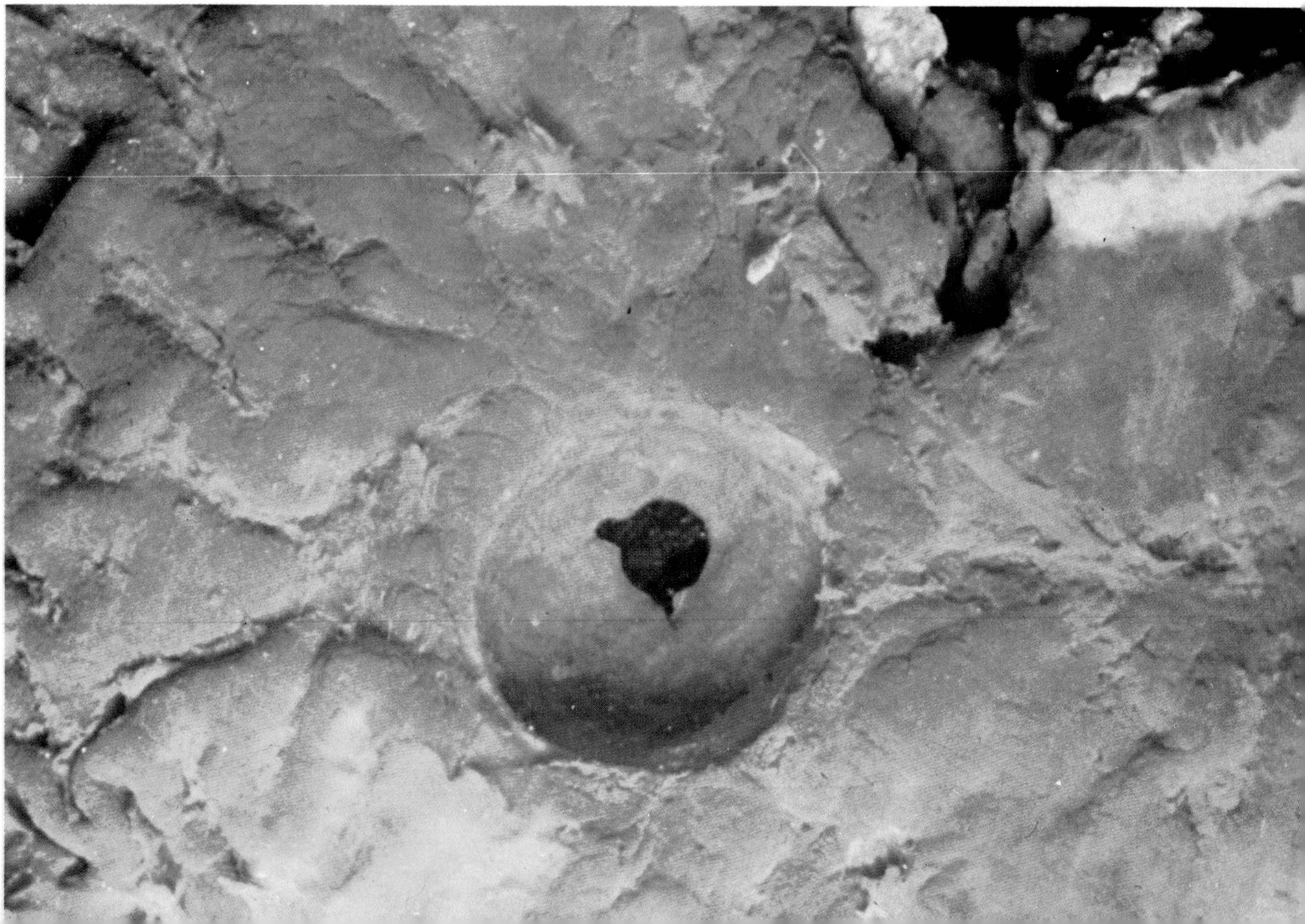

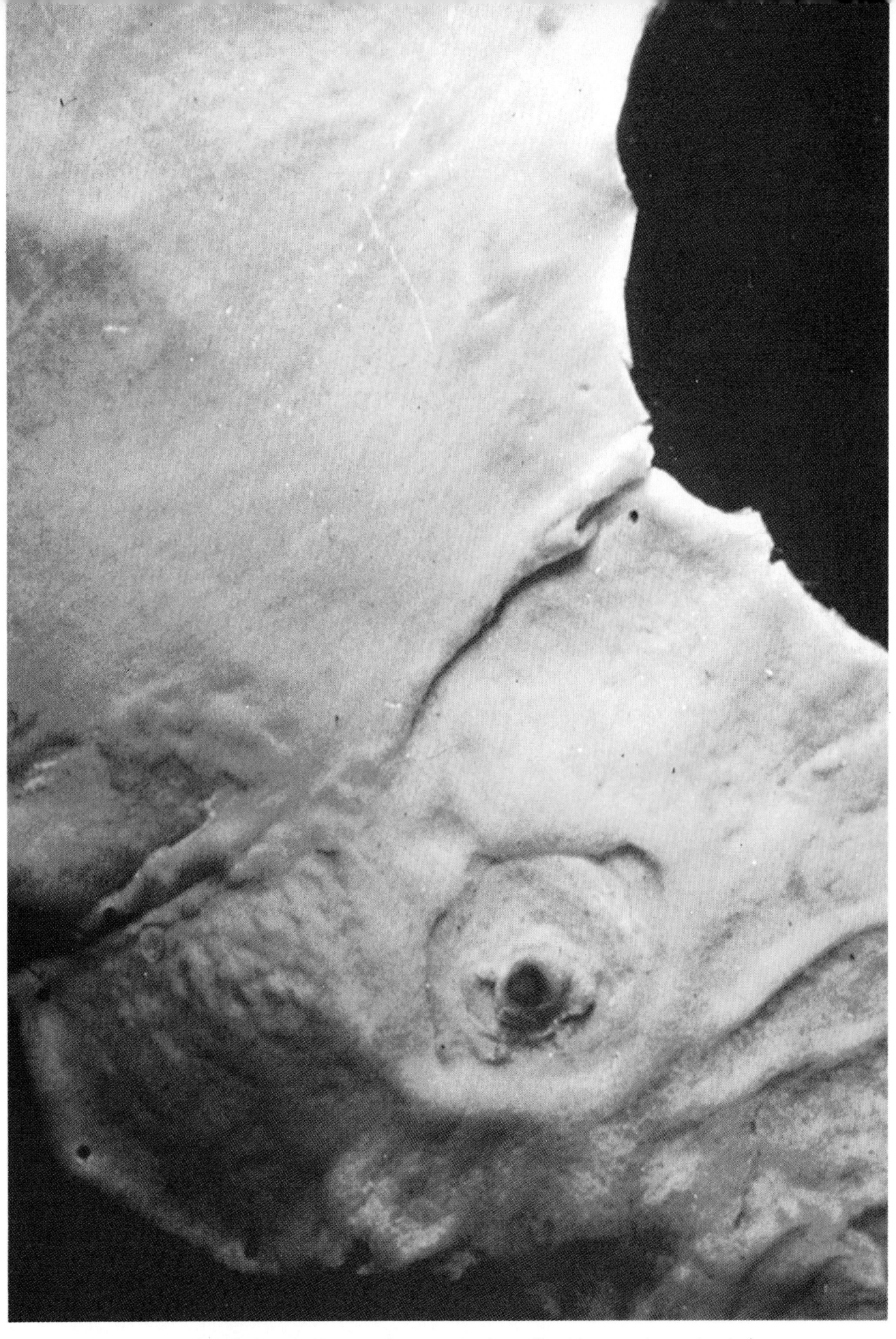

Approximately nine out of ten peptic ulcers, like this example, are located
in the first portion of the duodenum, rather than in the stomach.

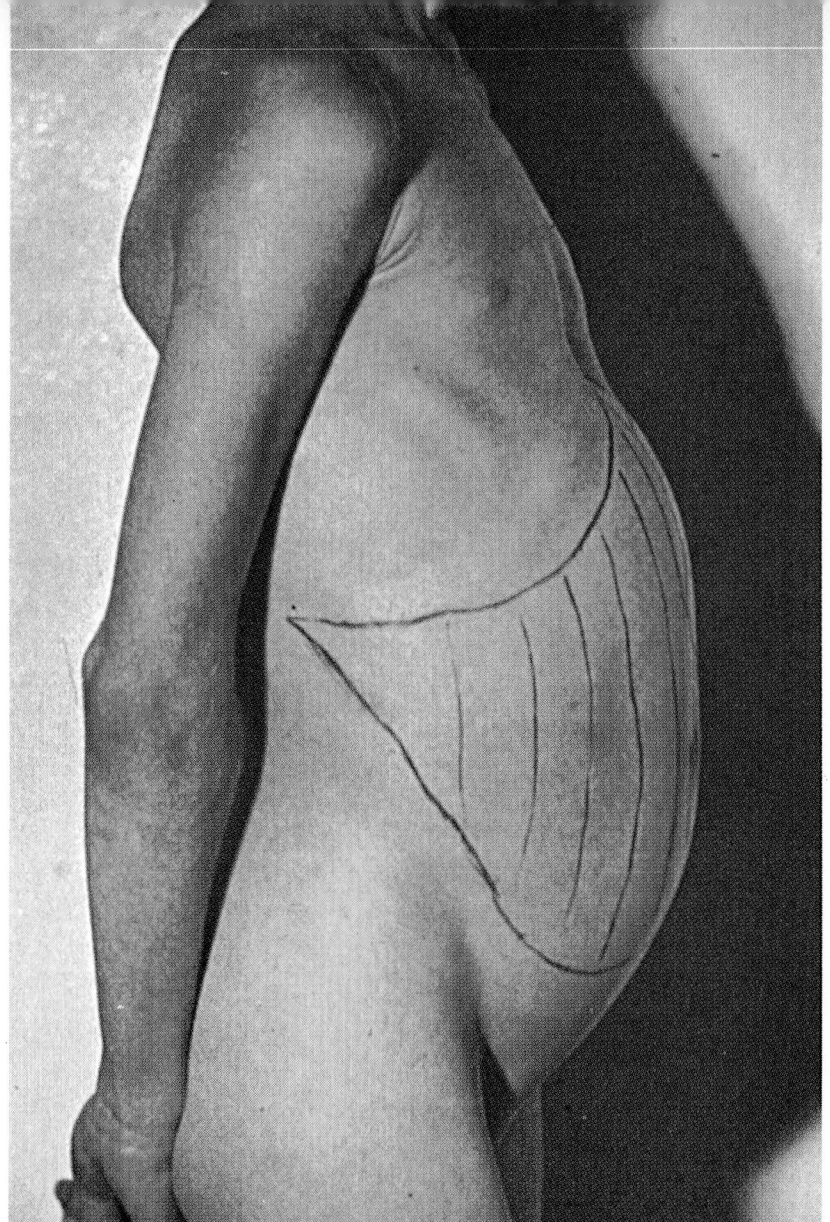

An enlarged spleen can be felt by the examining physician. In many instances, this condition is associated with an anemic disorder or with a malignant disease such as leukemia.

Rupture of the spleen, illustrated below, often results from a fall or from a severe blow to the abdomen.

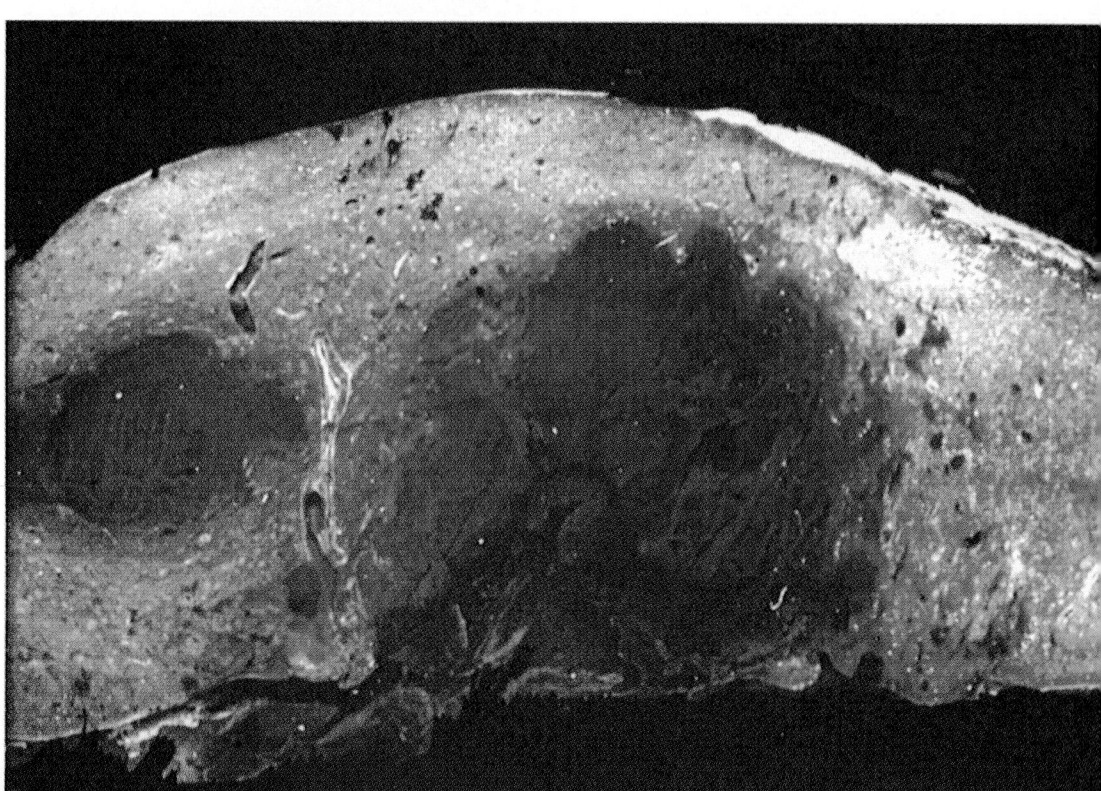

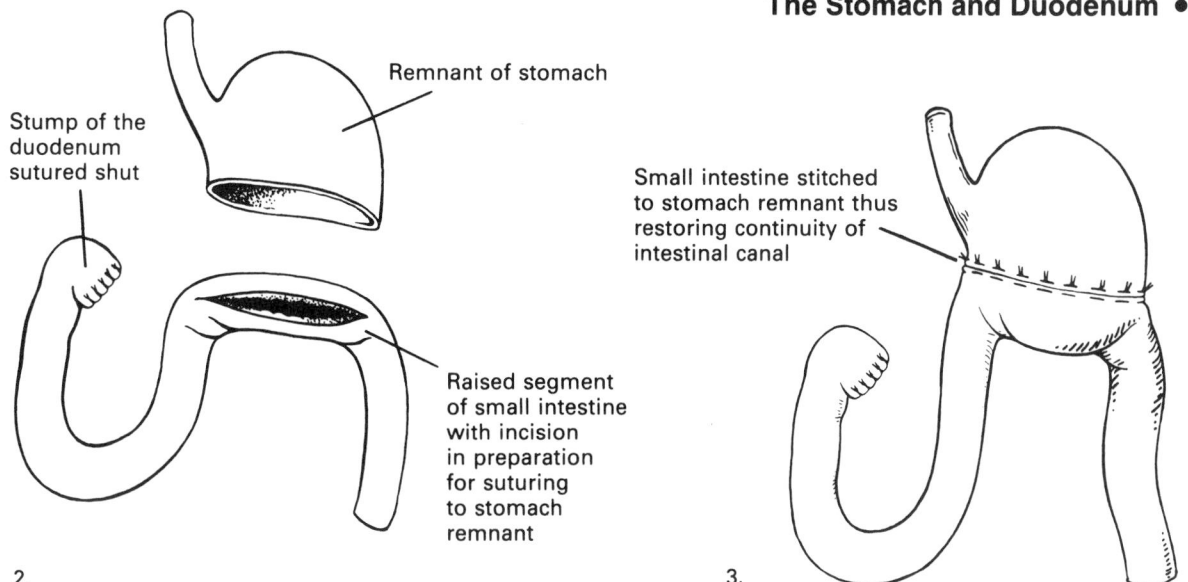

Stump of the duodenum sutured shut

Remnant of stomach

Raised segment of small intestine with incision in preparation for suturing to stomach remnant

2.

Small intestine stitched to stomach remnant thus restoring continuity of intestinal canal

3.

b. A vagotomy is performed, and the outlet of the stomach is altered so as to permit the regurgitation of bile from the alkaline duodenum into the stomach. This procedure is known as pyloroplasty.

c. A subtotal gastrectomy, as mentioned above.

d. A vagotomy is performed, and a short circuiting opening is made between the stomach and small intestine. This latter procedure is known as a gastrojejunostomy.

**Are all of the above operations equally successful in treating peptic ulcer?**

Although all of the above operations give satisfactory results, recent statistical studies seem to show that the operations associated with vagotomy give a somewhat higher cure rate than plain gastrectomy. This holds true for ulcers in the duodenum, but not for those located in the stomach.

**How long a period of hospitalization is usually required for operations for ulcer?**

Ten to fifteen days.

**Will special preoperative preparations be necessary?**

Yes. Patients are often admitted to the hospital a few days prior to surgery so that they can be prepared by liquid diet, washings of the stomach, intravenous medications, vitamins and—if they have lost much blood—transfusions.

**Are special nurses required after an operation for peptic ulcer?**

Yes, for several days.

**How long does it take to perform an ulcer operation?**

From two to five hours, depending upon the severity of the case and the type of operation performed. (Speed in surgery is not important.)

**What anesthesia is usually employed in ulcer operations?**

General inhalation anesthesia.

**What special postoperative treatments are necessary after ulcer operations?**

a. Liquid by mouth is withheld for two to three days, and food is not given for four to five days.

b. The patient is fed intravenously with glucose, proteins, minerals, and vitamins.

c. Stomach tubes are employed to keep the stomach or stomach remnant empty.

d. Antibiotics are sometimes given to prevent postoperative infection.

**What takes over the function of the stomach or duodenum when part of it is removed because of an ulcer?**

The remnant of the stomach dilates over a period of several months and, along with the small intestine to which it has been joined, a pouch is formed, which serves as an excellent receptacle for food.

**Do ulcers tend to recur after an operation has been carried out?**

They recur rarely—in less than 3 percent of cases.

**Can one ever return to completely normal eating after an ulcer operation?**

Yes, within a few months.

**What postoperative precautions must be followed after operations for ulcer?**

a. Do not eat too large quantities of food at one time.

b. Highly seasoned foods and alcoholic beverages should be kept at a minimum for several months postoperatively until one is sure that all ulcer symptoms have disappeared completely.

**What limitations on one's activities must be imposed after an ulcer operation?**

None, after the patient has convalesced completely. (This may require three to four months.)

**Does stomach removal for ulcer affect the span of life?**

No.

**Does stomach removal tend toward the development of anemia?**

Yes, in some cases. However, this can be treated successfully with medications to build up the blood.

**Is pregnancy permissible after an operation for peptic ulcer?**

Yes.

**How soon after an ulcer operation can one do the following:**

Bathe:
Ten to fifteen days.
Walk out on the street:
Ten to fifteen days.
Walk up and down stairs:
Ten to fifteen days.
Perform household duties:
Five to six weeks.
Drive a car:
Six weeks.
Resume sexual relations:
Five weeks.
Return to work:
Eight weeks.

**How often should one return for a periodic examination after an ulcer operation?**

Every four to six months.

**If a patient has had gastrectomy for duodenal ulcer, is the ulcer itself always removed?**

Not if it is technically too difficult to remove. Cure, in ulcer cases, is brought about by removing the acid-producing portion of the stomach, by

cutting the vagus nerve, which stimulates the production of acid, and by short-circuiting the flow of food so that it completely bypasses the duodenum. If this is done, the ulcer that has been left behind will heal very rapidly and will cause no symptoms.

**Can digestion be normal even without stomach acids and without part of the stomach?**

Yes. Approximately 10 percent of all people have little or no acid in their stomach. Also, it should be remembered that the major phase of digestion of foods takes place in the small intestine, not in the stomach.

## PYLORIC STENOSIS
*(Obstruction of the Outlet of the Stomach in the Newborn)*

**What is pyloric stenosis?**

An obstruction to the outlet of the stomach in infants during their first few weeks of life.

**What causes pyloric stenosis?**

An overgrowth of the muscle surrounding the pylorus.

**Are male infants affected more often than female infants?**

Yes. It is three times more common in males.

**How common is pyloric stenosis?**

It occurs approximately once in a thousand births.

**What are the symptoms of pyloric stenosis?**

a. Forceful vomiting, which sometimes shoots out of the mouth.
b. A lump, the size of a walnut, can usually be felt in the upper right portion of the abdomen.
c. Weight loss due to repeated vomiting.

d. X-ray findings demonstrating an obstruction to the passage of food from the stomach into the small intestine.

**What is the treatment for pyloric stenosis?**

The great majority of cases will require surgery. A small number can be treated successfully with antispasmodic drugs.

**How long should one wait before deciding to operate if symptoms persist?**

No longer than one to two weeks.

**What operative procedure is carried out?**

A small incision, two inches long, is made in the upper right portion of the abdomen. The pyloric portion of the stomach is grasped and the muscle fibers are cut. The mucous membrane lining is permitted to remain intact.

**How effective is surgery in the cure of pyloric stenosis?**

Practically all cases are cured by the operation described above.

**Is this operation dangerous?**

No. Recovery will take place in all cases, barring the exceptional complication that may accompany any surgical procedure.

**What type of anesthesia is used in operating upon pyloric stenosis?**

General inhalation anesthesia.

**How long a period of hospitalization is usually necessary?**

Five to seven days.

**Are special nurses required for the infant?**

No.

**How long does it take the wound to heal after an operation for pyloric stenosis?**

Seven to ten days.

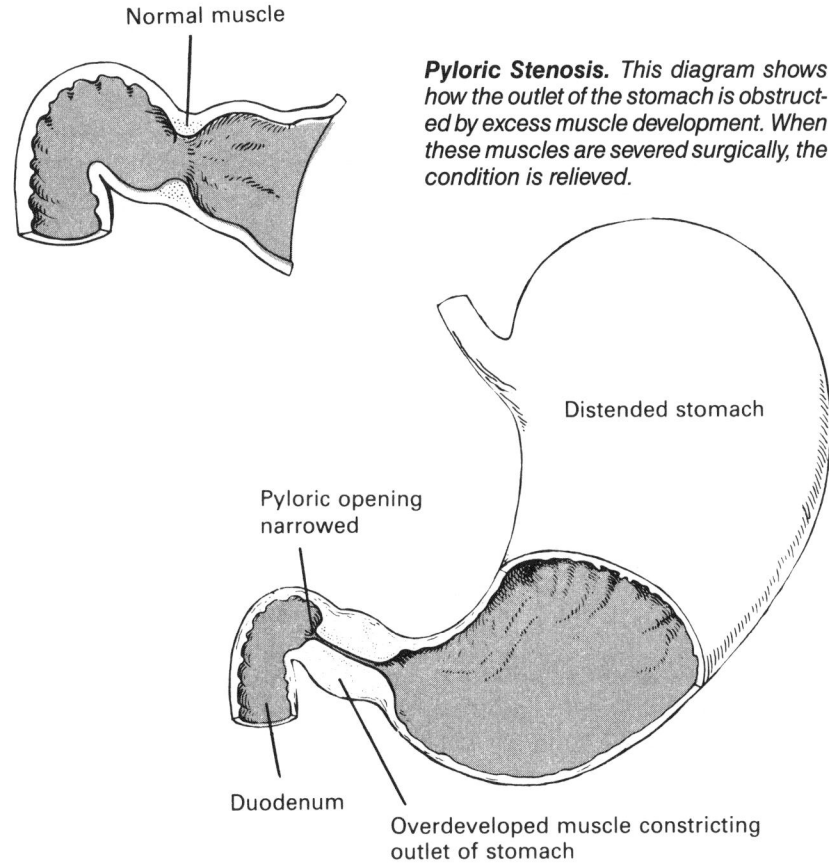

Normal muscle

*Pyloric Stenosis. This diagram shows how the outlet of the stomach is obstructed by excess muscle development. When these muscles are severed surgically, the condition is relieved.*

Distended stomach

Pyloric opening narrowed

Duodenum

Overdeveloped muscle constricting outlet of stomach

**How soon after surgery are feedings begun?**

Within twenty-four to forty-eight hours.

**Does pyloric stenosis, once operated upon, have a tendency to recur?**

No.

**Will the child live a completely normal life after pyloric stenosis?**

Yes. Development will not be impaired once surgical cure has been obtained.

**Does pyloric stenosis ever occur in older people?**

Yes, but this is a rare phenomenon.

## UPSIDE-DOWN STOMACH (Hernia of the Diaphragm)
*(See Chapter 30 on Hernia)*

## CANCER OF THE STOMACH

**What causes cancer of the stomach?**

In most instances, the cause is unknown. Some cancers are thought to have their origin in ulcers of the stomach.

**Are all tumors of the stomach cancerous?**

No. There may be tumors of the mucous membrane lining or of the muscle wall that are nonmalignant. The most common nonmalignant tumors are polyps of the mucous membrane, lipomas (fatty tumors), and myomas (tumors containing muscle tissue).

**Are nonmalignant tumors of the stomach curable?**

Yes. They can be removed surgically, either by local excision or by removing that portion of the stomach in which they grow.

**How common is cancer of the stomach?**

It is a frequently encountered type of cancer, but, for some unaccountable reason, its incidence has decreased considerably within the past twenty to thirty years.

**What age groups are most affected by cancer of the stomach?**

This is a disease most often found in middle age and in the later years of life.

**Does cancer of the stomach tend to run in families or to be inherited?**

No.

**Is there any way to prevent cancer of the stomach?**

The prompt removal of an ulcer in the stomach may prevent it from becoming cancerous. Also, cancer might be apprehended in its early stages if more people would visit their physician for a regular physical examination and if more people who have gastrointestinal symptoms would submit to thorough x-ray examinations.

**How is the diagnosis of cancer of the stomach made?**

By x-ray examination and by direct examination through an endoscope.

**What are the symptoms of cancer of the stomach?**

There are very few early symptoms. However, chronic indigestion, loss of appetite, slight weight loss, or pallor should stimulate one to seek medical advice.

**What is the treatment for cancer of the stomach?**

Prompt surgery with gastrectomy (the removal of all but a small remnant of the stomach).

**What special preoperative measures are necessary for cancer of the stomach?**

The same as for peptic ulcer.

**Are operations for cancer of the stomach very serious?**

Yes, but with modern advances in surgery, well over 90 percent will recover from their operation.

**How long a hospital stay is necessary for cancer of the stomach?**

Approximately two weeks.

**What type of anesthesia is used?**

General anesthesia used in conjunction with muscle relaxants and other drugs.

**How long does it take to perform an operation for cancer of the stomach?**

Two to five hours, depending upon whether the entire stomach is removed or only a portion of it is removed. Also, a great deal will depend upon the extent of spread and the technical problems that are encountered.

**Will a surgeon know whether a stomach ulcer is malignant when he views it at operation?**

Not always, but he will perform a gastrectomy nevertheless. The tissue will be submitted for microscopic examination, and this will tell the story within a few minutes. If the microscopic findings are not conclusive on immediate examination, the answer will be delayed for a couple of days until permanent microscopic sections have been checked.

**Are blood transfusions given during operations upon the stomach?**

Yes, in many cases.

**What is the usual postoperative course and what are the postoperative routines employed in cases of cancer of the stomach?**

Practically the same as those used after gastrectomy for ulcer, except that the patient is a good deal sicker after gastrectomy for cancer. (See the section on Peptic Ulcer in this chapter.)

**Are anticancer drugs ever helpful in prolonging the life of a patient who has undergone surgery for cancer of the stomach?**

Yes. A drug known as 5-FU, as well as other chemicals, sometimes brings about remission for several months or even years.

# CHAPTER 71
# THE THROAT

*(See also Chapter 39 on Lips, Jaws, Mouth, Teeth, and Tongue; Chapter 48 on Nose and Sinuses; Chapter 63 on Salivary Glands; Chapter 72 on Thyroid Gland)*

*Tonsils.* In this diagram, one tonsil is of normal size and the other one is enlarged because of infection.

Enlarged tonsil

Normal tonsil

## THE TONSILS AND ADENOIDS

### What are the tonsils, and where are they located?

The tonsils are two ovoid, glandlike structures measuring about one and a half inches long by three-quarters of an inch wide, imbedded in the sides of the throat just behind and above the level of the tongue.

### What is the normal appearance of the tonsils?

When normal, the tonsils are barely visible.

### What is the appearance of the tonsils when infected?

They may occupy a major portion of the pharynx and may actually meet in the midline. They can be seen as large reddened masses and, when acutely inflamed, yellow spots of pus can often be seen on their surface.

### What are the adenoids, and where are they located?

They consist of the same type of tissue as the tonsils and are located high up in the throat above the level of the soft palate. They cannot be easily seen on ordinary inspection of the throat. Normally, the adenoids are about half the size of the tonsils.

### What is the function of the tonsils and adenoids?

They are composed of lymphoid tissue and are thought to serve as a

*Adenoids.* Enlargement of the adenoids may lead to ear infections and often prevents breathing through the nose. In children adenoids are removed at the same time as tonsils.

Adenoids

barrier that localizes and gives immunity to infections that enter the body through the mouth or nose. They also serve to aid delayed immune responses.

### Since tonsils and adenoids are supposed to perform a useful function, why are they so frequently removed?

Because their function is lost when they become chronically infected. Under such circumstances, they act as a focus of infection and may lead to disease of other organs, such as the eyes, joints, muscles, kidneys, or even the heart.

### What are the symptoms of acute inflammation of the tonsils and adenoids?

Pain in the throat, high fever, and swelling of the glands of the neck. Infected adenoids may also cause infection of the sinuses, with obstruction of the air passages to the middle ear. This may eventually lead to ear infection and possible loss of hearing. With enlarged adenoids, the patient may develop into a mouth breather. If this condition is permitted to go uncorrected for a long period of time, facial changes may occur, with the upper lip being pulled upward and the face taking on a stupid, languid expression.

### When are tonsillectomy and adenoidectomy indicated?

Until recently, it was routine practice to recommend these operations for all children when they reached the age of three to five years. Now it is advised only when the tonsils have become chronically infected or when diseased adenoids give rise to nose or ear complications.

### What are the common causes of enlarged glands in the neck?

Acute infections of the tonsils, acute pharyngitis, infection of the adenoids, or infection of the sinuses.

### Are tonsils and adenoids always removed at the same time?

In children, it is customary to remove both the tonsils and the adenoids at the same time. However, in infants and young children with ear infection, it is occasionally advisable to remove adenoids without removing the tonsils. Since adenoid tissue tends to shrink after the tenth year of life, tonsillectomy is usually performed without removing the adenoids in adults.

### Are tonsillectomy and adenoidectomy dangerous operations?

These procedures are considered to be among the safest of all operations.

### What kind of anesthesia is used for these operations?

General anesthesia for children and local or general anesthesia for adults.

### What is the most favorable time of the year to remove tonsils and adenoids?

Any time of the year is satisfactory, except in allergic patients or children of allergic parents.

### Should allergic children, or those from an allergic family, undergo tonsillectomy or adenoidectomy?

Yes. However, the procedure should not be done in the hope of curing the allergy.

### Should children of allergic parents have tonsillectomy or adenoidectomy performed between April 1 and October 15?

No. It has been shown that tonsillectomy will increase their chances of developing into active hay fever patients during the following allergy season.

### Now that polio has been almost eradicated, have the restrictions been removed that govern the time of year when tonsillectomy should be performed?

Yes. Tonsils can be removed during any month of the year. Of course, if polio is present in a community, tonsillectomy will not be done during the months from April to November.

### What is the relationship of deafness to diseases of the tonsils and adenoids?

Enlarged and infected adenoids may cause recurrent middle ear infection and thus cause impairment of hearing. Also, adenoid tissue near the opening of the Eustachian tube, by mechanically obstructing the tube, may cause a faulty replacement of the air in the middle ear, thus interfering with hearing.

### Will removal of chronically infected adenoids and tonsils improve hearing in children?

Yes, if the deafness has been caused by the infected adenoid.

### How soon after an acute upper respiratory infection or an acute tonsillitis can tonsillectomy be performed?

At least two to three weeks should elapse. Usually, antibiotics are prescribed before and after such operations to minimize the chances of infection.

### If a child has been exposed to a contagious disease, should tonsillectomy be postponed?

Yes, until all chance of catching the disease has passed.

### Do acute infections of the tonsils require treatment?

Most definitely, yes. They should be strenuously treated with antibiotics. Failure to do this may result in bacteria getting into the bloodstream and affecting other parts of the body.

### Do abscesses ever form within the tonsil or near the tonsil?

Yes. Abscesses just behind or to the side of the tonsils are quite common. This is called a peritonsillar abscess or quinsy sore throat.

### What is the treatment for quinsy sore throat?

a. Removing the pus through a needle.
b. Incision and drainage of the abscess. This can often be done with a little local anesthesia in the surgeon's office. On the other hand, if the abscess is very large, it may be best to incise it in the hospital.

Antibiotics are administered following both of the above procedures.

### How is the diagnosis of peritonsillar abscess made?

The child will develop high fever, and on inspection it is noticed that there is a tremendous swelling and tenderness around the tonsil. There is also a characteristic voice change and an inability to open the mouth widely.

**Do adults ever develop peritonsillar abscess?**

Yes, but it is not nearly as common among them as it is among children.

**Does quinsy sore throat ever produce suffocation?**

Yes. If untreated, the entire back of the throat may become involved and may make it very difficult for air to reach the lungs. Also, the abscess may rupture spontaneously, and the pus may be breathed into the lungs, causing suffocation.

**What other diseases can result from a poorly treated case of acute tonsillitis?**

Rheumatic fever sometimes follows a streptococcal infection of the tonsils. Also, certain types of nephritis (kidney inflammation) can follow acute tonsillitis. In the rare case, the valves of the heart may become infected secondary to tonsillitis (endocarditis).

**Will most acute infections of the tonsils and adenoids clear up by themselves?**

Yes, but the chronic infections do not tend to clear up by themselves.

**What is the best method to prevent recurring attacks of tonsillitis?**

Remove the tonsils.

**Do tonsils and adenoids ever grow back once they have been removed?**

Yes, but only when they have not been removed completely.

**What are the definite indications for tonsillectomy and adenoidectomy?**

a. Obstruction to breathing.
b. Recurrent ear infections.
c. Recurrent sore throat.
d. When the tonsils are suspected of acting as a focus of infection for diseases in other organs.
e. Chronically infected tonsils or adenoids that no longer serve a useful function and are subject to recurrent acute infections.

**Are special preoperative measures necessary before removing the tonsils and adenoids?**

Some physicians will give antibiotics before this procedure in order to cut down on the possibility of infection. Other surgeons will prescribe Vitamin K to minimize the chances of bleeding postoperatively.

**Is it important to study a child's blood prior to removing his tonsils and adenoids?**

Yes. The child must be examined thoroughly to make sure he has no bleeding tendencies. This can be done on the day prior to, or the day of, the operation. Hemoglobin evaluation is also necessary, for if the child is very anemic, tonsillectomy will be postponed.

**Should children be told that they are going to have their tonsils removed?**

Yes. It is important that they be told the truth. If possible, children should see the recovery room several days prior to surgery. They should be told that the surgery is painless and that they will sleep through it. If it is to be performed in the surgeon's office, then the child should be told that his parents will be at his side when he awakens from the operation.

**Why is it that some surgeons perform tonsillectomy in their offices, while others insist upon hospitalizing their patients?**

If the surgeon has complete facilities, including beds for aftercare and the proper anesthetic equipment, he will often advocate that the operation be performed in his office. If the facilities in the surgeon's office are not equal to those in the hospital, the surgeon will probably advocate hospitalization. Office surgery is done only rarely today.

**What is the technique used in removing the tonsils and adenoids?**

The tonsillar tissue is separated from its bed and is snared off close to the tongue. Adenoids are removed with a knife attached to a basket. The entire procedure usually takes about a half hour to perform.

**Do stitches have to be removed after tonsillectomy and adenoidectomy?**

No.

**What are the usual aftereffects of these operations?**

Pain in the throat or ears, or both, may persist for a week or ten days after surgery. This pain is often aggravated by eating, drinking, or merely swallowing. This pain can be minimized and kept under reasonable control by the liberal use of pain-relieving medications.

**Do some children normally have a peculiar tone to their speech after removal of tonsils and adenoids?**

Yes. This should occasion no alarm as it will last for only a few weeks or, at the most, for a few months.

**How soon after surgery can a patient begin to talk?**

Even though it is painful, the sooner the patient begins to talk the better, as this will return the muscles of the throat to normal.

**How long must the patient remain in bed after tonsillectomy and adenoidectomy?**

One to two days.

**Do children require special nurses after these operations?**

The child should be watched for several hours after surgery to make sure he is breathing properly and that no excessive bleeding is taking place.

**How long a hospital stay is necessary after tonsillectomy?**

One day.

**How soon after operation can a child bathe?**

Five to seven days.

**How often does postoperative hemorrhage occur after tonsillectomy and adenoidectomy?**

This occurs in only one in twenty-five cases. Today's surgeons take much greater care in tying off bleeders in the tonsil bed, thus cutting down on the incidence of postoperative bleeding.

**What types of postoperative hemorrhages might be encountered?**

a. Immediate bleeding, which may occur shortly after the surgery and can be controlled quite readily before the child leaves the operating room or the surgeon's office.
b. The delayed type of postoperative bleeding occurs on the fifth to the eighth day after operation. This is due to the falling away or loosening of the scab that has formed at the operative site. A small vessel or capillary may be exposed, which forms a blood clot and keeps the vessel open and produces the bleeding.

**Is hemorrhage after tonsillectomy dangerous?**

No. However, certain rare cases will bleed excessively and must demand the attention of the surgeon. The surgeon can control the bleeding readily by removal of the clot and the application of pressure.

**How can hemorrhage after tonsillectomy be recognized?**

Most children normally vomit blood mixed with stomach juices several hours after operation. Thereafter, there should be no further blood seen either in the nostrils, in the mouth, or in the throat. If a child vomits after being taken home, and if the vomit contains blood, the doctor should be notified at once.

**Is any special postoperative diet required after these operations?**

No, except to avoid highly spiced or highly seasoned foods. It is suggested that on the first day the patient be given water, milk, ice cream, etc., in small quantities. On the second day, in addition, he may have cereal, malted milk, Jello, junket, pudding, custard, broth, etc. On the third and fourth days potatoes, eggs, toast, etc., may be added. On the fifth day, a normal diet may be resumed.

**When is it necessary to use antibiotics before or after tonsillectomy?**

When a child has had recurrent sore throats and colds without a free interval of two to three weeks, they should be given. In addition, it is now routine practice to give antibiotics for a week after surgery.

**Should an ice collar be used for the sore throat following tonsillectomy?**

No. It is of no value.

**When can the patient be taken out of doors after operation?**

About the fifth day, weather permitting.

**How soon can the child return to school after tonsillectomy?**

One week, if the temperature is normal.

**When should an adult return to full activity after tonsillectomy?**

Ten to fourteen days.

## PHARYNGITIS *(Sore Throat)*

**What is pharyngitis?**

An inflammation of the lining of the back wall of the throat due either to an irritant or to a bacterial infection.

**What are the symptoms of pharyngitis?**

Pain in the back of the throat, difficulty on swallowing, and fever, often accompanied by a feeling of malaise.

**Is sore throat always a disease entity in itself?**

No. It often is the beginning of an upper respiratory infection, such as a cold or influenza.

**Does pharyngitis often herald the onset of some other infection?**

Yes. There are innumerable diseases that begin with a sore throat.

**What is the meaning of the term streptococcus sore throat?**

While it is true that many cases of pharyngitis are caused by the streptococcus germ, many other bacteria and viruses can produce sore throats. The true streptococcus sore throat is an epidemiclike disease in the community, usually stemming from a common focus of infection, such as infected milk, etc.

**What are the symptoms of a true streptococcus infection of the pharynx?**

There is usually sudden onset, chills and fever, general weakness, headache, and severe prostration. The throat appears very red and swollen and has gray patches upon it. A culture of the germs infecting the pharynx will show the hemolytic streptococcus.

**What is the treatment of pharyngitis?**

This depends upon the cause. If it is bacterial in origin, antibiotics along with hot gargles and irrigations are prescribed.

**Is local treatment of much value in treating pharyngitis?**

No. However, in an isolated case, painting the back of the throat with silver nitrate may limit the spread of infection.

### Are the antihistaminic drugs of much value in the treatment of pharyngitis?

No, since the symptoms of infection will continue as soon as the drugs are discontinued.

### Are local medications such as lozenges, medicated chewing gum, and gargling of much value in the treatment of pharyngitis?

Although they may bring about temporary relief, they have no more than slight value. Most of their value is in the fact that they contain a local anesthetic agent.

### Should antibiotics be given for all cases of pharyngitis?

No. The giving of excess antibiotics may sensitize the patient to their use, so that they will not have nearly as much value when they are truly needed for a serious condition. It must be remembered that most cases of pharyngitis will clear up by themselves within a few days.

### What is the most soothing local medication for pharyngitis?

Warm gargles or irrigations containing salt and aspirin.

### What is chronic pharyngitis?

This is a thickening in the lining membrane of the pharynx associated with repeated attacks of acute pharyngitis or secondary to chronic irritating factors.

### What are some of the causes of chronic pharyngitis?

a. Repeated attacks of acute pharyngitis.
b. Excess tobacco smoking.
c. Excess use of alcohol.
d. Sinus infections.
e. Inhalation of irritating substances over a prolonged period of time.
f. Constitutional or generalized disease.

### What are the symptoms of chronic pharyngitis?

Dry and sore throat, with a tickling sensation requiring repeated hawking and coughing.

### Can a diagnosis of chronic pharyngitis be made on observation?

Yes. There is usually a thickening of the mucous membranes and an overgrowth of the lymphoid tissue.

### What is the treatment for chronic pharyngitis?

The primary aim is to remove the cause to prevent further harm. Local treatment with stimulating medications is given along with other measures to improve the local oral hygiene.

## THE LARYNX

### What is the larynx?

A semirigid framework of cartilages held together by ligaments. It is lined with mucous membrane that is continuous with the throat above and the trachea (windpipe) below.

### Where is the larynx located?

It forms a prominence in the neck commonly known as the Adam's apple.

### What are the chief functions of the larynx?

The chief functions are speech, respiration, and action of the epiglottis, which shunts food into the esophagus.

### How is speech created?

By the passage of air through the larynx while the position of the vocal cords is varied so as to change the size of the opening and the degree of tension of the cords themselves.

### How is the larynx concerned with respiration?

Air is permitted to enter the trachea and lungs by action of the laryngeal muscles, which keep the vocal cords apart.

### How does the larynx serve as a valve?

It has a valvular action that closes the entrance to the trachea to food or any foreign particles. This same action prevents the escape of air from the lungs when it is found necesary to hold one's breath.

### Can the larynx be studied and examined by a physician on direct inspection?

Yes. This is done by mirror visualization and is called indirect laryngoscopy. It can also be seen by direct laryngoscopy, wherein a lighted hollow metal tube is inserted into the mouth and behind the tongue down toward the larynx.

### What conditions can be noted by the physician when he views the larynx?

He can determine the presence or absence of infection; he can observe the action of the vocal cords to note whether they are functioning properly; he can detect the presence of growths within the larynx.

### What are the symptoms of acute laryngitis?

Acute laryngitis is due to an inflammation of the mucous membrane of the larynx and is characterized by a hoarse voice and pain and swelling in the region of the larynx. There may be rapid onset, or it may be in a less acute form.

### What causes acute infections of the larynx?

Any of the bacteria that can cause an infection elsewhere in the body.

### Can inflammation of the larynx be caused by irritating substances, such as smoke, gas, fumes, scalding steam, dust, etc.?

Yes.

## Is acute laryngitis usually a dangerous condition?

No. It usually appears as part of an upper respiratory infection and will run its course within a week to ten days.

## What are the dangers of laryngitis?

The ordinary case of laryngitis is not dangerous. However, since the larynx is the bottleneck of the airway (it being the narrowest passage space to the lungs), any decrease in the area caused by swelling or any compression may produce a serious obstruction to breathing.

## What is croup?

It is an acute inflammation of the larynx and may produce serious impairment of breathing in children. (See Chapter 32, on Infant and Childhood Diseases.)

## What is the treatment for acute laryngitis?

a. Rest the voice and do not attempt to speak.
b. Humidify the air, usually by steam inhalations.
c. Take heavy doses of the antibiotic drugs under the supervision of the physician.
d. If there is great difficulty in breathing, an oxygen tent may be necessary.
e. In emergency cases only, it may be necessary to do a tracheotomy to save life.

## What are the usual causes of hoarseness?

Any factor that prevents the normal meeting of the two vocal cords in the midline will cause a change in the voice. This may be a slight swelling of the mucous membrane, a foreign body, a tumor or paralysis of one of the vocal cords.

## What is the significance of prolonged or chronic hoarseness?

It indicates a disease of one or both of the vocal cords.

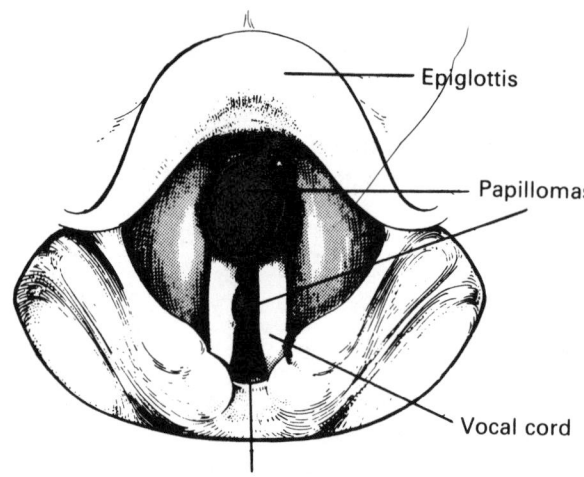

*Papilloma of the Vocal Cord. This diagram shows a warty growth known as a papilloma on one of the vocal cords and a larger one below the epiglottis. Such tumors cause persistent hoarseness. This type of tumor lends itself to easy surgical removal and cure.*

Epiglottis

Papillomas

Vocal cord

Air passage into trachea

## How soon should one consult his physician for hoarseness?

Any hoarseness that does not clear up within one to two weeks should be investigated by a physician.

## What are the chief causes of chronic hoarseness?

a. A chronic inflammation of the larynx.
b. A paralysis of one of the vocal cords.
c. A tumor of one of the vocal cords.
d. Pressure from a growth, such as a goiter, upon the larynx.
e. A tumor of the wall of the larynx.

# TUMORS OF THE LARYNX

## Are tumors of the larynx very common?

Yes. This is a very commonly encountered condition. Fortunately, most of these growths are benign.

## What is the most frequently encountered benign tumor of the larynx?

A papilloma of the vocal cord.

## How is the diagnosis of laryngeal tumor made?

The larynx is inspected by direct or indirect laryngoscopy. The surgeon can usually tell, from the appearance and location of the tumor, whether or not it is benign.

## How is a definite diagnosis of the type of laryngeal tumor made?

A small piece of the tumor tissue is removed through the laryngoscope and is examined under the microscope in the laboratory. This biopsy will tell whether the tumor is benign or cancerous.

## What are the common symptoms of a laryngeal tumor?

Hoarseness is the chief symptom and may be the only one. If the tumor becomes very large, which is unusual, it may obstruct the airway and result in difficult breathing. Less common complaints are coughing, pain, difficulty in swallowing, and a blood-tinged sputum.

## What is the treatment for benign laryngeal tumors?

They must be removed surgically. This can frequently be done in an office under local anesthesia through the laryngoscope. Occasionally, hospitalization is required and the tumor is removed under local or general anesthesia. Although the procedure may be unpleasant, it is not painful or serious.

## What are the results of surgery for benign laryngeal tumors?

Excellent. Most of these lesions are

polyps. Some have a tendency, once removed, to recur. Thus, removal may have to be done again.

### Is hoarseness cured by the removal of a benign laryngeal tumor?

Yes, but it is important to emphasize that the voice should not be used for two to three weeks following surgery.

### How frequent is cancer of the larynx?

It is a relatively uncommon disease, seen mainly in men over fifty years of age.

### What is the cause of cancer of the larynx?

The cause is unknown. However, the history of most patients with cancer of the larynx indicates that they have been heavy smokers or people who abuse their voice. Also, a history of drinking excessive quantities of straight alcohol is often obtained.

### How is a definite diagnosis of cancer of the larynx made?

By taking a piece of the tissue and submitting it to microscopic examination.

### What is the treatment for cancer of the larynx?

a. Cobalt or supervoltage x-ray radiation.
b. Surgical removal of the larynx.
c. A combination of radiation treatment and surgical removal of the larynx.

### Is removal of the larynx (laryngectomy) a serious surgical procedure?

Yes. However, in expert hands, operative recovery takes place in the vast majority of cases.

### Can a cure of cancer of the larynx be obtained?

Yes, provided the operation has been performed when the cancer is in a relatively early stage of development. Or, if x-ray therapy has been the treatment of choice, a cure can frequently be obtained if treatment is begun during the early stages of the tumor growth.

### Are blood transfusions given during operations for removal of the larynx?

Yes. Also, special nursing care is an absolute necessity, as patients who have undergone such operations have a tracheotomy tube, which must be carefully tended.

### How long a hospital stay is necessary following laryngectomy?

Usually two weeks, but sometimes as long as three or four weeks.

### Can people who have had their larynx removed talk again?

Yes, but the voice is markedly changed and speaking is accomplished only after they have received several weeks or months of special instruction.

### If the entire larynx has been removed, will people breathe normally or will they have to use a tracheotomy tube?

When a total laryngectomy has been performed, the patient must breathe through a tracheotomy tube placed in the neck.

### Can a useful voice be developed after a total laryngectomy?

Yes. This is accomplished by learning how to bring up air from the stomach. Also, there are electrical devices that act more or less in the same manner as a larynx.

## THE TRACHEA *(Windpipe)*

### What is tracheitis?

It is an inflammation of the mucous membrane lining of the trachea, extending from below the Adam's apple down into the lungs.

### What are the symptoms of an inflammation of the trachea?

a. A tightness and burning in the chest and under the breastbone.
b. A cough and wheezing.
c. The bringing up of sputum.
d. Fever, malaise.

### What are the causes of tracheitis?

It is most often seen as an accompaniment of an acute upper respiratory infection and can be caused by the usual causes of these conditions.

### Can tracheitis also be caused by irritants such as smokes, vapors, chemicals, and fumes?

Yes.

### What is the treatment for acute tracheitis?

The same as for the other upper respiratory infections that usually accompany it.

### Does tracheitis often appear as a forerunner of bronchitis or pneumonia?

Yes. Tracheitis is usually seen as part of a general respiratory infection.

## TRACHEOTOMY
*(Tracheostomy)*

### What is a tracheotomy?

It is an operation in which an artificial opening is made into the trachea through an incision in the neck below the level of the larynx.

### What conditions require tracheotomy?

a. Suffocation due to obstruction of the airway above or at the level of the larynx.
b. Postoperative conditions in which mucous secretions block the bronchial tubes, causing severe respiratory difficulties so that the patient is unable to expel the mucus voluntarily.

### What are the main symptoms of obstruction of the larynx?

a. Difficulty in breathing.
b. Pallor and restlessness.

*(continued)*

c. Bluish discoloration of the lips.

d. Rapid respiration and rapid pulse.

**What are the most common causes of obstruction of the larynx?**

a. Abscess formation.

b. Inflammation of the lining of the cartilages of the larynx.

c. Severe croup.

d. Acute inflammation involving the tissues surrounding the larynx. This may occur from neck infections extending from the floor of the mouth (Ludwig's angina).

e. Injuries or wounds of the larynx or nearby structures with swelling of the tissues composing the larynx.

f. A foreign body that gets stuck in the larynx. This occurs in children who sometimes swallow coins or peanuts, etc.

g. Burns of the larynx from scalding liquids or inhaling live steam.

h. Inhalation of severely irritating chemicals or vapors.

i. Paralysis of both vocal cords.

**What first aid should be given to someone choking from a foreign body in the larynx or trachea?**

If the foreign body cannot be

*Tracheotomy. This diagram shows how the trachea has been opened and a tube inserted in order to restore a free airway. This procedure is performed whenever there is danger of suffocation due to obstruction in the throat or larynx. When the obstruction has been relieved, the tube is removed, the hole will heal, and the patient will resume normal breathing through the nose.*

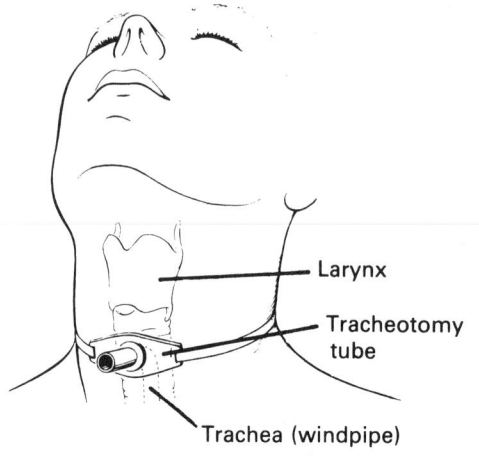

Larynx

Tracheotomy tube

Trachea (windpipe)

retrieved by inserting a finger into the throat, then the Heimlich maneuver should be tried. The victim should be grasped from behind with both arms surrounding the lower chest. The first-aider's fist, covered by his other hand, should be at a level just below the breastbone. Then with a sudden, forceful inward and upward thrust, the arms and hands are tightened. This will usually cause the foreign body to be dislodged and coughed up.

**When should a tracheotomy be performed?**

When the laryngeal obstruction has developed to such an extent that the patient is unable to breathe at all and life is obviously threatened.

**How is an emergency tracheotomy performed?**

If necessary, this operation can be done without anesthesia or any attempt at sterilization. In an emergency, to prevent total suffocation, a knife is inserted into the neck over the trachea in the midline just below the Adam's apple. Air is allowed to reach the lungs from a point below the obstruction.

**When an elective tracheotomy is performed, how is the opening into the trachea kept open?**

By insertion of a tracheotomy tube. This tube has a double lining, and the inner lining can be taken out as often as necessary to keep it clean and free of mucous collection.

**Should an endotracheal tube be placed in the upper trachea before performing an elective tracheotomy?**

Yes, This will be done by the anesthesiologist.

**When the tracheotomy tube is removed after the obstruction has disappeared, will the hole heal readily?**

Yes. Once normal breathing has been resumed and the tube re-

moved, the tracheotomy hole will close within a few days.

**Does a tracheotomy interfere with normal eating?**

No!

## BRANCHIAL CYSTS (*Gill Slits*)

**What are branchial cysts?**

They are pouches that persist as remnants from incompletely absorbed grooves seen in embryonic development.

**Where are branchial cysts usually encountered?**

They appear in the neck as remnants of improper and incomplete absorption of the gill slits during embryonic life.

**When are branchial cysts usually noted?**

During childhood or early adult life, an unusual opening may be seen on the side of the face or behind the ear or along the lateral aspect of the neck as far down as the collarbone.

**What is the treatment for branchial cysts or openings?**

If they show evidence of enlargement or if there is a discharge from an abnormal opening, they should be removed surgically.

**Are operations for removal of branchial cysts dangerous?**

No, but they may be complicated by the fact that the cyst may have to be traced far up into its opening in the throat.

**Do branchial cysts have a tendency to recur once they have been removed?**

If incompletely removed, they may recur, and this will require a secondary operation.

**Are branchial cysts common?**

No.

# CHAPTER 72

# THE THYROID GLAND

*(See also Chapter 4 on Adrenal Glands; Chapter 51 on Parathyroid Glands; Chapter 55 on Pituitary Gland)*

## Where is the thyroid located?

It is around the windpipe (trachea) in the lower portion of the front of the neck. Normally, it is made up of three portions, one lobe on each side of the windpipe and a connecting portion called the isthmus. Each lobe measures about two inches by one inch in diameter, and there is a mid-portion measuring a half to one inch in diameter, which crosses over the front of the windpipe.

## What is the function of the thyroid gland?

It is one of the most important organs in the body, as it regulates metabolism (the rate and manner in which we turn food into energy and expend that energy).

## Is the thyroid one of the endocrine glands?

Yes. It secretes the hormone called thyroxin.

## What is the function of the thyroid hormone?

It regulates the manner and rate at which the tissues utilize food and chemical substance for the production of energy. It is also concerned with the elaboration of body heat and muscular energy and body growth and development.

## What symptoms occur when there is an absence of the thyroid gland or when it functions underactively (hypothyroidism)?

a. Its incomplete development or absence at birth leads to a condition known as cretinism. This condition is characterized by markedly retarded mentality and a dwarfed body.
b. Milder inactivity and underfunction of the gland, either in adolescence or adult life, may lead to overweight, lack of energy, and a slowed mentality.

## What happens when there is persistent overactivity of the gland (hyperthyroidism)?

This condition may lead to bulging of the eyes, marked weight loss, sleeplessness, nervousness, irritability, excessive perspiration, and eventually serious heart damage.

## Is the cause for malfunction of the thyroid gland known?

It is thought that the disturbances in the function of this gland are caused either by the effect of the pituitary gland upon the thyroid or by disturbances within the thyroid gland itself.

## How does one determine activity of the thyroid gland?

a. By chemical tests known as T3 and T4.
b. By measuring the uptake of radioactive iodine by the thyroid gland.
c. Each year newer and more sophisticated laboratory tests are being evolved and used to assist the diagnosis when the aforementioned tests are either borderline or inconclusive.

## Is the basal metabolic rate useful in determining metabolic activity?

This breathing test has been abandoned because it has been found that the tests enumerated above are far more accurate in determining thyroid activity.

## Can one know the results immediately after taking one of the above thyroid tests?

No. It may take several days before the various tests are completed. Technically, some of the chemical and radioactive tests are difficult to carry out and to analyze.

## What is a thyroid scan?

It is a test in which the activity of the gland, as it absorbs the radioactive iodine, is shown by placing a scanner over the patient's gland. A scan is recorded on paper and can be readily interpreted.

## What is a goiter?

A goiter is a swelling or enlargement of the thyroid gland.

## What are the most common causes for enlargement of the thyroid?

a. Colloid goiter. This is a diffuse, even swelling of the gland and is usually unaccompanied by symptoms or evidence of changes in metabolism or in the patient's state of well-being. It is seen most commonly in young adults in regions where the iodine content of drinking water is low.
b. Nodular goiter. This is characterized by a lumpy, irregular swelling either as a single area in the gland or as multiple irregularities within the gland. There are two types of nodular goiter:
  1. The nontoxic goiter, which occurs in either sex at any time during adult life. These usually produce no symptoms, but they are dangerous because some 7 to 10 percent of them may, at some future time, turn into cancerous growths.
  2. Toxic goiter. These consist of small areas within the gland that cause overactivity of the entire gland.
c. Hyperthyroidism, or overactivity of the thyroid. This is often associated with a diffuse, smooth enlargement of the gland. This is the

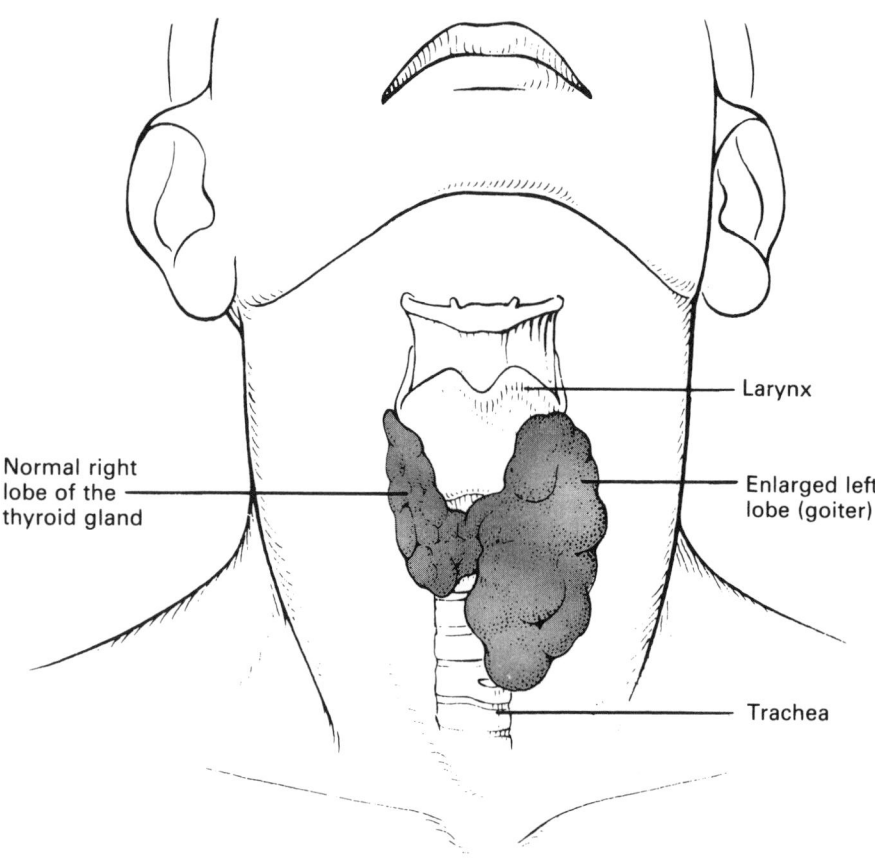

**The Thyroid Gland.** *This diagram shows a thyroid gland with a right lobe of normal size and a left lobe involved in goiter formation.*

Labels on diagram: Larynx, Normal right lobe of the thyroid gland, Enlarged left lobe (goiter), Trachea

type of goiter most often seen with bulging eyes, tremor, extreme nervousness, loss of weight, irritability, profuse sweating, and heart palpitation.

**Do goiters tend to run in families?**

No. However, the colloid goiter may appear in several children in the same family because they live in a vicinity where an iodine insufficiency exists.

**What is the treatment for the simple colloid goiter?**

In the early stages, a few drops of an iodine solution given by mouth may have curative results. Later on in the course of the disease, this form of treatment is of no value. In these instances, regulated doses of thyroid extract taken over a prolonged period of time may cause considerable shrinkage of the goiter.

**Is there any medical treatment for the toxic goiters that cause an elevation in thyroid activity?**

Yes. A great number of the cases of overactivity of the thyroid gland can be treated successfully, by medical means. This consists of the giving of iodine preparations in proper amounts and also the use of a group of medications, which curtail the production of thyroid hormone. This latter group of medications is called the antithyroid drugs. A third method of treatment, the giving of radioactive iodine in certain selected cases, is also successful in halting overactivity of the thyroid gland. If these methods of treatment fail, then surgical excision is advisable.

## THYROIDITIS *(Inflammation of the Thyroid)*

**What is thyroiditis?**

An inflammatory reaction within the gland, caused by bacteria, viruses, or autoimmune mechanisms. Autoimmune reactions are thought to be peculiar mechanisms whereby the individual starts to produce antibodies that attack his own tissues.

**Is thyroiditis a rare condition?**

No, it is more common than previously suspected.

**What are the symptoms of thyroiditis?**

Swelling of the thyroid, along with fever, pain, and tenderness in the neck over the region of the gland; also hoarseness, and discomfort upon swallowing.

**What is the treatment for thyroiditis?**

This varies in different types of cases. Many patients get well without treatment. In recent years cortisone has been used to alleviate the discomfort and limit the damage to the thyroid gland. Occasionally, antibiotics or x-ray therapy is used. Only occasionally is it necessary to perform surgery for complications of this condition.

## SURGERY OF THE THYROID GLAND *(Thyroidectomy)*

**When is it necessary to operate upon the thyroid gland?**

a. When the goiter presses upon the windpipe or causes continued hoarseness.

b. When the hyperthyroidism (overactivity of the gland) continues despite thorough treatment with iodine and the antithyroid drugs.

c. When the thyroid has one or more isolated nodules (lumps) that can be felt by the physician. Surgery is advised in these cases to forestall the development of cancer or the development of toxicity within one of these nodules.

### When is it possible to avoid surgery in thyroid disease?

a. When a simple colloid goiter responds satisfactorily to the intake of iodine.
b. When diffuse hyperthyroidism responds satisfactorily to the taking of the antithyroid drugs or to radioactive iodine.
c. When there is a recurrent hyperthyroidism after surgery and there is satisfactory response either to the antithyroid drugs or to radioactive iodine.

### Is special preparation necessary before a thyroid operation?

Yes, if the gland is overactive because of a goiter. In this event, the giving of proper doses of iodine and the antithyroid drugs will precede surgery in order to bring thyroid function down to normal. No special preparation is necessary before an operation upon a simple colloid goiter or a nontoxic nodular goiter.

### Is it possible to tell before operation whether a nodule in the thyroid is cancerous?

In the great majority of cases, the surgeon can make a correct diagnosis. However, the most accurate diagnosis can be made by the microscope after removal of the lump.

### What harmful effects can there be if a diseased thyroid is not operated upon?

a. An enlarged simple goiter may cause dangerous compression of the windpipe and an inability to breathe properly.
b. The continuation of the toxic effects of an overactive gland will cause serious and irreparable damage to the heart.
c. As mentioned previously, 7 to 10 percent of the small nodular goi-

ters may become cancerous if not removed.

### Do goiters often recur after surgery?

In occasional instances, a new nodule may form in the remnant of the gland left behind after surgery.

### Can anything be done to prevent a goiter from recurring?

Yes. The incidence of recurrence is diminished greatly by giving the patient thyroid pills each day. In order to assure that no recurrence takes place, it is necessary for the patient to take these pills indefinitely.

### Are thyroid operations dangerous?

No. They may be classified as simple major operative procedures with very little risk.

### Is this a painful operation?

No, although there may be a certain amount of discomfort in the neck for

a few days and some difficulty in swallowing for a few days after surgery.

### Are thyroid operation scars very noticeable?

Usually not. In many cases it is impossible to find a scar a year or two after operation. The surgeon will always attempt to make his incision in one of the natural skin lines of the neck.

### Does the surgeon usually remove the entire gland when performing a thyroid operation?

No, except when operating for a known cancer. It is customary to remove about 90 percent of the gland and to allow the remainder to carry on with normal thyroid function.

### Can the remnant of the thyroid, after surgery, carry out satisfactory thyroid function?

Yes. There is some regrowth of the

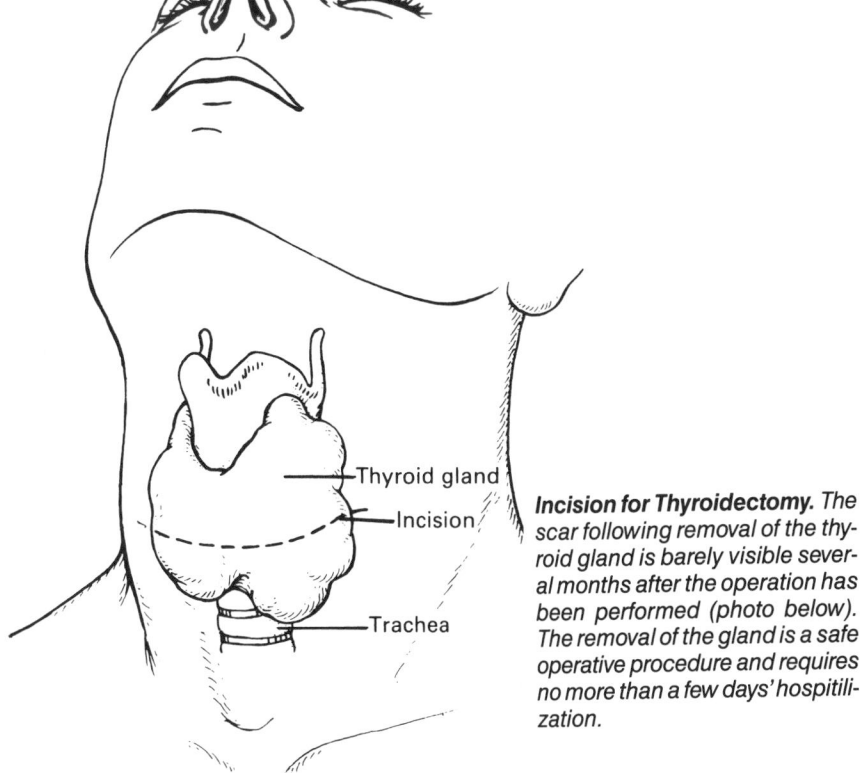

*Incision for Thyroidectomy. The scar following removal of the thyroid gland is barely visible several months after the operation has been performed (photo below). The removal of the gland is a safe operative procedure and requires no more than a few days' hospitilization.*

remnant of gland that permits perfectly normal thyroid function.

## How long does the operation take to perform?

Anywhere from three-quarters of an hour to two and a half hours, depending upon the size of the goiter and how much of the gland is to be removed.

## What anesthesia is used for thyroid operations?

A general inhalation anesthesia is used, along with intravenous medications.

## Are the wounds drained after thyroid operations?

Yes, and there may be leakage of serum for a few days postoperatively,

## Are special postoperative measures necessary?

Usually not, unless there was marked hyperthyroidism preoperatively. The patient is usually out of bed the day after surgery.

## What are the results of removing the thyroid gland?

In almost every type of thyroid operation the results are excellent, with disappearance of the symptoms within a few days.

## Does an overactive gland ever become underactive after surgery?

This does occur occasionally. In this event, the condition is controlled by the giving of thyroid pills.

## Will the bulging of the eyes disappear after thyroid surgery?

It may recede somewhat, but if there has been marked bulging before surgery, a good measure of it will remain.

## Will a patient with an overactive gland gain weight after surgery?

Yes.

## Will patients gain weight after removal of the thyroid?

Not if some of the gland has been left behind, not if thyroid pills are taken postoperatively, and not if the patient watches his diet.

## Does removal of the thyroid gland affect one's sex life?

No.

## How long a convalescent period is usually necessary after thyroidectomy?

Approximately three weeks.

## Are there permanent voice changes after a thyroid operation?

No. Occasionally, however, it is necessary to disturb the nerve going to the larynx when removing a thyroid. If this has been necessary, hoarseness or voice changes may result for several weeks or even months.

## Can one smoke immediately after thyroid surgery?

This is not advisable, since the throat may be sore after this operation.

## Can cancer of the thyroid be cured by surgery?

Many cancers of the thyroid have been permanently cured by removing the gland.

## How long a hospital stay is necessary for thyroid surgery?

Approximately four to seven days.

## How long does it take for a thyroid wound to heal?

Approximately one week.

## Can one return to a completely normal life after removal of the thyroid?

Yes.

## Are medications prescribed after a thyroid operation?

Yes, in most cases the patients are advised to take thyroid tablets for an indefinite period of time. This will help to prevent new lumps from forming within the gland.

## Can a woman permit herself to become pregnant after cure of a thyroid condition?

Yes.

## Should one return for periodic checkups after thyroid surgery?

Yes, about once every six months.

## How soon after thyroid surgery can one do the following:

Bathe:
    Seven days.
Walk out on the street:
    Five to six days.
Walk up and down stairs:
    Five to six days.
Perform household duties:
    Three weeks.
Drive a car:
    Three weeks.
Resume sexual relations.:
    Three weeks.
Return to work:
    Four weeks.
Resume all physical activities:
    Four to six weeks.

# CHAPTER 73

# TRANSPLAN- TATION OF ORGANS

*(See also Chapter 24 on Eyes; Chapter 29 on Heart; Chapter 37 on Kidneys and Ureters; Chapter 40 on Liver; Chapter 41 on Lungs)*

### Is it ever possible to transplant and replace worn-out organs or tissues?

Yes, in certain instances, tissues and organs can be grafted. Unfortunately most tissues transplanted from one individual to another, or to a human from an animal, will not survive more than a few days or weeks.

### Is it possible to transplant an organ or a tissue from one part of a patient's body to another?

This can often be carried out with good chances for permanent success.

### What are the most frequently transplanted tissues or organs?

By far the most commonly transplanted tissue is skin, but cartilage, bone, blood vessels, a kidney, or adrenal gland are sometimes transplanted from one part of the body to another. Hearts, livers, kidneys, corneas, and lungs have been transplanted from one individual to another.

### What is an autotransplant?

It is a graft of an organ or tissue from one part of the same body to another.

### What is a homotransplant?

It is a graft of an organ or tissue from one human to another.

### Is it technically possible to transplant an entire organ?

Yes, from the purely surgical point of view this is often feasible. There are now many cases on record in which an entire heart has been transplanted from one individual to another; there are also a large number of cases in which a kidney has been transplanted from one patient to another, and a small number of cases where a liver or lung has been transplanted.

### Do transplants from one individual to another always survive?

Unfortunately, no. The reason for this is that all humans have antibodies and immune bodies circulating in their bloodstreams. It is the function of these substances to protect the individuals from the invasion of foreign bodies. Foreign bodies usually consist of bacteria, viruses, or inert particles that enter the body through infection or a break in the normal tissue barriers, or through an injury or wound. The body of the host reacts the same way toward transplanted organs or tissues as it does toward any other kind of foreign body, and the protective cells within the host often bring about the ultimate destruction of the grafted tissue.

### What is this reaction of the host to the transplant called?

There are two popular names for this phenomenon, namely, the *rejection reaction* and *transplantation immunity*.

### Do all transplants from one individual to another die?

No. There have now been successful transplants of kidneys and heart transplants from one person to another. Also, segments of tissue such as the cornea (the thin, clear membrane covering the pupil of the eye) have been successfully transplanted in innumerable cases from one individual to another.

### Is it ever possible to have a successful graft of tissue from an animal to a human?

Yes. Animal cartilage has been frequently transplanted successfully in plastic surgery. Such cartilage is used to build up a receding chin or saddlenose. Recently, there are several reports in the medical literature of grafts of whole kidneys from chimpanzees or dogs that have survived for several months and up to two years.

### Is it ever possible to overcome the rejection or transplantation immunity?

Yes, a great deal of progress has been made within the past few years in this field. To overcome the rejection reaction it is necessary to temporarily immobilize or inhibit the antibodies of the recipient of the transplant. A substance known as *antilymphocytic globulin* has recently proved effective in this connection.

### What are some of the organs that technically can be transplanted from one human to another?

The heart, the lung, the liver, the kidney, the adrenal glands. Again it must be emphasized that the ability to perform a surgical procedure for transplantation does not guarantee that the transplanted organ will survive indefinitely.

### Is it necessary to protect the patient during the period when his antibodies and fighting mechanisms are inactive?

Yes. Large dose of antibiotics and steroid drugs such as cortisone are given. If this were not done, the patient would succumb to overwhelming infection.

## How does one attempt to overcome the rejection reaction to a transplanted organ?

a. Before grafting from one human to another, careful tissue matching is carried out. This matching is similar to that done before transfusing blood from one person to another. Tissues that are poorly matched are not grafted.

b. Chemicals are given such as Imuran and cortisone, which will temporarily suspend the ability of the recipient's antibodies to act against the organ.

c. It has been found that large doses of x-ray radiation to the area of the transplant or to the host's entire body will also temporarily inhibit the action of the antibodies and immune bodies.

d. In some cases it has been discovered that the removal of the thymus gland, beneath the breastbone, or the spleen will aid in the inhibition of the antibodies and thus allow a grafted organ to survive.

e. Antilymphocytic globulin (ALG) is administered.

f. A combination of the above forms of treatment is usually employed to overcome the reaction phenomenon so as to permit the transplanted organ to survive.

## Does a successfully transplanted organ always react normally in its new environment?

No. It has been discovered in animal experiments that sometimes healthy transplanted organs may develop the same disease as the structure it has replaced.

## Can diseased arteries and blood vessels be replaced with a transplant?

Yes, this is one of the most successful areas for grafts and transplants. However, it has been learned that the transplantation of nonliving substances such as Dacron and other plastic materials is more satisfactory than the use of living tissue.

## For what diseases of blood vessels are transplants advisable?

There are many conditions that are benefited by the use of grafts. Some of these are:

a. In certain cases of stroke, it has been found that the cause lies in arteriosclerosis of the carotid artery in the neck. This can be helped in many cases by coring out the narrow passageway of the carotid artery in the neck (endarterectomy) and by supplying a patch graft of Dacron or a segment of a vein.

b. There are many cases in which there is such marked arteriosclerosis of the aorta in the abdomen that insuffcient blood supply reaches the legs. In these cases, the abdominal aorta may be replaced with a Dacron tubular

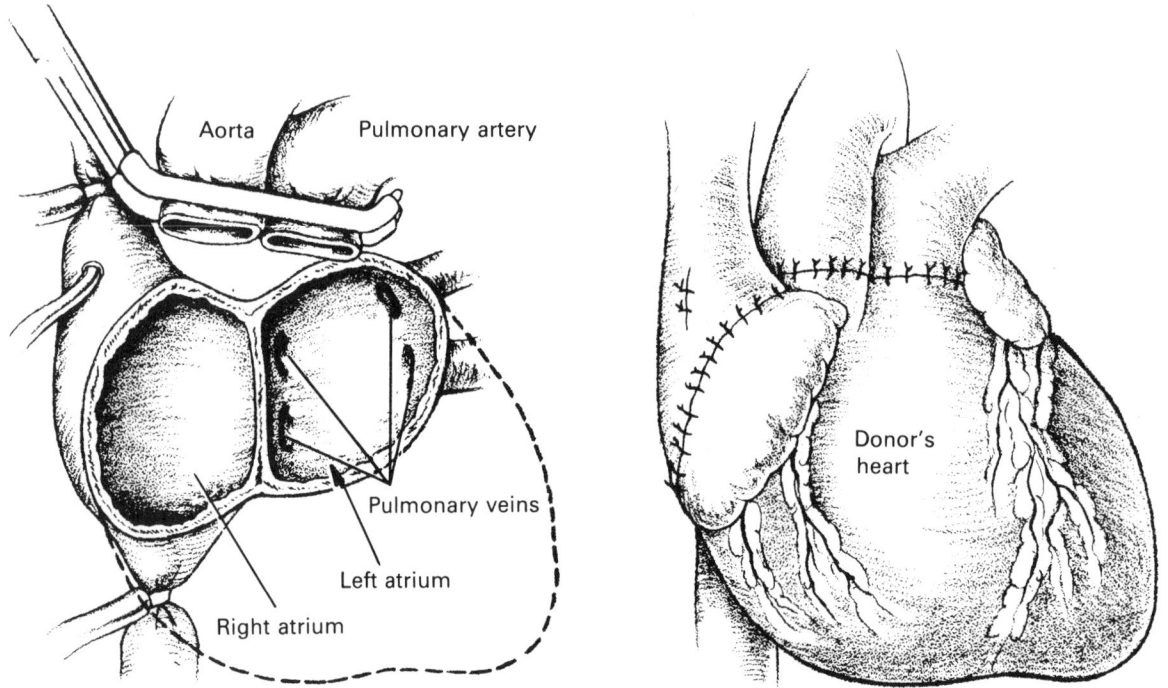

**Heart Transplant.** *In the drawing on the left, the major part of a diseased heart, shown by the dotted lines, has been cut away. The upper chambers of the heart and the main vein and arteries are left. As shown in the drawing below, they are all sutured to the new, or donor's, heart to which blood circulation and function are restored.*

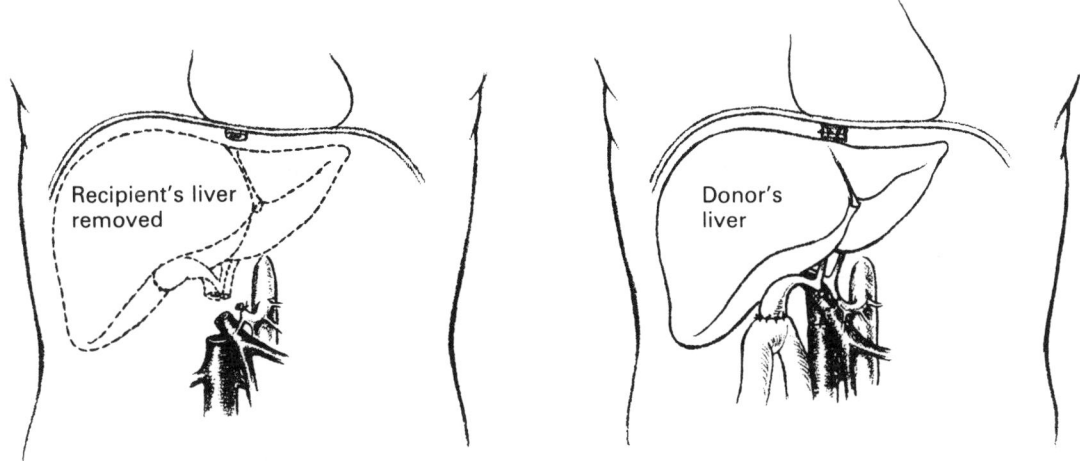

**Liver Transplant.** *In the drawing on the left, the dotted lines outline the patient's diseased liver, which is cut off from the main veins and arteries. In the drawing on the right, the donor's liver has been placed in position and sutured to the large blood vessel, and function is restored.*

graft, or its narrow passageway may be reamed out and a patch graft applied.

c. There are quite a large number of cases in which high blood pressure is due to arteriosclerosis and narrowing of the main artery to the kidney. In these cases, the renal artery can be cored out and a patch graft applied to it in order to broaden its passageway.

d. There are a large number of cases in which the circulation to the leg and foot is threatened by arteriosclerosis affecting the arteries in the pelvic region or in the thighs. In some of these cases, it is possible to bypass the narrowed blood vessels with a Dacron graft. When bypassing the arteries at the knee, most surgeons prefer to use a vein graft rather than a non-living graft.

e. An aneurysm of the aorta in the chest or abdomen is one of the most common reasons for the employment of a graft. An aneurysm is a bulging and blistering out with a thinning of the wall of an artery. If this is allowed to persist, the vessel may burst and may cause the patient's death. To overcome this, a Dacron tubular graft can be used to replace the diseased segment of aorta. (See Chapter 13, on Blood Vessel Surgery.)

f. Within recent years, it has been found that certain of the arteries within the abdomen that supply large segments of the intestinal tract may undergo arteriosclerosis, and in these cases a replacement with a Dacron graft is feasible.

g. In cirrhosis of the liver, a graft is often inserted between the superior

mesenteric vein and the vena cava. This procedure, known as a *mesocaval shunt,* is used in cases of cirrhosis. (See Chapter 40, on The Liver.)

**Can one look forward to a day when there will be an extension of the life span as a result of organ transplantation?**

There is no question but that within the next few decades the life span of many individuals will be prolonged by the successful transplantation and exchange of a healthy organ for a diseased one. Of course, in order for a patient to live extra years as a result of a transplant, other organs in his body must be in a relatively healthy state, for it is not possible to transplant all of the worn-out structures.

# CHAPTER 74

# TUBERCU-LOSIS

*(See also Chapter 41 on Lungs)*

## What is tuberculosis?

It is a communicable (contagious) disease caused by the tubercle bacillus, a germ that is transmitted from one person to another by "droplet infection," that is, by sneezing, coughing, or spitting.

## What progress has been made in the control of tuberculosis?

At the beginning of the twentieth century, it was the most common cause of death in the United States, with a mortality of about 200 per 100,000 persons per year. By 1961, it had fallen to sixteenth place among the causes of death with a mortality of only 5.4 per 100,000 persons per year.

## Does tuberculosis always affect the lungs?

No. It usually does, but it may also involve the skin, bones, joints, intestinal tract, kidney, bladder, genital organs, lymph glands, or the brain and nervous system.

## Are there different types of tubercle bacilli (germs)?

Yes. The human type, the bovine (cattle) type, and the avian (bird) type. This last type is very rare in human infections. The bovine type is now practically insignificant in this country because it has been almost completely eradicated by the pasteurization of milk and the eradication of tuberculosis among cattle. It still causes a considerable amount of disease in other countries where tuberculosis in cattle still exists. When this type of disease occurs in man, it is usually of the extrapulmonary (outside the lungs) variety, involving lymph glands, kidneys, intestines, bones, and joints.

## How do the tuberculosis germs enter the body?

Usually in three ways:
a. Inhalation of droplets or dust particles spread by coughing, sneezing, or spitting from tuberculosis patients.
b. Swallowing of material from contaminated foods and eating utensils, and drinking milk from tuberculous cows.
c. Rarely, by direct inoculation of the skin with some contaminated object.

## Is tuberculosis ever inherited?

No. Some population groups (American blacks, American Indians, Mexicans, etc.) seem to be more prone to acquire a severe, rapidly fatal form of the disease, but this is probably due to greater exposure opportunities among them, occasioned by poor living conditions and over-crowding. This occurs most often when they move into large cities after having lived in the country.

## Why is early recognition of a case of tuberculosis so important?

Because every new case of tuberculosis comes from an old case of tuberculosis!

## Is anyone immune to tuberculosis?

No. Anybody, rich or poor, can contract the disease, but it is more apt to occur under poor living conditions and in people whose general health is bad. It can spread easily from one member of a family to another, from a teacher to her pupils, from one pupil to another, and even by less close contacts, such as coughing, sneezing, spitting in public places, etc.

Children may be come infected by being kissed by parents or relatives who are unaware that they have the disease, or by carrying the germs to their mouths from contaminated eating utensils or toys.

## How can tuberculosis be prevented?

By following sensible rules of health: getting plenty of rest; eating nutritious foods; avoiding overcrowded living, playing, or traveling conditions; and by staying away from people who sneeze, cough, or spit. Also, by the examination of all contacts of a patient who has a positive tuberculin test and by treating those who are found to have active tuberculosis.

## Does age play any part in tuberculosis infection?

Yes. Infants up to the age of five years are more apt to get a severe, rapidly fatal type of the disease. Between the ages of five and fifteen, the incidence of fatal disease is at its lowest and gradually increases from then on. Young girls from fourteen to twenty are particularly susceptible. The greatest number of "chronic" cases occur in middle life (thirty to fifty years of age). When tuberculosis first occurs in the elderly, it may be acute and severe.

## Are there always early symptoms of tuberculosis?

No. Some people who are apparently perfectly well may have tuberculosis that can be detected only by x-ray examination, before any symptoms of the disease appear.

## What are the symptoms of tuberculosis?

The early warnings may be few, and they may progress and be disregarded unless they are properly evaluated and respected. They are:
a. Fatigue leading to exhaustion.
b. Loss of weight and energy.
c. Indigestion and loss of appetite.
d. Cough. This is often disregarded

and passed off as a "cigarette cough." Occasionally, the onset of the disease may be sudden and dramatic; it may start with a sudden hemorrhage from the lung or with acute pain in the chest due to pleurisy.

## How is tuberculosis diagnosed?

The most positive methods are the x-ray examination and the sputum examination. Physical examination with the stethoscope and examination with the fluoroscope may help establish the diagnosis, but they are rarely sufficient to determine a positive diagnosis.

## What is the tuberculin test?

It is a test used to see if there is a skin reaction to tuberculin, a product of the tubercle bacillus. A "positive" test means that the person has been infected at sometime during his life but does not tell whether the disease is active. Only the x-ray examination and sputum examination can determine whether or not the disease is active.

## Who should have tuberculin tests done routinely?

All children entering elementary school should be tested. Those found to react as positive should be x-rayed, and all their contacts should be examined for the purpose of discovering active cases. All children from twelve to thirteen years of age should be tested again; those found to be positive should receive preventive drug treatment.

## Is it important for apparently healthy people to have periodic x rays of the chest?

Yes. After the age of fifteen or sixteen, it is a good idea to have x rays made every few years. In that way, signs of disease in the lungs would be detected early.

Some people, such as student nurses and doctors and other employees working in hospitals where there are tuberculous patients, or anyone found to have a positive tuberculin test, should have a chest x ray every year.

## Is it important for young children to have periodic x rays?

No. The incidence of active lung tuberculosis among children up to the age of sixteen is very small. However, those who have been found to have positive tuberculin tests should have such x rays.

## What factors aside from poor living conditions lower one's resistance to tuberculosis infection?

Prolonged fatigue, alcoholism, severe illnesses—especially diabetes. Also, industrial exposure to silicone dust, such as in sandblasting, etc.

## What determines which of the positive tuberculin reactors will develop active disease?

The establishment of active infection depends upon the number and virulence of the invading germs and the degree of immunity or resistance of the patient. A large number of "strong" germs may overcome the resistance of a relatively immune person, or a small number of "weak" germs may be enough to cause infection in a susceptible individual or in one whose resistance has been lowered by malnutrition, alcoholism, etc.

## What is meant by a primary tuberculous infection?

It is the process that occurs following the first contact of the patient with the germ of tuberculosis. A small area of inflammation occurs (like a small patch of pneumonia), and the lymph glands in the region become inflamed too, but they wall off the spread of infection. Unless the infection is overwhelming, healing begins to take place, and scar tissue and, finally, calcium replace the inflamed portion of lung. The primary complex can then be recognized on the x ray

as a small area of calcification (chalky deposit) with some enlargement of the lymph glands.

As a result of the primary infection, the tuberculin skin test becomes positive. The positive skin test is really an allergic reaction to the tuberculin that has invaded the system.

## What happens to people once they have had a primary infection?

Nothing more happens to about nine out of ten such people. At some later date, a very small number develop active chronic pulmonary tuberculosis. This is the type usually seen in adults and may follow months or years after the primary infection.

## How may the primary type of tuberculosis be recognized?

There are usually no signs or symptoms except for some unexplained fever and weight loss. The x-ray finding of the "primary complex" may not appear until years later, when calcium has been deposited within the infected area. The change from a negative to a positive tuberculin skin reaction indicates that a tuberculosis infection has taken place somewhere in the body.

## Is the chronic form of lung tuberculosis due to flesh infection or to the breakdown of an old primary infection?

It may come about in either way.

## What course does chronic tuberculosis take?

It can follow either one of two courses. It can heal by scarring, or it can destroy lung tissue and cause involvement of other portions of the lung or spread to other parts of the body.

## Is the healing process ever complete in lung tuberculosis?

Probably not. Some bacteria deep in the diseased tissue may remain in a dormant state until such time as the patient's resistance is lowered and then resume their active destructive processes. However, healing can take place in one area while the disease is still active in other areas.

## How may other areas of the body become involved from lung tuberculosis?

The larynx, the throat, and the intestinal tract may become involved when the patient swallows sputum that has been coughed up from cavities through the bronchial tubes. On occasion, the disease may be spread by way of the bloodstream to other organs.

## What are the early signs and symptoms of chronic lung tuberculosis?

There may be no early signs, the first evidence often being the x-ray appearance of the disease. Some cases start like acute pneumonia, others like grippe or influenza, with fever, weakness, and malaise, which may persist for weeks. Most cases, however, begin very insidiously, with gradually increasing fatigue and weakness, loss of appetite, loss of weight, and low-grade fever. Cough and expectoration of sputum, sometimes bloody, may be early or late signs of the disease. Drenching night sweats may occur. Chest pain usually occurs only where the disease process is close to the pleural surface. Wheezing may occur if there is partial obstruction of the bronchial tubes with sputum.

## Can the doctor always diagnose tuberculosis of the lungs by examination alone?

Usually not. In early cases, the area of lung involved may be too small to give signs that can be recognized by physical examination. It is therefore very important to have a chest x ray in every case in which there is any suspicion of tuberculosis.

## Is the x-ray examination alone sufficient for a positive diagnosis of lung tuberculosis?

No. Many other diseases can cause x-ray shadows that are indistinguishable from those of tuberculosis.

## What procedure, aside from physical examination and x-ray examination, is most important for the positive diagnosis of pulmonary tuberculosis?

The sputum examination. When properly done, sputum examination is positive in over 90 percent of active cases.

## Suppose a patient does not expectorate any sputum. Can a positive diagnosis still be made?

Yes. If sputum is swallowed, it can be obtained by analysis of the stomach contents.

## If sputum examinations by the usual "smear" method are negative, does that definitely prove the absence of tuberculosis?

No. The sputum should then be cultured so that any germs present will grow out and multiply.

## What constitutes an "active" case of tuberculosis?

One in which sputum or gastric contents show the presence of the tuberculosis germs. Also, one in which the x rays reveal changes over a period of time.

## When is the disease considered to be inactive or arrested?

When the patient seems well and when the sputum is negative and the x rays are stable (show no change) over a prolonged period of time.

## What are some of the diseases that must be differentiated from pulmonary tuberculosis?

All lung diseases with cough, fever, and x-ray changes; these include the pneumonias, bronchiectasis, emphysema, lung abscess, tumors of the lung, the dust diseases, the diseases caused by yeasts and fungi, and sarcoidosis. Heart disease may cause secondary changes in the lungs, which may be confused with tuberculosis.

## How may tuberculosis spread from the lungs to cause disease in other parts of the body?

a. By direct spread along the bronchial tubes to involve the pleura and the larynx and by swallowing of sputum to involve the intestinal tract.

b. By way of the bloodstream to involve the entire body (generalized miliary tuberculosis)—the kidneys, liver, spleen, brain, testes, adrenal glands, and even the eyes.

## How does tuberculosis affect pregnancy?

It has no effect on the ability of the woman to carry to term or to have a normal delivery. Most patients, even with active disease, can carry to term and tolerate labor and delivery. (This does not mean that pregnancy is desirable in a patient with tuberculosis.)

## How does pregnancy affect tuberculosis?

Badly. If the disease has been inactive for over two years, pregnancy may be allowed fairly safely, but it should not be allowed if active disease is present or has been present within two years. Though the patient may tolerate pregnancy and delivery well, she must be watched very carefully after delivery, because that is when the disease is most likely to be reactivated.

## What is the outlook (prognosis) in a case of pulmonary tuberculosis?

This depends upon several factors:

a. The general health and resistance of the patient.

b. The nature and extent of the lung

involvement. The better the general health of the patient and the smaller the area of involvement, the better the outlook. The presence of cavities increases the seriousness of the disease. The larger the cavities, the more serious is the outlook.

The disease has a poorer prognosis in infancy and early childhood, and especially in adolescent girls.

With the newer drugs used in treatment, the outlook has improved tremendously in the past ten years.

## What is the best program for preventing the spread of tuberculosis in the community?

a. Mass x-ray surveys to pick up unknown cases.
b. Investigation of known contacts of active cases in the family or community.
c. Prevention of overcrowded living conditions and transportation.
d. Slum clearance.
e. Pasteurization of milk.
f. Control of tuberculosis in cattle.
g. Provision of adequate treatment facilities.

## What is BCG?

The initials stand for bacillus Calmette-Guérin. It is a vaccine that was developed in France. It is made from a weakened tubercle bacillus and is believed to have some value in producing immunity against tuberculosis in those with negative skin tests who are unavoidably exposed to the disease—doctors, medical students, nurses.

## What does BCG vaccination accomplish?

It converts nonreactors (people with negative tuberculin tests) to reactors; it gives them positive skin tests. It is believed that this causes the body to react in such a way as to localize the disease and promote healing if exposure has occurred.

## TREATMENT IN TUBERCULOSIS

## Is complete bed rest necessary in the treatment of pulmonary tuberculosis?

No. Excellent results are now achieved without complete bed rest. Limited physical activity is desirable during the early stages of treatment with the antituberculous drugs, but most patients are treated on an ambulatory basis.

## When is absolute bed rest necessary?

Critically ill patients and those with fever should be kept at complete bed rest, with meals in bed and bed baths. Bathroom privileges should be allowed as soon as the patient can tolerate a short walk.

## Is it all right for the patient to move about in bed, or must he lie "stock still"?

Nowadays, we feel that there is no objection to sitting up in bed, moving about, shaving, washing, reading, etc.

## How soon can the patient resume normal physical activity?

When sputum cultures have been converted to negative and when such symptoms as fever, cough, expectoration, and weight loss have subsided. However, drug treatment must be continued.

## Is climate important in treatment of pulmonary tuberculosis?

No. Formerly it was thought to be important, but now it is felt that as long as extremes of heat, cold, and altitude are avoided, it does not matter whether the patient is in the city or the country or in the north or the south.

## Is the tuberculous patient allowed to be out in the sun?

Yes, but undue exposure of the chest to direct sunlight to the point of sunburn is to be avoided because it increases the chances of hemoptysis (blood spitting) and reactivation of disease.

## Is there any specific diet for tuberculosis?

No. A well-balanced diet with enough calories to allow for a moderate gain in weight, along with a vitamin supplement, is desirable.

## For how long a time should the successfully treated patient take care of himself?

There is some danger of relapse for about five years after treatment is completed. Physical activity should be kept within bounds during this time. Rest periods during the day and adequate sleep at night are desirable.

## Should the patient with tuberculosis be allowed to smoke?

Since tobacco smoke (no matter what its dangers are in relation to cancer of the lung) is an irritating substance, it should be avoided by the patient who has or has had tuberculosis.

## How frequently should the patient who has recovered from the disease have x-ray examinations?

At least every six months, for several years. More frequent x rays are indicated in cases where there is a suspicion of residual disease.

## Is any particular drug, combination of drugs, or set dosage of drugs, used routinely in treatment?

No. Each case must be evaluated individually by the physician. Over varying periods of time, one, two, or even three antituberculous drugs may be used for any case.

## Is there any drug that *cures* tuberculosis?

No. However, there are several drugs

that when used properly are highly effective against the disease. Most tuberculous infections are arrested promptly by the administration of these drugs, and healing is accelerated by their prolonged use.

### Should every patient with active tuberculosis be treated with the antituberculosis drugs?

Yes. Whenever active disease is recognized, it should be treated. However, the particular drug or drugs, the problem of home or hospital care, and the duration of treatment must be individualized.

### What is the usual length of time that treatment is continued?

It is now thought that drug treatment should be continued for at least two years after the last positive culture is obtained. Cases with open cavities and negative sputum are treated for more prolonged periods. There are some who feel that drug treatment should be continued for an indefinite prolonged period.

### What are some of the effective drugs in the treatment of tuberculosis?

Those commonly used, either separately or in combination, are ethambutol, streptomycin, PAS (para-aminosalicylic acid), and INH (isonicotinic acid hydrazide). Several other drugs may also be employed in certain cases.

### How many cases relapse in tuberculosis?

Before the era of drug treatment,

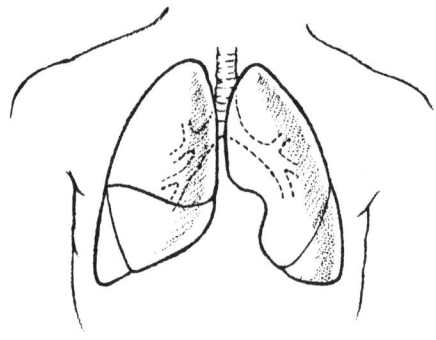

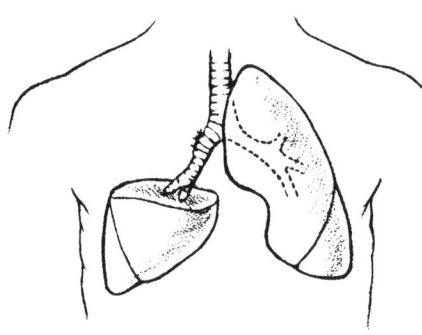

*Lobectomy.* The top drawing shows the two normal lungs with their bronchial tubes. In the bottom drawing, the diseased upper lobe of the right lung has been removed, and the bronchial tube has been left to maintain function in the lower lobe of the lung.

about 50 percent of arrested cases suffered relapses. Now, with modern, adequate treatment, only about 10 percent relapse.

### Since the drugs have been shown to be effective, how are the previous forms of treatment modified?

a. Hospitalization is usually not necessary.

b. Bed rest can be modified and the length of time shortened.

c. Collapse therapy can be almost completely dispensed with.

d. Surgery is seldom necessary.

e. It is still important to maintain adequate nutrition, to avoid respiratory irritants such as tobacco smoke, and to get adequate rest under the best possible living conditions.

### What does "pulmonary resection" mean?

The surgical removal of a portion of lung so as to actually remove the diseased tissue.

### Which cases may require surgery?

This decision must be based on mature medical and surgical judgment in each individual case. The cases considered are those with open cavities and positive sputum that have failed to respond to adequate medical treatment. Some cases with open cavities and negative sputum have been resected on the theory of preventing subsequent breakdown of diseased tissue in cavity walls.

### Is the surgical treatment of lung tuberculosis safe and effective?

Yes. When performed on suitable cases, the results are most encouraging.

### Why aren't most people with pulmonary tuberculosis treated surgically?

Because most cases get well without the need for surgery.

# CHAPTER 75

# UPPER RESPIRATORY DISEASES

*(See also Chapter 34 on Infectious and Virus Diseases; Chapter 41 on Lungs; Chapter 48 on Nose and Sinuses)*

## THE COMMON COLD

**What is the common cold?**
An acute inflammation and infection of the nose and the throat.

**What causes the common cold?**
A virus (a group of infecting agents, which are much smaller than bacteria; they are so small that they cannot be seen under an ordinary microscope).

**Is the common cold contagious?**
Extremely contagious.

**How is the common cold transmitted?**
By coughing, sneezing, or close contact with another person.

**What predisposes people toward catching a cold?**
a. A general weakness or rundown condition.
b. Enlarged infected tonsils or adenoids, which reduce the ability to stave off infections of the nose and throat.
c. Any other disorder of the mucous membranes or the upper respiratory tract.
d. Allergies of the nose and throat, which weaken local resistance.

**Is a common cold the same as grippe?**
No. The term grippe is no longer used. Grippe is now classified as an influenzal infection, commonly called "flu."

**What is the difference between the common cold and the flu?**
The flu is a more severe infection with higher temperature and is associated with muscular aches and pain varying in degree.

**Does the flu often start out as a common cold?**
Yes.

**What is the incidence of the common cold?**
It is the most frequently encountered of all medical conditions. Statistics estimate that one in eight people in this country currently has a cold!

**What other diseases have their onset as the common cold?**
Such illnesses as measles, whooping cough, and several other diseases of the upper air passages frequently start as a common cold. Also, hay fever and other allergies may masquerade as colds for a short time.

**What is the usual course of the common cold?**
An uncomplicated cold lasts from four to seven days. Minor complications may persist for a few days longer.

**How can one prevent the common cold?**
There is no sure method of prevention. Vaccines and cold injections are not of proven value, but both inactivated and live vaccines are under investigation, and combinations of viruses in vaccines are being studied as well. These may one day prove effective.

**Do vitamins help in preventing colds?**
Not specifically, although if the patient has a generally weakened condition, the taking of Vitamins A, C, and D may build up resistance to all types of infection, including the common cold.

**Are the antihistamine drugs of any value in preventing colds?**
Actually, they are not. They do tend to dry the nasal secretions and probably are somewhat effective in those mild allergic conditions that are mistaken for the common cold. They may also postpone the full-blown appearance of a cold for a day or two.

**Will the taking of large quantities of Vitamin C or fresh fruit juice be helpful in preventing colds?**
Although there are many advocates of these practices, most physicians believe they will not prevent colds.

**Are the antibiotic drugs of value in the treatment of the common cold?**
No. As a matter of fact, they may do harm because they may sensitize patients to their use. Then at some future date, when the patient is ill and really needs these drugs, they may be ineffective or the patient may not be able to take them.

**What is the best treatment for the common cold?**
Adequate rest at the very onset of the cold is probably the best treatment. By resting and by isolating himself, the patient not only helps himself, but prevents spread to others with whom he comes in contact. Simple remedies such as aspirin, nose drops, and antihistamine drugs, make the patient more comfortable, but actually have no specific curative effects. Drinking large quantities of fluids is advisable, as in any acute upper respiratory infection. If fever or a distressing cough develops, it is best to have a medical examination

to determine if a complication has set in.

## What are some of the complications of a cold?

Most common colds do not develop complications. However, since the nose and throat are lined by a membrane that extends into the sinuses and the ears, down into the trachea (windpipe), bronchial tubes, and lungs, any one or all of these organs may become involved. If the virus infection extends beyond the nose and throat, this may be followed by sinusitis, middle ear infections, laryngitis, tracheitis, bronchitis, and even pneumonia, as complications of the common cold.

## When are complications most likely to occur?

When the patient fails to take care of the common cold by adequate rest and treatment. Also, if the patient's resistance is low or he has had some other recent debilitating illness.

## Is it important to take the temperature when one has a cold?

Yes. This should be done three times daily. An elevated temperature may herald the beginning of a complication.

## How long should one wait after a cold to resume normal activities?

The patient should rest until he has had no symptoms and no fever for at least two full days.

## Having recovered from a cold, does a person develop any resistance against getting another one?

For a period of several weeks, yes. However, unfortunately, no permanent resistance develops.

## Is there any truth to the statement that one should "starve a cold" by not eating?

No. A normal light diet should be taken while one has a cold.

## Is there any truth to the statement that one should "feed a cold"?

No.

## Is the taking of a large quantity of whiskey helpful?

No.

## THE LARYNX
*(See also Chapter 71 on Throat)*

## What is the significance of hoarseness?

Hoarseness means that the larynx or voice box is involved by any one of a variety of conditions. Symptoms may vary from a slight huskiness of the voice to a complete loss of voice.

## What conditions can cause hoarseness?

a. Inflammation, such as the common cold, influenza, tonsillitis, bronchitis, whooping cough, diphtheria, etc.
b. Inhalation of irritating dust, fumes, tobacco smoke, or chemicals.
c. Nerve involvement of the vocal cord, secondary to pressure upon it from an enlarging mass in the neck.
d. A goiter that presses upon the nerves supplying the larynx, or an injury to the nerve secondary to an operation upon the thyroid.
e. Allergies that cause swelling of the larynx.
f. Benign tumors (fibromas) of the vocal cords.
g. Cancer of the vocal cords.

## What is croup?

It is an acute inflammation of the larynx with swelling of the vocal cords often accompanied by difficulty in breathing. (See Chapter 32, on Infant and Childhood Diseases.)

## What is laryngitis?

An inflammation of the voice box or larynx, usually caused by a virus or bacterial infection.

## Are there other causes for laryngitis?

Yes. Certain cases can be caused by a tuberculous infection, and others may be caused by a syphilitic infection of the larynx.

## What are the usual symptoms of acute laryngitis?

a. Slight to moderate fever.
b. Hoarseness or complete temporary loss of the ability to speak.
c. Pain in the throat.
d. A dry, hacking cough.

## What is the treatment for acute laryngitis?

a. Do not talk!
b. Drink large quantities of fluids, such as water, tea, and fruit juices.
c. If there is difficulty in breathing, take steam inhalations.
d. If the infection is severe, antibiotic drugs are sometimes prescribed.
e. Stay in bed until the temperature is normal for at least twenty-four to forty-eight hours.
f. Aspirin, or some similar drug, will often relieve accompanying aches and pains.

## Does the voice always return after an attack of laryngitis?

Yes. The inability to speak will last for only a few days.

## BRONCHIAL TUBES

## What is acute bronchitis?

A self-limited acute infection, usually occurring as a complication of the common cold or the flu.

## What is the usual course of acute bronchitis?

It runs a parallel course to the underlying infection and will clear up soon after the cold or the flu subsides.

## When is bronchitis most prevalent?

During the winter months. It is often

associated with exposure, chilling, and fatigue.

**What is the most common complication of bronchitis?**

Pneumonia.

**Is there a tendency for some people to get recurrent attacks of acute bronchitis?**

Yes. These people probably have a chronic source of infection, such as the sinuses or tonsils. Allergic individuals are also unusually susceptible to episodes of acute bronchitis.

**What is the outstanding symptom of bronchitis?**

A hacking, stubborn cough, with varying amounts of sputum being expectorated.

**Should coughing be stopped by medication when one has bronchitis?**

No. While coughing is a distressing symptom, it is also a beneficial one in that it gets rid of excessive mucous secretions that have accumulated in the bronchial tubes. Attempts should be made to keep the cough "loose" so that these secretions can be expectorated without difficulty.

**When does acute bronchitis become chronic bronchitis?**

Acute bronchitis should last no more than two to three weeks. If it has not been given the proper care and attention, it may persist longer and develop into a chronic infection.

**If acute bronchitis does not subside, what diseases should be looked for as possible complications?**

Pneumonia, tuberculosis, sinus infection, bronchiectasis (dilatation of the small bronchial tubes), emphysema, asthma, a foreign body in the lung, or even a lung tumor.

**Should one who has a persistent bronchitis or persistent cough be x rayed?**

Yes, by all means.

**Should smoking be permitted during any one of the upper respiratory illnesses such as a common cold, influenza, bronchitis?**

No. Tobacco smoke is particularly irritating to the lining membranes of the nose, throat, and bronchial tubes.

**What is a "cigarette cough"?**

This occurs commonly in the heavy smoker, but should not be interpreted as arising solely from the irritation of the tobacco smoke. Anybody, whether he is a heavy smoker or not, who coughs continuously should be investigated for an underlying lung or bronchial disease, as mentioned above.

**Is the quantity and character of sputum raised by coughing of importance in determining the extent or character of the underlying condition?**

Yes. In simple bronchitis the sputum is usually scant. In bronchiectasis, it is more profuse, thicker, and may be yellow or green in color. In lung abscess, it has a foul smell and may be bloody. In tuberculosis, it is usually blood tinged. In lung cancer, it may also contain blood.

**Does blood in the sputum always indicate tuberculosis or lung cancer?**

No. It also occurs in rather minor conditions, including plain acute bronchitis, sinusitis, etc.

**Does blood in the sputum always call for further careful investigation?**

Yes. This is a definite indication to see your physician.

## BRONCHIECTASIS

**What is bronchography?**

A procedure in which a liquid mixture is allowed to run down into the bronchial tubes so as to outline and fill them with an opaque substance. On x ray, excellent outlines of the large and small bronchial tubes will be demonstrated.

**What is bronchoscopy?**

It is a procedure in which an instrument (bronchoscope) is inserted into the throat, past the vocal cords, into the trachea, and down into the bronchial tubes.

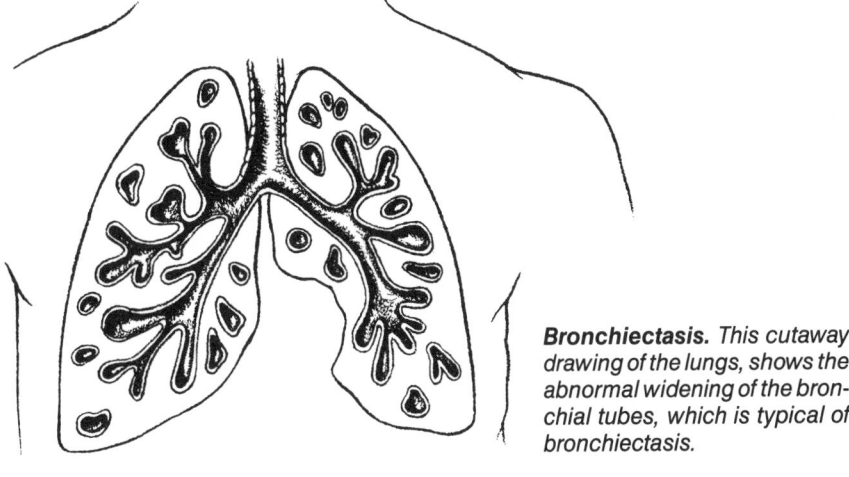

*Bronchiectasis.* This cutaway drawing of the lungs, shows the abnormal widening of the bronchial tubes, which is typical of bronchiectasis.

## What can be seen on bronchoscopy?

Bronchoscopy is of inestimable value in lung conditions in which the x ray and sputum examinations do not give a definite diagnosis. It may show the site of origin of bleeding; it may demonstrate foreign bodies that have been aspirated into the lungs; it may show a tumor in the bronchus, or the location of a cancer of the lung. It will also show the point of blockage of a bronchus.

## What other value has bronchoscopy?

Since suction can be carried out through a bronchoscope, it is used to remove pus and mucus from areas that are wholly or partially blocked by these substances. Also, pieces of tissue may be removed through the bronchoscope (biopsy material) for various laboratory examinations to determine the exact nature of an existing disease process. Sometimes, an area of ulceration or bleeding may be cauterized through a bronchoscope, thus effecting a cure.

## What is bronchiectasis?

It is a chronic disease in which the bronchial tubes are widened, either generally or in small localized areas.

## What are the forms of bronchiectasis?

a. Congenital bronchiectasis (existing from time of birth).
b. Acquired bronchiectasis.

## What are the symptoms and complications of bronchiectasis?

Chronic, long-standing cough, usually with profuse expectoration, asthma, thinning of the air sacs of the lungs (emphysema), hemorrhage from the bronchial tubes, lung abscess formation, or pneumonia.

## Can bronchiectasis be diagnosed by an ordinary x ray of the chest?

Not definitely. It may be necessary to pass a tube into the bronchial tubes

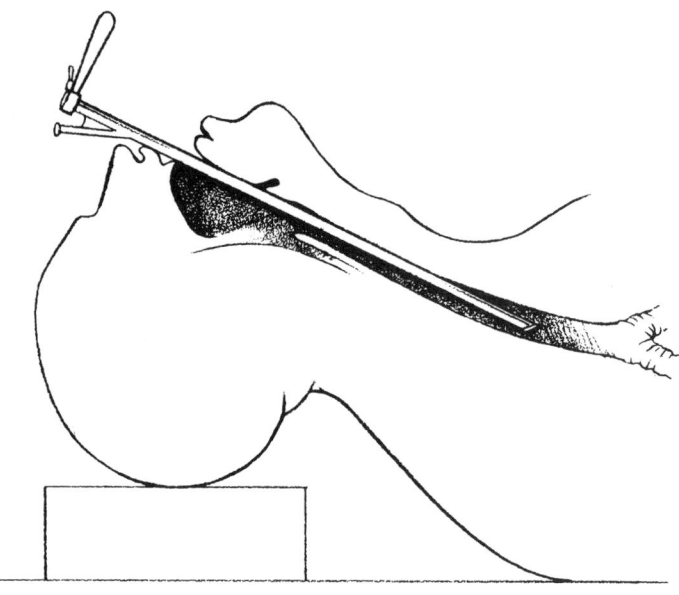

**Bronchoscopy.** *The drawing shows a side view of a bronchoscope in position. The metal tube allows a doctor to view the bronchi and make a definite diagnosis.*

(bronchoscopy) or to perform a bronchogram in order to clinch the diagnosis.

## What are the principles of treatment for bronchiectasis?

a. Maintenance of adequate drainage of the mucous secretions from the bronchial tubes. To accomplish this, the secretions must be loosened, and certain expectorant medications are given toward that end.
b. The giving of antibiotic drugs to control the infection.
c. The use of inhalations of various drugs, which may dilate and open the bronchial tubes.
d. Postural drainage (coughing in various positions with the upper part of the body dependent or hanging down over a bed or table) may be very helpful in ridding the bronchial tubes of pus and mucus. This type of exercise should be done several times a day.

## Is surgery ever indicated for bronchiectasis?

Yes, if the bronchiectasis is localized; that is, if there is widening in a small area of the lungs. In such an event, that portion of the lung can be removed successfully by surgery. Also, severe hemorrhage from bronchiectasis is an indication to remove that area of the lung.

## Is surgery for bronchiectasis dangerous?

Today, operations for removal of part or all of the lung (lobectomy or pneumonectomy) can be carried out safely by chest surgeons.

## What are the chances of recovery following surgery for bronchiectasis?

Well over 95 percent recover and are cured, provided all of the diseased portions of the lung are removed. The amount of lung tissue that can be removed safely can be determined by properly performed pulmonary function tests.

## How long a period of hospitalization is necessary?

See Chapter 41, on The Lungs.

# INFLUENZA

## What is "la grippe"?

It is an outmoded term to denote a condition known as influenza or flu;

that is, a highly contagious virus disease with fever, muscular aches and pains, cough, running nose, sore throat, and inflammation of the respiratory passages.

### Are the exact causes of influenza known?

The domestic type may be caused by at least two specific viruses, A and B, which have been isolated. There are undoubtedly many other virus strains that also produce this infection.

### What are the distinguishing features between the common cold and influenza?

Patients with influenza have more severe symptoms, including headache, lack of appetite, weakness, and higher temperature ranges (up to 103° F. or 104° F.) than those suffering from the common cold.

### How long does influenza usually last?

The acute phase with fever lasts from four or five days to a week or ten days, but is often followed by a period of weakness that may last for several weeks.

### What is the significance if fever continues longer than four to five days?

It probably signifies that a *bacterial* infection has been superimposed upon the *virus* infection.

### What are the main complications of influenza?

Bronchitis or pneumonia.

### Are there vaccines that will prevent influenza?

Yes. There are several different vaccines on the market, some of which have been shown to be effective against certain types of influenza but not against other types. Debilitated patients and aged patients should take influenza injections late in the fall.

### How often should these vaccines be repeated if they are to be given at all?

About once a year.

### Are the antibiotic drugs of value in the treatment of influenza?

Yes, but only to a certain extent. Their action is not to cure the virus infection, but rather to prevent secondary infections from taking hold. Thus, complications such as sinusitis, bronchitis, and pneumonia are much less likely to take place while the antibiotics are being used.

### What is the incubation period of influenza?

One to three days.

### Is there any specific method of diagnosing influenza?

Not really, except during an influenza epidemic, which occurs every few years.

### Does immunity result from an attack of influenza?

Yes, but it lasts no more than a few months.

### How long should one remain in bed with influenza?

At least forty-eight hours after the fever has come down and all medications have been discontinued. Longer periods of rest may be necessary if cough is a prominent symptom.

### How soon after an attack of influenza can one resume full activity?

Not until all the symptoms, including fatigue, weakness, and dizziness, have disappeared. Too early resumption of activity may lead to a relapse.

### Aside from the antibiotic drugs, what other measures should be used routinely for the treatment of influenza?

The same measures as are advo-cated for the common cold. (See the section on the Common Cold in this chapter.)

### Does the onset of cough during an attack of influenza necessarily indicate that pneumonia has set in?

No. Cough can occur when any part of the respiratory tract becomes irritated.

### When should the patient decide to call a physician when a respiratory illness occurs?

Physicians should be called when an elevated temperature persists for more than twenty-four hours.

## ASIATIC AND HONG KONG INFLUENZA

### What is Asiatic flu?

It is a variety of influenza, usually seen in widespread epidemics throughout the world, caused by a variant of the Type A influenza virus as well as by several other virus strains.

### What are the symptoms of Asiatic flu?

They are very similar to those of the more commonly known types of influenza and include weakness, chills, fever, headache, muscular pains, and, sometimes, intestinal symptoms.

### What is the course of the disease?

It usually lasts five to ten days and then subsides unless complications develop.

### Can an accurate diagnosis of this type of influenza be made?

Since the symptoms are those of the common variety, it cannot always be diagnosed specifically but will probably be classed with the usual types of flu. Positive diagnosis depends upon complicated laboratory studies, which are not carried out in the ordinary case.

### How is the disease spread?

By droplet infection from one patient to another, in the same way as in the ordinary type of flu.

### What is the incubation period?

Twenty-four to seventy-two hours.

### What are the complications of Asiatic flu?

Epidemics of influenza A seem to be associated with greater incidence of serious complications than those due to influenza B. The most common complications are viral pneumonias, bacterial pneumonias, tracheobronchitis, myocarditis (inflammation of the heart muscle), and certain neurologic complications, such as encephalitis and various forms of neuritis.

### Is it a serious disease?

No. Although the attack rate is very high, the disease is usually mild, and few people become seriously ill. Those most prone to its serious effects and complications are people with chronic heart, lung, and kidney disease, the older age group (over fifty-five), and pregnant women. Vaccination is highly recommended for these people.

### Is there any specific treatment?

There is no specific treatment for the disease itself, but antibiotics are of value in the prevention and treatment of complications.

## "SWINE" INFLUENZA

### What is "swine" flu?

It is a severe form of influenza thought to be quite similar to the disease that appeared in epidemic proportions during World War I. The disease is not transmitted to man by eating pork or pork products.

### Is there a likelihood of a swine flu epidemic recurring?

Experts in the field of contagious disease predict that an epidemic of swine flu may recur one day.

### Should one seek vaccination against swine flu?

No.

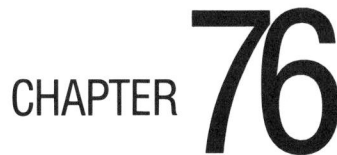

# CHAPTER 76

# THE URINARY BLADDER AND URETHRA

*(See also Chapter 25 on Female Organs; Chapter 37 on Kidneys and Ureters; Chapter 42 on Male Organs; Chapter 59 on Prostate Gland; Chapter 77 on Venereal Disease)*

### Where is the urinary bladder, and what is its function?

The bladder is a hollow, muscular organ situated at the bottom of the abdominal cavity behind the pubic bone. It is capable of changing size, depending upon the amount of urine it contains or expels.

The bladder receives urine from the kidneys via the ureters (which enter on either side) and expels the urine through the urethra, which connects with the outside. In the male, the neck of the bladder is in close proximity to, and surrounded by, the prostate gland.

The urethra in the male courses through the penis and is the same length as that structure. In the female, the urethra is short and terminates through a separate opening between the lips of the vulva.

## BLADDER INFECTION
### (*Cystitis*)

### Is cystitis a common disease?

Yes. It is perhaps the most prevalent disorder of the urinary tract. It occurs in children as well as in adults, and especially in females.

### What is the most frequent cause of cystitis?

A bacterial infection with such germs as the staphylococcus, streptococcus, colon bacillus, and *bacillus proteus*.

### How do bacteria reach the bladder?

From the outside through the urethra, from the kidneys, and from the intestinal tract.

### What are different forms of cystitis?

a. Acute.
b. Chronic.
c. Interstitial.

### What are the symptoms of acute cystitis?

The onset is usually sudden, characterized by frequent painful urination and not infrequently by the presence of pus and blood in the urine.

### What is the treatment for acute cystitis?

a. The administration of the appropriate sulfa or antibiotic drug.
b. The liberal intake of fluids.
c. Bed rest.
d. A bland diet, with special care to avoid highly seasoned foods and alcoholic beverages.
e. Sedatives to relieve pain or spasm.

### How long does an attack of acute cystitis usually last?

If treated promptly and adequately, the acute symptoms may subside within a few days. Some disability may persist for a week or two. The urine may take this amount of time to clear.

### What are the symptoms of chronic cystitis?

Essentially the same as for acute cystitis, except that the symptoms may be less severe, more prolonged, and may tend to recur. Patients with this condition usually have associated disease in other parts of the urinary tract.

### What is interstitial cystitis?

It is a form of chronic cystitis seen mainly in older women. This type of cystitis is characterized by marked thickening of the bladder wall and decreased bladder capacity.

### How does one make the diagnosis of cystitis?

By finding pus cells, bacteria, and blood in the urine, and by noting the symptoms listed above.

### Is it necessary to cystoscope all patients who have cystitis?

It is not necessary if the symptoms and infection subside quickly. However, if there have been recurring attacks, if there is blood in the urine, or if the condition has become chronic, the entire urinary tract should be studied by cystoscope as well as by other means. This is important in order to rule out disease more serious than cystitis. (See the section on Cystoscopy in this chapter.)

### What conditions within the urinary tract may produce cystitis?

a. An infection in the kidney.
b. A stone or tumor in the bladder.
c. Any obstructive condition within the urinary tract, such as an enlarged prostate, a cystocele, or narrowing of the urethra in a female.

## CYSTOSCOPY

### What is a cystoscopic examination?

One in which the interior of the bladder is viewed directly through a tubular metal instrument known as a cystoscope. Cystoscopes are equipped with lights and lenses, which permit excellent visualization of the inside of the bladder. In addition, the outlets of the ureters from the kidneys may

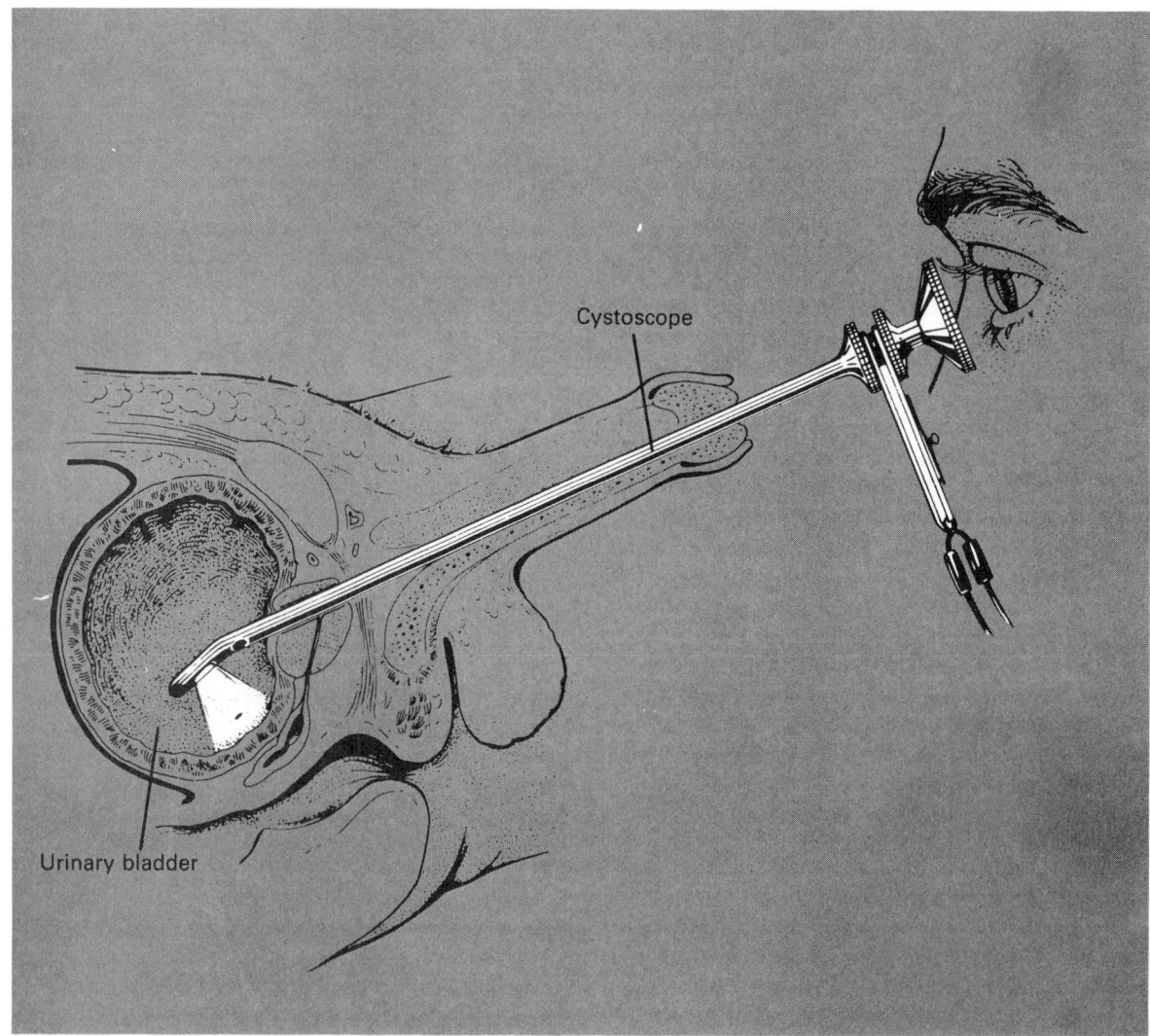

**Cystoscopy.** *This diagram shows a cystoscope being passed into the urinary bladder. By peering through this instrument, the urologist can see disease within the bladder. Tumors, portions of enlarged prostate glands, and bladder stones can often be removed through the cystoscope.*

be studied through this instrument, as may the internal size and configuration of the prostate gland.

### Is a cystoscopic examination painful?

In the female, it is virtually painless. In the male, there is some discomfort, but this can be minimized by using local anesthetic agents or general anesthesia. In children, cystoscopy is performed under general anesthesia.

### What are the aftereffects of cystoscopy?

Some temporary urinary discomfort and possibly some blood in the urine. There may also be a rise in temperature for a day or two.

### Is it necessary to be hospitalized for a cystoscopic examination?

Usually not. Most cystoscopic examinations can be done in the urologist's office. When catheters are to be placed through the cystoscope into

the ureters and up toward the kidneys, hospitalization is often advised. When such catheters are to be left in place for a few days, hospitalization is mandatory.

## BLADDER FISTULAS

### What is a bladder fistula?

An abnormal communication between the bladder and some neighboring organ such as the vagina, the intestine, the uterus, etc.

## What are the causes for the development of a bladder fistula?

It may result from a severe infection, a malignant growth, an injury secondary to a difficult labor, or as a complication of a surgical operation.

## What is the most commonly encountered bladder fistula?

A connection between the bladder and the large bowel, secondary to an inflammation of the large bowel (diverticulitis). Another frequently encountered fistula is one between the bladder and bowel, secondary to a tumor of the bowel.

## What are the symptoms of a bladder fistula?

If the fistula extends between the bladder and bowel, the patient will pass gas, feces, or food particles with the urine. If the fistula is between the bladder and vagina, the patient will leak urine from the vagina and will lose control over bladder emptying.

## What is the treatment for bladder fistulas?

This will depend upon the cause. Small fistulas that are secondary to injury or infection may heal spontaneously, or they will close by diverting the urine with a rubber catheter. Most fistulas, however, require surgical correction if a permanent cure is to be obtained. If the underlying cause is malignant disease, the primary growth as well as the involved portions of the bladder wall must be removed. If diverticulitis (inflammation of the colon) has produced the fistula, the diseased segment of the colon must be removed as well as the involved portion of bladder wall.

## Are operations for fistula serious?

Yes, but recovery is the general rule. In cases where malignant disease is the cause, extensive surgery may be indicated.

## Are bladder fistulas always cured on the first attempt?

No. Recurrence does take place in a small proportion of cases, and these must be reoperated to obtain a satisfactory result.

# BLADDER STONES (Calculi)

## Are stones often encountered on examination of the urinary bladder?

Yes.

## What causes bladder stones?

a. Those that form directly in the bladder are usually the result of poor emptying, with stagnation and pooling of urine.
b. Other stones may form as a result of a bladder disease such as chronic cystitis, a tumor, or diverticulum of the bladder wall.
c. Many bladder stones originate in the kidney and pass down into the bladder from above.

## What symptoms do bladder stones produce?

Frequent, painful, bloody urination. Occasionally, stones may cause sudden blockage of the urinary outlet, with resultant inability to void.

## How is a positive diagnosis of bladder stones made?

By x-ray examination or by direct visualization through a cystoscope.

## What is the treatment for bladder stones?

If small, they often pass spontaneously, without treatment. More often, however, they must be removed. This is accomplished either by opening the bladder surgically or by crushing the stones with a specially designed instrument, which is passed through a cystoscope. This latter procedure is called litholapaxy.

## When is litholapaxy performed?

When the stones are not too large or firm, and when there are not too many of them. Also, since this procedure is carried out through instrumentation and not by open operation, it is more applicable to those people who are unable to withstand major surgery.

## How are the stones removed from the bladder after they have been crushed?

By irrigation. In this manner, they are washed out of the bladder.

## When is an open operation (cystotomy) for removal of stones indicated?

When the stones are very firm and therefore cannot be crushed. When they are very numerous, stones should be removed surgically. If there is an enlargement of the prostate along with bladder stones, the surgeon may elect to do an open operation so that he can remove the prostate at the same time.

# TUMORS OF THE BLADDER

## Do tumors often form within the bladder?

Yes.

## Are most bladder tumors malignant?

It is thought that most are either malignant or potentially malignant.

## What are the benign tumors of the bladder?

These are wartlike growths known as papillomas.

## What are the symptoms of bladder tumors?

Painless bleeding on urination. Occasionally there is frequency of urination or the passage of infected urine when cystitis supervenes.

## How is the diagnosis of a bladder tumor made?

By visualization through a cystoscope. A piece of the tumor is removed through the cystoscope and is submitted for microscopic examination.

## What is the treatment for bladder tumors?

This will depend upon the size, location, and multiplicity of the tumor. Simple superficial tumors that do not interfere with the flow of urine from either kidney and are readily accessible are burned away by electrofulguration through a cystoscope. Large tumors, or ones that penetrate the wall of the bladder deeply, should be removed by cutting out that section of the bladder wall.

When the bladder is extensively involved by a highly malignant growth, it is necessary to remove the entire structure. This procedure is called a cystectomy. When this is done, some disposition must be made of the ureters to provide drainage of urine. Accordingly, the ureters are transplanted either to the skin (cutaneous ureterostomy) or a pouch is constructed from a segment of small intestine and the ureters are attached to this pouch. This procedure is known as an ileal bladder operation. Occasionally, the ureters are transplanted into the large bowel (ureterosigmoidostomy).

## How does one pass his urine when the ureters are transplanted into the large bowel?

Urine is passed through the rectum.

## How does the urine drain when the ureters are transplanted into the small intestine?

This segment of small intestine (the ileum) is brought out to the skin, and

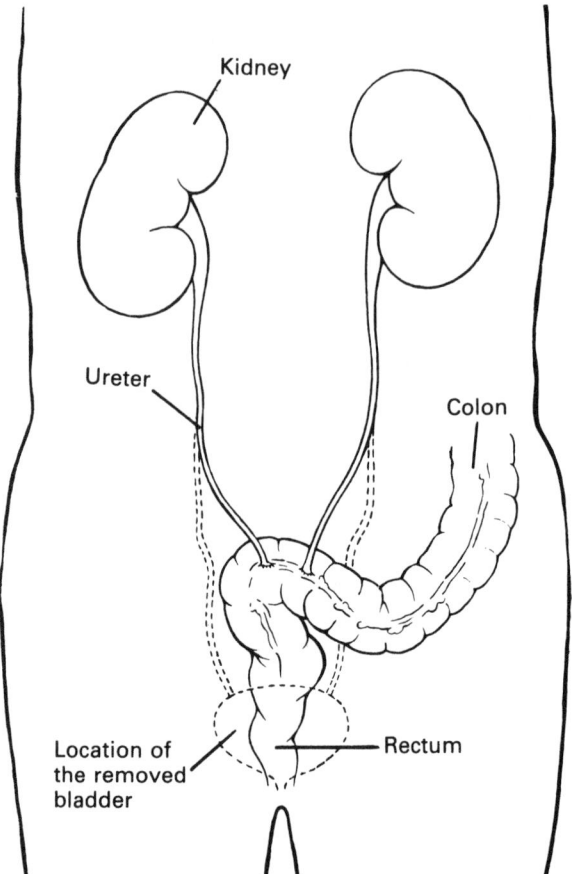

*Ileal Bladder Operation. In this operation, a segment of small intestine (ileum) is isolated from the rest of the bowel. One end of the ileum is closed tightly, and the other end is left open and is stitched to the skin. The ureters are implanted into this segment of bowel, and the urine drains into it and out to the skin. A special apparatus is attached to the opening of the ileum, which drains the urine into a plastic bag strapped to the leg.*

the opening is attached to a plastic bag, which fits snugly to the skin.

## Are operations for transplantation of the ureters and removal of the bladder serious?

Yes. They are of great magnitude, but it should be remembered that they are lifesaving procedures, performed in most instances to eradicate cancer.

## Is there any treatment other than surgery for bladder tumors?

Yes. X-ray therapy can be used in conjunction with surgery, but it is not very efficacious. Also, radium can be implanted into bladder tumors with occasionally successful results. Also, external cobalt irradiation has been used with some good results.

## How long a hospital stay is necessary for operations upon the urinary bladder?

Operations for the removal of bladder stones, tumors, etc., usually require two weeks of hospitalization. Operations for removal of the entire bladder may require a much longer hospital stay.

## Are blood transfusions necessary during operations upon the bladder?

Yes, if an extensive procedure is to be carried out.

## Are special nurses needed for major bladder operations?

Yes, for several days.

## What is the period of convalescence after a major bladder operation?

Approximately one month.

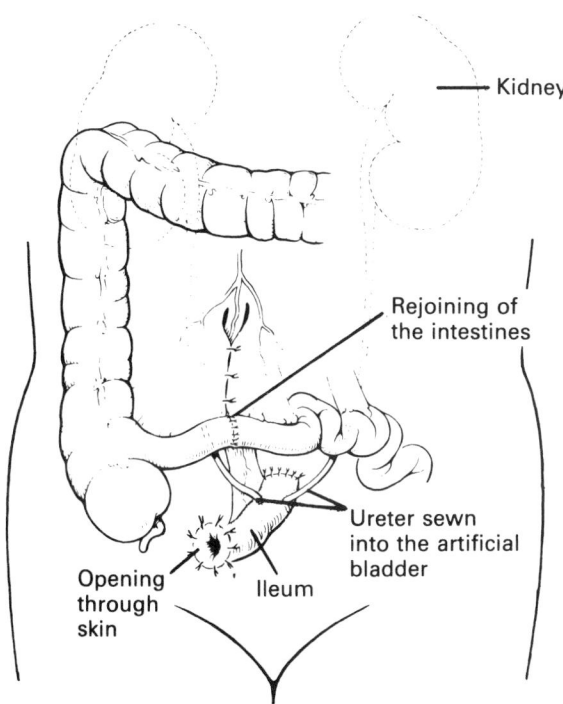

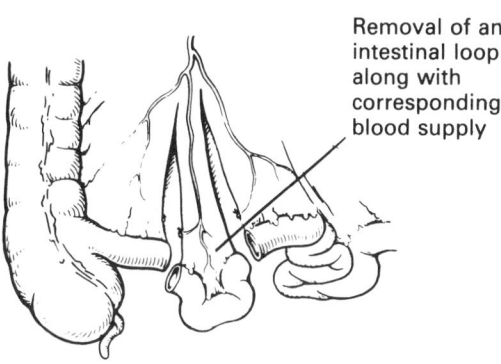

*Ureteral Transplant Operation.* This diagram shows the ureters being implanted into the large bowel after the urinary bladder has been removed for cancer. Operations more recently devised utilize a portion of small bowel for the implantation of the ureters (ileal bladder).

## THE URETHRA

### What is the urethra?

It is a tubular passageway leading from the bladder to the outside. Its sole function is to convey urine.

### Is the female urethra very different in construction from the male urethra?

Yes. The female urethra is very short, leading from the bladder to its exit between the minor lips of the vulva. The male urethra extends the entire length of the penis.

### What are the most common conditions affecting the urethra?

a. Strictures.
b. Caruncle.
c. Diverticulum.
d. Infections (gonorrhea, *Trichomonas*, nonspecific bacteria).

e. Congenital deformities, such as hypospadias and epispadias.

## Strictures

### What is a stricture of the urethra?

An abnormal narrowing in the canal, usually caused by scar tissue formation.

### What are the causes of strictures?

a. A birth deformity (congenital stricture).
b. Infection of the urethra, usually the end result of gonorrhea.

### What are the symptoms of stricture of the urethra?

a. Reduction in the size and force of the urinary stream.
b. Retention of urine, if the structure is extensive.
c. Recurrent attacks of cystitis.

### How is the diagnosis of stricture made?

By noting the obstruction to the passage of an instrument through the urethral canal and by noting a narrowed urinary stream.

### What is the treatment for urethral strictures?

a. Repeated dilatations by the passage of special instruments known as "sounds" or "bougies."
b. Cutting the stricture surgically.
c. In severe cases, plastic operations to reshape the urethra.

### If a stricture cannot be cured by dilatation or operation, what procedure is recommended?

Since these cases are accompanied by obstruction to the outflow of urine, a cystotomy must be performed in order to drain the urine. In this event, the urine will drain abdominally through a rubber tube, which is attached to a bottle. Fortunately, this situation does not often develop.

## Caruncles of the Urethra

### What is a caruncle of the urethra?

A small piece of overgrown tissue located at the opening of the urethra.

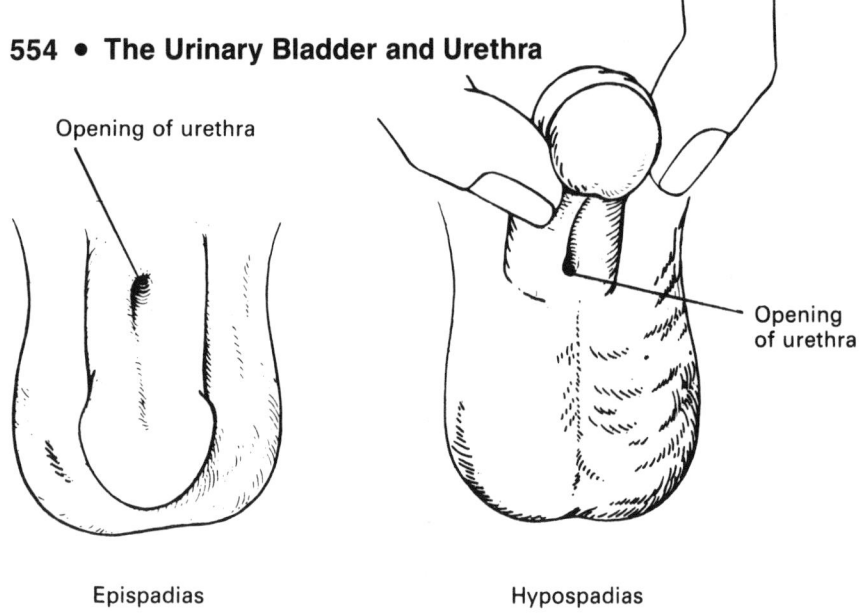

Opening of urethra

Opening of urethra

Epispadias

Hypospadias

*Above and below:*

**Epispadias and Hypospadias.** *These schematic illustrations show the normal channel of the urethra and two defects that sometimes occur at birth. Epispadias is the opening of the urethra on the upper side of the penis. Hypospadias is the opening of the urethra on the underside of the penis. These abnormalities can be eliminated by plastic surgery upon the penis.*

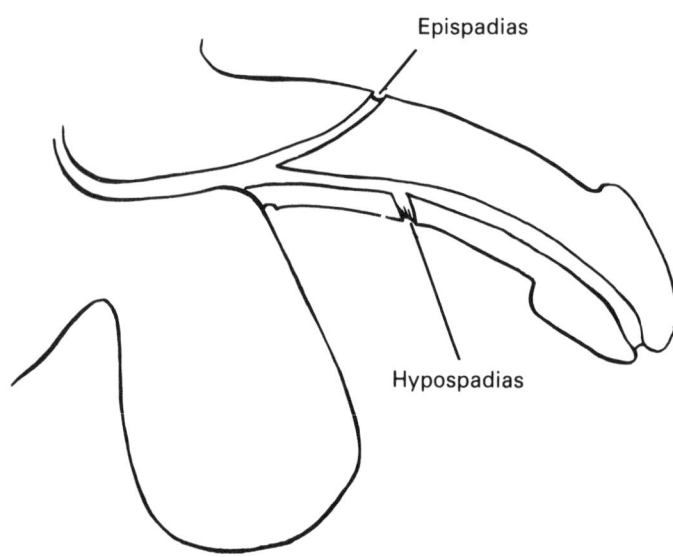

Epispadias

Hypospadias

It occurs exclusively in women and results from localized infection or chronic irritation.

### What are the symptoms of a caruncle?

There may be no symptoms at all, or the patient may experience pain when the caruncle is touched or when urine passes over it. Frequency of urination with discomfort and bleeding occurs in some cases.

### Is treatment always necessary for a caruncle?

No; only if it is large, painful, or causes symptoms.

### What is the treatment for a caruncle?

It should be excised surgically or removed by means of an electrocautery. Very small caruncles may be cauterized with chemical agents such as silver nitrate.

### Do caruncles have a tendency to recur?

Yes, but not after surgical removal.

## Diverticulum of the Urethra

### What is a diverticulum of the urethra?

It is a small outpouching of the urethral canal resulting from a birth deformity or secondary to infection in the wall of the urethra. It occurs almost exclusively in women.

### What are the symptoms of an urethral diverticulum?

a. Recurrent attacks of bladder infection.
b. Obstruction to the passage of urine.
c. Painful intercourse.
d. After voiding, the patient finds that she can produce more urine by pressing on the region of the diverticulum.

### What is the treatment for a diverticulum of the urethra?

Surgical removal, which will result in a cure.

## Infections of the Urethra

### Are infections of the urethra (the tube leading from the urinary bladder to the outside) very common?

Yes. They are seen with great frequency.

### What are the commonest causes of infection of the urethra?

a. Gonorrhea. (See Chapter 77, on Venereal Disease.)
b. Fungus infections such as *Trichomonas*.
c. Bacterial infections with germs such as streptococcus, staphylococcus, etc.
d. Chlamydia infections caused by an organism that is an intermediate form between viruses and bacteria.

### What are the symptoms of an infection within the urethra?

a. The appearance of a discharge from the penis or opening of the urethra above the vagina in the female.
b. Frequent, painful urination.
c. Pain in the genital region.
d. Appearance of blood or pus, or both, in the urine.

### How is a diagnosis of the cause of an urethral infection made?

a. By taking some of the discharge, smearing it onto a glass slide, staining it, and examining the slide under a microscope.
b. By culturing the discharge to see if bacteria will grow.

### Will microscopic examination of the discharge tell accurately what has caused the infection?

Yes.

### How does one get a *Trichomonas* infection of the urethra?

Through sexual intercourse, It is frequently transmitted back and forth from male to female in this manner.

### How does one get a chlamydia infection of the urethra?

It is transmitted through sexual intercourse.

### Can a chlamydia infection be cured?

Yes, by the giving of appropriate antibiotic medications.

### What is the treatment for an infection of the urethra?

This depends upon its cause. Fungal infections are treated with specific antifungal medications. Gonorrhea and bacterial infections are treated with specific antibiotic drugs.

While suffering from an urethral infection, a patient should do the following, in addition to taking medications:

a. Drink large quantities of liquids.
b. Abstain from sexual intercourse.
c. Avoid highly seasoned foods.
d. Avoid alcoholic beverages.

### Can urethral infections be cured?

Yes, but some are stubborn to overcome and require prolonged treatment.

## Hypospadias and Epispadias

### What are hypospadias and epispadias?

Birth deformities of the urethra, in which the urethra ends short of the tip of the penis. When the urethra ends on the underside of the penis, the condition is called hypospadias; when it opens on the top side, it is called epispadias.

### Are there varying degrees of these deformities?

Yes. In certain cases the urethra ends right near the tip of the penis, and no symptoms result. In the more severe types, the urethra may end near the very beginning of the penis; this will result in serious voiding difficulties.

### What is the treatment for hypospadias or epispadias?

Minor deviations from normal require no treatment; others require correction by plastic surgery. This is

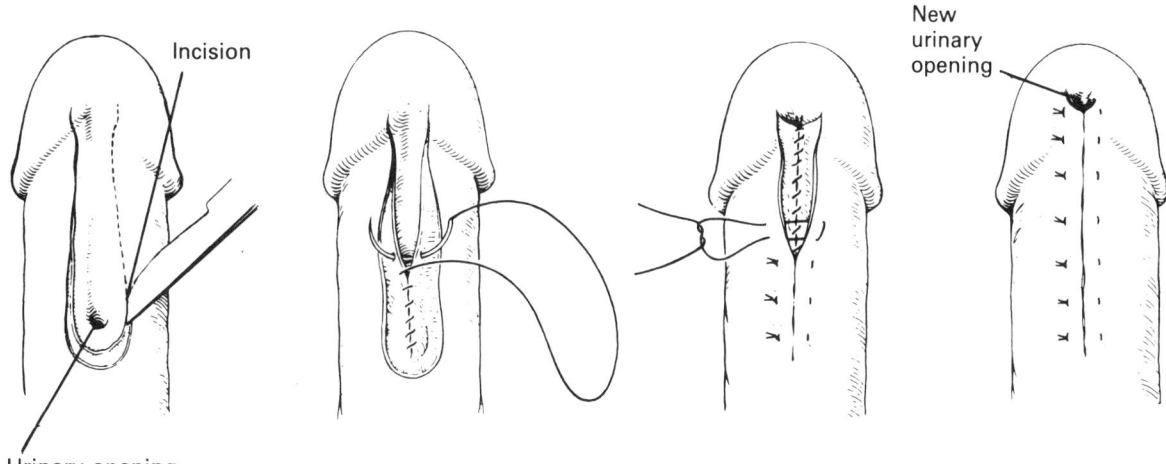

**Operation for Hypospadias.** Plastic surgery to correct this condition starts with an incision on the underside of the penis from a point below the urinary opening to the tip of the penis. A tube is rolled from the skin leading from the urethra to the tip of the penis. The tube is finally sutured, as is the incision. The drawing at the far right shows the operation completed.

often carried out in several stages and constitutes complicated techniques necessitating the services of a competent urologist.

## When is the best time to operate for hypospadias or epispadias?

During the first few years of life.

## How successful are these operations?

In most cases good results are obtained. However, when the results are unsatisfactory, reoperation can effect a cure. Some of these reoperative procedures are carried out years later, when the tissues have grown considerably and are easier to handle surgically.

## If the operations for hypospadias or epispadias are successful, will urinary and sexual function be normal?

Yes.

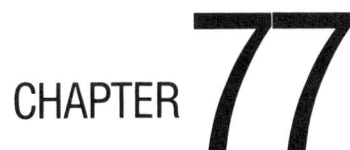

# CHAPTER 77

# VENEREAL DISEASE

*(See also Chapter 25 on Female Organs; Chapter 42 on Male Organs; Chapter 69 on Sterility, Fertility, and Male Potency; Chapter 76 on Urinary Bladder and Urethra)*

**What is a venereal disease?**

A condition that is contracted as a result of sexual contact or exposure.

**Is this the only way in which venereal disease can be contracted?**

No. Kissing, nursing, or even the simple handling of infected materials may cause a venereal infection such as syphilis.

**Can venereal diseases be contracted from unclean toilet seats?**

This is theoretically possible, but with the exception of gonorrhea in the female, it is a very rare occurrence.

**What venereal diseases are most prevalent?**

a. Gonorrhea.
b. Syphilis.
c. Herpes.
d. Chlamydia.

**What is the difference between gonorrhea and syphilis?**

Although both are venereal diseases, there is very little similarity. Gonorrhea is caused by an organism, which, in most instances, is localized to the genitals and is characterized by frequency of urination, painful swelling, and discharge from the region. Syphilis, on the other hand, is a disease that starts as a sore in the region of contact. It eventually spreads throughout the entire body and affects all the organs to a greater or lesser degree. In other words, gonorrhea is a localized disease; syphilis a generalized or systemic disease.

**Which condition is more serious, gonorrhea or syphilis?**

Syphilis is a much more serious condition, as it may ultimately produce grave damage to organs such as the brain, the heart, the liver, etc.

**Does gonorrhea ever affect organs other than the genitals?**

Yes. It may affect the eyes, and for this reason all newborns are given preventive eyedrops at birth. Occasionally, if untreated, gonorrhea may affect the joints, causing a specific type of arthritis. Very rarely, it may involve the lining of the brain or spinal cord, thus causing a specific type of encephalitis or meningitis.

**Will cleansing and taking a prophylactic treatment after exposure prevent venereal disease in all instances?**

No! The only sure way to avoid gonorrhea or syphilis is to avoid contact with infected individuals.

**Are prophylactic treatments helpful in preventing venereal infection?**

Yes, if taken properly, *immediately* after exposure. However, this procedure is never dependable or always available.

## SYPHILIS

**What causes syphilis?**

It is caused by a bacterial organism known as the *Treponema pallidum* (a spirochete).

**What is the incidence of syphilis in this country today?**

Seventy-seven out of every hundred thousand people develop syphilis each year according to the latest statistics.

**Is syphilis on the decline?**

It was until recently. Within the past year or two, however, there has been a marked increase in the incidence of syphilis due to increased promiscuous heterosexual and homosexual activity.

**Does everyone who is exposed to syphilis develop it?**

Not necessarily. There are factors, such as the state of activity of the disease, the type of exposure, contact, etc., that influence the likelihood of infection.

**Is there any natural immunity to syphilis?**

No.

**Can syphilis be inherited?**

Yes. Syphilis can be transmitted through the blood from parent to child. It is not, however, transmitted through the genes.

**How can one tell if he has syphilis?**

A sore, called a chancre, will appear several weeks after the initial exposure. It may be located on the genitals or on any other region of the body where contact has taken place with an infected person. The chancre is usually painless.

**Are there other ways to tell whether one has syphilis?**

Yes. There are several accurate blood tests that indicate whether the patient is infected. (The most common test has always been the Wassermann test, but this has been replaced within recent years by other, more sensitive tests.)

**What is a chancre?**

It is the primary lesion of syphilis. It is a small, painless sore, measuring no more than about a half inch in diameter. The chancre will appear on the penis, the female genitals, or at any other point of contact, such as the lips, etc.

### What happens to a chancre if it is permitted to go untreated?

It will persist for several weeks and then disappear spontaneously.

### What happens after the chancre disappears?

A month or two later a rash will appear on other parts of the body and a sore throat will develop. This is called the secondary eruption, or secondary stage of syphilis.

### What happens to this rash and sore throat if permitted to go untreated?

This, too, will disappear spontaneously within a few weeks.

### Does this mean that the patient is thereafter cured of his syphilis?

Emphatically not! The germs will live and travel throughout the entire body and may produce an active infection elsewhere at a later date, perhaps many years later.

### Will the blood test be positive even when there is no obvious evidence of syphilis?

Yes.

### Is there any way to prevent syphilis?

Yes, by avoiding exposure to a possible contact! Also, do not use personal utensils of unclean, potentially infected people.

### Is there any entirely safe method of protection during sexual exposure?

No. If one has contact with a person suffering from active syphilis, the chances are great that one will acquire the disease.

### Can a person have a positive blood test for syphilis without ever having

had any signs whatsoever of the disease?

Yes. It is possible that a person might have inherited syphilis. This is one of the most potent arguments in favor of subjecting all people to a blood test for syphilis.

### Is the blood test ever positive when the patient does not actually have syphilis?

Yes. This occurs only occasionally in situations in which people have high fever, or in certain other diseases.

### Is there any way of telling at birth whether a child has inherited syphilis?

Yes. A blood test can be taken from a sample of blood from the umbilical cord. More important, if neither parent has had the disease and their blood tests are negative, the child will not have the disease.

### If one or both parents has had syphilis that has been treated successfully, what are the chances of their child having syphilis?

If the parents have been cured of the disease, their children will be free of the disease.

### Are there any evidences during childhood that a child has inherited syphilis?

Yes, There are certain physical signs by which the physician will be able to make a diagnosis of inherited (congenital) syphilis.

### Can syphilis in a newborn child be treated successfully?

Yes.

### What are the dangers from untreated syphilis?

When untreated, syphilis will usually crop out years later with an active infection within a vital organ.

### What organs are most frequently

affected by late, or tertiary, syphilis?

a. The nervous system.
b. The heart.
c. The large blood vessels such as the aorta.
d. The liver.
e. The skin.

### What diseases are caused by syphilitic infection of the nervous system?

a. A form of insanity known as paresis.
b. Tabes (locomotor ataxia), a condition in which there is loss of sense of position in the extremities, making it extremely difficult to walk.

### What is the treatment for syphilis?

Syphilis can be treated very successfully today if treatment is begun early in the course of the disease. Penicillin and other antibiotic drugs have been found to produce cures in the vast majority of cases.

### Is it more difficult to cure syphilis in its secondary or tertiary stages?

Yes. Anyone with a primary lesion such as a chancre should go for immediate treatment. Results are much better when treatment is started early.

### Can the late complications of syphilis be treated effectively?

To a certain degree, but not nearly as effectively as in the early stages of the disease. Late complications can merely be arrested or prevented from getting worse.

### How early in the development of syphilis will the blood tests register as positive?

By the time the chancre has appeared, in about three weeks.

### When is syphilis most contagious?

During its primary and secondary stages, when there is a chancre, rash, or sore throat.

**Is syphilis contagious during the late stages (tertiary)?**

Almost never, except that at any stage of the disease a syphilitic parent can transmit it to the unborn offspring.

**Should a patient who has had syphilis ever get married?**

Yes, if the disease has been successfully treated and cured.

**What are the chances of a syphilitic patient transmitting the disease to his or her mate?**

If adequate treatment has been carried out, the chances are practically nil.

**How long does it take for full recovery from syphilis when it has been thoroughly treated?**

Before someone can be pronounced cured, he must be followed medically and found to be free of the disease for a period of at least two to three years.

**How soon after treatment has begun does the contagious aspect of syphilis disappear?**

Within a few days or, at the latest, weeks after penicillin injections have been started. Often, contagion disappears after the first few injections.

**How long can the germs of syphilis live in the open air or on plates or eating utensils, etc.?**

They die within a minute or two under such circumstances.

**Can one contract syphilis a second time after having been "cured" of an initial infection?**

Yes.

**Are any medications other than antibiotics effective in treating syphilis?**

Yes. In the rare case, when an individual is sensitive to the antibiotics, treatment can be effectively carried out by the older methods of utilizing arsenic and bismuth injections.

**Can arsenic and bismuth bring about cures in the average case of syphilis?**

Yes, but the method of treatment with these medications takes much longer and is more painful than treatment with the use of antibiotic drugs.

**Can one return to a completely normal life after having been treated successfully for syphilis?**

Yes.

**Are there any permanent limitations on activity after an episode of syphilis?**

No.

**Does syphilis ever cause death?**

Yes, particularly the late complications, such as syphilis of the brain or blood vessels.

**Should a woman with syphilis permit herself to become pregnant?**

Not until she has been fully treated and pronounced cured.

**Is syphilis thought to be a cause for repeated miscarriage and for stillbirths?**

Yes. Many physicians think that syphilis predisposes toward these conditions.

**How often should one return to his physician for a checkup after having been discharged from treatment for syphilis?**

At least once a year.

## GONORRHEA

**What is the most common cause for an infection of the urethra?**

Gonorrhea. Infections have increased tremendously in recent years since men have abandoned the use of the protective condom.

**Can gonorrhea be contracted in any way other then by sexual contact?**

This is an extremely rare occurrence, and when it does take place, it occurs in the female, not in the male.

**What are the symptoms of gonorrhea?**

a. The appearance of a creamy urethral discharge about a week to ten days following unprotected sexual relations. This discharge appears from the orifice of the penis or from the vulva in the female.
b. Frequent, painful urination.
c. Pus and blood in the urine.
d. Pain and swelling in the region of the external genitals.

**Does a discharge from the urethra always mean gonorrhea?**

No, it may be caused by a *Trichomonas* infection, or it may be caused by germs such as streptococci, staphylococci, Chlamydia, etc.

**How is a positive diagnosis of gonorrhea made?**

By actually visualizing the gonorrheal germ under the microscope or by culturing the discharge. This is accomplished by taking some of the pus from the urethra.

**Do gonorrhea and syphilis always occur together?**

No, but when one of these conditions is present, a thorough search should be made for the other.

**What is the treatment for gonorrhea?**

The antibiotic drugs, if used promptly and properly, will bring about a cure within a few days.

**How long does it take for antibiotic drugs to work?**

Their action is effective within twenty-four to forty-eight hours.

**Is it safe for a patient with gonorrhea to administer treatment to himself?**

Absolutely not. A chronic form of the disease may result if the patient attempts to treat himself by purchasing his own antibiotics. It is essential that these medications be given under the supervision of a physician.

**Do all gonorrhea germs respond satisfactorily to all antibiotics?**

No. The physician will frequently have to change the antibiotic in order to find the one that is most effective for the particular type of germ causing the infection.

**What are the complications from the improper treatment of gonorrhea?**

a. In men, a spread of the infection to the prostate gland, testicle, and/or epididymis.
b. A stricture of the urethra may result.
c. In women, a spread of the infection to the cervix, uterus, Fallopian tubes, and/or ovaries. Also, peritonitis may ensue from an extension of the infection to the abdominal cavity.

**Can gonorrhea cause sterility?**

Yes. In women, gonorrhea is the most frequent cause of sterility. In men, if the infection has involved the testicles or epididymis, sterility may sometimes take place.

**How can one prevent sterility in cases of gonorrhea?**

By prompt treatment by a competent physician.

**Does gonorrhea ever recur?**

Yes. In inadequately treated cases, the germ may lie dormant within the genital tract, only to flare up again.

**Can chronic gonorrheal infection be cured?**

Yes, by adequate treatment with antibiotics and, sometimes, by the performance of surgery to remove structures that have been destroyed by the gonorrheal infection, such as the Fallopian tubes, ovaries, etc.

**Does gonorrhea cause impotence?**

No.

## HERPES

**What is herpes?**

It is a virus infection of the skin or of the nerve endings in the skin, characterized by the appearance of many small superficial blisters.

**Are there various types of herpes?**

Yes, each caused by a different virus. They are:

a. Herpes simplex, also called a "cold sore." This type occurs about the lips.
b. Herpes zoster, also known as "shingles." This type occurs along the routes of superficial nerves in the head, neck, or torso.
c. Genital herpes, appearing on the penis or on the mucous membranes of the female genitals.

**Are cold sores or shingles contagious?**

No.

**Is genital herpes contagious?**

Yes, it is very contagious.

**How does one get genital herpes?**

It is transmitted through sexual contact, either through penis-vaginal contact or orogenital contact.

**Is genital herpes very common?**

Yes, and its incidence is greatly on the increase since sexual permissiveness has increased so markedly in recent decades.

**Will everyone who is exposed to a mate with genital herpes catch it?**

No. There are those who have a natural immunity to the condition. It has been found that people who had chickenpox in their childhood are particularly prone to genital herpes during adulthood.

**Does genital herpes tend to recur?**

Yes.

**What is the treatment for genital herpes?**

There is no specific treatment, but the condition will subside spontaneously within a week or two. The application of an antibiotic ointment to the sores might be beneficial.

**Is there any way to prevent genital herpes?**

If a male has herpes on his penis, he should refrain from intercourse until it has disappeared completely. A female is seldom aware that she has a herpes infection, and therefore she cannot avoid transmitting the condition during intercourse.

**Are there any permanent harmful effects from genital herpes?**

No proved harmful effects have been noted, although some investigators think that genital herpes might make a female somewhat more prone to uterine malignancy. This theory is questionable.

# CHAPTER 78
# VITAMINS

*(See also Chapter 5 on Aging; Chapter 20 on Diet; Chapter 33 on Infant Feeding; Chapter 57 on Pregnancy and Childbirth)*

## What are vitamins?

They are specific chemical compounds essential to normal body chemistry and health. They are not manufactured by the body itself but are obtained principally from foods.

## Do vitamins add calories to food intake?

No.

## Are vitamins essential to life?

Yes. However, people may live for long periods of time with insufficient vitamin intake before the deficiency diseases become apparent.

## How can one tell if he needs vitamins?

The signs and symptoms of vitamin deficiency may be extremely difficult to diagnose. Certainly, the patient himself cannot make an accurate diagnosis of a vitamin deficiency and therefore should not undertake to medicate himself by taking vitamins indiscriminately.

## Will the addition of vitamin pills to a normal diet increase the general resistance to disease?

No. If one's food vitamin intake is normal and vitamin absorption by the body is normal, taking additional vitamins in the form of pills will not increase resistance to disease.

## For how long a period of time must vitamins be taken in order to cure a deficiency?

If the deficiency has existed for a long time, it may take several weeks or longer for the body to attain a normal vitamin status. If the deficiency has been present for only a short time, adequate vitamin intake will probably start to have an effect immediately.

## What are the causes of vitamin deficiency?

a. Inadequate food intake or unbalanced food intake.
b. Inadequate vitamin absorption due to intestinal dysfunction or disease.
c. Poor vitamin metabolism due to disease processes within various organs of the body.
d. Unusual vitamin demands as would occur during sickness, pregnancy, periods of extraordinary growth, periods of stress or special activity, and when the patient is undergoing surgery.

## What diseases or conditions are caused by vitamin deficiency?

a. Vitamin A deficiency:
  1. Poor night vision.
  2. Dryness of the tissues of the eyes, skin, and respiratory tract.
  3. Reduced resistance to infection.
b. Vitamin $B_1$, or thiamine, deficiency:
  1. Beriberi, a severe deficiency disease characterized by extreme degrees of weight loss, loss of muscle strength, neuritis, mental confusion, and impairment of heart function.
  2. Minor deficiencies in Vitamin $B_1$ will lead to milder symptoms of weight loss, poor appetite, loss of strength, and damage to nerve tissues.
c. Vitamin $B_2$, or riboflavin, deficiency:
  Cracking of the skin at the angles of the mouth, scaly lesions in the folds of the skin, which extend from the angles of the nose to the lips. Also, irritation and redness of the lining of the mouth and tongue, with purplish discoloration.
d. Nicotinic acid deficiency:
  Pellagra, a severe deficiency disease characterized by sensitivity of exposed skin surfaces to sunlight. This causes skin rashes. Pellagra is also accompanied by gastrointestinal symptoms and mental instability and disorientation.
e. Folic acid deficiency:
  This condition will cause severe anemia of varying types.
f. Vitamin $B_6$, or pyridoxine, deficiency:
  Gastrointestinal symptoms, general weakness, nervousness, irritability, and nerve tissue damage can be caused by this vitamin deficiency.
g. Vitamin $B_{12}$ deficiency:
  This can create pernicious anemia and nerve tissue diseases such as neuritis.
h. Vitamin C, or ascorbic acid, deficiency:
  Scurvy, a severe deficiency disease characterized by marked degrees of weakness, accompanied by bleeding tendencies. This is characterized by widespread bruising and bleeding from the gums or other organs.
i. Vitamin D deficiency:
  Rickets, a severe deficiency disease in infants and children characterized by poor absorption of calcium from the diet with malformation of bone structures. This, in an advanced state, can lead to marked bowing of the legs or malformation of the pelvis or of the chest.
j. Vitamin E deficiency:
  It is thought by some investigators that a Vitamin E deficiency leads to diseases of red blood cells, diseases of the heart and blood vessels, and diseases of muscles and nerves. The exact role of Vitamin E has not yet been determined conclusively.
k. Vitamin K deficiency:
  This vitamin is concerned with the

manufacture of one of the important elements required in normal blood coagulation. Deficiency of Vitamin K, as seen in cases of jaundice, may lead to severe hemorrhage from the various mucous membrane surfaces of the body.

## Do deficiencies of the above vitamins always produce the characteristic diseases?

No. The most common finding today is that one is only mildly deficient in these vitamins. Thus, the full-blown disease will not be evident, but rather certain minimal symptoms of the disease may be present.

## Is vitamin deficiency usually limited to one vitamin?

Generally speaking, isolated vitamin deficiency is the exception rather than the rule. When vitamin deficiency exists, multiple vitamin deficiency is usually the case.

## Which foods are particularly rich in vitamin content?

a. Vitamin A:
Butter, eggs, milk, liver, fish, liver oils, green leafy vegetables, yellow vegetables.
b. Vitamin $B_1$ (thiamine):
Meat, whole grains, yeast, vegetables, liver, eggs.
c. Vitamin $B_2$ (riboflavin):
Dairy foods, meat, eggs.
d. Niacin:
Peanuts, liver, yeast, organ meats, wheat germ.
e. Vitamin $B_6$ (pyridoxine):
Meat, fish, grains, vegetables, liver, yeast.
f. Vitamin $B_{12}$:
Meat, liver, eggs, dairy products.
g. Vitamin C:
Oranges, lemons, grapefruit, and other citrus fruits, potatoes, cabbage, tomatoes, green peppers.
h. Vitamin D:
Fish liver oils, eggs, dairy products.
i. Folic acid:
Green vegetables, yeast, liver, kidneys.
j. Vitamin K:
A fat-soluble vitamin whose absorption depends greatly on normal fat absorption from the gastrointestinal tract.
k. Vitamin E:
Wheat germ, whole grains.

## What is meant by the minimum daily requirement of a vitamin?

The smallest amount that, when taken daily over a prolonged period of time, will prevent the development of a deficiency disease.

## What is meant by "therapeutic formula" vitamins?

This term applies to a combination of all of the known vitamins in doses usually adequate to prevent and treat disease from most vitamin deficiencies. It usually contains many times the daily requirements of the body.

## Is it possible to take an overdose of vitamins?

Yes. Severe toxic effects and sometimes permanent damage can be caused by overdose of certain vitamins, particularly Vitamins A and D.

## Should all people routinely take vitamin pills to maintain good health?

No. They should be taken only when there is a known or strongly suspected vitamin deficiency or dietary deficiency.

## Should people take vitamins on their own, or should they consult their physician before taking vitamins routinely?

Consult your physician. Most people, under the pressure of advertising, take an excess amount of vitamins. This is wasteful and in some instances may be harmful if an overdose is taken.

## When is it necessary to give vitamins by injection?

a. When oral intake is not possible, such as after certain types of surgery or in severe cases of gastrointestinal disorder.
b. When there is poor absorption of the vitamins from the intestinal tract.
c. When large initial doses are indicated in severe deficiencies and the physician wishes the patient to gain rapid absorption of large quantities of vitamins.

## What vitamins are routinely given to newborns?

Newborns usually obtain a daily supplement of Vitamins A, B, C, and D.

## Do growing children normally require extra vitamin intake in the form of pills?

Not if they eat a well-balanced diet. Vitamins should be added to the diet only on the advice of one's physician.

## Do elderly people require extra vitamins?

Recent research would indicate that most aged people can benefit from supplementary vitamins. This stems from the fact that their food intake of vitamin-rich substances is often reduced, their gastrointestinal absorption is impaired, and their metabolic processes are inadequate.

## What supplementary vitamins are usually given to pregnant women?

Because of increased needs for vitamins during pregnancy, it has become the practice to give expectant mothers Vitamins A, C, D, and B complex. Sometimes Vitamins E and K are added. Such vitamin intake should not be a substitute for a well-balanced diet.

## Should people who are obese and undergoing strenuous dieting take vitamins?

Yes. It is wise for such people to take

a multivitamin supplement containing most of the known vitamins.

### Are vitamins of value in quieting nervous people?

Only if the nervousness is due to a vitamin deficiency. This is rarely the case.

### Are vitamins valuable in treating anemia?

Very few types of anemia are caused by vitamin deficiency alone. However, where there is a vitamin deficiency along with anemia, vitamins may be given.

### Will the taking of extra vitamins reduce the incidence of colds or influenza?

There is insufficient scientific evidence to prove this. However, it is thought that people with vitamin deficiencies may be more susceptible to upper respiratory infection.

### Does the regular taking of mineral oil interfere with the absorption of vitamins?

It is doubtful whether the taking of mineral oil results in serious interference with vitamin absorption. In order to insure that this does not take place, it is wisest to take the vitamins several hours before or after taking the oil.

### Does it make much difference which brand of vitamin one purchases?

All vitamin manufacture and distribution is regulated by the provisions of the Pure Food and Drug Act. It is safe to purchase any brand of vitamins as long as the quantities contained in the prescription are clearly marked on the label.

### Will taking Vitamin A improve the eyesight?

No, unless the impaired eyesight is due to a proved Vitamin A deficiency.

### Are vitamins helpful in the so-called "general rundown condition"?

Only if there is an existing vitamin deficiency.

### Will the taking of vitamins tend to make one gain weight?

Not unless the diet has been previously deficient in vitamins and such deficiency has in some way led to poor appetite and inadequate food intake.

# CHAPTER 79
# X RAY

## What are x rays?

They are electromagnetic waves of very short length, which are created by passing a high-voltage electric current through a vacuum tube equipped with a metallic target for the electrons to strike against. X rays have a peculiar penetrative power through matter and living tissues. By passing these rays through the part of the body to be studied, shadows are created that can be recorded on photographic film. These shadows form certain patterns, varying according to the density of the particular tissue. The interpretation of these shadows is the task of the radiologist, who can, from his study, often make a specific diagnosis.

## What is a radiologist?

A radiologist is a physician who has had special education and training and is qualified in the use of x rays, radium, cobalt, and other radioactive substances for the diagnosis and treatment of diseases and abnormalities of the human body.

## What is an x-ray technician?

An x-ray technician is one who has had special training and experience in the use of x-ray apparatus for the purpose of taking x-ray films or giving x-ray therapy. He or she is also experienced in the technical processing of the exposed x-ray films.

## Can all the tissues of the body be visualized by x rays?

No. There are many soft tissues in the body that are not visualized by x rays upon direct study. This is due to the fact that these tissues absorb the same amount of x rays as the immediate surrounding tissues and therefore do not reveal contrast. However, with the aid of contrast media such as opaque dye or air, almost all parts of the body can be visualized.

## Is it safe for the x rays to be taken by a technician?

Yes. The x-ray technician is a person who has been specially trained to do x-ray technical work, and he or she does this work under the supervision of the radiologist. Most states require certification, registry, or licensing of the x-ray technician.

## Why do x-ray technicians stand behind screens or in another room when taking x rays?

These screens, or room walls, have lead shielding to protect the technician from the effects of scattered radiation, which has a cumulative effect over a period of time, even though this radiation may be in small amounts at each exposure.

## Is there any danger of getting a shock from an x-ray machine?

No. All present x-ray apparatus is fully shock-proof, as are the cables, etc.

## Is an x ray a true picture of the part of the body examined?

No. It is a projection of shadows as the x-ray beam goes through the various densities of the tissues. It is the interpretation of these shadows that makes the diagnosis.

## What is a xeroradiogram?

It is a special technique of x raying a patient in which the image is recorded on a sensitized paper rather than on x-ray film. Xeroradiography is now being employed widely in performing mammograms be-cause it affords an excellently detailed picture of the breast.

## Can x-ray moving pictures be made?

Yes. These are known as cineradiograms or cinefluorograms.

## Are x-ray films the property of the patient?

No. X-ray films are a part of the permanent record of a medical examination and, as such, are the property of the examining physician. State laws govern this factor. However, the patient is entitled to a report of the physician's findings or x-ray diagnosis.

## Can x-ray films of different patients get mixed up?

This is almost impossible, as films are imprinted with the patient's name and a specific number.

## What is a fluoroscope?

It is an x-ray apparatus, which reveals the image of the parts of the body studied upon a fluorescent screen; it also shows the movements of these parts.

## Why must the room be darkened during a fluoroscopic examination?

Because the images appearing upon the fluorescent screen will be much better visualized if the room is darkened to prevent light reflections upon the screen.

## What is an image intensifier?

It is a unit attached to the fluoroscope that greatly increases the brightness and improves the visual acuity of the ordinary fluoroscopic image. It also permits fluoroscopy in room light.

## Can photographs be taken from the fluoroscope?

Yes. Cinefilming and projection upon TV systems are also possible.

**Why does the radiologist wear rubber gloves and a rubber apron when performing fluoroscopy?**

Since he is constantly working in and around x rays, the cumulative effect can be harmful unless he protects himself from overexposure. The apron and gloves protect him because they contain lead, which is impervious to x rays.

**Is it possible to undergo too many fluoroscopic examinations?**

Yes. Overexposure is definitely bad for the patient. The amount of x rays one can safely receive is determined by the radiologist. He will safeguard your welfare at all times.

**Does one get an overdose of x rays from the usual methods of examination?**

No.

**Is it safe for a child to be fitted for shoes by a fluoroscopic machine?**

No. This is not advisable, as it may result in unnecessary exposure. Furthermore, there is no advantage to this method.

**What are "contrast media"?**

These are substances used to outline an organ or area in the body that has not sufficient density difference to be visualized by x rays alone. One of the most frequently used contrast media is barium. This will demonstrate the outline of the entire gastrointestinal tract.

**Is it safe if repeated x rays of the spine are taken?**

No. When such x rays are taken, there is a great deal of radiation directed toward the reproductive organs. The effect of this is cumulative and can be harmful if repeated too often.

**What effect can an overdose of x rays have upon the reproductive organs?**

a. If given in very large doses directly over the female organs, radiation can cause a stoppage of menstruation. This effect may be temporary or permanent and may cause sterility.

b. Small doses given repeatedly are thought to have an effect upon the eggs within the ovaries. Some investigators feel that this may lead to deformities in future offspring, even unto the second or third unborn generation.

c. An overdose in the region of the testicles may also cause sterility.

**If a small metal pin has been swallowed, will it show up in the x ray?**

Yes. Any metallic foreign body will be visible by x-ray examination.

**Can a piece of glass that has entered the body be seen on an x-ray film?**

Yes, if the glass has sufficient opacity. A very tiny piece that has the same density as the surrounding tissues may not be visible.

**Can wood that has entered the body be seen on an x-ray film?**

Only if it has a greater density than the surrounding tissues. Small slivers and splinters usually cannot be seen.

**Can air or other gases in various parts of the body be seen in the x rays?**

Yes, because they contrast with the denser surrounding tissues.

**What is a CAT, or CT, scan?**

A CAT (computerized axial tomography) scan, also called a CT scan, is a method of examination wherein the interaction of many x-ray beams throughout a slice of body tissue is analyzed by a computer. The result is a picture that permits the radiologist to study the images and to make remarkably accurate diagnoses of disease, even when the lesion is tiny in size. (This new technique is valued so highly that its inventor was awarded the Nobel Prize in medicine for 1979.)

**What is the advantage of a CAT scan over conventional x-ray studies?**

The scanning device enables the radiologist to see and diagnose very small tumors that would not be seen on ordinary x rays. Tumors and other abnormalities, too, in soft tissues such as the brain, the liver, the pancreas, the kidneys, the bladder, the adrenal glands, the pelvic organs, etc., can be spotted with the CAT scan.

**Is the CAT scanner able to take pictures of all parts of the body?**

Yes, but its greatest value is in lesions of the head, chest, abdomen, and vertebral column.

**Can the CAT scanner take hundreds of pictures in a brief time?**

Yes.

**Is the patient exposed to large doses of x rays during a CAT scan?**

No, because exposure time is so brief and the amount of radiation released by the machine is small.

**Should everyone undergo a CAT scan periodically?**

Such a procedure is unnecessary and wasteful. There are far too few CAT scan apparatus available, and their use should be devoted to those patients in whom one suspects a serious abnormality.

**Is it painful to undergo a CAT scan?**

No.

**Does it take long to perform a total body CAT scan?**

No.

**Can any physician interpret the findings of a CAT scan?**

No. It takes the expertise of a qualified radiologist to make diagnoses from CAT scans.

## Can a CAT scan demonstrate a brain tumor?

Yes. As a matter of fact, the original application of this technique was for the study of the brain. The CAT scan has revolutionized neurological diagnosis. Small brain tumors, brain cysts, hemorrhages into the brain, and many other abnormalities can be seen in great detail on a CAT scan.

## Does CAT scanning make sonography (ultra sound examination) unnecessary?

No. The two methods of investigation complement each other, resulting in the very highest degree of accurate diagnoses.

## Will a small foreign body in a bronchial tube show up on x ray?

If the foreign body is opaque, it will be seen directly. If not, its presence may be suspected by changes in the normal x-ray appearance of the lungs.

## What is a bronchogram?

It is a technique of visualizing the bronchial tubes by instilling an iodized oil into the trachea (wind-pipe). This oil is opaque to the x rays and will therefore outline the tubes on film.

## Are repeated routine chest x rays safe to perform?

Yes. The amount of radiation received is very small and the amount of scattered radiation reaching the reproductive organs is negligible. However, the amount of radiation must be controlled by the radiologist.

## Can an x ray of the chest reveal tuberculosis even when there are no symptoms?

Yes. Therefore, it is advisable for everyone to have a periodic chest x-ray examination.

## Can a chest x ray show cancer of the lung?

It will often reveal the presence of a lung tumor long before there are any symptoms.

## Can an x ray determine the size of the heart?

Yes. It will show the size, contour, and position of the heart.

## Can the inside of the heart be seen by x-ray examination?

Yes, through angiocardiography. This is carried out by instilling an opaque substance into the chambers of the heart by injection. The injection is made not by putting a needle into the heart but by feeding a long tube from a vessel in the arm into the heart.

## Can a deformity of the heart be seen on x rays?

Some defects can be revealed by direct studies. Other defects can be demonstrated by angiocardiography, through the injection of an x-ray opaque contrast medium.

## Can arteries be seen on x-ray films?

If they are hardened (sclerosed), they may be visible because of the accompanying calcium deposits. Most normal vessels are not opaque to the x rays but can be visualized by arteriograms. These are special x rays obtained by injecting an opaque substance directly into the arterial system.

## Can veins be seen on x rays?

No, but they can be visualized by injecting a substance that is opaque.

## Can lymphatic vessels be seen merely by taking an ordinary x ray?

No, but they *can* be visualized after injection of opaque contrast media directly into the lymph channel. This procedure is known as *lymphangiography*.

## Why must a patient take a barium mixture when the gastrointestinal tract is being x rayed?

Barium is used to outline the mucous membrane lining of the tract. Disease or abnormality will show up as a deformity or variation from the normal pattern.

## Why must the patient fast before stomach x rays are taken?

If food is in the stomach, it will distort the pattern that will be seen on the films when the opaque barium mixes with it.

## Why is it necessary to take so many views of the stomach?

The stomach and the rest of the intestinal tract are in constant motion. It is therefore essential to take many films from many angles in order to gain full knowledge of the contour and action of the stomach.

## Can a hernia of the diaphragm involving the upper end of the stomach be diagnosed by x ray?

Yes.

## Why is it sometimes necessary to take a laxative or an enema prior to x-ray examination?

This is done to eliminate gas or solid materials, which might obscure the view of the organ to be studied.

## Is the gall bladder seen on ordinary direct x-ray examination?

Usually not, unless it has calcium deposits in its wall.

## Are gallstones usually visualized on direct x-ray examination?

The majority of them do not appear on ordinary x-ray film. However, those that contain calcium are visualized.

## How are the gall bladder and gallstones visualized by x ray?

By a special test known as cholecystography. This consists of giving a special dye in the form of tablets the night before the x rays are to be taken. The dye appears in the gall bladder the next day, unless disease is present. If the gall bladder fails to visualize on the x-ray film, it is diseased. Sometimes, when the gall bladder is visualized by the dye, it will demonstrate the presence of stones, which will appear as negative shadows.

## If the gall bladder fails to visualize on x-ray film after the dye has been given, does this indicate the presence of disease?

Yes. In more than 95 percent of cases, this indicates a diseased organ.

## What is a cholangiogram?

It is the test used to visualize the bile ducts. It can be done by injecting certain dyes into the bloodstream; or, if the test is performed while the surgeon is operating upon the gall bladder, the dye is injected directly into the patient's ducts.

## Why is it important to visualize the bile ducts?

To determine whether the bile ducts contain any gallstones that must be removed. Also, to learn whether any abnormalities of the ducts are present.

## Can the kidneys be visualized on x-ray examination?

Yes, as they have sufficient density from the surrounding tissues to be revealed upon direct study.

## What is intravenous urography?

It is a study of the urinary tract after an opaque dye has been injected intravenously. This dye is excreted by the kidneys and therefore will cause the entire urinary tract to be visualized; by this method the diagnosis of malfunction, abnormality, or disease can be made.

## Can kidney stones by seen in x-ray studies?

The stones that are opaque to the x rays will be seen upon direct study. Those that are not opaque can be demonstrated in the urinary tract through intravenous urography, after which they may be seen as negative shadows.

## What is a cystogram?

It is an x-ray study of the bladder after an opaque substance has been instilled into it.

## Can breast cysts and tumors be seen by x rays?

Yes, in the great majority of instances. This process is known as *mammography*.

## How accurate are mammograms in diagnosing cancer of the breast?

Anywhere from 85 to 92 percent of the time.

## Does a negative mammogram mean that a woman requires no surgery for a lump in her breast?

Absolutely not! Since 8 to 15 percent of breast cancers cannot be seen on mammography, all suspicious lumps should be removed surgically and submitted for microscopic examination. Failure to do so will be very dangerous.

## Does a positive mammogram always mean that cancer is present?

No, in some 8 to 15 percent of cases, the mammographic findings may be that of a malignancy, but the surgical biopsy will reveal a benign, noncancerous growth.

## Is there danger of getting cancer from repeated mammography?

With modern equipment, the danger is very slight, as the amount of radiation the machine gives off is extremely small. It is thought that the risk is much greater in *not* having a mammogram if the surgeon is dealing with a patient who has a high risk for breast cancer. Moreover, one would require yearly mammograms over a ten-year period to increase the chances of cancer significantly.

## Who should undergo mammography?

a. Women whose mother, aunt, or sister has had breast cancer.
b. Women who have had a cancer of the opposite breast.
c. Women who have had repeated benign breast cysts or tumors.
d. Women who have lumps in their breast that the physician thinks might be malignant.

## Should all women have periodic mammograms?

No. These x rays are especially valuable in the situations mentioned above and in women past forty-five to fifty years of age.

## Can the uterus and Fallopian tubes be seen by x-ray examination?

Yes. This is done by instilling an opaque substance into these organs through the cervix; the films so obtained are called *hysterograms*.

## Will an x ray show a pregnancy?

Yes, but x rays have been largely replaced by sonography (ultrasound) except in some cases that are near full term.

## What is pelvimetry x ray?

This procedure is done to determine the measurements of the fetal head and maternal pelvis so as to ascertain whether a normal delivery will be possible. It may also demonstrate the need for a Cesarean section.

## Will an x ray show a fracture of any bone?

Yes, but it may require several different views or positions of the bone to reveal the fracture site. Such x rays will also show the position of the fractured fragments of the bone.

### Will an x ray be able to demonstrate the presence of muscle sprains, ligament injuries, or torn cartilages?

Not muscle sprains. Ligament injuries and torn cartilages may be determined by x ray with the aid of contrast media, such as air or opaque dye.

### What is arthrography?

It is the visualization of a joint space by x ray after the injection of a contrast medium into it.

### Will a bone infection be seen on x-ray examination?

Not in the early stage of its development. However, it will be revealed when the bone cells show some destruction.

### Will x rays show a bone tumor?

Yes.

### Why is it usually advisable to x ray the opposite extremity after an injury?

To be certain that what appears to be an abnormality is not a normal deviation, such as an accessory bone.

### What is myelography?

It is the x-ray examination of the spinal canal by means of introducing an opaque substance into the canal via spinal puncture. This will often demonstrate the presence or absence of a slipped disk or spinal cord tumor.

### Can congenital defects be seen by x-ray examination?

Yes, after the injection of a contrast medium into the heart through the blood vessels. This is known as angiocardiography.

## RADIATION THERAPY
### (X-ray Therapy)

### What is radiation therapy?

It is the treatment of diseases or tumors by the use of x ray, radium, or radioactive substances.

### What types of radiation therapy are used today?

X rays, high energy electron beams, cobalt, radium, cesium, iridium, radioactive iodine, radioactive gold, radioactive phosphorus, etc.

### Are newer types of radiation being discovered through development of atomic energy?

Yes. We can look forward to many new and beneficial types of radioactive substances and techniques of administration.

### What are the most common forms of radiation therapy?

X rays of various voltages, radium, and cobalt.

### What is a kilovolt?

It is a thousand volts.

### What does "mev" mean?

It means a million electron volts and usually is used to refer to multimillion volt x-ray apparatus.

### What is an "r"?

It is a roentgen, which is a unit used in measuring ionizing radiation dosage.

### What is a "rad"?

It is a unit of absorbed radiation dosage.

### Why must so many treatments be taken in radiation therapy?

When a lesion is being treated, the amount of rays needed to affect the lesion must be divided into a number of smaller doses, so as not to damage the normal tissues surrounding the lesion.

### Does radiation therapy cure?

Many conditions are completely cured by radiation therapy. In other cases, where the condition is beyond the stage of permanent cure, radiotherapy will often relieve the condition and extend life for many months or years. Pain and suffering are often relieved by the judicious use of radiation therapy.

### Are there any hazards from exposure to the rays during radiation therapy?

There are some, but they are negligible when treatment is for conditions less serious than malignancies. In malignancies, the risk is minimized since the radiation is given under the care of a radiologist or radiation therapist.

### Is radiation safe for the patient?

The radiologist or radiation therapist is an experienced and trained specialist, and under his care the patient is safe.

### Is the effect of x-ray treatments in children the same as in adults?

No. The younger the child, the greater is the possible harmful effect from radiation. Such therapy should be used only when necessary and upon the explicit advice of the radiologist.

### Is radiation therapy used for malignant conditions only?

No, it is of value and is used occasionally for some nonmalignant diseases or lesions.

### Does the patient feel any pain or discomfort while undergoing radiation therapy?

No. There is no sensation from the rays at the time of treatment.

### Why does the skin get red after a period of radiation treatments?

Because the skin reacts to the rays in a manner similar to the way it reacts to the sun. The reaction in some people is greater than in others. The reaction will subside after the therapy is finished.

### Does radiation therapy cause the hair in the area being treated to fall out?

If a large amount of therapy is given, the hair will fall out. In many cases, the hair will grow back.

### What is radiation sickness?

Some patients develop nausea, weakness, loss of appetite, and, possibly, vomiting after a series of treatments. This is called radiation sickness. It is controlled readily by appropriate medication and, if necessary, by adjusting therapy radiation dosages and frequency.

### How long does radiation sickness usually last after therapy has been discontinued?

Usually not longer than several days.

### Does radiation therapy destroy the normal cells around the diseased cells?

The diseased cells are more sensitive to the rays than the normal cells, and the therapy is so given as to destroy only the diseased cells. Normal cells recover from the temporary damaging effect of radiation.

### Can radiation therapy shrink a large thyroid gland that causes pressure in the neck?

It may diminish the size of the gland to some degree, but treatment by other medical or by surgical means is preferable.

### Are fibroids of the uterus treated by radiation therapy?

No.

### Can a cyst within the abdomen be treated effectively with x-ray therapy?

No. The cyst should be removed surgically.

### Can x-ray therapy remove warts?

Some can be treated adequately by means of x ray; others will require surgical removal. non-irradiation methods are preferable.

### Can x-ray therapy reduce the size of a keloid (an overgrown scar)?

Yes, in many instances. However, if treatment is to be effective, it must begin soon after the appearance of the keloid.

### Can x-ray therapy aid the patient with acne?

In certain carefully selected cases, it is beneficial, but other methods of treatment are preferable.

### Will x-ray therapy clear the pock marks in acne?

No. These marks are scars resulting from the acne and are best treated by other methods.

### Can x-ray therapy relieve obstruction of the eustachian tubes, which extend from the inside of the throat to the ears?

If such obstruction is caused by enlarged lymphoid tissue, x-ray or radium therapy often shrinks such tissue and relieves the obstruction of the ears. However, surgery is more advisable than irradiation for children.

### Should x-ray therapy be used to treat arthritis?

No.

### Is x-ray therapy of value for the treatment of bursitis?

Yes, in certain cases. It will reduce the inflammation and relieve the pain.

### Can x rays affect the reproductive system so that birth deformities may be more likely to occur in one's children or grandchildren?

Yes. This is a distinct possibility in a small number of cases when excessive doses of x ray are given. The chances of such an eventuality are minimal when x rays are controlled by competent radiologists.

### How is radium applied?

It is placed in tubes, needles, flat applicators (plaques), and is used as a gas, which is sealed in hollow gold containers ("seeds").

### What is radon?

It is a gas given off by radium when it breaks down. This gas is usually encapsuled in small gold "seeds," which are then implanted in tumors so as to produce maximal radiation effect locally.

### Is the effect of atomic fallout upon the human body similar to that of x rays or radium?

Yes.

### What are isotopes?

These are substances that have been made radioactive in atomic piles and are used as tracer chemicals or for radiation therapy.

### How many radioactive isotopes are in existence today?

There are more than nine hundred known isotopes.

### Are radioactive isotopes dangerous to handle?

Yes, very much so, and many precautions are taken to safeguard all personnel involved in the production, transportation, and use of all radio-active materials.

### Do isotopes lose their power in time?

Yes. Some are radioactive for a period of hours, and others for days, months, or years. The half-life period for some of the radioactive isotopes used in radiation therapy is as follows: gold, 64.6 hours; iodine, 8.1 days; iridium, 2.48 months; cobalt, 5.3 years.

## What is meant by "tagging" with an isotope?

Combining a substance such as a food or drug with a radioactive product so that the isotope can then be traced in the body with a radiation detection apparatus.

## Are radioactive isotopes used in industry?

Yes. They are used for purposes of tracing and testing. They are used in agriculture to produce better plant types.

## Which are the more commonly used isotopes?

Iodine 131, cobalt 60, gold 198, iron 59, phosphorus 32, cesium 137, and strontium 90.

## What is cobalt 60?

It is chemical cobalt, which has been made radioactive in an atomic pile; it gives off gamma rays similar to those from radium.

## What are the uses of the iodine isotope?

Iodine 131 has an affinity for the thyroid gland and is used as a tracer. In cases of overactivity of the thyroid, it will sometimes suppress its secretion and return the gland to a less active state. It is also used in certain cases of thyroid cancer and has been known to effect an occasional cure.

## What are the uses of phosphorus isotopes?

Phosphorus 32 is used as a tracer in much the same manner as other radioactive drugs, It has also proven effective in the treatment of certain blood diseases, such as leukemia and polycythemia.

## What is nuclear scanning?

It is the radiation scanning from the isotope tracer used for the particular gland or organ in which this isotope will settle. It will reveal either a normal outline or an abnormality.

## How is this done?

By means of a scintillation counter apparatus, which is affected by the local radiation coming from the isotope contained in the gland or organ.

## How is scanning performed?

The patient receives a small injection of a radioactive material and soon thereafter is placed under the machine, which records the radiation emanating from the organ where the radioactive material concentrates.

## What organs lend themselves to scanning?

The brain, thyroid gland, the lungs, the liver, kidneys, and bones.

## Can diseases be detected by use of nuclear scanning?

Yes, both tumors and other conditions can be diagnosed by scanning techniques.

## Are the radiation doses from nuclear scanning dangerous?

No. The doses given cause no harm.

## Can nuclear scans detect diseases other than tumors?

Yes. They may show blood clots in the lungs, abscesses in the lungs or liver, disturbances in blood flow, and the function of various organs, depending upon the diagnostic isotope that has been injected and on the method of detection used.

# DEFINITIONS OF
# MEDICAL TERMS

# A

**abarticulation,** joint dislocation.

**abasia,** inability to walk due to incoordination.

**abatement,** decrease in severity of pain or other symptom.

**abdomen,** area of body between thorax and pelvis.

**abdominoscopy,** examination of the abdominal cavity by an instrument.

**abduct,** to draw an extremity away from the body.

**aberration,** deviation from normal state or action.

**ablation,** removal or separation by surgery.

**abnormal,** variation from normal.

**abortion,** the termination of pregnancy, spontaneous or induced.

**abrade,** chafing of skin by friction.

**abrasion,** a scraping injury to the outer layer of skin.

**abscess,** a localized collection of purulent matter in any part of the body that may cause pain or swelling.

**abscission,** the removal of a growth by surgical means.

**absolute,** pure or perfect.

**absorb,** to take in by soaking up.

**abuse,** improper use, frequently cited in connection with drugs or alcohol misuse or mistreatment of children.

**acariasis,** a skin disease caused by a mite or acarid. See scabies.

**acclimation,** becoming accustomed to a different climate or situation.

**accomodation,** adjustment of the eye for seeing varied distances.

**accouchement,** act of delivery in childbirth or confinement.

**acetabulum,** the cavity in the hip bone which receives the head of the femur or thigh bone.

**acetic,** having properties of vinegar.

**acetic acid,** used as a reagent. An aqueous solution containing alcohol.

**acetone,** a volatile, colorless and inflammable liquid useful as a solvent; found in the blood and urine of diabetics.

**acetylcholine,** an acid found in various organs and tissues necessary for the transmission of nerve impulses.

**acetylicysalic acid,** used to relieve symptoms of pain and fever. Syn: aspirin.

**achalasia,** inability of muscles or sphincters to relax.

**ache,** a continued dull or severe pain.

**Achilles tendon,** connects the muscles of the calf of the leg to the heel bone.

**achlorhydria,** abscence of hydrochloric acid in stomach.

**acholic,** absence of bile.

**achondroplasia,** dwarfism caused by a defect in the formation of cartilage in which the trunk of the body is of normal size but the limbs are abnormally short.

**acroma,** an absence of normal pigmentation; albinism.

**achromatin,** found in a cell nucleus which lacks staining properties.

**acid,** a sour tasting compound containing hydrogen that easily combines with metals; also, informal term for the hallucinogenic drug LSD.

**acid-fast,** pertaining to bacteria which are not easily decolorized after staining but retain the red dyes.

**acidity,** a sour stomach due to an excess of hydrochloric acid.

**acidosis,** an accumulation of acids causing a disturbance in the acid-base balance of the body often seen in diabetic acidoses or renal disease.

**acne,** a disease of the sebaceous glands and hair follicles of the skin characterized by blackheads and pimples which usually occurs during adolescence.

**acoria,** ingestion of large amounts of food; gluttony.

**acoustic,** relating to hearing or sound.

**acoustics,** the science of sound.

**acquired,** originating outside the organism.

**acrid,** biting or irritating.

**acriflavine,** an orange granulated powder used as an antiseptic.

**acromegaly,** excessive growth of the extremities -- fingers, toes, jaw and nose; caused by an overactive pituitary gland.

**acromion,** the highest extension of the shoulder.

**acrophobia,** an abnormal fear of high places.

**ACTH,** a pituitary hormone; adrenocorticotropic hormone that stimulates a specific area of the adrenal glands.

**actin,** a muscle protein.

**actinodermatitis,** an inflammation to the skin caused by excessive exposure to the sun or X-rays.

**actinomcete,** a parasite that causes a fungus disease in animals; sometimes communicated to man.

**actinomycin,** an anti-bacterial substance effective against gram-positive organisms.

**acuity,** clarity of vision; sharpness.

**acupuncture,** method of treatment used for a variety of disorders by puncturing specific points on the body with long needles; a technique first used by the ancient Chinese.

**acute,** a sudden onset of an illness that is attended by a brief course and severe symptoms.

**adactyly,** congenital absence of digits of hands or feet.

**Adam's apple,** prominence on the front of throat produced by the thyroid cartilage.

**adaptation,** ability of an organism to adjust to its environment for survival.

**addict,** one who exhibits addiction.

**addiction,** the state of being physically or psychologically dependent on some agent such as drugs or alcohol.

**Addison's Disease,** a condition caused by underactive adrenal glands characterized by pigmentation of skin, weakness, fatigue, and digestive disturbances.

**additive,** a substance added to another to enhance its appearance, or nutritional value.

**adduct,** the movement of an extremity toward the body's main axis.

**adduction,** the movement of a limb, the trunk, or head toward the median axis of the body.

**adductor,** the muscle that adducts.

**adenalgia,** pain in a gland.

**adenectomy,** surgical removal of a gland.

**adenine,** white, crystaline substance found in plant and animal tissues; a decomposition product of nuclein.

**adenitis,** inflammation of lymph nodes or a gland.

**adenocarcinoma,** malignant tumor cells occurring in glandular tissue.

**adenofibroma,** benign tumor cells arising from connective tissue frequently found in the uterus.

**adenoids,** lymph glands in the upper pharynx which function to trap germs which can enlarge to the point of hindering nasal breathing.

**adenoidectomy,** the removal of the adenoids by excision.

**adenoiditis,** inflammation of the adenoids.

**adenoma,** a benign epithelial tumor in a gland.

**adenomatosis,** the development of multiple grandular growths.

**adenomyofibroma,** a fibroma containing muscular and glandular elements.

**adenopathy,** enlargement and morbid change of glands and lymph nodes.

**adenosarcoma,** a malignant tumor composed of both glandular and sarcomatous elements.

**adenosine,** derived from nucleic acid consisting of adenine and the pentose sugar D--ribose.

**adenosis,** abnormal development of a gland; gland disease.

**adenovirus,** virus causing disease of the upper respiratory tract.

**adermia,** absence of skin, congenital or acquired.

**adhesion,** the abnormal joining of structures or organs which have been separated by incision.

**adhesive,** adhering; sticky.

**adipose,** pertaining to fat accumulations in cells.

**adiposis,** an increase of fat in the body; obesity.

**adjuvant,** an additive to a drug which enhances the action of a principal prescription.

**adnerval,** near or toward a nerve.

**adnexa,** accessory parts of a structure or organ.

**adnexopexy,** attaching the fallopian tube and ovary to the abdominal wall.

**adolescence,** beginning of puberty until maturity.

**adrenal,** pertaining to the kidney or its function.

**adrenal gland,** an endocrine gland attached to the kidney.

**adrenalectomy,** excision of the adrenal glands.

**adrenalin,** epinephrine, a drug used as a heart and circulatory stimulant.

**adrenaline,** the hormone epinephrine.

**adrenergic,** activated by epinephrine.

**adrenocortical,** pertaining to the cortex of the adrenal gland./

**adrenocorticotropic hormone,** ACTH, an anterior pituitary hormone that stimulates the adrenal cortex of the adrenal glands.

**adsorb,** to attract and retain other substances.

**adsorption,** the action of a substance in attracting and retaining other materials to its surface.

**adult,** having reached full maturity.

**adventitia,** the outer coat of a structure or organ.

**aeration,** an exchange of carbon dioxide for oxygen by the blood in the lungs.

**aerobe,** a microorganism that lives and thrives only in the presence of free oxygen.

**aeroembolism,** an obstruction within the blood vessel by air or gas.

**aeroneurosis,** a nervous disorder occurring to aviators.

**aerophagia,** habitual air-swallowing.

**aerosol,** a drug or suspension that is dispensed in a fine spray.

**afebrile,** without fever.

**affect,** cognitive display of emotion reflecting a mental state.

**affective,** pertaining to the emotions.

**afferent,** transporting impulses toward a center.

**affinity,** a tendency to unite with another object or substance.

**afflux,** a sudden rush of blood to a part of the body.

**afterbirth,** after childbirth, the placenta and membranes that are expelled from the uterus.

**afterhearing,** sensations of sound heard after the stimulus has ceased.

**afterimage,** the persistence of images after the cessation of stimulus.

**afterpains,** cramplike pains after expulsion of placenta in the uterus.

**aftertaste,** a persistent taste after cessation of stimulus.

**agar,** a colloidal substance from red algae used in solid culture media for microorganisms; also used as a treatment for constipation.

**agensia,** an imperfect development; sterility.

**agglutination,** the clumping together of bacteria when exposed to immune serum; a process in wound healing.

**agglutinogen,** a substance that stimulates the production of agglutinin.

**aggregation,** a clumped mass of material such as platelets induced by agents.

**aglaucopsia,** inability to distinguish bluish-green and green tints.

**aglossia,** the absence of a tongue at birth.

**aglossostomia,** the absence of the tongue and mouth opening at birth.

**agnosia,** inability to comprehend sensory impressions.

**agonad,** an individual without sex glands.

**agoraphobia,** an extreme fear of open spaces.

**agranulocytosis,** a marked decrease in the number of granulocytes in the white blood cell count characterized by high fever and prostration.

**agraphia,** a loss of ability to express thoughts in writing.

**agromania,** morbid desire to live in solitude.

**ague,** intermittent malerial fever, characterized by fever, sweating, and chills.

**ahypnia,** insomnia; sleeplessness.

**AIDS,** or Acquired Immune Deficiency Syndrome, a generally fatal viral disease which attacks the body's immune system.

**ailurophobia,** unusual fear of cats.

**air embolism,** an obstruction of a blood vessel brought about by a bubble of air.

**akatamathesia,** inability to comprehend.

**akathisia,** motor restlessness due to anxiety.

**akinesia,** lacking muscular movement.

**ala,** resembling a wing; winglike appendage.

**alalia,** unable to speak because of vocal organs paralysis or defect.

**alanine,** a natural amino acid.

**albinism,** congenital absence of normal pigmentation; albino.

**albumin,** a water-soluble protein found in blood, milk, and the white of an egg.

**albuminuria,** albumin found in urine indicating a kidney disorder.

**alcohol,** organic compound which can be used as an astringent or antiseptic. Also a common name for ethyl alcohol found in alcoholic beverages.

**alcoholism,** an addictive disease characterized by a craving for alcohol which interferes with an individual's health, relationships, and economic functioning.

**aldehyde,** a colorless, flammable liquid resulting from the oxidation of a primary alcohol.

**aldosterone,** a hormone secreted by the adrenal cortex which regulates the electrolyte and water balance of the organism.

**aleukemia,** absence of white blood cells.

**aleukocytosis,** deficiency of white blood cell production.

**alexia,** inability to read; form of aphisia.

**algae,** various water plants, including the seaweeds.

**algesia,** increased sensitivity to pain.

**algogenic,** producing pain; lowering body temperature.

**algophobia,** unusual fear of pain.

**alienation,** a mental disorder; insanity.

**alimentary,** pertaining to nutrition and digestion.

**alkalemia,** abnormal alkalinity of the blood.

**alkali,** a caustic base such as sodium or potassium hydroxide that can neutralize acids to form salts.

**allele,** one of two alternative forms of a gene, dominant or recessive, which occupy the same locus on a designated pair of chromosomes that determine heredity.

**allergen,** any substance inducing hypersensitivity or allergy.

**allergist,** a specialist in allergies.

**allergy,** sensitivity to an allergen.

**allopathy,** a treatment based on producing a condition antagonistic to the condition being treated.

**allorhythmia,** an irregular heart beat or pulse that recurs regularly.

**allotropism,** possessing different forms of the same element with unlike properties.

**aloe,** a plant whose juices are used in pharmaceutical preparations.

**alopecia,** baldness; an absence of normal body hair.

**alum,** a crystaline substance used as an astringent and stypic.

**aluminosis,** chronic inflammation of the lungs due to aluminum-bearing dust.

**alveolar,** the cavities or sockets found in the jaw for the teeth.

**alveolus,** a small hollow; socket of a tooth; an air cell of the lungs.

**Alzheimer's Disease,** a mental disease causing deterioration similar to senility.

**A.M.A., American Medical Association.**

**amalgam,** an alloy containing mercury; mixture; blend.

**amara,** bitters.

**amarthritis,** inflammation of more than one joint.

**amaurosis,** loss of vision in which there is no evidence of pathology within the eye itself.

**ambidextrous,** one who is able to use either hand with equal proficiency.

**ambivalence,** simultaneous conflicting feelings or emotions toward a goal, person, or object.

**Amblyomma,** hard-bodied ticks.

**amblyopia,** dullness of vision without a detectable cause sometimes called "lazy eye".

**ambulatory,** able to move about and not confined to bed.

**ameba,** a single celled protozoan which moves about and absorbs food by completely surrounding it. Some amebae cause amebic dysentery in man. Also known as amoeba.

**amebiasis,** ulceration and infection of mucous membranes of the intestinal walls with Entameoba histolytica, the causative agent of amebic dysentery.

**amelioration,** the improvement of a condition.

**amelodentin,** pertaining to dentin or dental enamel.

**amenorrhea,** the absence or suppression of menstruation which is normal before puberty, after menopause, and during pregnancy or lactation.

**amentia,** feeble-mindedness or mental deficiency marked by mental confusion and subnormal intelligence.

**ametropia,** an abnormal condition of the eye in which vision is affected due to imperfect focus of images on the retina as in astigmatism, hyperopia, and myopia.

**amino acid,** one of a group of organic compounds containing both an amino and a carboxyl radical which are the building blocks of protein.

**aminopyrine,** an antipyretic and analgesic which has longer lasting effects in smaller doses than an antipyrine.

**aminuria,** accumulations of nitrogen-containing compounds found in the urine.

**amitosis,** cell division without changes in the nucleus or formation of chromosomes.

**amitriptyline,** an antidepressant drug.

**amniocentesis,** a surgical procedure which penetrates the uterus for aspiration of amniotic fluid to determine genetic defects.

**amnion,** the inner membrane which surrounds the fetus and holds the amniotic fluid.

**amniotic fluid,** the albuminous fluid within the amniotic sac which is colorless and functions to protect the floating fetus.

**amnionitis,** inflammation of the amnion.

**amoeba,** see: ameba.

**amorphous,** shapeless and having no specific form.

**amphetamine,** a drug used to stimulate the central nervous system. Misuse may lead to drug dependence.

**amphoteric,** showing or having opposite characteristics and capable of neutralizing both acids and bases.

**ampule,** a small container for hypodermic solutions.

**ampulla,** a dilatated end of a tubular structure such as a canal or duct.

**amputation,** the act of cutting off a limb or appendage by a surgical procedure.

**amusia,** loss of ability to produce or recognize musical sounds.

**A.M.W.A.,** American Medical Women's Association.

**amyelia,** absence of the spinal cord at birth.

**amygdaline,** shaped like an almond; pertaining to a tonsil.

**amylaceous,** resembling starch.

**amylase,** pancreatic and salivary juices with enzymes that convert starch into sugar.

**amyloid,** starchlike, translucent material formed in a variety of diseases and deposited intercellularly.

**amylolysis,** the conversion of starch into sugar by enzymes in the process of digestion.

**amylopsin,** an enzyme in pancreatic juice which converts starch into sugar maltose.

**amylum,** corn starch used as dusting powder.

**amyocardia,** weakness of the heart muscle.

**amyosthenia,** muscular weakness and lacking muscle tone.

**amyotrophy,** muscular wasting that is painful.

**amyxorrhea,** an absence of mucous secretion.

**ana,** used in medical ingredients meaning in equal proportions or of each.

**anabiosis,** restoration of life after an apparent cessation of vital processes.

**anabolism,** opposed to catabolism in the metabolic process by which the body substance is built up.

**anabolite,** a complex substance of anabolism.

**anadipsia,** intense thirst.

**anaerobe,** a microorganism that thrives without oxygen.

**anakusis,** total deafness.

**anal,** a ring, pertaining to the rectal opening; near the anus.

**analeptic,** drug that gives strength and is restorative.

**analgesic,** drug that relieves pain without loss of consciousness.

**anallergic,** not allergic or hypersensitive.

**analysis,** separation and or act of determining the compound parts of a substance; separation into compound parts; psychoanalysis involving diagnosis and treatment.

**analyst,** one who analyzes.

**anamnesis,** recollection; past history of a patient and his family.

**anaphase,** third stage in mitosis between metaphase in which longitudinal halves of chromosomes separate and move toward opposite poles.

**anaphia,** diminished sense of touch.

**anaphoresis,** insufficient activity of the sweat glands.

**anaphrodisia,** loss of sexual desire.

**anaphrodisiac,** a substance that represses sexual desire.

**anaphylaxis,** an increased sensitivity to a drug, so that a second dose brings about a severe reaction, severe enough to cause serious shock.

**anaplasia,** an alteration in cells which is believed to produce characteristics of tumor tissue.

**anaplastic,** restoring of an absent part.

**anarthria,** speechlessness resulting from the loss of the ability to articulate words.

**anasarca,** severe generalized edema.

**anastaltic,** very astringent.

**anastomosis,** the surgical formation of a passage between two normally distinct organs or spaces; the joining together of parts such as nerves or connective tissue fibers; the union of arteries or veins.

**anatomist,** one skilled in anatomy.

**anatomy,** the scientific study of structures of organisms.

**anconal,** pertaining to the elbow.

**ancylostomiasis,** infestation with hookworms which gain entrance into the body through the skin of the bare foot of a person causing inflammation, itching, allergic reactions, pneumonia-like symptoms, nausea, and diarrhea. Excessive blood loss leads to anemia.

**androgen,** a substance producing male characteristics, as testosterone.

**androgynous,** resembling an androgynoid and without definite sexual characteristics.

**androsterone,** a male hormone found in urine.

**anemia,** a reduction in hemoglobin, or in the volume of packed red blood cells. It occurs when hemoglobin is less than 13--14 gm. per 100 ml. for males or 11--12 gm. per 100 ml. for women.

**anemic,** having anemia.

**anencephaly,** an absence of brain and spinal cord, a congenital defect.

**anesthesia,** a lost sense of feeling due to disease or induced to permit the performance of surgery and other painful procedures.

**anesthesiology,** a branch of medicine which studies the administration of anesthetics.

**anesthetist,** a person trained to administer anesthetics.

**anesthetize,** to place under an anesthetic agent.

**aneurin,** thiamine, or Vitamin B1.

**aneurysm,** a widening of a blood vessel due to pressure on weakened tissues causing the formation of a sac of blood that may become clotted.

**angiasthenia,** a loss of tone in the vascular system.

**angiitis,** inflammation of the coats of either blood or lymph vessels.

**angina,** a choking, spasmodic, or suffocating pain that characterizes any disease.

**angina pectoria,** severe pain about the heart that radiates to the shoulder and down the left arm, usually caused by interference with the oxygen supply to the heart muscle.

**angiocardiogram,** a film produced by an X-ray of the heart and the great vessels after intravenous injection of a radiopaque solution.

**angiocarditis,** inflammation of the heart and the great blood vessels.

**angiography,** an examination of blood vessels and lymphatics by roentgen rays which are made visible by injection of a diagnostic solution.

**angiology,** the scientific study of blood vessels and lymphatics.

**angioma,** a tumor which is usually benign believed to be misplaced fetal tissue consisting of blood vessels and lymphatics.

**angiomyosarcoma,** a tumor consisting of a mass of blood vessels or lymphatics resembling elements of angioma, myoma, and sarcoma.

**angioneurectomy,** excision of blood vessels and nerves.

**angioplasty,** reconstruction of blood vessels by surgery.

**angiospasm,** excessive contractions of blood vessels.

**angiostaxis,** trickling of blood; oozing of blood as in Hemophilia.

**angiostenosis,** narrowing of a blood vessel.

**angulation,** angular loops which form in the intestine.

**anhidrosis,** deficiency of secretion of sweat.

**anhydremia,** deficiency of the normal fluid content in the blood.

**anhydrous,** without water.

**anhypnia,** insomnia.

**animation,** the quality of being alive, or active. (**suspended, a.** temporary suspension of vital activities).

**aniridia,** absence of the iris at birth.

**anisocoria,** inequality in size of the pupils, a normal condition or congenital.

**anisocytosis,** excessive variations in size of red blood cells indicating an abnormal condition.

**ankle,** the joint between leg and foot.

**ankylo-,** combining word form meaning bent or crooked.

**ankylocolpos,** pathological closure of the vagina.

**ankylosis,** partial or complete rigidity of a joint as a result of disease, injury, or surgical procedure.

**ankyroid,** hook-shaped.

**anlage,** the beginning of cell formation in an embryo which will develop specific tissue, organ, or part.

**annular,** ring-shaped.

**annulus,** a ring-shaped structure.

**anococcygeal,** refering to the anus and coccyx.

**anodyne,** a medication that relieves pain.

**anomalous,** irregular or abnormal.

**anomaly,** deviation from normal resulting from congenital or hereditary defects; a malformation.

**anoia,** idiocy.

**anomia,** inability to name objects or to recognize names of persons.

**anonychia,** without nails.

**anopheles,** widely distributed mosquitoes, many of which are vectors of malaria.

**anopsia,** defective vision resulting from strabismus, cataract, or refractive errors.

**anorexia,** loss of appetite for food.

**anorexia nervosa,** a lack or complete loss of appetite usually seen in girls and young women; sometimes the disease is accompanied by induced vomiting, emaciation, and amenorrhea. The psychophysiologic condition may also occur in males.

**anosmia,** absence of the sense of smell.

**anostosis,** defective development of bone.

**anovarism,** absence of the ovaries.

**anoxemia,** reduced oxygen level in the blood.

**anoxia,** absence of oxygen to body tissues despite adequate blood supply.

**ant-, anti-,** prefix meaning opposed to or counteracting.

**Antabuse,** trademark for disulfiram used in treatment of alcoholism.

**antacid,** an alkali that neutralizes acids in the stomach.

**antagonism,** opposition between similar muscles, medicines, or organisms.

**antagonist,** counteracting the action of anything.

**antalkaline,** neutralizing alkalinity.

**ante-,** prefix meaning before.

**antefebrile,** before a fever.

**anteflexion,** the foreward bending of an organ; the normal foreward bending of the uterus.

**antemortem,** occurring before death.

**antenatal,** before birth.

**antepartum,** before labor commences.

**anterior,** directed toward the front.

**anterolateral,** in front and situated to one side.

**anteversion,** tipping forward of an organ.

**anthelmintic,** an agent which is destructive to parasitic intestinal worms.

**anthemorrhagic,** medication for preventing hemorrhage.

**anthracosis,** a pneumoconiosis due to the inhalation of coal dust.

**anthrax,** a disease man contracts from animal hair or waste; a carbuncle; the disease may be of two forms, one on the skin and the other in the lungs. If untreated, anthrax may often be fatal.

**anthropo-,** prefix denoting relation to man.

**anthropogeny,** origin of man.

**anthropoid,** resembling man; tailless apes such as the gorilla, orangutan, and chimpanzee.

**anthropology,** the science of man in relation to origin, classification, race, physical and mental constitution, environmental and social relations, and culture.

**anthropometry,** the science of measuring the size, weight, and proportions of the human body.

**anthropophobia,** a morbid fear of a particular person, or of society. May be the onset of mental illness.

**anthypnotic,** hindering sleep.

**anti-,** prefix meaning against.

**antianaphylaxis,** desensitization to antigens.

**antiarrhythmic,** an agent alleviating cardiac arrhythmias.

**antibacterial,** destroying or hindering the growth of bacteria.

**antibiotic,** a substance produced by a microorganism which has the capacity to inhibit or destroy other microorganisms. Antibiotics are produced by bacteria and fungi and can be made synthetically.

**antiblennorrhagic,** a substance used to prevent or cure gonorrhea or catarrh.

**antibody,** a protein produced by the body in response to the presence of an antigen.

**anticholingeric,** an agent that blocks the passage of impulses through the parasympathetic nerves; parasympatholytic.

**anticoagulant,** acting to prevent clotting of blood; any substance which prevents or delays the coagulation of blood.

**anticonvulsive,** inhibiting or relieving convulsions.

**antidepressant,** acting to relieve or prevent depression.

**antidiuretic,** a substance that acts to suppress excretion of urine by the kidneys.

**antidotal,** acting as an antidote.

**antidote,** an agent which neutralizes poison or its effects.

**antiemetic,** an agent that prevents or alleviates nausea and vomiting.

**antienzyme,** an agent which inhibits enzymatic action; an enzyme produced by the body retarding the activity of another enzyme.

**antiepileptic,** an agent that combats epilepsy.

**antifebrile,** relieving fever.

**antigalactic,** an agent that suppresses the secretion of milk.

**antigen,** any substance which induces the formation of antibodies when bacteria or foreign blood cells are introduced into the body.

**antihistamine,** a substance which counteracts the effects of histamine such as used in treatment of allergies.

**antihypertensive,** reducing high blood pressure.

**antimalarial,** acting to relieve or prevent malaria, such as quinine.

**antimicrobial,** preventing or destroying the development of microbes.

**antimony,** a metallic element with a crystalline structure used in medicine.

**antimycotic,** preventing the growth of fungi.

**antiparkinsonian,** an agent used in treatment of parkinsonism.

**antipathy,** aversion or disgust; a chemical incompatibility.

**antiperistalsis,** the peristalic contractions moving toward the oral end of the gastrointestinal tract.

**antiphlogistic,** relieving inflammation.

**antiprothrombin,** anticoagulant.

**antipyretic,** an agent effective against fever.

**antipyrine,** an odorless, white crystalline powder used to reduce pain and fever.

**antiscabious,** relieving or preventing scabies.

**antiscorbutic,** effective against scurvy such as Vitamin C.

**antisepsis,** pertaining to sepsis, preventing the growth of germs.

**antiserum,** a serum containing antibodies specific for the antigen.

**antispasmodic,** relieving or preventing spasms.

**antitoxin,** a substance produced by the body capable of neutralizing a specific poison or toxin.

**antitussive,** an agent which relieves or prevents coughing.

**antivenin,** a substance used in treatment of animal venom poisoning.

**antiviral,** an effective agent inhibiting a virus.

**antivitamin,** an antagonistic substance which inhibits certain vitamins.

**antrum,** any nearly closed chamber or cavity in bones.

**anuresis,** a condition in which the kidneys fail to secrete urine.

**anuria,** failure to produce urine.

**anus,** outlet of the rectum leading from the bowel.

**anvil,** one of the three small bones of the middle ear between the stirrup and the hammer.

**anxiety,** an emotional feeling indicating uneasiness and apprehension; a psychological term.

**aorta,** the main artery arising from the left ventricle of the heart.

**aortic stenosis,** a narrowing of the aorta due to lesions of the wall with scar tissue from infection often seen resulting from rheumatic fever or embryonic anomalies.

**aortitis,** inflammation of the aorta.

**apandria,** an aversion to men.

**apaneuria,** impossibility of cloitus.

**apathetic,** indifferent; lacking interest.

**apathy,** sluggish; without feeling or emotion.

**aperient,** a mild laxative usually given at night on an empty stomach.

**aperitive,** an appetizer; a gentle purgative.

**aperture,** an opening.

**apex,** the extremity of anything; used to indicate the uppermost part of a body organ.

**aphagia,** inability to swallow.

**aphakia,** absence of crystalline lens behind the pupil of the eye.

**aphasia,** inability to express oneself through speech; a loss of verbal comprehension.

**aphemia,** loss of speech due to a central lesion.

**aphonia,** lack of voice with intact inner speech due to chronic laryngitis, hysteria, psychological problems, or diseases of the vocal cords.

**aphrasia,** inability in using connected phrases in speaking.

**aphrodisia,** extreme or morbid sexual passion.

**aphrodisiac,** a substance that excites sexual desire.

**aphtha,** a white spot or small ulcer occurring in the mouth.

**aphthous stomatitis,** recurring blister-like ulcers inside the mouth and on the lips; canker sores.

**aphylaxis,** absence of immunity.

**aplasia,** defective development of an organ or tissue.

**apnea,** temporary cessation of breathing due to reduction of stimuli to respiratory center; may occur during Cheyne-Stokes respiration.

**apocrine,** cells which lose part of their cytoplasm while functioning, especially mammary gland and certain sweat gland cells.

**apodal,** having no feet.

**apomorphine,** a morphine derivative used as an emetic and expectorant.

**aponeurosis,** a fibrous sheet of connective tissue which attaches muscle to bone or other tissues at insertion.

**apophysis,** a projection from a bone; an outward growth without a center of ossification.

**apoplectic,** pertaining to apoplexy.

**apoplexy,** sudden loss of consciousness followed by paralysis resulting from rupture of a blood vessel of the brain; a stroke.

**appendage,** anything attached to a larger part.

**appendectomy,** surgical removal of the vermiform appendix.

**appendicitis,** inflammation of the vermiform appendix.

**appendix,** an appendage; the vermiform appendix attached to the cecum.

**appestat,** a section of the brain, centrally located, controlling the appetite.

**appetite,** chiefly a desire for food, not necessarily hunger.

**apraxia,** loss of ability to carry out familiar purposeful movements without motor or sensory impairment.

**apyrexia,** absence of fever; nonfebrile period of an intermittent fever.

**aqua,** water; solution.

**aquaphobia,** unusual fear of water.

**aqueous,** containing water.

**aqueous humor,** watery transparent liquid produced by the iris, ciliary bodies, and cornea which circulates through the anterior and posterior chambers of the eye.

**arachnoid,** resembling a web.

**arachnoid membrane,** the thin, transparent center membrane that covers the brain and spinal cord.

**Aran-Duchenne disease,** muscular atrophy beginning in the extremities and progressing to other parts of the body; a progressive muscular atrophy.

**archiform,** bow-shaped.

**arcus,** an arc or arch.

**arcus senilis,** the opaque white ring which appears around the periphery of the cornea, seen in aged persons due to lipoid degeneration.

**areola,** a small area in a tissue; a small space between tissues that surrounds a skin lesion such as a boil; the colored circle surrounding the nipple; the part of the iris that surrounds the pupil.

**areolar,** containing small cavities in a tissue such as the glands lying beneath the breasts with ducts opening on its surface; connective tissue within the innerspaces of the body.

**ariboflavinosis,** a condition caused by a deficiency of riboflavin (Vitamin B2 or G).

**arnica,** a substance derived from plants used as an application to wounds.

**aromatic,** a drug or medicine having a fragrant odor.

**arrectores pilorum,** involuntary muscle fibers contracting under the influence of cold or fright and raising the hair follicles resulting in "goose-flesh".

**arrhythmia,** a disturbance of rhythm in the heartbeat.

**arrhythmic,** without regularity; abnormal rhythm of the heartbeat.

**arsenic,** a poisonous chemical element used in medicine and industry.

**ateria,** an artery.

**arterial,** pertaining to an artery or arteries.

**arterial bleeding,** bright-red blood pumped out of an artery, may be arrested by pressure on the proimal side of the blood vessel nearest the heart.

**arterialization,** changing venous blood to arterial by aeration.

**arteriogram,** a radiograph of arterial pulse.

**arteriography,** radiography of an artery or arterial system after injection of a contrast medium into the blood stream.

**arteriola, arteriole,** a minute artery, especially one which leads into a capillary at its distal end.

**arterioplasty,** surgical reconstruction of an artery.

**arteriosclerosis,** a thickening or hardening and loss of elasticity of the blood vessels and arteries.

**arteriospasm,** pain in an artery caused by spasms.

**arteriostenosis,** constriction of an artery.

**arteriovenous,** pertaining to both arteries and veins.

**arteritis,** inflammation of an artery.

**artery,** one of the many vessels carrying blood from the heart to the tissues of the body.

**arthralgia,** pain in a joint.

**arthritic,** pertaining to a joint; pertaining to arthritis; a person afflicted with arthritis.

**arthritis,** inflammation of the joints.

**arthrography,** an x-ray of a joint after injection with an opaque solution.

**arthropathy,** any joint disease.

**arthroplasty,** a surgical procedure upon a joint to make it function.

**arthrosclerosis,** stiffening of the joints, occurring especially in the aged.

**arthrosis,** a joint; degeneration of a joint.

**arthrosynovitis,** inflammation of the synovial membrane of a joint.

**articular,** pertaining to the joint.

**articulation,** connection of bones or joints; clearly enunciated speech; in dentistry, the contact relationship of the surfaces of the teeth.

**artifact,** artificially produced; a structure produced in a tissue or cell by staining.

**artificial,** not natural; formed in imitation.

**artificial insemination,** mechanical injection of seminal fluid within the vagina or cervix.

**artificial respiration,** maintaining respiratory movements by mouth-to-mouth breathing or by mechanical means.

**artus,** a joint or limb.

**arytenoid,** resembling a ladle, usually referring to the larynx and relating to cartilage or ligaments.

**arytenoiditis,** inflammation of arytenoid cartilage.

**asaphia,** inability to articulate normally due to a cleft palate.

**asbestosis,** lung disease caused by the inhalation of asbestos particles.

**ascaris,** infestation of an intestinal parasite.

**ascites,** excessive fluid accumulation in the peritoneal cavity or abdominal cavity.

**ascorbic acid,** Vitamin C which occurs naturally or may be produced synthetically.

**asepsis,** absence of germs; sterile, free from microorganisms.

**aseptic,** free from germs.

**asexual,** not sexual.

**Asiatic cholera,** an acute infectious disease of epidemic proportion.

**aspergillosis,** a condition produced by Aspergillus fungi producing mycotic nodules in the lungs, liver, kidneys, or on any mucous surface.

**aspermia,** lack of semen, or failure to ejaculate sperm.

**asperous,** minute, uneven elevations; roughness.

**asphyxia,** an interruption of effective gaseous exchange, oxygen and carbon dioxide, resulting in respiratory interference or suffocation.

**asphyxiate,** to cause asphyxia.

**aspirate,** to remove by suction; to inhale.

**aspiration,** to draw foreign bodies in or out by suction through the nose, throat, or lungs; withdrawal of fluid from a body cavity with an instrument called an aspirator.

**aspirin,** a derivative of acetylsalicylic acid used as an analgesic, antipyretic, and antirheumatic.

**astasia,** motor incoordination resulting in the inability to sit, stand, or walk normally.

**asteatosis,** an absence of sebaceous secretion.

**asternal,** not connected to the sternum.

**asthenia,** loss of strength; weakness originating in muscular or cerebellar disease.

**asthenic,** pertaining to asthenia.

**asthenopia,** tiring or weakness of eye muscles due to fatigue; painful vision.

**asthma,** a chronic condition characterized by difficulty in breathing and wheezing due to spasmodic bronchial contractions.

**asthmatic,** pertaining to asthma; one who suffers from asthma.

**astigmatic,** pertaining to astigmatism.

**astigmatism,** an imperfection of the eye caused by differences in curvature of the lens and refractive surfaces of the eye so that light rays are not focused properly on the retina.

**astragalus,** the talus, or anklebone of the foot.

**astraphobia,** unusual fear of lightening and thunderstorms.

**astringent,** styptic or contracting; an agent that has an astringent effect; a constricting or binding effect which checks hemorrhages and secretions.

**astrocyte,** a neuroglial cell resembling a star-shape, collectively named astroglia.

**astrocytoma,** a malignant tumor composed of astrocytes.

**asynergia,** incoordination between muscle groups.

**asynovia,** insufficient secretion of synovial fluid of a joint.

**asystole,** abnormal contractions of ventricles of the heart.

**atactilia,** inability to distinguish tactile impressions.

**ataractic,** a drug that produces ataraxia.

**atavism,** reappearance of a disease or abnormality experienced by an ancestor.

**ataxia,** muscular incoordination affecting voluntary muscular movements.

**atelectasis,** partial or total collapse of the lung; a condition in which lungs of a fetus remain unexpanded at birth.

**atelencephalia,** congenital anomaly, an imperfect development of the brain.

**atelocardia,** congenital anomaly, an incomplete development of the heart.

**atelocephalus,** having an incomplete head.

**atelocheilia,** incomplete development of the lip; harelip.

**atheroma,** a sebaceous cyst; a thickening of the wall of larger arteries.

**atherosclerosis,** localized accumulations of deposits of lipids within the inner surfaces of blood vessels, one of the causes of arterial occlusion.

**athetosis,** repeated involuntry, purposeless, muscular distortion involving the entire body, especially hands, fingers, feet, and toes.

**athlete's foot,** a fungus infection of the foot which is contagious; ringworm of the foot.

**athrombia,** defective blood clotting.

**athymia,** without emotion or feeling.

**atlas,** the first cervical vertebra which supports the head.

**atom,** the smallest particle of an element.

**atomizer,** a device for dispensing liquid into a fine spray.

**atonic,** lack of normal tone.

**atony,** flaccidy and lack of strength; lack of muscular tone.

**atopy,** a group of diseases of an allergic nature; an acquired or inherited hypersensitivity of the skin to an agent.

**atresia,** closure of a normal body opening or congenital absence of a body orifice such as anus or vagina.

**atrioventricular,** pertaining to an atrium and ventricle of the heart.

**atrium,** the auricles; receiving chambers of the heart.

**atrophic,** pertaining to or characterized by atrophy.

**atrophy,** degeneration of the body or of an organ or part.

**atropine,** an anticholinergic alkaloid which acts to block stimulation of muscles and glands and used as a smooth muscle relaxant; used to dilate the pupil of the eye.

**attenuation,** the act of thinning or weakening.

**attic,** the upper part of the tympanic cavity of the ear.

**audiogram,** a drawing of the audiometer.

**audiometer,** an instrument for testing the acuity of hearing.

**auditory nerve,** a sensory nerve of hearing leading to the brain; the eighth cranial nerve.

**aura,** a subjective feeling that precedes the onset of an attack, such as experienced in epilepsy or hysteria.

**aural,** pertaining to the ear; pertaining to an aura.

**aureomycin,** a trademark for chlortetracycline, an antibiotic.

**auricle, auricula,** the external ear; pina or flap; the atrium of the heart.

**auricular,** pertaining to an auricle or to the ear.

**auriscope,** an instrument for making an aural examination.

**aurotherapy,** treatment of rheumatoid arthritis using gold salts.

**auscultate,** to examine by listening to the sounds of the viscera.

**ascultation,** process of listening for sounds produced in the body cavities such as the chest and abdomen to detect abnormalities with a stethoscope.

**autism,** a self-centered mental state in which thoughts and behavior are not subject to correction by external information.

**autistic,** self-centered; living in a phantasy of wish fulfillment.

**autoclave,** an airtight apparatus used to sterilize materials by steam pressure for a specified length of time.

**autodigestion,** digestion of tissue by their own secretion.

**autogenous,** self-produced; originating within the body.

**autograft,** a tissue graft taken from one part of a person's body and transferred to another part of the same body.

**autohypnosis,** self-induced hypnosis.

**autoinfection,** infection by microorganisms present within one's own body.

**autoinoculation,** inoculation of organisms obtained from another part of the body.

**autointoxication,** poisoning within the body by toxic substances produced within the body.

**autolysis,** digestion of tissue or cells by ferment in the cells themselves, even after death.

**automatism,** automatic actions and behavior without conscious volition; the activity of tissues or cells spontaneously such as the movement of cilia or the contractions of smooth muscles or organs removed from the body.

**autonomic nervous system,** spontaneous control of involuntary bodily functions as part of the nervous system which innervates glands, smooth muscle tissue, blood vessels, and the heart.

**autophobia,** abnormal fear of being alone.

**autoplasty,** a replacement of diseased or injured parts with a graft taken from the patient's own body.

**autopsy,** dissection of a body after death to determine the cause of death; a postmortem examination of a body.

**autosome,** any non-sex-determining chromosome of which there are 22 pairs in man.

**autosuggestion,** suggestion or thought originating within one's self.

**autotoxemia,** self-poisoning due to absorption of a poisonous substance generated within the body.

**autotoxin,** a toxin generated within the body upon which it acts.

**avitaminosis,** a condition caused by a lack of vitamins in the diet; a deficiency disease.

**avivement,** a procedure to hasten wound healing by refreshing the edges of the wound.

**avulsion,** a forcible pulling away of a part or structure.

**axalein,** a red dye.

**axanthopia,** yellow blindness.

**axilla,** armpit.

**axion,** pertaining to the brain and spinal cord.

**axis,** a line, real or imaginary, that runs through the center of the body; the second cervical vertebra of the neck on which the head turns.

**axon, axone,** a process of a nerve cell which conducts impulses away from the cell body.

**azoospermia,** absence of spermatozoa from the semen.

**azotenesis,** a condition caused by an excess of nitrogen in the body.

**azoturia,** an increased accumulation of nitrogenous compounds in urine.

**azygous,** singled, not in pairs.

**azymia,** lack of an enzyme.

# B

**Babes-Ernst bodies,** metachromatic bodies seen in bacterial protoplasm.

**Babinski reflex,** backward flexion of the great toe when the sole of the foot is stroked, a normal reaction found in children up to one year of age. When the reflex is found in adults it indicates pyramidal tract involvement.

**bacillary,** relating to or being caused by bacilli, rod-like structures.

**bacillemia,** presence of bacilli in the blood.

**bacilluria,** bacilli in the urine.

**bacitracin,** an antibiotic effective against a wide range of infections.

**back,** posterior surface of the body; the region of the body from neck to pelvis.

**backbone,** vertebral or spinal column.

**bacteria, bacterium,** plant-like microorganisms without chlorophyll.

**bacterial,** pertaining to, or caused by bacteria.

**bactericidal,** being able to destroy bacteria.

**bactericide,** an agent capable of destroying bacteria.

**bacteriology,** the scientific study of bacteria.

**bacteriolysis,** destroying bacteria or dissolving them by a specific antibody.

**bacteriophagia,** destruction of bacteria by a virus capable of inducing lysis.

**bacterioscopy,** a microscopic examination of bacteria.

**bacteriostasis,** arresting bacterial growth.

**bacterium,** (singular of bacteria) single-celled microorganisms called Schizomycetes, having rod-shaped, round, or spiral bodies found in animal tissue, soil, and water.

**bacteriuria,** bacteria found in urine.

**bag-of-waters,** the amnion that surrounds the fetus.

**baker's itch,** eczema caused by yeast irritation.

**baker's leg,** knock-knee.

**balanitis,** inflammation of the glans penis.

**balanus,** the glans penis or glans clitoridis.

**barbiturate,** a salt used for its sedative effects; hypnotic.

**basal metabolism,** the process and measurement of cellular activity necessary to maintain life in the fasting and resting state based on oxygen requirements of the individual.

**Basedow's disease,** Graves's disease; exopthalmic goiter.

**basiphobia,** morbid fear of walking.

**basocytopenia,** a decrease of basophil leukocytes in the blood.

**basocytosis,** excess of basophil leukocytes in the blood.

**basophil,** applied to cells which are readily stained with basic dyes; a type of white blood cell.

**bathophobia,** extreme fear of looking downwards from high places.

**bathycardia,** a condition in which the heart is fixed in an abnormally low position.

**battarism,** stuttering.

**B complex,** see Vitamin B complex.

**bedsore,** see decubitus.

**bedwetting,** see enuresis.

**behavior,** conduct; the observable actions and activity of an individual.

**behaviorism,** a psychological theory based upon objective observation and measurable data, rather than subjective ideas and emotions.

**belch,** an involuntary escape of gas from the stomach through the mouth.

**belladona,** a poisonous plant from which a drug is manufactured to relieve spasmodic disorders; active principle of atropine.

**Bell's palsy,** paralysis of facial nerves and muscles; an acute inflammatory reaction causing distortion to facial muscles.

**belly,** stomach.

**bends,** a decompression illness caused by bubbles of nitrogen in the blood and tissues.

**benign,** not malignant.

**Benzedrine,** proprietary name for amphetamine; a central nervous system stimulant.

**benzocaine,** a nontoxic local anesthetic; found in an ointment.

**beriberi,** a deficiency caused by faulty nutrition and the lack of Vitamin B, uncommon in the United States.

**bicarbonate,** a salt containing two parts of carbonic acid and one part of a base.

**biceps,** a muscle with two heads; a major muscle in the upper arm and in the thigh.

**bicuspid,** premolar tooth; having two cusps; mitral valve between left atrium and left ventricle of the heart.

**bifid,** split into two parts; cleft or forked.

**bifocal,** having two foci as seen in eyeglasses that correct both near and far vision.

**bifurcate,** having two distinct branches; forked.

**bifurication,** a division into two branches.

**bilateral,** relating to two sides of the body.

**bile,** a bitter secretion of the liver which aids digestion.

**bile acids,** complex acids which occur as salts and which are important to the digestion of fats in the intestines.

**bile duct,** a tube which conveys the liver secretion as it leaves the gall bladder.

**biharzia,** a term used for Schistosoma, the human blood fluke.

**biliary,** pertaining to the bile or gallbladder or to the passages conveying bile.

**bilifulvin,** bilirubin mixed with other substances, resulting in a tawny pigment.

**bilious,** an excess of bile due to a disorder of the liver.

**bilirubin,** a reddish-yellow pigment in bile, also found in blood and urine.

**biliverdin,** a greenish pigment found in bile formed in oxidation of bilirubin.

**bilobate,** having two lobes.

**bilocular,** divided into two cells or compartments.

**bimaxillary,** afflicting both jaws.

**binocular,** pertaining to two eyes.

**binovular,** derived from two ova.

**bioassay,** determining the strength of a drug by observing its effects on test animals and comparing these effects with a standard substance.

**biocatalyst,** a biochemical that dissolves; an enzyme.

**biochemistry,** the scientific study of living things and the chemical changes that occur during vital processes.

**bioclimatology,** pertaining to the relations or effect of climate on living things.

**biodynamics,** the science of energy; biophysiology.

**biogenesis,** the origin of living organisms.

**biokinetics,** the science of movement occurring in the developing of organisms.

**biological,** pertaining to biology; medical preparations used in the treatment or prevention of disease such as serums and vaccines.

**biological block,** pertaining to the internal mechanism in living organisms that direct the rhythmic cycles of varied involuntary processes.

**biologist,** a specialist who studies biology.

**biology,** the scientific study of life and living things; the study of plants and animals.

**biometry,** the study and computation of life expectancy.

**bion,** any living organism.

**bionomy,** the science pertaining to vital functions within the organism.

**biophysics,** the scientific study of living organisms using the principles of physics.

**biopsy,** tissue excised from a living organism for examination under the microscope.

**biostatics,** vital statistics.

**biotics,** pertaining to the law of living things.

**biotin,** a component of the vitamin B complex of which the therapeutic value has not been proven.

**biotomy,** vivisection on living animals for physiological and pathological study.

**biotype,** a genotype; the basic constitution of an organism.

**biovular twins,** twins from two separate ova.

**biparous,** giving birth to twins.

**biramous,** having two branches.

**birth,** the act of being born.

**birth control,** the prevention of pregnancy; any method used to prevent conception such as artificial devices or drugs.

**birthmark,** a permanent mark from birth injury found on the skin of an infant; nevus.

**birth trauma,** the emotional stress experienced by an infant at birth which may be a source of neurosis as an adult according to psychoanalytic theory.

**bisexual,** having both sexes in one individual; hermaphroditic; possessing genital and sexual characteristics of both man and woman.

**bisferious,** having a double pulse; dicrotic.

**bismuth,** a silvery white metallic element; it is used in its salt form as an antiseptic, astringent, sedative, and in treatment of diarrhea.

**bistoury,** a small surgical knife, used for minor surgery.

**bitemporal,** referring to both temporal bones in the skull.

**bituminosis,** pneumoconiosis originating from inhalation of dust or soft coal.

**black death,** a contagious and malignant disease known as bubonic plague.

**blackhead,** a fatty deposit of dried sebum in a sebaceous gland.

**blackout,** a sudden temporary loss of consciousness and vision.

**blackwater fever,** a form of malaria characterized by a sudden rise in body temperature, enlarged liver and spleen, epigastric pain, vomiting, jaundice, dark bloody urine, and shock.

**bladder,** collecting sac for urine; a reservoir.

**bland,** mild or soothing; pertaining to diet in which irritating food is avoided.

**Blandin's glands,** glands near tip of tongue.

**blastocyst,** a group of undifferentiated cells, the bastula, which develop into an embryo; a stage in the development of an embryo which follows the morula.

**blastogenesis,** the transmission of characteristics from parents to offspring by genes.

**blastoma,** a granular tumor.

**blastomere,** one of the cells into which fertilized ovum separate into segments.

**blastomyces,** pathogenic yeastlike organisms producing disease.

**blastula,** an early stage in the development of an ovum that develops into an embryo.

**bleb,** a blister or pustule.

**bleeder,** one who bleeds an abnormal amount; see hemophilia.

**bleeding time,** a natural stoppage of bleeding from a wound or cut, usually about three minutes or less.

**blennorrhagia,** an accumulative amount of discharge from mucous membranes, esp. gonorrheal discharge from the genital or urinary tract; gonorrhea.

**blepharitis,** inflammation of the eyelids involving hair follicles and glands causing swelling, redness and crusting.

**blepharon,** the eyelid.

**blindness,** inability to see partially or totally; visual impairment as a result of disease, irritation, or accident.

**blind spot,** a region on the retina where the optic nerve enters the eye and that is insensitive to light.

**blister,** a collection of fluid under the skin due to pressure or injury.

**bloated,** an abnormal swelling beyond normal size.

**blood,** the fluid which circulates throughout the body carrying nourishment and oxygen to the cells and tissue, and, at the same time, takes away waste matter and carbon dioxide.

**blood bank,** a storing place and processing center for reserve blood kept for emergency transfusions.

**blood cell,** a minute chamber; a corpuscle in the blood; red or white corpuscle.

**blood clot,** a coagulated mass of blood cells which forms when blood vessels are injured.

**blood corpuscle,** a circulating cell in the blood; a red cell, erythrocyte, or a white cell, leukocyte.

**blood count,** determination of the number and type of red and white blood cells per cubic millimeter of blood.

**blood group,** a classification into which human blood can be based or grouped; blood groups are designated as O, A, B, and AB.

**bloodletting,** an old method for treating disease by opening a vein and allowing a person to bleed for the specific purpose to reduce blood volume and hence the amount of work required by the heart; phlebotomy.

**blood plasma,** the colorless fluid of the blood separated by centrifuging.

**blood poisoning,** a diseased condition caused by the entrance of toxins or microorganisms into the blood stream; toxemia; pyremia; septicemia.

**blood pressure,** the pressure existing against the inner walls of the large arteries at the height of the pulse when the heart contracts, systolic pressure, and when the heart relaxes, diastolic pressure.

**blood serum,** the clear liquid that separates from the blood when it is allowed to clot; blood plasma from which fibrogen has been removed.

**bloodshot,** excessive congestion of capillaries causing inflammation and redness of the eyes.

**blood smear,** a drop of blood spread on a slide for microscopic examination.

**blood sugar,** glucose circulating in the blood, normally 60--90 mg. per 100 ml. of blood.

**blood test,** test of blood sample to determine blood type or the contents (such as sugar) of the blood.

**blood transfusion,** a technique for transferring the blood from one individual to another directly without being exposed to air.

**blood type,** determining classification of blood according to blood groups such as O, A, B, or AB.

**blood vessel,** vessels of the body that transport blood; three major types of blood-vessel: artery, capillary, and vein.

**blotch,** usually a red or pink spot on the skin.

**blue baby,** an infant born with a bluish color due to a mixture of venous and arterial blood caused by a defect in the heart.

**boil,** a microbic infection of the skin; a furuncle.

**bolus,** a pill-shaped mass.

**bone,** the hard, dense connective tissue consisting of bone cells that form the skeleton.

**bone reflex,** a reflex action resulting from a tapping; actually a tendon or muscle response or reflex.

**borborygmus,** a rumbling sound in the bowels; intestinal flatus.

**boric acid,** an odorless, white, crystalline powder used as a mild antiseptic, especially for the eyes, mouth, and bladder. In large amounts taken by children it may be poisonous.

**botulinic acid,** a toxic substance found in putrid meat.

**botulism,** severe food poisoning containing the toxin produced by Clostridium botulinum.

**bougie,** an instrument for dilating canals and passages of the body.

**boulimia,** abnormal hunger sensation after a meal.

**bowels,** see intestines.

**bowleg,** an outward bending of the leg.

**brachialgia,** extreme pain in the arm.

**brachium,** pertaining to the upper arm from shoulder to elbow.

**brachycardia,** slowness of heartbeat.

**brachycephalic,** short headed.

**brachydactylia,** shortness of fingers.

**brachymetropia,** nearsightedness; myopia.

**bradycardia,** unusually slow heart action.

**bradykinesia,** extremely slow movements.

**bradyphagia,** slowness in eating.

**bradypnea,** abnormally slow breathing.

**bradyrhythmia,** slow pulse rate.

**bradyuria,** slowness in passing urine.

**brain,** a large mass of nerve tissue which fills the cranium of man and other vertebrates.

**brain fever,** meningitis.

**brain storm,** a temporary outburst of mental excitement often seen in paranoia.

**breakbone fever,** a sudden febrile disease of epidemic proportion.

**breast,** the upper anterior aspect of the chest; mammary gland.

**breath,** inhaled and exhaled air in act of respiration.

**breathing,** respiration; taking in air and exhaling carbon dioxide.

**breech,** the buttocks.

**breech presentation,** the appearance of the buttocks or feet first instead of the head in childbirth occurring in about 3% of all labors.

**bregma,** the junction of the coronal and sagittal sutures on the surface of the skull.

**Bright's disease,** a disease of the kidneys usually associated with faulty uric acid elimination and high blood pressure.

**broad-spectrum,** any antibiotic that is effective against a wide variety of bacteria.

**Brocca's area,** the speech center in the left hemisphere of the brain which controls the movements of the tongue, lips, vocal cords, or motor speech.

**bromides,** the salts of bromine used in medication as a sedative and a hypnotic.

**bromism, brominism,** state of poisoning due to prolonged use of bromides.

**bromomania,** psychosis induced by use of bromides.

**bromopnea,** an offensive breath.

**bronchadenitis,** inflammation of the bronchial glands.

**bronchi,** plural of bronchus; primary divisions of the thrachea.

**bronchial,** pertaining to the bronchi or bronchioles.

**bronchial tubes,** the bronchi that lead from the trachea or windpipe.

**bronchiectasis,** a condition arising from inflammed bronchial tubes, usually secreting large amounts of offensive, infectious pus.

**bronchiole,** the smallest branch of the bronchi within the lungs.

**bronchitis,** an inflammation of the membranes lining the bronchi.

**bronchopneumonia,** inflammation of the bronchi and lungs caused by various types of pneumococci, pathogenic bacteria as well as viruses, rickettsias, and fungi.

**bronchoscope,** an instrument for examination of the interior of the bronchi.

**bronchospasm,** contractions of the smooth muscles of the bronchi which occurs in asthma.

**bronzed skin,** characteristic of Addison's disease due to adrenal cortical insufficiency.

**brow,** the forehead; the prominence over the eyes.

**brucellosis,** an infectious disease which primarily affects cattle, swine, and goats but sometimes affects man; caused by bacteria Brucella.

**bruise,** a contusion; an injury produced by impact without skin breakage but causing blood vessels to rupture and discolor surrounding tissues.

**bruit,** a murmur or sound heard in auscultation by means of a stethoscope.

**bruxism,** the grinding of teeth while sleeping.

**bubo,** an inflamed or enlarged lymph node, especially in the groin or axilla.

**bubonic plague,** an acute, infectious disease, frequently fatal, caused by infected rats and ground squirrels who carry the rat-flea which ultimately infects man through its bite; the black death of the Middle Ages.

**buccal,** pertaining to the cheek or mouth.

**Buerger's disease,** a recurring inflammatory disease affecting the veins and arteries of the limbs, seen mostly in males between the ages of 15 and 50 years.

**bulbous,** bulb-shaped; swollen or enlarged.

**bulimia,** unusual hunger experienced a short time after eating a meal.

**bulla,** a large blister; a skin vesicle or bubble filled with a watery fluid; the dilated portion of the bony external meatus of the ear.

**bundle,** group of fibers; a bundle of fibers of the impulse-conducting system of the heart.

**bundle branch block,** formation of a heart block in which the two ventricles contract independently of each other.

**bunion,** inflammation and thickening of the bursa of the joint of the great toe resulting from chronic inflammation.

**burn,** injury to the tissues of the skin as a result of excessive high heat, chemical, or radio-active exposure; burns are classified according to the extent of damage to the layers of skin.

**bursa,** a sac lined with synovial membrane containing synovial fluid which acts as a lubricant and reduces friction between joints and surrounding structures.

**bursectomy,** surgical removal of the bursa.

**bursitis,** inflammation of a bursa.

**butacaine,** used as a local anesthetic.

**butalbital,** a sedative.

**buttocks,** the fleshy prominence formed by the gluteal muscles of the lower back which joins the thighs.

**bypass,** a shunt performed by surgery creating an alternate pathway for the blood to bypass an obstructed main artery.

**bysma,** a plug.

**byssinosis,** a pulmonary disease from inhalation of cotton dust.

**byssus,** growth of pubic hair.

# C

**cachet,** a wafer in which medicine is placed; capsule.

**cachexia,** a condition of malnutrition and wasting occurring in chronic illness in the later stages.

**cachinnation,** hysterical laughter.

**cadaver,** corpse; dead body.

**cadaverous,** resembling the appearance or color of a corpse.

**caduceus,** a symbol of the medical profession.

**caesarean,** see cesarean.

**caffeine,** an alkaloid found in coffee and tea which is used as a stimulant, diuretic, and as a treatment for headache.

**caffeinism,** chronic effects from excessive use of coffee causing heart palpitations, trembling, general depression, anxiety, insomnia, and agitated states.

**caisson disease,** a painful condition occurring in divers when air pressure is reduced too rapidly after coming to the surface causing nitrogen in the blood and tissues to be released as bubbles; the bends.

**calamine,** a pink, watery substance composed of zinc and iron oxides used externally as a protective astringent, skin lotion or ointment.

**calcaneus,** heel bone.

**calcar,** a spurlike process or projection.

**calcareous,** containing calcium carbonate; chalky.

**calcemia,** an excess of calcium in the blood.

**calcic,** pertaining to calcium or lime.

**calcicosis,** a pulmonary condition caused by inhaling dust from limestone, especially by marblecutters.

**calciferol,** vitamin D2 derived from ergosterol; used in treatment of rickets and hypocalcemic tetany.

**calcification,** the deposit of calcium in the tissues and bone.

**calcinosis,** an abnormal condition caused by deposits of calcium in tissues.

**calcipenia,** a calcium deficiency in the body.

**calcium,** a silvery white metallic element; the basic element of lime, necessary to skeletal structure and body function.

**calcium carbonate,** a white tasteless powder used as an antacid.

**calculus,** resembling a stone composed of mineral salts, found in kidneys, bladder, urethra, or other organs and ducts in the body under abnormal conditions.

**calf,** the fleshy part on the back of the leg below the knee.

**calibrator,** an instrument for measuring openings.

**calisthenics,** a systematic exercise routine for improving health, strength, and flexibility in movement.

**callus,** a thickening or horny layer of skin; the osseous material at the ends of a fractured bone and eventually replaced by new bone growth.

**caloric,** relating to heat or calories.

**calorie,** calory, a unit of heat; a measure of energy intake and output of the body; the amount of heat necessary to raise the temperature of one gram of water one degree centigrade.

**calorimeter,** an apparatus for determining the heat of the body.

**calosity, callositas,** the formation of thick skin due to pressure, friction, or irritation.

**calvaria,** human skull cap; cranium skull.

**calvities,** alopecia, baldness.

**calyx,** a cup-shaped organ or cavity such as the cup-like structure of the kidney pelvis.

**camphor,** a gum derived from an Asian evergreen tree used as a topical antipruitic.

**camphorated,** containing camphor.

**canal,** a passage or duct.

**canaliculus,** a tubular small channel or passage.

**cancellate,** latticelike or porous.

**cancer,** a malignant tumor; neoplasm; sarcoma or carcinoma characterized by abnormal growth of cells which spread to other tissues.

**cancerous,** pertaining to malignant growth.

**cancroid,** appearance of a cancer; skin cancer.

**cancrum,** a rapidly spreading cancer or ulcer.

**canine,** pertaining to upper and lower teeth between the incisors and molars of which there are four in number.

**canker,** a mouth ulcer; thrush; gangrenous inflammation of the mouth.

**canker sore,** an ulceration of the lips or mouth.

**cannabis,** the dried tops of hemp plants which produces euphoric states when used as a narcotic; hashish and marijuana.

**cannula,** a tube used for insertion into a duct or cavity for the purpose of withdrawing fluid or injecting medication into the body.

**cannular,** a hollow needle.

**cantharis,** a strong substance derived from crushed blister beetles used in medicine as a diuretic stimulant to reproductive or urinary organs; Spanish fly.

**canthectomy,** excision of a canthus.

**canthitis,** inflammation of the canthus.

**canthus,** the junction or angle of the upper and lower corner of both sides of the eyelids.

**capiat,** an instrument for removing foreign materials from body cavities, especially the uterus.

**capillaritis,** inflammation of the capillaries.

**capillarity,** action by which the liquid's surface is elevated or depressed at the point of contact with a solid.

**capillary,** minute blood vessel which connects the smallest arteries with the smallest veins.

**capital,** pertaining to the head.

**capitate,** head-shaped; having a rounded end.

**capitatum,** small capitate bone in the hand.

**capitellum,** the rounded projection or knob of the humerus articulating with the radial head.

**capsitis,** crystalline lens.

**capsula,** resembling a capsule; internal capsule of the brain.

**capsular,** referring to a capsule.

**capsulation,** enclosed within a capsule.

**capsule,** a covering usually of gelatin which envelops medication; a small membranous sac.

**caput,** head; upper part of an organ.

**carbohydrase,** an enzyme such as amylase and lactase that aids in the digestion of carbohydrates.

**carbohydrates,** a group of compounds including starches, sugars, celluloses, and gums; organic compounds composed of carbon, oxygen, and water, and classified as monosaccharides, disaccharides, and polysaccharides; carbohydrates provide 47% of calories in the diet and are one of the major sources of nourishment.

**carbolic acid,** used as an antiseptic and disinfectant derived from coal tar.

**carbon,** a nonmetallic element found in all living matter in various forms; coal is a common form, a diamond is a crystallized form, and in food it is a fuel which creates heat in animal life.

**carbon 14,** used in cancer research and archaeological studies.

**carbon dioxide,** an acid-tasting gas which is heavier than air and exhaled by all living animals; found in the atmosphere as a colorless, odorless non-combustible gas necessary to all plant life.

**carbon monoxide,** a colorless, odorless, tasteless, poisonous gas which is formed as a result of incomplete combustion and oxidation.

**carbon monoxide poisoning,** poisoning produced as a result of breathing in carbon monoxide gas and mixing with the hemoglobin of the blood which prevents oxygen from being carried to the tissues of the body causing difficult breathing, dizziness, pounding of the heart, headache, reddish color to face and chest, faintness, and nausea. If the victim can inhale fresh air, he will recover, but if not found in time convulsions, paralysis, and death may occur.

**carbuncle,** large boil.

**carcinogenic,** causing cancer.

**carcinoid,** a benign epithelial growth resembling a cancer.

**carcinoma,** a cancer; a malignant tumor which infiltrates connective tissues and spreads.

**carcinomatophobia,** extreme fear of carcinoma.

**carcinomatosis,** having a widespread dissemination of carcinoma throughout the body.

**carcinosarcoma,** pertaining to a mixed tumor of both carcinoma and sarcoma.

**cardia,** the region of the heart; the part of the stomach surrounding the esophagus.

**cardiac,** heart failure; having heart disease; referring to cardiac orifices surrounding the stomach; a heart medication.

**cardiac failure,** inability of the heart to pump blood in sufficient volume to meet body needs.

**cardiac hypertrophy,** enlargement of the heart.

**cardiasthenia,** weakness of the heart muscles with cardiac symptoms.

**cardiataxia,** very irregular heart contractions.

**cardiectomy,** a surgical procedure which involves the excision of the cardiac portion of the stomach.

**cardiogram,** record of electrical energy changes of the heart cycle.

**cardiograph,** apparatus for recording the heart cycle on a graph.

**cardiologist,** a specialist in the treatment and diagnosis of the heart.

**cardiology,** scientific study of the heart and its functions.

**cardioneurosis,** functional neurosis with cardiac symptoms such as rapid heart beat.

**cardiopathy,** any disorder or disease of the heart.

**cardiophobia,** extreme fear of heart disease.

**cardiopulmonary,** pertaining to the lungs and heart.

**cardiopyloric,** referring to both the cardiac and pyloric ends of the stomach.

**cardiosclerosis,** thickening and hardening of the cardiac tissues and arteries.

**cardiospasm,** spasm or contraction of the cardiac sphincter of the stomach when the esophagus fails to function properly.

**cardiosphygmograph,** an apparatus for recording movements of the heart and pulse.

**cardiotomy,** incision of the heart.

**cardiovalvulitis,** inflammation of the valves of the heart.

**cardiovascular,** pertaining to the heart and blood vessels.

**carditis,** inflammation of the heart muscles.

**caries,** decay and disintegration of bone or teeth.

**carminative,** a drug that will remove flatus from the gastrointestinal tract.

**carnal,** relating to the flesh.

**carnophobia,** abnormal fear to eat meat.

**carotene,** a yellow, orange, or red pigment found in some plants and animal tissues; stored in the liver and kidney and converted into Vitamin A in the body.

**carotid,** the main artery of the neck which divides into the left and right branch that transports the blood from the aorta to the head.

**carpal,** relating to the joint of the wrist.

**carpophalangeal,** pertaining to the carpus and the finger bones.

**carpus,** eight bones of the wrist.

**carrier,** an individual carrying disease germs without being infected himself; one who transmits a disease without suffering from it himself.

**car sickness,** motion sickness.

**cartilage,** dense connective tissue consisting of cells embedded in compact matrix but without blood vessels; gristle; the cartilage or elastic connective tissue composing the skeletal structures of the embryo is converted into bone after birth.

**cartilaginous,** pertaining to cartilage.

**caruncle,** an abnormal fleshy growth.

**cascara,** a laxative.

**caseation,** conversion of necrotic tissue into a cheese-like granular mass in some diseases; formation of casein during coagulation of milk.

**case history,** information about a patient's personal or family's history recorded during interview, used especially in social work, medicine, or psychiatry.

**casein,** the principle protein in milk occurring in milk curds.

**caseous,** resembling cheese.

**cassia,** used as a laxative derived from a plant in the form of senna.

**cast,** a mold made of plaster of Paris to hold a bone rigid and straight as in fractures, dislocations, and other serious injuries.

**castor oil,** a sticky oil used as a purgative derived from the castor bean.

**castrate,** to remove the testicles or ovaries.

**castration,** destruction or excision of the testicles or ovaries.

**castration complex,** morbid fear of castration.

**catabasis,** decline of a disease or illness.

**catabolic,** pertaining to catabolism.

**catabolism,** the breaking-down phase of metabolism in which complex substances are converted to simpler substances; the opposite of anabolism.

**catalepsy,** a neurosis characterized by a temporary loss of the senses and the power to move the muscles; trance-like.

**catalyst,** an agent that causes a chemical reaction or change.

**catamenia,** menses; periodic menstrual discharge from the uterus.

**catamnesis,** the medical history of a patient documented by the physician after the first examination including subsequent visits.

**cataphasia,** a speech disorder causing involuntary or constant repetition of the same phrase or word.

**cataphora,** lethargy with intermittent periods of waking.

**cataphoria,** a condition in which a downward turning of the visual axis of each eye continues after the visual stimuli have been removed.

**cataplasia,** degeneration change in which cells and tissues revert to earlier, more primitive conditions.

**cataplasm,** a poultice, usually with a medication.

**cataplexy, cataplexia,** resembling a stroke; sudden shock with a temporary loss of muscular weakness and muscle tone; often a result of emotional shock, sudden onset of an illness, or associated with narcolepsy.

**cataract,** a condition of the eye caused by a clouding of the crystalline lens or its capsule or both which prevents normal vision.

**catarrh,** inflammation of the mucous membranes with a discharge of mucus secretions, particularly from the upper respiratory tract.

**catatonia,** type of schizophrenia characterized by immobility and unresponsiveness; stupor; exhibiting fixed posturing and refusal to communicate.

**catatonic,** pertaining to catatonia.

**catatropia,** the downward turning of both eyes.

**catgut,** a cord or surgical thread that is sterile and absorbable used for tying or binding blood vessels, usually made of twisted sheep's intestine or silk.

**catharsis,** a purging of the bowels; in psychoanalysis, experiencing emotional release by recalling an event that precipitated a psychoneurosis; abreaction.

**cathartic,** pertaining to catharsis.

**catheter,** a tube of elastic, elastic web, rubber, glass, or metal used for evacuating or injecting fluids.

**catheterization,** inserting a catheter into a body channel or cavity.

**cathexis,** the attachment of emotional or mental energy to an idea or object.

**cauda,** taillike structure.

**caudad,** toward the tail or posterior direction of the body.

**caudal,** pertaining to any taillike structure; inferior in position.

**caudate,** having a taillike projection.

**caul,** the great omentum; membranous amnion covering the head of the fetus at birth.

**causalgia,** burning pain.

**caustic,** corroding and burning; an agent capable of destroying tissue.

**cauterization,** burning or cauterizing a part.

**cauterize,** to burn or sear with a cautery.

**cautery,** destroying tissue by application of electricity, heat, or corrosive chemicals.

**caval,** pertaining to the vena cava.

**cavernous,** containing hollow spaces.

**cavity,** hollow space; a hollow place within the body or one of the organs; hole in a tooth or a dental cavity.

**cecectomy,** surgical removal of part of the cecum or incision of the cecum.

**cecitis,** inflammation of the cecum.

**cecoileostomy,** an opening or stoma into the ileum.

**cecoptosis,** displacement of the cecum.

**cecostomy,** surgical creation of an artificial opening into the cecum.

**cecum,** a pouchlike formation at the beginning of the large intestine and bears at its lower end the vermiform appendix; any blind sac.

**celiac,** pertaining to the abdominal cavity.

**celiac disease,** a chronic intestinal disorder occurring in infants and children due to a dietary deficiency.

**cell,** a small enclosed chamber containing a nucleus within a mass of protoplasm which is the basic structure of all living things.

**cellular,** pertaining to, or composed of cells.

**cellulase,** an enzyme produced by snails or molluscs used in medicine to convert cellulose to celloboise; used as a digestive aid.

**cellulitis,** inflammation of connective tissues.

**celluloneuritis,** inflammation of nerve cells.

**cellulose,** a carbohydrate forming the framework of plants; plant fiber.

**cell wall,** boundary lying outside the cell membrane.

**cementum,** thin layer of bony tissue deposited by cementoblasts which form the dentine or outer surface of the root of a tooth.

**cenogenesis,** appearance of characteristics in a person which are absent in ancestors and which do not have a phylogenetic importance.

**cenotype,** common or original type.

**centigrade,** pertaining to a thermometer in which the boiling point is 100° and the freezing point is 0°.

**central nervous system,** abrr. CNS, brain and spinal cord, including nerves and end organs which control voluntary action; voluntary nervous system.

**centrifuge,** an apparatus used in testing corpuscles in the blood, and solids in urine by employing centrifuging force which hastens sedimentation.

**cephalad,** toward the head.

**cephalagia,** pain in the head; headache.

**cephalhematoma,** a swelling of the subcutaneous tissues containing blood, frequently found on the head of a newborn infant a few days after delivery.

**cephalic,** pertaining to the head.

**cephalitis,** encephalitis; inflammation of the brain.

**cephalometer,** an instrument for measuring the head.

**cephalonia,** enlarged head marked by idiocy.

**cera,** wax.

**cerebellar,** pertaining to the cerebellum.

**cerebellitis,** inflammation of the cerebellum.

**cerebellospinal,** relating to the cerebellum and spinal cord.

**cerebellum,** posterior portion of the brain which controls voluntary muscular movements, equilibrium, and posture.

**cerebral,** pertaining to the cerebrum or brain.

**cerebral hemorrhage,** resulting from a ruptured blood vessel in the brain associated with disease, accident, or high blood pressure.

**cerebral palsy,** brain damage, usually occurring at birth, characterized by incoordination of muscular activity, spasms, and abnormal speech.

**cerebritis,** inflammation of the brain.

**cerebromalacia,** softening of the brain.

**cerebromeningitis,** inflammation of the brain and its membranes.

**cerebrosclerosis,** hardening of the brain, esp. of the cerebrum.

**cerebrospinal,** pertaining to the brain and spinal cord.

**cerebrospinal fluid,** a watery substance produced by the choroid plexuses in the lateral ventricles situated at the base of the brain which acts as a cushion protecting the brain.

**cerebrum,** the largest part of the brain consisting of the left and right hemisphere being united by the corpus callosum and the anterior and posterior commissures.

**cerumen,** earwax.

**cervical,** pertaining to the neck of the womb.

**cervicitis,** inflammation of the cervix.

**cervitamic acid,** crystalline ascorbic acid; Vitamin C.

**cervix,** narrow part of the uterus; part of an organ resembling a neck.

**cervix vesicae,** the neck of the bladder.

**cesarean,** abdominal operation to remove an infant from the womb; cesarean section.

**cestode,** belonging to the subclass Cestoda; a parasitic tapeworm found in the alimentary tract.

**cestoid,** resembling a tapeworm.

**cetrimonium bromide,** a quaternary ammonium compound used as an antiseptic and detergent; applied topically to the skin as a disinfectant.

**chafe,** injury by friction or rubbing.

**chalazion,** a sty; small, hard sebaceous cyst developing on the eyelids.

**chancre,** a syphilitic ulcer usually occurring two or three weeks after infection.

**chancroid,** a nonsyphilitic soft veneral ulcer, highly contagious.

**change of life,** menopause; climacteric.

**chapped skin,** skin which becomes dry, split, and cracked due to overexposure to a harsh environment and decreased activity of glands in the surrounding area.

**charting,** recording the progress of an illness or disease which also gives information about the patient and his treatment; a clinical chart or record.

**chauffage,** treatment with a cautery at low heat that is applied close to the tissue.

**cheek,** fleshy portion of either side of the face below the eyes; pertaining to the mucous membranes within the inner surface of the mouth.

**cheekbone,** zygomatic bone.

**cheilitis,** inflammation of the lip.

**cheilosis,** a condition of the lips characterized by dry scaling, fissures, and reddened appearance at the angles of the mouth, resulting from Vitamin B deficiency.

**cheirospasm,** writer's cramp; spasms of the muscles of the hand.

**chemical,** pertaining to chemistry.

**chemocautery,** application of a caustic substance in cauterization.

**chemoprophylaxis,** prevention of a disease by drugs or chemical agents.

**chemosis,** edema of the conjunctiva of the eye.

**chemosurgery,** destruction of diseased tissue by chemical agents for therapeutic purposes.

**chemotaxis,** movement of living cells in response to a chemical stimulus.

**chemotherapy,** treatment of disease by chemical agents.

**cherophobia,** extreme fear of and aversion to gaiety.

**chest,** the thorax which encloses the ribs.

**Cheyne-Stokes respiration,** irregular type of arrhythmic breathing occurring in acute illness or in certain acute diseases of the central nervous system, heart, lungs, and occasionally involving intoxication.

**chiasm,** a crossing of tendons or nerves; a structure in the forebrain formed by fibers of the optic nerves.

**chickenpox,** varicella; a highly contagious disease characterized by vesicular eruptions on the skin and mucous membranes.

**chiggers,** a six-legged reddish mite larva which burrows beneath the skin producing wheals, intense itching and sever dermatitis.

**chilblain,** inflammation, swelling, and itching of the ears, fingers, and toes produced by frostbite.

**childbed,** puerperal period in childbearing.

**childbirth,** process of giving birth; parturition.

**chill,** shaking of the body when affected by cold temperatures or occurring with certain diseases such as malaria; shivering.

**chiropodist,** podiatrist; one who treats foot irregularities.

**chiropractic,** manipulative treatment based on the theory that all diseases are caused by interference with spinal nerves and can be treated by adjusting the spinal column.

**chiropractor,** one who practices chiropractic manipulation.

**chirospasm,** see cheirospasm.

**chloasma,** discoloration of pigment in skin occurring in yellowish brown patches or spots.

**chloral,** an oily, bitter tasting substance derived from chlorine and alcohol.

**chloral hydrate,** colorless crystalline substance used as a sedative and hypnotic.

**chloramphenicol,** a broadspectrum antibiotic made synthetically used especially to treat typhoid fever.

**chloride,** a salt of hydrochloric acid.

**chlorinated,** treat with chlorine.

**chlorinated lime,** used in solution as a bleach and as an antiseptic derived from calcium hypochlorite.

**chlorine,** a yellowish-green irritating gas used in compounds as a bleaching agent and germicide; a poisonous gas which can cause severe damage to the mucous membranes of the respiratory passages and cause death if inhaled in excessive amounts.

**chloroform,** colorless, heavy liquid with a sweet taste and ethereal odor used as a solvent, general anesthetic, locally in liniments, and internally as a carminative or a sedative.

**chloroma,** green cancer of the cranial bones; a greenish colored malignant tumor found in myeloid tissue.

**Chloromycetin,** trademark for chloramphenicol, an antibiotic.

**chloromyeloma,** multiple growths in bone marrow.

**chlorophyll,** green coloring matter found in plants and which acts in the manufacture of simple carbohydrates.

**chloropsia,** vision in which all things appear green.

**chlorosis,** iron deficiency anemia.

**chlorpromazine,** a major tranquilizer used in treatment of psychotic states; trademark name is Thorazine; used as an antiemetic.

**chlorpropamide,** an oral hypoglycemic used to treat mild diabetes.

**chlortetracycline,** a broad-spectrum antibiotic which destroys strains of streptococci, staphylococci, pneumococci, rickettsiae, and some viruses; trademark name is Aureomycin.

**choke,** to interrupt respiration by obstruction or by constriction about the neck; strangle; spasm of the larynx; suffocate.

**cholangitis,** inflammation of the bile ducts.

**cholecystectomy,** surgical removal of the gallbladder.

**cholecystitis,** acute or chronic inflammation of the gallbladder.

**cholesystography,** examination of the gallbladder by x-ray.

**cholecystolithiasis, cholelithiasis,** the formation of gallstones in the gallbladder.

**cholecystopathy,** any gallbladder disease.

**cholecystotomy,** incision of gallbladder to remove gallstones.

**choledochitis,** inflammation of the common bile duct.

**choleic,** pertaining to the bile.

**cholelithotomy,** surgical removal of gallstones.

**cholemia,** presence of bile pigments in the blood causing jaundice.

**cholera,** an acute, infectious disease caused by Vibrio cholerae, characterized by diarrhea, severe cramps of muscles, vomiting, and exhaustion.

**choleretic,** an agent that increases bile production.

**choleric,** quick-tempered; easily irritated.

**cholesteatoma,** a small, pearl-like tumor occurring in the brain.

**cholesterol,** fatty, steroid alcohol found in animal tissues, occurring in egg yolk, oils, fats, and organ tissues; constitutes the largest portion of gallstones; most of the cholesterol is synthesized in the liver, and it is important to bodily metabolism.

**choline,** an amine found in plant and animal tissues which is important to normal fat and carbohydrate metabolism.

**cholinergic,** pertaining to nerve endings which produce acetylcholine which is important in the transmission of nerve impulses.

**chondral,** pertaining to cartilage.

**chondroma,** a slow growing cartilaginous tumor.

**chondromalacia,** abnormal softening of cartilage.

**chondropathy,** any disease of the cartilage.

**chorda,** referring to a chord, string, or tendon.

**chorditis,** inflammation of the vocal cord.

**chorea,** muscular twitching of the limbs; known as St. Vitus' dance or Sydenham's chorea, a disease of the central nervous system; Huntington's chorea is a hereditary form marked by mental deterioration.

**chorion,** the outermost embryonic membrane from which chornionic villi develop and connect with the endometrium from which the fetal part of the placenta forms.

**chorionic,** pertaining to the chorion.

**chorioretinitis,** inflammation of the choroid and retina.

**choroid,** the vascular coat of the eye between the sclera and retina.

**choroiditis,** inflammation of the choroid membrane.

**chromatelopsia,** color blindness.

**chromatid,** either of the two chromosomal bodies resulting from cell division, each drawn to a different pole.

**chromatin,** the specific portion in the nucleus of a cell that stains readily with basic dyes, and is considered to carry hereditary characteristics in the genes.

**chromatosis,** pathological skin pigmentation.

**chromaturia,** abnormal color of the urine.

**chromocystoscopy,** examination of kidney functions by use of dyes.

**chromoscopy,** examination of renal function by color of urine after dyes have been administered; testing for color vision.

**chromosomal,** pertaining to chromosomes.

**chromosome,** found in all plant and animal cells; a structure in the nucleus containing threads of DNA responsible for transmitting genetic information; there are 23 pairs of chromosomes in man.

**chronic,** recurring or occurring over a long period of time; in reference to a disease that is not acute.

**chyle,** a milklike substance found in the intestinal lymphatic vessels, produced during digestion, especially fats.

**chylopoiesis,** the formation of chyle.

**chylothorax,** chyle in the pleural cavity or chest.

**chylous,** pertaining to chyle.

**chyme,** the liquid mixture of partially digested food and gastric juices during digestion found in the stomach and small intestine after a meal.

**chymotrypsin,** an enzyme found in the intestine combined with trypsin which hydrolyzes protein to peptones.

**cicatrix,** healed wound; scar.

**cilia,** hairlike projections that arise from epithelial cells as found in bronchi, which transport mucus and dust particles upward; eyelashes.

**ciliary,** pertaining to eyelashes and to eye structures such as ciliary body.

**ciliary body,** consists of ciliary processes and ciliary muscle that extends from the iris base to the choroid.

**cillosis,** spasmodic twitching of the eyelid.

**cinchona,** a tree or shrub whose bark is the source of quinine.

**cinchonism,** poisoning resulting from overdoses of cinchona or quinine, characterized by headache, deafness, dizziness, and ringing of the ears.

**circulation,** movement of blood through the blood vessels of the body maintained by the pumping action of the heart.

**circulatory,** pertaining to circulation.

**circumcision,** the cutting around or removal of the foreskin of the penis.

**cirrhosis,** inflammation of an organ characterized by degenerative changes, particularly the liver.

**cirrhotic,** affected with or pertaining to cirrhosis.

**cirsectomy,** surgical removal of a part of a varicose vein.

**cirsotomy,** treatment for varicose veins with multiple incisions.

**citric acid,** an acid derived from citrus fruits used to flavor pharmaceuticals; important to metabolism.

**citric acid cycle, Kreb's cycle,** involved and complicated reactions pertaining to the oxidation of pyruvic acid in metabolism and converting it into energy for the body.

**clamp,** used for surgical procedures to compress a part or structure such as a blood vessel.

**clap,** see gonorrhea.

**claudication,** lameness; limping due to severe pain in the muscles of the calf resulting from decreased blood flow.

**claustrophobia,** an obsessive, intense fear of closed spaces.

**clavicle,** collarbone; a curved bone which joins the sternum and the scapula.

**clavicular,** pertaining to the clavicle.

**clavus,** a corn.

**cleft palate,** a congenital malformation in the roof of the mouth which forms a communicating opening between the mouth and the nasal cavities.

**cleidorrhexis,** bending or fracturing the clavicles of the fetus to ease delivery.

**cleptomania,** the impulsive act of stealing.

**climacteric,** menopause; cessation of a woman's reproductive period; corresponding period in a male characterized by decreased sexual activity.

**clinic,** a medical center for examination, diagnosis, and treatment for non-hospitalized patients.

**clinical,** pertaining to a clinic; pertaining to actual observation and treatment of patients.

**clinician,** a specialist in clinical procedures such as a clinical physician, teacher, or nurse; practicing physician.

**Clinistix,** trademark for glucose oxidase reagent strips to test urine for glucose.

**clitoris,** an organ of the female genitalia; an erectile structure located beneath the anterior part of the vulva.

**clonic,** alternate contraction and relaxation of muscle groups in rapid succession.

**clonicity,** condition of being clonic.

**clonus,** opposite of tonus.

**Clostridium,** a genus of spore-bearing anaerobic, rod-shaped bacteria commonly found in soil and in the intestinal tract of animals and man; frequently found in wound infections and the primary cause of gangrene and tetanus.

**clot,** coagulated blood or lymph; a thrombus.

**clotting time,** see coagulation time.

**clouding of consciousness,** state of mental confusion characterized by disorientation of time and place, amnesia, and decreased reaction time due to illness.

**cloudy swelling,** degeneration of tissues which become swollen and turbid.

**clubbed fingers,** broadening and rounding of the fingertips due to swelling, often seen in children with congenital heart disease and adults with pulmonary disease of long duration.

**club-foot,** congenital foot deformity.

**clumping,** see agglutination.

**clunes,** buttocks.

**clysis,** injection of a cleansing fluid for washing out blood in a cavity.

**C.N.S.,** see central nervous system.

**coagulability,** being capable of forming clots.

**coagulant,** an agent responsible for coagulation.

**coagulate,** cause a clot or to become clotted.

**coagulation,** process of clotting.

**coagulation time,** period of time required for blood to clot or coagulate which is indicated when fibrin appears in tiny threads; normal clotting time is between 3 to 7 minutes.

**coagulum,** clump of clotting blood.

**coarctate,** pressed together; to tighten.

**coarctation,** compression of vessel walls; narrowing or tightening.

**coarctotomy,** division of a stricture by incision.

**coat,** a layer in the wall of an artery.

**cobalt,** a chemical element; cobalt 60 is a radioisotope of cobalt used in radiation therapy.

**cocaine,** a bitter alkaloid obtained from coca plants used in medicine as a local anesthetic and as a narcotic.

**cocarcinogenesis,** the development of cancer in preconditioned cells.

**coccidia,** sporozoa which are commonly found in epithelial tissue of the intestinal tract, the liver, and other organs in the body.

**coccygeal,** pertaining to the coccyx.

**coccygectomy,** removal of the coccyx by surgery.

**coccygodynia,** pain in the coccyx and the surrounding area.

**coccyx,** usually referring to the last four bones of the spine which attach to the sacrum.

**cochlea,** a cone-shaped, winding structure in the inner ear containing the organ of corti which is the receptor for hearing.

**cochleitis,** inflammation of the cochlea.

**cocoid,** resembling a cocus.

**coconscious, coconsciousness,** a conscious objective state in which subconscious impressions may rise to the surface and influence the stream of consciousness.

**cocoa butter,** a fat obtained from cocoa seed used as a lubricant in pharmaceuticals.

**cocus,** a spherical bacterium; organisms of the genus staphylococcus, and micrococcus.

**codeine,** an alkaloid from opium or synthetically produced, used as an analgesic and hypnotic sedative.

**cod liver oil,** a fixed oil obtained from cod fish livers used for its Vitamin A and D.

**cohabitation,** sexual intercourse; living together.

**coherent,** sticking together; being logically consistent.

**cohesion,** the process of sticking together; adhering; causing particles to unite.

**coitus,** sexual intercourse; copulation.

**colchicum,** a drug derived from the Colchicum seed used to relieve symptoms of gout.

**cold,** common viral infection of the respiratory mucous membranes causing symptoms of nasal congestion, headache, coughing, body aches, fatigue, fever, and chills.

**cold sore,** a fever blister particularly around the mouth caused by herpes simplex virus.

**colectomy,** excision of part of the large intestine or colon.

**colic,** spasms accompanied by abdominal pain; pertaining to the colon; occurring in infants, especially in the first few months of life.

**colicstitis,** cystitis caused by Eschericia coli.

**colitis,** inflammation of the colon.

**collagen,** a substance composed of white fibers of connective tissue found in the skin, tendons, cartilage, and bone; a body protein composed of connective tissue fibers.

**collapse,** a sudden caving in of the walls of an organ; an extreme loss of vital functioning of organ systems producing shock or breakdown.

**collarbone,** the clavicle.

**collecting tubules,** small ducts which receive urine from the renal tubules.

**Colles' fracture,** fracture of the distal end of the radius (just above the wrist bone).

**colliculus,** small anatomical mound.

**collodion,** a substance applied to the skin which forms a very thin protective layer.

**colloid,** a gelatinous protein found normally in thyroid secretion.

**colloma,** colloid degeneration found in cancerous tissue.

**collutory,** used as a gargle or mouth wash.

**collyrium,** a neutral solution used as an eyewash.

**coloboma,** an eye defect, usually due to an abnormal closure of the fetal fissure which may affect any part of the eye.

**colon,** the section of the large intestine between the cecum to the rectum.

**color blindness,** a hereditary condition in which a person is totally or partially unable to distinguish between certain primary colors; chromatelopsia.

**colostomy,** a surgical procedure that provides an opening between the colon and the abdominal wall creating a stoma.

**colostrum,** the first secretion of the breasts after childbirth before lactation commences, within a two to three day period, containing high protein and immunity factors for the newborn.

**colotomy,** incision of the colon.

**colpalgia,** vaginal pain.

**colpitis,** vaginitis.

**colpocystitis,** inflammation of both the bladder and vagina.

**copocystocele,** prolapse of the bladder into the vagina.

**colpohysterectomy,** excision of the uterus through the vagina.

**coloplasty,** plastic repair involving the vagina.

**colpoptosis,** prolapse of the vagina.

**colporrhapy,** suturing the vaginal wall for the purpose of narrowing it.

**colposcope,** an instrument for examining the cervix and vagina.

**coma,** a state of abnormal unconsciousness from which a person cannot respond to external stimuli due to illness or an injury; stupor.

**comatose,** pertaining to coma.

**comedo,** a blackhead caused by dried sebum blocking a duct in the skin.

**comminute,** breaking into pieces such as a shattered bone.

**comminution,** comminuting or reducing to fine particles.

**commissure,** joining together of corresponding structures such as lips or eyelids; a band of nerve fibers coming together.

**communicable disease,** transmission of a disease from one person to another either directly or indirectly.

**compensation,** making up for some abnormality.

**complemental,** adding something that is deficient.

**complex,** a group of associated ideas which are usually unconscious, believed to be influencing factors of abnormal attitudes and mental states.

**complication,** a complex state in which disease or accident is added to an existing illness without being related specifically.

**compos mentis,** sane; of sound mind.

**compound,** a substance composed of two or more parts.

**compound fracture,** bone which is broken and pierces the skin.

**compress,** a soft pad, moist or dry, applied to a part of the body with pressure to prevent hemorrhage, or to apply medication, heat or cold.

**compression,** being pressed together.

**compulsion,** an insistent, repetitive, and unwanted urge to perform an irrational act; state of being compelled.

**compulsive,** exhibiting repetitive patterns of behavior.

**concave,** a rounded, hollowed out surface, or cavity.

**concavity,** a concave surface.

**concavoconvex,** being concave on one side and convex on the other side; pertaining to the lens of the eyes.

**conceive,** to become pregnant; to form a mental image or an idea.

**concentration,** increasing in strength of a substance by evaporation.

**concept,** a mental image of an idea.

**conception,** the beginning of pregnancy when the ovum is fertilized by a sperm forming a zygote.

**concha,** a structure resembling a shell; the pinna or outer ear; one of the three bones on the nasal cavity.

**conchitis,** inflammation of a concha.

**concretion,** a calculus; an inorganic mass found in a body cavity or tissues.

**concubitus,** sexual intercourse, copulation, coition.

**concussion,** an injury resulting from a collision or impaction with an object; partial or complete loss of bodily functions resulting from a violent shock or a blow to the head.

**conditioned reflex,** acquired response through repetition and training.

**condom,** a thin rubber sheath to be worm over the penis during sexual intercourse to prevent impregnation or veneral disease.

**condyle,** a rounded projection at the end of a bone which articulates with another bone.

**condylectomy,** excision or removal of a condyle.

**condyloma,** a wartlike lesion on the skin occurring on the mucous membranes or external genitals or near the anus.

**confabulation,** an unconscious replacing of imaginary experiences due to memory loss, seen principally in organic mental disorders.

**confinement,** period of childbirth or puerperal state.

**confusion,** disturbance in orientation to time, place, or person; a psychological evaluation pertaining to a disordered consciousness.

**congenital,** present at birth, including conditions arising from fetal development or the birth process that are not hereditary.

**congest,** to cause an abnormal amount of blood to accumulate in an organ.

**congestion,** the presence of an excess amount of fluid in an organ or in tissue.

**congestive,** pertaining to congestion.

**conization,** excision of a cone of tissue pertaining to the cervix.

**conjugate,** paired; working together; an important measurement in the diameter of the pelvis.

**conjugation,** a coupling.

**conjunctiva,** mucous membranes lining the eyelids and covering the anterior surface of the eyeball.

**conjunctivitis,** inflammation of the conjunctiva.

**connective tissue,** primarily functions to support or bind together bodily tissues, organs, and parts; other functions include food storage, blood formation, and defensive mechanisms.

**consanguinity,** kinship; blood relationship.

**conscience,** associated with superego; a person's set of moral values which controls his behavior and performance.

**conscious,** being aware of one's existence and having the ability to respond subjectively to stimuli; awake.

**consciousness,** awareness; being conscious.

**consolidation,** the process of becoming solid, referring to a condition in the lungs due to an accumulation of fluid in acute pneumonia.

**constipation,** irregular, difficult, or sluggish defecation.

**constitution,** the functional habits and physical properties of the body; a disposition, temperament, or condition of the mind.

**constitutional,** pertaining to the whole body.

**constriction,** a narrowing of a part or opening.

**consultant,** acting in an advisory capacity.

**consultation,** two or more specialists who deliberate about diagnosis and treatment of a client.

**consumption,** pertaining to tuberculosis; wasting away of the body.

**consumptive,** one afflicted with tuberculosis.

**contact,** one who has been exposed to a contagious disease; touching of two bodies.

**contact lens,** a thin concave disk which fits on the convex surface of the eyeball and floats on the fluid of the eye, helpful in correcting impaired vision.

**contagion,** the process of spreading a disease from one person to another by direct or indirect contact.

**contagious,** a readily transmitted disease either directly or indirectly from one person to another; communicable.

**contaminate,** the act of soiling or exposing to infectious germs into normally sterile objects; render impure by contact or mixture.

**continence,** the practice of self-restraint in sexual indulgence.

**contortion,** a spasmodic twisting or writhing of the body; distortion.

**contraception,** the prevention of conception.

**contraceptive,** an agent or device to prevent conception or impregnation.

**contraction,** a shortening or drawing up of a muscle; a shrinking.

**contracture,** a permanent contraction or shortening of a muscle due to spasm, fibrosis of tissues, or paralysis.

**contraindication,** a condition or circumstance that indicates that a form of treatment of medication is inappropriate in a specific case.

**contralateral,** affecting the opposite side of the body.

**contuse,** to injure or wound by bruising.

**contusion,** an injuring to the skin without breaking the flesh; a severe bruise.

**convalescence,** a recovery period after an illness, operation, or injury.

**convalescent,** pertaining to convalescence; a patient who is recovering from an illness, operation, or injury.

**convergence,** coordinating the movements of both eyes toward a common point.

**convex,** having an elevated or rounded surface.

**convexoconcave,** having one convex and one concave surface, especially the lens.

**convolute,** rolled or coiled up, as a scroll.

**convolution,** a folding or coiling of anything which is convoluted; the many folds on the surface of the brain or the intestines.

**convulsant,** medication or a drug which causes convulsions.

**convulsion,** severe involuntary muscle contractions with a temporary loss of consciousness due to many causes.

**convulsive,** pertaining to, characterized by convulsions.

**Coombs' test,** used in the diagnosis of several forms of hemolytic anemias.

**coprolalia,** abnormal desire to use obscene words in ordinary conversion.

**coprophagy,** ingesting of feces.

**coprophilia,** abnormal attraction to feces and defecation.

**coprophobia,** an abnormal disgust of filth and feces.

**coprostasis,** fecal impaction.

**copulation,** sexual coitus, or the act of copulating.

**coracoid process,** pertaining to the upper anterior surface of the scapula.

**Coramine,** trademark for nikethamide used as a respiratory stimulant.

**cord,** the umbilical cord; stringlike structures such as vocal cords, the spinal cord, or the spermatic cord.

**cordate,** heart-shaped.

**corectomy,** surgical removal of the iris.

**corium,** the dermis; the layer of skin immediately beneath the epidermis which contains vascular connective tissue, nerve endings, hair follicles, sebaceous glands, sweat glands, and smooth muscle fibers.

**corn,** a horny and thickened area of the skin which may be either soft or hard depending on its location on the foot due to pressure or friction.

**cornea,** the transparent membrane covering the iris and pupil of the eye.

**corneal,** pertaining to the cornea.

**corneitis,** inflammation of the cornea.

**corneous,** horn-shaped.

**cornification,** conversion of stratified squamous epithelium cells into keratin, or horn.

**corona,** resembling a crown.

**coronal,** pertaining to corona; referring to the suture which joins the parietal and frontal bones in the skull.

**coronary,** pertaining to a circle or crown.

**coronary arteries,** two arteries which supply blood to the heart muscles.

**coronary occlusion,** closure or blockage of one of the coronary arteries.

**coronary thrombosis,** clotting of blood in the blood vessels which supply the heart; a common cause of myocardial infarction.

**coroner,** a county officer who investigates any death from unknown causes or violent crimes.

**corpulence,** obesity.

**corpulent,** being stout, fat, obese.

**corpus,** principle part of an organ; any mass or body.

**corpuscle,** any minute rounded body; a blood cell.

**corpusculum,** corpuscle.

**corpus luteum,** a yellowish endocrine substance secreted by the ovary after the rupture of a Graafian follicle and the release of ovum; during pregnancy the corpus luteum persists in secreting the hormone progesterone.

**corrode,** to wear away by chemical action.

**corrosion,** disintegrating; the process of corroding.

**corrosive,** an agent that is destructive to the tissues.

**cortex,** outer portion of an organ, the brain, and the adrenal glands.

**cortical,** pertaining to the cortex.

**corticosteroids,** hormones produced by the adrenal glands.

**cortin,** a hormone secreted by the adrenal cortex.

**cortisone,** a hormone extracted from the adrenal cortex of the adrenal gland and also prepared synthetically, important to fat metabolism.

**coryza,** nasal catarrh resulting from inflammation of the mucous membranes; common head cold.

**costa,** rib.

**costae,** the rib cage composed of twelve ribs on each side.

**costal,** pertaining to the ribs.

**costalgia,** pain in a rib, or intercostal spaces.

**costive,** constipated.

**costoclavicular,** pertaining to the ribs and clavicle.

**costovertebral,** the joining of a rib to a vertebrae.

**cough,** a more or less violent expulsion of air from the lungs in an attempt to expel an irritant from the respiratory tract.

**counterirritant,** the application of an agent to reduce or relieve another irritation.

**courses,** menses.

**cowperitis,** inflammation of the Cowper's glands.

**Cowper's glands,** two composed tubular glands the size of a pea beneath the bulb of the urethra in males.

**cowpox,** pustular eruptions of milk cows on areas of udder and teats resembling smallpox in man; when virus is contained in vaccine and given to humans against smallpox, it offers some degree of immunity against the disease.

**coxa,** the joint in the hip or hip bone.

**coxalgia,** pain in the hip.

**cramp,** a spasmodic, involuntary contraction of a muscle or group of muscles with pain.

**cranial,** pertaining to the cranium or skull.

**cranial nerves,** originating in the brain; there are twelve pairs of cranial nerves.

**craniectomy,** excision of part of the skull.

**craniometry,** the science of skull measurement.

**cranioplasty,** plastic repair on the skull.

**craniopuncture,** an exploratory procedure in which the skull is punctured.

**cranium,** including all of the bones of the head that enclose the brain.

**crapulent, crapulous,** excessive drinking of alcohol; intoxication.

**creatine,** a nitrogenous compound synthesized in the body which serves as a source of high energy phosphate.

**Crede's method,** a procedure used in obstetrics whereby the placenta is expelled by employing a downward pressure on the uterus through the abdominal wall; treatment of the eyes of the newborn with 1% silver nitrate solution immediately after birth for prevention of infection.

**cremaster,** one of the fascialike muscles suspending the testicles and spermatic cord.

**cremation,** burning of dead bodies by heat.

**crepitant,** a crackling sound; making a grating sound.

**cresol,** a substance used as a disinfectant derived from coal tar.

**crest,** a ridgelike formation on a bone.

**cretin,** one afflicted with cretinism.

**cretinism,** a congenital affliction caused by abnormal thyroid secretion, characterized by stunted physical and mental development.

**crevice,** a small fissure or crack.

**cribbing,** swallowing air.

**cribriform,** sievelike; having many small openings.

**cribriform plate,** a thin, perforated bone in the skull through which many nerve filaments pass.

**cricoid cartilage,** the lowermost, ringlike cartilage of the larynx.

**crinogenic,** stimulating secretions in a gland.

**crisis,** the turning point of a disease marked by a sudden decrease in high temperature to normal; a turning point in illness for better or worse.

**cross-eye,** esotropia.

**cross-matching,** testing before transfusion to determine blood compatibility.

**croup,** a disease occurring in children characterized by inflammation of the respiratory passages causing difficult breathing, laryngeal spasm, coughing, and sometimes exudation due to the formation of a membrane.

**crowning,** stage in delivery when the fetal head appears at the opening of the birth canal.

**crural,** pertaining to the leg or thigh.

**crus,** the leg.

**crush syndrome,** renal failure following the severe crushing of the lower extremities.

**crust, crusta,** a scab; an outer covering.

**crutch,** used to support the body weight in walking. A staff which extends from the armpit to the ground.

**cryanesthesia,** the inability to perceive cold.

**cryesthesia,** having an abnormal sensitivity to cold.

**cryocautery,** cold cautery; a device used for application of solid carbon dioxide.

**cryogenic,** pertaining to low temperatures.

**cryosurgery,** the application of extreme low temperatures to destroy or remove diseased tissue.

**cryotherapy, crymotherapy,** the therapeutic use of cold.

**crypt,** a small sac or cavity which extends into epithelial or glandular surfaces.

**cryptogenetic,** of unknown origin.

**cryptorchidism,** a condition in which the testicles fail to descend into the scrotum.

**crystalline,** resembling a crystal; clear.

**crystalline lens,** the lens of the eye behind the pupil.

**crystaluria,** the appearance of crystal formations in the urine.

**crystalluridrosis,** urinary elements appearing on the skin as crystallized sweat.

**cubital,** pertaining to the forearm.

**cubitus,** elbow; forearm; ulna.

**cuboid,** referring to the outermost bone of the tatsal or instep bones which connect with the 4th and 5th metatarsus.

**cul-de-sac,** a blind cavity or pouch.

**culdoscopy,** a visual examination of the female viscera of the pelvic cavity through an endoscope introduced into the vagina.

**Culex,** a genus of mosquitoes found throughout the world which are vectors of malaria producing organisms.

**culture,** a mass of microorganisms growing in a culture medium in the laboratory.

**cumulative,** increasing in effect or amount; an accumulation of drugs by successive additions or dosages.

**cupula,** an inverted cup-shaped cap or dome over a structure.

**curare, curari,** an extract obtained from tropical plants used as an arrow poison by South American Indians; used in anesthesia to control convulsions, spasms, and for skeletal muscle relaxation.

**curet, curette,** a spoon-shaped instrument used in scraping a cavity to remove foreign matter or a diseased surface.

**curettage,** scraping of a cavity with a curette.

**curie,** a standard unit of radioactivity.

**curietherapy,** radium therapy.

**cusp,** a point of a crown of a tooth.

**cuspid,** a canine tooth, of which there are four; a cuspidate tooth.

**cuspidate,** having cusps.

**cutaneous,** pertaining to the skin.

**cuticle,** a layer of solid or semisolid nonliving skin that surrounds fingernails and toenails.

**cutis,** the skin.

**cyanemia,** dark blue-colored blood.

**cyanide,** a fast-acting poison.

**cyanocobalamin,** Vitamin B12.

**cyanopsia,** objects appear tinged with blue due to a defect in vision.

**cyanosis,** a bluish, slatelike, or dark purple skin color due to excessive concentration of reduced hemoglobin in the blood.

**cyanotic,** pertaining to cyanosis.

**cycle,** a series of events or a sequence of movements.

**cyclic,** pertaining to cycles.

**cyclitis,** inflammation of the ciliary body or ciliary region of the upper eyelid.

**cyclomate,** an artificial sweetener with no nutritional value.

**cycloplegia,** paralysis of the ciliary muscles.

**cyclothyme,** one afflicted with cyclothymia.

**cyclothymia,** a cyclic disorder of the mind characterized by recurring and alternating periods of sadness and elation.

**cyesis,** pregnancy.

**cyst,** a pouch or closed sac under the skin or in the body which contains fluid, semifluid, or solid matter.

**cystadenoma,** a tumor containing cysts.

**cystalgia,** a painful urinary bladder.

**cystectomy,** removal of a cyst; removal of the gallbladder; excision of the urinary bladder or part of it.

**cystic,** pertaining to a cyst; pertaining to the urinary bladder, or to the gallbladder.

**cystic fibrosis,** a disease occurring in childhood involving the exocrine glands resulting in pancreatic insufficiency and chronic respiratory disease; believed to be hereditary.

**cystitis,** inflammation of the bladder.

**cystocele,** a protrusion of the urinary bladder into the vagina.

**cystocolostomy,** a surgical procedure that creates a permanent communication between the gallbladder and the colon.

**cystoid,** resembling a cyst; bladderlike.

**cystolith,** having a calculus or stone in the urinary bladder.

**cystolithectomy,** excision of calculus from the bladder.

**cystoma,** a cystic tumor.

**cystoplasty,** plastic repair upon the bladder.

**cystoscope,** an instrument for examining the bladder.

**cystoscopy,** examination of the bladder with a cystoscope.

**cystospasm,** a spasmodic contraction of the urinary bladder.

**cystostomy,** surgical procedure of the urinary bladder to make an opening.

**cytobiology,** biology of the cells.

**cytoblast,** a cell nucleus.

**cytochemistry,** the scientific study of the structure and chemistry of living cells.

**cytochromes,** iron-containing compounds found in animal and human tissue which play an important role in cellular respiration.

**cytogenesis,** the origin and development of cells.

**cytokalipenia,** a deficiency of potassium in the body.

**cytokinesis,** the movement of cytoplasm into two parts during cell division.

**cytology,** the study of the structures and functions of cells.

**cytolysis,** the destruction or degeneration of cells.

**cytoplasm,** the protoplasm of a cell not including the nucleus.

**cytosine,** a component of nucleic acid common to both DNA and RNA.

**cytoscopy,** a diagnostic microscopic examination of cells.

**cytotropism,** the movement of cells in response to external stimuli.

**cytula,** the impregnated ovum.

**cyturia,** the presence of various cells in the urine.

## D

**dacrocystitis, dacryocystitis,** inflammation of the lacrimal or tear sac.

**dacryadenitis, dacroadenitis,** inflammation of a lacrimal (tear) gland.

**dacryocele,** protrusion of a lacrimal (tear) sac.

**dacryocystotomy,** surgical operation of the lacrimal sac.

**dacryolith,** a calculus or stone in the tear duct.

**dacryorrhea,** excessive flow of tears.

**dactyl,** a finger or toe.

**dactylitis,** inflammation of a finger or toe.

**dactylography,** the study of fingerprints.

**dactylology,** communicating by sign language made with the hands and fingers.

**dactylolysis,** loss or amputation of a finger or toe.

**dactylomegaly,** abnormally large fingers or toes.

**dactylus,** referring to a finger or toe; a digit.

**daltonism,** color blindness, especially in differentiating between red and green.

**D and C,** pertaining to dilatation of the cervix and curettage of the uterus.

**dandruff,** dry scales of epidermis forming on the scalp which shed, sometimes due to seborrheic dermatitis.

**dandy fever,** an acute febrile disease which occurs in the tropics; dengue.

**dartos,** a fibrous layer beneath the skin of the scrotum.

**darwinian ear,** a congenital deformity of the helix of the ear.

**deaf,** lacking the sense of hearing.

**deaf-mute,** unable to hear or speak.

**deafness,** complete or partial loss of hearing.

**deamination,** the removal of the amino group from a compound.

**dearterialization,** changing arterial to venous blood by deoxygenation.

**death rattle,** a rattling sound heard in the throat of the dying.

**debilitant,** drug to reduce excitement.

**debilitate,** producing weakness or debility.

**debility,** weakened condition of the body and loss of bodily function; feebleness.

**debridement,** the removal of foreign matter or dead tissue from a wound.

**decalcification,** the removal of lime salts from bones; loss of bone calcium.

**decalcify,** softening of bone by removal or loss of calcium or its salts.

**decannulation,** to remove a cannula or tube.

**decant,** to pour off liquid with sediment remaining in the bottom of the flask or container.

**decapitation,** beheading; to remove the head from the body.

**dechloridation, dechlorination,** decrease sodium chloride in the body by the removal of salt from the diet.

**decibel,** a unit of sound measuring intensity and volume.

**decidua,** the endometrium when conception occurs which divides itself into three layers enveloping the impregnated ovum.

**decidual,** pertaining to the decidua.

**deciduoma,** a uterine tumor containing decidual tissue.

**deciduous,** shedding at a particular stage of growth, especially of temporary teeth.

**decimeter,** one-tenth of a meter.

**declinator,** an instrument used in surgery to retract or hold apart the dura matter.

**decline,** a declining period of a disease or illness.

**decoloration,** bleaching or the removal of color.

**decompensation,** the ability of the heart or other organs in the body to maintain adequate functioning; a term used in psychiatry which implies the failure of defense mechanisms resulting in disintegration of personality.

**decomposition,** decaying process.

**decompression,** removal of pressure, or removing of air pressure from a chamber; a normal bodily adjustment to atmospheric pressure.

**decongestant,** a substance or drug that reduces congestion and swelling, especially in nasal passages.

**decontamination,** rendering free of contamination as in an object or person contaminated by poisonous gas or radioactive substances.

**decortication,** removal of the surface layer from structures or organs.

**decrepit,** wasted or worn down by the infirmities caused by the aging process.

**decrepitude,** senile breaking down.

**decubation,** recovery stage of an infectious disease.

**decubitus,** a bedsore; a pressure wound.

**decussate,** crossing of parts.

**decussation,** crossing of structures or nerves which form an X; chiasma.

**defecation,** evacuation of the bowels, or the expulsion of fecal matter.

**defective,** imperfect; physically or mentally deficient.

**defeminization,** loss or absence of female sexual characteristics.

**deferens,** to carry away, as in ductus deferens, excretory duct of the testicles.

**deferent,** to carry downward.

**deferentitis,** inflammation of the ductus deferens.

**defervescence,** subsidence of fever to normal body temperature.

**defibrillation,** terminating atrial or ventricular fibrillation or irregular heart muscle contractions.

**deficiency disease,** any disease caused by a dietary insufficiency.

**defluvium,** sudden loss of air.

**defluxion,** a flowing down of a copious discharge of any kind.

**deformation,** disfiguration or malformation.

**deformity,** a malformation or misshapen part of the body or organ; a distortion of the body or part of the body which may be acquired or congenital.

**degenerate,** a sexual pervert; to deteriorate.

**degeneration,** impairment or deterioration of an organ or its parts.

**deglutition,** act of swallowing.

**degradation,** act of degrading; conversion of a chemical compound to one less complex.

**degustation,** act of tasting.

**dehiscence,** bursting open; separation of the layers of a surgical wound.

**dehydrate,** to lose moisture or water.

**dehydration,** excessive loss of body fluids or water; the process of dehydrating.

**déjà vu,** a sensation that what one is seeing is a repetition of a previous experience.

**dejecta,** feces.

**dejection, dejecture,** feeling of being downcast; a state of mental depression; excretment.

**delacrimation,** a constant overflow of tears.

**delactation,** cessation of lactation; weaning.

**deleterious,** injurious or harmful to health or well-being.

**delinquent,** antisocial, criminal, or illegal behavior, especially significant in a minor exhibiting such behavior.

**deliquescence,** liquefaction of salts by absorption of water from the air.

**delirious,** pertaining to delirium.

**delirium,** a temporary disorientation, usually accompanied by illusions and hallucinations due to various causes such as fever, intoxication, or trauma.

**delirium tremens,** an acute mental disorder characterized by delirium, trembling, great anxiety, mental distress, sweating, and gastrointestinal symptoms, caused by excessive alcohol consumption.

**delivery,** giving birth; parturition.

**delomorphous,** having a definite form or shape.

**deltoid,** referring to a large triangular muscle which covers the shoulder prominence.

**delusion,** a false belief which is firmly maintained despite obvious evidence to the contrary.

**delusional,** pertaining to delusions.

**demented,** out of one's mind; insane.

**dementia,** mental deterioration; organic loss of intellectual functioning.

**dementia praecox,** schizophrenia; an obsolete descriptive term for schizophrenia.

**demineralization,** abnormal loss of mineral salts from the body by excessive secretion and excretion.

**demonomania,** obsolete term for an irrational belief that one is possessed by demons or evil spirits.

**demulcent,** a substance that will soothe and soften the skin.

**demyelinate,** to remove the myelin sheath from a nerve or nerves.

**denatured,** to change the nature of a substance; to render unfit for human consumption without impairing usefulness for other purposes, as alcohol.

**dengue,** an infectious tropical disease carried by mosquitoes characterized by fever and severe pain in the joints and muscles.

**dental,** pertaining to the teeth.

**dental caries,** decay of the teeth.

**dentalgia,** toothache.

**dental hygienist,** one trained to clean teeth, provide instruction on general tooth care, and assist a dentist.

**dentate,** notched, or toothed.

**denticle,** a small tooth; projecting toothlike point.

**dentifrice,** a substance for cleaning teeth.

**dentin, dentine,** the main hard tissues of a tooth enclosing the pulp which is covered by enamel on the crown and cementum on the roots.

**dentist,** a practioner who cares for and treats the gums and teeth.

**dentistry,** the branch of medicine which is concerned with the care of teeth, and with the prevention, diagnosis, and treatment of diseases of the teeth and gums.

**dentition,** the teeth in situ or in the dental arch.

**dentures,** false teeth; artificial teeth.

**denudation,** act of denuding; removal of a protective covering.

**denutrition,** malnutrition.

**deodorant,** an agent that masks offensive odors.

**deodorize,** to remove offensive and foul odors.

**deossification,** loss of mineral elements from bone.

**deoxidation,** process of depriving or reducing oxygen.

**deoxycholic acid,** a crystalline acid found in bile.

**deoxyribonuclease,** an enzyme produced by some streptococci.

**deoxyribonucleic acid,** see DNA.

**depersonalization,** a neurosis characterized by feelings of unreality and lost sense of personal identity; a lessened sense of one's perception of self, may occur in a mild form in a normal person.

**depilate,** to remove or pluck out hair.

**depilation,** the process of removing hair.

**depilatory,** a substance used for hair removal.

**deplete,** to empty or relieve, as in blood letting or purging.

**deplumation,** loss of eyelashes due to illness or disease.

**deposit,** collecting of matter in an organ part, or in an organism; sediment.

**depraved,** one perverted or abnormal; deteriorated.

**depressant,** a substance that depresses any functional body activity; an agent that depresses; sedative.

**depressed,** pertaining to depression.

**depression,** a depressed region or hallow; lowering of a body part or vital function; a morbid sadness, melancholy, or lack of hope.

**depressomotor,** an agent which retards muscular movements.

**depressor,** a device for depressing the tongue or a body part.

**depurate,** an agent that purifies.

**deradentis,** inflammation of a lymph gland in the neck.

**derangement,** a mental disorder.

**dereistic,** day dreaming.

**derm, derma,** true skin, beneath the epidermis.

**dermal,** pertaining to the true skin.

**dermatitis,** inflammation of the derma.

**dermatoautoplasty,** grafting of skin taken from the patient's own body.

**dermatogen,** an antigen produced from a skin disease.

**dermatoid,** resembling skin.

**dermatologist,** a skin specialist.

**dermatology,** the branch of medicine concerned with the skin and its diseases.

**dermatomycosis,** a skin infection caused by fungi; athlete's foot.

**dermatomyositis,** inflammation of the skin and muscles.

**dermatone,** an instrument used for cutting thin sections of skin for transplants.

**dermatoneurosis,** skin disease caused by a nervous disorder.

**dermatophobia,** morbid fear of contracting a skin disease.

**dermatophyte,** a plant parasite which infects the skin of animals and man causing diseases such as eczema and ringworm; a parasitic plant fungus.

**dermatoplastic,** pertaining to the grafting of skin.

**dermatorrhea,** excessive secretion from sebaceous glands.

**dermatosis,** any skin disease.

**dermis,** see derm, derma.

**desensitization,** to lessen hypersensitivity reactions by giving subsequent injections of an antogen; in treatment of phobias, a patient is intentionally exposed to emotionally distressing stimuli.

**desiccant,** a medication which causes drying.

**desiccate,** to dry up.

**desmalgia,** pain in a ligament.

**desmectasis,** stretching of a tendon.

**desmitis,** inflammation of a ligament.

**desmoid,** resembling a ligament; a very tough and fibrous tumor.

**desmology,** science of ligaments and tendons.

**desmotomy,** incision of a ligament.

**desquamate,** shedding of the epithelium.

**desquamation,** shedding of skin or cuticle.

**detelectasis,** collapse of an organ.

**deteriorate,** to become worse, to degenerate.

**determinism,** the theory that nothing in a person's emotional or mental life results by chance alone but rather from specific causes known or unknown.

**detoxify,** to decrease the toxic properties of a substance; to remove the effects of a toxic drug.

**detritus,** any degenerative or broken down tissue.

**detrusor urinae,** the longitudinal muscular layer of the bladder that helps to excrete urine.

**detumescence,** the subsidence of a swelling or of erectile tissue.

**deutencephalon,** the interbrain.

**deuteranopia,** defective color vision, especially an inability to distinguish between green and red.

**deviant,** varying from a normal standard or condition.

**deviated septum,** a congenital or acquired cartilaginous partition between the nostrils or septum.

**devitalize,** to weaken; to deprive of life or vitality.

**devolution,** degeneration as in catabolism.

**dexter,** pertaining to the right side.

**dextral,** pertaining to the right side.

**dextrocardia,** the heart positioned on the right side of the chest.

**dextrose,** a simple form of sugar, also known as glucose or grape sugar; a constituent of corn syrup and honey.

**dextrosuria,** the presence of dextrose in the urine.

**diabetes,** any one of various diseases which indicate the body's inability to handle glucose.

**diabetes insipidus,** a disease characterized by the excretion of excessive amounts of pale urine with no sugar or albumin, and extreme thirst, weakness, and dry skin.

**diabetes millitus,** a disorder of carbohydrate metabolism characterized by an elevated blood sugar and the presence of sugar in the urine, resulting from decreased insulin production or utilization.

**diabetic,** pertaining to one afflicted with diabetes.

**Diabinese,** trademark for chlorpropamide which is used in selected patients for management of diabetes mellitus.

**diagnosis,** recognition of diseases based on examination, and microscopic and chemical results of laboratory findings.

**diagnostic,** pertaining to diagnosis.

**diagnostics,** the science concerned with diagnosis of diseases.

**dialysis,** the passage of small molecules or solute through a membrane; a procedure used to purify colloidal substances enclosed in a thin membraneous sac, and exposing to water or solvent which continually circulates outside the sac.

**dialyze,** to loosen or separate by a dialyzer.

**dialyzer,** a membrane used in performing dialysis such as a coiled cellophane tube.

**diameter,** measured by a straight line passing through the center of a circle or body surface and connecting opposite points on its circumference.

**diapason,** a tuning fork used in diagnosing diseases of the ear.

**diapedesis,** the passage of blood cells outward through unruptured capillary walls.

**diaphane,** translucent membrane of a cell.

**diaphoresis,** excessive or profuse perspiration or sweating.

**diaphoretic,** pertaining to profuse perspiration; an agent which increases perspiration.

**diaphragm,** a membraneous partition separating the abdominal and thoracic cavity which serves in inspiration and expiration; any separating membrane; female contraceptive placed over the cervix.

**diarrhea,** an abnormal evacuation of the intestines characterized by watery and frequent stools.

**diarthric,** pertaining to two or more joints.

**diarthrosis,** an articulation in which the bones move freely; a synovial or hinged joint.

**diarticular,** pertaining to two joints.

**diastalsis,** a foreward movement due to a wave of inhibition before a downward contraction of the intestines.

**diastase,** an enzyme or ferment found in plant cells of grains and malt, and in the digestive juice which converts starch into sugar.

**diastasis,** an injury to a bone occurring during surgery in which an epiphysis is separated; pertaining to the rest period of the cardiac cycle between the diastole and the systole.

**diastole,** the normal period of dilatation of the heart, especially the ventricles.

**diastolic,** pertaining to the diastole of the heart; referring to diastolic pressure; it is the point of the greatest cardiac relaxation.

**diathermia,** diathermy.

**diathermic,** being permeable by heat waves.

**diathermic surgery,** the application of high frequency heat to remove tissue as in cauterization.

**diathermy,** therapeutic use of heat within the body in treatment of disease or injury.

**diathesis,** a constitutional perdisposition to certain diseases.

**dichotomy, dichotomization,** dividing into two parts, or dividing into pairs.

**dichromasy,** partial colorblindness.

**diachromatic,** perceiving only two colors.

**dicliditis,** inflammation of a cardiac valve.

**dicoria,** double pupil in each eye.

**dicrotic,** having one heartbeat for two arterial pulsations; a double pulse.

**dicrotism,** the state of having a double pulse.

**Dicumarol,** trademark for bishydroxycoumarin, an anticoagulant used in treatment of intravascular clotting.

**didactylism,** having only two digits on a hand or foot.

**didelphic,** having a double uterus.

**didymitis,** inflammation of the testicle.

**diencephalon,** second portion of the brain which includes the epithalamus, thalamus, metathalamus, and hypothalamus.

**diet,** one's nutritional intake; a prescribed food exchange adapted for a particular health problem; to eat sparingly according to prescribed rules to reduce body weight.

**dietetic,** pertaining to diet.

**dietetics,** science of nutrition and diet.

**dietitian,** one trained in dietetics and nutritional needs and who is part of the treatment team in hospitals and institutions in charge of diets.

**dietotherapy,** the regulation of diet in the treatment of disease.

**differential blood count,** microscopic determination of the number and variety of white and red blood cells in a cubic millimeter of a blood specimen.

**differential diagnosis,** a diagnosis of symptoms of two or more diseases by comparison.

**differentiation,** pertaining to distinct differences between individuals, groups or objects.

**diffuse,** irregular spreading or scattering of a substance; to pass through a tissue or substance.

**diffusion,** the process of becoming diffused; widely spread.

**digest,** to undergo digestion.

**digestion,** the process of converting food by enzymatic action into chemical substances and assimilation into the body.

**digestive tract,** the system responsible for the conversion of food in the body which includes the mouth, pharynx, esophagus, stomach, small intestine, large intestine, and accessory glands.

**digit,** a finger or toe.

**digital,** pertaining to digits.

**digitalis,** a drug obtained from common foxglove, or Eurasian herbs used in powdered form as tablets or capsules which acts as a heart stimulant and indirectly as a diuretic.

**digitalism,** a condition caused by the poisonous effects produced by digitalis.

**digitalization,** the administration of the drug digitalis in scheduled dosages designed to produce and maintain optimal therapeutic results.

**digitate,** having digitlike appendages.

**digitoxin,** a cardiotoxic, bitter-tasting glycoside obtained from Digitalis purpurea used as a heart stimulant and in treatment of congestive heart failure.

**Dilantin,** trademark for phenytoin used as an anticonvulsant in the treatment of epilepsy.

**dilatation,** enlargement or expansion of an organ or vessel; expansion of an opening with a dilator.

**dilation,** see dilatation.

**dilator,** an instrument used to dilate or stretch muscles, cavities, or openings.

**dilute,** rendering less potent by mixing with water.

**dilution,** process of diluting a substance; weakening the strength of a substance.

**dimercaprol,** a metal antagonist used as an antidote in heavy metal poisoning which is effective against arsenic, gold, and mercury poisoning.

**diminution,** act of reducing.

**dimpling,** a retracting of the subcutaneous tissue in the formation of a dimple which occurs in certain carcinomas.

**dinical,** vertigo.

**Diodoquin,** trademark for diodohydroxyquin used as an antiamebic drug.

**diopsimeter,** an apparatus for exploring the visual field.

**diopter,** something that can be seen through such as a lens with refractive power with focal distance of 1 meter; one diopter is used as a unit of measurement in refraction.

**dioptometer,** an instrument for measuring ocular refraction and accommodation.

**dioptric,** pertaining to refraction of light.

**dioxide,** a compound consisting of two atoms of oxygen and another element such as carbon dioxide.

**dipeptidase,** an enzyme that converts dipeptids into amino acids by hydrolysis.

**dipeptide,** a derived protein by hydrolysis.

**diphasic,** having two phases.

**diphtheria,** an acute infectious disease affecting the mucous membranes of the nose, throat, or larynx with symptoms of fever, pain, and respiratory obstruction; toxins produced by the causative organism Corynebacterium diphtheriae may also cause myocarditis and neuritis.

**diphtheritic,** pertaining to diphtheria.

**diphyodont,** having two sets of teeth, as in man.

**diplegia,** a paralysis of similar parts occuring on both sides of the body.

**diplococcus,** gram positive bacteria occurring in pairs.

**diploe,** cancellated tissue between the inner and outer walls of the skull bones.

**diploetic, diploic,** pertaining to the diploe.

**diploid,** having two sets of chromosomes, as in somatic cells.

**diplophonia, diphonia,** producing two different voice tones at the same time in speaking.

**diplopia,** having double vision.

**dipsomania,** having an uncontrollable craving for alcoholic beverages.

**dipsophobia,** abnormal fear of drinking alcohol.

**dipsosis,** abnormal thirst.

**disaccharide,** any of the group of sugars in carbohydrates yielding two monosaccharides in hydrolysis.

**disarticulation,** separation or amputation through a joint.

**disc, disk,** a round, platelike structure or organ such as the fibro-cartilaginous disc between two vertebrae in the spinal column.

**disease,** any interruption of the normal function of any body organ, part, or system that presents an abnormal or pathological body state.

**disinfect,** to free from infection or destroy bacteria by physical or chemical means.

**disinfectant,** a chemical agent which kills bacteria; germicide.

**disjoint,** to separate bones from their natural positions in a joint.

**dislocate,** to move out of position or joint.

**dislocation,** the act of dislocating.

**dismemberment,** amputation.

**disorganization,** state of being disorganized or confused.

**disorientation,** being disoriented; inability to perceive one's self in relation to time, place, or person; a state of confusion.

**dispensary,** clinic for free dispensation of medicines or medical treatment; a place in which medicines are dispensed.

**displacement,** a defense mechanism in which an emotion is transferred unconsciously from its original object to one more acceptable; removal from the normal or usual position such as a body part.

**disposition,** a natural tendency or aptitude within a person; having susceptibility to disease.

**dissect,** to divide or cut apart tissues for the purpose of anatomical study; to separate tissues of a cadaver.

**dissection,** referring to the cutting of parts or tissues and studying of same.

**dissector,** one who dissects such as an anatomist.

**disseminated,** to scatter or spread over a wide area.

**dissociation,** a state of being separated; a defense mechanism through which emotional attachment is separated from an object, idea, or situation, usually an unconscious process.

**dissolution,** the process of dissolving of one substance into another; liquefaction; death.

**dissolve,** to cause a solid substance to pass into solution.

**distal,** farthest point from the medial line or center of the body.

**distemper,** an infectious disease of animals.

**distend,** to swell up, stretch out, or to become inflated.

**distill,** to purify by vaporization of heat, condensing a volatile substance.

**distillation,** the process of purifying a liquid by vaporizing it and then condensing the substance.

**districhasis,** the growing of two hairs from the same follicle.

**distrix,** the splitting of ends of the hairs.

**disulfiram,** a drug used in treatment of alcoholism to deter ingestion of alcohol by producing an unpleasant reaction, nausea, and vomiting.

**diuresis,** abnormal secretion of urine.

**diuretic,** an agent which increases urinary output.

**divagation,** incoherent speech.

**divergent,** radiating or separating in different directions.

**diver's paralysis,** an occupational disease occurring after working under high air pressures and returning too suddenly to normal atmospheric pressure; the bends.

**diverticula,** pertaining to diverticulum; a pouch or sac in the walls of a canal or cavity.

**diverticulitis,** inflammation of the diverticulum.

**diverticulosis,** the presence of diverticula without inflammation.

**divulsion,** the act of pulling apart.

**divulsor,** an apparatus for dilation of a part.

**diztgotic twins,** fraternal twins, who are the product of two ova.

**dizziness,** state of being dizzy; foolish; vertigo.

**DNA,** deoxyribonucleic acid, a complex protein found in all cells, considered the chemical basis of heredity; a nucleic acid found in chromosomes consisting of a long chain molecule of repeated combinations of four basis (two purines, adenine and guanine, and two pyrimadines, thymine and cystosine).

**doctor,** one licensed to practice medicine and graduated from a college of medicine, dentistry, or veterinary medicine.

**dolichocephalic,** a long head; having a skull with a long front to back diameter.

**dolichoderus,** having a long neck.

**dolichomorphic,** having a thin, long body type.

**dolor,** pain, sorrow.

**dolorific,** producing pain.

**dolorus,** expressing pain, or grief.

**domatophobia,** morbid fear of being in the mouse; pertaining to a form of claustrophobia.

**dominant,** exerting control or influence; in genetics, the expression of a trait or characteristic which is inherited from one parent and excluding a contrasting trait from the opposite parent; a dominant allele or trait.

**donor,** a person who furnishes blood for transfusion or an organ for transplant.

**dorophobia,** morbid aversion to touching animal fur.

**dorsad,** toward the back.

**dorsal,** pertaining to the back; thoracic.

**dorsalgia,** pain in the back.

**dorsiflect,** bending backward.

**dorsiflexion,** backward flexion, as in bending backward either a hand or foot.

**dorsolateral,** pertaining to the back and the side.

**dorsosacral,** pertaining to the lower back.

**dorsum,** pertaining to the back or posterior surface of a body part.

**dosage,** the determination and regulation of the amount of medicine to be given at one time.

**dose,** a prescribed amount of medication to be taken at one time.

**dosimeter,** a device for measuring doses of radiation or X-rays.

**dosimetry,** a scientific determination of radiation; measurement of doses.

**dotage,** feeblemindedness or senility of old age.

**double vision,** seeing two images of an object at the same time.

**double-blind,** in reference to a study in which neither the administrator nor the subject knows which treatment the subject is getting.

**douche,** a stream of hot or cold water directed against a body part or cavity used for hygenic or medicinal purposes, especially the vagina.

**DPT,** diptheria-pertussis-tetanus vaccine.

**Down's Syndrome,** a common form of mental retardation caused by a chromosomal abnormality; mongolism.

**drainage,** the withdrawal of fluids and discharges from a cavity or wound.

**dram, drachm, dr.,** a unit of liquid measure of the apothecaries system, containing 60 minims; a unit of weight equal to 60 grains, 1/8 ounce of the apothecaries' system.

**Dramamine,** trademark for dimenhydrinate, effective in the prevention and treatment of nausea, vomiting, and vertigo associated with surgery, motion sickness, and radiation sickness.

**dreams,** images that occur during sleep.

**dressing,** a protective covering for treatment of a wound caused by disease or injury to aid the healing process.

**drip,** to fall in drops; a slow injection of glucose or saline a drop at a time; intravenously.

**drive,** the urge or force that activates and motivates animals and man.

**drop foot,** inability to raise the foot upwards due to paralysis, of dorsal flexor muscles.

**dropsy,** a condition characterized by generalized accumulation of fluids in the tissues and cavities; see edema.

**drug,** a medicinal substance used internally or externally in treatment of disease or for diagnostic purposes.

**drug addiction,** a physical dependence on a drug caused by excessive or continued use of habit-forming drugs.

**druggist,** pharmacist.

**drum,** the middle ear; the tympanic membrane which serves to separate the tympanic cavity from the exterior acoustic meatus.

**duct,** a narrow tube or channel which serves to convey secretions from a gland.

**ductless,** having no duct, or secreting internally; see endocrine glands.

**ductule,** a small duct.

**ductus arteriosus,** the fetal blood vessel which communicates between the pulmonary artery and the aorta.

**dumb,** unable to speak; mute.

**duodenal,** pertaining to the duodenum.

**duodenectomy,** an operation excising all or part of the duodenum.

**duodenitis,** inflammation of the duodenum.

**duodenostomy,** a surgical procedure of making a permanent opening into the duodenum through the abdominal wall.

**duodenum,** the first segment of the small intestines connecting with the pylorus of the stomach and extending to the jejunum.

**dural,** pertaining to the dura mater, the outermost covering of the brain and spinal cord.

**durematoma,** an accumulation of blood between the arachnoid and dura membranes.

**dwarf,** an undersized human being.

**dwarfism,** being abnormally small in size.

**dynamia,** having vital energy or an ability to combat disease.

**dynamometer,** an apparatus for measuring muscular strength.

**dynamoscopy,** to examine the muscles by auscultation.

**dysacousia, dysacousma,** discomfort caused by loud noises, or having a hypersensitivity to sounds.

**dysarthrosis,** disease or deformity of a joint.

**dyscrasia,** a disordered condition of the body; an abnormal condition of the blood.

**dysenteric,** pertaining to dysentery.

**dysentery,** any of a group of intestinal disorders characterized by inflammation and irritation of the colon, with diarrhea, abdominal pain, and the passage of mucous or blood.

**dysergia,** incoordination in voluntary muscular movements.

**dysfunction,** impairment or absence of total function of the body or an organ.

**dysgenesis,** defective development, or malformation.

**dysgenics,** research study into causative factors in degeneration or deterioration in offspring.

**dysgerminoma,** a slow-growing, malignant tumor of the ovary; the seminoma is the counterpart in testicular neoplasm.

**dysgraphia,** inability to write due to a brain lesion; writer's cramp.

**dyskinesia,** any of a number of diseases which produce defective voluntary movements; impairment of normal movement.

**dyslexia,** difficulty in reading and visual confusion resulting from a brain lesion; inability to comprehend written language due to a central lesion.

**dysmenorrhea,** painful menstruation.

**dyspepsia,** indigestion due to any one of many causes.

**dysphagia,** difficulty in swallowing.

**dysphemia,** stuttering; a speech disorder.

**dysphonia,** any voice impairment causing difficulty in speaking; hoarseness.

**dysphoria,** restlessness; having a feeling of unrest and depression without cause.

**dysplasia,** abnormal growth of tissue, as in pathology; irregular growth in size, shape, and structure of cells.

**dyspnea,** difficult and labored breathing; shortness of breath, which may be accompanied by pain.

**dystonia,** impairment of muscle tone or tonicity.

**dystrophy,** defective nutrition; any disorder due to poor nutrition marked by degeneration of the muscles.

**dysuria,** painful urination.

# E

**ear,** the organ of hearing and equilibrium composed of three different sections: the external, middle, and internal ear.

**earache,** pain in the ear usually caused by inflammation.

**eardrum,** the tympanic membrane.

**earwax,** cerumen.

**eburnation,** changes in bone structure causing a hardening of bone into an ivory-like mass.

**ecbolic,** an agent which hastens labor or abortion by causing the uterine muscles to contract.

**eccentric,** deviating from a center; peripheral; peculiar or abnormal behavior.

**ecchondroma,** a cartilaginous tumor of slow growth.

**ecchymosis,** a hemorrhagic, non-elevated, irregularly-formed discolored area of the skin caused by the seepage of blood beneath the epidermis.

**eccrinology,** the study of glandular secretions.

**eccyesis,** extrauterine pregnancy.

**ecderon,** pertaining to the epidermis or outer portion of the skin.

**ecdysis,** the sloughing off or shedding of skin; desquamation.

**echidin,** the venom of poisonous snakes.

**Echinococcus,** a genus of tapeworms whose larvae may develop in mammals and form cysts, especially in the liver.

**echinosis,** a change in the appearance of blood corpuscles such as losing their smooth outlines; crenation of red blood cells.

**echolalia,** uncontrollable senseless repetition of words spoken by others.

**eclampsia,** a major toxemia occurring in pregnancy or childbirth characterized by high blood pressure, albuminuria, decreased urine formation, edema, convulsions, and coma.

**eclectic,** choosing from a wide variety of sources what appears to be the best.

**ecmnesia,** forgetfulness of recent events, as seen in senility.

**ecologist,** a specialist in ecology.

**ecology,** the study of the physiology of organisms as affected by environmental factors.

**ecomania,** extreme humbleness in the presence of those in authority but having a dominating and irritable attitude toward family members; manifested in chronic alcoholism.

**ecphoria,** reestablishment of a memory trace.

**ecthyma,** an infection of the skin as a result of neglected treatment of impetigo.

**ectiris,** the external part of the iris.

**ectoblast,** ectoderm, the outer layer of cells in a developing embryo; from this outer layer, the epidermis, nails, hair, skin glands, nervous system, external sense organs, and the mucous membrane of the mouth and anus are derived.

**ectodermosis,** ectodermatosis, a disorder or illness resulting from congenital maldevelopment of organs.

**ectogenous,** developing from outside a body structure, as infection from pathogenic bacteria.

**ectomere,** any of the cells forming the ectoderm.

**ectomorphic,** having body structures that are slightly developed characterized by linearity and leanness; referring to body tissues derived predominantly from the ectoderm.

**ectoparasite,** pertaining to a parasite living outside the host's body.

**ectopia,** displacement of an organ or structure.

**ectopic pregnancy,** a pregnancy occurring in the abdominal cavity of a fallopian tube.

**ectoplasm,** the outer portion of the cell protoplasm.

**ectopotomy,** surgical removal of the fetus in ectopic pregnancy.

**ectopy,** displacement or malposition.

**ectoretina,** outer portion of the retina.

**ectotoxemia,** introduction of a toxin into the blood.

**ectromelia,** congenital absence of a limb or limbs.

**ectropic,** pertaining to complete or partial turning outward of a part such as eversion of the eyelid.

**ectropion,** eversion of a part or edge, especially of an eyelid.

**eczema,** an inflammatory condition of the skin which may be acute or chronic, characterized by itching or burning, tiny papules and vesicles, oozing, crusting, and scaling; dermatitis.

**eczematous,** resembling eczema.

**edema,** swelling of body tissues due to an excessive accumulation of fluid in connective tissue or a serous cavity.

**edematous,** pertaining to edema.

**edentia,** without teeth.

**edulcorant,** sweetening.

**edulcorate,** to sweeten; to wash out acids, or salts.

**EEG,** electroencephalogram.

**effect,** a result or consequence of an action.

**effector,** a motor nerve ending having the efferent process terminate in a muscle or gland cell.

**effemination,** having feminine qualities in a man.

**efferent,** conducting impulses from the brain or spinal cord to muscles, glands, and organs.

**effervescence,** the formation of bubbles of gas rising to the surface of a liquid; to show exhilaration or excitement.

**efflorescence,** a rash, eruption, or redness of the skin.

**effluvium,** a noxious or foul exhalation.

**effusion,** the escape of fluid into a cavity, as the pleural space.

**egersis,** extremely alert; abnormal wakefulness.

**egest,** excrete or discharge from the body.

**egesta,** excrement or waste matter eliminated from the body.

**egestion,** eliminating undigested matter.

**egg,** a female gamete or egg; a female reproductive cell before fertilization.

**ego,** the conscious part of the psyche that maintains its identity and tests reality; in psychoanalysis, the ego mediates between the id and the superego.

**egocentric,** self-centered and withdrawing from the external world; having most of one's thoughts and ideas centering on self.

**ego ideal,** an unconscious perfection or desired standard of character usually identified with significant others or esteemed and admired persons.

**egoism,** an overevaluation of self; self-seeking personal advantage at the expense of other people.

**egomania,** egotism developed to a pathological degree.

**egotism,** an overevaluation of self.

**egotist,** a boastful and self-centered person.

**eidoptometry,** measuring visual acuteness.

**eighth cranial nerve,** the acoustic nerve.

**eikonometry,** determining distance of an object by measuring the image produced by a lens with an instrument.

**ejaculation,** the sudden ejection of seminal fluids from the male reproductive organs.

**ejaculatio precox,** premature ejaculation.

**EKG,** electrocardiogram.

**elastin,** an albuminoid material forming the main constituent of yellow elastic tissue found in tendons and cartilage.

**elation,** emotional excitement, or joyous emotion; euphoria.

**elbow,** the joint of the arm and forearm.

**Electra complex,** the suppressed, unresolved libidinal feelings a daughter has for her father, accompanied by strong feelings of jealousy toward her mother.

**electroanesthesia,** a local anesthesia injected into tissues by electricity.

**electrocardiogram,** a record of heart action by an electrocardiograph.

**electrocardiograph,** an apparatus used for recording variations in heart muscle activity.

**electrocardiography,** the study and recording of electrocardiograms produced by an electrocardiograph of the heartbeat.

**electrocatalysis,** chemical decomposition using electricity.

**electrocautery,** cauterization by means of an instrument containing a platinum wire heated by a current of electricity.

**electrocoagulation,** coagulation of tissue using a high frequency electric current.

**electroconvulsive,** using electric current to induce convulsions in treatment of mental illness.

**electroencephalogram,** a record of electrical activity in various areas of the brain.

**electroencephalograph,** an instrument for recording electrical activity of the brain.

**electroencephalography,** the study of changes in electrical fluctuations of the brain made by an electroencephalograph.

**electrohemostasis,** stopping of hemorrhage by electrocautery.

**electrolysis,** the destruction of a chemical compound by an electric current passing through it; the removal of body hair by electric current.

**electrolyte,** a solution which is capable of conducting electricity.

**electrolytic,** pertaining to electrolysis, or to an electrolyte.

**electromassage,** application of electrization in massage.

**electromyogram,** a graphic record of muscle contraction resulting from electrical stimulation.

**electromyography,** the preparation, study, and interpretation of an electromyogram.

**electronarcosis,** inducing narcosis or anesthesia by the application of electricity which is used in treatment of mental illness.

**electropathology,** the study of electrical reaction of muscles and nerves as a means of determining a diagnosis.

**electroretinograph,** an apparatus for measuring the electrical responses of the retina using light stimulation.

**electroshock,** shock induced by an electric current used in treatment of mental illness.

**electrosurgery,** surgery performed by electricity.

**electrotherapy,** treatment of disease by use of low-intensity electricity.

**electuary,** a medicinal substance mixed with a powdered drug and honey or syrup to form a paste.

**elephantiasis,** a chronic disease due to a tropical infection characterized by inflammation and obstruction of the lymphatics, and hypertrophy of the skin and subcutaneous tissues, affecting the lower extremities and the scrotum most frequently.

**elinguation,** surgical removal of the tongue.

**elixir,** a sweetened, aromatic alcoholic liquid used in oral preparations.

**elytrocleisis,** surgical closure of the vagina.

**elytrotomy,** surgical incision into the vaginal wall.

**emaciate,** to become extremely thin or lean; wasting.

**emaciation,** wasting of flesh; the state of growing extremely thin.

**emaculation,** removal of spots from the skin.

**emasculation,** removal of the testicles; castration.

**embalming,** a procedure to retard decomposition in treatment of the dead.

**embedding,** a process by which a piece of tissue is fixated in a medium such as paraffin to keep it intact during cutting into thin sections for microscopic examination.

**embolic,** pertaining to or caused by embolism.

**embolism,** an obstruction of a blood vessel by a clot of blood or foreign substance.

**embolalia,** including meaningless words or phrases in a spoken sentence.

**embolus,** a plug or clot of blood present in a blood or lymphatic vessel having been brought from another vessel and obstructing the circulation within the smaller vessel.

**emboly,** invagination of one part into another such as the formation of the gastrula by the bastula.

**embradure,** to widen an opening.

**embrocation,** fomentation, such as the application of heat and moisture to a diseased or bruised part of the body; a drug rubbed into the skin.

**embryectomy,** the removal of an extrauterine embryo by excision.

**embryo,** the offspring of any organism in the process of development from the fertilized ovum; prenatal development of a mammal between the ovum and the fetus; in humans, the stage of development between the second week to the eighth week after conception.

**embryogeny,** study of the origin or development of the embryo.

**embryology,** the science of the development of the individual organism during the embryonic stage.

**embryoma,** a dermoid cyst; a tumor consisting of embryonic germ tissue but devoid of organization.

**embryonic membrane,** derived from the zygote but outside the embryo, an additional embryonic structure in vertebrates providing additional nutritive and protective value.

**emesis,** vomiting.

**emetic,** an agent or substance to induce vomiting.

**emetine,** a white powdered alkaloid derived from ipecac with emetic properties used as an antiamebic.

**eminence,** a projection or bony prominence.

**emissary,** providing an outlet.

**emissary veins,** small veins which penetrate the skull carrying blood from the sinuses.

**emission,** an involuntary discharge of semen by the male, particularly during sleep.

**emmenagogue,** a medicine that stimulates menstrual functioning.

**emmenia,** the menstrual flow.

**emmenic,** pertaining to the menses.

**emmeniopathy,** any menstrual dysfunction.

**emmetropic,** normal vision.

**emollient,** an agent that softens and soothes the skin.

**emotion,** a mental state or strong feeling accompanied by physical bodily changes; any intense state of mind such as hate, love, anger, joy, or grief which precipitates physiological changes.

**empathy,** an attempt to identify one's feelings with those of another; having understanding and recognition of another's feelings.

**emphysema,** a distention caused by accumulated air in tissues or organs; pulmonary emphysema, a disease of the lungs due to overdistention of lung tissues and atrophic changes such as loss of elasticity and thinning of lung tissues.

**emphysematous,** pertaining to emphysema.

**empiric,** based on experience and observation.

**empirical,** pertaining to empiric, or based on experience.

**Empirin,** trademark for acetylsalicylic acid, phenacetin, and caffeine combined in a tablet used as an analgesic and antipyretic compound.

**empyema,** accumulation of pus in certain cavities of the body such as the chest cavity.

**emulsify,** to make into an emulsion.

**emulsion,** a mixture of two liquids not mutually soluble, one being divided into droplets and dispersed throughout the other.

**enamel,** the hardest substance in the body forming a white, dense covering for the crown of the teeth.

**enanthesis,** a skin eruption or rash originating from internal disorders or diseases.

**enarthritis,** inflammation of a ball-and-socket joint.

**enarthrosis,** any ball-and-socket joint.

**encanthis,** a new growth at the inner angle of the eye.

**encelialgia,** abdominal pain; belly-ache.

**endoderm,** inner layer of cells of an embryo.

**endosteitis,** inflammation of the medullary cavity of a bone.

**endosteum,** the membrane lining the medullary cavity of the bone which contains the marrow.

**endothelial,** pertaining to the endothelium.

**endothelioma,** a malignant growth of the endothelial lining of blood vessels.

**endothelium,** a lining formed of epithelial cells which line the blood and lymphatic vessels, heart, and the serous body cavities.

**endothermy,** surgical diathermy.

**endotoscope,** an instrument to examine the ear; and ear speculum.

**endotoxin,** bacterial toxin present within the body of a bacterium, liberated only when the bacterium disintegrates.

**end plate,** the terminal mass of a motor nerve ending which joins a skeletal muscle fiber.

**enema,** introduction of water or solution into the rectum and colon to evacuate the contents of the lower intestines, or as a means of introducing nutrients or medicine for therapeutic purposes.

**energy,** having the ability to work or take part in any activity.

**enervation,** weakness; lack of energy or strength.

**engorged,** distended with blood.

**engorgement,** the state of being engorged or distended; vascular congestion.

**engram,** the lasting impression of a physical experience upon nerve cells.

**enomania,** a craving for alcohol; delirium tremens.

**enophthalmus, -mos,** recession of the eyeball into its orbit.

**ensiform,** sword-like structure of the lower part of the sternum.

**enstrophe,** turning inward, especially of the eyelids.

**enteral,** pertaining to the small intestine.

**enteralgia,** pain in the intestines; colic or intestinal cramps.

**enterectomy,** surgical excision of part of the intestines.

**enteric,** pertaining to the intestines.

**enteric fever,** typhoid fever.

**enteritis,** inflammation of the intestines, usually of the small intestines.

**enterocele,** intestinal hernia; posterior vaginal hernia.

**enterocinesia,** movement of the intestines; peristalsis.

**enterococcus,** any streptococcus found in the intestines of man.

**enterocolitis,** inflammation of the intestines and colon.

**enterocolostomy,** surgical joining of the small intestine to the colon.

**enteroenterostomy,** surgical joining between two segments of the intestine after a diseased portion has been excised.

**enterogastritis,** inflammation of the intestines and of the stomach.

**enterogenous,** originating in the intestines.

**enterohepatitis,** inflammation of both large and small intestines and the liver.

**enterlith,** an intestinal calculus.

**enterology,** the study of the large and small intestines.

**enteromegalia, enteromegaly,** abnormal enlargement of the intestines.

**enteron,** the alimentary canal with specific reference to the small intestine.

**enteropathy,** referring to intestinal diseases.

**enteroplasty,** surgical plastic repair of the intestine.

**enteroplegia,** paralysis occurring in the intestines.

**enterospasm,** painful peristaltic movement in the intestines; resembling colic.

**enterostenosis,** narrowing of the intestine; a stricture.

**enterostomy,** creating a permanent opening into the intestine through the abdominal wall by a surgical procedure.

**entoderm,** see endoderm.

**entopic,** pertaining to the eyeball.

**entoptoscopy,** examining the interior of the eye.

**entropion,** turning inward of the edges of the lower eyelid.

**enucleate,** to remove the entire tumor or structure without rupturing; to remove the nucleus of a cell.

**enuresis,** being incontinent, involuntary complete or partial discharge of urine.

**environment,** external surroundings which influence an organism.

**enzygotic,** developing from the same ovum.

**enzyme,** a complex colloidal substance produced by living cells which induces chemical changes in another substance without being changed; a catalyst in the metabolism of organisms.

**enzymology,** the science that studies enzymes and enzymatic activity.

**eonism,** sexual perversion, as in transvestism of the male.

**eosin,** an acid dye used for diagnostic purposes and microscopic examination.

**eosinophil,** a cellular structure that stains readily with eosin dye.

**epencephalon,** the anterior portion of the embryonic hindbrain which develops into the pons and cerebellum.

**ependyma,** membrous lining of cerebral ventricles and the spinal cord's central canal.

**ephedrine,** an alkaloid, usually produced synthetically, known for its therapeutic properties as a bronchodilator in treatment of asthma, and for its constricting effects on the nasal passages in colds.

**epicardia,** the abdominal part of the esophagus which extends from the diaphragm to the stomach.

**epicardiac,** pertaining to the epicardium.

**epicardium,** the visceral layer of the pericardium which forms a serous membrane surrounding the outer layer of the heart wall.

**epicranium,** soft section covering the cranium.

**epicritic,** extreme sensitivity of the skin in discriminating between varying degrees of sensation produced by touch or temperature.

**epidemic,** infectious disease affecting many people at the same time and in the same region; a contagious disease widely diffused and quickly spreading and of high morbidity.

**epidemiology,** the study of epidemic diseases.

**epidermal,** pertaining to the epidermis.

**epidermatoplasty,** grafting with pieces of skin.

**epidermis,** outer layer of skin.

**epidermitis,** inflammation of the epidermis.

**epididymis,** a small, oblong structure resting upon and beside the posterior section of the testes.

**epididymitis,** inflammation of the epididymis.

**epidural space,** outside of the dura matter of the brain or spinal cord.

**epigastric,** the upper region of the abdomen, pertaining to the epigastrium.

**epigastrium,** region over the pit of the stomach or belly.

**epiglottis,** the thin, lid-like structure behind the posterior section of the tongue which covers the entrance of the larynx when swallowing.

**epilation,** removal of hair by the roots.

**epilepsy,** an episodic disturbance of the brain function characterized by a loss of consciousness, sensory disturbance, and generalized convulsions; three major types of epilepsy are: grand mal, petit mal, and focal seizures.

**epileptic,** one who is afflicted with epilepsy.

**epileptoid,** resembling or similar to epilepsy.

**epimysium,** a fibrous sheath of connective tissue surrounding the skeletal muscle.

**epinephrine,** a hormone produced by the adrenal medulla which is a powerful stimulant of the sympathetic nervous system, and a potent vasopressor which acts on the cardiovascular system and stimulates the myocardium to increase cardiac output; other medicinal uses include increasing metabolic activity, relaxing bronchioles in treatment of asthma, and inducing uterine contractions.

**epinephritis,** inflammation of the adrenal gland.

**epineurium,** the connective tissue sheath around the trunk of a nerve.

**epiphora,** abnormal excessive flow of tears.

**epiphylaxis,** to increase defensive powers within the body.

**epiphyseal,** pertaining to an epiphysis.

**epiphysis,** the end part of a juvenile long bone separated by cartilage from the main shaft but which later becomes a part of the larger bone through ossification.

**epiphysitis,** inflammation of an epiphysis, mostly of the hip, knee, and shoulder in infants.

**epiploic,** pertaining to the omentum.

**episiotomy,** surgical cutting of the vaginal opening to avoid the tearing of tissues in childbirth.

**epistasis,** a substance which rises to the surface like scum instead of sinking; the checking of a discharge; in heredity, a presence of a determining gene which prevents another gene not allelomorphic to it from expressing itself.

**epistaxis,** hemorrhage from the nose.

**episternum,** upper part of the sternum.

**epithelial,** pertaining to the epithelium.

**epithelioma,** malignant tumor consisting of epithelial cells; a carcinoma.

**epithelium,** the cellular layer forming the epidermis of the skin and internal and external covering of mucous and serous membranes.

**equilibrium,** a balance between opposing forces.

**equivalent,** equal in force or value.

**erection,** a distended state of an organ or part, especially in erectile tissue when filled with blood; becoming rigid.

**erector,** muscle that raises another part.

**eremophobia,** morbid fear of being alone.

**erepsin,** an enzyme found in intestinal juice which causes a peptide-splitting action.

**erethism,** excessive irritability or excitement.

**ereuthrophobia,** morbid fear of blushing.

**ergograph,** a device for recording muscle contractions and measuring the amount of work done.

**ergonovine,** an alkaloid derived from ergot, also produced synthetically; used to prevent hemorrhage after childbirth and to relieve migraine.

**ergophobia,** abnormal dread of working.

**ergosterol,** found in animal and plant tissues, and also derived from yeast, ergot, and other fungi; resembles cholesterol, and may be converted into Vitamin D by ultraviolet radiation.

**ergot,** a drug derived from fungi used to cause contractions of the uterus and control hemorrhage after childbirth.

**ergotamine,** a crystalline substance derived from ergot, used to treat migraine and to stimulate uterine contractions.

**ergotism,** poisoning resulting from excessive use of ergot, or from infected rye or wheat by fungus Claviceps purpurea, producing symptoms marked by spasms, cramps, or dry gangrene.

**erogenous,** sexual excitability; producing sexual desire.

**eroticism,** excessive libido; a condition of intense but normal sexual desire.

**erotomania,** abnormal, unrestrained libido.

**erotopathia,** any perverted sexual impulse.

**erotophobia,** an aversion to sexual love.

**erubescence,** a reddening of the skin, as in blushing.

**eructation,** bringing up of gas from the stomach; belching.

**eruption,** the appearance of a skin rash which accompanies a disease such as measles; the breaking through of a tooth through the gum.

**erysipelas,** an infectious disease of the skin due to infection with Streptococcus pyogenes characterized by fever and vesicular and bulbous lesions.

**erysipeloid,** a contagious dermatitis resembling erysipelas.

**erythema,** unusual redness of the skin caused by capillary congestion, resulting from inflammation, as in heat or sunburn.

**erythrism,** unusual redness of hair with a ruddy-colored skin.

**erythroblast,** a nucleated cell which possesses hemoglobin; the precursor of the erythrocyte.

**erythrocyte,** a mature red blood corpuscle, or cell.

**erythrocythemia,** an increase in the number of erythrocytes in the blood.

**erythrocytosis,** an abnormal increase in the number of red blood corpuscles.

**erythrodermia, erythroderma,** abnormal redness of the skin over a large area.

**erythromycin,** an antibiotic effective against many gram-positive organisms, used in treating amoebic and other diseases.

**erythropoiesis,** producing red blood corpuscles.

**eschar,** a sloughing or crusting which forms on the skin after cauterization or a burn.

**esophagismus,** spasms of the esophagus.

**esophagitis,** inflammation of the esophagus.

**esophagoscope,** a device used to examine the esophagus.

**esophagus,** the muscular canal extending from the pharynx to the stomach, approximately 9 inches in length.

**esophoria,** a tendency for the visual lines to converge.

**esophoric,** pertaining to esophoria.

**esotropia,** a marked turning inward of one eye toward that of the other causing crossed eyes.

**ester,** the combination of an organic acid with an alcohol; esters usually have fruity or flowery odors in liquid form.

**esterase,** an enzyme that catalyzes the hydrolysis of esters.

**esthesioneurosis,** loss of feeling in a body part without any apparent organic lesion.

**estradiol,** a hormone found in the ovary with estrogenic properties used in treatment of estrogen deficiency.

**estriol,** a hormone found in the urine of pregnant women.

**estrogen,** an estrogenic hormone produced by the ovarian follicle and other structures, responsible for the development of secondary female characteristics and changes in the epithelium of the vagina and the endothelium of the uterus; the natural estrogens include estradiol, estrone, and estriol.

**estrone,** a female sex hormone found in urine of pregnant women, used in the treatment of estrogen deficiencies.

**estrum, estrus,** the recurrent period of sexual receptivity in mammals called ''heat.''

**ether anesthetic,** a thin, colorless, highly volatile, and highly inflammable liquid widely used for general anesthesia and having a great margin of safety.

**ethmoid,** sievelike, cribriform plate which forms the nasal fossae and part of the floor of the skull.

**ethmoidal,** pertaining to the ethmoid bone.

**ethmoidectomy,** surgical removal of ethmoid cells.

**ethmoiditis,** inflammation of the ethmoidal cells causing headache, pain between the eyes, and nasal discharge.

**ethmoid sinus,** air spaces inside the ethmoid bone.

**etiology,** the study of any of the causes of diseases or abnormal body states.

**eucalyptus,** an oily substance derived from fresh plant leaves used as an expectorant and antiseptic.

**eugenics,** the scientific study of inheritance and the improvement of the human offspring.

**eunuch,** one with testicles removed; castrated male.

**euphoria,** feeling of mild elation and a sense of well-being.

**euplastic,** healing quickly and organizing well, as in tissue repair.

**eupnea,** normal respiration.

**eupraxic,** normal functioning.

**eustachian tube,** the auditory tube that connects the middle ear with the pharynx.

**eustachitis,** inflammation of the eustachian tube.

**euthanasia,** known as mercy killing; the ending of life for those who have an incurable disease or condition.

**evacuant,** an agent which promotes evacuation; cathartic.

**evacuate,** to discharge or expel, especially from the bowels.

**evacuation,** the process of evacuating.

**evagination,** the protrusion of an organ or part of an organ from its natural place.

**eversion,** a turning inside out, or turning outward.

**evert,** to turn outward; to turn inside out.

**evisceration,** the removal of viscera, contents of a cavity, or internal organs.

**evolution,** a developmental process from a rudimentary to a more complex state.

**evulsion,** a forcible extraction, or the act of tearing away of a part.

**exacerbation,** an increase in the severity of symptoms in a disease.

**exaltation,** a state of mind characterized by excessive or abnormal feelings of joy, optimism, elation, self-importance, or personal well-being.

**examination,** the process of inspecting the body and its products as a means of diagnosing a disease or as to physical fitness.

**exanthema,** any eruptive disease accompanied by inflammation of the skin, fever, or rash, as in measles or smallpox.

**exanthrope,** any cause of a disease originating externally.

**exarteritis,** inflammation of the outer coat of an artery.

**exarticulation,** amputation of a limb, or partial removal of a joint.

**excipient,** a substance such as jelly or sugar which is added to a drug to give it more consistency.

**excise,** to cut off or remove.

**excision,** the act of cutting out or removing, as in removing an organ or part of an organ.

**excitability,** susceptible to being stimulated.

**excitant,** an agent producing excitation of vital functions of the brain.

**excitation,** the condition of being excited, stimulated, or irritated.

**excitor,** a nerve which stimulates to greater activity.

**excoriate,** to abrade or wear off the surface of the skin or cuticle.

**excoriation,** the abrasion of the skin or the coating of an organ caused by disease or injury.

**excrement,** excreta, feces, or dejecta.

**excreta,** waste material expelled from the body.

**excretion,** the elimination of waste materials from the body.

**excretory,** pertaining to excretion.

**exenteration,** the surgical removal of the internal organs; evisceration.

**exercise,** physical exertion for health improvement; voluntary muscle activity.

**exfoliation,** the falling off of dead tissue in scales.

**exhalation,** breathing outward; the opposite of inhalation.

**exhaustion,** state of being extremely fatigued; weariness; the using up of a supply of something.

**exhibit,** to administer, as a drug or medicine; to show.

**exhibitionism,** an abnormal compulsion to expose the genitals to the opposite sex; a psychoneurosis.

**exhibitionist,** one with an abnormal impulse to exhibit the genitals to attract attention.

**exhumation,** disinterment of a body, or corpse.

**exocrine,** external secretion of a gland; excretion which reaches epithelial tissue or a duct.

**exodontia,** dentistry concerned with tooth extraction.

**exodontist,** one who practices exodontics.

**exoenzyme,** an enzyme that functions outside the cell which secretes it.

**exogastritis,** inflammation of the peritoneal coat of the stomach.

**exogenous,** originating outside an organ.

**exometritis,** inflammation of the peritoneal coat of the uterus.

**exophoria,** visual axes diverging outward.

**exophthalmia,** an abnormal protrusion of the eyeballs.

**exormia,** any skin rash.

**exoserosis,** an oozing or discharge of exudate.

**exostosis,** a bony growth projecting from the surface of a bone capped by cartilage.

**exoteric,** developing outside the body.

**exotoxin,** a toxin excreted by a microorganism into its surrounding medium.

**expectorant,** an agent having the quality of liquefying sputum or phlegm.

**expectoration,** ejecting or expelling mucus or phlegm from the lungs and throat; spitting.

**expiration,** the process of breathing out air from the lungs.

**expire,** to exhale; to die.

**exploration,** examining of an organ, part of an organ, or a wound by various means.

**exploratory,** pertaining to exploration.

**expulsion,** the act of expelling.

**exsanguinate,** to deplete of blood; bloodless;

**exsanguination,** the process of draining blood from a part.

**exsanguine,** anemic.

**exsection,** to cut out; excision.

**exsiccation,** the process of drying by heat.

**extima,** the outermost layer of blood vessels.

**extirpation,** to cut out totally; removal by the roots.

**extraction,** pulling out a tooth; the process of removing the active part of a drug.

**extrasystole,** an abnormal or premature contraction of part of the heart.

**extrauterine,** occurring outside the uterus.

**extravasate,** to escape into the tissues from a blood vessel.

**extravasation,** an escape of blood into the surrounding tissues; process of being extravasated.

**extravascular,** occurring outside a vessel.

**extremity,** a limb of the body; a terminal part of a structure.

**extrinsic,** originating externally.

**extroversion,** the direction of one's energy or attention turned outward from the self and toward objects.

**extrude,** to push out of a normal position.

**extrusion,** the process of being extruded, as in a tooth being pushed out of alignment.

**extubation,** removal of a tube.

**exudate,** the accumulation of fluid or pus in a cavity.

**exudation,** abnormal oozing of fluids, as in inflammatory conditions.

**eye,** the organ of vision; a globular structure consisting of three coats: the retina, uvea, and sclera with the cornea; the three layers enclose two cavities. The anterior cavity is divided by the iris into an anterior chamber and a posterior chamber which are filled with a watery aqueous humor. The cavity behind the lens is much larger in proportion and is filled with a jelly-like substance vitreous humor.

**eyebrow,** the ridge containing hair above the eye.

**eyedrops,** ophthalmic solutions for the treatment of eye disorders.

**eyeglass,** a lens for aiding impaired sight.

**eyelash,** a cilium or stiff hair on the edge of the eyelid.

**eyelid,** a movable protective fold of skin which covers the eyeball.

**eyesight,** having the ability to see.

**eyestrain,** fatigue of the eye due to excessive use or to an uncorrected visual defect.

**eyetooth,** a cuspid or upper canine tooth.

# F

**fabella,** small fibrocartilages which develop in the head of the large muscle of the leg, or gastrocnemius.

**face,** the anterior or front part of the head from the forehead to the chin.

**facet, facette,** a small smooth surface on a bone.

**facial,** pertaining to the face.

**facies,** a specific surface of an organ or body structure; face.

**faciocephalalgia,** a neuralgia affecting the face and head.

**facioplasty,** plastic surgery of the face.

**facioplegia,** facial paralysis resulting from a stroke, or injury.

**factitious,** artificial or not natural; contrived.

**faculty,** having the ability to function.

**faint,** syncope; to feel weak and about to lose consciousness; temporary loss of consciousness.

**fainting,** the loss of consciousness.

**falcate,** sickleshaped; hooked.

**fallectomy,** excision of part of the fallopian tube.

**fallopian tube,** one of two tubes or ducts which extend laterally from the uterus to the ovary, and that function to convey the ova from the ovary to the uterus.

**fallostomy,** a surgical procedure to create an opening of the fallopian tube.

**Fallot, tetralogy of,** stenosis of the pulmonary artery which is a congenital defect occurring in newborns.

**fallotomy,** surgical division of the fallopian tubes.

**false ribs,** the lower five ribs which are not directly attached to the sternum.

**falx,** a sickle-shaped structure.

**familial,** common to the same family.

**family,** members of a group descended from a common progenitor.

**fantasy,** mental images which satisfy unconscious wishes or desires.

**faradism,** an interrupted current of electricity used to stimulate muscles and nerves.

**farcy,** a form of glanders which is a contagious infection in animals that may be communicated to man.

**farsighted,** clarity of vision at a distance.

**fascia,** a fibrous membrane of connective tissue supporting, and separating muscles and body organs.

**fascicle, fasciculus,** a small bundle of muscle fibers or nerves; a synonym for tract.

**fasciectomy,** surgical removal of strips of fascia.

**fasciola,** a small group of nerve or muscle fibers.

**fascioplasty,** plastic repair on a fascia.

**fasciotomy,** surgical incision and separation of a fascia.

**fascitis,** inflammation of a fascia.

**fastidium,** aversion to eating.

**fastigium,** the highest point of the 4th ventricle of the brain; the period of maximum temperature during the development of acute, infectious diseases.

**fasting,** going without nourishment.

**fat,** obese; corpulent; oily consistency; a group of organic compounds composed of carbon, oxygen, and hydrogen.

**fatigue,** a feeling of weariness resulting from excessive mental or physical exertion; temporary loss of capacity to respond to stimulation.

**fauces,** a passage leading from the mouth to the pharynx or throat cavity.

**faucial,** pertaining to the fauces.

**faucitis,** inflammation of the fauces.

**faveolus,** a depression on the skin.

**favus,** a contagious skin disease which may spread all over the body and scalp which is characterized by yellowish crusts resembling honeycomb.

**febricula,** a mild fever of short duration.

**febrifacient,** fever producing.

**febrifuge,** an agent which lessens fever such as an antipyretic.

**febrile,** pertaining to a fever.

**fecal,** pertaining to feces.

**feces,** excreta, dejecta, stools; waste products of the body discharged through the anus.

**feculent,** containing feces; having sediment.

**fecundation,** fertilization; impregnation.

**fecundity,** having the ability to produce offspring.

**feeblemindedness,** mental deficiency.

**fellatio,** oral stimulation of the penis.

**felon,** a purulent infection of the deeper tissues of the distal phalanx of a finger.

**feminism,** having female characteristics by the male.

**feminization,** adopting female characteristics.

**femoral,** pertaining to the femur or the thigh bone.

**femur,** the thigh bone which extends from the hip to the knee.

**fenestra,** a window-like open area in the inner wall of the middle ear covered by a membrane.

**fenestration,** surgical operation creating an artificial opening into the labyrinth of the ear.

**fermentation,** decomposition of complex substances by the action of anaerobic microorganisms' enzymatic conversion.

**ferric,** pertaining to iron; containing iron.

**ferrotherapy,** therapeutic use of iron compounds.

**ferrous,** pertaining to iron.

**ferruginous,** containing the color of iron rust; pertaining to iron.

**fertile,** capable of reproduction.

**fertility,** the ability to produce offspring.

**fertilization,** fecundation; impregnation of a sperm cell and an ovum.

**fester,** to become suppurate.

**fetal,** pertaining to a fetus.

**fetalism,** the retention of fetal structures after delivery.

**fetation,** pregnancy.

**feticide,** intentional destruction of a fetus.

**fetid,** having an offensive or foul odor.

**fetish,** an object or body part which excites the libido or sexual interest.

**fetishism,** belief that an object has certain power, or it is symbolically endowed with special meaning, especially that of a beloved person; the attraction of an object is associated with libido gratification and sexual desire.

**fetor,** an offensive odor such as halitosis; stench.

**fetus,** the developing young in utero of humans from the eighth week after fertilization.

**fever,** an elevation of body temperature above 98.6°F; pyrexia; characteristic of a disease such as typhoid fever or yellow fever in which the body temperature is abnormally elevated.

**fiber,** a threadlike structure as in a nerve fiber; the axonal part of a neuron; in nutrition, pertaining to constituents found in a diet.

**fibra,** pertaining to a fiber.

**fibralbumin,** globulin.

**fibremia,** fibrin formation which causes embolism or thrombosis in the blood.

**fibril,** an extremely fine filament or fiber.

**fibrillar,** pertaining to fibrils.

**fibrillation,** elements composed of fibrils; a quivering of muscle fibers which are uncoordinated; rapid and tremulous action of the heart.

**fibrillolytic,** dissolution of fibrils.

**fibrin,** a whitish, elastic protein formed by the action of thrombin on fibrinogen which forms a network of red and white blood cells and platelets, causing a clot.

**fibrinogen,** a soluble protein in the blood which through the action of thrombin and calcium ions is converted into fibrin, responsible for the clotting of the blood.

**fibrinogenic, fibrogenous,** producing fibrin.

**fibrinolytic,** pertaining to the dissolution of fibrin.

**fibrinopenia,** a deficiency of fibrin and fibrinogen in the blood.

**fibroadenoma,** fibrous tissue adenoma, a benign tumor occurring in the breasts of young women.

**fibroangioma,** a fibrous tissue angioma, usually benign.

**fibroblast,** a cell from which connective tissue is developed.

**fibrocyst,** a fibrous tumor with cystic degeneration.

**fibrocystic,** consisting of fibrocysts.

**fibroid,** a fibroid tumor.

**fibroma,** a fibrous benign tumor, slow in growth.

**fibromatosis,** having multiple fibromas developing simultaneously.

**fibrosarcoma,** a malignant tumor consisting of connective tissue, primarily.

**fibrosis,** an abnormal fibrous tissue formation.

**fibrositis,** inflammation of white fibrous connective tissue anywhere in the body.

**fibrous,** resembling fibers.

**fibula,** the outer and smaller bone of the leg, or calf bone, connecting the ankle to the knee.

**fibulocaneal,** pertaining to the fibula and calcaneus.

**filaria,** a threadlike worm.

**filariasis,** a disease caused by a long filiform worm which may be found in the lymphatic ducts, circulatory system, and connective tissues of man, causing inflammation, fibrosis, or blockage of the lymph flow that results in edema.

**filtration,** passage of a liquid through a semipermeable membrane such as a filter.

**filum,** a threadlike structure.

**fimbria,** resembling fringe.

**finger,** a digit of the hand.

**first aid,** emergency treatment given to persons who have been injured in an accident or have an acute illness prior to regular medical care.

**first cranial nerve,** olfactory nerve.

**fissure,** a natural division, cleft, or furrow in body organs such as the brain; an ulcer; a crack or break in tooth enamel.

**fistula,** an abnormal passage or duct between two internal organs, or between an internal organ to the body surface.

**fistulous,** pertaining to a fistula.

**fit,** a sudden attack or convulsion.

**fixation,** holding in a fixed position; arresting psychosexual development at an early stage, often resulting from childhood trauma.

**flaccid,** absence of muscular tone; relaxed; flabby.

**flagellum,** hairlike processes on the extremities of protozoa and bacteria.

**flatfoot,** an abnormal flatness of the arch of the foot causing the sole to rest upon the ground.

**flatulence,** excessive gas in the stomach and the alimentary canal.

**flautus,** gas formed in the digestive tract and expelled through the anus.

**flavedo,** yellowish pigment of the skin; jaundice.

**fleam,** an instrument used in venesection.

**flection, flexion,** to bend, as in bending a limb.

**fletcherism,** excessive chewing of small amounts of food.

**flexibility,** being capable of being bent without breaking; adaptability.

**flexor,** a muscle that bends a joint.

**flexure,** a bend, or curvature to a structure.

**flight of ideas,** skipping from one idea to another in a continuous stream of talk.

**floaters,** visual spots caused by deposits in the vitreous of the eye, occurring as benign degenerative changes.

**floating kidney,** a kidney displaced from its normal position in the body.

**floating ribs,** the 11th and 12th ribs which do not directly connect with the sternum.

**flora,** normal bacteria living in the intestines or the skin of humans; plant life.

**fluid,** liquid; gaseous substance.

**fluid ounce,** eight fluidrams.

**fluidram,** measure of liquid capacity equal to one-eight part of a fluid ounce.

**fluke,** any of several parasitic worms in man.

**fluor albus,** a whitish discharge from the uterus or vagina; leukorrhea.

**fluorescein,** a red crystalline substance used in diagnostic examination of the eye to detect corneal lesions or foreign bodies.

**fluoridation,** addition of fluorides to drinking water as a means of preventing tooth decay.

**fluoride,** any binary compound of fluorine, especially with a radical.

**fluorine,** a gaseous, nonmetallic element found in the soil in combination with calcium which is important to plant and animal life.

**fluoroscope,** an apparatus that permits visual observation of the deep structures of the body on a fluorescent screen.

**fluoroscopy,** the use of a fluoroscope for medical examination and diagnosis.

**fluorosis,** chronic fluorine poisoning often caused by an excess of fluoride in drinking water.

**flush,** sudden reddening to the skin; blushing; flushing a body cavity or part with water.

**flutter,** a rapid pulsation or regular movement, especially of the heart.

**flux,** an excessive evacuation or discharge of fluid matter from the body or a cavity; diarrhea.

**focal,** pertaining to a focus.

**focus, foci,** point at which convergent light rays or sound waves intersect; that part of the body or organ in which a disease is localized.

**folic acid,** a B- vitamin important in the diet of humans used in treatment of pernicious and macrocytic anemia, and gastrointestinal disorders.

**follicle,** a small secretory cavity, sac, or gland.

**follicle-stimulating hormone,** a pituitary hormone that stimulates estrogen secretions and the production of Graafian follicles in the female; the follicle-stimulating hormone (FSH) in males stimulates the seminiferous tubules to produce sperm more rapidly.

**follicular,** pertaining to a follicle.

**folliculin,** the oophorin hormone produced by the ovarian follicles.

**folliculitis,** inflammation of a follicle.

**fomentation,** the application of heat and moisture to relieve pain or inflammation.

**fomes,** any material or substance on which infectious disease-producing agents may be transmitted.

**fontanel, fontenelle,** the soft spot of an infant's head lying between the cranial bones of the skull.

**food,** any nutritive taken into the body which provides a source of energy for physical activity, growth support, and maintenance of body tissue repair.

**food allergies,** allergic reactions to certain foods in one's diet caused by a sensitivity to one or more foods ingested; the most common foods that cause sensitivity are: eggs, lettuce, milk, spinach, strawberries, and tomatoes.

**food poisoning,** an acute digestive disorder due to ingesting foods which contain poisonous substances.

**foot,** the terminal part of a leg.

**foot-and-mouth disease,** Aphthous fever, a disease of cattle characterized by ulcers in the mouth, the hooves, teats, and udder, which can be transmitted to man.

**footdrop,** a condition in which the foot falls in a planter-flexed position caused by paralysis of flexor leg muscles.

**foramen,** an opening or communication between two cavities of an organ, or a perforation in a bone through which vessels or nerves pass.

**foramen magnum,** a perforation in the occipital bone through which the spinal cord unites with the medulla oblongata.

**foramen ovale,** an opening between the left and right cardiac atria that normally closes after birth.

**forceps,** a two-pronged instrument resembling a pair of tongs used for holding or extracting.

**forearm,** the section of the arm between elbow and wrist.

**forebrain,** the part of the brain which develops from the anterior portion of the embryonic brain, comprising the diencephalon and telencephalon.

**forehead,** the brow above the eyes.

**forensic medicine,** legal aspects of medicine.

**foreskin,** the fold of skin or prepuce which covers the glans of the penis.

**formaldehyde,** a pungent, colorless gas used in solution as a disinfectant, preservative, astringent, and fumigant.

**formalin,** an aqueous solution of formaldehyde with the addition of methanol.

**formication,** a creeping sensation as if ants were crawling upon the body; form of paresthesia.

**formula,** a prescription of ingredients with proportions in the preparation of medicine.

**formulary,** book of formulas.

**fornication,** voluntary sexual intercourse on the part of an unmarried person.

**fornix, fornices,** a vault-like band of a fibrous formation connecting the cerebral lobes; an arch-like space formed by such a structure.

**fossa,** a hollow or depressed area in the body.

**fossette,** a small, deep corneal ulcer; a small fossa.

**fourchet, fourchette,** a transverse fold of mucous membrane connecting the posterior ends of the labia minora which forms the margin of the vulva.

**fovea,** a small pit or depression, often indicating the central fovea of the retina.

**Fowler's position,** a semi-sitting position with the back rest elevated or the head of the patient placed on several pillows to relieve dyspnea.

**fracture,** a break or rupture, especially in a bone.

**fragilitas,** a brittleness or fragility.

**fragility,** state of being brittle or frail.

**fragmentation,** breaking into small pieces.

**fraternal twin,** derived from two separate fertilized ova.

**freckle,** a small, localized brownish spot on the skin, often due to exposure to the sun.

**fremitus,** palpation of vibratory tremors felt through the chest wall.

**frenum,** a membranous fold which connects two parts, one more or less restrained in movement, as in the underside of the tongue.

**frenzy,** state of violent mental agitation; wild excitement; delirium.

**Freudian,** pertaining to Sigmund Freud, founder of psychoanalysis, and to his theories regarding the causes and treatment of neurosis and psychosis.

**friable,** easily pulverized or broken down into crumbs.

**friction,** act of rubbing.

**frigidity,** usually applied to the inability to respond to sexual desire or sexual stimuli; coldness.

**frontal,** pertaining to the forehead or the bones forming the forehead.

**frontal lobe,** the anterior portion of the cerebral hemisphere, the cerebrum.

**frostbite,** damage occurring by the freezing of part of the body such as nose, fingers, or toes causing numbness.

**frottage,** rubbing; massage; sexual gratification by rubbing against a person of the opposite sex.

**frotteur,** one who practices frottage.

**fructose,** fruit sugar; levulose.

**FSH,** see follicle stimulating hormone.

**fugue,** physical flight from home on a hysterical impulse; a state of personality dissociation accompanied by amnesia.

**fulguration,** destruction of tissue by electricity.

**fulminating,** pain occurring with rapidity and severity.

**fumigation,** exposing to poisonous fumes or gases for the purpose of destroying living organisms such as vermin; disinfecting of rooms by gases.

**functional,** pertaining to function and not to structure.

**functional disease,** one not organic but in which there is a pathological alteration in the functioning of an organ.

**fundus,** referring to the base part or body of a hollow organ; the part most remote from its opening.

**fungicide,** a bactericide which destroys fungi.

**fungoid,** resembling fungus.

**fungus, fungi,** any of a group of eukaryotic protists such as yeasts, molds, or mushrooms that subsist on organic matter.

**funiculus,** small structure resembling a cord; small bundle of nerve fibers; umbilical or spermatic cord.

**funny bone,** outer part of the elbow where part of the ulnar nerve passes by the internal codyle of the humerus.

**furfur,** dandruff.

**furfuraceous,** resembling dandruff; flaky or scaling.

**furuncle,** a boil.

**furunculosis,** a condition marked by the presence of boils on the skin.

**fusiform,** spindle-like structures.

**Fusobacterium,** a genus of gram-negative anaerobic bacteria normally found in the mouth and large intestines, and in necrotic lesions.

**fusospirillosis,** Vincent's angina caused by fusiform bacilli and spirochetes.

# G

**gag,** a device to hold the mouth open; to retch or to cause to retch or vomit.

**gait,** a manner of moving on foot or walking.

**galactacrasia,** an abnormal condition occurring in the composition of milk from the breast.

**galactan,** a carbohydrate which forms galactose upon hydrolysis.

**galactemia,** an abnormal milky condition of the blood.

**galactic,** pertaining to flow of milk.

**galactidrosis,** sweat that appears milklike.

**galactischia,** suppression of the secreting ducts and the flow of milk.

**galactophore,** a milk duct.

**galactophoritis,** inflammation of a milk duct.

**galactorrhea,** excessive flow of milk after cessation of nursing.

**galactstasis,** cessation of breast milk secretion.

**galeophobia,** morbid aversion to cats.

**gall,** pertaining to the gallbladder bile.

**gallbladder,** a pear-shaped organ containing bile produced in the liver, located beneath the right lobe of the liver.

**gallstone,** a stonelike mass formed in the gallbladder or bile ducts.

**galvanism,** the use of direct electric current to the body for therapeutic purposes.

**galvanometer,** an apparatus that measures current strength using electromagnetic action.

**galvanopalpation,** the testing of nerve sensibility of the skin by galvanic current.

**galvanopuncture,** the use of needles to complete an electric current.

**galvanoscope,** a device which detects the direction of a galvanic current.

**gamete,** a male or female reproductive germ cell that unites to form an offspring; the spermatozoon or ovum.

**gametocyte,** an oocyte or spermatocyte.

**gametogenesis,** the formation of gametes.

**gamic,** sexual, especially as applied to eggs after fertilization.

**gamma globulin,** a blood protein containing antibodies, given by injection as a prophylactic measure against measles, poliomyelitis, and infectious hepatitis.

**gamma rays,** extremely short-wave length rays which penetrate radioactive material and reduce the cell nucleus; used in radiotherapy.

**gamogenesis,** sexual reproduction.

**gamophobia,** a psychoneurotic fear of being married.

**ganglial,** pertaining to a ganglion.

**gangliectomy, ganglionectomy,** surgical removal of a ganglion.

**ganglioma,** a tumor of a lymphatic gland; swelling which occurs in lymphoid tissue.

**ganglion,** a knot-like mass of nervous tissue consisting of nerve-cell bodies, located outside the brain or spinal cord; a cystic tumor which develops on a tendon, sometimes occurring on the back of the wrist due to strain.

**ganglionitis,** inflammation of a ganglion.

**gangrene,** necrosis or a gradual deterioration of an area of tissue resulting from interference of the blood supply to that part of the body.

**gargle,** a solution for washing the throat or mouth; to wash the mouth or throat by holding a liquid preparation in the mouth and agitating it with expired air from the lungs.

**gargoylism,** Hurler's syndrome, characterized by a form of dwarfism accompanied by mental deficiency, damaged vision, and grotesque facial features.

**garrot,** a form of tourniquet.

**gaseous,** having the nature of gas.

**gastralgia,** periodic pain in the stomach without gastric lesion.

**gastrectomy,** surgical removal of part or the whole of the stomach.

**gastric,** pertaining to the stomach.

**gastric ulcer,** a peptic ulcer of the stomach.

**gastrin,** a hormone secreted by the glands in the pyloric end of the stomach which stimulates the secretion of gastric acid and pepsin in the cardiac end of the stomach; it is a weak stimulant of pancreatic enzymes and gallbladder contraction.

**gastritis,** inflammation of the stomach mucous membranes.

**gastrocele,** hernia of the stomach.

**gastrocnemius,** the large muscle in the calf of the leg.

**gastrocolic,** pertaining to the colon and the stomach.

**gastrocolic reflex,** the peristaltic waves produced in the colon by the ingestion of food into an empty stomach.

**gastrocolitis,** inflammation of the stomach and colon.

**gastrocolostomy,** surgical joining of the stomach to the colon.

**gastroduodenal,** pertaining to the stomach and the duodenum.

**gastroduodenitis,** inflammation of the stomach and the duodenum.

**gastroenteric,** pertaining to the stomach and the intestine.

**gastroenteritis,** inflammation of the stomach and the intestine.

**gastroenteroptosis,** displacement downward of the stomach and the intestines.

**gastroenterostomy,** a surgical joining of the stomach wall to the small intestine.

**gastroesophageal,** pertaining to the stomach and the esophagus.

**gastrogavage,** feeding through a tube passed into the stomach.

**gastrointestinal,** pertaining to the stomach and the intestines.

**gastrojejunostomy,** surgical joining between the stomach and jejunum.

**gastrology,** the study of structures, functions, and diseases of the stomach.

**gastromalacia,** a softening of the walls of the stomach.

**gastronephritis,** inflammation of both the stomach and the kidneys at the same time.

**gastroparalysis,** paralysis of the stomach.

**gastropathy,** any disorder of the stomach.

**gastrophrenic,** referring to the stomach and the diaphragm.

**gastroplegia,** see gastroparalysis.

**gastroptosia,** abnormal falling of the stomach, usually involving the displacement of other organs.

**gastrorrhagia,** excessive bleeding from the stomach.

**gastroscope,** an instrument for examining the interior of the stomach.

**gastroscopy,** examination of the stomach and abdominal cavity with a gastroscope.

**gastrosia,** excessive secretion of hydrochloric acid in the stomach.

**gastrostaxis,** an oozing of blood from the mucosa of the stomach.

**gastrotomy,** incision of the abdominal or stomach wall.

**gatophobia,** fear of cats.

**gauze,** a thin fabric used as a bandage applied to wounds.

**gavage,** a tube passed through the nares, pharynx, and esophagus into the stomach for feeding purposes, or forced pumping of the stomach contents.

**gene,** a unit of heredity located at a specific position on a chromosome which determines characteristics in the offspring from a parent.

**generic,** pertaining to a genus of a drug name, not a trademark.

**genetic,** pertaining to the science of genetics; referring to genes.

**genetics,** the science concerned with individual differences of related organisms and the study of heredity.

**genial,** pertaining to the chin.

**genicular,** pertaining to the knee.

**geniculate,** bent as a knee; pertaining to the ganglion of the facial nerve.

**genitals, genitalia,** organs of the reproductive system, especially the external organs.

**genitourinary,** pertaining to the genital and urinary organs.

**genotype,** the basic hereditary constitution of the individual in a combination of genes.

**gentian violet,** a dye derived from coal tar used as a stain in bacteriology, cystology, and histology; therapeutic uses include an anti-infective and an anthelmintic agent.

**genupectoral position,** knee-chest position.

**genu varum,** bowleg.

**genyplasty,** plastic surgery on the chin.

**geotragia,** practice of eating earth, clay, or chalk.

**gereology,** the science concerned with old age.

**geriatrics,** the branch of medicine concerned with the problems and diseases of aging.

**germ,** a microorganism that causes disease; an early embryonic stage.

**German measles,** rubella, a viral infection with a rash and fever of short duration.

**germicide,** an agent destructive to germs.

**germinal,** pertaining to a germ or reproductive cells, egg or sperm; germination.

**germinal disk,** blastoderm, or disk of cells from which the embryo develops.

**germination,** the stage of development of an impregnated ovum into an embryo.

**germ layer,** one of three embryonic layers of cells: ectoderm, endoderm, mesoderm.

**gerontology,** the scientific study of the aging process.

**gestation,** period of fetal development in the womb.

**gestosis,** any disorder of pregnancy such as toxemia.

**giantism, gigantism,** abnormal growth or development of the body or its parts.

**giddiness,** dizziness, vertigo, or a sensation of reeling.

**gingivitis,** inflammation of the gums.

**girdle,** an area around the waist; cingulum; a structure which resembles a belt or band.

**glabella,** the flat surface of the frontal bone or the area of the face between the eyebrows.

**glabrous,** smooth and bald.

**gland,** specialized secretory cells in a structure or organ; a gland may be ductless or endocrine whose secretions directly enter the blood or lymph system, or a gland maybe exocrine, having ducts which transport the secretions to an epithelial surface.

**glanders,** a contagious disease found in horses which is communicable to man.

**glandular,** consisting of, or pertaining to glands.

**glans,** bulbous end of the penis; head of the clitoris; goiter; a gland.

**Glauber's salt,** a crystalline salt used as a purgative.

**glaucoma,** an eye disease characterized by increased intraocular pressure resulting in degeneration of the optic nerve and gradual loss of vision.

**gleet,** a purulent discharge from the urethra resulting from chronic gonorrhea.

**glenoid,** resembling a socket.

**gliadin,** a protein found in the gluten of wheat or rye.

**glial,** pertaining to glia or neuroglia.

**glioma,** a tumor consisting predominantly of neuroglia.

**globin,** a protein formed from hemoglobin.

**globulin,** a simple protein insoluble in water.

**globus hystericus,** a sensation of a lump in the throat occurring in hysteria or other neuroses.

**glomerulitis,** inflammation of the glomeruli.

**glomerulonephritis,** nephritis with inflammation of the capillary loops in the renal glomeruli which may frequently follow other infections.

**glomerulus,** a small rounded mass of capillary loops eclosed within the Bowman's capsule of a renal tubule and which serves as a filter in the formation of urine.

**glossa,** tongue.

**glossal,** pertaining to the tongue.

**glossitis,** inflammation of the tongue.

**glottis,** an opening at the upper part of the trachea and between the vocal cords responsible for the modulation of the voice; the vocal apparatus of the larynx.

**glucagon,** a hormone secreted by the alpha cells of the islets of Langerhans in the pancreas which functions in response to hypoglycemia and to stimulate the growth hormone.

**glucogenic,** producing glucose.

**glucohemia,** sugar in the blood.

**glucose,** a monosaccharide or dextrose found in certain foods such as nuts; an end product in the metabolism of carbohydrates and the chief source of energy for the body.

**glucosuria,** excessive amount of sugar in the urine.

**glutamic acid,** an amino acid formed in the hydrolysis of proteins; in the form of monosodium glutamate it is used as a salt substitute.

**gluteal,** pertaining to the buttocks, or gluteal muscles.

**gluten,** protein found in cereals and bread.

**glycemia,** sugar or glucose present in the urine.

**glycerin,** a clear, syrupy liquid, soluble in alcohol and water, used in medication preparation.

**glycerol,** transparent, syrupy liquid formed by hydrolysis of fats.

**glycine,** a crystalline amino acid derived from gelatin and from other proteins.

**glycogen,** a storage form of carbohydrate found in the liver and muscles.

**glycogenesis,** the formation of glycogen from glucose in the body.

**glycolysis,** the breakdown of carbohydrates in living organisms by enzymatic action.

**glycolytic,** pertaining to the hydrolysis of sugar.

**glyconeogenesis,** formation of carbohydrates from fat or protein.

**glycosemia,** excessive sugar in the blood.

**glycoside,** a substance derived from plants which hydrolyze into sugars.

**glycosuria,** sugar in the urine.

**gnathalgia,** pain in the jaw.

**gnathitis,** inflammation of the jaw.

**goiter,** an enlargement of the thyroid gland causing a swelling to the front part of the neck.

**gomphosis,** a conical process which is inserted into a socket in an immovable joint.

**gonad,** female or male reproductive gland that produces gametes; the sex glands in the embryo before differentiation.

**gonadal,** pertaining to a gonad.

**gonadotrophin,** gonad-stimulating hormone.

**gonarthritis,** inflammation of knee joint.

**gonococcus,** organism causing gonorrhea, Neisseria gonorrhoeae.

**gonorrhea,** a contagious, catarrhal disease of the genital mucous membranes of both males and females.

**gonorrheal,** pertaining to gonorrhea.

**goose flesh,** erection of skin papilae resulting from exposure to cold, shock, or fear.

**gout,** a metabolic disease characterized by acute arthritis and inflammation of the great toe, diagnosed by excessive accumulation of uric acid in the bloodstream.

**graft,** a section of skin, muscle, bone, or nerve tissue inserted into a similar substance by surgical means.

**gram,** basic unit of mass, equivalent to 15.432 grains.

**gramicidin,** an antibiotic obtained from soil bacillus, effective against gram-positive bacteria.

**gram-positive,** pertaining to organisms that will retain the gentian violet color when stained; gram-negative organisms will not retain the violet color when stained.

**Gram's method,** a method for staining organisms for identification under a microscope.

**grand mal,** severe epileptic attack characterized by convulsions, stupor, and temporary loss of consciousness.

**granulation,** new tissue formed in the process of healing; granular projections formed on the surface of an open wound.

**granule,** a very small grainlike body or structure.

**granulocyte,** a white blood cell or granular leukocyte.

**granuloma,** a granular growth consisting of epithelial and lymph cells which occur in diseases such as leprosy, yaws, and syphilis.

**granulomatosis,** multiple granulomas.

**granulose,** soluble part of starch.

**graphobia,** unusual fear of writing.

**graphorrhea,** the writing of meaningless words or phrases.

**gravel,** small calculi of crystalline dust which form in the kidneys or bladder.

**gravid,** being pregnant.

**gravida,** a pregnant woman.

**gray matter,** a grayish color nervous tissue; the term is applied to the gray portions of the central nervous system which include the cerebral cortex, basal ganglia, brain nuclei, and the gray spinal cord columns.

**green sickness,** anemia found in adolescent girls resulting from a poor diet.

**gripe, grippe,** sudden onset of an infectious disease characterized by fever, fatigue, headache, back pain, and phlegm from the respiratory tract.

**gripes,** severe intermittent pain in the bowels.

**gristle,** cartilage.

**groin,** the hollow on either side of the body between thigh and trunk; inguinal region.

**growth,** to develop or increase in size; abnormal cell or tissue growth, as in a tumor.

**gullet,** the esophagus; passage to the stomach.

**gum,** fleshy tissue covering the jaws' alveolar parts and the necks of the teeth.

**gumboil,** a gum abscess.

**gumma,** a soft tumor characteristic of the tertiary stage of syphilis.

**gustation,** taste sensation stimulated by gustatory nerve endings in the tongue.

**gustatory,** pertaining to sense of taste.

**gut,** bowel; intestine.

**gutta,** a drop.

**guttate,** a drop-like spot, as in certain skin lesions.

**guttur,** throat.

**guttural,** pertaining to the throat.

**gymnophobia,** unusual aversion to looking at a naked body.

**gynecologist,** a specialist in gynecology, or who specializes in diseases of women.

**gynecology,** the science of the diseases of women, especially of the genital, urinary, or rectal organs.

**gynecomania,** abnormal sexual desire in the male.

**gynecomastia,** unusually large breasts in the male.

**gynephobia,** aversion to female companionship.

**gyrus,** one of the ridges or convolutions of the cerebral hemisphere of the brain.

# H

**habit,** a pattern or action which becomes automatic following constant repetition; a predisposition or characteristic of a person's mental makeup; clothing characteristic of a function, as a priest; bodily temperature; an addiction to drug, alcohol, or tobacco usage.

**habit chorea or spasm,** voluntary spasmodic movement of muscles that has become involuntary, as blinking of the eyes, coughing, or scratching.

**habitual,** acting in a repeated manner from force of habit.

**habitus,** attitude or physical appearance that indicates a tendency to certain diseases or abnormal conditions.

**hachement,** massaging with chopping strokes with the edge of the hands.

**hacking,** strokes with the edge of the hand.

**hair,** threadlike outgrowth from the skin.

**hairball,** a mass of hair in the stomach.

**halation,** blurring of vision due to a strong light shining in one's eyes from the direction of the object being viewed.

**halazone,** a disinfectant for drinking water.

**Haldol,** trademark for haloperidol, a psychotropic drug used in treatment of psychosis.

**half-life,** the time in which the radioactive atoms associated with an isotope are reduced by half through decay.

**halisteresis,** the lack of calcium in bones.

**halitosis,** foul or offensive breath.

**halitus,** exhalation of vapor; the breath.

**hallucination,** false sensory perception in the absence of an actual external cause.

**hallucinogen,** a chemical substance or narcotic used to produce fantastic visions and hallucinations.

**hallucinogenic,** pertaining to a hallucinogen.

**hallucinosis,** an abnormal condition marked by persistent hallucinations.

**hallux,** the great toe.

**hallux flexus,** see hammer toe.

**hallux valgus,** great toe displacement toward other toes.

**hallux varus,** great toe displacement away from other toes.

**halogen,** any of the group of elements astatine, bromine, chlorine, flourine, and iodine which form salt when combined with metal.

**haloid,** resembling salt in composition.

**halothane,** used as a general anesthetic.

**ham,** the region behind the knee; commonly used for buttock, hip, or thigh in which the hamstring muscles are located.

**hamartoma,** a benign tumor composed of a new growth of mature cells on existing blood vessels; a tumor resulting from faulty development of the embryo.

**hammer,** common name for malleus, a bone in the middle ear.

**hammer toe,** deformity of the toe due to abnormal dorsal flexion.

**hamstring,** one of three muscles on the posterior part of the thigh which flex the leg and adduct and extend the thigh.

**hamulus,** a hooked-shaped structure.

**hand,** terminal part of the arm attached to the wrist.

**hangnail,** a partly detached piece of skin at the base or side of the fingernail.

**haphalgesia,** sensation of pain when touching objects.

**haphephobia,** an aversion to being touched by others.

**haploid,** having half the normal number of chromosomes following the division of germ cells in gametogenesis.

**hairlip,** a congenital defect resulting from faulty fusion of the vertical fissure of the upper lip, often involving the palate; cleft lip.

**haunch,** hips and buttocks.

**haut-mal,** grand mal seizure at its height.

**hay fever,** an allergy to air-borne pollens marked by inflammation of mucous membranes of the nose and upper air passages, catarrh, watery eyes, headache, asthmatic symptoms, and other symptoms similar to a head cold.

**head,** caput; the part of the body above the neck containing the brain.

**headache,** diffused pain in the head.

**heal,** to cure or restore to health; to make whole.

**healing,** the process of restoring to a normal or improved condition.

**health,** a state of having a sound or active body and mind; a sense of well-being and the absence of disease.

**healthy,** enjoying or being in a state of good health.

**hearing,** the ability to perceive sound.

**hearing aid,** a small device to amplify sound waves for those with impaired hearing.

**heart,** a hollow muscular organ that maintains the circulation of blood throughout the body, consisting of four chambers: the lower chambers are the left and right ventricles and the upper chambers are the left and right auricles.

**heart attack,** a sudden decrease in the flow of blood to the heart muscle resulting in impaired heart functioning often caused by an embolism or by chronic high blood pressure.

**heart block,** an impairment of the conductile tissue of the heart, specifically the S-A node, A-V node, bundle of His, and Purkinje fibers which fail to conduct normal impulses resulting in altered heart rhythm.

**heartburn,** a sensation of burning in the esophagus behind the lower part of the sternum, sometimes accompanied by an acid-tasting liquid in the mouth.

**heart disease,** any pathological or abnormal condition of the heart.

**heart failure,** an inability of the heart to maintain sufficient circulation resulting in cessation of the heart beat.

**heart-lung machine,** an apparatus through which the circulation of the blood is maintained and oxygenated while the heart is opened during surgery.

**heart murmur,** an abnormal heart sound which is detected by a stethoscope, usually indicating either a functional or structural defect.

**heat,** a warm sensation; high temperature; a form of energy; sexual excitement in lower animals; to make hot.

**heat exhaustion,** a condition caused by prolonged exposure to high temperatures combined with fatigue; characterized by dizziness, faintness, nausea, sweating, and general weakness.

**heatstroke,** a condition due to excessive exposure to high temperatures or the sun, occurs especially with those who are debilitated or who have been drinking alcoholic beverages, resulting in symptoms of dizziness, nausea, weakness, spots before the eyes, ringing in the ears, reddened and dry skin, rapid pulse, and collapse.

**hebephrenia,** a schizophrenic disorder characterized by disorganized thinking, regressive behavior, giggling, hypochondrial complaints, and bizarre delusions and hallucinations.

**hebephrenic,** pertaining to hebephrenia.

**hebetic,** pertaining to puberty.

**hebetude,** mental slowness; dullness.

**hebosteotomy,** an enlargement of the pelvic diameter by surgery to facilitate delivery.

**hectic fever,** a fever that occurs with an organic disease such as pulmonary tuberculosis or kidney or liver abcess.

**hedonism,** preoccupation with pleasure.

**helcoid,** resembling an ulcer.

**helicoid,** resembling a helix or spiral.

**heliencephalitis,** inflammation of the brain due to sunstroke.

**heliotherapy,** therapeutic application of sunlight in treatment of disease.

**helix,** the whole circuit of the external ear structure.

**helminth,** worm-like animal including flatworms, spiney-headed worms, threadworms or roundworms, and segmented or tapeworms.

**helminthiasis,** the presence of parasitic worms.

**helminthic,** pertaining to worms; that which expels worms.

**helminthicide,** a worm-expelling agent.

**helminthology,** the study of intestinal parasitic worms.

**helminthophobia,** a pathological dread of worms, or delusion of being infested by worms.

**heloma,** callosity, or corn.

**helosis,** having corns.

**helotomy,** removal of corns by surgery.

**hemacytometer, hemocytometer,** an apparatus for counting blood corpuscles.

**hemadostenosis,** contraction of blood vessels.

**hemal,** pertaining to the blood or blood vessels.

**hemangioma,** a tumor consisting of blood vessels.

**hemarthrosis,** the effusion of blood into a joint.

**hematemesis,** the vomiting of blood.

**hematherapy,** the infusion of fresh blood in the treatment of disease.

**hematic,** referring to blood; a treatment for anemia.

**hematidrosis,** excreting bloody sweat.

**hematimeter,** an apparatus used in counting blood corpuscles in a cu. mm. of blood.

**hematin,** the reddish iron-containing pigment of hemoglobin.

**hematinic,** pertaining to blood; a medicine which increases the hemoglobin level in the blood.

**hematinuria,** hematin in the urine.

**hematocolpos,** blood accumulation in the vagina.

**hematocrit,** a centrifugal apparatus used to determine the percentage of red blood cells in whole blood; the volume percentage of erythrocytes or red blood cells in blood.

**hematodyscrasis,** pathological blood condition.

**hematogenesis,** the formation of blood corpuscles.

**hematogenous,** produced by the blood; disseminated by means of the blood stream.

**hematology,** the branch of medicine concerned with blood diseases.

**hematoma,** a swelling of blood which occurs in an organ or tissue resulting from ruptured blood vessels.

**hematometra,** hemorrhage in the uterus.

**hematomyelia,** hemorrhage of blood into the spinal cord.

**hematoperitoneum,** effusion of blood into the peritoneal cavity.

**hematophobia,** abnormal fear of the sight of blood.

**hematopoiesis,** formation of red blood cells.

**hematorrhea,** profuse bleeding.

**hematosalpinx,** retained menstrual flow in the fallopian tube.

**hematoscopy,** blood examination.

**hematosis,** the development of red blood cells in the formation of blood; blood oxygenation in the lungs.

**hematospermia,** bloody semen.

**hematostatic,** arresting the flow of blood in a hemorrhage; retaining blood in a part.

**hematothorax,** presence of blood in the chest cavity.

**hematozoon,** a parasitic organism in the blood.

**hematuria,** blood in the urine.

**heme,** hematin.

**hemeralopia,** day blindness; difficulty in seeing during the day.

**hemialgia,** pain in one-half of the body.

**hemic,** pertaining to blood.

**hemicrania,** affecting one side of the head, usually a migraine headache.

**hemiplegia,** paralysis affecting one side of the body.

**hemisphere,** either of two sides of the cerebellum or cerebrum.

**hemispheric,** pertaining to a hemisphere.

**hemocytoblastoma,** a tumor consisting of embryonic blood cells.

**hemocytology,** the scientific study of blood cells.

**hemocytometer,** an instrument used to determine the number of blood cells in the blood.

**hemoglobin,** the red oxygen-carrying pigment of red blood cells.

**hemolysin,** an agent or substance in a serum which dissolves red blood corpuscles.

**hemolysis,** destruction of red blood corpuscles with the liberation of hemoglobin.

**hemophilia,** an inherited blood disease of males characterized by defective coagulation and an abnormal tendency to bleed.

**hemophiliac,** a person afflicted with hemophilia.

**hemophobia,** morbid fear of the sight of blood.

**hemophthalmia, hemophthalmus,** escape of blood inside the eye.

**hemoptysis,** the spitting of blood; blood-stained sputum.

**hemorrhage,** excessive or profuse bleeding; an abnormally heavy flow of blood from a ruptured blood vessel.

**hemorrhagenic,** producing hemorrhage.

**hemorrhagic,** pertaining to hemorrhage.

**hemorrhoid,** a swelling or dilated blood vessel in the anal area.

**hemorrhoidectomy,** surgical excision of hemorrhoids.

**hemostasis,** interruption of blood flow; a stopping of bleeding; stagnation of blood.

**hemostat,** a device or drug which stops the flow of blood.

**hemostatic,** checking bleeding or hemorrhage.

**hemostypic,** an astringent to stop bleeding.

**hemothorax,** a blood fluid present in the pleural cavity due to inflammation of the lungs, as in pneumonia.

**hepar,** the liver.

**heparin,** a complex blood anticoagulant present in many body tissues, especially in the liver and lungs; an agent used in prevention and treatment of embolism and trombosis, obtained from domestic animals.

**heparinize,** therapeutic treatment with heparin to prolong blood clotting time.

**hepatic,** pertaining to the liver.

**hepatitis,** inflammation of the liver.

**hepatogenic,** being produced in the liver.

**hepatography,** liver roentgenography.

**hepatologist,** one who specializes in diseases of the liver.

**hepatology,** the study of the liver and its diseases.

**hepatoma,** a tumor of the liver.

**hepatomegaly,** an enlargement of liver.

**hepatopathy,** liver disease.

**herbivorous,** a vegetarian living on plants; an animal that eats plants.

**hereditary,** genetically transmitted from one's ancestry.

**heredity,** the genetic transmission of individual traits and characteristics from parent to offspring.

**hermaphrodite,** having genital and sexual characteristics of both male and female.

**hermaphroditism,** a condition characterized by the presence of both male and female sexual characteristics and genitalia.

**hernia,** a protrusion of an organ or part of an organ through the cavity wall that encloses it; rupture.

**hernial,** pertaining to a hernia.

**herniated disk,** the protrusion or rupture of a disk between the vertebrae, especially involving the lumbar vertebrae of the spinal column.

**herniation,** development of a hernia.

**heroin,** a morphine derivative altered to increase its potency and used to relieve pain and induce sleep; an addictive narcotic.

**herpes,** an inflammation of the skin and mucous membranes marked by vesicles or blisters appearing in clusters, which often spreads.

**herpes simplex,** a viral disease which produces clusters of blisters around the mouth or genital regions that cause itching and localized congestion. The lesions dry up within a 10-14 day period and form yellowish crusts that shed.

**herpes zoster,** an infectious, inflammatory skin disease; shingles.

**herpetic,** pertaining to herpes.

**herpetiform,** resembling herpes.

**hertergenous,** differing species or sources; dissimilar elements in contrast to homogeneous.

**heterologous,** consisting of abnormal cell tissue.

**heterology,** an abnormality; differing from the normal structure of growth.

**heteropathy,** an abnormal reaction to an irritation.

**heterophasia,** the expression of nonsensical words instead of those intended.

**heterophthalmia,** a difference in the color of the iris of each eye.

**heteroplasty,** the procedure of grafting with skin tissue from another person or animal to repair skin lesions.

**heterosexual,** having sexual desire for the opposite sex.

**heterosexuality,** sexual attraction for the opposite sex.

**heterotopy,** displacement of an organ or a portion of the body.

**heterotropia,** a defect of the eyes; not having normal bifocal vision.

**heterozygosity,** the state of having one or more pairs of unlike genes.

**heterozygote,** a person who has one or more different alleles in regard to a given character.

**hexachlorophene,** a bactericidal and bacteriostatic compound used as a local antiseptic and detergent in emulsions, soaps, and other skin applications.

**hexadactylism,** having six fingers or six toes.

**hexamine,** a substance used as a disinfectant of the urinary tract.

**hiatus,** any natural cleft or opening, as the opening in the diaphragm for the passage of the esophagus.

**hiatus hernia,** a protrusion of part of the stomach upward through the esophageal hiatus of the diaphragm.

**hiccough, hiccup,** a spasmodic closure of the glottis following a sudden involuntary intake of breath causing an abrupt, sharp sound, or inspiratory cough.

**hidrosis,** excessive perspiration; profuse sweating.

**high blood pressure,** hypertension; abnormally high pressure in the arteries at the height of the pulse wave.

**hilus,** a depression or an organ at the point where ducts, nerves, or vessels enter or emerge.

**hindbrain,** the posterior part of the brain composing the pons, cerebellum, and the medulla oblongata.

**hindgut,** the embryonic entodermal tube which develops into the alimentary canal including the ileum, colon, and rectum.

**hip,** upper portion of the thigh; hip joint on either side of the pelvis.

**hipbone,** innominate bone.

**hip joint,** ball-and-socket joint between the femur and hipbone.

**Hippocrates,** ancient Greek physician referred to as "the father of medicine," born in 460 B.C.

**Hippocratic oath,** an oath taken by graduating physicians which embodies a practicing code of ethics.

**hirsute,** hairy or shaggy; roughly hairy.

**hirsutism,** abnormal condition marked by the excessive growth of hair, sometimes in unusual places as on the face of a woman.

**histaminase,** an enzyme distributed throughout the body which inactivates histamine.

**histamine,** a bodily substance that naturally occurs whenever there is tissue damage or allergic reactions; an amine produced by the putrefactive action of bacteria; may also be synthetically produced.

**histidase,** an enzyme produced in the liver that converts histidine to urocanic acid.

**histogenesis,** the origin and development of tissue.

**histologist,** one who studies the microscopic structure of tissue.

**histology,** the scientific study of tissue, esp. their microscopic structure.

**histolysis,** the disintegration and breaking down of tissues.

**histone,** simple proteins derived from cell nuclei which yield certain amino acids resulting from hydrolysis.

**histoplasmosis,** a respiratory disease caused by Histoplasma capsulatum, a fungus, which produce pulmonary calcifications, sometimes mistaken for tubercular calcifications. The usually fatal infection is marked by emaciation, irregular fever, decrease in white blood cells, and enlarged spleen.

**hives,** an eruption of uncertain origin marked by itchy wheals; urticaria.

**hoarseness,** difficulty in speaking due to a harsh, rough voice, as with cold symptoms or flu.

**Hodgkin's disease,** a progressive disease causing an enlargement of the lymph glands, spleen, liver, and kidneys.

**holarthritis,** inflammation of many of the joints; polyarthritis.

**homeopathy,** a method of treating a disease by administering minute doses of a drug that normally causes symptoms similar to those of the disease.

**homeostasis,** a state of equilibrium of the internal environment of the organism; self-regulating maintenance of the metabolic or psychologic processes which are necessary for survival.

**homeostatic,** pertaining to homeostasis.

**homergic,** having the same effect.

**homicide,** murder; the killing of one human being by another, involving acts of manslaughter, murder, accidental killing, and justifiable homicide.

**homogeneity,** state of being uniform in composition or nature.

**homogeneous,** having the same quality or uniformity throughout; belonging to the same kind or type.

**homogenesis,** the reproduction and development of offspring similar to the parents in each subsequent generation.

**homogenetic,** pertaining to homogenesis; having a common origin.

**homograft,** an organ or tissue grafted from an individual or animal to another of the same species, but of a different genotype.

**homologous,** any organ or part which corresponds in structure and in origin.

**homology,** state of being homologous, or similar in structure and origin.

**homosexual,** one sexually attracted to another of the same sex; a homosexual person.

**homosexuality,** exhibiting sexual desire toward persons of the same sex.

**homozygosity,** having identical alleles in referring to a given character.

**homozygote,** an individual possessing like pairs of genes for any hereditary characteristics.

**hookworm disease,** a condition produced by a nematode parasite present in the intestinal tract of man and other vertebrates causing severe anemia, listlessness, and general weakness. The most common port of entry is by walking on infected soil in bare feet, and once the microscopic worms are in the body they quickly invade the heart and lungs.

**hormone,** a chemical substance secreted by the endocrine glands which is conveyed throughout the body and serves to regulate the activity of certain cells or organs.

**host,** any organism that nourishes another organism such as a parasite.

**hot flashes,** a condition which occurs commonly during menopause characterized by vasodilation in the skin of head, neck, and chest with a sensation of suffocation and profuse sweating.

**hot line,** a 24-hour telephone service which provides assistance for people who are in a crisis situation and have a need to reach a mental health professional.

**humerus,** the upper bone of the arm between the shoulder and the elbow.

**humor,** any fluid or semifluid produced in the body.

**humoral,** pertaining to body substances or fluids.

**humpback,** a curvature of the spine; kyphosis.

**hunchback,** a person with kyphosis.

**Huntington's chorea,** an inherited disease involving the central nervous system.

**hyaline,** a glassy, translucent nitrogenous substance.

**hyaline cartilage,** the typical smooth, translucent cartilage which covers bone surfaces that articulate with other bones.

**hyaline membrane disease,** a thin membrane inside the lung of the newborn fetus which interferes with normal respiration.

**hyaluronic acid,** mucopolysaccharide (polymer) found in connective tissue which holds cells together and acts as a protective agent; also found in synovial fluid, skin, and vitreous humor.

**hyaluronidase,** an enzyme which increases connective tissue permeability by breaking down the molecular structure of hyaluronic acid; an enzyme present in the testes, other tissues, and semen.

**hybrid,** a heterozygous individual; the offspring of parents who differ in one or more distinct traits.

**hybridization,** production of hybrids.

**hydatid, hydatid cyst;** a cyst-like structure formed in the tissues by tapeworm larva, especially in the liver of man and certain animals.

**hydatid mole, hydatidiform mole,** a degenerative process occurring in the chorionic villi, characterized by many cysts resembling a bunch of grapes, and rapid growth of the uterus with hemorrhage.

**hydradenitis,** inflammation of a sweat gland.

**hydradenoma,** a tumor of a sweat gland.

**hydragogue,** producing a watery discharge from the bowels; a drug which acts as a cathartic causing a watery evacuation of the bowels.

**hydrarthrosis,** serous accumulation in a joint cavity, with swelling.

**hydrated,** chemical combination of a substance with water.

**hydration,** act of hydrating.

**hydremia,** excess of watery fluid in the circulating blood.

**hydriatics,** the application of water in treatment of disease.

**hydroa,** a chronic skin disease with bullous eruptions.

**hydrocarbon,** a compound made up of hydrogen and carbon.

**hydrocele,** an accumulation of serous fluid in a saccular cavity, especially the scrotum.

**hydrocephalus,** an abnormal enlargement of the head due to an increased accumulation of cerebrospinal fluid resulting from developmental anomalies, infection, injury, or brain tumors.

**hydrochloric acid,** an aqueous solution of hydrogen chloride, a strong highly corrosive acid which is used in industry and medicine; found in gastric juices in the stomach in a diluted and neutralized form which converts pepsinogen into pepsin.

**hydrocortisone,** an adrenal cortical steroid which has life-maintaining properties; used in synthetic preparations for inflammations, allergies, pruritus, shock, bursitis, rheumatoid arthritis, and many other diseases.

**hydrogen peroxide,** a colorless liquid with an irritating odor used as a mild antiseptic, germicide, and cleansing solution.

**hydrolysis,** any reaction produced by combining water with a salt to produce an acid and a base, or a chemical decomposition in which a substance is broken down into simpler compounds by taking up elements of water, as the conversion of starch into maltose.

**hydrometer,** an apparatus which measures the specific gravity of fluids.

**hydromyelocele,** a protrusion of a membraneous sac containing cerebrospinal fluid through a spina bifida.

**hydronephrosis,** an accumulation of urine in the kidney causing swelling due to an obstruction of the ureter, with atrophy of the kidney.

**hydropericarditis,** serous effusion around the heart with inflammation.

**hydroperitoneum,** an accumulation of fluid in the abdominal cavity.

**hydrophobia,** rabies, a disease resulting from a rabid animal bite; abnormal fear of water.

**hydrops,** edema or dropsy.

**hydrotherapy,** the application of water in treatment of disease.

**hydrothorax,** increased swelling of the chest due to the effusion of serous fluid into the pleural cavity.

**hydroureter,** an accumulation of urine or fluid causing distention of the ureter due to obstruction.

**hydruria,** increased water content of urine with decreased solids; polyuria.

**hygiene,** the study and practice of certain rules or principles for the purpose of maintaining health and cleanliness.

**hygenic,** pertaining to hygiene.

**hygienist,** a specialist in hygiene, as in the dental profession.

**hygroscopy,** determination of the quantity of moisture in the atmosphere by a hygroscope.

**Hygroton,** trademark for chlorthalidone, a diuretic.

**hymen,** a membranous fold of tissue covering the vaginal orifice.

**hyoid,** the U-shaped bone between the root of the tongue and larynx.

**hyosine,** scopolamine in some sedative medication.

**hyoscyamine,** an anticholinergic alkaloid obtained from solanaceous plants used as a sedative, mydriatic, antispasmodic, and analgesic.

**hyperacidity,** excessive gastric acidity.

**hyperactive,** pertaining to hyperactivity or hyperkinetic.

**hyperactivity,** abnormal and excessive activity; hyperkinesia.

**hyperacusis,** having an exceptionally acute sense of hearing.

**hyperalgesia,** extreme sensitivity to pain.

**hyperkinesia,** excessive motor activity.

**hyperaphia,** extreme sensitivity to touch.

**hyperbilirubinemia,** an excessive amount of bilirubin in the blood.

**hypercalcemia,** an excessive amount of calcium in the blood.

**hyperchromic,** excessive pigmentation.

**hyperchromia,** an abnormal increase in the hemoglobin in each red blood cell, with a decrease in the number of red blood cells.

**hyperemesis,** an abnormal amount of vomiting.

**hyperemesis gravidarum,** toxemia of early pregnancy marked by excessive vomiting.

**hyperemia,** an unusual amount of blood or congestion in a part which gives rise to reddened areas on the skin.

**hyperesthesia,** an increased sensibility to external stimuli, an oversensitivity to pain, touch, cold, or heat.

**hyperglocosuria,** excessive sugar in the urine.

**hyperglycemia,** excessive increase of blood sugar, as in diabetes.

**hyperinsulinism,** an excessive amount of insulin in the blood, producing hypoglycemic symptoms.

**hyperinvolution,** a reduction in size below normal of the uterus after parturition; a reduction in size below normal of an organ following hypertrophy.

**hyperkeratosis,** an overgrowth of the cornea; excessive development of the horny layer of the skin; keratosis.

**hypermenorrhea,** abnormal flow or frequency of menstrual periods.

**hypermetropia,** farsightedness; hyperopia.

**hypermyatrophy,** abnormal muscle wasting.

**hypermyotonia,** excessive muscle tonus.

**hypernephroma,** malignant tumor of the kidney.

**hypernoia,** excessive imagination or mental activity.

**hyperopia,** defect in eyesight in which the focal point falls behind the retina resulting in farsightedness.

**hyperosmia,** hypersensitivity to odors.

**hyperparathyroidism,** overactivity of the parathyroid glands.

**hyperpiesia,** having extremely high blood pressure.

**hyperpituitarism,** excessive pituitary gland activity resulting in increased growth hormone which produces gigantism and acromegaly.

**hyperplasia,** increased size of a tissue or organ due to excessive proliferation of cells.

**hyperpnea,** increased respiratory rate with deeper breathing or panting, such as a normal state after exercise.

**hyperpyretic,** pertaining to elevated body temperature; hyperpyrexia.

**hyperpyrexia,** a high fever.

**hypersecretion,** an excessive increase in secretion.

**hypersensitivity,** an abnormal sensitivity to a stimulus, as in drug reactions; allergic.

**hypertension,** persistently high arterial blood pressure.

**hyperthermia,** an unusually high body temperature.

**hyperthymia,** having excessive emotion, or morbid sensitivity.

**hyperthyroidism,** excessive thyroid gland activity characterized by goiter, increased metabolic rate, rapid pulse, psychic disturbances, excitement, and other symptoms.

**hypertonia,** an abnormal tension of the muscles or arteries.

**hypertonicity,** excess tonus of the muscle; intraocular pressure.

**hypertrichiasis,** an abnormal growth of hair.

**hypertrophy,** an enlargement of an organ or structure as a result of functional activity and not due to an increase in the number of cells.

**hypervitaminosis,** a condition caused by an excesive ingestion of vitamins, especially Vitamin A and D.

**hyperventilation,** an increased or forced respiration which results in carbon dioxide depletion with accompanied symptoms of lowered blood pressure, vasoconstriction, and faintness.

**hypesthesia,** a lessened sensation to touch.

**hyphidrosis,** a decrease in the amount of perspiration.

**hypnagogic,** inducing sleep; pertaining to dreams just before loss of consciousness.

**hypnogenesis,** producing sleep.

**hypnogenic zones,** certain areas on the body which produce sleep when stimulated, as in the elbow.

**hypnoidal,** pertaining to a mental state between sleep and waking, similar to sleep.

**hypnolepsy,** irresistible sleep; narcolepsy.

**hypnophobia,** pathological aversion to falling asleep.

**hypnosis,** a subconscious state of mind accompanied by an abnormal sensitivity to respond to impressions or verbal suggestions which allows the subject to be induced into a trance or dream state.

**hypnotic,** any agent that induces sleep, or dulls the senses.

**hypnotism,** the science concerned with hypnosis.

**hypnotist,** one trained in hypnosis.

**hypoblast,** inner cell layer or entoderm.

**hypochondria,** an abnormal concern about health issues and false belief of being afflicted with some disease.

**hypochondriasis,** preoccupation with the body and abnormal fear of diseases.

**hypochondrium,** the abdominal portion beneath the lower ribs on each side of the epigastrium.

**hypocythemia,** a deficiency in the number of red blood cells.

**hypodermic,** administered beneath the skin such as an injection into the subcutaneous tissue.

**hypodermic syringe,** a hollow tube, usually with a hollow needle used to inject a solution or medication under the skin; it may be administered subcutaneously, intramuscularly, intraspinally, or intravenously.

**hypodermis,** subcutaneous tissue.

**hypogastric,** pertaining to the hypogastrium.

**hypogastrium,** the area below the naval and between the right and left inguinal areas.

**hypogenitalism,** underdeveloped genital organs.

**hypoglossal,** underneath the tongue.

**hypoglossal nerve,** a mixed nerve which carries afferent and efferent impulses that give rise to tongue movements.

**hypoglycemia,** a deficiency of blood sugar marked by fatigue, restlessness, malaise, irritability, and weakness.

**hypohidrosis,** diminished perspiration or sweating.

**hypokalemia,** abnormal depletion of potassium in the circulating blood producing muscle weakness, tetany, and postural hypotension.

**hypokinesia,** diminished motor activity.

**hypomania,** a mild degree of mania without behavioral change.

**hypomenorrhea,** a deficient menstrual flow.

**hypometropia,** myopia; shortsightedness.

**hypophyseal,** referring to the pituitary gland.

**hypophysectomy,** excision of the hypophysis or pituitary gland.

**hypophysis,** the pituitary body.

**hypophysitis,** inflammation of the pituitary gland.

**hypopituitarism,** a condition resulting from diminished pituitary secretion of hormones.

**hypoplasia,** incomplete development of an organ or tissue.

**hypopnea,** abnormally slow depth and rate of respiration.

**hypopyon,** a condition seen in corneal ulcer in which purulence occurs in the anterior chamber of the eye in front of the iris.

**hyposecretion,** diminished amount of secretion.

**hyposensitive,** exhibiting reduced ability to respond to external stimuli.

**hypostasis,** a sedimentation; poor circulation in a body part or organ.

**hypostatic,** pertaining to hypostasis.

**hypotension,** abnormally low blood pressure.

**hypothalamus,** part of the diencephalon; the gray matter in the floor and walls of the third ventricle of the brain.

**hypothermia,** subnormal body temperature, below 37°C, or between 78 and 90°F.

**hypothymia,** a decreased emotional response.

**hypothyroidism,** a condition caused by a thyroid secretion deficiency marked by lowered basal metabolism, and cretinism.

**hypotonia,** reduced muscle tone or activity.

**hypotonic,** pertaining to decreased muscle tone or tension.

**hypovolemia,** a diminished blood supply.

**hysterectomy,** surgical excision of the uterus, either through the abdominal wall or through the vagina.

**hysteria,** a psychological state characterized by lack of control over emotion, abnormal self-consciousness, anxiety, simulated bodily symptoms, and impairment of both motor and sensory functions.

**hysterogenic,** producing hysteria.

**hystero-oophorectomy,** surgical excision of the uterus and one or both ovaries.

**hysterotomy,** incision of the uterus; a caesarean operation.

**I**

**iatric,** pertaining to medicine or the physician.

**iatrogenic,** caused by the treatment of a physician, resulting in an adverse condition in a patient.

**iatrology,** medical science.

**ichor,** a watery, fetid discharge from an ulcer or a wound.

**ichorrhemia,** septic blood poisoning caused by ichorous matter.

**Ichthyol,** trademark, used as an astringent, antiseptic, and to relieve pruritis.

**ichthyosis,** any of many skin disorders characterized by dryness, and scaliness, giving rise to eczema; a congenital skin disorder characterized by a thick, scaly skin resembling fish-skin.

**ICTH,** interstitial cell stimulating hormone, a male hormone which stimulates testosterone production in the interstitial cells of the testes.

**icteric,** pertaining to jaundice.

**icteroid,** resembling jaundice.

**icterus,** bile pigments causing jaundice in the tissues, membranes, and secretions of the body.

**id,** in Freudian theory, the unconscious part of the personality that deals with instinctive desires or libinal energy of the individual; a biological germ structure carrying hereditary qualities.

**idea,** a concept, or mental imge.

**ideation,** the thinking process, or the formation of mental images.

**identical twins,** twins exactly alike which originate from a single fertilized ovum.

**identification,** a defense mechanism, usually unconscious, by which a person identifies himself with another, such as a hero.

**idiocy,** mental deficiency; severe mental retardation.

**idiopathic,** pertaining to idiopathy.

**idiopathy,** usually in reference to disease without a known cause; a spontaneous disease.

**idiosyncrasy,** individual peculiarities; a quality which makes a person react differently and distinguishes him from others; an unusual susceptibility to a drug.

**idiosyncratic,** pertaining to idiosyncrasy.

**idiot,** severe mental retardation; an uncouth or foolish person.

**idiot savant,** one who is severely mentally retarded, yet has an outstanding mental ability developed to an unusually high degree, as in mathematics or music.

**ileac,** pertaining to the ileum.

**ilectomy,** excision of the ileum.

**ileitis,** inflammation of the ileum.

**ileocecal,** pertaining to the ileum and cecum.

**ileocecum,** referring to both the ileum and cecum.

**ileocolic,** relating to the ileum and colon.

**ileocolostomy,** surgical forming of a passage between the ileum and the colon.

**ileostomy,** the creation of a passage through the abdominal wall into the ileum by a surgical procedure.

**ileum,** the lower third portion of the small intestine between the jejunum and the cecum.

**ileus,** an obstruction of the small intestine.

**iliac,** pertaining to the ileum.

**ilium,** the haunch bone, or the wide upper part of the innominate bone; hip bone.

**illness,** having an ailment, or a deviation from a normal healthy state.

**illusion,** an inaccurate perception, or the misinterpretation of a real experience or sensation.

**illusory,** based on deceptive perception.

**image,** a mental picture with a likeness to a real object.

**imagery,** imagination; mental images that are products of the imagination.

**imago,** the unconscious, idealized mental image of an important person from one's early childhood.

**imbalance,** lack of balance, as in glands or muscles.

**imbecile,** mental deficiency, having an intelligence quotient between 25 and 50 or of about age seven.

**immature,** not fully developed; having not reached full growth potential.

**immiscibility,** state of being immiscible.

**immiscible,** that which cannot be mixed together such as liquids, especially oil and water.

**immobilization,** a part or limb that is immovable; fixed; to immobilize.

**immobilize,** to restrain movement, as by a cast on the arm or leg.

**immune,** able to resist disease; protected from certain diseases by vaccination.

**immunity,** having resistance, or being immune to injury, poisons, foreign proteins, or certain invading organisms.

**immunization,** the process of obtaining immunity to a specific disease; active immunity with a specific agent to stimulate an immune response, or passive immunity by administering serum from immune persons.

**immunize,** to render immune.

**immunochemistry,** the study of immunology as it relates to physical chemical aspects.

**immunogenetics,** the study of genetic factors which control individual immune responses, and how it affects succeeding generations.

**immunogenic,** inducing immunity to a particular disease.

**immunology,** the scientific study of immunity to specific diseases.

**immunosuppressive,** being capable of inhibiting immune responses, as the rejection of a transplant by the body.

**immunotherapy,** passive immunization of an organism by the administration of antibodies in serum or gamma globulin.

**immunotoxin,** an antitoxin.

**immunotropic,** enhancing immune response mechanisms.

**impacted,** a firmly wedged tooth in the jawbone which prevents it from emerging from the gum; in obstetrics, referring to twins being wedged firmly together preventing complete enlargement of either before delivery; accumulation of feces in the rectum.

**impaction,** condition of being impacted.

**impalpable,** not detectable by the touch.

**imparidigitate,** having an uneven number of fingers or toes.

**impedance,** self-induced resistance.

**imperception,** inability to perceive; faulty perception.

**imperforate,** having no opening.

**impermeable,** not allowing the passage of fluids; impenetrable.

**impetigo,** an inflammatory skin disease which may be highly contagious, marked by pustules that become crusted and rupture.

**implant,** a tissue graft, a pellet of medicine, or a radioactive substance.

**implantation,** the attachment of a blastcyst to the lining of the uterus which occurs within six to seven days after fertilization of the ovum; the grafting of an organ or tissue into the body.

**impotence,** the inability of male copulation.

**impotent,** unable to copulate; sterile.

**impregnate,** to fertilize or make pregnant; to saturate.

**impregnation,** the fertilization of an ovum.

**impression,** a depression in the surface; the effect produced upon the mind; a dental imprint of the jaw and teeth.

**impulse,** an instinctual urge; neural transmission through nerve fibers by electrochemical process.

**impulsive,** impelling emotional or involuntary behavior.

**inactivate,** to render inactive.

**inactivation,** destruction of biological activity.

**inactive,** being out of use or sluggish; not active; inert.

**inanition,** a condition of exhaustion due to lack of nourishing food which is essential to the body.

**inappetence,** lack of appetite or craving for food.

**inarticulate,** unable to express oneself verbally; not jointed.

**in articulo mortis,** at the time of death.

**inassimilable,** unable to be used as nourishment by the body.

**inborn,** innate characteristics which are inherited or acquired before birth; congenital or being acquired during fetal development.

**inbred,** producing offspring closely related.

**incest,** sexual intercourse between close blood relations.

**incidence,** the number of new cases of a disease or other condition in a given population and within a specific time period.

**incipient,** beginning, or about to appear.

**incise,** to cut into with a surgical instrument.

**incision,** surgical process of cutting with a knife.

**incisor,** one of the eight cutting teeth located in the upper and lower jaw.

**inclusion,** being enclosed.

**inclusion bodies,** stainable bodies present in the nucleus or cytoplasm of a viral-infected cell; negri bodies.

**incoherent,** not understandable or disorganized and rambling, as in thoughts or language.

**incompatible,** not capable of being mixed in solution; antagonistic or mutually unsuited.

**incompetence,** inability to function realistically or properly; a legal status determined by the court.

**incontinence,** unable to control the elimination of feces or urine.

**incoordination,** inability to produce rhythmic and coordinated muscular movements due to disturbances in tone or harmony between muscle groups.

**incrustation,** the formation of crusts or scabs.

**incubation,** the period between infection of a disease and the appearance of symptoms.

**incubator,** an apparatus for regulating and maintaining a suitable temperature, oxygen, etc. for the survival of premature infants; apparatus for cultivating bacteria or for artificially hatching eggs.

**incubus,** a nightmare; a heavy burden.

**incurable,** not able to be cured; an individual with terminal cancer.

**incus,** the middle of three ossicles in the ear that is shaped like an anvil.

**index,** the forefinger; a ratio between a given measurement compared with a fixed standard.

**indication,** a sign that points to the cause or treatment of a disease.

**indigestion,** failure of complete digestion usually marked by abdominal discomfort after meals.

**indisposition,** a disorder or temporary illness.

**indole,** a crystalline compound found in feces that is largely responsible for odor.

**indolent,** sluggish; inactive.

**induced,** to cause or produce, as in induced labor.

**induction,** the process of inducing, as an abortion; electric current generated by electricity when near a charged body; the interaction between an embryonic cell and inductive cells adjacent to it.

**indurate,** to become hardened; callous.

**induration,** the act of hardening; a specific area of hardened tissue.

**inebriant,** something that intoxicates.

**inebriate,** intoxicate; to make drunk.

**inebriation,** state of being intoxicated; drunkenness.

**inert,** inactive; sluggish.

**inertia,** inactivity; tendency to remain in repose.

**in extremis,** near death; reaching the point of death.

**infant,** a child under two years of age.

**infanticide,** the killing of an infant.

**infantile,** pertaining to infancy.

**infantile paralysis,** poliomyelitis.

**infantilism,** failure of development pertaining to the mind and body; failure to attain maturation.

**infarct,** a necrotic area of tissue following cessation of the blood supply.

**infarction,** the development of an infarct, as in myocardial infarction.

**infect,** to contaminate with pathogenic organisms.

**infection,** the condition in which the body is penetrated by a pathogenic agent such as a virus.

**infectious,** pertaining to a disease which is capable of being transmitted due to a microorganism, either by direct or indirect contact.

**infectious hepatitis,** inflammation of the liver caused by a virus which produces jaundice, nausea, and abdominal pain.

**infectious mononucleosis,** a contagious viral disease characterized by constant fatigue, and other symptoms which include fever, headache, sore throat, swollen glands, jaundice, and stomach irritability.

**infecundity,** sterility in women.

**inferior,** beneath; lower placement.

**inferiority complex,** manifested feelings of inferiority either real or imagined evolved from physical or social inadequacies that produce anxiety.

**infertile,** not productive; unable to produce offspring.

**infertility,** being sterile or barren.

**infestation,** harboring parasites which do not multiply within the body in contrast to infection which does multiply and spread.

**infirm,** feeble, or weak.

**infirmary,** a hospital or a place for the care of the sick or infirmed.

**infirmity,** having an illness or debility; state of being infirmed; feebleness or weakness.

**inflammation,** a tissue or organ reaction to injury or irritation characterized by pain, heat, swelling, redness, and possible loss of function.

**inflammatory,** a sudden onset marked by inflammation and heat.

**influenza,** a contagious viral infection marked by head and back pain, catarrh of the respiratory or gastrointestinal tract; grippe.

**infra-auxillary,** below the axilla, or armpit.

**infraclavicular,** below the collarbone.

**infracostal,** below a rib.

**infraction,** incomplete fracture of a bone in which the two parts do not become displaced.

**inframammary,** below the mammary gland.

**infraorbital,** beneath the orbit of the eye.

**infrapubic,** below the pubis.

**infrared rays,** invisible heat rays beyond the red end of the visible spectrum.

**infrascapular,** below the shoulder blade.

**infrasternal,** below the sternum.

**infundibulum,** a funnel-shaped passage; a tube which connects the frontal sinus cavity with the middle nasal cavity.

**infusion,** introduction of a solution into a vein.

**ingesta,** substances taken into the body through the mouth such as food.

**ingestion,** the process of taking food into the gastrointestinal tract.

**ingrowing,** growing inward.

**inguinal,** pertaining to the groin region.

**inhalant,** a medicinal preparation which may be inhaled.

**inhalation,** the process of breathing medicated vapors or oxygen into the nose and lungs; act of drawing in of breath.

**inhalator,** an apparatus used for administering vaporized medication by inhalation, or for breathing in oxygen.

**inherent,** belonging to something naturally; intrinsic.

**inheritance,** hereditary factors transmitted and blended in the offspring.

**inherited,** characteristics received from one's ancestors.

**inhibition,** the act of repressing or the state of being restrained; commonly applied to the unconscious defense against the sex instinct; suppression.

**inhibitor,** something which inhibits.

**inject,** to introduce a solution into the body tissue or cavity with a syringe.

**injection,** forcing a fluid or liquid into a body tissue or cavity using a sterile needle and syringe; injections into the skin may be subcutaneous, intramuscular, or intraveneous.

**inlet,** a passage which leads to a cavity.

**innate,** inborn, or hereditary.

**innervate,** the supply of nerves to an organ or part of the body; to stimulate through the nerves.

**innervation,** stimulating a body part through the action of nerve fibers, or nervous energy; the functioning of the nervous system.

**innocent,** benign, not malignant.

**innocuous,** harmless; inoffensive.

**innominate artery,** the right artery arising from the aortic arch.

**innominate bone,** the hip bone consisting of the ilium, ischium, and pubis which form the pelvis.

**innominate veins,** the right and left vein from the jugular and subclavian veins which form the superior vena cava.

**inoculability,** being susceptible of infection transmitted by inoculation.

**inoculate,** to inject a virus or bacteria into the body to cause a mild disease as a prevention against certain diseases and to build immunity.

**inoculation,** the act of injecting serum to induce antibody formation.

**inoculum,** a substance introduced into the body by inoculation.

**inoliomyoma,** a tumor consisting of smooth muscle tissue.

**inoma,** a fibrous tumor.

**inoperable,** unsuitable for excision without danger of death.

**inquest,** postmortem examination to determine legally the medical cause of death; act of inquiry.

**insane,** unsound mind; mentally deranged.

**insanitary,** unhealthy; pertaining to filth.

**insanity,** a legal term for mental derangement or mental illness; mental incompetence; unable to distinguish "right from wrong".

**insatiable,** incapable of being satisfied.

**insemination,** discharge of seminal fluid into the vagina; fertilization of an ovum.

**insensibility,** the state of being insensible.

**insensible,** unconscious; incapable of sensory perception.

**insensitive,** lacking feeling or physical sensation.

**insertion,** the place of muscle attachment to a bone allowing movement; the act of implanting.

**insidious,** a gradual and deliberate development; a slow developing disease that does not exhibit early symptoms.

**insight,** self-understanding.

**insipid,** without taste; lacking animation or spirit.

**in situ,** in its normal position.

**insolation,** exposure to the rays of the sun for brief periods, as a treatment of certain skin disorders; heat therapy; heat- or sunstroke.

**insoluble,** incapable of being dissolved.

**insomnia,** disturbances in sleep patterns; chronic inability to sleep.

**inspection,** to visually examine the external surface of the body.

**inspersion,** sprinkling with powder or a solution.

**inspiration,** inhalation; pertaining to breathing air into the lungs; a state of being inspired.

**inspiratory,** pertaining to breathing in, or inspiration.

**inspissate,** to thicken by absorption of liquid content or by evaporation.

**inspissated,** being thickened by absorption, evaporation, or dehydration.

**inspissation,** the process of diminishing fluidity and increasing thickness.

**instep,** the upper surface of the foot or the arch, in front of the ankle.

**instillation,** dispensing a liquid drop by drop.

**instinct,** an inborn drive or innate urge characteristic of a species necessary for self-preservation, and which satisfies basic biological needs.

**instinctive,** unlearned responses determined by instinct.

**instrumentation,** the use of instruments, or work resulting from their use.

**insudation,** an accumulated substance derived from the blood, as in a kidney.

**insufficiency,** being inadequate for its function or purpose.

**insuffiate,** to blow a medicated substance into a cavity such as lungs; to blow air into the lungs.

**insufflation,** the process of insuffiating.

**insufflator,** a device used for insuffiation.

**insula,** any round cutaneous body.

**insulin,** a pancreatic hormone secreted by the beta cells of the islets of Langerhans essential for oxidation and utilization of blood sugar. A sterile preparation of insulin is used in the treatment of diabetes mellitus.

**insulinemia,** the presence of too much insulin in the blood.

**insulin shock,** a condition resulting from an overdose of insulin which causes the blood sugar level to drop below normal, producing symptoms of hypoglycemia such as increased hunger, thirst, excitability, rapid pulse, flushing, pallor, sweating, fainting, convulsions, and coma.

**insuloma,** a tumor of the islets of Langerhans.

**insusceptibility,** having immunity.

**integration,** constituting a whole; assimilation.

**integument,** a covering such as skin; the skin.

**integumentary,** pertaining to a covering consisting of dermis or epidermis.

**intellect,** having the mental capacity to comprehend ideas and to exercise judgment; the capacity for knowledge.

**intellectual,** pertaining to the mind, or possessing intellect.

**intellectualization,** a defense mechanism that uses reasoning as a defense against conscious confrontation with unconscious conflict and its distressing mental tension.

**intelligence,** having the capacity to learn, to comprehend relationships, and to reason with facts and propositions.

**intelligence quotient,** (I.Q.), a numerical rating of intelligence, determined by dividing one's mental age, derived through intelligence test scores, by one's chronological age, then by multiplying by 100.

**intemperance,** excessive usages of anything.

**intensive,** relative to the degree or extent of activity.

**interaction,** the process of two or more things acting on each other.

**interarticular,** situated between two joints.

**interatrial,** situated between the atria of the heart.

**interbrain,** diencephalon.

**intercellular,** between the cells.

**interchondral,** between the cartilage.

**interclavicular,** between the clavicles.

**intercostal,** between the ribs.

**intercourse,** coitus; the sexual act; social contacts.

**intercurrent,** intervening; a disease that occurs during another illness.

**interdental,** between the teeth.

**interdigital,** between the fingers or toes.

**interdigitation,** fingerlike processes that interlock.

**interfemoral,** between the thighs.

**interlobar,** between lobes.

**intermenstrual,** between menstrual periods.

**intermission,** a temporary cessation of symptoms of a disease.

**intermittent fever,** an absence of symptoms between attacks of fever, as in malaria.

**intermittent pulse,** a pulse in which a beat is dropped at intervals, as in cardiac exhaustion.

**intermuscular,** between muscles.

**intern, interne,** a medical graduate assisting in a hospital as a resident physician or surgeon.

**internal medicine,** the branch of medicine concerned with diseases not usually treated by surgery.

**internist,** one concerned with internal diseases, and not a surgeon.

**internuncial,** serving as a connecting medium.

**interosseous,** between bones.

**interosseus,** a muscle lying between bones.

**interpalpebral,** between the eyelids.

**interparietal,** between walls; between the parietal bones; between the parietal lobes on the cerebrum.

**intersex,** a person having both male and female characteristics.

**interspace,** an area between two similar parts, as between ribs.

**interstice,** a gap or space in a tissue or an organ.

**interstitial,** placed between; pertaining to interstices or gaps between the cellular structures.

**interventricular,** between two ventricles.

**intervertebral,** between two adjacent vertebrae.

**intestinal,** pertaining to the intestine.

**intestinal juice,** a chemical liquid produced by the intestinal mucosa.

**intestine,** the alimentary canal which is divided into the small intestine and the large intestine extending from the pylorus to the anus.

**intima,** the innermost lining of a structure, as a blood vessel.

**intolerance,** the inability to endure pain; the side effects of drugs or foods.

**intoxicant,** an agent which intoxicates.

**intoxication,** the state of being intoxicated or drunk; being poisoned by a toxic substance.

**intra-abdominal,** within the abdomen.

**intra-arterial,** within the arteries.

**intra-articular,** within a joint.

**intra-atrial,** within the atrium of the heart.

**intracellular,** within cells.

**intracranial,** within the skull.

**intracutaneous,** within the substance of the skin or layers.

**intracutaneous test,** a test to determine allergic sensitivity.

**intradermal,** between the layers of the skin.

**intradural,** within the dura matter.

**intraglandular,** within a gland.

**intra-intestinal,** within the intestine.

**intramammary,** within the breast.

**intramastoiditis,** inflammation of the antrum and mastoid process.

**intramural,** within the substance of a wall or hollow cavity.

**intramuscular,** within a muscular substance.

**intranasal,** within the nasal cavity.

**intraocular,** within the eyeball.

**intraoral,** within the mouth.

**intraorbital,** within the orbit of the eye, or eye socket.

**intraosseous,** within the substance of a bone.

**intraperitoneal,** within the peritoneal cavity.

**intrapleural,** within the pleural cavity.

**intrapsychic,** originating within the mind such as conflicts; mental origin or basis.

**intrapulmonary,** within the lung.

**intrathoracic,** within the thorax.

**intratracheal,** introduction into the trachea.

**intrauterine,** within the uterus.

**intravascular,** within a blood vessel.

**intravenous,** within a vein.

**intraventricular,** within a ventricle.

**intravital,** occurring during life.

**intrinsic,** belonging within or pertaining essentially to a part.

**intrinsic factor,** a substance produced from gastrointestinal mucosa of animals which increases the absorption of Vitamin B complex in humans.

**introitus,** an opening into a cavity such as the vagina.

**introjection,** a defense mechanism in which external objects are taken within oneself symbolically.

**introspection,** looking into one's own mind.

**introversion,** a preoccupation with oneself with little interest in the outside world; turning inside out of a part or organ.

**introvert,** one whose interests are turned inward and away from reality.

**intubation,** the introduction of a tube into a body cavity, as into the larynx.

**intumesce,** to swell or enlarge.

**intumescence,** the process of enlarging.

**intussusception,** the prolapse of one part of the intestine into another part adjacent to it; a growth of new cells by receiving nutrients and its transformation into protoplasm.

**intussuscipiens,** that part of the intestine which contains the intussusceptum.

**inulin,** a starch of certain plants which yield fructose upon hydrolysis, used in renal function testing.

**in utero,** within the uterus.

**invagination,** folding of one part within another structural part, as in intestines; intussusception.

**invalid,** a weak and sickly person.

**inversion,** the turning inside out of an organ, especially the uterus; homosexuality; a chromosomal aberration resulting in a change in the sequence of genes.

**invertase,** an enzyme found in intestinal juice.

**invertebrate,** having no backbone.

**in vitro,** observable in a test tube or within an artificial environment.

**in vivo,** within a living organism.

**involuntary,** working independently of conscious control.

**involution,** a turning inward; the process of decreasing the size of the uterus after delivery; a degeneration of the internal organs with the aging process.

**iodide,** a compound of iodine.

**iodine,** a chemical element composed of a black, crystalline substance, essential to the body for synthesis of thyroxine, a thyroid hormone.

**iodism,** a poisonous condition occurring with prolonged use of iodine or its compounds.

**iodoform,** a yellowish crystalline substance with an offensive odor used as an antiseptic.

**iodopsin,** photosensitive violet pigment present in the retinal cones which are important for color vision.

**ipecac,** dried roots of the plant impecacuanha used in treatment against amebic dysentery; other uses are as an expectorant, emetic, and diaphoretic.

**iridemia,** hemorrhaging from the iris.

**iridocyclectomy,** surgical removal of part of the iris and of the ciliary body.

**iridocystectomy,** surgical procedure to form an artificial iris.

**iridotomy,** surgical incision of the iris without removal of a piece.

**iris,** the pigmented contractile membrane forming the portion of the eye containing the pupil.

**iritis,** inflammation of the iris.

**iron,** a chemical element essential for the formation of hemoglobin in the body, and the prevention of certain forms of anemia.

**irradiate,** to treat with radiation.

**irradiation,** the therapeutic use of roentgen rays, radium rays, ultraviolet and other radiation for healing purposes.

**irrational,** lacking reason or understanding.

**irrigate,** to wash out with water or solution.

**irrigation,** to cleanse a canal or cavity with the injection of fluids.

**irritability,** the state of being excitable; a condition in which an organism, organ, or body part responds excessively to stimuli.

**irritant,** that which causes irritation; an agent which produces local inflammation and gives rise to irritation.

**irritation,** a condition which produces unusual sensitivity in part of the body.

**ischemia,** temporary and localized anemia due to restricting circulation to a part.

**ischial,** pertaining to the ischium.

**ischium,** the lower portion of the hip bone.

**ischuria,** suppression or retention of urine.

**islets of Langerhans,** clusters of beta cells which produce insulin in the pancreas.

**isoagglutinin,** an antibody serum which agglutinates blood cells.

**isogamete,** a gamete or sex cell which conjugates with a similar cell and reproduces; a gamete of the same size as another with which it unites to form a zygote.

**isoleucine,** an amino acid containing fibrin and other proteins essential in the diets of man.

**isomer,** a compound which has the same molecular formula in each chemical substance but differing in chemical and physical properties resulting from different arrangements of the atoms in the molecule.

**isomeric,** pertaining to isomer arrangements.

**isometric,** pertaining to, or having equal dimensions.

**isometric exercises,** physical exertion of muscles that does not involve motion, achieved by setting one muscle against another.

**isometropia,** having the same refraction in the two eyes.

**isosthenuria,** a decreased variation of specific gravity of urine in renal dysfunction.

**isothermal,** having an equal degree of heat.

**isotonic,** of equal tone or tension, as in muscles; pertaining to a solution in the body having the same osmotic pressure.

**isotope,** a chemical element having the same atomic number as another, but differing in atomic mass.

**isotropic,** possessing the same properties in every direction such as conduction.

**isthmitis,** inflammation of the throat or fauces.

**isthmus,** a narrow connection between two cavities.

**itch,** an irritation of the skin that induces a desire to scratch; pruritus; scabies.

**iter,** a tubular passageway.

**ivy poisoning,** a dermatitis caused by poison ivy contact with the skin.

**ixodic,** caused by ticks.

# J

**jacket,** a covering for the trunk or thorax made of plaster of Paris or leather bandage, used to immobilize the spine or to correct certain deformities.

**jactition,** extreme restlessness marked by tossing to and fro during an acute illness; convulsive movements.

**jargon,** chattering, unintelligible language or speech pattern; paraphasia.

**jaundice,** a yellow tinge to the skin and sclera of the eyes caused by an increase in bile pigment resulting from excess bilirubin in the blood due to obstruction of the bile ducts, excessive red blood cell destruction, or disturbances in liver cell function.

**jaw,** one of two bones that form the framework of the mouth.

**jecur,** the liver.

**jejunectomy,** surgical removal of part or all of the jejunum.

**jejunitis,** inflammation of the jejunum.

**jejunocolostomy,** surgical creation of a communication between the jejunum and the ileum.

**jejunoileitis,** inflammation of the jejunum and ileum.

**jejunojejunostomy,** surgical joining between two portions of the jejunum after the removal of the diseased part.

**jejunotomy,** surgical incision of the jejunum.

**jejunum,** the middle section of the small intestine extending from the duodenum to the ileum.

**jerk,** an abrupt muscular movement; reflex action to a stimulus.

**joint,** a junction or union between two bones such as at the elbow; an articulation between two bones or cartilage.

**Jolles test,** a test to determine the presence of biliary pigments in urine.

**jugal,** pertaining to the malar or zygomatic or bony arch of the cheek.

**jugular,** pertaining to the throat.

**jugular veins,** the large veins at the front of the throat which receive the blood from the head, brain, and face and returns it to the heart.

**jugulate,** to quickly stop or arrest a process or disease by therapeutic intervention such as a tracheotomy.

**juice,** body secretions.

**junction,** coming together of two parts as a nerve with a muscle.

**junctura,** an articulation or suture of bones.

**juvenile,** pertaining to youth; immature; young.

**juxtaposition,** a side by side position.

# K

**Kahn's test,** a blood test for detecting syphilis.

**kakotrophy,** malnutrition.

**kalium,** potassium.

**kaliuresis,** presence of potassium in the urine.

**kaolin,** a mineral clay used as an adsorbent in the coating of pills and in kaolin mixture with pectin.

**karyogenesis,** the formation and development of a cell nucleus.

**karyokinesis,** division of the nucleus of a cell at an early stage of mitosis.

**karyoplasm,** the substance of the nucleus in a cell.

**karyosome,** chromatin mass within the nuclear network.

**karyotype,** complete characteristics of a cell's nucleus including its size, form, and chromosome number.

**katabolism,** catabolism, the opposite of anabolism.

**katotropia,** the tendency for the eyeball to drop downward; a turning downward.

**keloid,** scar formation consisting of dense tissue.

**keloidosis,** a formation of keloids.

**kelotomy,** operation for a strangulated hernia through the tissues of the constricting part or neck.

**kenophobia,** extreme fear of empty spaces.

**keratalgia,** a neuralgia of the cornea.

**keratectasia,** the conical protrusion of the cornea of the eye.

**keratectomy,** surgical excision of part of the cornea.

**keratiasis,** the formation of multiple horny warts on the skin.

**keratin,** a scleroprotein present in skin, hair, nails, and horny formations.

**keratitis,** inflammation of the cornea.

**keratoconjunctivitis,** inflammation of the cornea and the conjunctiva of the eye.

**keratoderma,** the horny layer of the skin; the cornea.

**keratodermatitis,** inflammation of the horny layer of the skin.

**keratodermia,** hypertrophy or thickening of the horny layer of the skin, especially on the palms of the hands and soles of the feet.

**keratogenous,** producing horny tissue development.

**keratoid,** resembling horn or corneal tissue layer of the skin.

**keratoma,** a callosity, or horny growth of tissue.

**keratome,** a surgical knife for incising the cornea.

**keratometer,** a device for measuring the curves of the cornea.

**keratonosis,** any disease of the horny layer of skin which is nonflammatory.

**keratoplasty,** plastic surgery on the cornea.

**keratosis,** any growth of horny tissue development on the skin.

**keratotomy,** surgical incision of the cornea.

**kernicterus,** a form of jaundice, icterus neonatorum, occurring in infants due to high levels of bilirubin in the blood resulting in severe neural symptoms and degeneration of parts of the brain.

**ketamine,** a general anesthetic which is rapid-acting.

**ketoacidosis,** acidosis caused by an accumulation of ketone bodies in the blood.

**ketogenesis,** the production of ketones or acetone within the body, especially in diabetes.

**ketol,** an organic compound formed in the intestine and pancreas during digestion and decomposition of protein.

**ketone,** a substance or an organic compound containing the carbonyl group (CO), as acetone.

**ketone bodies,** any acetone, B-hydroxybutyric acid, or acetoacetic acid produced during the oxidation of fatty acids and found in the blood and urine, especially in diabetics.

**ketosis,** an accumulation of ketone bodies in the body.

**kidney,** one of two glandular, bean-shaped organs situated at the back of the abdominal cavity which excrete urine (consisting of 95% water and 5% of solids).

**kinanesthesia,** the loss of perceptive power in sensations of movements.

**kinesalgia,** painful muscular movement.

**kinesia,** motion sickness.

**kinesis,** motion.

**kinesthesia,** sense of muscle movement.

**kinetotherapy,** treatment that employs active and passive movements, as in physiotherapy.

**kinesiology,** the science concerned with anatomy and muscular movement.

**kinesioneurosis,** a functional disorder manifested by tics and spasms which affect external muscles.

**kleptomania,** impulsive stealing

**kleptomaniac,** one afflicted with kleptomania.

**klieg eye,** inflammed conjunctiva, increased lacrimation and photophobia due to long periods of exposure to intense lights.

**Kline test,** a microscopic test for the presence of syphilis.

**knee,** pertaining to the knee joint between the thigh and the lower leg.

**kneecap,** the patella.

**knee jerk reflex,** a contraction of the quadriceps muscle which causes an involuntary kick when a sharp striking blow to the ligament patellae is applied by an instrument.

**knock-knee,** inward curvature of the legs which cause the knees to knock together when walking.

**knuckle,** the rounded end of the phalangeal joint of a finger.

**Korsakoff's syndrome,** a disease characterized by psychosis, polyneuritis, delirium, insomnia, illusions and hallucinations, as a sequel to chronic alcoholism.

**kraurosis,** a dryness and hardening of the skin and mucous membranes.

**kymograph,** a device for recording variations in motion and blood pressure changes.

**kyphosis,** a humpback; an abnormal backward curving of the spine.

**kyphotic,** humpback or hunchbacked.

**kysthitis,** inflammation of the vagina.

**kysthoptosis,** a prolapse of the vagina.

# L

**labia,** lips; the lips of the vulva.

**labial,** pertaining to lips.

**labia majora,** two folds of adipose tissue covered with pigmented skin and hair on the outer surface and free from hair on the inner surface which lie on either side of the vaginal opening.

**labia minora,** two thin folds of mucous membrane located within the labia majora on either side of the vaginal opening.

**labile,** unsteady; fluctuating.

**labium,** a lip-like structure; lip.

**labor,** delivery; parturition; childbirth.

**labyrinth,** the inner ear consisting of the vestibule, the cochlea, the semicircular canals or bony labyrinth, and the membranous labyrinth.

**labyrinthectomy,** surgical removal of the labyrinth.

**labyrinthine,** pertaining to the labyrinth; intricate.

**labryrinthitis,** inflammation of the labyrinth.

**lac,** any milklike medical substance.

**lacerate,** to tear, or to make a ragged gash of the flesh.

**laceration,** the process of tearing, as a tearing injury to the vaginal opening by childbirth.

**lacrima,** pertaining to tears or tearing.

**lacrimal,** characterized by tears, or pertaining to organs that produce tears.

**lacrimal gland,** a gland which secretes tears, located in the orbit of the eye.

**lacrimation,** a discharge of tears.

**lacrimonasal,** pertaining to the lacrimal sac and nose.

**lacrimotomy,** surgical incision of the lacrimal duct or gland.

**lactagogue, galactagogue,** a substance that stimulates alveoli of the mammary glands to secrete milk.

**lactalbumin,** a protein in human milk.

**lactation,** secretion of milk; breast feeding.

**lacteal,** pertaining to milk; relating to intestinal lymphatics which transport chyle.

**lactescense,** becoming milky, or resembling milk.

**lactic,** pertaining to milk.

**lactic acid,** a syrup-like, colorless substance formed by fermentation of sugars by microorganisms which occur naturally in sour milk; it is also formed during muscular activity by breaking down glycogen; medical uses of lactic acid are found in antiseptics and dietary products.

**lactiferous,** the process of secreting and conveying milk.

**lactiferous ducts,** referring to the ducts of the mammary gland.

**lactifuge,** an agent used to cause cessation of milk secretion in the mammary glands.

**lactin,** pertaining to lactose, a sugar of milk.

**lactobacillus,** a rod-shaped, gram-positive bacteria that produce lactic acid from carbohydrates and which cause milk to sour.

**lactogenic,** inducing lactation, the secretion of milk.

**lactose,** a sugar derived from milk which yields glucose and galactose upon hydrolysis, used as a sweetening substance in foods.

**lactosuria,** milk sugar in the urine.

**lacuna,** a minute hollow found in bones where osteoblasts lie; a gap found in cartilage or bone consisting of bone cells.

**lacus lacrimalis,** the inner portion of the eye where tears accumulate.

**lagophthalmos, lagophthalamus,** incomplete closure of the eyelids.

**la grippe,** an acute infectious respiratory or gastrointestinal disease; influenza.

**laliatry,** speech disorder therapy.

**lallation,** infantile speech or babbling; stammering; the constant use of ''i'' instead of ''r.''

**lalopathy,** any speech disorder.

**lalophobia,** extreme reluctance to communicate verbally due to stammering.

**laloplegia,** a paralysis caused by a stroke which affects speech muscles but not tongue action or movements.

**lalorrhea,** an abnormal flow of speech.

**lamella,** a gelatinous disk inserted under the lower eyelid used as a medicinal application to the eye.

**lamina,** a thin layer of membrane; pertaining to either flattened side of the vertebral arch.

**laminectomy,** surgical removal of the posterior vertebral arch.

**laminitis,** inflammation of the lamina.

**lance,** a surgical instrument; to incise with a lancet.

**lancet,** a pointed surgical instrument with two sharp edges.

**lanolin,** a greasy, purified substance obtained from sheep's wool used as a base in ointments or lotions that are beneficial to the skin.

**lanuginous,** a lanugo or wooly covering, as in the human fetus immediately after birth.

**lanugo,** a downy hair covering the body of a fetus.

**lapactic,** cathartic; laxative.

**laparocystotomy,** surgical incision through the abdomen for removal of a cyst or an extrauterine fetus.

**laparoenterostomy,** a surgical creation of an opening through the abdominal wall into the intestine.

**laparotomy,** an abdominal operation; surgical opening of the abdomen.

**laryngalia,** neuralgia of the larynx.

**laryngeal,** pertaining to the larynx.

**laryngectomy,** surgical removal of the larynx.

**laryngismus,** laryngeal spasm.

**laryngitic,** pertaining to or resulting from laryngitis.

**laryngitis,** inflammation of the larynx.

**laryngography,** a description of larynx movements as recorded by a laryngographic device.

**laryngologist,** a specialist in laryngology.

**laryngology,** the branch of medicine concerned with the treatment of diseases of the larynx.

**laryngoparalysis,** paralysis of the muscles of the larynx.

**laryngopharyngeal,** pertaining to both the larynx and the pharynx.

**laryngopharyngitis,** inflammation of both the larynx and the pharynx.

**laryngopharynx,** the lower part of the pharynx which extends into the larynx and esophagus.

**laryngoplasty,** surgical repair of a defect of the larynx.

**laryngoscope,** an instrument with a tiny light used to examine the larynx.

**laryngoscopy,** an examination of the interior of the larynx by an instrument.

**laryngospasm,** spasm of the muscles of the larynx.

**laryngostomy,** operation to make a permanent opening through the throat into the larynx.

**laryngotomy,** surgical operation of the larynx.

**laryngotracheotomy,** a surgical procedure in which upper tracheal rings and the larynx are incised to form an artificial airway.

**larynx,** the enlarged upper portion of the trachea or organ of voice, composed of nine cartilages and the vocal cords.

**laser,** a device that transfers light frequencies into an extremely intense beam of radiation which is capable of emitting immense heat when focused, used in surgery, in diagnosis, and in research.

**Lasix,** trademark for furosemide used as a diuretic and to prevent the accumulation of fluid in the body.

**lassitude,** weakness; listlessness; exhaustion.

**latent,** hidden; present in a concealed form but capable of becoming manifest; potential.

**latent content,** the unconscious meaning associated with thoughts or actions, especially applied to dreams or fantasies.

**latent period,** the period in disease from the time of infection to the appearance of symptoms∞ psychoanalytic theory, a period of psychosexual development.

**lateral,** situated to the side, or directed to the side.

**lateroflexion,** flexion or bending to one side.

**lateropulsion,** the tendency to fall to one side involuntarily due to cerebellar and labyrinthine disease.

**lateroversion,** a tendency to turn to one side.

**laudanum,** tincture of opium.

**laughing gas,** nitrous oxide gas.

**lavage,** the washing out of a cavity or organ, as in the stomach in poisoning.

**lax,** without tension.

**laxative,** a gentle purgative or cathartic.

**lead colic,** severe abdominal pain due to lead poisoning.

**lead poisoning,** an acute condition of poisoning from large doses of absorbed lead, as in children who eat paint chips, the absorbed lead affects the brain, nervous and digestive systems, and the blood; a condition among workers exposed to lead products in industry.

**lecithin,** derived from glycerin, a fatty substance found in the blood, bile, brain, egg yolk, nerves, and animal tissue and which yield stearic acid, glycerol, phosphoric acid, and choline upon hydrolysis.

**leech,** a blood-sucking water worm once used as a means of blood- letting, now abandoned; a device used for drawing blood.

**leg,** the lower extremity; that part of the body extending from the knee to the ankle.

**leiomyoma,** a smooth muscle tissue tumor.

**leiomyosarcoma,** a malignant smooth muscle tumor.

**lema,** the dried secretion of the meibomian glands which collects in the inner corners of the eye.

**lens,** the crystalline lens behind the pupil of the eye that focuses light rays on the retina; a piece of glass or other transparent material so shaped as to converge or scatter light rays.

**lenticular,** lens shaped; pertaining to a lens.

**lentiginous,** a freckle; covered with tiny dots.

**lentitis,** inflammation of the crystalline lens of the eye.

**leper,** one afflicted with leprosy.

**leprosy,** an infectious disease caused by a microorganism, once believed to be incurable, marked by a gradual onset of symptoms such as general malaise, headache, chilliness, mental depression, numbness in various body parts, ulcerations, tubercular nodules, and loss of fingers and toes.

**leprous,** afflicted with leprosy.

**leptocephalus,** one possessing an abnormally small head.

**leptomeninges,** the two delicate structures that cover the brain and spinal cord.

**leptopellic,** having an abnormally narrow pelvis causing labor to be difficult or impossible indicating need for cesarean section.

**Leptospira,** disease infecting spirochetes which are thin, hooked- end, aerobic bacteria that sometimes infect man.

**leptospirosis,** a condition resulting from Leptospira infection, marked by lymphocytic meningitis, hepatitis, and nephritis occurring in combination or separately.

**lesbian,** a female homosexual.

**lesion,** an abnormal localized tissue formation; a wound resulting from disease or injury.

**lethal,** causing death; fatal; deadly.

**lethargic,** relating to lethargy; sluggish; stupor; inclined to sleep.

**lethargy,** a condition characterized by drowsiness, indifference or inattention.

**leucine,** an amino acid derived from protein digestion which is present in all body tissue and is essential for normal growth and metabolism.

**leucinuria,** the presence of leucine in the urine.

**leucitis,** inflammation of the sclera.

**leucovorin,** folinic acid used in treatment of megaloblastic anemias caused by a deficiency in folic acid.

**leukanemia,** leukemia existing with anemia.

**leukemia,** a progressive and fatal disease characterized by rapid and abnormal growth of leukocytes in the blood-forming organs of the body such as bone marrow, spleen, and lymph nodes, and the presence of immature white blood corpuscles in the circulating blood; cancer of the blood.

**leukemic,** pertaining to leukemia.

**leukemoid,** resembling leukemia symptoms but caused by another condition.

**leukoblast,** a cell that gives rise to a leukocyte.

**leukoblastosis,** an excessive growth of immature white blood corpuscles.

**leukocyte,** white blood cells or corpuscles of which there are two types: granulocytes, containing granules in cytoplasm, and agranulocytes, lacking granules in cytoplasm. The leukocytes are scavengers and are essential to fight invading bacteria within the body.

**leukocythemia,** a condition marked by excessive white blood corpuscles in the body, and an enlarged spleen, lymphatic glands, and bone marrow; leukemia.

**leukocytic,** pertaining to leukocytes.

**leukocytogenesis,** the formation of white blood corpuscles or leukocytes.

**leukocytolysis,** the dissolution or destruction of white blood cells.

**leukocytopenia,** an abnormally low white blood cell number in the circulating blood.

**leukocytosis,** an increased number of white blood cells in the blood usually indicating an infection, or it may occur due to hemorrhage, surgery, coronary occlusion, malignant tumors, some intoxications, pregnancy, and toxemias.

**leukoderma,** usually an acquired condition marked by a localized deficiency of pigmentation in the skin rendering a patchy effect.

**leukoma,** a white, corneal opacity.

**leukopenia,** an abnormal decrease in white blood cells, below 5,000 per cu. mm.

**leukoplakia,** white patches which form on the mucous membranes of the cheek or tongue that may become malignant.

**leukorrhea,** an abnormal condition marked by a white or creamy- yellowish discharge from the vagina resulting from acute inflammation and infection by Trichomonas vaginalis.

**leukosis,** excessive growth of leukocyte-producing tissue.

**levator,** a muscle that raises a body part; an instrument used to lift depressed portions such as part of the skull.

**levitation,** a sensation that one is being lifted gently or moving through the air without physical support, as in a dream state.

**levulose,** fruit sugar; fructose which is present in honey and many fruits, used in medicinal preparations.

**libidinous,** marked by intense sexual desire or lust; salacious.

**libido,** sexual drive; innate drives and instincts that motivate human behavior; the energy force associated with pleasure seeking and sexual instinct.

**lichen,** any of various forms of eruptive skin diseases which have small, firm, and closely set papules.

**lid,** eyelid.

**Lieberkuhn crypts,** tubular glands present in the intestinal wall.

**lien,** the spleen.

**lienitis,** inflammation of the spleen.

**lientery,** diarrhea with undigested food in the fecal matter.

**ligament,** a strong fibrous band of connecting tissue which binds the articular ends of bones to limit motion or to hold body organs in place.

**ligamentous,** pertaining to a ligament.

**ligate,** to apply or bind, as with a ligature.

**ligation,** the application of a ligature.

**ligature,** any material that binds, such as a band, thread, or wire, used for tying blood vessels; the process of tying.

**limb,** an extremity, an arm or leg; a limblike appendage of a structure.

**limbus,** the rim or edge of a part.

**limen,** the edge, or threshold.

**liminal,** barely noticeable; pertaining to the threshold, as in consciousness.

**lingua,** the tongue, or resembling a tongue.

**lingual,** pertaining to the tongue.

**liniment,** a liquid medicine containing oil, alcohol, or water for external use, applied by friction to the skin as treatment for sprains.

**linin,** a threadlike substance that connects the chromatin granules in the cell nucleus.

**linitis,** an inflammation of the gastric cellular tissue.

**linkage,** in genetics, two or more genes which tend to remain together in the same chromosome in the formation of gametes.

**lip,** the soft structure around the mouth, or a formation bordering an opening or groove.

**liparous,** obese; fat.

**lipase,** a fat-splitting digestive enzyme occurring in the pancreas, liver, and found in the blood and which breaks down fat into fatty acids and glycerol.

**lipemia,** an accumulation of fat in the blood.

**lipid,** any group of fats which are water-insoluble.

**lipidosis,** a disease of faulty lipid metabolism in which an abnormal accumulation of lipids form in the body, as in Tay-Sachs disease, Gaucher's disease, and Niemann-Pick disease.

**lipogenic,** producing fat.

**lipoid,** resembling fat.

**lipolysis,** the dissolution or breaking down of fat into fatty acids and glycerol.

**lipoma,** a benign fatty tumor.

**lipomatosis,** excessive fat deposits in the tissues; obesity.

**lipomatous,** pertaining to lipoma.

**lipometabolism,** metabolism of fat.

**lipoprotein,** a simple protein combined with a lipid.

**lipothymia,** fainting; syncope.

**lipotropic,** having an affinity for fat utilization, therefore decreasing fat deposits in the liver.

**lipuria,** fat in the urine.

**liquefacient,** a liquefying drug that causes solid deposits to be converted into liquid.

**liquescent,** becoming liquid.

**liquor amnii,** referring to the amniotic fluid which is a clear, watery substance that surrounds the fetus in the amniotic sac.

**lithiasis,** the formation of calculi and concretions, as gallstones.

**lithium,** a metallic element in its salt form used in the treatment of manic and hypomanic states of excitement, as in manic-depressive illness.

**lithogenesis,** the formation of calculi.

**litholysis,** disintegration or dissolution of calculi.

**lithotomy,** surgical incision into the bladder for removal of a stone.

**lithotripsy,** the crushing of a stony formation in the bladder or urethra.

**lithotrite,** a device used for crushing stone in the bladder.

**lithuresis,** the passage of calculi or crushed stone by urination.

**litmus paper,** a chemically treated blue paper which turns red by acids, but remains blue in alkali solutions, used to indicate the presence of acid in urine testing.

**liver,** the largest organ of the body, a reddish-brown glandular structure situated on the right side beneath the diaphragm and which secretes bile and aids metabolic functioning.

**livid,** cyanotic or bluish color to skin; discoloration.

**lividity,** the condition of being discolored or livid.

**lobar,** pertaining to a lobe of the lungs.

**lobe,** the globular part of an organ with well-defined boundaries; lower portion of the ear without cartilage.

**lobectomy,** the removal of a lobe of any organ or gland by surgical excision.

**lobotomy,** incision of a lobe; the severing of nerve fibers, disconnecting the diencephalon and sectioning the white matter of the brain, used in treatment of mental disturbances.

**lobular,** consisting of small lobes.

**lobule,** a small lobe.

**lochia,** a discharge of blood, mucus, and tissue from the uterus during the first few weeks after childbirth.

**locomotion,** moving from one place to another; moving the body.

**locomotor,** pertaining to locomotion.

**locomotor ataxia,** a form of sclerosis which affects the posterior columns of the spinal cord; tabes dorsalis. Charcot's arthropathy.

**loculus,** a small cavity.

**logagnosia,** a form of aphasia; word blindness.

**logagraphia,** unable to express ideas in writing.

**logamnesia,** forgetfulness, or unable to recognize spoken or written words.

**logomania,** excessive and continuous flow of speech with a repetitive quality.

**logorrhea,** a condition marked by incoherent and excessive talking seen in the insane.

**loin,** portion of the back between thorax and pelvis.

**lordosis,** an abnormal inward curvature of the spine.

**lordotic,** pertaining to lordosis.

**LSD,** lysergic acid diethylamide.

**lubricant,** an agent which makes the skin soft and smooth.

**lucid,** clarity of mind; rational.

**lues,** a pestilent disease, especially syphilis.

**lumbago,** dull back pain across loin region caused by sudden chilling of overheated lumbar muscles.

**lumbar,** pertaining to the loins.

**lumbar vertebrae,** referring to five bones of the spinal column extending from the sacrum to the thoracic vertebrae.

**lumbosacral,** pertaining to both the lumbar vertebrae and the sacrum.

**lumbricalis,** one of the muscles of either the hand or foot resembling a wormlike structure.

**lumen,** the space or cavity within a tube or tubular structure or organ; a unit of light; a hollow of a tube.

**lunatic,** one who is insane or mad.

**lungs,** one of two cone-shaped structures which function as respiratory organs responsible for providing oxygen for the body and discharging waste products.

**lunula,** the pale crescent at the root of fingernails.

**lupiform,** resembling lupus.

**lupus,** any of the skin diseases caused by tubercle bacilli characterized by lesions with raised edges and depressed centers that become scarlike when the scales shed.

**lupus erythematosus,** a chronic inflammation of the skin characterized by reddish macules that scale and drop off; the lesions form a butterfly pattern over the bridge of the nose and cheeks, occurring predominantly in females between puberty and menopause.

**luteal,** pertaining to the corpus luteus, the cells, or the hormone.

**lutein,** a yellowish pigment from the corpus luteum, lipochromes, fat cells, and egg yolk.

**luteinization,** the process involving the development of the corpus luteum within the ruptured graafian follicle.

**luteinizing hormone,** a substance secreted by the pituitary gland that stimulates the reproductive organs and the development of the corpus luteum.

**luteoma,** a tumor of the ovary containing lutein cells.

**luxation,** a dislocation.

**lying-in,** puerperal period; puerperium; confinement.

**lymph,** a transparent, opalalescent liquid composed of plasma and white cells found within the lymphatic vessels. The fluid is collected from the body tissues and returned to the blood through the lymphatic system.

**lymphadentitis,** inflammation of the lymph nodes or glands.

**lymphatic,** pertaining to lymph, or the lymphatic vessels.

**lymph cell,** a lymphocyte.

**lymph node, lymph gland,** a rounded body of glandular tissue found at intervals throughout the lymphatic system, varying in size from a pinhead to an olive, which produce lymphocytes and monocytes.

**lymphoblast,** immature cells that become lymphocytes.

**lymphocyte,** a white blood corpuscle or leukocyte which participates in the body's immunity.

**lymphocytic,** referring to lymphocytes.

**lymphocytoma,** a malignant lymphoma or tumor.

**lymphocytosis,** a condition in the blood that involves an excess of lymphocytes above normal range.

**lymphogranuloma,** Hodgkin's disease; inflammed lymph nodes, as in venereal disease.

**lymphogranulomatosis,** infection of the lymphatic system; Hodgkin's disease.

**lymphoid,** resembling lymph or tissue of the lymphatic system.

**lymphoma,** any malignant disorder of the lymphoid tissue.

**lymphopoiesis,** the formation of lymphocytes or lymphatic tissue.

**lymphosarcoma,** a malignant tumor of lymphoid tissue, but not including Hodgkin's disease.

**lyse,** to cause disintegration of cells; the process involving lysis.

**lysergic acid,** a crystalline ergot derivative composing the base of LSD.

**lysine,** an amino acid derived from protein digestion, essential for growth and repair.

**lysis,** gradual decline of a fever or disease, opposite of crisis; destruction to a cell or substance by an influencing agent.

**Lysol,** trademark, used as a disinfectant and antiseptic.

**lysozyme,** an antibacterial enzyme present in tears, saliva, and various body fluids.

# M

**macerate,** to soften by soaking or steeping.

**maceration,** the softening of a solid or tissue by soaking.

**macrocardius,** abnormal heart enlargement.

**macrocephaly,** an excessively large head.

**macrochelia,** excessively large lips.

**macrocolon, megacolon,** enlargement of the colon.

**macrocyte,** an abnormally large red blood corpuscle.

**macrocytic,** pertaining to a macrocyte.

**macrocytosis,** an excess of macrocytes, being greater in number than normal.

**Macrodantin,** trademark for nitrofurantoin used in treatment of urinary tract infection caused by Escherichia coli.

**macrodontia,** abnormally large size of one or more teeth.

**macrogamete,** the larger female gamete which is fertilized by the smaller male gamete; pertaining to the female reproductive cell.

**macroglossia,** excessively large tongue.

**macromastia,** excessively large breasts.

**macrophage,** a large phagocytic cell derived from monocytes present in loose connective tissues and various body organs which become active when stimulated by inflammation.

**macroscopy,** examination of an object with the naked eye.

**macula, macule,** a small colored spot on the skin.

**maculation,** the development of macules on the skin.

**maculopapular,** having both macules and papules.

**mad,** mentally deranged; irrational; suffering from rabies.

**madarosis,** the loss of eyelashes or eyebrows.

**magnesium,** a mineral element found in soft body tissue, muscle, bone and teeth essential to the proper functioning of the body. An excellent source of magnesium is found in nuts, whole-grain products, dry beans and peas, and dark green vegetables.

**maidenhead,** hymen.

**mal,** sickness or a disorder.

**mala,** cheek; cheekbone.

**malacia,** abnormal softening of body tissue or organs.

**maladjusted,** an inability to adjust one's desires or needs to the environment often causing anxiety.

**malady,** illness.

**malaise,** generalized uneasiness or discomfort, as a preliminary condition of disease; morbid discontent.

**malar,** pertaining to the cheekbone, or cheek.

**malaria,** a febrile, infectious disease caused by a protozoan parasite found in red blood cells, injected by a mosquito bite and characterized by periodic attacks of chills, fever, sweating, which may cause progressive anemia and enlargement of the spleen.

**malformation,** deformity or abnormal structure, especially congenital.

**malign,** malignant.

**malignancy,** condition of being malignant.

**malignant,** virulent and becoming worse, or resisting treatment, as in cancerous growths which threaten to produce death.

**malinger,** to pretend to be ill, usually to gain sympathy or to escape work.

**malleal,** pertaining to the malleus.

**malleolus,** the projections on either side of the ankle joint.

**malleus,** one of the three bones in the middle ear shaped like a hammer.

**malnutrition,** insufficient or faulty nutrition due to lack of necessary food ingestion, improper absorption, or any other disorder of nutrition.

**malocclusion,** imperfect closure or meeting of opposing teeth caused by abnormal growth of the upper or lower jaw.

**malodor,** an offensive stench or odor.

**malodorous,** ill-smelling, fetid, or putrid.

**malpighian layer,** the innermost layer of the epidermis which replaces the outer cells of the skin.

**malposition,** an abnormal placement of a body part.

**malpractice,** wrong and injurious treatment implying neglectful or illegal performance of duty by one in a practicing position, as a physician, surgeon, lawyer, or public servant.

**malpresentation,** an abnormal position of the fetus over the pelvic inlet, as in breech, or scapula.

**Malta fever,** brucellosis, an infectious disease transmitted from animals to man, marked by swelling of joints and spleen, excessive perspiration, weakness, and anemia.

**maltase,** a salivary and pancreatic enzyme which converts maltose to glucose by hydrolysis.

**maltose,** a disaccharide found in malt, malt products, and seed sprouts, formed by the hydrolysis of starch; primarily used as a sweetener.

**mamma,** mammary glands, or breasts.

**mammary,** pertaining to the breasts or glands which secrete milk formed in the lactiferous ducts during lactation.

**mammilla,** the nipple of the breast; a nipple-like process or proturberance.

**mammillary,** resembling a nipple, or concerning a nipple.

**mammogram,** radiography of the mammary gland.

**mammography,** a study of the mammary structures by X-ray photography to detect cancer.

**mammotomy,** surgery of a breast.

**mandible,** the lower portion of the jaw.

**mandibular,** pertaining to the lower jaw bone.

**manducation,** chewing of food, mastication.

**maneuver,** a skillful procedure, as in manipulation of the fetus and placenta to aid in delivery.

**mania,** intense excitement; madness; violent passion or desire.

**manic-depressive,** one afflicted with alternating attacks of mania and depression; cyclic affective psychosis.

**manifestation,** the appearance of symptoms of a disease that determine diagnosis.

**manifest content,** the remembered content of a dream including events and images.

**manubrium,** the upper portion of the sternum which articulates with the clavicle and the first pair of costal cartilages.

**manus,** hand.

**manustupration,** masturbation.

**marasmus,** emaciation or wasting of flesh, especially in infants.

**marijuana, marihuana,** an intoxicating drug usually in cigarette form, illegally used in the U.S.

**marrow,** soft tissue consisting of red or yellow marrow occupying the inner cavities of long bones responsible for blood cell and hemoglobin production.

**masculine,** having male characteristics.

**masochism,** sexual perversion in which pleasure is derived from physical or psychological pain inflicted upon another, or being abused; any pleasure obtained from the abuse of another which gives sexual gratification to the recipient.

**masochist,** one addicted to masochism.

**massage,** methodical manipulation of the body applied by kneading or rubbing the bare skin to stimulate circulation or increase flexibility.

**masseter,** the principle muscle of the mouth which is used in mastication and closing of the mouth.

**masseur,** a man trained in massage techniques.

**masseuse,** a woman trained to practice massage.

**mastadenitis,** inflammation of the mammary gland.

**mastadenoma,** a benign breast tumor.

**mastalgia,** breast pain.

**mastectomy,** surgical excision of the breast.

**mastication,** chewing of food.

**masticatory,** pertaining to mastication; a substance chewed to promote salivary secretion.

**mastitis,** inflammation of the breast occurring mostly in women during lactation.

**mastodynia,** pain in the breast.

**mastoid,** pertaining to the mastoid process located in the temporal bone behind the ear.

**mastoidal,** pertaining to the mastoid.

**mastoidalgia,** pain in the mastoid.

**mastoidectomy,** surgical removal of mastoid cells.

**mastoiditis,** inflammation of any of the mastoid process.

**mastopexy,** surgical correction of large, drooping breasts.

**mastoptosis,** pendulous or sagging breasts.

**masturbation, manustupration,** self production of an orgasm by manipulation of the genitals.

**materia medica,** scientific study concerned with all drugs used in the treatment of diseases, their origin, ingredients, preparation, dosage, and uses.

**maternal,** pertaining to a mother.

**maternity,** the state or condition of motherhood.

**matter,** pus; any substance that occupies space such as gas, liquid, or solid.

**maturation,** maturing or ripening, as a graafian follicle.

**mature,** fully developed.

**maturity,** the state of being mature.

**maxilla,** the upper jawbone.

**maxillary,** referring to the jawbone.

**M.D.,** Doctor of Medicine.

**measles,** a highly infectious viral disease, usually occurring in childhood, characterized by reddish skin eruptions appearing on the face which rapidly increase in size and spread to the trunk and extremities, elevation of temperature, loss of appetite, and bronchitis; rubeola.

**meatus,** a passage or opening; a duct in the body; opening of the nose or ear.

**meconium,** the first fecal discharge of a newborn infant, usually tarry colored, consisting of salts, mucilaginous amnii, mucous, bile, and epithelial cells; also: opium.

**media, medium,** pertaining to the middle, as in the wall of an artery.

**mediad,** in the median line of the body, or central plane.

**medial, median,** pertaining to the middle.

**mediastrinum,** a median partition of the chest cavity from the sternum backward; a septum between two main portions of an organ; the pleural folds and space between the right and left lung.

**mediate,** between two parts or sides.

**medicable,** expectation of cure; treatable.

**Medicaid,** medical aid for the disabled or needy of any age not eligible for social security benefits, sponsored by federal, local, and state governments.

**medical,** pertaining to medicine.

**medicament,** a remedy or substance for healing wounds; medication.

**Medicare,** a Federal insurance program financed by social security which provides medical care for the aged.

**medication,** the administration of remedies, medicine, or drugs for the treatment of diseases or the healing of wounds.

**medicine,** any drug or remedy; the science of diagnosis and treatment of diseases and care of the injured; nonsurgical means of treatment of diseases; the science of preserving health.

**medulla,** the marrow; medulla oblongata; the inner surface of an organ or part of an organ.

**medulla oblongata,** the lower portion of the brain stem, or enlarged part of the spinal cord in the cranium.

**medullary,** pertaining to the marrow or inner portion.

**megacardia,** an enlargement of the heart.

**megacephalic,** enlargement of the head.

**megacephaly,** the condition of having an enlarged head or megacephalic.

**megacolon,** extreme enlargement of the colon.

**megalomania,** a mental disorder characterized by extreme preoccupation with delusions of power, greatness, or goodness.

**meiosis,** the process of nuclear cell division of mature reproductive cells in which the number of chromosomes are reduced to half their original number before the cell divides in two, or from diploid to the haploid.

**melancholia,** a major affective disorder characterized by worry, anxiety, agitation, great depression, severe insomnia, and inhibition of activity; many of the observable symptoms are similar to the depressed phase of manic-depressive psychoses.

**melancholy,** an abnormal state of despondency or dejection; an overelaboration of sadness and grief.

**melanemia,** an unnatural dark pigment in the blood.

**melanidrosis,** black colored sweat.

**melanin,** the black or brown compounds which are the chief pigments produced by melanoblasts located in the deepest layers of the skin. Many factors influence skin melanin pigments such as exposure to the sun, radiation therapy, hormone deficiency, and some types of Vitamin B deficiency.

**melanism,** excessive amounts of black or dark pigment in the skin, hair, and eyes.

**melanoleukoderma,** having mottled skin.

**melanoma,** any tumor which is composed of melanin-pigmented cells; a malignant melanoma.

**melanomatosis,** the formation of widespread melanomas on or beneath the skin.

**melanopathy,** a diseased condition of the skin marked by dark pigmented areas.

**melanosis,** an abnormal deposit of black pigments in the skin found on different parts of the body.

**melanosis lenticularis,** a very rare skin disorder which appears in early youth marked by various pigmented areas, ulcers, and atrophy.

**melanotic,** blackish discoloration; pertaining to melanosis.

**malenuria,** dark pigments present in urine.

**melissophobia,** abnormal aversion or fear of bee or wasp stings.

**melitemia,** the presence of sugar in the blood; glycemia.

**melitis,** inflammation of the cheek.

**membrane,** a thin layer of tissue which lines a cavity or canal, covers organs, or separates one structure from another.

**membranoid,** resembling a membrane.

**membranous,** pertaining to a membrane, or relating to the nature of a membrane.

**membranous labyrinth,** the inner ear which is also called labyrinth because of its complicated shape. The membranous labyrinth within the bony labyrinth consists of the utricle and saccule inside the vestibule, the cochlear duct inside the cochlea, and the membranous semicircular canals inside the bony structures.

**menarche,** the onset of menses, normally between ages 10--17.

**Mendel's laws,** the fundamental rules which govern the transmission of genetic traits based on experiments with the common garden pea (Pisum sativum).

**Meniere's disease,** a usually progressive disease of the labyrinth characterized by a hearing loss, ringing in the ears, dizziness, and a sensation of fullness or pressure.

**meningeal,** pertaining to the meninges.

**meninges,** relating to the three membranes enveloping the spinal cord and brain including the dura mater, pia mater, and the arachnoid.

**meningioma,** a tumor in the meninges.

**meningitis,** inflammation of the membranes of the brain or spinal cord, especially of the arachnoid or pia mater.

**meningocele,** congenital hernia in which the meninges protrude through an opening of the skull or spinal column.

**meningococcus,** the microorganism, Neisseria meningitidis, that causes cerebral meningitis.

**meningoencephalitis,** inflammation of both the brain and its membranes.

**meningoencephalomyelitis,** inflammation of the brain, the spinal cord, and their membranes.

**meningomyelitis,** inflammation of the spinal cord and its membranes.

**meniscectomy,** surgical removal of meniscus cartilage of the knee.

**meniscus,** a crescent-shaped interarticular fibrocartilage found in joints, as in the knee joint; concavo-convex lens.

**menopausal,** pertaining to menopause.

**menopause,** the cessation of the menses; climacteric, or change of life for women between ages 45--50.

**menorrhagia,** excessive or profuse bleeding during the menstrual period.

**menorrhea,** normal menstruation; free flowing menstruation.

**menses,** monthly menstruation; monthly flow of blood from the female genital tract.

**menstruate,** the process of discharging blood from the uterus.

**menstruation,** the periodic discharge of blood and mucus from the uterus occurring at regular intervals of approximately 28 days during a woman's life from puberty to menopause.

**menstruum,** a solvent or a medium.

**mensuration,** the act of measuring.

**mental,** relating to the mind.

**mental age,** the age of a person's mental ability which may be determined by mental tests.

**mental deficiency,** mental retardation; subnormal intellectual functioning, present at birth or which may develop during early childhood, affecting areas of learning, social adjustment, and maturation.

**mentality,** one's mental capacity or mental power; intellectuality.

**mentum,** the chin.

**meperidine,** a synthetic narcotic used as an analgesic and sedative.

**meprobamate,** a tranquilizing drug used to relieve anxiety and mental tension.

**merbromin,** trademark Mercurochrome, used as an antiseptic and a germicide.

**mercuric chloride,** a compound of mercury, highly poisonous, useful as a disinfectant, fungicide, antiseptic, and preservative.

**mercuric oxide,** a yellowish powder used in ointments.

**mercury,** a metallic element soluble in hydrochloric acid, useful in two salt forms, mercurous and mercuric, in germicides.

**mercury poisoning,** acute poisoning due to ingestion marked by severe abdominal pain, vomiting, watery and bloody diarrhea, diminished urinary output, and digestive tract ulceration; chronic form of mercury poisoning due to absorption through the skin and mucous membranes by inhalation, and ingestion which causes inflamed tongue, bleeding gums, loosening of teeth, tremors, incoordination and other various symptoms.

**Merthiolate,** trademark for thimersol used as an antiseptic and germicide.

**mesarteritis,** inflammation of the middle coat of an artery.

**mescaline,** a crystalline alkaloid drug obtained from mescal cactus which causes hallucinations.

**mesencephalon,** the middle portion of the brain, or midbrain.

**mesenchyme,** a network of embryonic mesodermic cells that develop into connective tissues, blood and lymphatic systems, heart, and cartilage and bone.

**mesenteric,** pertaining to the msentery.

**mesenteritis,** inflammation of a mesentery.

**mesentery,** a fold of membranous tissue which attach and support various organs to the body wall such as the peritoneal fold connecting the small intestine to the posterior abdominal wall.

**mesial,** pertaining to the middle.

**mesial plain,** a median plane or division of the body longitudinally into symmetrical parts.

**mesmerism,** an early term for hypnosis, named after Anton Mesmer (1733--1815) which now means therapeutic hypnotism.

**mesmerize,** to hypnotize; to facinate.

**mesoblast,** the mesoderm, or an early stage in the development of the middle layer of the mesoderm.

**mesocardia,** a location of the heart in the middle plane of the thorax.

**mesocolic,** pertaining to the mesocolon.

**mesocolon,** the mesentery or peritoncal fold that connects the colon to the posterior wall of the abdomen.

**mesoderm,** the middle layer of the primary embryonic layers lying between the ectoderm and the entoderm.

**mesometritis,** inflammation of the uterine muscular structures.

**mesomorph,** a body type which is well-proportioned, muscular, and of medium height.

**mesomorphic,** having characteristics of mesomorphs.

**mesonephroma,** a malignant tumor found in the female genital tract, or in the ovary.

**mesonephros,** an excretory organ of the embryo.

**mesosternum,** the middle portion of the sternum.

**mesothelium,** a layer of cells derived from the mesoderm which forms the lining of the embryonic cavity.

**metabolic,** pertaining to metabolism.

**metabolism,** all physical and chemical changes within the organism involving energy and material transformations, and including two fundamental processes, anabolism (building-up process), and catabolism (breaking down process).

**metabolite,** any product of metabolic functions.

**metabolize,** to be transformed by metabolism.

**metacarpal,** pertaining to the metacarpus; a bone of the hand between the fingers and wrist.

**metacarpus,** the bony structure of the hand between the fingers and the wrist.

**metaphase,** the second stage of mitosis or cell division in which chromosomes align across the equatorial plane of spindle fibers prior to separation.

**metaplasia,** a change of one kind of tissue into a form that is abnormal for that tissue.

**metamorphosis,** a change in form or structure; in pathology, a change that is degenerative.

**metapsychology,** speculative psychology concerned with mental processes that reach beyond empirical verification.

**metastasis,** the movement of bacteria or diseased body cells from an organ or body part to another part of the body, usually applied to malignant cells spread by the lymphatics or blood stream.

**metastatic,** pertaining to metastasis.

**metatarsal,** a bone of the metatarsus or foot.

**metatarsus,** the portion of the foot between the tarsus or ankle and the phalanges or toes; including the five bones of the foot.

**metencephalon,** anterior portion of the hindbrain which consists of the cerebellum and pons; that part of the brain vesicles formed by a specialization of the hindbrain in the development of the embryo.

**meteorism,** formation of gas or flautus resulting in distention of the abdomen or intestines.

**methadone,** a synthetic compound with actions similar to morphine which is habit-forming; the hydrochloride is used as a potent analgesic and weak sedative, also used as an antitussive in tuberculosis, bronchiectasis, whooping cough, bronchogenic carcinoma, and congestive heart failure; used in treatment of addiction as a withdrawal substitute for morphine.

**methemoglobin,** present normally in the blood in small amounts, but becomes toxic when a larger portion of hemoglobin is converted into methemoglobin by the oxidation of iron, giving the blood a dark-brown color and decreasing its function to carry oxygen.

**methenamine,** a urinary antiseptic.

**methionine,** an essential amino acid important to nutrition.

**metopic,** pertaining to the forehead.

**metopian,** that part of the forehead between the frontal eminences.

**metra,** the uterus.

**metralgia,** pain in the uterus.

**Metrazol,** trademark for pentamethylenetetrazol used in treating certain heart conditions and as a respiratory stimulant.

**metrectomy,** surgical excision of the uterus; hysterectomy.

**metritis,** inflammation of the uterus.

**metrocarcinoma,** cancerous uterine tumor.

**metrocystosis,** the formation of many uterine cysts.

**metropathy,** any uterine disease.

**metroptosis,** a dropped uterus.

**metrorrhagia,** excessive or profuse bleeding from the uterus not associated with menses.

**microbe,** a microorganism, bacteria, or germ which produces disease.

**microbic,** referring to microbes.

**microbiologist,** a specialist in microbiology.

**microbiology,** the scientific study of microorganisms.

**microcephalic,** pertaining to a small head below 1350 cc.

**microcephaly, microcephalism,** an abnormal small head, a congenital anomaly, as seen in idiocy.

**micrococcus,** belonging to gram-positive bacteria of the Micrococcaceae family which are globular or oval and produce certain diseases in man.

**microcyte,** a small red blood cell less than 5 microns in diameter occurring in certain anemias.

**micron,** measurement of a unit of length equal to one millionth of a meter.

**microorganism,** a bacteria, or minute living structure which cannot be seen with the naked eye.

**microscope,** an optical apparatus which magnifies minute structures and microorganisms.

**microscopic,** pertaining to a microscope; visible only by means of a microscope.

**microscopy,** a microscopic examination, as in viewing specimens under a glass slide.

**microsome,** a minute particle or granule present in cell protoplasm.

**microtome,** a device for cutting thin sections of tissue for microscopic examination.

**micturate,** to discharge urine; urinate.

**micturition,** urination, or voiding of urine.

**midbrain,** mesencephalon, which lies below the inferior surface of the cerebrum and above the pons, consisting mainly of white matter.

**middle ear,** consisting of the tympanic membrane and a cavity containing the incus, malleus, and stapes.

**midriff,** the diaphragm.

**midwife,** a woman who practices midwifery; one who assists at childbirth.

**midwifery,** the art of assisting at childbirth or delivery.

**migraine,** sudden attacks of headache which usually affect the vision and may cause nausea, vomiting, constipation or diarrhea, resulting from constriction of the cranial arteries affecting one side of the head.

**miliaria,** an acute inflammation of the sweat glands causing vesicles to appear on the skin due to obstruction and the retention of sweat.

**miliaria rubra,** prickly heat, or heat rash.

**miliary,** resembling millet seeds; small nodules on the skin due to excessive exposure to heat.

**milieu,** pertaining to environment.

**milium,** a tiny pink and white vesicle or nodule appearing beneath the skin due to the retention of a fatty secretion of the sebaceous gland.

**milk,** an opaque white secretion of the mammary glands for feeding the young.

**milk fever,** a fever appearing with the beginning of lactation following childbirth, resulting from an infection.

**milk leg,** an inflammation of the iliac or femoral vein which causes pain and swelling, often a complication of childbirth.

**milk tooth,** a temporary or deciduous tooth occurring in childhood.

**milligram,** one-thousandth of a gram; abbreviated mg.

**millimeter,** one-thousandth meter; abbreviated mm.

**millicron,** one-thousandth of a micron; one-millionth of a millimeter.

**mind,** the psyche; having integrated brain functioning resulting in one's ability to perceive, comprehend, reason, and process information in an intelligent manner.

**miosis,** an abnormal contraction of the pupils.

**miotic,** an agent that produces contraction of the pupil.

**misanthropy,** hatred of mankind.

**miscarriage,** spontaneous abortion; referring to the interruption of pregnancy usually between the fourth month and viability.

**miscegenation,** marriage or sexual union between mixed races; inbreeding between different races.

**miscible,** having mixing capability; able to be mixed with separation.

**misogamy,** a hatred or fear of marriage.

**misogyny,** an aversion to women.

**misologia,** hatred for mental work.

**misoneism,** an aversion to new ideas; conservatism.

**misopedia,** an abnormal dislike for children.

**mithridate,** an antidote against poisoning.

**mithridatism,** acquiring immunity to a poison by taking small amounts and gradually increase dosages.

**mitochondria,** threadlike structures in cell cytoplasm.

**mitosis,** indirect cell division involving complex changes in the nucleus in a continuous process divided into four phases: prophase, metaphase, anaphase, and telephase.

**mitotic,** pertaining to mitosis.

**mitral,** pertaining to the bicuspid valve in the heart that prevents the blood in the left ventricle flowing back to the left auricle.

**mittelschmerz,** pain between menstrual periods at the time of ovulation.

**modality,** a method of application of any therapeutic agent.

**molar,** broad surfaced tooth for grinding, one of three on both sides of the upper and lower jaw.

**mole,** nevus; a congenital discolored spot on the skin which is slightly elevated.

**molluscum,** any slightly infectious skin disease marked by the formation of cutaneous tumors.

**mongolism,** Down's syndrome, a congenital mental deficiency.

**mongoloid,** a person with characteristics of mongolism.

**moniliasis,** candidiasis; an infection of the mucous membranes or skin caused by yeastlike fungi.

**moniliform,** resembling a string of beads.

**monoamine,** a molecule from one amino group, as serotonin, dopamine, and norepinephrine.

**monocular,** affecting one eye; pertaining to a single lens.

**monocyte,** a phagocytic leukocyte with a nucleus shaped like a kidney which is formed in bone marrow and which constitutes part of the important defense mechanism of the body.

**monocytosis,** having an excess of monocytes in the blood.

**monodactyly,** having only one digit on a foot or hand.

**monomania,** a mental illness marked by a morbid preoccupation with one idea or activity.

**monomaniac,** a person afflicted with monomania.

**monomelic,** affecting only one limb.

**mononuclear,** having a single nucleus.

**mononucleosis,** having an excess of monocytes in the blood stream; an infectious mononucleosis is an acute disease caused by the Epstein-Barr virus marked by fever, sore throat, general lymph node enlargement, and an abnormal increase of mononuclear leukocytes.

**monoparesis,** paralysis of one part of the body.

**monophobia,** pathological fear of being alone.

**monoplegia,** paralysis of one limb or one group of muscles.

**mons pubis,** the pubic eminence.

**morbid,** pertaining to, or being affected by disease; referring to an unhealthy mental state.

**morbidity,** the state of being diseased.

**morbiliform,** resembling measles with skin eruptions.

**morgue,** a public mortuary where dead bodies are held until identified or buried.

**moribund,** dying, or a state of dying.

**morning sickness,** nausea and vomiting that affects some women during the early stages of pregnancy.

**moron,** an adult who is feebleminded or mentally deficient, whose mental intellect corresponds to that of a normal child between ages 7--12 years.

**morose,** a gloomy or sullen disposition.

**morphia,** morphine.

**morphine,** an alkaloid found in opium used as an analgesic and sedative.

**morphinism,** habitual or excessive use of morphine which results in a morbid disposition.

**morphinomania,** madness resulting from the habitual use of morphine; a morbid and uncontrolled desire for morphine.

**morphogenesis,** various changes occurring during the development of an organism or part of the body.

**morphology,** the study of structure and form of organisms without regard to function.

**mortal,** causing death; destined to die; human.

**mortality,** state of being mortal; statistical death rate.

**morula,** a solid mass of cells formed by cleavage of a fertilized ovum.

**mosaic,** in genetics, a person exhibiting mosaicism.

**mosaicism,** two or more cell lines which are distinct karyotypically or genotypically and are derived from a single zygote.

**motility,** having spontaneity of movement; capable to perform voluntary movements.

**motion sickness,** a condition marked by nausea, vomiting, and dizziness caused by rhythmic, irregular, or jerky movements, as in sea sickness.

**motor,** a muscle, nerve, or center that conveys an impulse which produces movement.

**Motrin,** trademark for ibuprofen used as an anti-inflammatory agent, and possesses analgesic and antipyretic properties.

**mouth,** the cavity or first portion of the digestive system, consisting of the hard palate, teeth, tongue, and cheeks; essential part for speaking, and is an alternate breathing passage.

**mouth-to-mouth resuscitation,** a life-saving procedure to induce artificial respiration of an apneic victim by pressing the nostrils together to close the airway and at the same time blowing directly into the mouth and lungs using short, repeated, and regular breaths.

**movement,** motion or the act of moving; evacuation of the bowels.

**mucilage,** a gummy, aqueous preparation or glue used as an adhesive.

**mucin,** a glycoprotein which is the chief component of mucous secretions.

**mucocutaneous,** pertaining to an area where the skin and mucous membranes come together.

**mucoid,** a glycoprotein which is similar to mucin but differing in solubility.

**mucoprotein,** protein, containing polysaccharides, which is present in all connective and supporting tissues in the body.

**mucopurulent,** containing mucous and pus.

**mucosa,** referring to mucous membrane.

**mucoserous,** composed of both mucous and serum.

**mucosin,** mucin present in viscous, and sticky mucus.

**mucous,** resembling or pertaining to mucus; secreting mucus.

**mucous membranes,** membranes that secrete mucus.

**mucoviscidosis,** the disease cystic fibrosis of the pancreas.

**mucus,** a viscid secretion of the glands and mucous membranes, consisting of mucin, leukocytes, various salts, and desquamated cells.

**multigravida,** a woman pregnant for the third time or more.

**multipara,** a woman who has had two or more viable fetuses.

**multiparous,** having borne more than one child.

**multiple sclerosis,** MS, a progressive and degenerative disease of the central nervous system which is not contagious, marked by tremors, muscular weakness, speech disturbances, and visual complaints.

**mumps,** an acute contagious disease occurring mainly in childhood marked by swelling of the large salivary glands in front of the ears, but may involve the meninges and testes in postpubertal males.

**mural,** pertaining to the wall in any cavity of the body.

**murmur,** an abnormal heart sound which has a blowing or rasping quality.

**muscle,** an organ which produces body movement within an animal by contraction, composed of bundles of fibers of different lengths, breaths, and thicknesses.

**muscular,** pertaining to muscles; composed of muscle; having well-developed muscles.

**muscular dystrophy,** a progressive disease in which deterioration and atrophy of the muscles cause wasting and symmetrical weakening, believed to be inherited.

**musculature,** involving the muscular arrangement of the body or of a part.

**musculoskeletal,** comprising the skeleton and the muscles.

**mutant,** a living organism that is a product of genetic mutation.

**mutate,** to alter or change.

**mutation,** a permanent change in genetic material; an individual exhibiting such a change.

**mute,** one who is unable to speak.

**myalgia,** having muscle pain; muscular pain.

**myasthenia,** muscular debility or weakness.

**myasthenia gravis,** a neuromuscular disorder without atrophy, characterized by progressive fatigue and exhaustion of the muscular system.

**myatrophy,** muscle wasting.

**mycete,** a fungus.

**Mycobacterium,** a gram-positive bacteria found in swimming pools which causes granuloma.

**mycology,** the scientific study of fungi.

**mycosis,** a disease caused by fungi.

**mycotic,** pertaining to mycosis.

**Mycostatin,** trademark for nystatin used for fungus infections.

**mydriasis,** dilatation of the pupils.

**mydriatic,** an agent that dilates the pupil of the eye.

**myelencephalitis,** inflammation of the brain and the spinal cord.

**myelencephalon,** the posterior part of the embryonic hindbrain from which the medulla oblongata and the lower portion of the fourth ventricle develop.

**myelin,** the whitish fatlike substance that surrounds the axon of myelinated nerve fibers.

**myelinic,** pertaining to myelin.

**myelinization,** the formation of the myelin sheath around the axon.

**myelin sheath,** a segmented wrapping of a double layer of Schwann cells surrounding some nerve fibers.

**myelitis,** inflammation of the spinal cord or bone marrow.

**myelocyte,** a cell intermediate between a promyelocyte and a metamyelocyte in development of leukocytes found in red bone marrow.

**myeloencephalitis,** inflammation of the spinal cord and brain.

**myelography,** radiography of the spinal cord after an injection of a radiopaque substance into the subarachnoid space.

**myeloid,** pertaining to or resembling bone marrow; referring to the spinal cord; resembling myelocytes but not developing from bone marrow.

**myeloma,** a tumor originating in hematopoietic cells of bone marrow.

**myocardiograph,** an instrument for tracing heart movements.

**myocarditis,** inflammation of the myocardium.

**myocardium,** the thickest and middle layer of the wall of the heart, or muscle of the heart.

**myogenic,** originating in muscle.

**myoglobin,** a protein of hemoglobin in muslces, composed of one polypeptide chain and one hemp group, and carrying more oxygen and less carbon monoxide.

**myograph,** an apparatus used to measure muscular contraction.

**myology,** the study of muscles and their accessory structures such as bursae and synovial membrane.

**myoma,** a tumor consisting of muscular tissue.

**myomatous,** pertaining to a myoma.

**myoneural,** concerned with both muscles and nerves.

**myopia,** nearsightedness; defective vision in which objects can only be seen clearly when very close to the eyes.

**myopic,** pertaining to myopia.

**myositis,** inflammation of voluntary muscle tissue.

**myospasm,** spasm of a muscle or group of muscles.

**myotomy,** dissection of muscular tissue.

**myringa,** tympanic membrane.

**myringitis,** eardrum inflammation.

**myringoscope,** a device used to examine the eardrum.

**myxedema,** a condition causing nonpitting edema with abnormal deposits of mucin in the tissues, accompanied by a blunting of the senses and intellect due to hypothyroidism.

**myxoma,** a tumor consisting of connective tissue cells and mucous.

**myxorrhea,** an excessive flow of mucus.

**myxovirus,** a group of related viruses which produce influenza, mumps, and measles.

# N

**nacreous,** a pear-like, iridescent luster in certain bacterial clusters.

**nail,** the horny cutaneous cell structure on the dorsal end of fingers and toes forming flat plates.

**nalorphine,** used as an antagonist of morphine and in treatment of narcotic overdose.

**nanism,** dwarfism; an abnormal small stature.

**nape,** the back of the neck.

**naprapathy,** a treatment of disease based on the assumption that an illness is due to faulty ligament functioning which may be corrected or adjusted by massage and manipulation of joints and muscles.

**narcissism,** self-love, or being interested in one's self, as opposed to the love of another person. An excess of narcissism interferes with relationships, but some degree of self-love if considered normal.

**narcolepsy,** an uncontrollable desire to sleep for brief periods.

**narcosis,** a state of unconsciousness, stupor, or insensibility produced by a chemical or narcotic drug.

**narcotic,** a drug which produces sleep; used in moderate doses, a central nervous system depressant which relieves pain and induces sleep; used in excessive doses, produces unconsciousness, stupor, coma, and even death.

**narcotized,** to become unconscious under the influence of a narcotic.

**naris,** nares; nostril or nostrils.

**nasal,** pertaining to the nose.

**nascent,** having just come into existence; being born.

**nasofrontal,** pertaining to the nasal and frontal bones.

**nasolabial,** pertaining to the nose and lip.

**nasolacrimal,** pertaining to the nose and tear ducts and glands.

**nasology,** the study of the nose and its diseases.

**nasopalatine,** pertaining to both the nose and palate.

**nasopharyngeal,** pertaining to the nose and pharynx.

**nasopharyngitis,** inflammation of the nasopharynx.

**nasopharynx,** that portion of the pharynx situated above the soft palate.

**natal,** pertaining to birth.

**natality,** birth rate.

**nates,** the buttocks.

**natural selection,** Darwin's theory of evolution which accounts for the origin of species. Because of limited food supply and a struggle for existence those genetic species which have particular characteristics tend to survive.

**naturopathy,** the therapeutic use of natural forces such as air, heat, light, massage, and water.

**nausea,** having an upset stomach and the inclination to vomit.

**nauseant,** causing one to feel nauseated; affecting nausea.

**nauseate,** to cause nausea.

**nauseous,** affecting or producing nausea, disgust, or loathing.

**navel,** the depression in the center of the abdomen; the umbilicus.

**navicular,** boat-shaped; a wrist or ankle bone.

**nearsightedness,** myopia; seeing clearly only objects that are near.

**nearthrosis,** an artificial joint due to a broken bone.

**nebula,** a corneal opacity; an oily liquid prepared for atomizer usage.

**nebulizer,** an apparatus which produces a fine spray such as an atomizer.

**neck,** that part of the body which connects the head to the trunk; a constricted part of an organ.

**necrobiosis,** a gradual degeneration and death of certain tissues or cells.

**necrophilia,** a pathological attraction to dead bodies or death.

**necrophobia,** morbid fear of death or dead bodies.

**necropsy,** autopsy; examination of a corpse.

**necrose,** to become necrotic.

**necrosis,** death of cells or bone caused by enzymatic degradation surrounding tissues which are healthy.

**necrotic,** pertaining to death of a portion of tissue.

**negative,** lacking confirmation of a disease by testing results, as a negative diagnosis; showing resistance.

**negativism,** opposition to advice; an opposite behavior to one appropriate in a specific situation.

**Neisseria,** a gram-positive bacteria, causing gonorrhea.

**nematode,** a roundworm belonging to Nematoda, a parasitic phylum whose hosts may be man, animals, or domestic plants.

**nematology,** the study of nematodes.

**Nembutal,** trademark for pentobarbital sodium used as a hypnotic and sedative prior to anesthesia and to control convulsions.

**neoantigen,** an intranuclear antigen present in cells which are infected by oncogenic viruses.

**neogenesis,** regeneration of tissues.

**neomycin,** a broad-spectrum antibiotic effective against various gram-negative organisms, used in skin infections, wounds, burns, and ulcers which form in the urinary tract, ear, eye, skin, and for preoperative preparation of the skin.

**neonatal,** pertaining to the newborn infant.

**neonate,** a newborn infant.

**neophobia,** an aversion to all unknown things or new scenes or circumstances.

**neoplasia,** the formation of new tissues or a neoplasm.

**neoplasm,** any new abnormal growth of tissue in the body; a tumor.

**neoplastic,** pertaining to neoplasm.

**neoplasty,** surgical restoration of tissue or parts.

**Neo-synephrine hydrochloride,** trademark for phenylephrine useful in raising blood pressure, as a decongestant, and as a mydriatic.

**nephralgia,** pain in a kidney.

**nephralgic,** pertaining to renal pain.

**nephrectomy,** excision of a kidney.

**nephric,** pertaining to the kidney or kidneys.

**nephrism,** various symptoms caused by chronic kidney disease.

**nephritic,** pertaining to nephritis; referring to a kidney.

**nephritis,** inflammation of the kidney.

**nephrolith,** a stone or calculus in the kidney.

**nephrolithiasis,** the presence of renal calculi.

**nephrolithotomy,** surgical removal of a kidney stone.

**nephroma,** a tumor of the kidney or its tissue.

**nephron,** the structural and functional unit of the kidney, approximately a million and a quarter nephrons in each kidney.

**nephropathy,** kidney disease.

**nephrosis,** a kidney disease marked by degenerative lesions of the renal tubules without inflammation.

**nerve,** a white cord-like structure comprising nerve fibers which conduct and convey impulses from the brain and spinal cord throughout the body.

**nerve cell,** a neuron.

**nerve fiber,** an enlongated thread-like process, or axon, which conducts impulses.

**nerve impulse,** an excitatory process occurring in nerve fibers by the introduction of a stimuli.

**nervous,** easily excited or agitated; pertaining to a nerve.

**nervous breakdown,** signifying any mental disorder that affects an individual's normal activities such as depression, psychosis, or neurosis.

**nervousness,** excitability or mental unrest.

**nervous system,** consisting of a network of nerve cells responsible for controlling body functions including ganglia, spinal cord, nerves, and brain; CNS, or central nervous system which acts to regulate and coordinate bodily activities and initiate responses that help the body to adjust to environmental changes.

**neural,** pertaining to a nerve or nerves; the nervous system.

**neuralgia,** sharp pain along the course of a nerve or several nerves.

**neural tube,** a tubular formation of nerve tissue in the embryo from which the brain and spinal cord develop.

**neurasthenia,** a condition following depressed states from prolonged emotional tension marked by weakness, exhaustion, headache, sweating, polyuria, ringing ears, vertigo, double vision, fear, irritability, poor concentration, insomnia, and many other symptoms.

**neuraxitis,** encephalitis.

**neurectomy,** excision of a nerve or part of a nerve.

**neurectopia,** an abnormal position of a nerve.

**neurilemma,** a thin membranous sheath surrounding a nerve fiber.

**neurinoma,** a peripheral nerve tumor.

**neuritis,** inflammation of a nerve or nerves accompanied by impaired reflexes.

**neuroblastoma,** a hemorrhagic malignant tumor involving nerve ganglia.

**neurocirculatory,** pertaining to circulation and the nervous system in the body.

**neurocrine,** relating to hormonal influence on nervous activity.

**neurodermatitis,** severe irritation and itching of the skin due to a nervous disorder.

**neurodynia,** pain in a nerve.

**neurofibril,** any of the delicate fibrils found in nerve cells which extend into the axon and dendrites.

**neurofibroma,** a tumor of peripheral nerves found in connecting nerve tissue.

**neurofibromatosis,** a conditioned marked by various sizes of tumors on peripheral nerves, muscles, bones, and skin.

**neurogenic,** beginning in a nerve or nerve tissue.

**neurogenous,** developing in the nervous system.

**neuroglia,** delicate connective tissue which supports the structure of nervous tissue in the central nervous system.

**neuroglial,** pertaining to neuroglia.

**neuroglioma,** a tumor consisting of neuroglial tissue.

**neuroleptic,** an antipsychotic drug.

**neurologist,** a specialist in neurology.

**neurology,** the branch of medicine concerned with the nervous system.

**neurolysin,** an agent which destroys neurons.

**neurolysis,** the cutting of a nerve sheath to relieve tension; stretching a nerve to reduce tension; dissolution of nerve tissue.

**neuroma,** a new growth composed of nerve cells and nerve fibers.

**neuromalacia,** an abnormal softening of the nerves.

**neuromuscular,** pertaining to both nerves and muscles.

**neuromyopathic,** affecting the nervous system and muscles including the heart.

**neuron,** a nerve cell, or any of the conductive cells of the nervous system.

**neuronal,** relating to neurons.

**neuropathology,** the study of the diseases of the nervous system.

**neuropathy,** any disease of the peripheral nervous system.

**neuropharmacology,** the science concerned with the effects of drugs on the nervous system.

**neurophysiology,** the physiology of the nervous system.

**neuroplasty,** surgical repair of nerves.

**neuropsychiatry,** the branch of medicine concerned with neurology and psychiatry.

**neurosis,** an emotional disorder characterized by anxiety arising from unresolved and unconscious conflicts, considered to be less severe than psychoses because personality disorganization and distortion of reality are not manifested.

**neurosurgery,** surgery performed on the nervous system.

**neurosyphilis,** syphilis involving the central nervous system.

**neurotherapy,** treatment of nervous disorders.

**neurotic,** pertaining to one affected with neurosis; relating to nerves; an unusually nervous person.

**neurotomy,** surgical cutting of nerves.

**neurotoxin,** a poisonous substance which is destructive to nerve cells and tissue.

**neurotripsy,** crushing of a nerve by surgery.

**neurovascular,** pertaining to the nervous and vascular systems.

**neutral,** neither acid or alkaline.

**neutrophil,** a leukocyte that stains readily with neutral dyes.

**nevocarcinoma,** a malignant melanoma developing from a mole.

**nevoid,** resembling a nevus.

**nevose,** marked with nevi or moles.

**nevus,** a congenital circumscribed malformation of the skin which is not caused externally; a birthmark.

**newborn,** recently born infant.

**Niacin,** trademark for nicotinic acid essential to the body.

**nicotine,** a poisonous alkaloid found in tobacco used as an insecticide, and in veterinary preparations as an external parasitide.

**nicotinic acid,** from the complex Vitamin B group consisting of a crystalline compound occurring in various animal and plant tissues, used for its curative property in pellagra, poor peripheral circulation, and high cholesterol levels in the blood.

**nictitation,** the act of winking; blinking of the eyelids.

**night blindness,** defective vision in the dark due to lack of visual purple in the rods of the retina, or to regenerative slowness after being exposed to light.

**nightmare,** a terrifying and anxiety provoking dream.

**nightwalking,** somnambulism; a state of walking habitually in one's sleep.

**nipple,** mammilla papilla, a protuberance from the mammary gland from which the lactiferous ducts discharge milk in the female; any similarly shaped structure.

**nit,** the egg of a louse.

**niter,** potassium nitrate or sodium nitrate.

**nitrate,** a salt of nitric acid.

**nitric acid,** a corrosive, poisonous liquid in concentrated form widely used in industry and in the manufacture of medicinal preparations.

**nitrogen mustard,** used in therapeutic mustard compounds important in treating some diseases.

**nitroglycerin,** a vasodilator used in treatment of angina pectoris; also used in making dynamite or rocket propellants by treating glycerol with nitric and sulfuric acids.

**nitrous oxide,** a gas used as a general anesthetic and analgesic, especially during dental procedures and surgery; laughing gas.

**noctalbuminuria,** an excessive amount of albumin voided in urine at night.

**nocturia,** excessive urination at night; enuresis or bed-wetting.

**node,** a knot or swelling; a constricted area; a tiny rounded structure; a lymph gland.

**nodose,** knotlike projections at intervals; having nodes.

**nodular,** resembling nodules.

**nodule,** a tiny node; an aggregation of small cells.

**nodulose,** having nodules or small knots.

**nodus,** a node.

**noma,** a progressive gangrenous condition of the mouth and cheek spreading from the mucous membranes to cutaneous surfaces, occurring in malnourished children.

**nomenclature,** classified system of anatomical structures, organisms, and names signifying the genus and species of animals and plants.

**nonipara,** a woman who has delivered nine viable fetuses.

**nonunion,** the failure of a fracture to heal, especially the ends of a bone that do not unit.

**nonviable,** not capable of living; inadequate development.

**norepinephrine,** a hormone secreted by the adrenal glands, a powerful vasopressor, and used to restore blood pressure in hypotensive conditions.

**normal,** a standard; natural and proper functioning.

**nose,** the projection on the face that contains the nares, the nasal cavity, olfactory nerve endings, and functions in speech, respiration, and sense of smell.

**nosebleed,** epistaxia.

**nosology,** scientific classification of diseases.

**nosomania,** an assumption that one has some special illness or disease; hypochondriasis.

**nosomycosis,** a fungal disease; mycosis.

**nosophobia,** morbid fear of sickness.

**nostril,** one of either of the nares.

**notalgia,** back pain.

**notochord,** a rod-shaped primitive groove of the embryo which develops into the vertebral column.

**Novocain,** trademark for procaine hydrochloride used as a local anesthetic.

**noxious,** injurious to health; hurtful.

**nubility,** being able to marry or marriageable, said of a girl at puberty; the final stage of sex development.

**nucleate,** having a nucleus.

**nucleic acid,** an organic compound found in cells, especially the nucleus, which is important to heredity and the control of cell metabolism. It is composed of phosphoric acids, bases from purines or pyrimidines, carbohydrates, and sugars.

**nucleolus,** a small rounded body within the cell nucleus in which the synthesis of RNA takes place.

**nullipara,** a female who has never given birth to an infant.

**nulliparous,** having never borne an infant.

**numb,** having no feeling or sensation in a body part.

**numbness,** a state of lacking sensation in a part of the body; lacking the power to move; state of being numb.

**nurse-midwife,** a person trained in the two disciplines of nursing and midwifery, and having received certification from the American College of Nurse-Midwives.

**nutation,** involuntary nodding of the head.

**nutrient,** a substance that provides nourishment, as in a component of food.

**nutriment,** nourishment that serves to sustain the body by promoting growth and replacement of worn-out cells.

**nutrition,** the process of ingesting food and utilizing it in the growth, repair, and maintenance of body activities.

**nutritionist,** one who specializes in scientific study of nutrition.

**nutritious,** providing nourishment.

**nutritive,** pertaining to nutrition and the process of assimilating food substances.

**nyctalgia,** pain occurring during the night.

**nyctalopia,** poor vision in a faint light or at night; night blindness.

**nyctophilia,** an unusual preference for night.

**nyctophobia,** morbid fear of darkness.

**nympha,** small fold of mucous membrane which form the inner lips of the vulva.

**nymphomania,** an abnormal and excessive need for sexual intercourse in females.

**nystagmus,** involuntary rapid eye movements.

**nyxis,** paracentesis, or puncturing the abdominal cavity for the removal of fluid to relieve the pressure of ascites; piercing.

# O

**oarialgia,** pain in an ovary.

**obduction,** scientific examination of a dead body to learn cause of death; autopsy.

**obese,** extremely corpulent; fat; overweight.

**obesity,** a condition of the body in which an abnormal amount of fat accumulates beyond body requirements.

**oblique,** a slanting or diagonal direction; involvement of two muscles of the eye, the abdomen, the head, and the ears which run at an angle, not laterally.

**obsession,** an uncontrollable need to dwell on a thought or an emotion, or to behave in a specific way.

**obsessive,** pertaining to obsession.

**obstetric,** pertaining to obstetrics or midwifery.

**obstetrician,** a physician who attends women during pregnancy, labor, and puerperium.

**obstetrics,** the branch of medicine concerned with prenatal care and puerperium.

**obstipation,** extreme constipation which is resistive to treatment and cure, usually caused by an obstruction.

**obturate,** to obstruct or to close.

**obturator,** any obstruction that closes an opening, as a plate or disk that closes an abdominal opening.

**obtusion,** a deadening of normal sensations.

**occipital,** pertaining to the occiput or the back part of the head.

**occipital bone,** concerning the bone in the lower posterior portion of the skull between the parietal and temporal bones in the head.

**occipitocervical,** pertaining to the occiput and the neck.

**occipitofacial,** relating to both the occiput and face.

**occipitomental,** pertaining to the occiput and chin.

**occipitoparietal,** pertaining to the occiput and parietal bones.

**occipitotemporal,** pertaining to the occiput and temporal bones.

**occiput,** the back part of the skull.

**occlusion,** the state of being occluded or closed; referring to closely fitting opposing teeth in the upper and lower jaw.

**occlusive,** pertaining to occlusion or closing up.

**occult,** hidden or concealed from view, as a hemorrhage.

**occult blood,** a minute amount of blood that can only be detected by a microscope or chemical means.

**occupational disease,** a functional disease caused by one's occupation, such as writer's cramp.

**occupational therapy,** a method of rehabilitative treatment using activities to encourage a physically or mentally disabled person to aid his own recovery by performing light work, physical exercise, creative arts, cooking, crafts, or vocational training.

**ochlophobia,** abnormal fear of crowds.

**ocular,** pertaining to the eye; concerned with the eye or vision; the eyepiece of a microscope.

**oculist,** one who specializes in diseases of the eye; ophthalmologist.

**oculomotor,** referring to movements of the eye.

**oculomotor nerve,** the third cranial nerve which originates in the ventral part of the midbrain and extends to the external eye muscles.

**oculomycosis,** any of the fungal eye diseases.

**oculus,** the eye.

**adontalgia,** a toothache.

**odontectomy,** excision or the removal of a tooth.

**odontitis,** inflammation of a tooth.

**odontoblast,** connective tissue cells that line the tooth pulp outer surface and form deposits of dentin on teeth.

**odontoid,** resembling a tooth.

**odontologist,** a dentist or dental surgeon.

**odontology,** dentistry; the study of teeth, as they relate to health, growth, diseases and structure.

**odontoma,** a tumor arising from dental tissues.

**odontonecrosis,** extensive tooth decay.

**odontopathy,** diseases of teeth.

**odontophobia,** unusual aversion to the sight of teeth; morbid fear of dental surgery.

**odontorrhagia,** hemorrhaging from a socket after tooth extraction.

**odontosis,** development or eruption of teeth.

**odontotherapy,** special treatment of diseased teeth.

**oedipal,** pertaining to the Oedipus complex.

**Oedipus complex,** Freudian concept; abnormal intense love of a child for a parent of the opposite sex manifested by envy and aggressive feelings toward the parent of the same sex, most commonly love of a son for his mother.

**oikomania,** a nervous disorder caused by unhappy home surroundings.

**oikophobia,** an abnormal dislike of the home.

**ointment,** a soft fatlike substance used in external preparations and having an antiseptic quality.

**olecranal,** pertaining to the olecranon.

**olecranoid,** resembling the olecranon or elbow joint.

**olecranon,** the large bony projection of the ulna forming the elbow joint.

**olfaction,** the process of smelling; the sense of smell.

**olfactology,** the study of the sense of smell.

**olfactory,** referring to the sense of smell.

**olfactory nerves,** the first pair of cranial nerves consisting of sensory fibers which conduct impulses from the mucosa of the upper part of the nasal cavity to the brain.

**olfactory organ,** the nose consisting of hair cells with receptors in the mucosa of the upper part of the nasal cavity which are extremely sensitive to delicate odors.

**oligemia,** deficiency of blood volume in the body.

**oligocholia,** a lack of bile.

**oligocythemia,** decreased number of red blood cells than normal.

**oligogalactia,** a deficient milk secretion.

**oligohemia,** an insufficiency of circulating blood in the body.

**oligohydramnios,** an abnormal small amount of amniotic fluid.

**oligohydruria,** urine that is highly concentrated.

**oligopnea,** having infrequent respirations.

**oligospermia,** a deficient number of spermatozoa in seminal fluid.

**oliguria,** insufficiency in the amount of urine produced.

**omental,** pertaining to the omentum.

**omentectomy,** surgical removal of a portion of the omentum.

**omentitis,** inflammation of the omentum.

**omentum,** a double fold of peritoneum which extends from the stomach to the abdominal viscera.

**omphalic,** pertaining to the umbilicus.

**omphalitis,** inflammation of the umbilicus.

**omphalocele,** a protrusion of a portion of the intestine through an abdominal defect in the wall at the umbilicus occurring at birth.

**omphalos,** umbilicus or navel.

**omphalotomy,** cutting the umbilical cord at birth.

**onanism,** coitus interruptus, or withdrawal during intercourse before ejaculation; masturbation.

**oncogenesis,** producing tumors.

**oncology,** the branch of medicine concerned with the study of tumors.

**onychauxis,** nail hypertrophy.

**onychectomy,** surgical removal of a finger or toe nail.

**onychia,** inflammation of a nail bed frequently causing nail loss.

**onyx,** a fingernail or toenail.

**onyxis,** ingrown nails.

**oocyte,** an early stage of the ovum before maturation.

**oogenesis,** the formation and development of the ovum after a series of cell divisions beginning with the primordial germ cells in the ovary.

**oogenetic,** pertaining to oogenesis.

**oophorectomy,** excision or surgical removal of an ovary; ovariectomy.

**oophoritis,** inflammation of an ovary.

**operable,** subject to surgical treatment with a reasonalbe chance of safety.

**ophidism,** poisoning caused by snakebite.

**ophthalmalgia,** pain the eye.

**ophthalmia,** inflammation of the eye or its membranes.

**ophthalmic,** belonging to the eye.

**ophthalmologic,** pertaining to ophthalmology.

**ophthalmologist,** a medical physician who practices ophthalmology.

**ophthalmology,** science of the eye; study of eye anatomy, physiology, and diseases.

**ophthalmopathy,** any of the eye diseases.

**ophthalmoplasty,** plastic surgery of the eye or the surrounding appendages.

**ophthalmoplegia,** paralysis of the eye musculature.

**ophthalmoscope,** an instrument used to examine the interior of the eye or the retina.

**opiate,** any medicine derived from opium; sleep inducing.

**opiomania,** an abnormally intense craving for opium.

**opisthotonos,** a tetanic spasm in which the feet and head are bent backwards and the body arched forward, sometimes seen in meningitis and tetanus.

**opium,** dried juice obtained from unripe poppy capsules, used in medicine for its narcotic and analgesic effect.

**opsonin,** an antibody that causes bacteria to become more susceptible to phagocytic destruction.

**optic,** pertaining to the eyes.

**optical,** pertaining to vision.

**optic disk, optic disc,** the area in the retina known as the blind spot where the optic nerve enters.

**optician,** a specialist who makes optical lenses or eyeglasses for correcting visual defects.

**optic nerve,** the second cranial nerve which functions as the sense of sight, one of a pair.

**optics,** the scientific study of light and vision.

**optometer,** an instrument which measures the eye's refractive power.

**optometrist,** one trained to measure the eye's refractive powers and to fit eyeglasses to correct defects in vision.

**optometry,** an examination and measurement of refractive powers of the eye and the correction of visual defects with eyeglasses.

**oral,** pertaining to the mouth.

**oralogy,** the study of oral hygiene and diseases of the mouth.

**orbit,** the bony cavity which holds the eyeball.

**orbital,** concerning the orbit of the eye.

**orchialgia,** pain in the testis.

**orchidectomy,** surgical removal of a testicle.

**orchioplasty,** plastic surgery of a testis or testes.

**orchitis,** inflammation of a testis.

**orderly,** a male hospital employee who attends especially to male needs.

**organ,** a body part that performs a specific function.

**organelle,** a specialized part of cell strucutre, such as a mitochondrion or ''power plant'' within a cell.

**organic,** pertaining to an organ; having an organized structure; pertaining to substances produced by living organisms; denoting chemical materials containing carbon.

**organism,** any living plant, animal, or unicellular bacteria, yeasts, or protozoa.

**organoplexy,** the reattachment of an organ by surgical fixation.

**organotherapy,** treatment of diseases by endocrine gland preparations and extractions from animals.

**orgasm,** a state of culminated sexual excitement; the apex of sexual intercourse.

**orientation,** the ability to comprehend one's self with regard to time, place, and person.

**orifice,** the entrance or outlet of a body cavity; foramen, meatus, or opening.

**Orinase,** trademark for tolbutamide used to treat uncomplicated, mild, or stable diabetes mellitus that has some functioning islet cells.

**ornithosis,** a disease found in birds and domestic fowl which may be transmitted to man.

**oropharynx,** the space between the soft palate and the upper epiglottis.

**orthocephalic,** having a head with a height and length index between 70--75.

**orthodontia,** the science of dentistry concerned with correcting teeth irregularities, malocclusion, and facial abnormalities.

**orthodontist,** a dentist who specializes in orthodontia.

**orthogenics,** eugenics, or the science that is concerned with the improvement of hereditary qualities in the human race.

**orthognathics,** the study of the causes and treatment of malposition of jaw bones.

**orthopedics,** the branch of surgery dealing with the skeletal system in preservation and restoration of its articulations, and structures.

**orthopedist,** an orthopedic surgeon.

**orthopnea,** difficulty in breathing except in an erect sitting position or standing, associated with cardiac diseases, pulmonary edema, severe emphysema, pneumonia, angina pectoris and several other conditions that affect respiration.

**orthopsychiatrist,** one specialized in orthopsychiatry.

**orthopsychiatry,** the branch of psychiatry concerned with the study and treatment of human behavior in the clinical setting and which emphasizes preventive techniques that provide healthy emotional growth of children.

**orthoptic,** promoting normal binocular vision.

**orthoptics,** treatment with ocular exercises to correct strabismus.

**orthoscope,** an apparatus for examining the eyes which uses a layer of water that neutralizes corneal refraction.

**orthoscopic,** pertaining to the correction of vision.

**orthoscopy,** an examination using an orthoscope.

**orthotonos, orthotonus,** muscular spasm which fixes the head, body, and limbs in a straight and rigid line.

**os,** a body opening; the mouth; a bone.

**oscheitis,** inflammation of the scrotum.

**oscillograph,** an instrument which records electric vibrations of the heart activity or blood pressure.

**oscillography,** a process which records alternating current waves.

**oscilloscope,** an electronic instrument that presents visual changes of electrical variations on the fluorescent screen of a cathode-ray tube.

**osmics,** the science concerned with the sense of smell.

**osmidrosis,** a condition in which body perspiration has a strong offensive odor.

**osmose,** subject to osmosis.

**osmosis,** the movement or diffusion of a solution through a selectively permeable, or a semipermeable membrane from an area of higher density to an area of lesser density. In the human body the cell membranes are selectively permeable which permits oxygen, blood, and nutrients to pass through cells by the process of osmosis. Waste products are removed from the blood in the kidneys through the same process of osmosis.

**ossa,** bones.

**osseous,** bonelike, or bony.

**ossicle,** a small bone, as in the middle ear.

**ossicula auditus,** the three small bones in the middle ear: incus, malleus, and stapes.

**ossiculectomy,** surgical excision of one of the ossicles of the middle ear.

**ossiferous,** forming or producing bone; bonelike tissue.

**ossify,** to form bone, or to turn into bone.

**osteal,** pertaining to bone.

**ostectomy,** surgical removal of a bone or part of a bone.

**osteectopia,** displacement of a bone.

**osteitis,** inflammation of bone.

**osteoarthritis,** a degenerative disease of the joints, especially those which bear the bodies weight.

**osteoarthropathy,** any disease of the joints or bones.

**osteoarthrosis,** a chronic bone disease which is noninflammatory.

**osteoblast,** arising from a fibroblast cell which matures and produces bone.

**osteoblastic,** pertaining to the bone-forming osteoblast.

**osteclasis,** the fracture or refracture of a bone by surgical means to correct deformity in the bone.

**osteoclast,** a large multinuclear cell present in growing bone and which functions to absorb and remove osseous tissue in the formation of canals; an instrument used for refracturing bone.

**osteodermia,** formation of bony tissue in the skin.

**osteodystrophia,** bone development that is defective.

**osteodystrophy,** defective bone formation.

**osteogen,** a substance from which bone is formed within the inner periosteal layer.

**osteoid,** resembling bone.

**osteology,** the branch of anatomy concerned with bones and the structure of bones.

**osteoma,** a bony tumor, or a bone-like structure which develops on a bone.

**osteomalacia,** softening of the bones.

**osteometry,** study of bone measurements.

**osteomyelitis,** inflammation of the bone marrow, or of both the bone and marrow.

**osteopath,** one trained in osteopathy.

**osteopathic,** pertaining to osteopathy.

**osteopathy,** any bone disease; the branch of medicine based on the theory that the body is able to make its own remedies against disease with favorable environmental conditions and good nutrition; its therapeutic procedure involves manipulation of the bony framework and muscles for correction or cure.

**osteophyte,** a bony outgrowth from the surface of a part.

**osteophytic,** pertaining to an osteophyte.

**osteoplastic,** pertaining to bone repair.

**osteoplasty,** plastic surgery of the bones to correct a defect.

**osteoporosis,** loss of bone calcareous matter and increased bone porosity.

**osteosclerosis,** abnormal density or hardening of the bone.

**osteoseptum,** the bony portion of the septum of the nose.

**osteotome,** a bevelled chisel for surgical cutting through bones.

**osteotomy,** surgical procedure for cutting through a bone, or excising part of it.

**ostium, ostial,** a mouth, orifice, or a small opening.

**otalgia,** pain in the ear.

**otantritis,** inflammation of the mastoid antrum.

**otectomy,** surgical removal of the middle ear contents.

**otic,** pertaining to or concerning the ear.

**otitis,** inflammation of the ear.

**otocleisis,** an occlusion of the auditory tube.

**otolaryngologist,** a specialist in otology, rhinology, and laryngology.

**otolaryngology,** the division of medicine concerned with the ear, nose, and throat.

**otolith,** a minute calcareous body in the inner ear composed of calcium carbonate.

**otologist,** one trained in diseases of the ear.

**otology,** the science of the ear, its diseases, and functions.

**otopharyngeal,** pertaining to both the ear and the pharynx.

**otopharyngeal tube,** eustachian tube, the passage between the tympanic cavity and the pharynx.

**otosalpinx,** referring to the eustachian tube or otopharyngeal tube.

**otoscope,** an instrument used for an ear examination.

**otoscopy,** the auscultation of the ear with an otoscope.

**ovarian,** pertaining to the ovary.

**ovariectomy,** excision of an ovary or part of it; oophorectomy.

**ovariohysterectomy,** surgical removal of the ovaries and uterus.

**ovariotomy,** incision into an ovary, as in an ovarian tumor procedure to excise it.

**ovaritis,** inflammation of an ovary.

**ovary,** one of two reproductive glands in females which produce ova and sex hormones.

**overexertion,** excessive physical activity to the point of exhaustion.

**overextension,** hyperextension; extension beyond a reasonable point.

**overriding,** having one end of a fracture slipping past the other part.

**overweight,** exceeding one's normal weight by 10--15%; obese.

**oviduct,** fallopian tube, one of two tubes which extend laterally from the ovary to the uterus and which transport the ovum from the ovary to the uterus.

**ovular,** pertaining to an ovum.

**ovulate,** to release an ovum from one of the ovaries.

**ovulation,** the periodic process of ovulating.

**ovule,** an immature ovum within a graafian follicle.

**ovum,** an egg, or female reproductive cell, capable of developing into a new organism of the same species after fertilization.

**oxygen,** an odorless, colorless gas essential to respiration of most plants and animals, which constitutes approximately 20% of the atmosphere's total volume, and is necessary to support combustion.

**oxygenate,** to saturate or combine with oxygen.

**oxygen tent,** an air-tight enclosure that allows the oxygen content of air to be raised above normal to aid the respiration of a patient.

**oxygen therapy,** the administration of oxygen for treating conditions resulting from a lack of oxygen such as arterial anoxia from pneumonia, pulmonary edema, breathing obstruction, or congestive heart failure.

**oxyhemoglobin,** the combined arterial blood of hemoglobin and oxygen.

**oxytocic,** an agent used to accelerate childbirth; a drug which stimulates uterine contractions.

**oxytocin,** a pituitary hormone that stimulates uterine contractions.

**ozena,** a disease of the nose marked by a thick mucopurulent discharge with an offensive odor.

**ozone,** a form of oxygen with three atoms to a molecule which is irritating and toxic to the respiratory system.

**ozostomia,** a foul breath; halitosis.

# P

**pabulum,** food or nourishment.

**pacemaker,** the sinuauricular node which sets the pace of cardiac rhythm situated in the right atrium which controls the heartbeat; an artificial cardiac pacemaker, as a small electronic device.

**pachycephaly,** abnormal thickness of the skull bones.

**pachydermatous,** having an unusual thickness of the skin.

**pachydermia,** excessive thickening of the skin; elephantiasis.

**pachymeningitis,** inflammation of the dura mater in the brain.

**pachyvaginitis,** a chronic condition of the vaginal walls in which they become abnormally thickened.

**packing,** the filling of a wound or cavity with gauze or similar material.

**pagetoid,** resembling Paget's disease.

**Paget's Disease,** Osteitis Deformans; a progressive, chronic disorder of bone metabolism which causes a thickening of bones, predominantly in the skull and shin.

**pain,** a sensation of agony, or suffering due to the stimulation of certain nerve endings; emotional suffering such as grief.

**painful,** a feeling of pain; distressing.

**painter's colic,** a condition marked by colic accompanying lead poisoning resulting in vomiting, abdominal pain, prostration, paralysis, and collapse.

**palatable,** savory, or agreeable to taste.

**palatal,** pertaining to the palate.

**palate,** the partition which separates the nasal and oral cavities in the roof of the mouth.

**palatitis,** inflammation of the palate.

**palatoglossal,** pertaining to the palate and tongue.

**palatognathous,** a congenital cleft palate.

**palatoplasty,** plastic repair of the palate to correct a cleft.

**palatoplegia,** paralysis the musculature structure of the palate.

**palatum,** palate.

**palilalia,** an abnormal condition in which words and phrases are repeated with increasing rapidity.

**palindromia,** a relapse, or recurrence of an illness or disease.

**palingraphia,** an abnormal condition in which written letters or words are repeated.

**palinphrasia,** an abnormal repetition of words and phrases in speaking.

**pallial,** pertaining to the cerebral cortex or brain.

**palliate,** to sooth; to relieve symptoms.

**palliative,** a drug that affords relief; something that soothes pain.

**pallid,** having no color; pale; wan.

**pallidum,** the globus pallidus of the cerebral hemisphere.

**pallium,** the cerebral cortex.

**pallor,** a paleness to the skin.

**palm,** the hollow surface of the hand.

**palmar,** referring to the palm of the hand.

**palmar reflex,** a grasping reflex found in newborn infants which is more developed in some than in others. It persists for 4 or 5 months then gradually disappears.

**palpable,** able to be touched, or easily perceived.

**palpation,** the act of examining with the hand; the application of fingers to the surface of the body to assist in diagnosing its condition.

**palpebra,** the eyelid.

**palpebral,** pertaining to the eyelid, or situated near it.

**palpitate,** to cause to throb or pulsate intensely, especially associated with the heart; abnormally rapid throbbing or fluttering involving the heart.

**palpitation,** an abnormal rapid or irregular heart beat, usually subjective.

**palsy,** a temporary or permanent paralysis or loss of ability to control movement; a person so disabled.

**paludism,** malaria; swamp fever.

**panaris,** infection and inflammation around a fingernail, or toenail.

**panacea,** a solution or remedy to cure all diseases; a cure-all.

**panarthritis,** inflammation in all joints.

**pancreas,** an elongated gland situated behind the stomach which secretes digestive enzymes and produces insulin.

**pancreatalgia,** pain in the pancreas.

**pancreatectomy,** surgical excision of the pancreas or a portion of it.

**pancreatic,** pertaining to the pancreas.

**pancreatic juice,** contains digestive enzymes produced in the tubuloacinar units of the pancreas, important in carbohydrate metabolism.

**pancreatin,** a substance derived from the pancreas of hogs and cattle containing the enzymes amylase, protease, and lipase which is used as an aid to digestion.

**pancreatitis,** inflammation of the pancreas.

**pandemic,** pertaining to an epidemic of a disease which affects a major portion of a country or the world.

**panagenesis,** a theory by Darwin, now abandoned, which states that each cell of a parent is represented in the reproductive cell, and is capable of reproducing itself in the offspring.

**panhidrosis, panidrosis,** perspiration over the entire body surface.

**panhysterectomy,** surgical removal of the entire uterus including the cervix uteri.

**panic,** an overwhelming fear that produces extreme anxiety; a sudden unreasonable, contagious fear that produces mass flight.

**pannus,** superficial vascular tissue growth arising from the conjunctiva into the cornea of the eye.

**panophobia, panphobia,** a fear of everything; a vague apprehension.

**pansinusitis,** inflammation involving all the nasal sinuses.

**pant,** to gasp or breathe quickly, especially after physical exertion; pant or panting during the second stage of labor under direct supervision of a trained person which allows the woman to have some control over expulsion of the fetus.

**pantalgia,** pain felt over the whole body.

**papilla,** a tiny nipple-shaped protuberance found on the elevations of the tongue and on the fingertips; the mesodermal papilla surrounding the hair bulb; the optic disc.

**papillary,** resembling or referring to a papilla; pertaining to the nipple of the breast.

**papillectomy,** surgical excision of a papilla.

**papillitis,** inflammation and swelling of the optic disc.

**papilloma,** a benign skin tumor consisting of hypertrophied papilla.

**papillomatosis,** the condition of having multiple papillomas.

**Pap Smear,** a microscopic examination of cells collected from the vagina for early detection of cervical or uterine cancer.

**papule,** a small elevated lesion of the skin.

**papulopustular,** having both papules and pustules.

**papulosis,** marked by multiple papules.

**para,** a woman who has given birth to one or more viable offspring.

**para-anesthesia,** the loss of feeling in the lower part of the body, or two corresponding sides of the body.

**parabiosis,** the union or fusion of two individuals, as conjoined twins.

**paracentesis,** a puncture of a cavity for the aspiration of fluid, as in dropsy.

**paracephalus,** a congenital defective head and imperfect sense organs in a fetus.

**parachlorophenol,** used in dentistry as a local anti-infective.

**parachromatopsia,** color blindness.

**paracusis,** defective sense of hearing.

**paracystitis,** inflammation of the tissues surrounding the urinary bladder.

**paradenitis,** inflammation in tissues surrounding a gland.

**parageusia,** dysfunction in the sense of taste.

**parahepatitis,** inflammation of parts adjacent to the liver.

**paralalia,** an abnormal speech defect marked by producing a vocal sound different from one desired, or speaking with sound distortion.

**paralambdacism,** unable to sound the letter ''l'' and substituting another letter for it.

**paraldehyde,** a colorless liquid polymer characterized by an unpleasant odor used as a sedative and hypnotic in medicinal preparations.

**paralexia,** a condition in which one is unable to comprehend printed or written words and transposes words or syllables into meaningless combinations; dyslexia.

**paralogia,** a disorder of reasoning ability; psychosis.

**paralysis,** an impairment of motor function in one or more parts of the body due to a lesion; an impairment of sensory function which causes a loss of voluntary motion.

**paralysis agitans,** a progressively slow form of Parkinson's disease marked by masklike facies, fine hand tremors, slowing of voluntary muscle movement, shuffling gait, peculiar posturing, weakness, and other symptoms.

**paralytic,** pertaining to paralysis; a person with paralysis.

**paralyze,** to affect with paralysis, or to cause a temporary or permanent loss of muscular movement or sensation.

**paramastitis,** inflammation surrounding the breast.

**paramedic,** one who performs adjunctive professional medical duties.

**paramenia,** an abnormal or difficult menstrual period.

**paramnesia,** the sensation of remembering something which has never actually existed or occurred.

**paranephritis,** inflammation of the adrenal gland; inflammation of connective tissues which surround the kidney.

**paranephros,** one of two adrenal glands.

**paranesthesia,** see para-anesthesia.

**paranoia,** a rare mental disorder marked by elaborate and systematized delusions of grandeur and persecution, a condition which does not appear to interfere with the rest of a person's thinking and personality.

**paranoiac,** one affected with paranoia.

**paranoid,** a term applied to persons who are overly suspicious and who harbor grandiose or persecutory delusions, or ideas of reference; resembling paranoia.

**paranoid schizophrenia,** a mental disorder characterized primarily by persecutory or grandiose delusions, but frequently associated with hallucinations.

**paraphasia,** a type of aphasia in which wrong words are employed in senseless combinations.

**paraphobia,** mild form of phobia.

**paraphonia,** an unusual weakness in the sound of one's voice; a partial loss of the voice.

**paraphrasia,** a disordered arrangement of spoken words.

**paraplegia,** paralysis of the lower trunk and the lower limbs.

**paraplegic,** pertaining to paraplegia; one affected with paraplegia.

**parapsoriasis,** slow developing, persistent skin disorder marked by scaly red lesions.

**parapsychology,** the study of metapsychic phenomena which deal with psychical actions and experiences that fall outside the scope of physics or physical law, as telepathy, clairvoyance, etc.

**parasalpingitis,** inflammation of the tissues around a fallopian tube.

**parasite,** any animal or plant that lives inside or upon the body of another living organism, often at a disadvantage to the host; symbiosis.

**parasitic,** concerning a parasite.

**parasitism,** the condition of being infected with parasites.

**parasitize,** to infect or be infected with a parasite.

**parasitology,** the scientific study of parasites.

**parasitosis,** a disease resulting from parasitism.

**parastruma,** an enlargement of the parathyroid gland resulting from a goiterlike tumor.

**parasympathetic nervous system,** a subdivision of the autonomic nervous system. Fibers which originate from nuclei in the midbrain, medulla, and sacral region of the spinal cord, pass through the cranial and sacral nerves. Some of the effects of the parasympathetic system are: constriction of pupils, slowing of heart rate, contraction of smooth muscles, increased glandular secretions, and the constriction of bronchioles.

**parasynovitis,** inflammation of tissues surrounding the synovial sac.

**parathyroid,** one of four tiny endocrine glands, pea-size, located on the lower back portion of the thyroid gland that secretes the hormone parathormone responsible for calcium-phosphorous metabolism.

**paprathyroidal,** pertaining to the parathyroid glands.

**parathyroidectomy,** surgical removal of one or more of the parathyroid glands.

**paratyphoid,** an infection resembling typhoid fever caused by bacteria Salmonella.

**paregoric,** a mixture containing a derivative of opium, anise oil, camphor, alcohol, benzoic acid, and glycerin, used in treatment of diarrhea.

**parencephalitis,** inflammation of the cerebellum.

**parencephalon,** the cerebellum.

**parenchyma,** the functioning cells of an organ.

**parenteral,** situated or occurring outside of the digestive tract, as by injection through an alternate route or means.

**paresis,** an imcomplete paralysis; a weakness of an organic origin.

**paresthesia,** an abnormal tactile sensation, often described as creeping, burning, tingling, or numbness.

**paretic,** pertaining to paresis.

**paridrosis,** any disordered condition involving the secretion of perspiration.

**paries, parietes,** the enveloping wall of any hollow organ.

**parietal,** pertaining to the wall of a cavity.

**parietal bone,** one of two bones forming the top portion and sides of the skull.

**Parkinson's disease,** a chronic, slowly progressive nervous disorder characterized by muscular rigidity, tremors, drooling, restlessness, peculiar involuntary movements, shuffling gait, chewing movements and protrusion of the tongue, blurred vision, and other neurological symptoms.

**parkinsonism,** Parkinson's disease.

**parodontitis,** inflammation of the tissues around a tooth.

**parodynia,** a difficult or abnormal delivery; labor pains.

**paroniria,** terrifying abnormal dreaming.

**paroniria ambulans,** sleepwalking.

**paronychia,** infection of the tissues around the base of a nail.

**parorexia,** a perversion of the appetite marked by a craving for strange foods.

**parosmia,** an abnormal sense of smell.

**parotid,** pertaining to the parotid gland; near the ear.

**parotidectomy,** surgical removal of a parotid gland.

**parotid gland,** one of two salivary glands on other side of the face in front of each ear.

**parotiditis,** inflammation of a parotid gland; mumps.

**parous,** having given birth to at least one offspring.

**paroxysm,** a sudden, intense attack, or recurrence of symptoms; a seizure or spasm.

**paroxymal,** pertaining to paroxysms.

**parrot fever,** psittacosis; a disease occurring in parrots and other domestic birds that is transmitted to man, which resembles pneumonia accompanied by fever, cough, and enlargement of the spleen; ornithosis.

**parturient,** pertaining to birth or giving birth, as a woman in labor.

**parturition,** the birth process; labor; childbirth.

**parulis,** an abcess of the gum, especially beneath a tooth socket.

**parvule,** a tiny pill, granule, or pellet.

**passive,** not active; submissive.

**pasturization,** a process of heating a liquid such as milk for a definite period of time and at a moderate temperature in order to destroy specific bacteria which is undesirable.

**Pasteur treatment,** a method of treatment for preventing rabies by a series of injections with a virus of gradually increasing strength.

**pastille,** a medicated lozenge for irritated mucosa of the throat and mouth; a small cone of aromatic paste used to fumigate or disinfect the air by burning it within a room.

**patch test,** a skin test to determine sensitivity.

**patella,** kneecap.

**patellar,** pertaining to the kneecap.

**patellar reflex,** an involuntary jerk of the leg following a tapping of the patellar ligament with an instrument; knee jerk reflex.

**pathetic,** the causing or arousing of emotions such as pity or sorrow.

**pathogen,** a microorganism that causes disease.

**pathogenesis,** the development of disease; the pathogenic reactions occurring in the development of disease.

**pathogenic,** causing disease.

**pathogenicity,** having the ability to produce morbid changes or disease.

**pathognomonic,** specifically characteristic of a disease; denoting one or more symptoms indicative of a disease.

**pathological,** pertaining to the causes of a specific disease.

**pathologist,** a specialist trained in pathology.

**pathology,** the scientific study of the nature and causes of disease, and changes in function and structure; manifestations of a disease.

**pathophobia,** morbid fear of disease.

**patient,** a person who is receiving medical treatment; one who is enduring pain without complaining.

**pavor nocturnus,** night terror such as nightmares during sleep occurring in children and the aged.

**peccant,** producing disease; morbid; pathogenic.

**pectoral,** pertaining to the chest or breast; an expectorant which relieves respiratory tract disorders.

**pectoralgia,** pain in the chest.

**pectoral girdle,** the arch formed by the collarbone and the shoulder.

**pectoralis,** pertaining to the breast or chest; one of the four muscles of the breast.

**pectus,** the chest; breast; thorax.

**pedal,** referring to the foot.

**pedatropy,** marasmus; a wasting disease occurring in children; Tabes mesenterica, tuberculosis of mesenteric glands in children.

**pederasty,** coitus between males through anal intercourse, especially with young boys; sodomy.

**pediatrician,** a physician who specializes in pediatrics.

**pediatrics,** the branch of medicine concerned with children and their development, and the care and treatment of children's diseases.

**pedicle,** a footlike, narrow structure; a bony process which forms the root of the vertebral arch.

**pedicular,** pertaining to pediculosis.

**pediculosis,** being infected with lice.

**pedodontia, pedodontics,** the branch of dentistry concerned with the teeth and mouth care of children.

**pedodontist,** a dentist trained in pedodontics.

**peduncle,** a stemlike collection of nerve fibers that attaches a new growth such as a nonsessile tumor which hangs free on a stalk; a band connecting structures of the brain.

**peduncular,** relating to a peduncle.

**pedunculation,** developing a stalk or peduncle.

**pelioma,** a livid cutaneous spot; ecchymosis.

**peliosis,** a condition marked by purple patches on the skin and mucous membranes; purpura.

**pellagra,** a disease caused by niacin deficiency which affects the skin, digestive system, and nervous system.

**pellagrin,** one afflicted with pellagra.

**pellagroid,** resembling pellagra.

**pellicle,** a thin membrane; a film which forms on the surface of liquids.

**pellucid,** translucent; limpid or clear.

**pelvic,** pertaining to the pelvis.

**pelvimeter,** an apparatus for measuring the pelvis.

**pelvis,** the lower portion of the body trunk formed by the innominate bones, the sacrum, and the coccyx.

**pemphigus,** a condition marked by successive crops of watery blisters eruting on the skin and mucous membranes which disappear leaving pigmented areas.

**pendulous,** to hang or swing freely.

**penetrometer,** an instrument which measures the penetrating power of x-rays and radiation.

**penicillin,** one of a group of antibiotics semisynthesized from various molds, especially from the genus Penicillum, effective against most gram-positive bacteria and certain gram-negative forms, also effective against some forms of mold, spirochetes, and rickettsias by inhibiting bacterial growth.

**penicillium,** a genus of fungi, often found in mold forms of bluish color on cheese, bread, and fruit.

**penile,** pertaining to the penis.

**penis,** the male organ for urination and copulation, a pendulous structure that is suspended from the front and the sides of the pubic arch.

**penitis,** inflammation of the penis.

**pentobarbital,** a barbiturate acid derivative, the sodium salt is effective as a hypnotic and sedative, or as an analgesic; Nembutal sodium, a trademark, reduces responsiveness to external stimuli and is often used as a sedative prior to anesthesia.

**pentylenetetrazol,** a bitter, white powder used in preparation of a compound that is effective as a respiratory stimulant in certain circulatory conditions, and as a convulsant analeptic.

**peotomy,** excision of the penis.

**pepsin,** the primary enzyme of gastric juice that reduces protein to proteoses and peptides; an extract obtained from the glandular layer of the stomachs of hogs, sheep, or cows, used as a digestive aid.

**pepsinogen,** the inactive form of pepsin, the proteolytic enzyme in gastric juice which is converted to the active form by hydrochloric acid.

**peptic,** concerning digestion; relating to pepsin; a medicine that aids digestion.

**peptic ulcer,** an ulcer found in the lower part of the esophagus, in the stomach, in the duodenum, or in the gastrojejunostomy.

**peptidase,** any of a group of proteolytic enzymes that hydrolyze peptides or peptones into amino acids.

**peptide,** the linkage of two or more amino acid units by hydrolysis.

**peptone,** a derived protein produced by partial hydrolysis of native protein by the action of pepsin and trypsin.

**peptonize,** the process of converting a native protein into peptone.

**peracute,** very acute.

**per anum,** through the opening of the anus; by way of the anus.

**Percodan,** trademark for a fixed preparation of oxycodone hydrochloride and oxycodone terphthalate with aspirin, caffeine, and phenacetin.

**percuss,** to perform percussion by tapping a body part for diagnostic purposes.

**percussion,** the process of striking or tapping a part of the body with quick, sharp blows in diagnosing a condition of the underlying parts by sound.

**percussor,** an instrument used for percussion.

**percutaneous,** performed through the skin, as in the application of ointment by rubbing into the skin.

**perflation,** the process of blowing air into a cavity in order to expand its walls or to expel its contents.

**perforans,** perforating or penetrating, as of nerves or muscles.

**perforation,** the act of puncturing a hole, as caused by ulceration; any hole made through a substance or part.

**perfusion,** the passage of fluids through the blood vessels of an organ; the pouring of a fluid through an organ or tissue.

**periadenitis,** inflammation of tissues surrounding a gland.

**periarterial,** surrounding an artery.

**periarteritis,** inflammation of the outer coats of an artery.

**peribronchitis,** inflammation of all tissues around the bronchi or bronchial tubes.

**pericardiac, pericardial,** pertaining to the pericardium.

**pericardiectomy,** surgical removal of part or all of the pericardium.

**pericardiotomy,** incision of the pericardium.

**pericarditis,** inflammation of the pericardium.

**pericardium,** the fibroserous sac that envelops the heart and the roots of the great blood vessels.

**pericecal,** surrounding the cecum.

**pericecitis,** inflammation of the tissues situated around the cecum.

**perichondral,** relating to the perichondrium.

**perichondrium,** a membrane of fibrous connective tissue covering all cartilage except at synovial joints.

**pericolic,** around the colon.

**pericolitis,** inflammation of the area surrounding the colon.

**perichonchal,** around the concha of the ear.

**pericorneal,** around the cornea of the eye.

**pericranium,** the periosteum or membranous covering of the skull.

**pericystitis,** inflammation of the tissues around the urinary bladder.

**peridental,** surrounding a tooth or part of it.

**perihepatitis,** inflammation of the peritoneal capsule of the liver and the tissues of the surrounding area.

**perimeter,** the outer margin of a body; a device for measuring the visual field.

**perimetrium,** the peritoneum covering the uterus.

**perimetry,** the circumference of the body; the measurement of the scope of the field of vision using a perimeter.

**perineal,** pertaining to the perineum.

**perineorrhaphy,** the repair of a laceration in the perineum following childbirth.

**perineotomy,** surgical incision of the perineum to facilitate childbirth.

**perineum,** the area between the anus and the vulva in the female, or between the scrotum and the anus in a male.

**perineurium,** the connective tissue sheath surrounding the bundle of fibers in peripheral nerves.

**period,** the menses; the time it takes for a disease to run its course.

**periodic,** occurring at intermittent intervals.

**periodontal,** pertaining to the periodontium around a tooth.

**periodontics,** the branch of dentistry concerned with diseases of the periodontium and their treatment.

**periodontist,** a dentist trained in periodontics.

**periodontitis,** inflammation of the periodontium.

**periodontium,** the surrounding supportive tissues around a tooth, including the bone and gum.

**perionychia,** iniflammation around a finger or toe nail.

**perionychium,** the epidermis bordering a finger or toe nail.

**periosteal,** pertaining to the periosteum.

**periosteotomy,** surgical incision into the periosteum.

**periosteum,** the fibrous membrane which forms a covering of bones containing numerous blood vessels for nouorishment, and a supporting structure for the attachment of muscles, and ligaments.

**periostitis,** inflammation of the periosteum.

**periotic,** around the ear; pertaining to certain bones that protect the internal ear, and constituting a portion of the temporal bone.

**peripheral,** pertaining to an outer surface.

**periprostatitis,** inflamed tissues surrounding the prostate gland.

**perisalpingitis,** inflammation of the peritoneal coat surrounding the oviduct.

**peristalsis,** normal contraction and relaxation of the hollow tubes of the alimentary canal which slowly moves the contents along for variable distances.

**peristaltic,** pertaining to peristalsis.

**perisystole,** the interval preceding the systole in the cardiac rhythm.

**peritheli022,** a tumor of the perithelial layer of the blood vessels.

**perithelium,** the fibrous outer layer, composed of connective tissue, of the smaller blood vessels and capillaries.

**peritoneal,** relating to the peritoneum.

**peritoneum,** the thin, serous membrane which lines the entire internal surface of the abdominal cavity and envelops the viscera.

**peritonitis,** inflammation of the peritoneum.

**peritonsillar,** around a tonsil.

**permanent teeth,** the teeth which develop at the second dentition that supplant the milk teeth.

**permanganate,** a purple salt which contains potassium, manganese, and oxygen, used in solution as a disinfectant and an oxidizer.

**pernicious,** fatal; destructive; very harmful.

**pernicious anemia,** a severe and often fatal blood disease caused by a progressive decrease in red blood cells resulting in muscular weakness, gastrointestinal disorders, and neural disturbances.

**peroneal,** pertaining to the fibula.

**peroral,** by mouth; given by mouth.

**per os,** by mouth.

**peroxide,** a compound containing more oxygen than other oxides of the element, for example, the peroxides of hydrogen, sodium, and nitrogen.

**perspiration,** the secretion of sweat; sweating.

**perspire,** to sweat; to excrete fluid of perspiration through the skin.

**pertussis,** an infectious disease marked by catarrh and cough; whooping cough.

**perversion,** deviation from normal, as in sexual perversion or desire.

**pervert,** one who is perverted, esp. sexually.

**pervious,** capable of being penetrated; permeable; passing through.

**pes,** resembling a foot; serving as a foot; foot.

**pessary,** a device placed into the vagina to support and correct the uterus or rectum; a medicated vaginal suppository; a contraceptive device.

**pestiferous,** infectious; producing a pestilence; noxious.

**pestilence,** a widespread contagious disease that is usually of epidemic proportion and deadly, specifically bubonic plague.

**pestilential,** producing an infectious and deadly disease; destructive.

**petechia,** a tiny red spot occurring on the skin caused by a small amount of escaping blood.

**petrolatum,** a semisolid, purified mixture obtained from petroleum used in ointment preparations which protect and soothe the skin.

**petrosal,** pertaining to the petrous portion of the temporal bone.

**phagedena,** a sloughing and eroding ulcer that spreads.

**phagocyte,** a leukocyte which has the ability to destroy bacteria by ingesting or absorbing the harmful cells.

**phagocytic,** concerning phagocytosis.

**phagocytosis,** the destruction and absorption of bacteria and particles by phagocytes.

**phagomania,** an abnormal craving for food.

**phakitis,** inflammation of the crystalline lens of the eye.

**phalacrous,** baldness.

**phalangeal,** pertaining to a phalanx.

**phalangitis,** an inflammation of one or more digits.

**phalanx,** any of the bones of the fingers or toes.

**phallic,** pertaining to the phallus, or penis.

**phallitis,** an inflammation of the phallus or penis.

**phallus,** the penis.

**phantasy,** daydream; imaginary possibilities.

**phantom limb,** an illusion that a limb still exists after amputation.

**pharmaceutical,** pertaining to drugs or to a pharmacy.

**pharmaceutics,** the science of preparing pharmaceutical preparations.

**pharmacist,** one licensed to prepare, sell, or dispense drugs, and to fill prescriptions of physicians.

**pharmacodynamics,** the scientific study of drug actions and effects upon the body.

**pharmacognosy,** the branch of pharmacology concerned with natural drugs and possible medicinal substitutes.

**pharmacologist,** one who specializes in pharmacology.

**pharmacology,** the science concerned with drugs, including origin, chemistry, nature, effects, and uses of drugs.

**pharmacopoeia,** an authoritative book on official listings of drugs and drug standards, such as the United States Pharmacopeia.

**pharmacy,** the branch of health science that deals with preparation, dispensing, and proper usage of drugs; a drug store.

**pharyngeal,** relating to the pharnyx.

**pharyngitis,** inflammation of the pharyngitis.

**pharyngology,** the branch of medicine that studies the larynx and its diseases.

**pharyngoparalysis,** paralysis of the musculature of the pharynx.

**pharynx,** the membraneous tube that connects the mouth and the esophagus.

**phase,** a stage of development; a distinct stage in mitosis.

**phenacaine,** a crystalline compound used in its hydrochloridic form to anesthetize the eye for removal of foreign particles and to relieve discomfort of laceration in the cornea.

**phenacetin,** an analgesic.

**phenobarbital,** a white crystalline substance used as a hypnotic, sedative, and antispasmodic.

**phenolphthalein,** a crystalline compound used as a laxative.

**phenoluria,** excretion of phenols in the urine.

**phenotype,** the physical appearance of a person, or the traits exhibited.

**phenylketonuria,** see PKU.

**phial,** a vial; a small container for medicine.

**phimosis,** a narrowness of the preputial orifice that prevents the foreskin from being pushed back over the glans penis.

**phlebitis,** inflammation of a vein.

**phlebotomist,** one trained to open a vein for blood letting.

**phlebotomy,** the practice of opening a vein for the letting of blood in treatment of disease.

**phlegm,** a thick mucus which is secreted in respiratory passages.

**phlegmatic,** one sluggist in temperament; apathetic.

**phlyctena,** a tiny watery blister or pustule.

**phlyctenular,** resembling a pustule; pertaining to vesicles.

**phlyctenule,** a tiny blister or vesicle, as on the cornea or conjuctiva.

**phobia,** an abnormal or exaggerated fear, usually illogical.

**phonation,** the utterance of vocal sounds.

**phonatory,** pertaining to utterance of vocal sounds.

**phonetics,** the science of speech and the pronunciation of words.

**phonic,** concerning the voice, speech, or sound.

**phosphatase,** an enzyme which catalyzes the hydrolysis of phosphoric esters secreted by the liver and important to the metabolism of carbohydrates.

**phosphocreatine,** an important form of high-energy phosphate found in muscle tissue; the source of energy in muscle contraction.

**phospholipid,** any group of lipids that contain phosphorus, including lecithin and cephalin, found in living cells, especially nerve tissue.

**photalgia,** pain in the eye caused by intense light.

**photic,** pertaining to light.

**photochemotherapy,** treating with drugs that react to sunlight or ultraviolet radiation.

**photodermatitis,** an abnormal skin condition caused by overexposure to light, especially from the sun.

**photophobia,** an abnormal intolerance to light.

**photopia,** vision in day-light.

**photopsia,** an appearance of flashes of light, occurring in certain retinal, optic, or brain conditions.

**photopsin,** a protein found in the cones of the retina that combines with retinal to produce photochemical pigments responsible for color vision.

**photoreceptor,** a receptor, or a nerve end-organ that is sensitive to light.

**photosensitive,** an abnormal sensitivity to sunlight, occasionally seen in certain drug reactions.

**phototherapy,** exposure to the sun or artificial light rays in treatment of disease. Ultraviolet phototherapy is effective in preventing dangerous levels of bilirubin in low birth weight infants with increased jaundice conditions.

**phrenalgia,** pain in the diaphragm; melancholia.

**phrenasthenia,** mental deficiency, or feeblemindedness.

**phrenic,** pertaining to the mind or to the diaphragm.

**phrenology,** the study of the shape of the skull as supposedly indicative of mental powers and character.

**phylaxis,** the active bodily defense against infection.

**physiatrics,** the branch of medicine concerned with physical therapy, and use of light, heat, electricity, and massage in the diagnosis and treatment of disease; physiotherapy.

**physic,** the art of medicine and healing; a cathartic; general drugs; to purge.

**physical,** pertaining to the body; relating to material things; pertaining to physics.

**physician,** one trained and legally qualified to practice medicine after being licensed by an appropriate board; a doctor who practices medicine as distinguished from one specializing in surgery.

**physics,** the study of natural forces and phenomena, and properties of energy and matter.

**physiognomy,** the face or quality of countenance as indicative of moral or mental character; the facial expression and bodily appearance used in diagnosis.

**physiological,** pertaining to physiology; normal; concerning functions of the body.

**physiologist,** one who specializes in physiology.

**physiology,** the science concerned with the functions of the living organism, its organs, and its parts; the science of the functioning of all structures in the human body.

**physiotherapy,** the treatment of disease by physical therapy.

**physique,** the organization, development, and structures of a body; body build.

**physostigmine,** an alkaloid obtained from the Calabar bean, used as a topical myotic in glaucoma.

**pial,** pertaining to pia mater.

**pia mater,** the highly vascular membrane forming the innermost of the three coverings which envelop the brain and spinal cord. The inner coverings consist of membranes, called meninges, which are composed of three distinct layers of tissue: the dura matter, the arachnoid membrane, and the pia mater.

**pica,** an unnatural craving for substances that are not food such as clay, chalk, or ashes; a depraved appetite.

**pigeon breast,** an abnormal projection of the sternum and the area surrounding the sternum resulting in a malformation of the chest, often seen in rickets.

**pigment,** coloring substance in the tissues or cells.

**pigmentary,** concerning a pigment.

**pigmentation,** a deposit of coloring matter or pigments.

**pigmented,** colored by a deposit of pigment.

**pilar, pilary,** pertaining to the hair; covered with hair.

**piles,** hemorrhoids.

**pill,** medicine in a small globular or oval shaped mass to be swallowed; a tablet.

**pilose,** covered with hair; hairy.

**pilosis,** an excessive growth of hair.

**pilosity,** hairiness.

**pimple,** a tiny elevation of the skin with an inflamed base which may form pus; pustule.

**pineal,** pertaining to the pineal body.

**pineal body,** a small, cone-shaped body in the brain believed to be an endocrine organ which secretes a hormone that stimulates the adrenal cortex; pineal gland.

**pink eye,** acute conjunctivitis; contagious inflammation of the eyelids affecting man and some animals; a non-infectious, sporadic condition of the conjunctiva caused by irritation from various agents.

**pinna,** the auricle, or the external part of the ear.

**pinnal,** pertaining to the pinna.

**pinworm,** a nematoid worm which infects the intestines; formerly called oxyuris.

**pisiform,** resembling a pea, or pea-shaped bone of the wrist; the smallest carpal bone.

**pitting,** the formation of pits or depressions in the skin, as in smallpox.

**pituitary,** pertaining to the pituitary gland; a substance prepared from the posterior portion of animal pituitary glands used as an antidiuretic and as a vasoconstrictor; the hypophysis cerebri.

**pituitary gland,** a small, grayish colored, oval-shaped endocrine gland attached to the base of the brain which secretes a number of hormones that regulate many bodily processes including growth, reproduction, and metabolic activities; referred to as the ''master gland'' of the body.

**pituitrin,** an extract derived from posterior lobes of the pituitary glands of cattle used to stimulate contraction of blood vessels, peristalsis in intestines, and uterine contractions to facilitate labor.

**pityriasis,** a skin disease marked by irregular scaly patches and shedding of branlike scales, occurring in humans and some domestic animals.

**PKU,** phenylketonuria, a metabolic hereditary disorder resulting in faulty metabolism of phenylalanine which causes mental retardation.

**placebo,** an inactive preparation given merely to satisfy the patient's demand; used in experimentation and research of the effectiveness of genuine drugs in controlled studies.

**placenta,** the flatlike organ attached to the wall of the uterus through which the fetus receives nourishment and oxygen, and passes off metabolic waste products.

**placental,** pertaining to the placenta.

**placentation,** the formation and attachment of the placenta to the wall of the uterus; the process or events following implantation of the embryo and the development of the placenta.

**placentitis,** inflammation of the placenta.

**plague,** a widespread contagious disease with a high mortality rate; a virulent, infectious, and acutely febrile disease caused by the Pasteurella pestis bacteria, transmitted to man by fleas from rodents; bubonic plague.

**planomania,** pathological desire to wander and to be free of social restraints.

**planta,** the sole of the foot.

**plantar,** pertaining to the sole of the foot.

**plantar wart,** a painful wart occurring on the bottom of the foot.

**plaque,** a rounded patch on the skin or on a mucous surface; a blood platelet.

**plasma,** the liquid part of the blood or lymph; cell protoplasm outside the nucleus.

**plasmin,** a proteolytic enzyme in the blood which causes fibrin breakdown and has the ability to dissolve blood clots.

**plasmolysis,** the dissolution and shrinkage of cytoplasm within a living cell caused by excessive water loss by osmosis.

**plaster cast,** a firm dressing made of gauze and plaster of Paris which is used to immobilize an injured part of the body, as in bone fractures.

**plastic,** capable of building tissue; material that can be molded.

**plastic surgery,** surgery utilized to restore and repair external defects, malformation, injured bones, body organs, and tissue by grafts of bone or tissues.

**platelet,** a minute disk-shaped structure found in the blood important in clotting of the blood, and in stimulating phagocytic action of leukocytes.

**platycephalic,** having a wide skull with a flattened top.

**platyhelminthes,** a group of worms or phylum having a flattened body, including tapeworms, planarians, and flukes.

**platypodia,** flatfeet.

**platyrrhine,** having a wide nose in proportion to length.

**plethora,** an excess blood volume; congestion.

**plethoric,** pertaining to plethora.

**pleura,** a serous membrane lining the walls of the thorax and enclosing the lungs.

**pleural,** pertaining to the pleura.

**pleuralgia,** pain in the pleura, or in the side.

**pleurectomy,** surgical removal of part of the pleura.

**pleurisy,** inflammation of the pleura, frequently accompanied by respiratory difficulties and fever.

**pleuritic,** pertaining to pleurisy.

**pleuropneumonia,** inflammation of the pleura and of the lungs.

**plexor,** a small hammer with a soft rubber head used in percussion for diagnostic purposes.

**plexus,** a network of vessels or nerves; a complicated network of interlacing parts.

**plica,** a fold.

**plicate,** folded or braided.

**plication,** a process by which folds are stitched in an organ's wall to decrease its size.

**plumbism,** a chronic condition caused by lead poisoning.

**pneumatogram,** a record made by a pneumatograph.

**pneumatograph,** an apparatus for registering respiratory movements.

**pneumatometer,** an apparatus which measures the quantity of air involved in inspiration and expiration.

**pneumobacillus,** the bacillus Klebsiella pneumoniae which causes pneumonia.

**pneumococcal,** pertaining to pneumococci.

**pneumococcus,** bacterium Diplococcus pneumoniae which produces lobar pneumonia and various infectious diseases.

**pneumoconiosis,** any lung disease due to an occupation, such as by inhaling dust particles, mineral dust, or coal dust.

**pneumogastric,** pertaining to the lungs and the stomach; pneumogastric nerve, or vagus nerve.

**pneumoencephalography,** a radiographic examination of the fluid- containing structures of the brain after cerebrospinal fluid is withdrawn by a lumbar puncture and replaced by injecting air or a gas.

**pneumoenteritis,** inflammation of the lungs and intestine.

**pneumomyelography,** a radiography of the spinal canal after the withdrawal of spinal fluid and the injection of air or gas.

**pneumonectomy, pneumectomy,** surgical excision of part or all of a lung.

**pneumonia,** inflammation of the lungs caused by microbes, chemical irritants, dusts, or allergy, characterized by chills, fever, chest pain, cough, purulent sputum often spotted with blood.

**pneumonic,** pertaining to the lungs; having pneumonia.

**pneumothorax,** the presence of air or gas in the pleural space which may occur spontaneously due to trauma, or deliberately introduced in collapsing a lung.

**pock,** a pustule on the skin in an eruptive disease, as in smallpox.

**poockmark,** a depressed scar on the skin made by smallpox or other disease.

**podagra,** pain in the great toe caused by gout.

**podalgia,** pain in the feet.

**podiatrist,** chiropodist; one who specializes in podiatry.

**podiatry,** a specialized field concerned with the care or the foot, including its anatomy, medical and surgical treatment, and its diseases.

**pogoniasis,** an excessive growth of the beard, especially on women.

**poison,** an agent or substance which may cause structural damage or functional disorders when introduced into the body by ingestion, inhalation, absorption, or injection.

**polio,** poliomyelitis.

**polioencephalitis,** inflammatory lesions of the brain involving the gray matter.

**poliomyelitis,** a viral disease of the gray matter of the spinal cord marked by fever, sore throat, headache, vomiting, and frequently stiffness of the neck and back.

**pollex,** the thumb.

**pollex pedis,** the great toe; hallux.

**pollution,** the act of making foul or impure, as air, soil, or water.

**polyarteritis,** a condition in which the body is affected by multiple sites of inflammatory and destructive lesions in the arteries.

**polyarthritis,** inflammation of several joints at the same time.

**polychromatic,** having many colors.

**polyclinic,** a hospital or clinic which treats all kinds of injuries and diseases.

**polycythemia,** a condition in which the total cell mass of the blood is abnormally increased; excessive red blood cells; erythrocytosis.

**polypolydactylism,** the presence of more than normal numbers of fingers or toes.

**polydipsia,** abnormal thirst, or having an excessive desire to drink.

**polydysplasia,** abnormal development of several organs, systems, or tissues.

**polyesthesia,** the feeling that several points on the body were touched on application of one stimulus to a single point.

**polygalactia,** excessive secretion of milk.

**polygenic,** pertaining to the belief that humans have their origin from more than one ancestral line.

**polygraph,** an apparatus for recording blood pressure, pulse, respiration, and electrical resistance of the skin all at the same time; lie-detector.

**polynuclear, polymorphonuclear,** having many-shaped nuclei.

**polyp, polypus,** protruding mass of tissue growth from a mucous membrane, commonly found in the nose, uterus, and rectum; a tumor with a footlike structure.

**polyphagia,** excessive eating.

**polyphagous,** eating many different kinds of food.

**polyphobia,** morbid fear of many things.

**polyplegia,** paralysis of several muscles.

**polypnea,** abnormally heavy panting or breathing.

**polyposis,** formation of multiple polyps.

**polyptome,** a surgical instrument for excision of a polyp.

**polyspermia,** excessive secretion of seminal fluid; polyspermy.

**polyspermy,** the fertilization of an ovum by more than one mature male germ cell, or spermatozoon.

**polythelia,** the presence of more than one nipple on a mammary gland or breast.

**polyunsaturated,** denoting a fatty acid, or pertaining to animal or vegetable fats having more than one double bond in its hydrocarbon chain; linoleic acid.

**polyvalent,** multivalent, as in vaccine which has several strains of antibodies.

**pons,** a broad band of nerve fibers in the brain which connects the lobes of the cerebrum, medulla, and cerebellum; pons Varolio.

**popliteal,** pertaining to the area behind the knee; the ham.

**pore,** a tiny opening in skin or tissue.

**porosis,** the formation of cavities or pores in repair of bone fractures; callus formation in bone repair.

**porosity,** state of being porous.

**porous,** having many open spaces or pores.

**porphyrin,** any of a group of metal-free pyrrole derivatives, occurring in protoplasm, forming the basis of animal and plant respiratory pigments.

**porphyrinemia,** presence of porphyrin in the blood.

**porphyrinuria,** excretion of porphyrin in the urine.

**portal,** concerning an entrance to an organ; pertaining to the porta hepatis, or the fissure of the liver.

**portal vein,** the large vein which carries blood from the stomach, intestine, pancreas, and spleen to the liver.

**position,** a placement of the body, or a bodily posture, as in supine, prone, or standing position.

**posology,** the system of dosage of medicines.

**postauricular,** located behind the auricle of the ear.

**postcibal,** after eating; postprandial.

**posterior,** situated at the back; behind; coming after.

**postmortem,** subsequent to death, as an autopsy.

**postnasal,** occurring behind the nose, as postnasal drip.

**postnatal,** occurring after birth of a newborn.

**postpartum,** after childbirth, referring to the mother.

**postprandial,** after a meal; postcibal.

**postulate,** something taken for granted without proof; a fundamental principle.

**posthumous,** occurring after death, which is said of a child delivered by cesarean section after death of the mother.

**postural,** pertaining to or affected by posture.

**posture,** an attitude or carriage of the body.

**potable,** fit to drink.

**potassium,** a mineral element which is the main cation of intracellular fluid in the body. It functions with sodium and chloride to regulate osmotic pressure and acid-base balance; in combination with calcium and magnesium ions, it is essential for normal muscle excitability, especially the heart muscle; and it is necessary in the conduction of nerve impulses.

**potassium permanganate,** a dark crystalline compound used as a topical anti-infective, an astrigent, and oxidizing agent.

**potency,** the quality of being strong or potent; ability to perform coitus; strength.

**potion,** a dose of liquid medicine.

**Pott's disease,** caries of the vertebrae caused by tubercular infection resulting in the destruction and compression of vertebrae marked by curvature of the spine.

**pouch,** a pocket-like space or sac.

**poultice,** a soft, moist dressing made of hot linseed, bread, mustard, or soap and oil which is applied to the skin to relieve inflammation, and to hasten the excretion of pus.

**pox,** an eruptive or pustular disease, usually caused by a virus, such as chicken pox.

**practical nurse,** a nurse who is not a graduate registered nurse but who has sufficient professional training and skills to provide care for the ill.

**practitioner,** one who practices medicine; physician.

**preanesthetic,** a drug given to ease the induction of a general anesthetic.

**precancerous,** preceding the development of a carcinoma.

**precipitant,** an agent that causes precipitation.

**precipitation,** the process by which a substance is made to separate from another in a solution and settle in solid particles to the bottom.

**precipitin,** an antibody formed in the blood that causes certain proteins to precipitate when it unites with its antigen.

**precocious,** exhibiting mature mental development at an unusually early age.

**preconscious,** in reference to thoughts that are not in immediate awareness but that may readily be recalled.

**precursor,** something that precedes.

**predigestion,** a partial digestion of food by artificial means to make it more readily digestible.

**predisposition,** having a tendency to develop certain diseases, acquired or hereditary.

**pregnable,** vulnerable.

**pregnancy,** state of being pregnant.

**prpregnant,** being with child; the condition of having a developing fetus in the womb.

**prehensile,** adapted for grasping or seizing.

**prehension,** the act of graspping.

**premature,** happening before the proper time, as a premature infant.

**premaxilla,** the incisive bone.

**premaxillary,** situated in front of the maxilla, or upper jaw.

**premedical,** pertaining to preparatory professional studies in medicine.

**premedication,** preliminary medication which produces narcosis prior to administering general anesthesia.

**premolar,** in front of a molar tooth, or teeth.

**premorbid,** occurring before the development of a disease.

**prenatal,** previous to birth.

**preoperative,** preceding an operation or surgery.

**prepuce,** foreskin.

**preputium,** pertaining to the prepuce.

**presbyatrics,** geriatrics.

**presbyopia,** defect of vision involving loss of accommodation in which near objects are seen less distinctly than those at a distance, occurring in advancing age.

**presbyopic,** pertaining to presbyopia.

**prescription,** a written order for dispensing medication which is signed by a physician.

**presenile,** resembling senility but occurring in early or middle life.

**presentation,** in obstetrics, the manner in which the fetus is presenting itself at the mouth of the uterus and which can be determined by the examining finger, such as breech, cephalic, or scapula.

**pressor,** stimulating or increasing the activity of a function, as a nerve or an elevation of blood pressure.

**pressure sore,** bed sore; decubitus ulcer.

**presystole,** the period of time before the systole of the heart beat.

**preventive,** pertaining to a vaccine or medicine that wards off disease; prophylactic.

**prickly heat,** a noncontagious eruption of the skin causing red pimples that itch and tingle, usually in hot weather.

**primary lesion,** an original lesion from which a second one develops.

**primary sore,** the initial sore or hard chancre of syphilis.

**primipara,** a woman who has given birth to her first child, or who is parturient for the first time.

**primiparity,** the condition of having given birth to only one child.

**probang,** a flexible slender rod with a ball, sponge, or tuft at one end used to remove matter from the esophagus or larynx or to apply medicine.

**probe,** a slender instrument for exploring wounds, body cavities, or passages.

**procaine,** a compound which uses hydrochloride salt in solution for a local anesthetic as a nerve block, and for spinal anesthesia.

**process,** a bony prominence or protuberance; a series of steps or events leading to a specific result.

**procreant,** pertaining to procreation.

**procreate,** to beget; to reproduce.

**procreation,** the act of producing offspring; reproduction.

**proctalgia,** pain in the anus or rectum.

**proctectomy,** surgical removal of the anus or rectum.

**proctology,** the branch of medicine dealing with rectal and anal disorders.

**proctoplasty,** plastic repair of the anus or rectum.

**proctoscope,** an instrument with illumination for inspecting the interior of the rectum.

**proctoscopy,** an examination of the lower intestine with a proctoscope.

**proctostomy,** surgical creation of an artificial opening into the rectum.

**prodrome,** a symptom which indicates an approaching disease.

**professional nurse,** one who is licensed by the state board of examiners, and who works with doctors in a hospital or various other settings. The professional nurse plays an important role as a member of a treatment or surgical team.

**progeria,** premature senility usually occurring in childhood, marked by wrinkled skin, baldness, and hardened arteries.

**progestational,** referring to changes in the uterus when the corpus luteum is preparing the endometrium for the fertilization and growth of the ovum.

**progesterone, progestin,** the hormone excreted by the corpus luteum which prepares the uterus for reception and development of the fertilized ovum. Some synthetic and natural agents are called progestins and are used in treatment of menstrual disorders.

**prognathous,** marked by jaws which project forward beyond the face.

**prognosis,** a prediction of the probable course and outcome of a disease.

**prognostic,** pertaining to prognosis.

**progressive,** advancing forward; gradually increasing in severity of symptoms.

**prolactin,** a hormone that stimulates lactation.

**prolamin,** any of a group of simple proteins found in the seeds of grain such as wheat or oats.

**prolan,** a hormone present in the urine of pregnant women which allows early diagnosis of pregnancy.

**prolapse,** falling down, or downward displacement of a part or an organ.

**proliferation,** the rapid growth and reproduction of similar forms, as cells.

**proline,** an amino acid made in the body necessary to protein synthesis which is a basic constituent of collagen.

**promazine,** a phenothiazine used in the form of hydrochloride salt as a major tranquilizer in psychomotor states of anxiety and agitation.

**promontory,** a projecting bodily protuberance.

**pronation,** the act of lying with the face downward, or in a prone position; the position of turning the hand so that the palm faces downward.

**pronotor,** a muscle of the forearm that pronates the palm.

**prone,** lying with the face downward and lying horizontally.

**propagation,** reproduction.

**prophage,** an intracellular lysogenic bacterial virus that provides protection to its host from active viruses.

**prophase,** the first stage in cell reduplication in mitosis.

**prophylactic,** an agent that wards off disease; pertaining to prophylaxis.

**prophylaxis,** a preventive measure or treatment; the prevention of disease.

**proprietary,** a medicine protected against free competition by a trademark or patent.

**proprioceptor,** a sensory nerve ending originating chiefly in muscles, tendons, and the labyrinth that are concerned with movements and position of the body.

**protosis,** a bulging of the eyes; a forward displacement of an organ.

**propulsion,** a tendency for the body to bend forward while walking, characteristic in paralysis agitans; festination.

**prosection,** a programmed dissection for the purpose of demonstration of the anatomic structures of cadavers.

**prosencephalon,** forebrain.

**prosopoplegia,** facial paralysis.

**prostatalgia,** pain in the prostate gland.

**prostate gland,** a gland that surrounds the male urethra at the neck of the bladder and which contributes to the secretion of semen.

**prostatic,** pertaining to the prostate gland.

**prostatitis,** inflammation of the prostate gland.

**prostatocystotomy,** incision of the bladder and prostate.

**prostatomegaly,** an enlargement of the prostate gland.

**prostatovesiculectomy,** surgical excision of the prostate gland and seminal vesicles.

**prosthesis,** an artificial part substituted for a missing part of the body, such as an arm or leg.

**prosthodontics,** the branch of medicine which constructs artificial teeth or oral structures to replace missing or injured parts; prosthodontia.

**prosthodontist,** one trained in prosthodontics.

**prostrate,** lying with the body extended; to exhaust.

**prostration,** extreme exhaustion, or lack of energy.

**protamine,** basic proteins found in the sperm of some fish used as an antidote to heparin overdosage.

**protanopia,** inability to distinguish reds and greens; red blindness.

**protease,** any proteolytic enzyme that assists in hydrolysis of peptide linkages in the digestive action on proteins; peptidase.

**protein,** found in all cells, and constitutes about 15% of human body weight; any of a group of complex organic compounds that contain carbon, hydrogen, oxygen, nitrogen, and sulfur.

**proteinase,** any enzyme that hydrolyzes proteins, as pepsin and rennin.

**proteinic,** pertaining to protein.

**proteinuria,** an excess accumulation of serum proteins in the urine.

**proteolysis,** the hydrolysis of protein into simpler compounds such as polypeptides.

**proteolytic,** pertaining to proteolysis.

**proteose,** a class of compounds produced by partial degradation of proteins by hydrolysis.

**prothrombin,** a complex globulin protein in the blood important to coagulation.

**protodiastole,** pertaining to the first of four phases of ventricular diastole.

**protopathic,** responding solely to gross stimuli such as pain.

**protoplasm,** the primary living matter which composes all vegetable and animal cells and tissues.

**protoplasmic,** pertaining to protoplasm.

**protozoan,** a microscopic, one-celled organism.

**protozoology,** the science of protozoans, a division of zoology.

**proud,** flesh, pertaining to flesh which is characterized by an excessive granulation in wounds and ulcers.

**provitamin,** a substance such as ergosterol that can form a vitamin when acted upon by the body.

**proximal,** nearest to the point of reference.

**pruritogenic,** causing itching or pruritus.

**pruritus,** an intense, chronic itching, as in the anal region.

**pseudesthesia,** a subjective sensation which occurs without an appropriate stimulus, such as a pain felt in an amputated limb.

**pseudocyesis,** false pregnancy.

**pseudoplegia,** paralysis due to hysteria.

**pseudopregnancy,** a condition in which all symptoms of pregnancy appear to be present but without being substantiated; false pregnancy; pseudocyesis.

**psilocybin,** a hallucinogen derived from the mushroom Psilocybe mexicana.

**psittacosis,** an infectious viral disease occurring in birds that may be transmitted to humans that causes pulmonary disorders, chills followed by fever, headache, nausea, constipation, and epistaxis; parrot fever.

**psoriasis,** a chronic skin disease of various characteristics such as the formation of red scaly patches or flat-topped papules that cause itching.

**psychasthenia,** an emotional disorder marked by obsessions, compulsions, anxiety, doubts, feelings of inadequacy, and phobias.

**psyche,** the mind and all its mental processes both conscious and subconscious.

**psychedelic,** pertaining to any of several drugs that induce hallucinations, intensification of perception of the senses, psychotic states, and heightened awareness. The most commonly used psychedelics are LSD, marijuana, mescaline, psilocybin, and morning-glory seeds.

**psychiatric,** pertaining to psychiatry.

**psychiatrist,** a physician who specializes in the treatment of mental disorders, or psychiatry.

**psychiatry,** the medical science concerned with the origin, diagnosis, treatment and prevention of mental illness.

**psychic,** pertaining to the mind.

**psychoanalysis,** a psychologic method or theory of human development and behavior originated by Sigmund Freud that provides a system of psychotherapy which analyzes the subconscious thoughts in order to determine and eliminate physical and mental disorders.

**psychoanalyst,** a psychiatrist who has training in psychoanalysis.

**psychoanalytic,** pertaining to psychoanalysis.

**psychobiology,** the science concerned with the interaction between the mind and body as being an integrated unit in the formation and functioning of the personality.

**psychodrama,** a technique of group psychotherapy in which individuals dramatize roles enabling them to increase awareness of their emotional problems.

**psychodramatic,** pertaining to psychodrama.

**psychodynamics,** a systemized theory of human behavior and the role of unconscious motivation.

**psychogenesis,** the origin and development of the mind; the causation of a symptom or illness by mental or psychic factors as opposed to organic ones.

**psychogenetic,** pertaining to a disease which has its origin in the mind.

**psychogenic,** of mental origin; having a psychological origin.

**psychokinesis,** the alteration of motion directed by thought processes.

**psycholepsy,** sudden alteration of moods.

**psychological,** pertaining to the study of the mind.

**psychologist,** one who specializes in psychology.

**psychology,** the science concerned with mental processes and the behavior in man and animals.

**psychometry,** the science dealing in testing and measuring psychologic ability, efficiency, potential, and functioning.

**psychomotor,** pertaining to motor effects of the cerebral or psychologic functioning; causing voluntary movement.

**psychoneurosis,** a neurosis of a functional nature characterized by anxiety, phobias, compulsions, obsessions, and physical complaints without physical cause; neurosis.

**psychoneurotic,** one suffering from psychoneurosis.

**psychoparesis,** weakness of the mind.

**psychopath,** one lacking moral sensibility, but possessing normal intelligence; a mentally unstable person.

**psychopathic,** pertaining to a mental disorder; relating to treatment of mental disorders; abnormal.

**psychopathology,** the study of the causes and processes of mental disease or abnormal behavior.

**psychopathy,** any mental disease, especially one characterized by a defective personality.

**psychopharmacology,** the science of drugs as they relate to mental and behavioral effects on emotional states; the use of drugs to modify psychological symptoms.

**psychophysics,** the study of mental processes in relation to physical processes; the study of the relation between stimuli and the effects they produce.

**psychophysiology,** the physiology of the mind; the correlation between the body and mind.

**phychosis,** a major mental disorder of organic or emotional origin, often characterized by regressive behavior, inappropriate mood, lack of impulse control, delusions, hallucinations, loss of contact with reality, and a disintegration of personality.

**psychosomatic,** referring to illnesses in which bodily symptoms are of mental or emotional manifestation.

**psychosomatic medicine,** the branch of medical science emphasizing mental factors as the cause of functional and structural changes in disease processes.

**psychosurgery,** surgery of the brain to relieve certain symptoms in mental illness, as a lobotomy.

**psychotherapeutic,** pertaining to psychotherapy.

**psychotherapist,** one trained in psychotherapy.

**psychotherapy,** a treatment or method based primarily upon the verbal and nonverbal aspects of communication with a patient, as distinguished from the use of drugs or other measures of treatment.

**psychotic,** pertaining to psychosis; one exhibiting psychosis.

**psychotropic,** a term applied to drugs that have a special action upon the mind or psyche.

**psychrophobia,** an abnormal fear or sensitivity to cold.

**psychrotherapy,** treatment of disease by application of cold.

**ptamic,** that which causes sneezing.

**ptarmus,** spasmodic sneezing.

**pterygoid,** shaped like a wing; pertaining to the two large processes of the sphenoid at the base of the skull.

**ptilosis,** the loss of eyelashes.

**ptomaine,** any of a class of nitrogenous organic bases which become toxic resulting from the action of putrefactive bacteria produced in animal and vegetable matter.

**ptosis,** a drooping of the upper eyelid caused by paralysis of the levator muscle; the prolapse of any organ of the body.

**ptotic,** pertaining to ptosis.

**ptyalism,** excessive secretion of saliva; salivation.

**ptyaloith,** a salivary concretion or stone.

**puberal,** concerning puberty.

**puberty,** the period in life during which the secondary sex characteristics begin to develop and either sex becomes capable of sexual reproduction.

**pubes,** the pubic region; the anterior region of the innominate bone covered with pubic hair; os pubis.

**pubescence,** one arriving at puberty; the covering of fine hair on the body.

**pubescent,** reaching puberty.

**pubic,** pertaining to the pubes.

**pubis,** pubic bone, or the innominate bone.

**pudendal,** relating to the external female genitalia, or genitals. pudendum, external female genitals; vulva.

**puerile,** childlike.

**puerilism,** childish behavior exhibited by an adult; immature behavior.

**puerperal,** pertaining to puerperium.

**puerperal fever,** septicema following childbirth.

**puerperium,** the state of a woman immediately following childbirth, usually a period of 3 to 6 weeks.

**pulmometry,** determination of the capacity of the lungs with a pulmometer.

**pulmonary,** pertaining to the lungs.

**pulmonary artery,** an artery which conveys venous blood directly from the heart to the lungs.

**pulmonary vein,** any of four veins conveying oxygenated blood directly from the lungs to the heart.

**pulmonectomy,** surgical removal of part or all of a lung's tissue; pneumonectomy.

**pulmonic,** pertaining to the lungs.

**pulmonitis,** inflammation of the lung; pneumonia.

**pulmotor,** a mechanical apparatus for inducing artificial respiration by forcing oxygen into the lungs or to expel the lung contents, as in asphyxiation or drowning.

**pulp,** the soft part of an organ; referring to dental pulp in the interior of a tooth.

**pulpy,** resembling pulp.

**pulsation,** the process of rhythmic beat, as in the heart and blood vessels; pulse.

**pulse,** the rate or rhythm of the heart contractions causing the arteries to contract and expand at regularly throbbing intervals; the pulsation of the radial artery at the wrist.

**pulsimeter,** an instrument for measuring the frequency and force of a pulse; sphygmometer.

**pulverization,** the crushing of any substance into tiny particles. pulverulent, resembling powder; fine powder; dusty.

**pulvis,** a powder.

**pump,** an apparatus used to transfer or to remove fluids or gases by suction or pressure.

**puncture,** a hole or wound made by a sharp pointed device; to make a hole with a pointed instrument.

**pupil,** the round contractile orifice or opening at the center of the iris.

**pupillary,** concerning the pupil of the eye.

**purgative,** a substance that evacuates the bowels; a cathartic.

**purge,** a drug that causes evacuation of the bowels; to evacuate the bowels by means of a purgative.

**purpura,** a condition of the skin marked by purple or livid spots caused by tiny hemorrhages that invade the tissues.

**purpuric,** pertaining to purpura.

**purulent,** consisting of matter or pus; resembling pus.

**pus,** a yellowish-white product of inflammation composed of a thin albuminous fluid and leukocytes or particles of their remains.

**pustulant,** causing pustules or blisters; a pustulant medication or agent.

**pustular,** pertaining to or having the nature of a pustule; covered with pustules.

**pustulation,** the formation of pustules.

**pustule,** a small, elevated pus-containing lesion of the skin; any circumscribed, flat, or rounded protruberance found on the skin resembling a pimple or blister with an inflammed base and containing pus.

**putrefaction,** the process of putrefying; the enzymatic decomposition of animal or vegetable matter, producing a foul- smelling compound.

**putrefy,** to undergo putrefaction.

**putrescence,** the process of undergoing putrefaction; becoming putrid.

**putrescine,** a polyamine found in decaying meat products.

**putrid,** decayed or rotten; putrefied.

**pyelitis,** inflammation of the renal pelvis.

**pyelocystitis,** inflammation of the renal pelvis and the bladder.

**pyelogram,** the x-ray film produced by pyelography.

**pyelography,** a radiography of the kidneys and ureter after an injection of a contrast solution or dye.

**pyelonephritis,** inflammation of the whole kidney due to a bacterial infection.

**pyelonephrosis,** any disease of the kidney and its pelvis.

**pyelotomy,** surgical incision of the kidney.

**pyemia,** septicemia or blood poisoning caused by pyogenic bacteria.

**pyknic,** having a shorot, thick, and stocky body build.

**pyknometer,** an apparatus for determining the specific gravity of fluids.

**pylephlebitis,** inflammation of the portal vein.

**pylic,** pertaining to the portal vein.

**pyloric,** pertaining to the pylorus.

**pylorus,** the opening between the stomach and the duodenum; used to refer to the pyloric part of the stomach.

**pyoderma,** any purulent disease of the skin.

**pyogenic,** producing pus; pertaining to the formation of pus.

**pyorrhea,** a bacterial gum infection with a copious discharge of pus.

**pyostatic,** a drug that arrests suppuration.

**pyothorax,** an accumulation of pus in the pleural cavity; empyema.

**pyramidal,** pertaining to drugs which have an accumulative effect; resembling a pyramid; see extrapyramidal.

**pyretic,** pertaining to fever.

**pyrexia,** a fever; a febrile condition.

**Pyridium,** a brick-red powder used to treat infections of the genitourinary tract; trademark for phenazopyridine hydrochloride.

**pyridoxine,** one of the forms of Vitamine B6 used in its salt form to treat a deficiency of B6 in the body; sometimes used in treatment of myasthenia gravis.

**pyromania,** an obsessive preoccupation with fires or the compulsion to set them.

**pyrosis,** heartburn.

**pyrotic,** caustic; burning.

**pyuria,** the presence of pus in the urine.

# Q

**Q-fever,** an acute infectious disease marked by fever, headache, muscular pains, chills, and loss of appetite, caused by rickettsia and transmitted by inhaling infected dust or drinking contaminated milk. Common among those who handle hides and animal products; Queensland fever.

**q-sort,** an assessment of personality in which the subject (or one who observes) indicates the degree to which a standardized set of descriptive statements are representative of the subject.

**quack,** one who pretends to have experience in medicine, as in diagnosis and treatment of disease; charlatan.

**quackery,** the methods used by a quack.

**quadrant,** a fourth of a circle; the four regions of the abdomen which are divided for diagnostic purposes.

**quadriceps,** having four heads, as in the large quadriceps muscle in front of the thigh.

**quadripara,** a woman who has produced four viable offspring.

**quadripartite,** having four parts.

**quadriplegia,** paralysis affecting all four limbs.

**quadroon,** the offspring of a white person and a mulatto; an individual having one-quarter Negro heritage.

**quadruplet,** being one of four children born to the same mother and of one birth.

**quarantine,** a period of detention or isolation to prevent the spread of a communicable disease.

**quartan,** recurring every fourth day, as in quartan fever.

**Queensland fever,** see Q-fever.

**quenching,** to suppress or extinguish by immersing in water.

**querulent,** fretful or complaining.

**quickening,** the first noticeable movement of the fetus in utero.

**quinidine,** a crystalline alkaloid isomer of quinine used to treat abnormal cardiac arrythmias.

**quinine,** a bitter-tasting alkaloid, obtained from the bark of cinchona trees, used in its salt form to treat malaria; quinine is used as an analgesic, antipyretic, oxytocic, cardiac depressant, and for other various treatments.

**quinsy,** an inflammation of the tonsils and the formation of abscess of the peritonsillar tissue.

**quintipara,** a woman who has had five viable offspring.

**quintuplet,** one of five offspring produced at one labor.

**quotidian,** occurring daily; recurring daily fever.

**quotient,** a number derived at by division.

**Q-wave,** a downward wave of an electrocardiogram that is associated with the contractions of the heart ventricles.

# R

**rabbetting,** interlocking of the splintered edges of a bone fracture.

**rabbit fever,** Tularemia.

**rabic,** pertaining to rabies.

**rabid,** being affected with rabies; relating to rabies.

**rabies,** an acute viral disease that produces infection of the central nervous system marked by paralysis of the muscle of deglutition, glottal spasm, manic behavior, convulsions, tetany, and respiratory paralysis. May be communicated by a bite of a rabid animal, often fatal to man without proper treatment.

**racemose,** resembling a cluster or bunch of follicles which are divided and subdivided, as in a gland.

**rachialgia,** pain in the spine.

**rachianesthesia,** spinal anesthesia.

**rachicentesis,** lumbar puncture to determine the pressure of fluid and to obtain fluid for examination.

**rachidial, rachidian,** pertaining to the spinal column.

**rachigraph,** a device that outlines the curves of the spine.

**rachiometer,** a device that measures spinal curvatures.

**rachiopathy,** any disease of the spine.

**rachioplegia,** spinal paralysis.

**rachiotome,** an instrument used to divide the vertebrae.

**rachiotomy,** surgical incision of the vertebral column.

**rachis,** vertebral or spinal column.

**rachitis,** rickets.

**radectomy,** surgical excision of the root of a tooth.

**radial,** pertaining to the radius bone of the arm.

**radiate,** to spread from a common center.

**radiation,** emission of rays from a central point; a treatment for certain disease using a radioactive substance.

**radiation syndrome,** an illness due to exposure of a body part to ionizing radiations from radioactive substances marked by anorexia, headache, nausea, vomiting, and diarrhea.

**radical,** directed to the origin to eliminate the cause of a disease; treatment by surgical excision, usually by the total eradication of diseased tissues.

**radicle,** the smallest branches of a nerve or blood and lymph vessels.

**radicular,** pertaining to a root or radicle.

**radiculitis,** inflammation of the spinal nerve roots.

**radioactive,** pertaining to radioactivity.

**radioactivity,** the ability of a substance to emit alpha rays, beta rays, and gamma rays that undergo spontaneous disintegration.

**radiobiologist,** a specialist in radiobiology.

**radiobiology,** the scientific study concerned with the effects of radiant energy or radioactive material on living tissue or organisms.

**radiocystitis,** inflammation of the bladder following roentgen rays or radium treatment.

**radiodermatitis,** inflammation of the skin caused by roentgen rays or radium treatment.

**radiodiagnosis,** the use of x-ray in diagnosis.

**radioelement,** an element possessing radioactive power.

**radiograph,** a film produced by radiography.

**radiography,** the production of film records of internal structures of the body for diagnostic purposes; roentgenography.

**radioisotopes,** radioactive forms of chemicals used in research and in the diagnosis and treatment of certain diseases; radioactive isotopes.

**radiologist,** one specializing in radiology.

**radiology,** the branch of science concerned with roentgen rays, radium rays, and other forms of radiation and their medical uses; the process of photographing organs or bones for diagnostic purposes.

**radiolucency,** the quality of being partly or wholly permeable to radiant energy.

**radionecrosis,** disintegration of tissue exposed to radium or x-rays.

**radioneuritis,** neuritis caused by exposure to radiant energy.

**radioresistance,** resistance to radiation by certain tumors or tissues.

**radiosensitive,** the ability to be destroyed by radiation, as a tumor by x-rays.

**radiosurgery,** the use of high-energy radioactive particles in treating cancer or other diseased tissues.

**radiotherapist,** one who specializes in radiotherapy.

**radiotherapy,** treatment of disease by radioactive elements such as radium or thorium.

**radiothermy,** short-wave diathermy.

**radioulnar,** pertaining to the radius and ulna.

**radium,** a radioactive element found in minerals used in radiography for treating cancer.

**radius,** a bone in the forearm on the thumb side; a line from the center of a circle to a point on its circumference.

**radix,** root, as of a spinal or cranial nerve.

**rage,** being violently angry.

**ragocyte,** a cell often found in the joints of one suffering from rheumatoid arthritis.

**rale,** an abnormal respiratory sound heard on auscultation indicating a pathologic condition; death rattle.

**ramification,** a branching.

**ramiform,** branchlike; having the form of a branch; ramal.

**ramose,** having many branches.

**ramulose,** having many tiny branches.

**ramus,** a branch of an artery, nerve, or vein.

**ranula,** a tumor or cyst beneath the tongue, caused by obstruction and subsequent swelling of a glandular duct.

**ranular,** pertaining to a ranula.

**rape,** sexual intercourse with a female without her consent; stupration.

**raphe,** the line of union or seam of the two symmetrical parts or halves of an organ.

**rarefaction,** a condition of becoming less dense.

**rash,** a temporary eruption on the skin which may be in the form of red spots or patches.

**raspatory,** a file or rasp used in surgery.

**ratbite fever,** an infectious disease transmitted to humans by the bite of an infected rat, marked by recurring fever, skin eruptions, and muscular pain; sodoky.

**ratio,** proportion.

**ration,** a fixed allowance of food and drink for a certain period of time.

**rational,** having a sound mind; logical or reasonable; sane.

**rauwolfia,** any group of trees or shrubs from the genus Rauwolfia from which numerous alkaloids are derived for medicine, such as reserpine which is used as an antihypertensive and sedative.

**rave,** irrational verbalization; to talk irrationally, as in delirium; to be furious or raging.

**reaction,** a response of an organism to a stimulus; counterreaction; the specific effect caused by the action of chemical agents; a chemical transformation of one substance into another substance; the emotional state that is manifested in a particular situation.

**reaction formation,** a defense mechanism by which a person assumes an attitude or behavior that is the opposite of the impulse harbored, usually operating unconsciously.

**reactivation,** the act of causing something to become active again, especially the reactivating of an immune serum which has lost its potency.

**reactive,** the ability to respond to a stimulus.

**reagent,** a substance used to produce a chemical reaction in order to detect, measure, or produce other substances.

**reagin,** an antibody.

**recall,** to remember; the act of bringing a memory into consciousness.

**rebound,** the act of rebounding; resilience.

**receptor,** the ending of an afferent neuron that is sensitive to stimuli.

**recess,** a small cavity or indentation.

**recessive,** a tendency to recede; a hidden trait or recessive character, as opposed to a dominant character.

**recidivation,** recurrence of a disease; relapse; the repetition of a crime or offense.

**recidivist,** one who tends to relapse or return to crime; a mentally ill patient who has repeated relapses.

**recipe,** a prescription of a physician.

**recrement,** secretions, such as saliva, which are reabsorbed into the blood stream.

**recrudescence,** the recurrence of disease after abatement or remission.

**rectal,** pertaining to the rectum.

**rectalgia,** proctalgia; pain in the rectum.

**rectectomy,** surgical excision of the rectum or anus; proctectomy.

**rectitis,** an inflammation of the rectum; proctitis.

**rectocele,** the protrusion of the posterior wall of the vagina with the anterior wall of the rectum into the vagina.

**rectocolitis,** inflammation of the rectum and colon.

**rectoscope,** proctoscope.

**rectostenosis,** a narrowing or stricture of the rectum.

**rectum,** the lower portion of the large intestine between the sigmoid flexure and the anal canal.

**rectus,** any straight muscle.

**recumbent,** lying down or reclining position.

**recuperate,** to be restored to normal health; to recover.

**recuperation,** the restoration to normal health.

**recurrence,** the return of symptoms of an illness or disease.

**recurrent,** returning at intervals, as a fever; relapse.

**red blood cell,** a blood corpuscle containing hemoglobin; erythrocyte.

**reduce,** to restore to a normal place, as the ends of a fractured bone; to lose weight.

**reduction,** the process of restoring a dislocated bone to its normal place.

**reflector,** an apparatus which reflects light or sound waves.

**reflex,** a reflected action, or an involuntary response to a stimulus, such as a movement.

**reflex arc,** impulses which travel from receptors to effectors between the point of stimulation and the responding organ in a reflex action; neural pathway.

**reflexogenic,** producing or causing a reflex action.

**reflexograph,** an instrument for charting a reflex.

**reflexophil,** characterized by exaggerated reflex activity.

**reflux,** a backward flow; regurgitation.

**refraction,** the bending of a light ray as it passes from a medium of one density to another of different density.

**refractory,** stubborn or obstinate; resistant to ordinary treatment, as in some diseases; resisting stimulation.

**regeneration,** regrowth, repair, or restoration of part of the body or of damaged tissues.

**regimen,** a method of therapy to improve or restore health.

**region,** a particular division or area of the body.

**regional,** pertaining to particular regions or areas of the body.

**registered nurse,** a professional nurse who receives a license to practice nursing after completing a training period of 3-5 years depending on the school of nursing and passing an examination by a state or provincial board of examiners. Specialization usually requires a master's degree which prepares a nurse for teaching, supervision, or administration.

**regression,** reverting to an earlier or more infantile pattern of behavior; returning to a prior status in physical or mental illness.

**regurgitate,** to pour forth; to vomit.

**regurgitation,** the act of regurgitating; a backflow of blood through a defective valve of the heart.

**rehabilitation,** the process of restoring to health or activity, as one physically handicapped.

**rehalation,** a rebreathing process sometimes employed in anesthesia.

**rehydration,** replacement of the water or fluid content to a body or a substance that has undergone dehydration.

**reimplantation,** replacement of a structure or tissue in the original site from which it was previously lost.

**reinfection,** a recurrence of an infection by the same agent or bacteria.

**reinforcement,** strengthening; in behavioral science, the presentation of a stimulus (either a reward or punishment) which elicits a response.

**reinforcer,** that which produces reinforcement, such as a stimulus.

**reinoculation,** a repeated inoculation with the same organism.

**relapse,** recurrence of an illness or disease; to slip or slide back.

**relapsing fever,** a tropical disease resulting from spirochetal infections transmitted by head lice, body lice, and ticks marked by intermittent attacks of high fever.

**relaxant,** an agent that relaxes tension, especially in muscles.

**relaxation,** a reduction of tension; the act of relaxing.

**relief,** the removal of distressing or painful symptoms.

**REM,** rapid eye movements, the dream phase during the sleep cycle.

**remediable,** capable of being remedied.

**remedial,** curative; intended to improve certain skills.

**remedy,** anything that cures a disease or illness; a curative medication, application, or treatment; to restore to the natural state or condition.

**remission,** an abatement of symptoms of a disease or pain.

**remit,** to abate or relax.

**remittent,** a temporary easing; having periods of abatement and returning.

**renal,** pertaining to the kidneys.

**reniform,** having a kidney-shaped form or structure.

**renin,** a proteolytic enzyme secreted by the juxtaglomerular cells of the kidney, which is a powerful vasoconstrictor.

**renopathy,** any disease of the kidney.

**reposit,** to replace surgically.

**repositor,** an instrument used in surgery to return a displaced organ to its original position.

**repress,** to reject or force out of consciousness, as impulses or fears.

**repressed,** affected by repression; marked by repression.

**repression,** the act of repressing, restraining, or inhibiting; a defense mechanism in which one banishes unacceptable ideas or impulses from conscious awareness.

**resect,** to surgically excise a portion of an organ or a structure.

**resection,** surgical excision of a segment of a structure or a portion of an organ.

**reserpine,** an alkaloid of rauwolfia which acts centrally on the vasomotor center to decrease peripheral vasoconstriction, used as an antihypertensive and as a tranquilizer for extremely agitated patients.

**residual,** pertaining to that which is left as a residue; that which remains behind; an aftereffect of experience which influences later behavior.

**residue,** remainder; that which remains after removal of another substance.

**resilience,** having the quality to bounce back; elasticity; flexibility.

**resilient,** elastic; rebounding; coming back to original shape.

**resolution,** disappearance of a disease, inflammation, or tumor.

**resolve,** to return to normal.

**resolvent,** an agent that causes dispersion of inflammation.

**resonance,** the act of resounding; the sound produced by tapping the chest or by percussion of a body cavity.

**resonant,** pertaining to resonance.

**respiration,** the act of respiring; breathing; inspiration and expiration in exchange of oxygen and carbon dioxide.

**respirator,** a mechanical apparatus used to aid breathing; a device for giving artificial respiration or promoting pulmonary ventilation.

**respiratory,** pertaining to respiration.

**respiratory system,** includes the lungs, pleura, bronchi, pharynx, larynx, tonsils, and the nose.

**respirometer,** a device that determines the nature of respiration.

**response,** a reaction resulting from a stimulus.

**rest,** refreshing repose of the body due to sleep; the freedom from activity or bodily exertion; a remnant of embryonic tissue that persists in the adult organism.

**restiform,** twisted or shaped like a rope.

**restitution,** returning to an original position or to a former state; the spontaneous turning of the fetal head either to the left or right after it has extended through the vagina.

**restorative,** causing a return to health or to consciousness; a remedy or substance that is effective in the regaining of health or strength.

**restore,** to bring back to health, or consciousness.

**restraint,** to forcibly control; state of being hindered.

**resuscitate,** to restore life to one apparently dead.

**resuscitation,** the process of restoring life to one who has stopped breathing; the act of bringing one back to full consciousness. CPR or cardiopulmonary resuscitation, in which the heart and lung action is reestablished after cardiac arrest or apparent death or loss of consciousness resulting from electric shock, drowning, respiratory obstruction, and various other causes. The two important components of CPR are artificial ventilation and cardiac massage.

**resuscitator,** one who initiates resuscitation; a device used for producing respiration in persons who have stopped breathing.

**retardation,** delayed development; subnormal general intellectual and physical activity due to impairment of social adjustment or of maturation, or both; mental retardation.

**retarded,** one who exhibits retardation.

**retch,** to strain, as in vomiting.

**retching,** an involuntary effort to vomit.

**rete,** a network of blood vessels.

**retention,** the process of holding back or retaining in the body materials which are normally excreted, such as urine.

**retial,** pertaining to a rete.

**reticular,** having a netlike structure; resembling a net.

**reticulation,** formation of a network.

**reticulocyte,** an immature red blood corpuscle containing a network of granules; a young erythrocyte or red blood cell.

**reticulocytosis,** an excessive amount of reticulocytes in the peripheral blood.

**reticulum,** a small network of protoplasmic cells or structures.

**retiform,** reticular.

**retina,** the innermost coat of the eyeball which receives images formed by the lens, and transmits these images to the brain by the optic nerve.

**retinal,** pertaining to the retina.

**retinene,** an orange-yellow pigment formed in the retina resulting from the action of light on rhodopsin (visual purple pigment) used in dark adaptation.

**retinitis,** inflammation of the retina.

**retinoscope,** an apparatus used for measuring refractory errors.

**retinoscopy,** an examination of the retina to determine refractory errors.

**retinosis,** any nonflammatory, degenerative condition of the retina.

**retractile,** able to be drawn back.

**retractility,** the capability of retraction.

**retraction,** drawing back; the condition of being drawn back.

**retractor,** an instrument for holding open the edges of a wound; a muscle that retracts.

**retral,** posterior; at the back.

**retrobuccal,** pertaining to the back part of the mouth.

**retrocedent,** returning or going backward.

**retroflex,** to bend backward.

**retroflexion,** a bending backward of an organ.

**retrograde,** going backward; decline or deterioration; catabolic.

**retrogress,** to revert.

**retrogression,** return to an earlier and less complex state; degeneration; decline or deterioration.

**retrogressive,** degenerative changes; changes to a lower complexity, such as atrophy, degeneration, or necrosis.

**retroinfection,** the infection of a mother communicated by the fetus in the uterus.

**retrolental,** behind the lens of the eye.

**retrolingual,** behind the tongue.

**retromammary gland,** behind the mammary gland.

**retromandibular,** behind the lower jaw.

**retromastoid,** behind the mastoid process.

**retronasal,** concerning the back of the nose.

**retroocular,** behind the eye.

**retroparotid,** behind the parotid gland.

**retroperitoneal,** behind the peritoneum.

**retroperitoneum,** the space behind the peritoneum.

**retroperitonitis,** inflammation of the retroperitoneal space.

**retropharyngeal,** behind the pharynx.

**retropharyngitis,** inflammation of the posterior region of the pharynx.

**retroplasia,** degeneration of tissues into a more primitive structure.

**restrospect,** to reflect, or look back in thought.

**retrospection,** by thought, to look back into the past; a survey of past experiences.

**retrospective falsification,** an unconscious distortion of past experiences to conform to the emotional needs of the present.

**retrosternal,** behind the sternum.

**retrovaccination,** vaccination with a virus obtained from a calf inoculated with a smallpox virus which was first obtained from a human.

**retroversion,** a state of being turned back; bending backward, as part of an organ, especially the uterus.

**reversion,** return to a previously existing form or condition; the expression of traits possessed by a remote ancestor; atavism.

**revulsion,** the act of drawing blood from one part of the body to another in diverting disease; counterirritant.

**revulsive,** an agent causing revulsion; a counterirritant.

**rhagades,** painful fissures appearing at the corner of the mouth or anus, caused by movement or infection.

**rhegma,** a rupture, or fracture.

**rheum,** a catarrhal or watery discharge.

**rheumatic,** pertaining to rheumatism.

**rheumatic fever,** a systemic inflammatory disease which varies in severity, duration, and frequently followed by heart disease, usually occurring in young adults or children.

**rheumatism,** pain, swelling, and deformity of joints causing stiffness, or limitation of motion.

**rheumatoid,** resembling rheumatism.

**rheumatoid arthritis,** an inflammation of the joints causing stiffness, swelling, pain, and cartilaginous hypertrophy.

**rheumic,** pertaining to rheum.

**rhexis,** the rupture of a blood vessel, or an organ.

**Rh factor,** Rhesus factor, first detected in the blood of Rhesus monkeys; inherited antigens in red blood cells of most humans who have a Rh positive blood type and, due to a blood transfusion or pregnancy, are capable of destroying red blood cells in one who is typed Rh negative, such as a newborn infant.

**rhinal,** pertaining to the nose; nasal.

**rhinalgia,** pain in the nose; nasal neuralgia.

**rhinencephalon,** the portion of the brain concerned with olfactory impulses.

**rhinitis,** inflammation of the nasal mucous membranes.

**rhinolaryngology,** the branch of science concerned with the structures and diseases of the nose and larynx.

**rhinologist,** one who specializes in the diseases of the nose.

**rhinology,** the study of the nose and its diseases.

**rhinopathy,** any disease of the nose.

**rhinophonia,** having a nasal tone in speaking.

**rhinoplasty,** plastic surgery of the nose.

**rhinopolyp,** a polyp of the nose.

**rhinopolypus,** a nasal polyp.

**rhinorrhagia,** a nosebleed; epistaxis.

**rhinorrhea,** a thin, watery discharge from the nose.

**rhinoscope,** a speculum used in nasal examination.

**rhinoscopy,** an examination of the nasal passages with a rhinoscope.

**rhizomelic,** concerning the roots of the extremities, such as the hips and shoulders in man.

**rhizotomy,** the surgical section of a root, as a nerve or tooth.

**rhodogenesis,** the formation or regeneration of visual purple that has been bleached by light.

**rhodophylaxis,** the ability of the retina to form or regenerate rhodopsin (visual purple).

**rhodopsin,** visual purple, a photosensitive red pigment in the outer segment of retinal rods important to night vision.

**rhombencephalon,** a primary division of the embryonic brain from which the metencephalon and myelencephalon are formed.

**rhoncal, rhonchial,** pertaining to rhoncus or rattle in the throat.

**rhonchus,** a rale or rattling in the throat; a snoring sound; a dry, coarse rale that occurs in the bronchial tubes because of a partial obstruction.

**rhubarb,** an extract made from roots and rhizome of Rheum officinale (rhubarb), used as a cathartic and astringent.

**rhypophagy,** eating of filth.

**rhypophobia,** a morbid disgust to the act of defecation or filth.

**rhythm,** a measured time or movement which occurs at regular intervals, as the action of the heartbeat.

**rhythmic,** pertaining to a rhythm; rhythmical.

**rhytidectomy,** plastic surgery for the excision of wrinkles.

**rhytidosis,** wrinkling of the skin; wrinkling of the cornea.

**rib,** a bone or cartilage that forms the chest cavity and protects certain vital organs.

**riboflavin,** a water-soluble vitamin of the B complex family found in milk, muscle, liver, kidney, eggs, malt, and algae, essential to man; Vitamin $B_2$.

**ribonucleic acid,** RNA which is a nucleic acid containing ribose found in cytoplasm in all cells.

**ribose,** a monosaccharide sugar present in ribonucleic acid (RNA).

**ribosome,** a large particle containing RNA and protein present in the cytoplasm of cells.

**ricin,** a poisonous white powdery substance made from the castor bean used in medicine as an agglutinin.

**ricinoleic acid,** an organic acid found in castor oil in the form of glyceride which is used as a laxative.

**ricinus,** the castor oil plant from which ricin and castor oil are derived used as a cathartic or lubricant.

**rickets,** a disease occurring in infancy and childhood due to a deficiency of Vitamin D, marked by bone distortion and softening, muscle pain, and sweating of the head.

**rickettsia,** a genus of the Rickettsiaceae which is transmitted by lice, ticks, fleas, and mites to humans from animals causing diseases, as typhus.

**ridge,** a narrow, elevated edge or border.

**rigidity,** stiffness; immovability; inability to bend.

**rigor,** chill preceding a fever; a state of stiffness as in a muscle.

**rigor mortis,** stiffening of muscles of a dead body.

**rima,** a slit, fissure, or crack.

**rimose,** filled with fissures or cracks.

**rimula,** a minute fissure or slit, especially of the brain or spinal column.

**ring,** a round organ or band which encircles an opening.

**Ringer's solution,** an aqueous solution used intravenously in conditions of dehydration and for improving circulation.

**ringworm,** a disease caused by fungi which appears in ring formations or patches on various parts of the body, especially on the scalp.

**risus,** laughter.

**risus sardonicus,** a peculiar grin caused by muscle spasms, as seen in tetanus.

**R.N.,** registered nurse.

**RNA,** ribonucleic acid.

**roborant,** a tonic; strengthening.

**Rocky Mountain spotted fever,** an infectious disease caused by a parasite, Rickettsia rickettsii, which is transmitted to man by a wood tick, resulting in fever; pain in the bones and muscles, prostration, skin eruptions, and chills.

**roentgen,** the unit of measurement of radiation that is used internationally, pertaining most commonly to x-rays.

**roentgenogram,** the film made by x-rays.

**roentgenography,** the x-ray pictures of internal body structures.

**roentgenologic,** pertaining to roentgenology.

**roentgenologist,** one who specializes in roentgenology.

**roentgenology,** the study of x-rays and technical application to medical diagnosis and therapy.

**roentgenoscope,** an apparatus which has a fluorescent viewing screen; fluoroscope.

**roentgenoscopy,** examination by means of roentgen rays.

**roentgenotherapy,** treatment of a disease by roentgen rays.

**rongeur,** a surgical instrument for cutting or removing small fragments of bone or tissue.

**root,** proximal end of a nerve; that portion of an organ that is implanted in tissues, such as a tooth, hair, or nail.

**Rorschach test,** a projective technique which seeks to determine personality traits and emotional conflicts by an analysis of subjective responses to a standard series of ten ink blots.

**rosacea,** a chronic disease of the skin, usually involving the nose, cheeks, and forehead, marked by flushing, papules, and acne-like pustules.

**rose fever,** rose cold, an allergy attributed to inhalation of rose pollen in the early part of summer.

**roseola,** a rose-colored rash from various causes.

**rotation,** the process of turning on an axis; in obstetrics, the twisting or turning of the fetal head as it follows the curves of the birth canal as it descends.

**roughage,** indigestible, rough material such as fibers, and cellulose which are found in certain fruits and cereals that stimulate peristalsis.

**rouleau,** a grouping of red blood cells arranged like a roll of coins.

**roundworm,** a nematode which is a parasite that thrives in the intestines.

**rubedo,** blushing; a temporary redness of the skin, especially the face.

**rubefacient,** an agent that reddens the skin; causing reddening of the skin.

**rubella,** German measles; an acute viral infection that resembles measles, but runs a shorter course, marked by a pink macular rash, fever, lymph node enlargement, and sometimes, a sore throat and drowsiness may occur.

**rubeola,** measles, rubella.

**rubescent,** growing red, or reddish; ruddy.

**rubor,** redness due to inflammation.

**rudimentary,** undeveloped; imperfectly developed.

**ruga,** a ridge, crest, or fold, especially of mucous membrane.

**rugose,** marked by wrinkles; ridged.

**rumination,** the casting up of food, or regurgitation, to be chewed the second time, as in cattle; preoccupation of the mind.

**rump,** the buttock; gluteal region.

**rupia,** a skin eruption marked by large cutaneous elevations, usually occurs in the third stage of syphilis.

**rupophobia,** morbid aversion to dirt or filth.

**rupture,** hernia; a tearing apart, as of an organ.

**rutilizm,** red-headedness.

**Rx,** symbol; a simple method for writing ''take'', ''recipe'', or prescription; treatment.

**rytidosis,** the contraction of the cornea preceding death which causes wrinkling of its surface.

## S

**sabulous,** sandy or gritty.

**sac,** a baglike structure or organ; a pouch.

**saccate,** having the form of a pouch or sac; contained within a sac.

**saccharide,** one of the carbohydrates containing sugar; a sugar substitute.

**sacchariferous,** yielding sugar.

**saccharification,** the conversion into sugar.

**saccharin,** a white, crystalline compound which is several hundred times sweeter than sucrose, used as a non-nutritive sweetener.

**saccharine,** resembling sugar; sugary consistency.

**saccharolysis,** chemical splitting up of sugar.

**saccharolytic,** pertaining to saccharometer.

**saccharometer,** saccharimeter, an optical instrument used to determine the strength of sugar solutions by measuring a plane of polarized light rotations after it passes through a sugar solution.

**saccharomycetes,** a genus of yeasts, including brewers' yeast, used in the fermentation of sugar.

**saccharomycetic,** pertaining to yeast fungi.

**saccharomycosis,** any of several diseases caused by yeast fungi.

**saccharum,** sugar.

**sacciform,** shaped like a pouch or sac.

**saccular,** resembling a sac.

**sacculate,** having saclike expansions; containing saccules.

**saccule,** a little sac; applied to the smaller of two sacs in the membranous labyrinth of the ear.

**sacculocochlear,** relating to both the saccule and cochlea.

**sacculus,** a saccule.

**sacrad,** toward the sacrum.

**sacral,** pertaining to the sacrum.

**sacralgia,** pain in the sacrum.

**sacrectomy,** surgical removal of part of the sacrum.

**sacrocoxitis,** inflammation of sacroiliac joint.

**sacrodnia,** pain in the sacrum region.

**sacroiliac,** pertaining to the sacrum and the ilium; relating to the juncture of the hipbone and the lower spine.

**sacrolumbar,** pertaining to the sacrum and the loins.

**sacrosciatic,** pertaining to the sacrum and the ischium.

**sacrospinal,** pertaining to the sacrum and the spinal column.

**sacrospinalis,** pertaining to the large muscle on either side of the spinal column which extends from the sacrum to the head.

**sacrotomy,** surgical removal of part of the sacrum.

**sacrouterine,** pertaining to the sacrum and uterus.

**sacrum,** part of the vertebral column between the lumbar and coccygeal regions.

**sadism,** a pathological condition in which pleasure is derived from inflicting physical or psychological pain on others; a perversion or sexual deviation when it is necessary to inflict pain upon another in order to obtain sexual gratification.

**sadist,** one who finds pleasure in inflicting pain on others.

**sadistic,** pertaining to sadism.

**sadomasochism,** the derivation of pleasure from inflicting physical or mental pain upon others or on oneself.

**sagittal,** resembling an arrow; pertaining to the suture that unites the parietal bones of the skull; referring to a plane that divides a body into two halves.

**Saint Vitus's dance,** involuntary muscular movements; chorea.

**salacious,** lustful.

**salicylate,** a salt of salicylic acid.

**salicylic acid,** a powder which is soluble in water, used as a food preservative, and in medicine as an analgesic and an antipyretic. Salicylic acid is too irritating internally to be used by itself, but is widely used in the preparation of acetylsalicylic acid (aspirin).

**salify,** combining an acid with a base to form a salt; to infuse with a salt.

**saline,** consisting of salt; containing chemical salt, as an alkali metal; salty.

**saline solution,** sodium chloride and distilled water in a solution; an isotonic solution.

**salinometer,** an instrument that measures the amount of salt present in a solution.

**saliva,** the slightly acid fluid secreted by the glands of the mouth that serves as the first digestive enzyme, ptyalin. The saliva begins the digestive process of converting starches into various dextrins and to some maltose. Final hydrolysis of these products breakdown to glucose is completed in the small intestine.

**salivary,** pertaining to saliva.

**salivary calculus,** a minute stone in a salivary duct.

**salivary glands,** the three pairs of glands in the oral cavity that contribute to the formation of saliva: parotid glands, submaxillary glands, and sublingual glands.

**salivation,** the process of secreting saliva; ptyalism.

**salivatory,** producing the secretion of saliva.

**Salk vaccine,** a vaccine against poliomyelitis produced from inactivated poliomyelitis virus, given by injection or orally on a sugar cube.

**Salmonella,** any rod-shaped bacteria belonging to the family Enterobacteriaceae that cause food poisoning, intestinal inflammation, or genital-tract diseases.

**salmonellosis,** infestation with Salmonella bacteria which cause food poisoning.

**salpingectomy,** surgical removal of a fallopian tube.

**salpingemphraxis,** an obstruction of an eustachian tube; an obstruction of a fallopian tube.

**salpingian,** concerning the eustachian tube, or an oviduct.

**salpingitis,** an inflammation of a fallopian tube, or eustachian tube.

**salpingocele,** a herniated protrusion of an oviduct.

**salpingocyesis,** a pregnancy in an oviduct; tubal pregnancy.

**salpinx,** pertaining to the fallopian or eustachian tube.

**salsoda,** a crystalline sodium carbonate which is used as a cleaning agent, or water softener.

**salsalate,** an analgesic and anti-inflammatory agent.

**salt,** sodium chloride; common table salt.

**saltation,** leaping, jumping, or dancing, as in chorea; conduction along myelinated nerves; in genetics, a mutation.

**saltatory,** characterized by leaping, jumping, or dancing.

**salt-free diet,** a diet with no more than two grams of salt.

**salubrious,** healthful; promoting good health; wholesome.

**salutary,** healthful; curative; promoting health.

**Salvarsan,** a yellowish arsenical powder used in treatment of syphilis; trademark; rarely used since the development of penicillin.

**salve,** a thick, soothing ointment or cerate.

**sanative,** having a healing quality; curative.

**sanatorium, sanitarium,** an institution for the treatment of diseases, for convalescents, or patients with mental disorders.

**sanatory,** healing; hygienic; conducive to health.

**sand-blind,** having imperfect eyesight.

**sandfly,** flies of the family Psychodidae, a biting fly inhabiting the seashore; a fly of the genus Phlebotomus which is a blood-sucking species that transmits sandfly fever and various other diseases affecting the skin, nasal cavity, or visceral organs such as the liver or spleen.

**sandfly fever,** usually a three-day fever produced by a mild virus transmitted by the sandfly from the genus Phlebotomus papatasii, similar to dengue fever.

**sane,** of sound mind; able to anticipate and judge one's action; having reason; rational.

**sanguicolous,** a parasite inhabiting the blood.

**sanguifacient,** making blood, or forming blood.

**sanguiferous,** conducting blood, as the circulatory system.

**sanguine,** abounding in blood; pertaining to blood; hopeful.

**sanguineous,** bloody; abounding in blood; relating to blood.

**sanguinolent,** tinged with blood; containing blood.

**sanies,** a fetid serous discharge from a wound or ulcer, containing pus tinged with blood.

**sanious,** pertaining to sanies.

**sanitarian,** a person skilled in public health science and sanitation.

**sanitary,** promoting health; clean; healthful.

**sanitation,** the use of measures to promote conditions favorable to health.

**sanitization,** the process of being made sanitary.

**sanitize,** to disinfect, or to sterilize.

**sanity,** rationality; soundness of mind; reasonableness.

**sap,** any fluid of a living structure essential to life.

**saphena,** small saphenous or the great saphenous veins of the leg.

**saphenous,** pertaining to certain arteries, nerves, or veins.

**saphenous nerve,** a branch of the femoral nerve that follows the long saphenous vein in the lower leg.

**sapid,** savory or very tasty.

**sapiens,** referring to modern man, Homo sapiens.

**sapor,** that which affects the sense of taste.

**saporific,** imparting a taste; pertaining to sapor.

**sapphism,** lesbianism.

**sapremia,** a toxic condition of the blood produced by putrefactive bacteria.

**saprodontia,** tooth decay.

**saprogen,** any bacteria produced by putrefaction, or causing it.

**saprogenic,** resulting from putrefaction or causing it.

**saprophilous,** living on decaying substances, such as bacteria.

**saprophyte,** any organism living upon decaying matter.

**saprophytic,** relating to a saprophyte.

**sarcitis,** inflammation of muscle tissue.

**sarcoid,** tuberculoid; resembling a sarcoma tumor; sarcoidosis.

**sarcoidosis,** a chronic, progressive granulomatous reticulosis of any organ or tissue marked by the presence of tubercle-like lesions, generally affecting the skin, lymph nodes, lungs, and bone marrow.

**sarcology,** the branch of medicine concerned with the study of soft body tissues.

**sarcoma,** a malignant tumor originating in connective tissue, bone, or muscle.

**sarcomatoid,** resembling a sarcoma.

**sarcomatosis,** a condition in which many sarcomas develop at various sites in the body; sarcomatous degeneration.

**sarcous,** belonging to flesh or muscle.

**sardonic laugh, sardonic grin,** a spasmodic affectation of the muscles of the face, giving the impression of laughter; risus sardonicus.

**sartorius,** a narrow, ribbon-shaped muscle of the thigh, the longest muscle in the body which aids in flexing the knee, and in rotating the leg to a cross-legged position.

**satiable,** capable of being satisfied.

**satiety,** a fullness or gratification; completely satisfied.

**saturated,** unable to hold any more in solution of a given substance; referring to an organic compound in which only single bonds exist between carbon atoms.

**saturation,** the state of being saturated.

**saturnine,** morose or gloomy; pertaining to the absorption of lead, as in lead poisoning.

**saturnism,** lead poisoning.

**satyriasis,** an exaggerated sexual desire in males.

**saxitoxin,** a neurotoxin produced by poisonous mussels, clams, and plankton; gonyaulax poison.

**scab,** a crust formation of a superficial sore or wound.

**scabicide,** a substance lethal to Sarcoptes scabiei.

**scabies,** a contagious skin disease caused by the itch mite, Sarcoptes scabiei, resulting in intense itching and eczema.

**scabious,** pertaining to scabies.

**scabrities,** a condition of the skin marked by a roughened and scaly appearance; a sand-like roughness of the inner surface of the eyelids.

**scala,** a ladder-like structure, as the spiral passages of the cochlea.

**scald,** a burn to the flesh or skin caused by hot liquid or steam.

**scalene,** pertaining to the scalenus.

**scalenus,** one of the three muscles located in the vertebrae of the neck and attached to the first two ribs; known as scalenus anterior, medius, and posterior.

**scall,** a scalp disease marked by scaly eruptions.

**scalp,** the skin covering the cranium; hairy integument of the upper part of the head.

**scalpel,** a straight, small, sharp-bladed surgical knife used in dissection and surgical procedures.

**scaly,** resembling scales.

**scan,** an image produced by a sweeping beam of radiation.

**scanner,** an apparatus that inspects and detects certain conditions of the body, as in ultrasonography.

**scanning speech,** pronunciation of words in syllables in a slow and hesitating manner, usually a symptom of disease involving the nervous system.

**scaphocephalic,** having a deformed head, resembling a boat's keel.

**scaphoid,** the boat- shaped bone of the carpus on the radial side; navicular bone.

**scaphoiditis,** inflammation of the scaphoid bone.

**scapula,** the large, flat bone of the shoulder; shoulder blade.

**scapulalgia,** pain in the shoulder blade region.

**scapular,** pertaining to the shoulder blade.

**scapulectomy,** surgical removal of part or all of the shoulder blade.

**scar,** the mark left on the skin by a healing wound or sore.

**scarification,** having many small superficial punctures or scratches in the skin over a part, as for introduction of vaccine.

**scarificator, scarifier,** an instrument with many sharp points.

**scarlatina,** mild form of scarlet fever.

**scarlatiniform,** resembling scarlet fever.

**scarlet fever,** a contagious disease characterized by sore throat, fever, rash, and rapid pulse, usually occurring in children.

**scatacratia,** fecal incontinence.

**scatemia,** intestinal toxemia in which chemical poisons are absorbed from retained fecal matter.

**scatology,** the study and analysis of waste products for diagnostic purposes.

**scatophagy,** the eating of feces.

**Schick test,** test for susceptibility to diphtheria.

**Schiller's test,** a test for superficial cancer of the cervix.

**schistoprosopia,** congenital fissure of the face.

**Schistosoma,** a genus of blood flukes which cause infection in man by penetration of the skin while coming in contact with infected waters; schistosomiasis.

**schistosomiasis,** infection with Schistosoma.

**schistothorax,** congenital fissure of the chest or thorax.

**schizogenesis,** reproduction by fission.

**schizoid,** resembling schizophrenia; referring to a person with a schizoid personality.

**schizomycete,** an organism of the class of Schizomycetes, a group of plant organisms belonging to fungi.

**schizomycetous,** pertaining to schizomycetes.

**schizont,** a stage in the development of the malarial parasite following the trophozoite in which its nucleus divides into smaller nuclei.

**schizonychia,** splitting of fingernails and toenails.

**schizophasia,** muttered or disordered speech of the schizophrenic.

**schizophrenia,** any of a large group of severe emotional disorders, usually of psychotic proportion, characterized by disturbances of thought, mood, and behavior, such as misinterpretation of reality, delusions and hallucinations, ambivalence, inappropriate affect, and withdrawn, bizarre, or regressive behavior.

**schizophrenic,** one afflicted with schizophrenia.

**schizotrichia,** splitting of the hair at the ends.

**sciatic,** pertaining to the ischium or hip.

**sciatic nerve,** the largest nerve in the body extending from the sacral plexus on either side of the body down the back of the thigh and leg.

**sciatica,** inflammation of or injury to the sciatic nerve and its branches; severe pain in the leg along the course of the sciatic nerve.

**scirrhoid,** pertaining to a hard scirrhus or carcinoma.

**scirrhoma,** a hard tumor or carcinoma; scirrhus.

**scirrhous,** hard like a scirrhus; knotty.

**scirrhus,** a hard, cancerous tumor caused by an overgrowth of fibrous tissue.

**scissor leg,** an abnormal crossing of both legs in walking due to adduction of both hips.

**sclera,** the white outer coat of the eye which extends from the optic nerve to the cornea; sclerotica.

**scleradenitis,** inflammation and hardening of a gland.

**scleral,** pertaining to the sclera.

**sclerectasia,** a protrusion of the sclera.

**sclerectoiridectomy,** surgical removal of part of the sclera and iris as a treatment for glaucoma.

**sclerencephalia,** sclerosis of the brain.

**scleriasis,** progressive hardening of the skin.

**scleritis,** inflammation of the sclera.

**scleroderma,** a disease that causes the skin to become hard and rigid.

**sclerodermatitis,** a skin inflammation accompanied by thickening and hardening.

**scleroid,** having a hard texture.

**scleroma,** sclerosis; a hardened patch or induration of nasal or laryngeal mucous membranes.

**sclerose,** to become hardened.

**sclerosis,** a hardening of tissue or a part, due to excessive growth of fibrous connective tissue.

**sclerotic,** pertaining to the sclera of the eye; affected with or pertaining to sclerosis.

**sclerous,** hard; indurated; bony.

**scolex,** the round, attachment organ of a tapeworm; the larva of a tapeworm.

**scoliosiometry,** measurement of spinal curvature.

**scoliorachitic,** relating to scoliosis or rickets.

**scoliosis,** a lateral curvature of the spine.

**scoliotic,** pertaining to scoliosis.

**scoop,** a surgical spoon-shaped instrument used in extracting the contents of cysts or cavities.

**scopolamine,** an anticholinergic alkaloid obtained from the Scopolia carniolica plant, used as a sedative, mydriatic, cycloplegic.

**scopophobia,** a morbid fear of being seen.

**scorbutic,** pertaining to or affected with scurvy.

**scorbutus,** a disease casued by a deficiency of vitamin C; scurvy.

**scotodinia,** vertigo accompanied by faintness and black spots before the eyes.

**scotoma,** a blind gap in the visual field.

**scotomatous,** pertaining to scotoma.

**scotometer,** an instrument for diagnosing and measuring areas of depressed vision in the visual field.

**scotophobia,** an aversion or fear of the dark.

**scotopia,** night vision; the adaptation of the eye to the dark.

**scotopsin,** a protein that combines with retinene to form rhodopsin, important to the adjustment of vision for darkness.

**scratch,** a superficial injury or mark on the skin produced by scraping with a fingernail or a rough or sharp surface.

**screen,** a structure used in fluoroscopy on which light rays are projected for diagnostic purposes.

**screening,** an examination of a large segment of a population to detect a particular disease.

**screwworm,** the larva of a two-winged fly that deposits its eggs in wounds or in the nose; the larva, then, thrives upon the tissue of the host.

**scrobiculate,** marked with furrows or pits.

**scrobiculus,** a small groove, furrow, or pit.

**scrofula,** a condition of primary tuberculosis of the lymph glands of the neck characterized by swelling and degeneration.

**scrofuloderma,** a skin disease characterized by suppurating abscesses on the chest, neck, and in the axilla and groin area. The condition responds to ultraviolet light and chemotherapy.

**scrofulous,** pertaining to scrofula.

**scrotal,** pertaining to the scrotum.

**scrotectomy,** surgical excision of part of the scrotum.

**scrotitis,** inflammation of the scrotum.

**scrotocele,** hernia of the scrotum.

**scrotum,** the external double pouch that contains the testicles.

**scruple,** 20 grains of the apothecaries' unit of weight; one-third of a dram.

**scurf,** a desquamation of the skin, or a flaking of dry scales resembling dandruff.

**scurvy,** a deficiency disease due to the lack of vitamin C, marked by anemia, swollen and bleeding gums, livid skin patches and exhaustion.

**scutiform,** shaped like a shield.

**scutulum,** shoulder blade; scapula.

**scutum,** any shield-shaped bone; thyroid cartilage.

**scyphoid,** shaped like a cup.

**seasickness,** motion sickness; nausea, and vomiting due to unusual motion.

**sebaceous,** pertaining to or secreting sebum.

**sebaceous cyst,** a swelling beneath the skin due to a blockage of a duct or gland filled with sebaceous material.

**sebaceous gland,** an oil- secreting gland of the skin.

**sebiferous,** producing fatty or sebaceous matter.

**sebiparous,** secreting or producing sebum.

**seborrhea,** a functional disease of the sebaceous glands marked by an excessive increase of sebaceous secretion.

**seborrheic,** pertaining to seborrhea.

**sebum,** the fatty secretion of the sebaceous glands of the skin.

**secobarbital,** a short-acting barbiturate used as an hypnotic and sedative prior to anesthesia; also used to control convulsions; trademark name, Seconal.

**secondary sex characteristic,** any manifest characteristic due to the effect of gonadal secretions of hormones, such as the development of beards in males, and the development of mammary glands in females at puberty.

**second-degree burn,** a burn marked by blistering and redness without destruction of the epidermis.

**secretagogue,** an agent that causes secretion of glands; stimulating secretion.

**secrete,** to separate from the blood; to produce secretion.

**secretin,** a hormone secreted by the duodenal and jejunal mucosa which aids digestion; it also stimulates secretion of pancreatic juice and bile.

**secretion,** the cellular process of releasing a specific product; any substance produced by secretion of glands.

**secretory,** pertaining to secretion; a secretory organ or gland.

**section,** the act of separating by cutting, as in surgery; a segment of material for microscopic examination.

**sector,** a separate part; an area of the body.

**secudines,** afterbirth.

**sedation,** the act of alleviating distress, pain, or tension by administering a sedative.

**sedative,** a tranquilizer; an agent allaying irritability or excitement; quieting.

**sedentary,** habitually sitting; inactive; staying in one locale.

**sediment,** the material settling at bottom of a liquid.

**sedimentation,** a formation of sediment; settling out of sediment.

**sedimentator,** a centrifuge apparatus for separating sediment from urine.

**segment,** a part of a whole, especially of an organ; a division or section.

**segmental,** pertaining to a portion; resembling segments.

**segmentation,** a division into parts that are similar.

**segregation,** separating; in genetics, the separation of paired genes into different gametes during meiosis.

**seismotherapy,** sismotherapy, treatment of disease by vibratory or mechanical massage.

**seizure,** a sudden attack of a disease or of a symptom; a convulsion, or epileptic attack, heart attack, or a stroke.

**selectivity,** the degree to which a single dose of medicine produces the desired effect.

**self-antigen,** the ability of the body's tissues to stimulate autoimmunity.

**self- destruction,** the destruction of oneself, as in suicide.

**self- hypnosis,** self-induced hypnosis, often used to overcome bad habits or to accomplish a specific feat.

**self-limited,** influenced by one's own peculiarities; a disease that runs a precisely limited course.

**self-tolerance,** individual tolerance of immunity to self-antigens.

**semeilogy,** the study of symptoms; symptomatology.

**semeiotic,** pertaining to symptoms or signs; symptomatic.

**semen,** the viscous secretion at ejaculation in the male containing spermatozoa.

**semicanal,** a passage or channel open at one end.

**semicircular canals,** three small tubular canals in the labyrinth of the ear responsible for maintaining equilibrium.

**semilunar,** resembling a half-moon, or a crescent shape.

**semilunar bone,** crescent shaped bone of the carpus or wrist.

**semilunar valves,** the valves of the aorta and pulmonary artery.

**seminal,** pertaining to semen.

**seminal vesicle,** one of two sac-like glands lying in back of the bladder of the male, which join the ductus deferens on each side.

**semination,** insemination; introduction of semen into the vagina.

**seminiferous,** producing or carrying semen.

**semipermeable,** permeable only to certain molecules, as a membrane that permits passage of a solvent but not the solute.

**semisynthetic,** produced by chemical manipulation of substances that occur naturally.

**senescence,** the process of aging, or growing old.

**senile,** pertaining to old age; decline of mental faculties.

**senilism,** premature aging, or old age.

**senility,** the physical and mental deterioration that accompanies old age.

**senna,** any of various leguminous herbs, shrubs, or trees of the genus Cassia, the dried leaves of which are used as a cathartic.

**senopia,** an improvement of vision in the aged usually a sign of incipient cataract.

**sensation,** an impression produced by impulses through the sense organs; the power of feeling or sensing; an awareness of stimulus to the nervous system.

**sense,** perceived through the nervous system or a sense organ; the normal power of understanding.

**sense organ,** any organ of the body that transmits impulses to the brain, such as the nose, ear, eye, and skin; receptor.

**sensibility,** an ability to feel or perceive; sensitivity.

**sensitive,** able to respond to stimuli; unusually responsive to stimulation; reacting quickly.

**sensitivity,** the quality of being sensitive; the state of being acutely affected by the action of a chemical or other agents.

**sensitization,** a condition of being made sensitive to certain stimulus; the exposure of a person to a specific antigen by repeated injections of it, as a serum; anaphylaxis.

**sensorimotor,** being both sensory and motor.

**sensorineural,** pertaining to a sensory nerve.

**sensorium,** the sensory nerve center in the cerebral cortex that receives and coordinates impulses sent to individual nerve centers; the special sensory perceptive powers and their integration in the brain; having a clear, accurate memory together with a correct orientation for time, place, and person; consciousness.

**sensory,** pertaining to sensation.

**sensuous,** pertaining to the senses; appealing to the senses; readily affected through the senses or susceptible to influence.

**sentient,** capable of sensation.

**sepsis,** the presence of pathological microorganisms or their toxins in the blood; a state of poisoning of the system caused by the spread of infection through the blood.

**septal,** pertaining to a septum.

**septate,** divided by a septum.

**septectomy,** surgical removal of a septum or part of it.

**septic,** pertaining to sepsis.

**septicemia,** blood poisoning, or a systemic disease caused by the presence of pathological microorganisms or their toxins in the bloodstream.

**septicemic,** pertaining to septicemia.

**septic sore throat,** an inflammation of the throat caused by streptococcus bacteria, accompanied by fever and prostration.

**septicophlebitis,** septic inflammation of a vein.

**septimetritis,** septic inflammation of the uterus.

**septometer,** an instrument that measures the width of the nasal septum.

**septonasal,** pertaining to the nasal septum.

**septotome,** an instrument used for surgical cutting of a section of the nasal septum.

**septotomy,** surgical incision of the nasal septum.

**septum,** a dividing membrane or partition; a partition of tissue.

**septuplet,** one of seven children born of one pregnancy.

**sequel, sequela,** the consequence of an illness or disease; a morbid condition occurring as a consequence of another condition.

**sequestration,** the formation of sequestrum; isolation of a patient.

**sequestrectomy,** surgical excision of a sequestrum.

**sequestrum,** a portion of dead bone which has separated from sound bone due to necrosis.

**seroalbuminuria,** the presence of serum albumin in the urine.

**serocolitis,** inflammation of the serous coat of the colon.

**seroculture,** bacterial culture on blood serum.

**seroenteritis,** inflammation of the serous coat of the intestine.

**serohepatitis,** inflammation of the peritoneal covering of the liver.

**serologist,** one who specializes in serology.

**serology,** the science concerned with the nature and reactions of blood serum.

**serolysin,** a bacterial substance occurring in blood serum.

**serosa,** serous membrane, as peritoneum, pleura, and pericardium.

**serositis,** inflammation of a serous membrane.

**serotherapy,** therapeutic measure in treatment of disease by injecting blood serum, either human or animal, containing antibodies.

**serotonin,** a hormone and neurotransmitter found in certain cells that causes muscle contraction and vasoconstriction.

**serous,** resembling serum; producing or containing serum.

**serous membrane,** any thin membrane lining a serous cavity such as the peritoneum.

**serpiginous,** creeping; having a wavy border.

**serpigo,** a creeping eruption, especially ringworm.

**serum,** any serous fluid that moistens the surfaces of serous membranes; the fluid portion of the blood after coagulation; serum from the blood of an animal that has been rendered immune to some disease, given by inoculation as an antitoxin; consisting of plasma minus fibrogen.

**serum albumin,** a simple protein found in blood serum.

**serum globulin,** a plasma protein that may be separated into three blood fractions, alpha, beta, and gamma globulin responsible for the body's resistance to certain infections.

**serum sickness,** an eruption of purpuric spots accompanied by pain in the limbs and joints following a serum injection.

**sesamoid,** a small nodular bone that is embedded in a tendon or joint capsule; sesamoid bone, resembling a sesame seed.

**setaceous,** bristle-like; resembling a bristle; bristly, or hairy.

**seventh cranial nerve,** the facial nerve.

**sex,** the distinctive characteristics which differentiate between males and females; activities related to sexual attraction; sexual reproduction; sexual intercourse.

**sex chromosome,** a chromosome that carries sex-linked traits, as determined by the presence of the XX (female) or XY (male) genotype in somatic cells.

**sex hormone,** a hormone that affects the growth or function of the sexual organs and the development of secondary sex characteristics in males and females.

**sex-linked,** transmitted by a gene which is located on the X chromosome.

**sexological,** pertaining to sexology.

**sexologist,** one specializing in sexology.

**sexology,** the study of sexual behavior in humans.

**sextuplet,** one of six children born at the same birth.

**sexual,** pertaining to sex.

**sexual intercourse,** copulation; coitus; sexual relations.

**sexuality,** state of having sex; the collective characteristics differentiating between the male and female; the constitution of a person relating to sexual behavior and attitudes.

**sexual organs,** genitalia; genitals.

**shaft,** the long slender portion of a long bone.

**shakes,** shivering due to a chill; fine vibrations of the hands, often seen in chronic alcoholics.

**shaking palsy,** a basal ganglion disease marked by progressive rigid tremulousness, affected gait, muscular contraction and weakness, often seen in Parkinson's disease.

**shank,** leg, or shin; tibia.

**sheath,** a tubular encasement or enveloping structure.

**shedding,** loss of deciduous teeth; casting off the top layer of the epidermis or skin.

**shell shock,** a form of psychoneurosis, often seen during military service and in training camps; war neurosis.

**shield,** a protective covering.

**Shigella,** a genus of nonmotile, gram- negative rods belonging to the family Enterobacteriaceae, which produce digestive disturbances ranging from mild diarrhea to dysentery.

**shin,** the anterior edge of the tibia or leg, between the ankle and the knee; shinbone.

**shingles,** a viral infection involving the central nervous system causing eruption of acute, inflammatory vesicles or blisters on the skin along peripheral nerves which are painful; herpes zoster.

**shiver,** slight tremor; involuntary shaking, as with cold, fear, or excitement.

**shivering,** an involuntary shaking or tremor of the body, as with cold.

**shock,** a sudden debilitating disturbance of bodily functions resulting from acute peripheral circulatory failure due to hemorrhage, severe trauma, burns, dehydration, infection, surgery, or drug toxicity. Outstanding symptoms of shock are: prostration, pallor, perspiration, rapid pulse, pulmonary deficiency, coldness of skin, and often anxiety.

**shock therapy,** a treatment in mental illness involving three different types: electric shock therapy, insulin shock therapy, or metrazol shock therapy.

**shortsightedness,** unable to see distant objects clearly; myopia, or nearsightedness.

**shoulder,** joining of the clavicle and scapula, where the arm joins the trunk.

**shoulder-blade,** scapula.

**shoulder dislocation,** displacement of the shoulder joint caused by falling on an outstretched arm.

**shoulder girdle,** the bony semicircular band which forms an arch, serving as supporting structure for the upper extremities.

**show,** appearance of a discharge of blood prior to labor; menstruation.

**shudder,** temporary convulsive shaking of the body resulting from fright, fear, or anxiety; tremor.

**shunt,** to turn to one side or to bypass; a passage between two blood vessels or between two sides of the heart that has an abnormal opening in its wall partition; a surgical creation of an anastomosis.

**sialaden,** a salivary gland.

**sialadenitis,** inflammation of a salivary gland.

**sialadenocus,** tumor of a salivary gland.

**sialagogic,** pertaining to sialagogue.

**sialagogue,** an agent that increases the flow of saliva.

**sialaporia,** a deficiency in saliva secretion.

**sialemesis,** vomiting caused by excessive secretion of saliva.

**sialine,** concerning saliva.

**sialism, sialismus,** excessive secretion of saliva; ptyalism.

**sialoadenectomy,** surgical removal of a salivary gland.

**sialoadenitis,** an inflammation of a salivary gland; sialadenitis.

**sialoaerophagia,** swallowing of saliva and air.

**sialoangitis,** inflammation of a salivary duct.

**sialocele,** a salivary cyst.

**sialolith,** a salivary calculus, or stone.

**sialolithiasis,** formation of several salivary calculi, or stones.

**sialoncus,** a tumor under the tongue caused by obstruction of a salivary duct.

**sialorrhea,** ptyalism.

**sialosis,** the flow of saliva; ptyalism.

**Siamese twins,** any twins born joined together, usually at the hips or buttocks; twins congenitally united.

**sib,** a blood relative; kinsman descended from a common ancestor; sibling.

**sibilant,** hissing or whistling.

**sibling,** offspring of the same parents; a brother or sister.

**sibship,** brothers and sisters of the same family group.

**siccus,** dry.

**sick,** not well; affected by disease; nauseous.

**sickle cell,** an abnormal crescent-shaped red blood cell.

**sickle cell anemia,** a hereditary form of anemia in which the presence of crescent-shaped red blood cells causes a crystallization of the hemoglobin within the cells, resulting in the clogging of blood vessels. This disease affects about 1 in 500 American Negroes and is marked by severe anemia, jaundice, abdominal, muscular, and joint pains, skin ulcerations, formation of bilirubin gallstones, and many other complications.

**sicklemia,** sickle cell anemia.

**sickly,** not robust; habitually indisposed; in poor health.

**sickness,** state of being affected with disease; illness.

**side effect,** an unintended secondary reaction to medication; an effect that is aside from the desired effect of a treatment.

**siderocyte,** a red blood corpuscle that contains iron in a form other than hematin.

**sideroderma,** a disorder of iron metabolism that causes a bronze discoloration of the skin.

**sideropenia,** iron deficiency in the blood or the body.

**sideropenic,** pertaining to sideropenia.

**sideroscope,** a device used to find metal particles in the eye.

**siderosis,** a form of pneumoconiosis caused by dust or fumes containing iron particles being inhaled, as in occupations such as arc-welding.

**siderous,** pertaining to or containing iron.

**sigh,** deep inspiration preceded by an audible, slower expiration; suspirium.

**sight,** the act of seeing; having the faculty of vision.

**sightless,** blind.

**sigmoid,** shaped like the letter S; pertaining to the sigmoid colon.

**sigmoidectomy,** surgical excision of all or part of the sigmoid colon.

**sigmoid flexure,** the lower segment of the descending colon between the crest and the rectum, shaped like the letter S.

**sigmoiditis,** inflammation of the sigmoid colon.

**sigmoidoscope,** an endoscope with an illuminated end used for examination of the sigmoid flexure.

**sgimoidoscopy,** examination of the sigmoid colon with a sigmoidoscope.

**sigmoidostomy,** a surgical creation of an artificial opening from the sigmoid colon to the body surface.

**sign,** any existing evidence of an abnormal nature in the body or of an organ.

**signa,** meaning "mark", used in writing prescriptions; designated "S" or "sig"

**signature,** that part of a prescription which gives instructions for use of medication.

**sign language,** hand signs or gestures used as a substitute for speech by the deaf.

**silicon,** a nonmetallic element found in soil which occurs in traces in skeletal structures such as teeth and bone.

**silicone,** any organic compound in which all or part of the carbon has been replaced by silicon, used in preparations of oils, greases, synthetic rubber, and resins.

**silicosis,** a lung condition caused by inhalation of dust of stone, sand, or flint containing silica, resulting in nodular, fibrotic changes in the lungs.

**silicotic,** pertaining to silicosis.

**silver nitrate,** a chemical element which is used as a local anti- infective, or prophylaxis of opthalmia neonatorum, a purulent conjunctivitis in the newborn.

**silver protein,** silver made colloidal in combination with protein, used in solutions as an active germicide.

**simple,** not complex; something not mixed or compounded; being deficient in intellect; a medicinal herb, or plant.

**simple fracture,** fracture without torn ligaments or broken skin; bone fracture without complications.

**simulate,** to feign illness or disease.

**simulation,** feigning disease or symptoms of a disease.

**simulator,** one who simulates; malingerer; something that simulates.

**sinapism,** a mustard plaster.

**sincipital,** pertaining to the sinciput.

**sinciput,** upper and front portion of the head.

**Sinequan,** trademark for doxepin hydrochloride used in treatment of psychoneurosis to alleviate symptoms of anxiety, tension, depression, sleep disturbances, guilt, fear, apprehension, worry, and lack of energy.

**sinew,** a tendon of a muscle.

**singuitus,** hiccup.

**sinister,** on the left side; left.

**sinistral,** pertaining to the left side; left-handed.

**sinistraural,** hearing better with the left ear.

**sinistrocardia,** a displacement of the heart to the left side of the medial line of the body.

**sinistrocerebral,** pertaining to or situated in the left cerebral hemisphere.

**sinistrocular,** having stronger vision in the left eye.

**sinistromanual,** left-handed.

**sinistropedal,** using the left foot more than the right; left-footed.

**sinistrotorsion,** a turning or twisting to the left, as of the eye.

**sinuitis,** sinusitis; inflammation of a sinus.

**sinuous,** winding or bending in and out.

**sinus,** a cavity, recess, or passage, as in bone; dilated channel or vessel for venous blood; any cavity having a narrow opening leading to an abscess.

**sinusal,** pertaining to a sinus.

**sinusitis,** inflammation of a sinus, especially of a paranasal sinus.

**sinusoid,** resembling a sinus.

**sinusotomy,** surgical incision of a sinus.

**sitiergia,** hysterical refusal to take food, probably related to anorexia nervosa.

**sitiology,** the science of nutrition; dietetics.

**sitomania,** periodic bulimia; excessive hunger, or abnormal craving for food.

**sitophobia,** an abnormal repugnance to food, either generally or to certain selective dishes.

**sitosterol,** any of a group of sterols from closely related plants used in varying combinations as an anticholesterolemic substance in the synthetic production of steroid hormone drugs.

**sitotherapy,** treatment by diet.

**situs,** a position, or the site of a body part or organ.

**sitz bath,** a bath in which to sit with water covering the hips; hip bath.

**skeletal,** pertaining to the skeleton.

**skeleton,** the bones of the body collectively, forming the framework. The human body consists of 206 bones.

**Skene's glands,** glands which lie inside of the posterior floor of the urethra in the female.

**skenitis,** inflammation of the Skene's glands or paraurethral ducts.

**skiagram,** an X-ray picture; roentgenograph.

**skiagraph,** an object made visible by a shadowed outline; a radiograph.

**skiagraphy,** the process of taking pictures with roentgen rays; radiography.

**skiameter,** an apparatus that determines differences in density and penetration of roentgen rays.

**skiascope,** an apparatus that examines by fluoroscope errors of refraction in the eye by observing movement of shadow and light; retinoscope.

**skiascopy,** shadow test of the eye to determine the refractive error; fluoroscopic examination of the body.

**skin,** the external covering of the body consisting of two layers, the epidermis and the corium. In the skin of the palms of the hands and soles of the feet there are five layers of epidermis.

**skin graft,** a viable section of skin transplanted in skin grafting.

**skin grafting,** the grafting of skin from another part of the body, or from a donor, to repair a defect or to replace skin that has been destroyed, as by burns.

**skleriasis,** progressive patches of hardened skin; scleroderma.

**skin test,** injected substances beneath the skin or applied to the surface of the skin to determine allergic sensitivity; scratch test; Schick test.

**skull,** the cranium; bony framework of the head.

**sleep,** a periodic and normal loss of consciousness in which bodily functions are reduced since the body and mind are at rest.

**sleeping sickness,** an infectious disease, usually fatal, marked by fever, drowsiness, increased lethargy, muscular weakness, weight loss, and cerebral symptoms caused by a parasitic protozoan, Trypanosoma gambiense, introduced into the blood by the bite of a tsetse fly; encephalitis lethargica.

**sleep walking,** walking in one's sleep; somnambulism.

**sling,** a support, usually out of a triangular cotton cloth or material, for an injured upper extremity.

**slipped disk,** a displaced vertebral disk that causes pressure on the spinal nerve, creating extreme pain.

**slough,** to cast off or shed; necrotic (dead) matter separated from living tissue.

**sloughing,** formation of slough or dead matter; the separating of necrosed tissue from living tissue.

**slow,** mentally dull; having a retarded pulse; bradycardia.

**smallpox,** an acute viral disease marked by fever, macules and papules that leave small depressed scars on the skin; variola.

**smear,** a specimen prepared on a slide for microscopic study.

**smegma,** a cheesy secretion of sebaceous glands, consisting of desquamated epithelial cells found under the labia minora and the foreskin.

**smegmatic,** pertaining to the smegma.

**smegmolith,** a calcareous mass in the smegma.

**smell,** to perceive by stimulation of the olfactory nerves or olfactory sense; to render an offensive or pleasant odor.

**smelling salts,** ammonium carbonate used for resuscitation and stimulation.

**snapping hip,** a hip joint that slips with a snap due to displacement over the great trochanter of a tendinous band.

**snare,** a surgical device for excision of polyps, tumors, and other growths by encircling them at the base with a wire loop and closing the loop.

**sneeze,** to emit air forcibly through the mouth and nose by involuntary spasmodic contractions of muscles of expiration, due to irritation of nasal mucosa.

**Snellen's chart,** used to test visual acuity.

**snore,** noisy breathing during sleep through the mouth which causes a vibration of the uvula and soft palate.

**snoring rale,** a sonorous, low-pitched rale resembling a snore.

**snow blindness,** an irritation to the conjunctiva of the eye caused by reflection of the sun on the snow.

**snuffles,** catarrhal discharge from nasal mucous membranes while breathing, especially in infants with congenital syphilis.

**soap,** a chemical compound formed by an alkali acting on fatty acid, used for cleansing purposes.

**SOAP,** a process of recording progress notes in a problem-oriented assessment of data obtained subjectively from a patient.

**sob,** to weep with convulsive movements of the throat, involving a sudden inspiration accompanied by spasmodic closure of the glottis, resulting in a wail-like cry.

**socialization,** the process by which society integrates the individual and the way in which one learns to behave in a socially acceptable way.

**sociobiology,** the study that proposes that all human behavior has a biological basis and is controlled by the genes.

**sociogenic,** imposed by society.

**sociologist,** one who specializes in sociology.

**sociology,** the scientific study concerned with social relationships, social organization, and group behavior in contrast to individual behavior.

**sociometry,** the study of measurement of human social behavior.

**sociopath,** an individual with an antisocial personality; a psychopath.

**socket,** a hollow or cavity into which a correspondent part fits.

**soda,** usually applied to sodium bicarbonate, sodium hydroxide, or sodium carbonate.

**soda lime,** combined mixture of sodium hydroxide or caustic soda and calcium hydroxide or slaked lime, used in the production of ammonia and the absorption of moisture; combined mixture of calcium hydroxide with sodium or potassium, or both, used as an absorbent of carbon dioxide in equipment, such as in oxygen therapy.

**sodium bicarbonate,** used in the production of baking powder and as an antacid.

**sodium chloride,** common table salt.

**sodium citrate,** used as an anticoagulant in blood transfusions.

**sodium iodide,** used in preparation of a compound resembling potassium iodide.

**sodium salicylate,** a compound powder used as an analgesic and antipyretic.

**sodium sulfate,** used as a mild cathartic and diuretic; Glauber's salts.

**sodomy,** unnatural sexual intercourse; anal intercourse; bestiality; fellatio.

**soft palate,** soft part of the palate.

**solar,** pertaining to the sun.

**solar plexus,** a network of nerves behind the stomach and situated at the upper part of the abdomen in front of the aorta from which sympathetic fibers pass to the visceral organs.

**sole,** the undersurface or bottom part of the foot.

**soleprint,** a footprint used in hospitals to identify newborn infants.

**solution,** process of dissolving; a homogeneous mixture of one or more substances; a rupture or separation; termination of an illness.

**solvent,** any substance which has a dissolving effect upon another substance.

**soma,** the body as distinguished from the mind or psyche; body tissues distinguished from germinal tissues.

**somatic,** pertaining to the body, as somatic symptoms.

**somatic cells,** any of the body cells that compose various organs and tissue except reproductive cells or germ cells.

**somatogenic,** originating in the body.

**somatology,** the study of anatomy and physiology; the study of the structure, functions, and development of the human body.

**somatopathy,** bodily dysfunction as distinguished from mental dysfunction.

**somatoplasm,** the protoplasm of the body cells as distinguished from that of germ plasm.

**somatopleure,** the embryonic layer formed by ectoderm and somatic mesoderm.

**somatopsychic,** pertaining to both body and mind; relating to a physical disorder which manifests mental symptoms.

**somatopsychosis,** any mental dysfunction symptomatic of bodily disease.

**somatotherapy,** treatment focused at relieving or curing bodily ills.

**somatotrophic,** influencing body cells and stimulating growth.

**somatotype,** a particular body build based on a theory that certain types of body build are associated with personality types, such as endomorphy, mesomorphy, actomorphy.

**somesthetic,** sensibility to bodily sensations.

**somite,** any embryonic segment alongside the neural tube, forming the vertebral column and various organs.

**somitic,** pertaining to a somite.

**somnambulate,** walking while asleep.

**somnambulism,** the state of walking during sleep; a hypnotic state in which the individual has full possession of the senses but no subsequent memory.

**somnambulist,** one subject to somnambulism.

**somniferous,** producing or inducing sleep, as a narcotic or soporific.

**somniloquism,** habitual talking in one's sleep.

**somnolence,** unusual drowsiness; sleepiness.

**somnolentia,** inclined to sleep; drowsiness, or somnolence; a lack of natural sleep with disorientation and anxiety.

**sonorous,** a deep resonant sound.

**sonovox,** an electronic device used for transmitting sounds to be emitted through the mouth by a person whose larynx has been removed.

**sopor,** a very deep sleep; stupor.

**soporiferous,** producing sleep; soporific.

**soporose,** soporous, pertaining to profound sleep; coma.

**sordes,** undigested food in the stomach.

**sore,** any lesion of the skin or mucous membranes; tender or painful.

**sore throat,** inflammation of the pharynx; laryngitis; pharyngitis; tonsillitis.

**souffle,** a soft, blowing sound heard through a stethoscope in auscultation, as any cardiac or vascular murmur.

**sound,** the effect produced in the auditory organs by sound waves or certain vibrations; a noise, which is normal or abnormal, heard within the body; an instrument for exploring and detecting by sound any foreign body within a cavity.

**space,** an area, region, or cavity of the body; delimited area; the universe beyond earth.

**Spanish fly,** a blister beetle used in medicine as a counter-irritant or diuretic.

**sparganosis,** infestation with a variety of Sparganum.

**Sparganum,** the larva of tapeworms, especially of the genus Dibothriocephalus.

**spargosis,** distention of the female mammary glands with milk; swelling and thickening of the skin; elephantiasis.

**spasm,** a sudden, abnormal, involuntary muscular contraction; a transitory constriction of a passage or orifice; spasms may be clonic, described as alternating contraction and relaxation of involuntary muscles, or they may be tonic, described as sustained involuntary muscle contraction.

**spasmodic,** occurring in spasms; relating to the nature of a spasm.

**spastic,** characterized by spasms; a hypertonic state of muscles producing rigidity and awkward movements; an individual exhibiting spasticity, as occurs in cerebral palsy.

**spasticity,** hypertension of the muscles, or sustained increased muscular tension.

**spay,** to remove female sex glands, usually said of animals.

**specialist,** a medical practitioner who limits his practice to a particular branch of medicine or surgery.

**specialty,** the specific field of a specialist.

**specific,** pertaining to a species; restricted in application or effect to a particular function or structure; a drug indicated for a particular disease; pertaining to special affinity of an antigen for its corresponding antibody.

**specimen,** a small sample to determine the nature of the whole, as a small quantity of urine for diagnostic purposes or a segment of tissue for microscopic examination.

**spectacles,** a pair of lenses to aid defective vision or to protect the eyes from light rays or dust particles.

**spectroscope,** an instrument used for developing and analyzing spectra.

**spectrum,** a series of wavelengths of electromagnetic radiation obtained by refraction and diffraction of a ray of white light. The visible spectrum consists of the colors red, orange, yellow, green, blue, indigo and violet. The invisible spectrum includes rays such as X-ray, infrared, ultraviolet, cosmic, etc.; a measurable range of activity of bacteria which are affected by an antibiotic.

**speculum,** an instrument for examining canals or for opening a body orifice to permit visual inspection.

**speech,** the power to express thoughts and ideas by articulated vocal sounds and words.

**sperm,** semen; spermatozoon; reproductive seminal fluid in males.

**spermacrasia,** lack of spermatozoa in the semen.

**spermatemphraxis,** an obstruction that prevents the discharge of seminal fluid.

**spermatic,** pertaining to the semen; seminal.

**spermatic cord,** the cord suspending the testis within the scrotum, and which contains the blood vessels, lymphatics, nerves, and ductus deferens.

**spermatid,** a cell developed from a spermatocyte which becomes a mature reproductive cell or spermatozoon.

**spermatism,** the ejaculation of semen, voluntary or involuntary.

**spermatocele,** a cystic tumor of the epididymis which contains spermatozoa.

**spermatocyte,** a primary male germ cell that develops from the division of a spermatogonium and then itself divides into spermatids which give rise to spermatozoa.

**spermatogenesis,** the formation of mature spermatozoa.

**spermatogenic,** pertaining to the origin and development of spermatozoa.

**spermatogonium,** a primitive germ cell that gives rise to the spermatocyte.

**spermatoid,** resembling spermatozoa.

**spermatology,** the study of seminal fluid.

**spermatolysis,** the destruction of spermatozoa.

**spermatopathy,** any disease of sperm cells or their secreting glands or ducts.

**spermatorrhea,** involuntary discharge of semen without orgasm.

**spermatozoic,** pertaining to spermatozoa.

**spermatozoon,** the mature germ cell which is formed in the seminiferous tubules of the testes.

**spermaturia,** discharge of semen with urine.

**spermiogenesis,** the second stage in the formation of spermatozoa, in which the spermatids are transformed into functional spermatozoa.

**sphenoid,** wedge-shaped or cuneiform.

**sphenoid bone,** the large bone at the base of the skull which is wedge-shaped.

**spherocyte,** an erythrocyte which is spheroid in shape but more fragile, occurring in certain hemolytic anemias.

**spheroid,** having a body shaped like a sphere.

**spheroidal,** resembling a sphere.

**sphincter,** a ringlike, or circular muscle which closes a natural passage, as the anus.

**sphincteral,** pertaining to a sphincter.

**sphincteralgia,** pain in the anal sphincter muscles; pain in a sphincter muscle.

**sphincterectomy,** surgical excision of a sphincter.

**sphincteritis,** inflammation of a sphincter.

**sphincterotomy,** surgical incision of a sphincter.

**sphygmogram,** tracing of the pulse produced by a sphygmograph.

**sphygmograph,** an instrument which records differences of pulse in disease and health.

**sphygmoid,** resembling the pulse.

**sphygmomanometer,** an instrument for determining the blood pressure in an artery.

**sphygmomanometric,** pertaining to the blood pressure in an artery.

**sphygmometer,** an instrument that measures the pulse rate; sphymograph.

**sphygmophone,** an instrument which makes the pulse beat audible.

**sphygmoscope,** an instrument which makes the pulse beat visible.

**sphygmotonometer,** an instrument which measures the elasticity of arterial walls.

**sphygmous,** pertaining to the pulse.

**sphygmus,** a pulse.

**spica,** a reverse spiral bandage with turns crossing each other, resembling a spike of wheat.

**spicule,** a tiny, needle-shaped body.

**spiculum,** a sharp, small spike.

**spiloma,** a mole or skin discoloration; nevus.

**spina bifida,** the protrusion of the spinal membranes due to a defective closure of the bony encasement of the spinal cord which is a developmental anomaly.

**spinal,** pertaining to the backbone or spine.

**spinal column,** the vertebral column which encloses the spinal cord, consisting of thirty-two bones.

**spinal cord,** the ovoid column of nervous tissue extending through the spinal canal which serves as a center for spinal reflexes and a conducting pathway of impulses to and from the brain.

**spine,** the vertebral column.

**spinobulbar,** pertaining to the spinal cord and the medulla oblongata.

**spinocerebellar,** pertaining to the spinal cord and the cerebellum.

**spinose,** spinous, pertaining to the spine; spinelike.

**spinous process,** the prominence at the posterior part of each vertebra.

**spireme,** the continuous threadlike figure formed by the chromosome material during prophase of meiosis.

**spirillemia,** the condition caused by the presence of spirilla bacteria in the blood from the genus Spirillum.

**Spirillum,** a genus of gram-negative bacteria that causes fever in man resulting from a rat-bite.

**spirit,** any volatile liquor or a solution of volatile liquid in alcohol; alcohol.

**spirochete,** a slender threadlike bacteria which is spiral in shape that is from the genus Spirocheta causing diseases, as syphilis and yaws.

**spirochetosis,** infection caused by spirochetes.

**spirograph,** an instrument for recording respiratory movements.

**spiroid,** resembling a spiral.

**spirometer,** an instrument that determines the air capacity of the lungs; pneometer, pneumatometer.

**spirometry,** measurement of the air capacity of the lungs.

**spirophore,** a device used for artificial respiration; iron lung.

**spit,** saliva; to expectorate spittle; expectoration; sputum.

**spittle,** saliva; digestive fluid of the mouth.

**splanchna,** intestines or viscera.

**splanchnemphraxis,** obstruction of any internal organ, such as intestines.

**splanchnic,** pertaining to viscera or intestines.

**splanchnicectomy,** surgical excision of part of a splanchnic nerve.

**splanchnic nerves,** three nerves from the thoracic sympathetic ganglia that control the viscera.

**splanchnicotomy,** surgical procedure of incising a splanchnic nerve.

**splanchnology,** the branch of medicine concerned with the study of the viscera or intestines.

**splanchnopathy,** any diseased condition of the viscera.

**splayfoot,** flatfoot; talis valgus.

**spleen,** a spongy, glandlike organ situated in the upper part of the abdomen posterior and inferior to the stomach, important to blood formation, blood storage, blood filtration, and formation of antibodies.

**splenadenoma,** enlargement of the spleen due to hyperplasia of its pulp.

**splenalgia,** pain in the spleen.

**splenectasis,** enlargement of the spleen.

**splenectomy,** surgical removal of the spleen.

**splenectopia,** displacement of the spleen; floating spleen.

**splenic,** pertaining to the spleen.

**splenitis,** inflammation of the spleen.

**splenius,** a compress or bandage; a broad, flat, band-like muscle of the upper dorsal region and the back and side of the neck, which serves in rotating the head and neck.

**splenocele,** hernia of the spleen.

**splenoma,** a tumor of the spleen.

**splenomegaly,** an abnormal growth of the spleen; enlargement of the spleen.

**splint,** a rigid appliance made of bone, wood, metal, or plaster used to fixate a fractured or dislocated bone or to protect an injured part of the body.

**splinting,** application of a splint to fixate a fractured or dislocated bone; in dentistry, a fixed restoration of two or more teeth into a rigid unit; rigidity of muscles which occurs as a means of avoiding pain caused by movement.

**spondylalgia,** pain in the vertebrae.

**spondylitis,** inflammation of the vertebrae.

**spondylopathy,** any disorder of the vertebrae.

**spondylosyndesis,** a surgical formation of joining two vertebrae.

**spondylotomy,** surgical removal of part of the vertebral column.

**sponge,** a porous, absorbent mass of gauze or cotton surrounded by gauze used in surgery to mop up fluids; an elastic fibrous skeleton of certain marine animals.

**spontaneity,** the quality of being spontaneous; behavior or activity that is spontaneous.

**spontaneous,** occurring voluntarily, as arising from one's own impulses.

**spontaneous fracture,** fracture resulting from the state of the bone and causing little or no injury.

**sporadic,** intermittent; occurring singly and widely scattered.

**spore,** an oval, refractile body formed within bacteria, as in Bacillus and Clostridium, which is resistant to environmental changes and difficult to destroy.

**spot,** a small blemish or macula; scar; birthmark.

**spotted fever,** any various eruptive fevers: Typhus, Tick fever, Cerebrospinal meningitis, or Rocky Mountain spotted fever.

**sprain,** the wrenching of a joint without producing dislocation.

**sprue,** a chronic malabsorption syndrome applied to three closely related conditions: namely, tropical sprue, idiopathic steatorrhea (nontropical), and celiac. Tropical sprue and nontropical sprue affect adults. Celiac disease is limited to children, but all three conditions involve the mucosa of the small intestine resulting in impaired food absorption. Symptoms are diarrhea, bulky and foul stools which are usually greyish in color, weakness, loss of weight, and other conditions.

**spud,** a spadelike bladed surgical instrument used to dislodge foreign substances.

**spur,** a sharply pointed bony projection; calcar.

**sputum,** spittle; any mixed matter with saliva that is expectorated through the mouth.

**squama,** a thin, scaly platelike structure.

**squint,** strabismus; to partly close the eyes, as in excess light.

**stabile,** resistant to change; stable; fixed.

**stability,** the quality of being stable.

**stable,** fixed; resistant to change; steady.

**staccato speech,** jerky pronunciation of words and syllables; scanning speech.

**stage,** a time period in the course of disease.

**stagnation,** the cessation of motion; stasis.

**stain,** a dye or reagent used in staining specimen for microscopic examination.

**stamina,** endurance; having strength to endure conditions resulting from disease, fatigue, or privation.

**stammer,** speech disorder marked by involuntary pauses while speaking; stuttering.

**standard,** an established measurement or model of authority to which other similar things should conform.

**stanch,** to stop the flow of blood from a wound.

**stapedectomy,** surgical removal of the stapes in the ear.

**stapedial,** pertaining to the stapes.

**stapes,** the stirrup, one of the three small bones in the middle ear.

**staphyle,** the fleshy mass hanging from the soft palate; uvula.

**staphylectomy,** surgical excision of the uvula; staphylotomy.

**staphylitis,** inflammation of the uvula, or staphyle.

**staphylococcus,** any organism of the genus Staphylococcus causing body infection.

**Staphylococcus aureus,** a species commonly present on the skin and mucous membranes of the nose and mouth that causes inflammation and suppurative conditions such as boils, carbuncles, and internal abscesses.

**staphylohemia,** the presence of staphylococci in the blood.

**staphylorrhaphy,** suture of a cleft palate.

**starch,** any of a group of polysaccharides found in plants that are able to be hydrolyzed by water in the body into maltose and then into glucose which provide heat and energy for humans.

**stasis,** stoppage of the flow of blood, urine, or the contents of the intestines due to illness, or disease.

**stasophobia,** abnormal fear of standing up.

**stat,** at once.

**state,** condition of a patient; situation.

**statistics,** numerical facts pertaining to a certain subject, such as vital statistics which present human natality, morbidity, and mortality in a given population.

**status,** a condition or state.

**statutory rape,** sexual intercourse with a female under legal age of consent.

**steapsin,** a fat-splitting enzyme of the pancreatic juice; lipase.

**stearate,** salt or ester of stearic acid.

**stearic acid,** a fatty acid found in solid animal fats and in a few vegetable fats used in producing lubricants, cosmetics, and medicine preparations.

**steariform,** resembling fat.

**stearodermia,** a disease of the sebaceous glands of the skin.

**stearrhea,** an excessive secretion of sebum or fat.

**steatitis,** inflammation of adipose tissue.

**steatoma,** a lipoma; a fatty mass found within a sebaceous gland.

**steatopathy,** disease of the sebaceous glands of the skin.

**steatopygia,** abnormal fat accumulation of the buttocks.

**steatorrhea,** excessive secretion of sebaceous glands; fatty stools caused by pancreatic diseases.

**stegnosis,** checking an excess secretion or discharge; closing a passageway; constipation.

**stellate,** star-shaped; radiating from a center.

**stenocephaly,** an abnormal narrowness of the head.

**stenosed,** narrowed or constricted.

**stenosis,** narrowing of a body opening or passage.

**stenotic,** pertaining to stenosis.

**stereoarthrolysis,** surgical formation of a new movable joint in cases of bony ankylosis.

**stereognosis,** having the ability to recognize the form and nature of objects by touch.

**sterile,** barren; not fertile; aseptic; free from living microorganisms.

**sterility,** state of being sterile.

**sterilization,** complete destruction of all microorganisms; any procedure rendering an individual incapable of reproduction.

**sterilizer,** an appliance for sterilizing especially medical instruments, such as an autoclave or steam-pressure cooker.

**sternal,** pertaining to the sternum.

**sternalgia,** pain in the sternum.

**sternocostal,** pertaining to the sternum and ribs.

**sternohyoid,** pertaining to the sternum and hyoid bone.

**sternoid,** resembling the sternum.

**sternum,** the narrow, flat bone in the median line of the thorax; breastbone.

**sternutatory,** an agent that causes sneezing; inducing sneezing.

**steroid,** a group of fat-soluble organic compounds which includes many hormones, cardiac aglycones, bile acids, and sterols.

**sterol,** any of a group of substances which are related to fats and belong to the lipids found in animals or plants.

**stertor,** laborious breathing or snoring due to obstruction of the air passages.

**stertorous,** pertaining to laborious breathing or sonorous respiration; a snoring sound.

**stethoscope,** an instrument used in auscultation of sounds produced in the body, which consists of rubber tubing in a Y shape.

**stethoscopic,** pertaining to a stethoscope.

**stethoscopy,** examination by menas of the stethoscope.

**sthenia,** normal strength.

**sthenic,** active, vigorous, and strong.

**stigma,** a mark or pupuric lesion on the skin; any mental or physical peculiarity that helps to identify or diagnose a specific disease or condition.

**stigmatic,** pertaining to a stigma; marked with a stigma.

**stigmatism,** marked by the presence of stigmata; a condition of the eyes in which the rays of light are accurately focused on the retina.

**stilbestrol,** diethylstilbestrol, a synthetic estrogen.

**stilet, stilette,** a very small, sharp-pointed instrument used for probing; a wire used to pass through a flexible catheter.

**stillbirth,** the birth of a dead fetus.

**stillborn,** dead at birth.

**stimulant,** any agent that produces a transient surge of energy and strength of activity.

**stimulate,** to increase functional activity.

**stimulation,** the act of stimulating or that of being stimulated.

**stimulus,** any agent that produces functional or tropic reaction in a receptor, organ, or irritable tissue.

**sting,** a sharp sensation due to a prick, wound, astringent, or tiny pointed organ of bees, wasps, and certain other insects.

**stirrup,** stapes in the middle ear.

**stitch,** a sudden, temporary pain; a suture.

**stoma,** a mouthlike opening which is kept open to allow drainage.

**stomach,** the large musculomembranous pouch which is the principal organ of digestion extending from the esophagus to the duodenum, and consisting of a fundus, or cardiac part, a body, and a pyloric part.

**stomachalgia,** pain in the stomach.

**stomachic,** a medicine which aids functional activity of the stomach.

**stomatitis,** inflammation of the mouth.

**stomatology,** the branch of medicine concerned with diseases and treatments of the mouth.

**stomatomycosis,** any disease of the mouth caused by fungi.

**stomatopathy,** any disorder of the mouth.

**stomatoplasty,** plastic repair of the mouth.

**stomodeum,** the ectodermal depression in the embryo which becomes the front part of the mouth.

**stone,** a calculus.

**stool,** fecal discharge from the bowels.

**strabismus,** a squint; a disorder of vision due to the turning of one or both eyes so that both cannot be directed at the same point at the same time; cross-eyed.

**strabometer,** a device for measuring the degree of strabismus.

**strabotomy,** section of an ocular tendon, a surgical procedure used in treatment of strabismus.

**strain,** to overexercise; overexertion or overstretching of musculature; to filter.

**strangulated,** congestion by restriction, or hernial stricture.

**strangulation,** a choking or arrest of respiration by an obstruction of the air passages.

**strangury,** a condition in urination marked by slow and painful discharge of urine.

**stratification,** an arrangement in layers.

**stratum,** a layer.

**Streptobacillus,** a genus of gram-negative bacteria which are grouped together to form a chain, the causative agent of Haverhill fever.

**streptococcus,** spherical bacteria from the genus Streptococcus, usually resembling long chains which are nonmotile, some of which are dangerous pathogens of man causing infection.

**streptokinase,** a proteolytic enzyme present in hemolytic streptococci which break down blood clots and fibrinous material.

**streptomycin,** an antibiotic derived from soil fungus.

**streptosepticemia,** septicemia resulting from infection by streptococci.

**stress,** a forcibly exerted influence or pressure; any adverse stimulus that tends to disturb the homeostasis of an organism, such as a physical, mental, or emotional stressor.

**stressor,** an agent or condition capable of producing stress.

**stria,** a streak line, or ridge; a narrow band or stripe; in anatomy, the longitudinal collections of nerve fibers found in the brain.

**stria atrohica,** fine pinkish or purplish, scarlike lesions that later become white found on the skin of the abdomen, breasts, thighs, and buttocks, caused by weakening of elastic tissues associated with obesity, tumor, or pregnancy (striae gravidarum).

**stricture,** an abnormal contraction or narrowing of a passage, or duct; stenosis.

**stridor,** a harsh or high-pitched respiratory sound, caused by an obstruction of the air passages.

**stroke,** a sudden attack or affliction, such as apoplexy or paralysis.

**stroma,** supporting tissue or matrix around an organ.

**Strongylus,** a genus of nematode parasites which inhabit man and many animals producing serious pathological conditions.

**strophanthin,** a white, crystalline glucoside obtained from the dogbane plant family, used as a stimulant in certain heart diseases.

**struma,** an enlargement of the thyroid gland; goiter.

**strychnine,** a poisonous alkaloid derived from plants.

**strychninism,** chronic strychnine poisoning induced by overdosing.

**stump,** the distal part of a limb after amputation.

**stupe,** a hot, wet cloth for external application which may be medicated.

**stupefactive,** an agent that produces stupor.

**stupor,** partial or complete unconsciousness, or deadened sensibility, mental apathy, or reduced responsiveness.

**stuporous,** affected with stupor, or reduced responsiveness.

**stuttering,** a speech disorder marked by spasmodic repetition of sounds, especially consonants.

**sty, stye,** an inflammatory enlargement of a sebaceous gland on the eyelid near the edge.

**stylet,** a wire placed into a catheter or cannula to render it stiff, used as a probe to remove debris.

**styloid,** resembling a pillar; pertaining to the styloid process of the temporal bone.

**stype,** a tampon of cotton.

**styptic,** contracting a blood vessel; an astringent that checks a hemorrhage; hemostat; astringent.

**subacute,** somewhat acute; between acute and chronic, but having some acute features.

**subarachnoid,** between the arachnoid and the pia mater.

**subcartilaginous,** below the cartilage.

**subclavian,** below the clavicle.

**subclavian artery,** the main artery of the arm at the base of the neck beneath the clavicle.

**subclavian vein,** the main vein beneath the clavicle leading to the arm.

**subclinical,** pertaining to disorders without clinical manifestations.

**subconscious,** not clearly conscious; existing beyond consciousness.

**subcortex,** the substance of the brain underlying the cortex.

**subculture,** pertaining to a culture of bacteria derived from another culture; a culture derived from another culture.

**subcutaneous,** beneath the skin; an injection introduced beneath the skin.

**subduct,** to draw downward.

**subfebrile,** somewhat feverish, less than 101°F.

**subglossal,** below the tongue.

**subiliac,** below the ilium.

**subject,** an individual or animal subjected to treatment, observation, or experiment; a corpse for dissection.

**subjective,** perceived only by the subject or person, and not by the examiner.

**sublatio retinae,** detachment of the retina.

**sublimation,** a defense mechanism operating outside of conscious awareness in which unacceptable instinctual drives are exhibited in a personal and social acceptable way.

**subliminal,** below the threshold of sensation; subconscious.

**sublingual,** situated beneath the tongue.

**submaxilla,** mandible.

**submaxillary,** below the maxilla or lower jaw.

**submaxillary gland,** a salivary gland.

**submicroscopic,** a size too small to be seen with a microscope.

**subnormal,** less than normal intelligence.

**subocular,** situated beneath the eye.

**suborbital,** beneath the orbit of the eye.

**subpharyngeal,** beneath the pharynx.

**subphrenic,** below the diaphragm.

**subscapular,** below the scapula.

**subscription,** the directions for compounding ingredients in a prescription.

**subsidence,** gradual abatement of symptoms of a disease.

**substantia alba,** the white substance of the brain.

**substantia cinerea,** the gray matter of the brain and spinal cord.

**succorrhea,** an excessive flow of any body secretion or of a digestive fluid.

**succus,** fluid produced by a living tissue.

**succussion,** shaking of a patient to determine the presence of either fluid or gas in a body cavity.

**suckle,** to nurse from a breast.

**sucrase,** an enzyme in the intestinal juice.$ sucrose, a crystalline compound obtained from sugar cane, sugar beet and other sources which is hydrolyzed in the intestine to glucose and fructose.

**sudation,** sweating.

**sudatorium,** a hot-air bath to induce sweating.

**sudor,** perspiration, or sweating.

**sudoriferous,** conveying or producing sweat; secretion of perspiration.

**sudorific,** a drug that causes sweating.

**suffocate,** to asphyxiate; to smother; to choke by stopping respiration.

**suffocation,** the stoppage of respiration; asphyxiation.

**sugar,** a sweet carbohydrate belonging to one of two groups, either diasaccharides or monosaccharides; sucrose.

**suggestibility,** being susceptible to suggestion.

**suggestion,** an idea that is introduced to an individual from without.

**suicidal,** pertaining to or suggesting suicide.

**suicide,** taking one's own life; one who intentionally takes his own life.

**sulcate,** sulcated, furrowed or grooved.

**sulcus,** a slight depression or fissure, as of the brain.

**sulfa drugs,** any of the sulfonamide group which possesses bacteriostatic properties; sulfonamides.

**sulfanilamide,** a crystalline compound derived from sulfanilic acid, used for its potent antibacterial action.

**sulfur,** a colorless chemical element existing in several forms, used most commonly in pharmaceutical preparations and, in a dry form, as an insecticide and rodenticide.

**sunburn,** dermatitis caused by prolonged exposure to the sun's rays; to be affected with sunburn; actinodermatitis.

**sunstroke,** a condition due to excessive exposure to rays of the sun or extreme heat.

**superciliary,** pertaining to the eyebrow.

**supercilium,** the eyebrow.

**superego,** that part of the personality associated with morals, standards, ethics, and self-criticism; part of the psyche which is derived from the id and the ego that acts as a mediator of the ego; the conscience.

**superfecundation,** fertilization of two or more ova during the same menstrual cycle by two separate acts of coitus.

**superfetation,** the occurrence of a second conception after one already existing, resulting in two fetuses in the womb at the same time, but of different ages.

**superficial,** situated on or near the surface of the skin.

**superficies,** an outer surface.

**superinduce,** to bring on in addition to something that already exists.

**supernormal,** beyond what is normal; beyond average human intellect.

**supernumerary,** in excess of a normal number.

**supersaturate,** to saturate more of an ingredient than can be contained in a solution.

**supinate,** to turn the hand so that the palm faces upward; to rotate the foot and leg outward; to assume a position of supination.

**supination,** turning of the palm or foot upward; lying flat upon the back.

**supinator,** a muscle that produces the motion of turning the palm and hand upward.

**supplemental,** adding something to supply a need.

**suppository,** a semi-solid mass in the form of a cone for introduction into the rectum, vagina, or urethra where it dissolves; a vehicle for medicine to be absorbed.

**suppress,** to conceal; to restrain from course of action.

**suppression,** the act of suppressing; conscious effort to conceal unacceptable impulses, thoughts or feelings.

**suppurant,** the production of pus; any agent that causes the formation of pus.

**suppuration,** the formation of pus.

**suppurative,** producing the generation of pus; a drug that produces pus formation.

**supraliminal,** above the threshold of consciousness; conscious.

**supramaxilla,** the upper jawbone.

**supraorbital,** located above the orbit of the eye.

**suprarenal,** above the kidney; pertaining to an adrenal gland.

**suprascapular,** situated above the scapula or shoulder blade.

**sura,** the calf of the leg.

**sural,** pertaining to the calf of the leg.

**surdity,** deafness.

**surdomute,** a deaf-mute; one who is deaf and dumb.

**surface,** the exterior of the body.

**surgeon,** a specialist in surgery.

**surgery,** the branch of medicine concerned with operative procedures for correction of deformities, repair of injuries, diagnosis and cure of diseases, and the relief of suffering and prolongation of life in humans; a room where surgery is performed.

**surrogate,** a substitute; a thing or person who takes the place of something or someone.

**susceptibility,** the quality of being susceptible; capacity for feeling emotions; sensitiveness.

**suspend,** to cease temporarily.

**suspension,** a condition of cessation, as of animation or pain or of any vital process; a treatment of spinal disorders by suspending a patient by supporting the chin and shoulders.

**suspensory ligament,** any of a number of ligaments that support anatomical parts, such as the ring-shaped fibrous tissue which holds the lens of the eye.

**suspiration,** a sigh; the act of sighing.

**sustentacular,** supporting or sustaining.

**sustentation,** sustenance, or support of life.

**susurrus,** a soft murmuring sound; whisper; murmur.

**suture,** a stitch or stitches that unite the edges of a wound; the material used in stitching a wound; the line of union between the skull bones.

**swab,** a small bit of cotton or gauze applied to one end of a slender stick which is used for wiping or cleansing or as an applicator for medication.

**sweat,** perspiration; the substance secreted by the sweat glands.

**sweat glands,** tubular glands found on all surfaces of the body except the lips, glans penis, and inner surface of prepuce.

**sweating,** the process of excreting sweat.

**swelling,** a temporary enlargement of a body part; an abnormal protuberance; a tumor.

**swoon,** to faint.

**sycoma,** a large, soft wart.

**sycosis,** an inflammation of hair follicles of the beard and scalp.

**syllepsis,** impregnation; pregnancy or conception.

**sylvian aqueduct,** a narrow passage from the 3rd to 4th ventricle; aqueduct of Sylvius.

**symbion, symbiont,** an organism which lives with another in a state of symbiosis.

**symbiosis,** the living together of two different organisms in a close association with both benefiting from the relationship.

**symbolia,** having the ability to recognize the nature of objects through the sense of touch.

**symbolism,** a condition in which everything that occurs is interpreted as a symbol of the patient's own thoughts.

**symmelus,** a fetus with fused legs and one to three feet, or no feet.

**symmetrical,** pertaining to symmetry.

**symmetry,** correspondence in arrangement, form, and size of parts found on the opposite side of an axis.

**sympathectomy,** resection or interruption of some part of the sympathetic nervous system.

**sympathetic nervous system,** autonomic nervous system which stimulates the heartbeat, dilates the pupils, and contracts the blood vessels, and, in general, functions in opposition of the parasympathetic nervous system.

**sympathin,** a neurohormonal mediator of nerve impulses at the synapses of sympathetic nerves.

**symphysion,** most anterior point of the alveolar process of the lower jaw.

**symphysis,** line of fusion of two bones which are separate in early development, such as the mandible.

**symptom,** a condition that results or accompanies an illness or a disease from which a diagnosis may be made.

**symptomatic,** relating to a symptom or symptoms.

**symptomatology,** the branch of medicine concerned with symptoms; all of the symptoms of a given disease.

**synapse,** the junction where neural impulses are transmitted, either between two neurons or a neuron and an effector by the release of a chemical neurotransmitter, as acetylcholine or norepinephrine.

**synapsis,** a stage in meiosis in which homologous chromosomes from the male and female pronuclei pair off.

**synaptic,** pertaining to a synapse or synapsis.

**synarthrosis,** a fibrous joint in which two bones that unite cannot move freely; fixed articulation.

**synchilia,** congenital joining of the lips.

**synclonus,** a successive clonic contraction of various muscle groups; muscular tremors.

**syncope,** loss of consciousness; faint; generalized cerebral ischemia causing temporary unconsciousness.

**syncytium,** a multinucleated mass of protoplasm which is not divided into definite cell structures.

**syndactyl,** a fusion between adjacent digits of the hand or foot, so that they are more or less webbed together.

**syndesis,** synapsis; arthrodesis.

**syndesmosis,** connection of bones by ligaments formed by fibrous connective tissue other than a joint articulation.

**syndesmotomy,** surgical incision of a ligament.

**syndesmus,** a ligament.

**syndrome,** symptoms that occur together; complexus of symptoms.

**syneresis,** the contraction of a gel causing it to separate from the liquid, as a shrinkage of fibrin from a colloidal gel.

**synergetic,** cooperative action of muscles working together.

**synergism,** any cooperative action of two agents that produce more effective results which neither alone could produce, such as two drugs.

**synergy,** combined action of two or more organs or muscles; coordinated action.

**synesthesia,** a sensation in one area of the body from a stimulus applied to another area; a subjective sensation of another sense than the specific one being stimulated, as a sound which produces a visual sensation of color.

**syngamy,** sexual reproduction; the union of female and male gametes to form a zygote in fertilization.

**synostosis,** union between adjacent bones by the formation of osseous material.

**synovia,** the transparent lubricating fluid secreted by the synovial membranes present in joints, cavities, bursae, and tendon sheaths.

**synovitis,** inflammation of the synovial membrane.

**synthesis,** the process which involves the formation of a complex substance from a simpler compound, as in the synthesis of protein from an amino acid.

**synthetic,** artificially prepared; relating to synthesis.

**syphilis,** a venereal disease caused by Treponema pallidium, transmitted by direct sexual contact or in utero, marked by lesions which involve any body organ. The disease usually has three degenerative stages that occur over the course of many years; leus venera.

**syphilogy,** the study of syphilis and its treatment.

**syringe,** a small, tubular device for injecting fluids or withdrawing them from a blood vessel or cavity.

**syringitis,** inflammation of the eustachian tube.

**syringomyelia,** a disease of the spinal cord in which fluid accumulates in the cavities, replacing the nerve tissue and causing muscle atrophy and spasticity.

**syringotome,** a surgical instrument used in operating, as an incision of a fistula.

**syssarcosis,** muscular articulation of bones, as of the hyoid and patella.

**systaltic,** contracting and dilating of the heart alternately; pulsating.

**system,** organized grouping of related structures that act together for a common purpose; a method of practice based on specific principles; the human body as an anatomical whole.

**systemic,** pertaining to a specific system of parts; affecting the entire bodily system or the body as a whole.

**systole,** the period of contraction of the heart, especially of the ventricles; opposed to diastole.

**systolic,** pertaining to systole.

**systremma,** cramp in the calf muscles of the leg.

**syzygium,** a partial fusion of two structures.

**syzygy,** the fusion of two organs with each remaining distinct.

## T

**tabella,** medicated material that is formed into a small disk; lozenge, tablet, or troche.

**tabes,** a gradual wasting or emaciation in any chronic disease.

**tabes dorsalis,** a late form of syphilis involving the degeneration of the spinal cord and sensory nerve trunks, causing muscular incoordination, intense pain, disturbances in sensation, and eventual paralysis.

**tabetic,** pertaining to or afflicted with tabes or tabes dorsalis.

**tablature,** separation or division of the cranial bones into inner and outer tables.

**tablet,** a small disk containing a solid dose of medicine.

**taboparesis,** general paralysis associated with tabes.

**tache,** a blemish, spot, or freckle on the skin.

**tachistoscope,** an apparatus used to test visual perception by exposing an object or group of objects to view for a selected brief period of time.

**tachography,** a recording of the movement and speed of the blood flow.

**tachyarrhythmia,** tachycardia associated with irregularity of normal heart rhythm.

**tachycardia,** an abnormal rapid heart rate, usually between 160-190 per minute.

**tachylalia,** speaking extremely rapidly.

**tachyphagia,** rapid eating.

**tachyphrasia,** extreme volubility of speech, often accompanying a mental disorder.

**tachyphrenia,** mental hyperactivity.

**tachypnea,** extremely rapid respiration.

**tactile,** pertaining to the sense of touch; touch.

**tactile corpuscles,** numerous elongated bodies that enclose the endings of afferent nerve fibers which serve as receptors for touch or for slight pressure beneath the epidermis of the finger tips, toes, soles, palms, lips, nipples, and tip of the tongue.

**tactometer,** a device that measures tactile sensibility.

**tactus,** touch.

**taenia,** a bandlike structure; a tapeworm.

**taeniacide,** an agent that is lethal to tapeworms.

**taeniasis,** infestation with tapeworms of the genus Taenia.

**Tagement,** trademark for cimetidine, used to decrease gastric acid secretion.

**talalgia,** pain in the heel or ankle.

**talc,** talcum powder, used as a dusting powder.

**talipea,** a congenital deformity of the foot; clubfoot.

**talipomanus,** clubhand.

**talocalcaneal,** pertaining to the talus and calcaneus.

**talofibular,** pertaining to the talus and fibula.

**talpa,** mole.

**talus,** the anklebone; the ankle.

**Talwin,** trademark for pentazocine used as an analgesic, anti-inflammatory, and antipyretic agent.

**tampon,** a pack, pad, or plug of cotton used in surgery to control hemorrhage or to absorb secretions, as produced in the nose or vagina; to plug with a tampon.

**tannin,** an acid substance found in the bark of certain plants and trees and in coffee and tea, used as an astringent, for burns, as an antidote for various poisons, and as a hemostatic; tannic acid.

**tantalum,** a noncorrosive chemical element used in replacement of cranial defects, for prosthetic appliances, and for fine sutures.

**tantrum,** a violent outburst of temper, anger, or rage.

**tap,** to drain of body accumulations of fluid by paracentesis.

**tapeinocephaly,** a flattening of the top of the skull or head.

**tapetum,** a layer of cells which cover a structure; a stratum in the human brain which is composed of fibers; a membranous layer, as in the retina.

**tapeworm,** a parasitic intestinal worm belonging to the class Cestoda, having a flat or bandlike form, characterized by having larval and adult stages in separate hosts.

**taphophobia,** a morbid fear of being buried alive.

**tarantism,** a nervous affection marked by manic or hysterical fits of dancing, melancholy, or stupor, believed to be attributed to the bite of a tarantula.

**tarantula,** a large, venomous spider feared by many, but relatively harmless.

**tardive,** late or tardy.

**tardive dyskinesia,** a serious side effect of antipsychotic drugs marked by grimacing, choreiform movements of the arms, fingers, ankles, and toes, and tonic contractions of the muscles of the neck and back, usually irreversible.

**target,** an area or an object toward which something is directed.

**tarsal,** pertaining to the tarsus of the foot.

**tarsalgia,** pain in the tarsus.

**tarsalia,** referring to the tarsal bones.

**tarsectomy,** surgical excision of the tarsus or tarsal bone.

**tarsectopia,** dislocation of the tarsus.

**tarsitis,** inflammation of the tarsus; inflammation of the upper eyelid.

**tarsometatarsal,** pertaining to the tarsus and metatarsus.

**tarsoplasty,** plastic surgery of an eyelid.

**tarsotibial,** pertaining to the tarsus and the tibia.

**tarsotomy,** surgical incision of the tarsal cartilage of an eyelid, or the tarsus of the foot.

**tarsus,** the proximal part of the foot; instep; the collection of bones between the tibia and metatarsus; the connective tissue plate along the edge of the eyelid.

**tartar,** the hard yallowish substance deposited on the teeth, mainly composed of calcium phosphate.

**tastant,** any salt capable of gustatory excitation that stimulates the sense of taste.

**taste,** the ability to distinguish flavor by the sense of taste; taste sensation occurs through stimulation of gustatory nerve endings in the tongue. Four distinguished qualities are: sweet, sour, salty, and bitter.

**taste bud,** a tiny end organ located on the surface of the tongue which mediates the sensation of taste.

**taxis,** the replacement of a displaced structure; reduction of a herniated tumor by manipulation, not by incision; the response of a mobile organism to a stimulus.

**taxonomy,** an orderly classification of organisms into categories according to correct or suitable names.

**Tay-Sachs disease,** an inherited disease that destroys the nervous system, caused by a lipid metabolism disorder which is always fatal. Tay-Sachs disease results from the absence of the enzyme hexosaminidase which is responsible for the breakdown of fat.

**tears,** a saline fluid secreted by the lacrimal glands that moistens the surface and cleanses the eyes of foreign particles.

**tease,** to pull apart or separate gently with very fine needles before microscopic examination.

**teat,** the nipple of a mammary gland.

**technic,** technique; expertness in performing the details of a procedure or operation.

**technician,** one skilled in specific technical procedures.

**technologist,** a technician who is highly trained and certified.

**tectocephaly,** having a roof-shaped cranium.

**tectum,** a roof-shaped structure.

**teeth,** hard, bony projections in the jaw. There are 32 permanent teeth, 16 in each jaw.

**teething,** the process of eruption of the teeth.

**tegmen,** a covering or integument.

**tegmental,** pertaining to the tegmentum.

**tegmentum,** a covering or roof; referring to the cerebral peduncle dorsal, a portion of the midbrain.

**tegument,** a natural covering of skin.

**tegumental,** pertaining to the skin.

**teichopsia,** attacks of temporary blindness, marked by zigzag lines appearing in the visual field, sometimes accompanying headache and mental or physical strain.

**tela,** a weblike structure.

**telalgia,** pain felt at a distance from its stimulus; pain referred.

**telangiectasis,** dilatation of the capillaries and other small blood vessels which cause an angioma of macular appearance, such as a birthmark in young children, or as caused by alcoholism, exposure to cold weather, diseases, and infections. May occur on the face, thighs, or nose.

**telangitis,** inflammation of the capillaries.

**telencephalic,** pertaining to the telencephalon.

**telencephalon,** endbrain; the anterior division of the forebrain.

**teleneuron,** a nerve ending.

**teleopsia,** a disturbance in vision in which objects appear to be farther away than they actually are.

**telepathy,** the communication of thought by means of extrasensory perception.

**telesthesia,** telepathy; the ability to respond to a stimulus beyond the usual range of perception.

**telesystolic,** pertaining to the termination of cardiac systole.

**telolemma,** the membrane covering the motor end plate in a striated muscle fiber.

**telomere,** pertaining to the ends of the chromosomes which have specific properties, such as having polarity that prevents reunion with any fragments after the chromosome has been broken.

**telophase,** the last of four stages of mitosis, and of two divisions of meiosis.

**temperament,** the combination of qualities, physical and mental, that determine personality.

**temperature,** heat or cold expressed in terms of a specific scale. Normal body temperature is 98.6° F and 37° C.

**temple,** the flattened area on either side of the forehead.

**temporal,** pertaining to the temple; pertaining to time; temporary.

**temporal bone,** one of the two bones on either side of the head.

**temporalis,** a muscle in the depression of the temporal bone which elevates the mandible.

**temulence,** intoxication; drunkenness.

**tenaculum,** a hooklike instrument used to grasp and hold parts in surgery or dissection.

**tenalgia,** pain in a tendon.

**tenderness,** sensitiveness to pain when pressure is applied to the skin.

**tendinitis,** inflammation of a tendon.

**tendinous,** resembling tendons; composed of tendons.

**tendon,** a fibrous cord of connective tissue by which a muscle is attached to a bone or cartilage.

**tenesmus,** painful straining in defecating or urinating.

**tenia,** taenia, a flat band of soft tissue; a tapeworm of the genus Taenia.

**teniacide,** an agent that is lethal to tapeworms.

**teniafuge,** an agent that expels tapeworms.

**tennis elbow,** radiohumeral bursitis; epicondylitis; pain caused by overexertion of the arm.

**tenodesis,** surgical fixation of the end of a tendon to a bone.

**Tenon's capsule,** a thin connective tissue that envelops the eyeball behind the conjunctiva.

**tenontitis,** inflammation of Tenon's capsule; tendinitis.

**tenophyte,** a growth in a tendon.

**tenotomy,** surgical section of a tendon.

**tensile,** pertaining to tension; capable of being stretched.

**tension,** the act of stretching or being stretched or strained.

**tensor,** any muscle that stretches or tightens a body part.

**tent,** a fabric covering placed over a patient's head for administering oxygen or vaporized medication.

**tentative,** a diagnosis which is subject to change because of insufficient data; experimental.

**tenth nerve,** vagus nerve.

**tentum,** the penis.

**tenuity,** the condition of being thin.

**tenuous,** slender or thin.

**tephromyelitis,** inflammation of the gray matter of the spinal cord.

**teras,** a deformed fetus; a monster.

**teratology,** the science dealing with monstrosities and malfomations of fetuses.

**teratoma,** congenital tumor that contains embryonic elements of the three primary germ layers, as teeth or hair; dermoid.

**teratoid,** resembling a monster.

**terebration,** the act of boring; boring pain; trephining.

**teres,** round and smooth; long and cylindrical.

**term,** parturition; a definite period; the normal nine months of pregnancy.

**terminal,** pertaining to an end; a termination, or ending.

**terminology,** the vocabulary of a science; nomenclature.

**Terramycin,** trademark for the oxy derivative of tetracycline, used as an antibiotic effective against rickettsias and some viruses.

**tertiary syphilis,** the third stage of syphilis and the most advanced stage.

**test,** an examination or trial; a chemical reaction; reagent.

**testectomy,** surgical removal of a testicle.

**testicle,** one of two oval-shaped glands of reproduction in the male; testis.

**testicular,** pertaining to the testis.

**testitis,** inflammation of the testicle or testicles.

**testosterone,** the principal male hormone responsible for secondary male sex characteristics.

**tetanic,** pertaining to tetanus.

**tetanoid,** resembling tetanus.

**tetanus,** an infectious disease, often fatal, caused by the neurotoxin of Clostridium tetani, marked by painful spasms of the voluntary muscles, especially those of the lower jaw and neck; lockjaw.

**tetany,** a condition characterized by painful muscle spasms, which are irregular and intermittent, usually occurring in the extremities due to an inability to utilize calcium salts.

**tetracycline,** a drug obtained naturally from certain soil bacilli of the genus Streptomyces or produced synthetically, used as an antibiotic.

**tetrad,** an arrangement of four chromosomes during meiosis by splitting off paired chromosomes.

**tetralogy of Fallot,** a congenital malformation of the heart involving pulmonic stenosis. As the infant grows, the pulmonary blood flow cannot increase causing right ventricular hypertrophy and shunting of blood from the right to the left ventricle, producing cyanosis. Growth of the child is poor, symptoms of fatigue, polycythemia and clubbing of the hands appear at the time cyanosis, a blue discoloration to the skin from lack of oxygen, becomes evident; a series of four congenital heart defects.

**tetraparesis,** muscular weakness present in all four extremities.

**tetraplegia,** quadriplegia.

**tetraploidy,** having four sets of chromosomes.

**tetter,** any of many cutaneous diseases, as impetigo, herpes, ringworm, and eczema.

**textural,** pertaining to the structure of tissues.

**thalamencephalon,** the part of the brain containing the optic thalami and the pineal gland.

**thalamus,** the region of the brain concerned with many bodily functions which lies between the hypothalamus and epithalamus, the center for sensory impulses to the cerebral cortex.

**thalidomide,** a sedative and hypnotic that causes serious congenital anomalies in the fetus when taken during early pregnancy.

**thanatoid,** resembling death.

**thanatology,** the science concerned with death and dying.

**thanatophoric,** lethal or deadly.

**thanatos,** in psychoanalysis, death instinct.

**theca,** a caselike structure or sheath.

**thecal,** pertaining to a sheath.

**thecitis,** inflammation of the sheath of a tendon.

**thelalgia,** pain in the nipples.

**theleplasty,** plastic surgery on a nipple.

**thelitis,** inflammation of a nipple.

**thelium,** a nipple or papilla.

**thenar,** the fleshy part of the hand below the thumb; palm.

**theobromine,** an alkaloid found in cacao seeds which have properties similar to caffeine, used as a smooth muscle relaxant, a diuretic, and as a myocardial stimulant and vasodilator.

**theophobia,** a morbid fear of God.

**therapeutic,** pertaining to therapeutics; curative.

**therapeutics,** the science of healing; scientific treatment of diseases and the application of remedies.

**therapeutist,** one skilled in therapeutics; a therapist.

**therapy,** the treatment of disease or a pathological condition.

**therm,** a unit of heat.

**thermal,** pertaining to heat.

**thermoanesthesia,** inability to distinguish between heat and cold.

**thermocauterectomy,** excision by thermocautery.

**thermocautery,** cautery by a heated wire or point.

**thermogenesis,** the production of heat within the body.

**thermogram,** a graphic record of variations of temperature.

**thermograph,** an instrument used for recording variations of temperature.

**thermolabile,** changed easily by heat; unstable.

**thermolysis,** a heat loss from the body due to evaporation; a chemical dissociation caused by heat.

**thermomassage,** the use of heat in massage.

**thermometer,** an instrument to measure heat.

**thermophile,** an organism that thrives in elevated temperatures.

**thermophore,** an apparatus for retaining heat.

**thermoplegia,** sunstroke; heatstroke.

**thermostable,** not destroyed by heat.

**thermotaxis,** the regulation and normal adjustment of the body to temperature; the movement of an organism toward or away from the stimulation of temperature or heat source.

**thermotherapy,** the therapeutic use of heat in treatment of disease.

**thermotropism,** the property within organisms to respond to heat stimulus.

**thiamine,** a B-complex vitamin compound found in animal and plant foods, dry yeast, and wheat germ which are the richest natural resources, essential to man for normal metabolism of both fats and carbohydrates; vitamin $B_1$.

**thigh,** that part of the leg between the knee and the hip.

**thighbone,** femur.

**thigmesthesia,** sense of touch; tactile sensibility.

**thimerosal,** used as a germicide and an antiseptic.

**thinking,** the process of forming concepts and images in one's mind.

**thiopental,** a short-acting barbiturate used in its salt form intravenously or rectally to induce general anesthesia.

**thiouracil,** an antithyroid drug used in treatment of hyperthyroidism, thyroiditis, and thyrotoxicosis which reduces the production of thyroid gland hormones.

**third cranial nerve,** regulates eye movements.

**third-degree burn,** implies a destruction of the full thickness of the skin, often of underlying fat, muscles and even bone, giving a pale white or charred appearance to the skin.

**thirst,** a craving for fluids, especially water.

**thoracentesis,** a puncture through the chest wall for tapping or removal of fluids; pleurocentesis.

**thoracic,** pertaining to the chest.

**thoracic duct,** the main lymphatic vessel of the body, which originates at the cisterna chyli on the abdomen.

**thoracostomy,** an opening of the chest wall for drainage or for an enlarged heart.

**thoracotomy,** surgical cutting into the chest wall.

**thorax,** the area between the base of the neck and the diaphragm.

**Thorazine,** trademark for chlorpromazine, a major tranquilizer used to treat severely excited psychiatric patients.

**threadworm,** term commonly applied to the pinworm which inhabits the intestines.

**three-day fever,** a viral disease which resembles dengue, transmitted by the sandfly.

**threonine,** one of the essential amino acids.

**threshold,** that point at which an effect is produced by a stimulus.

**thrill,** a vibration felt on palpation; to produce a sensation of tingling, as in excitement.

**throat,** the passage that extends from the nose and mouth to the lungs; pharynx; fauces.

**throb,** pulsating movement, as a heart beat,; palpitation.

**throbbing,** a pulsation, beating, or rhythmic movement.

**throe,** a severe pain, especially the sharp pain in childbirth.

**thrombin,** the enzyme that produces coagulation of the blood, resulting from the activation of prothrombin; a preparation used as a topical hemostatic that controls capillary bleeding.

**thromboangitis,** inflammation of a blood vessel.

**thrombocyte,** a blood platelet which aids in coagulation.

**thromboembolism,** an embolism carried by the blood from the site of origin to block another vessel.

**thrombogenesis,** clot formation.

**thrombolysis,** dissolution or breaking up of a thrombus.

**thrombophlebitis,** inflammation of a vein caused by a thrombus formation.

**thromboplastic,** acceleration of the formation of clots in the blood.

**thromboplastin,** a lipoprotein that promotes the conversion of prothrombin to thrombin.

**thrombosis,** formation of a thrombus.

**thrombotic,** pertaining to thrombosis.

**thrombus,** a blood clot that obstructs a blood vessel or a cavity of the heart.

**thrush,** a disease of the oral mucous membranes that forms whitish patches which become ulcerated, usually in infants and young children, caused by Candida albicans.

**thumb,** the first digit of the hand on the radial side.

**thylacitis,** inflammation of the sebaceous glands of the skin.

**thymectomy,** surgical removal of the thymus gland.

**thymic,** pertaining to the thymus gland.

**thymion,** a wart.

**thymin,** a hormone-like substance secreted by the thymus gland that impairs neuromuscular transmission.

**thymine,** a pyrimidine base found in DNA.

**thymitis,** inflammation of the thymus gland.

**thymocyte,** a lymphocyte produced by the thymus gland.

**thymolysis,** dissolution of thymus tissue.

**thymolytic,** thymus tissue destruction.

**thymoma,** a tumor arising from lymphoid or epithelial tissues of the thymus gland.

**thymus,** a ductless gland situated in the upper thoracic cavity, necessary in early life for the development of immunological functions, and which undergoes involution in adults.

**thyroadenitis,** inflammation of the thyroid gland.

**thyrocele,** a goiter.

**thyrochondrotomy,** surgical incision of the thyroid cartilage.

**thyroid,** a gland, in the neck, that partially surrounds the thyroid cartilage and upper rings of the trachea; thyroid secretions consist of two hormones, thyroxine and triiodothyronine, which help to regulate the metabolic rate, the growth process, and tissue differentiation. Thyroid extract is composed of dried thyroid glands of ox and sheep.

**thyroid cartilage,** the principal cartilage of the larynx which forms a v-shaped structure known as the Adam's apple.

**thyroidectomy,** surgical removal of part or all of the thyroid gland.

**thyroiditis,** inflammation of the thyroid gland.

**thyroptosis,** a displaced thyroid gland, partially or completely into the thorax.

**thyrotome,** a surgical instrument for excising the thyroid cartilage.

**thyrotoxicosis,** a disorder caused by an overactive thyroid gland; Graves' disease.

**thyroxine,** an iodine-containing hormone that is secreted by the thyroid gland responsible for increasing the rate of cell metabolism.

**tibia,** shinbone.

**tibial,** pertaining to the tibia.

**tic,** an involuntary, repetitive, compulsive movement of certain muscles of the face and shoulders.

**tic douloureux,** facial neuralgia accompanied by convulsive twitching.

**tick,** a parasitic mite or acarid of the genus Ixodes which buries its head into the skin of the host to suck blood, often transmitting diseases.

**tick fever,** an infectious disease transmitted by the bite of a woodtick; Rocky Mountain spotted fever.

**tilmus,** picking at bedsores in delirious patients.

**tincture,** diluted alcoholic solution used in preparation of a drug or a chemical substance, such as ginger, benzoin, guaiac, and others.

**tinea,** any of many different superficial fungal infections of the skin; ringworm.

**tinnitus,** a ringing or buzzing sound in the ear.

**tissue,** a grouping of similarly specialized cells that perform certain specific functions.

**titillation,** sensation produced by tickling, as in the throat; state of being tickled.

**titubation,** a staggering walk with shaking of the head and trunk, usually due to cerebellar diseases.

**tocology,** obstetrics.

**toe,** a digit of the foot.

**Tofranil,** trademark for imipramine preparations used to alleviate depression associated with specific mental conditions.

**toilet,** the cleansing and dressing of a wound.

**tolbutamide,** an oral hypoglycemic drug used to control uncomplicated, mild, stable diabetes mellitus in those who have some functioning islet cells; trademark name, Orinase.

**tolerance,** having the ability to endure without injury or effect.

**tolerate,** to resist the action of drugs or toxins.

**tolmentum,** a network of blood vessels found within the cortex of the brain and the cerebral surface of the pia mater.

**tomography,** a method of producing images of cross-sections of the body.

**tonaphasia,** the loss of recall of a tune due to cerebral lesions.

**tone,** having normal tension and vigor in muscles; tonus; a quality of sound or vocal production.

**tone deafness,** inability to distinguish musical pitch.

**tongue,** the freely moving muscular organ situated in the floor of the mouth which functions in mastication of food, taste, and in speech production.

**tongue tie,** a congenital shortening of the frenum which restricts tongue movement.

**tonic,** restoration of normal muscle tone; characterized by tension or contraction; an agent or remedy.

**tonicity,** the normal elastic tension of living muscles, arteries, etc.; in body fluid physiology, the effective osmotic pressure equivalent; tone.

**tonography,** recording the changes in intraocular pressure due to sustained pressure on the eyeball.

**tonometer,** a physiological instrument that measures the tension of the eyeball.

**tonometric,** pertaining to a tonometer or tonometry.

**tonometry,** measurement of tension of the eyeball.

**tonsil,** a rounded mass of lymphoid tissue, one on either side of the pharynx, which acts as a filter to protect the body from infection or invasion of bacteria.

**tonsillar,** pertaining to a tonsil.

**tonsillectomy,** surgical excision of a tonsil.

**tonsillitis,** inflammation of the tonsils.

**tonus,** the normal state of tension in muscles; a continuous contraction of a muscle.

**tooth,** one of the hard processes situated in the jaw which serves for biting and mastication of food.

**toothache,** pain in a tooth or area around the tooth.

**tophus,** a deposit of sodium biurate formed in the fibrous tissue near a joint, especially in gout.

**topical,** pertaining to a definite area; applied to a particular part of the body.

**topography,** a description of a specific part of the body.

**tormen,** a twisting or griping pain in the intestines.

**torpor,** sluggishness; abnormal inactivity; apathy.

**torporific,** causing torpor.

**torque,** rotary force; in dentistry, the rotation of a tooth on its axis by use of an orthodontic instrument.

**torsion,** the act of twisting, or state of being twisted.

**torso,** the trunk of the body, which excludes the head and limbs.

**torticollis,** wryneck; torsion of the neck caused by the contracted state of cervical muscles.

**tortuous,** full of many twists and turns.

**torulus,** a papilla or small elevation in the skin.

**torus,** a rounded swelling; a bulging or protuberant part.

**touch,** tactile sense; palpation by touching with the fingers.

**tourniquet,** a band that is placed tightly around a limb for the temporary arrest of circulation or hemorrhaging in the distal region.

**toxalbumin,** poisonous albumin or protein.

**toxanemia,** toxemia.

**toxemia,** the spread of bacterial toxins by the bloodstream, marked by fever, diarrhea, vomiting, quickened or depressed pulse and respirations, prostration.

**toxemia of pregnancy,** a specific hypertensive disease of pregnancy or of early puerperium (six week period after childbirth).

**toxic,** pertaining to a toxin or poison; poisonous.

**toxicant,** any toxic agent, or poison.

**toxicity,** having a toxic or poisonous quality; state of being toxic.

**toxicoderma,** a skin disease caused by poison.

**toxicogenic,** producing toxic or poisonous products.

**toxicologist,** one who specializes in the field of poisons and treatments.

**toxicology,** the science concerned with poisons, their effects, and antidotes.

**toxicosis,** any abnormal diseased condition due to poisoning or toxic action.

**toxin,** any organic poison of animal or plant origin; any poisonous substances produced by pathogenic organisms that cause disease in other living organisms.

**toxin-antitoxin,** a nearly neutral mixture of diphtheria toxin with an antitoxin, used for immunization against diphtheria.

**toxinic,** pertaining to a toxin.

**toxipathy,** any disease due to a poison.

**toxiphobia,** morbid fear of being poisoned.

**toxoid,** toxic properties of a toxin destroyed by a chemical agent, but still capable of inducing the formation of antibodies.

**toxoplasmosis,** a disease of the nervous system caused by Toxoplasma gondii, a parasitic protozoan, of which there is a congenital form and an acquired form.

**trabecula,** a supportive strand of connective tissue, which resembles a small beam extending from a structural part, as from a capsule into the enclosed organ.

**trabecular,** pertaining to a trabecula.

**trachea,** the windpipe; the membranous tube extending from the larynx to the bronchi.

**tracheal,** pertaining to the trachea.

**tracheitis,** inflammation of the trachea.

**tracheobronchial,** related to both the bronchi and the trachea.

**tracheobronchoscopy,** inspection of the trachea and bronchi with a bronchoscope.

**tracheoscopy,** inspection of the interior of the trachea with a laryngoscope.

**tracheostomy,** an incision of the trachea for the creation of an opening through the neck; used also for the insertion of a tube to relieve obstruction of the upper airway and to facilitate breathing or ventilation.

**tracheotome,** a surgical instrument for incising the trachea.

**tracheotomy,** surgical incision of the trachea.

**trachitis,** tracheitis, inflammation of the trachea.

**trachoma,** a contagious disease involving the conjunctiva and cornea of the eyes caused by Chlamydia trachomatis, marked by formation of granulations or tiny rounded growths.

**trachomatous,** pertaining to or affected with trachoma.

**tract,** a specific area of the body, especially of a system of related organs; a bundle of nerve fibers within the brain or spinal cord which compose a functional unit.

**traction,** the act of pulling or drawing.

**tractus,** a path or tract.

**tragus,** a cartilaginous projection in front of the external meatus of the ear.

**trait,** a distinguishing quality of an individual; a characteristic.

**trance,** an unconscious or hypnotic condition or state.

**tranquilize,** to render tranquil.

**tranquilizer,** drugs used in treatment of anxiety states, mental disorders, and neuroses.

**transcription,** synthesis of RNA using a DNA template.

**transect,** to cut across or divide.

**transection,** cross section.

**transference,** the unconscious transfer of attitudes and feelings to others that once were associated with parents, siblings, or significant others in forgotten childhood experiences; in psychiatry, the patient shifts any affect from one idea to another, or from one person to another by unconscious identification. Transference in the patient-physician relationship may be negative or positive.

**transformation,** the change of one tissue into another; degeneration.

**transfuse,** to transfer blood or blood components from one person into another directly into the blood stream.

**transfusion,** the process of transfusing.

**transillumination,** examination of a cavity or organ by the passage of a strong light through a body structure.

**translocation,** in genetics, the attachment of a fragment of one chromosome to another that is nonhomologous.

**transmigration,** the process of passing across or through, especially passage of white blood cells through the capillary membranes into the surrounding tissues; the passage of an ovum from the ovary to the uterus.

**transmission,** the transfer of disease from one individual to another; transfer of hereditary characteristics or traits.

**transmutation,** the process of evolution in which one species changes into another; change of properties of one substance into another.

**transpiration,** the discharge of moisture, air, or vapor through the skin or a membrane; perspiration.

**transpire,** to excrete perspiration through the pores in the skin.

**transplant,** a transfer of tissue in a graft to be transplanted from another person or from one body part to another site.

**transplantation,** the grafting of tissue or an organ from one person to another; grafting from one part of the body to another part.

**transudation,** a substance that has transuded; a fluid that has extruded from a tissue.

**transude,** to ooze through the pores of a membrane.

**transverse,** extending from side to side; lying crosswise.

**transverse colon,** that part of the colon that extends crosswise the abdominal cavity.

**transversectomy,** surgical removal of the transverse vertebral process.

**transverse process,** the right and left lateral projections from the posterior part of vertebra.

**transvestism,** the condition of finding sexual pleasure by wearing clothing appropriate to the opposite sex.

**transvestite,** one who has an uncontrollable compulsion to dress in clothing appropriate to the opposite sex.

**trapezium,** a bone in the wrist which is the first bone in the distal row of eight carpal bones.

**trapezius,** a large, flat triangular muscle that covers the posterior surface of the neck and shoulder serving to raise and lower the shoulder.

**trauma,** an injury or wound; an emotional shock causing injury to the subconscious which may have a lifelong effect.

**traumatic,** pertaining to trauma.

**traumatism,** an abnormal condition of the system produced by an injury or trauma.

**treatment,** the care and management of a patient; the application of medicinal remedies or surgery in combating disease or pathological conditions; therapy.

**tremble,** involuntary shaking or quivering.

**tremor,** involuntary quivering or shaking from fear, fever, or general weakness.

**tremulous,** marked by shaking, quivering, or trembling.

**trench fever,** recurrent fever caused by Rickettsia pediculi spread by body lice.

**trench foot,** a condition of the feet resembling frostbite, due to exposure to wet and cold for long periods, seen in trench warfare.

**trench mouth,** infection involving the tonsils and floor of the mouth caused by Vincent's bacillus, marked by inflammation, painful swelling, and ulceration; Vincent's angina.

**trepan,** to trephine.

**trephine,** a form of surgical trepan for removing a circular disk of skull bone; an instrument for removing a circular portion of cornea.

**trepidation,** trembling involuntary movements of the limbs due to fear or anxiety.

**treponema,** a spirochete of the genus Treponema, some of which are pathogenic and parasitic for man, as the organism that causes syphilis.

**triceps,** having three heads, as a triceps muscle that extends the lower arm.

**trichiasis,** an inversion of eyelashes that causes irritation by rubbing against the cornea of the eyeball.

**trichina,** a parasitic worm sometimes present in the muscular tissues of man as an encysted larva of the genus Trichinella.

**trichinosis,** a disease caused by Trichinella spiralis which is ingested into the system through eating pork insufficiently cooked. Symptoms include diarrhea, pain, nausea, fever, and later swelling of muscles, edema, stiffness, and many other conditions.

**trichinous,** infected with trichinae.

**trichoid,** resembling hair; hairlike.

**trichologia,** the pulling out of hair by some patients.

**trichomadesis,** abnormally premature loss of hair on the scalp.

**trichome,** a hairlike structure.

**trichomegaly,** a congenital condition marked by excessive hair growth of eyelashes and eyebrows associated with dwarfism, mental retardation, and degeneration of retina pigmentation.

**trichomoniasis,** an infection caused by Trichomonas vaginalis resulting in vaginitis and urethritis, marked by inflammation and persistent discharge with pruritus.

**trichoptilosis,** a splitting of the ends of hairs.

**trichorrhea,** an abnormally rapid falling of hair.

**trichromatic,** normal color vision in which one is able to see the three primary colors.

**trichromic,** able to distinguish only three colors of the spectrum of seven colors.

**tricrotic,** pertaining to three sphygmographic waves to one beat of the pulse.

**tricuspid,** having three cusps, as a tooth having three points or cusps; the tricuspid valve of the heart.

**tricuspid valve,** serving to prevent the back flow of blood from the right auricle into the right ventricle.

**trifacial,** pertaining to the 5th pair of cranial nerves; trigeminal.

**trigeminal neuralgia,** facial neuralgia; tic douloureux.

**trigone,** referring to the triangular space at the base of the bladder.

**triorchidism,** having three testes.

**triplegia,** paralysis involving three extremities.

**triplet,** one of three children produced at one birth.

**trismus,** a motor disturbance affecting the trigeminal nerve causing spasms of the masticatory muscles and difficulty in opening the mouth; an early symptom of tetanus.

**trisomy,** having an additional chromosome of one type in a diploid cell.

**trituration,** a reduction to a powdery substance by grinding or by friction, especially in a mixture of a medicinal preparation.

**trocar,** a surgical instrument with a sharp-tipped rod used to insert a cannula that serves to draw off body fluid from a cavity.

**trochanter,** a prominence on the upper part of the femur.

**troche,** a medicinal preparation that dissolves in the mouth.

**trochlea,** a pulley-shaped structure that provides a smooth surface over which tendons pass or with which other structures articulate.

**trochlear,** resembling a trochlea; pullylike.

**trochoides,** a pivot joint.

**trombiculiasis,** being infested with mites of the genus Trombicula.

**trophic,** pertaining to nutrition.

**trophoblast,** the outer edge of cells of the blastocyst that attaches the fertilized ovum to the uterine wall, and develops into the placenta and membranes serving to nourish and protect the developing embryo.

**tropic,** having to do with a turning or a change.

**true ribs,** the upper seven ribs on each side that articulate directly with the sternum attached by cartilages.

**trunk, truncus,** the main part of the body to which the head and limbs are attached.

**truss,** a device for retaining a reduced hernia which may be composed of elastic, canvas, or metallic material.

**truth serum,** a drug such as scopolamine, used to induce a state in which a patient or subject will talk unrestrainedly.

**trypanosoma,** a genus of parasitic flagellate protozoa present in the blood of man and other vertebrates, transmitted by insect vectors causing serious diseases, as sleeping sickness.

**trypanosomiasis,** any of the several diseases caused by a species of Trypanosoma; sleeping sickness.

**trypsin,** a proteolytic enzyme formed in the intestine from the action of enterokinase on trypsinogen which is secreted by the pancreas capable of converting proteins into proteoses, peptones, and polypeptides.

**trypsinogen,** a pancreatic juice converted into trypsin by enzyme action.

**tryptic,** relating to trypsin.

**tryptophan,** an amino acid in proteins necessary for tissue growth and repair; an essential amino acid necessary for human metabolism.

**tsetse,** a fly of Africa, genus Glossina, which transmits diseases, as sleeping sickness in man and domestic animals.

**tubal,** pertaining to a tube, especially the fallopian tube.

**tubal pregnancy,** a pregnancy occurring in one of the oviducts.

**tube,** any hollow, cylindrical organ or vessel.

**tubercle,** a minute rounded elevation on a bone; pertaining to a small rounded nodule of the skin; pertaining to tuberculosis.

**tuberculation,** the formation of many tubercles.

**tuberculin,** a sterile substance prepared from tubercle bacillus, used to determine the presence of a tuberculosis infection.

**tuberculin test,** a test to determine the presence of tuberculous infection based on a positive reaction to tuberculin.

**tuberculosis,** an infectious disease due to Mycobacterium, marked by the formation of tubercles and caseous necrosis in the tissues of an organ. The lung is the major site of the infection in man.

**tuberculous,** pertaining to or being affected with tuberculosis.

**tuberosity,** a protuberance or elevation of a bone.

**tubule, tubular,** a small tube.

**tubulus,** a tubule, or minute canal.

**tularemia,** a disease of rodents which is transmitted to man, by handling infected animals or by insects, causing intermittent fever and swelling of the lymph nodes.

**tumescence,** swelling; being swollen.

**tumis,** swollen; edematous.

**tumor,** an abnormal swelling, usually from inflammation; morbid enlargement; neoplasm; an uncontrolled new tissue growth in which the cells multiply or proliferate rapidly.

**tunic,** a coat or covering.

**tunica,** a tunic; a membrane covering or lining a body part or organ.

**turbidity,** a cloudiness or sedimentation in a solution.

**turbinal,** scroll-like structure; a turbinate bone.

**turbinate,** having a shape like a top; the spongy turbinate bone of the nasal concha.

**turbinectomy,** surgical excision of the turbinate bone.

**turgescence,** a swelling or distention of a part.

**turgescent,** growing turgid or swollen.

**turgid,** distended or swollen.

**turgor,** a condition of being turgid; normal fullness.

**twelfth cranial nerve,** one of a pair of cranial nerves extending to the base of the tongue; hypoglossal nerve.

**twilight sleep,** a state of partial anesthesia in which pain sensation is greatly reduced.

**twin,** one of two offspring born at the same birth.

**twinge,** afflicted with sudden, sharp pain or pains.

**twitch,** a spasmodic muscle contraction producing a jerking action; a brief contraction of muscles that is involuntary.

**tyloma,** a callosity.

**tympanectomy,** surgical excision of the tympanic membrane.

**tympanic,** pertaining to the tympanum; bell-like; resonant.

**tympanic membrane,** a membrane separating the tympanum or middle ear from the external ear; eardrum.

**tympanites,** distention or swelling of the abdomen resulting from a collection of air or gas in the peritoneal cavity.

**tympanitis,** pertaining to tympanites; bell-like quality.

**tympanum,** the middle ear cavity in the temporal bone.

**tympany,** a tympanic or bell-like percussion sound.

**type,** the general or prevailing character of a disease, a person, or a substance.

**typhlology,** the study of blindness, its causes and treatment.

**typhoid,** an infectious disease caused by the bacillus Salmonella typhosa, marked by intestinal inflammation and ulceration, usually acquired through ingestion of food or drink; typhoid fever; resembling typhus.

**typhomania,** delirium present with typhoid fever.

**typhus,** an acute infectious disease marked by high fever, severe nervous symptoms, macular eruptions of reddish spots, and severe headache, caused by Rickettsia prowazeki and transmitted to man by body lice; typhus fever.

**tyrosinase,** ferment that acts on tyrosine.

**tyrosine,** naturally occurring amino acid found in most proteins; a product of phenylalanine metabolism which is a precursor of thyroid hormones.

**tyrosinuria,** the presence of tyrosine in the urine.

**tyrosis,** the curdling of milk; the cheesy vomitus of infants; tyromatosis.

# U

**uaterium,** a medicinal preparation for the ear.

**uberous,** fertile; prolific.

**ulalgia,** pain in the gums.

**ulatropia,** recession or shrinking of the gums.

**ulcer,** an open lesion of the skin or mucous membrane produced by the casting off of necrotic tissue, sometimes accompanied by pus formation.

**ulcerate,** to become ulcerous.

**ulceration,** the process of ulcerating.

**ulcerous,** pertaining to an ulcer; marked by ulcer formations.

**ulcus,** an ulcer.

**ulectomy,** surgical removal of scar tissue; gingivectomy.

**ulitis,** gingivitis; inflammation of the gums.

**ulna,** the long bone in the forearm between the wrist and the elbow, on the side opposite to the thumb.

**ulnad,** toward the ulna.

**ulnar,** relating to the ulna, to the ulna nerve, or the ulna artery.

**ulocarcinoma,** carcinoma or cancer of the gums.

**ulorrhagia,** bleeding gums.

**ulosis,** the formation of scar tissue.

**ulotrichous,** pertaining to short, wool-like hair.

**ultramicroscope,** a dark field microscope having powerful side illumination.

**ultrasound,** pertaining to frequencies greater than 20,000 vibrations per second.

**ultrastructure,** that structure visible only under the ultramicroscope and electron microscope.

**ultraviolet,** beyond the visible spectrum at its violet end.

**ultraviolet rays,** extremely hot invisible rays converted into heat by the ozone layer which protects life on earth. The therapeutic effects include heat production, pigmentation of the skin, aid in production of vitamin D, bactericidal effects, and various metabolism effects.

**ultravirus,** any filterable virus that can be demonstrated by inoculation test.

**umbilectomy,** surgical removal of the navel.

**umbilical,** pertaining to the navel or umbilicus; located centrally, like a navel.

**umbilical cord,** the cord that connects the placenta with the fetus.

**umbilicate,** pertaining to or shaped like a navel or umbilicus.

**umbilicus,** navel.

**unciform,** hook-shaped.

**unciform bone,** a hook-shaped bone of the wrist.

**uncinariasis,** hookworm disease; ancylostomiasis.

**uncinate,** hooked; hook-shaped.

**uncinus,** shaped like a hook.

**unconscious,** lacking awareness of the environment; insensible; that part of personality which contains complex feelings and drives of which we are unaware, and which are not accessible to our consciousness.

**unconsciousness,** state of being unconscious.

**unction,** application of a salve or ointment; an ointment.

**unctuous,** having a greasy or oily quality.

**uncus,** any structure that has a hook-shape; the anterior end of the hippocampal gyrus of the brain that is hook-shaped.

**undersized,** having a stature less than normal or average.

**underweight,** having a weight deficiency; the weight is at least 10 percent less than the average weight for persons of the same age, sex, height, and body build.

**undifferentiated,** primitive.

**undine,** a small flask for irrigating the eye, usually made of glass.

**undulation,** a wavelike motion; fluctuating; pulsating.

**undulatory,** pertaining to undulation.

**ungual,** pertaining to the nails.

**unguent,** an ointment.

**unguiculate,** having nails or claws; clawlike.

**unguis,** a finger nail or toe nail.

**unhealthy,** lacking health and not vigorous of body.

**uniaxial,** having one axis.

**unicameral,** having one cavity.

**unicellular,** composed of a single cell, as a protozoan.

**unicornous,** having a single cornu.

**uniglandular,** affecting only one gland.

**unilateral,** affecting one side.

**unilocular,** having only one chamber.

**uninucleated,** mononuclear.

**union,** a juncture, as of broken bone.

**uniovular,** developed from one germ cell or ovum; monozygotic.

**unipara,** primipara; having one pregnancy.

**uniparous,** producing one ovum or one child at a time.

**unipolar,** having a single pole; pertaining to a nerve cell having a single process.

**unipotent,** pertaining to a cell having the ability to develop into only kind of structure.

**unisexual,** pertaining to only one sex.

**unit,** one portion of a whole; one of anything.

**unitary,** referring to a single object or person.

**unmyelinated,** the absence of a myelin sheath around some nerve fibers.

**unsaturated,** having the ability to absorb more of a solute; referring to compounds in which two or more atoms are connected by double or triple bonds.

**unsex,** to castrate; deprive of gonads.

**unstriated,** pertaining to smooth muscles which have no striations.

**urachus,** an epitheloid cord surrounded by fibrous tissue connecting the apex of the urinary bladder with the umbilicus.

**uracil,** a component of pyrimidine found in nucleic acid.

**uracrasia,** a disordered condition of urine; enuresis.

**uraniscus,** palate.

**uranoplasty,** surgical repair of a cleft palate.

**uranoschisis,** cleft palate.

**urarthritis,** gouty arthritis.

**urate,** a salt of uric acid.

**uratemia,** urates in the blood.

**uraturia,** urates in the urine.

**urea,** the diamide of carbonic acid which is found in urine, blood, and lymph, and is the chief nitrogenous end-product of protein metabolism in the body.

**ureapoiesis,** the formation of urine.

**ureameter,** a device that determines the amount of urea in urine; ureometer.

**urease,** an enzyme which catalyzes the decomposition of urea into ammonium carbonate.

**urelcosis,** the ulceration of the urinary tract.

**uremia,** a toxic condition produced by excessive by-products of protein metabolism in the blood, causing symptoms of nausea, vomiting, vertigo, convulsions, dimness of vision, and coma.

**uremic,** pertaining to uremia.

**uresis,** the excretion of urine from the bladder; urination; voiding.

**ureter,** one of two tubes 10 to 12 inches long which extend from the kidneys to the posterior surface of the bladder.

**ureteralgia,** pain in the ureter.

**ureterectasis,** dilatation or stretching of the ureter.

**ureterectomy,** surgical excision of the ureter.

**urethra,** a passage which carries the urine from the bladder to the outside of the body.

**urethralgia,** pain in the urethra.

**urethratresia,** an occlusion of the urethra which prevents the passage of urine.

**urethrectomy,** surgical excision of the urethra.

**urethremphraxis,** a urethral obstruction; urethrophraxis.

**urethritis,** inflammation of the urethra.

**urethrorrhagia,** hemorrhaging from the urethra.

**urethroscope,** an instrument used to examine the interior of the urethra.

**urethroscopy,** visual inspection of the urethra by means of a urethroscope.

**urgency,** a sudden, involuntary need to urinate.

**uric,** pertaining to urine.

**uric acid,** a crystalline acid found in urine occurring as an end-product of purine metabolism.

**urinal,** a vessel used to collect urine, especially for bedridden patients.

**urinalysis,** a chemical analysis of urine.

**urinary,** pertaining to secreting or containing urine.

**urinary bladder,** the distensible receptacle for urine before it is voided.

**urinary organs,** pertaining to the structures of the urinary system, such as the kidneys, ureters, bladder, and urethra; urinary tract.

**urinate,** to discharge urine; void; to cast out waste material.

**urination,** the process of urinating.

**urine,** the fluid secreted from the blood by the kidneys, which is collected in the bladder and discharged by the urethra.

**urinemia,** uremia, the contamination of the blood with urinary constituents.

**uriniferous,** transporting or carrying urine.

**uriniferous tubules,** renal tubules extending from the Bowman's capsule of the kidney and serving to transport urine.

**urinometer,** an instrument that determines the specific gravity of urine.

**urinous,** resembling urine.

**urobilin,** brown-colored pigment formed by the oxidation of urobilinogen, found in stools or in urine after exposure to air.

**urobilinogen,** a colorless compound found in the intestines by reduction of bilirubin.

**urochrome,** the yellowish coloring matter in urine, closely related to urobilin.

**urocyst,** urinary bladder.

**urocystitis,** inflammation of the urinary bladder; cystitis.

**urogenital,** pertaining to the urinary and genital organs.

**urography,** X-ray of the urinary tract or part of it after the introduction of radiopaque substance.

**urolith,** a urinary calculus.

**urologist,** one who specializes in disorders of the urinary organs.

**urology,** the branch of science concerned with the study, diagnosis, and treatment of diseases of the urinary tract; urinology.

**urometer,** urinometer.

**uroncus,** a swelling due to retention of urine.

**uropathy,** any disease or condition of the urinary tract.

**uropoiesis,** formation of urine.

**uropyoureter,** an infected ureter with an accumulation of urine and pus.

**urorrhagia,** excessive secretion of urine; polyuria.

**uroschesis,** retention of urine.

**urticant,** producing itching or urticaria.

**urticaria,** hives or wheals which are either redder or paler than the surrounding area and are often attended by itching.

**uteralgia,** pain in the uterus.

**uterine,** pertaining to the uterus.

**uteritis,** inflammation of the uterus.

**uteroplasty,** plastic repair of the uterus.

**uterotomy,** surgical incision of the uterus.

**uterus,** the hollow muscular organ in females that serves the developing embryo after fertilization of the ovum; the womb.

**utricle,** one of two small sacs in the labyrinth of the inner ear.

**utricular,** pertaining to the nature of the utricle; having a utricle or utricles.

**utriculitis,** inflammation of the utricle.

**uvea,** the middle layer of the eye, composed of the ciliary muscle, the choroid, and the iris.

**uveitis,** inflammation of the uvea.

**uvula,** the small tissue projection extending from the middle of the soft palate in the throat.

**uvulectomy,** surgical excision of the uvula; cionectomy.

**uvulitis,** inflammation of the uvula.

**uvulotomy,** excising the uvula or part of it.

## V

**vaccigenous,** to produce vaccine.

**vaccin,** pertaining to vaccine.

**vaccinate,** to inoculate with vaccine to provide immunity.

**vaccination,** the act of vaccinating with a vaccine by injection into the body.

**vaccine,** a suspension of killed microorganisms for prevention of infectious diseases.

**vaccinia,** a viral disease in cattle which is transmissible to man by inoculation of vaccinia virus used to induce antibody formation against smallpox.

**vacciniform,** having the nature of vaccinia or cowpox.

**vacciniola,** a secondary skin eruption sometimes following vaccinia.

**vaccinogenous,** producing vaccine.

**vacuolar,** possessing vacuoles.

**vacuolation,** the formation of vacuoles.

**vacuole,** a clear space within the cell protoplasm filled with air or fluid.

**vacuous,** empty.

**vacuum,** a space exhausted of its air or gaseous content.

**vagal,** pertaining to the vagus nerve.

**vagina,** a sheathlike structure; the canal within females between the vulva and the uterus.

**vaginal,** pertaining to the vagina, or any sheath.

**vaginalitis,** inflammation of the tunica of the testicles.

**vaginate,** to enclose in a sheath; enveloped by a sheath.

**vaginectomy,** surgical removal of the tunica of a testicle; excision of the vagina or part of it.

**vaginismus,** painful muscular spasms of the vagina.

**vaginitis,** inflammation of the vagina.

**vaginodynia,** pain in the vagina; colpopexy.

**vaginoplasty,** surgical repair of the vagina.

**vaginoscope,** an instrument used for inspecting the vagina.

**vaginoscopy,** visual examination of the vagina by a vaginoscope.

**vaginotomy,** incision of the vagina; colpotomy.

**vagus,** the 10th cranial nerve, a mixed nerve which has both motor and sensory functions.

**valence,** the degree of the combining power of an element or radical.

**valeric acid,** an acid extracted from the roots of the valerian plant, used in medicine.

**valetudinarian,** one seeking to recover health; invalid.

**valgus,** denoting a position, as being bent outward or twisted.

**valine,** an amino acid derived from the hydrolysis of proteins, essential for human metabolism.

**Valium,** trademark for diaezepam, used for management of anxiety disorders.

**vallate,** rim-shaped; a rim around a depression.

**vallecular,** a furrow or crevice, as on the back of the tongue.

**valval,** pertaining to a valve.

**valvate,** furnished with valves; resembling a valve.

**valve,** a membranous fold within a hollow organ that prevents a backward flow of fluid passing through it, as the entrance to the aorta from the left ventricle of the heart.

**valvotomy,** surgical incision into a valve.

**valvular,** pertaining to a valve.

**valvulitis,** inflammation of a valve.

**vapor,** a gaseous state of a substance; medicinal substance that is administered in the form of vapor which is inhaled.

**vaporization,** converting a liquid or solid into a vapor for inhalation as treatment for respiratory ailments.

**varicella,** chicken pox.

**varices,** dilated veins; plural of varix.

**variciform,** varicose.

**varicocele,** a varicose enlargement of the spermatic cord veins.

**varicocelectomy,** surgical removal of a portion of the scrotum to remove a varicocele.

**varicose,** distended or swollen veins; pertaining to varices.

**varicose veins,** veins that are enlarged and twisted, commonly found on the leg and thigh.

**varicosity,** a condition of being varicose; a varix; varicose vein.

**varicotomy,** a condition of being varicose; a varix; varicose vein.

**varicotomy,** surgical removal of a varix or varicose vein.

**varicula,** a varix of the conjunctiva of the eye.

**variola,** smallpox.

**variolate,** resembling a smallpox lesion; to vaccinate with smallpox virus.

**varioloid,** resembling smallpox; a mild form of smallpox.

**varix,** an abnormal, tortuous dilatation of a vein; varicose vein.

**varus,** denoting a deformity of the bone; bent inward; bowlegged.

**vas,** a duct or vessel.

**vascular,** pertaining to blood vessels.

**vascularity,** the condition of being vascular.

**vasculitis,** inflammation of a blood vessel; angiitis.

**vasculum,** a very small vessel.

**vas deferens,** the duct which transports sperm from the testis.

**vasectomy,** surgical removal of all or part of the vas deferens.

**Vaseline,** trademark for a translucent semisolid petroleum jelly used in medicinal preparations and for other purposes.

**vasifactive,** forming new vessels.

**vasiform,** resembling a tubular structure.

**vasitis,** inflammation of the vas deferens.

**vasoconstrictor,** causing a narrowing of blood vessels; an agent that causes constriction of blood vessels.

**vasodepression,** the lowering of blood pressure.

**vasodepressor,** an agent that produces vasodepression.

**vasodilatation,** dilatation of small arteries and arterioles.

**vasodilator,** causing relaxation or widening of blood vessels; an agent or nerve that dilates the blood vessels.

**vasoinhibitor,** a drug that depresses vasomotor nerves.

**vasoligation,** a surgical procedure involving the vas deferens which renders sterility.

**vasomotor nerves,** those nerves distributed over muscular coats of blood vessels which cause contraction or dilation of the inner diameter.

**vasoparesis,** partial paralysis or weakness of vasomotor nerves.

**vasopressor,** an agent which stimulates the contraction of the muscular tissue of blood vessels, such as adrenalin.

**vasosection,** surgical cutting of a vessel, especially the vas deferens.

**vasospasm,** spasm of any vessel.

**vasostimulant,** exciting vasomotor action.

**vasotomy,** surgical incision of the vas deferens.

**vasotrophic,** concerned with the nutrition of blood vessels.

**vastus,** great, referring to muscles.

**vector,** a carrier which transfers an infective microorganism from one host to another, usually an insect or tick.

**vegetarian,** one who eats no animal products, but lives on food of vegetable origin.

**vegetation,** an abnormal fungoid growth in the nasopharynx; a morbid outgrowth on any part, especially wartlike projections.

**vehicle,** an inactive substance used in a medicinal preparation for transporting the active ingredient; an excipient.

**vein,** a vessel carrying unaerated blood to the heart, excluding the pulmonary vein.

**veinlet,** small vein or venule.

**velamen,** a covering membrane, or skin covering.

**velar,** pertaining to velum, or veil.

**vellication,** spasms or twitching of muscular fibers.

**velum,** a veil-like structure.

**vena,** a vein.

**vena cava,** pertaining to either of two large veins that empties into the right atrium of the heart.

**venenous,** poisonous.

**venereal disease,** (VD); any disease contracted by sexual intercourse from an infected individual.

**venereologist,** one who specializes in venereology.

**venereology,** the branch of medicine concerned with the study and treatment of venereal diseases.

**venesection,** phlebotomy.

**venipuncture,** puncture of a vein for intravenous feeding, to administer medication, or for obtaining a blood specimen.

**venom,** poison or a toxic substance secreted by snakes, insects, or other animals.

**venomous,** poisonous.

**venous,** pertaining to the veins.

**vent,** an opening in any cavity.

**venter,** the abdomen or belly; a hollowed cavity.

**ventilation,** the process of supplying a room with a continuous flow of fresh air; oxygenation of the blood; the expression of feelings and thoughts in crisis intervention; abreaction.

**ventricle,** a small cavity, especially one of the two lower chambers of the heart; one of the connecting cavities of the brain.

**ventricose,** corpulent; big-bellied or a protruding abdomen; swelled out.

**ventriculus,** a ventricle; hollow organ, as the stomach.

**venula,** a small vein; venule.

**venule,** any of the small vessels from the capillary plexuses that join to form veins.

**vergence,** turning of one eye with reference to the other; convergence or divergence.

**vermicide,** an agent that is lethal to intestinal parasitic worms.

**vermicular,** resembling a worm in appearance or movement.

**vermiform,** having a wormlike shape.

**vermiform appendix,** a small tube opening into the cecum with its other end closed, varying from three to six inches long.

**vermifuge,** an agent that expels parasitic intestinal worms.

**vermin,** an external noxious parasitic animal or insect.

**verminous,** pertaining to, or infested with worms or vermin.

**vermis,** a worm.

**vernix caseosa,** a sebaceous covering consisting of exfoliations of outer skin layer, lanugo, and secretions from the sebaceous glands which envelops a fetus at birth, rendering a white, cheesy appearance to the skin of the newborn, believed to have beneficial protective properties.

**verruca,** a wart; a wartlike elevation.

**verrucose, verrucous,** having little warts on the surface.

**version,** the spontaneous or manual turning of the fetus in the uterus at childbirth.

**vertebra,** any of the 33 bones composing the vertebral or spinal column, of which there are: 7 cervical, 12 thoracic, 5 lumbar, 5 sacral, and 4 coccygeal vertebrae.

**vertebral,** pertaining to a vertebra or the vertebrae; spinal column.

**vertebrate,** having a backbone or spinal column; any member of the Vertebrata, animals having a vertebral column.

**vertebrectomy,** surgical excision of a vertebra.

**vertex,** the top of the head; the crown of the head.

**vertical,** pertaining to the top of the head; upright.

**vertigo,** a condition of dizziness.

**vesica,** the bladder.

**vesical,** pertaining to the urinary bladder.

**vesicant,** producing blisters; a substance that produces blisters.

**vesication,** the process of forming blisters.

**vesicle,** a sac containing fluid; a bladderlike cavity; a small blister; a small bladder.

**vesicocele,** a hernia of the bladder.

**vesicular,** pertaining to vesicles; composed of small saclike bodies or blisters.

**vesiculation,** the formation of vesicles.

**vesiculectomy,** surgical excision of the complete or part of a vesicle, usually the seminal vesicle.

**vesiculitis,** inflammation of a vesicle.

**vessel,** any tube, duct, or channel conveying fluid, such as blood.

**vestibular,** pertaining to a vestibule.

**vestibule,** any cavity or channel forming an entrance to another space.

**vestibulogenic,** arising from a vestibule of the ear.

**vestibulotomy,** surgical incision of the vestibule of the ear.

**vestige,** a small degenerate structure which functioned in the embryo or in a past generation.

**vestigial,** rudimentary.

**viable,** capable of sustaining an individual existence; having the ability to develop and grow after birth.

**vial,** a small bottle, usually containing medicine for administering as an injection.

**vibration,** rapidly moving to and fro; oscillation.

**vibrator,** a device used to produce a vibrating massage.

**vibratory,** causing or producing vibration.

**vibrissae,** long coarse hairs located in the vestibule of the nose in man.

**vicarious,** taking the place of another.

**villi,** minute vascular processes on the free surface of a membrane.

**villiferous,** having tufts of hair or villi.

**villiform,** resembling villi.

**villose,** covered with villi.

**villus,** a small hairlike vascular process on a free surface of a membrane.

**Vincent's angina,** a painful inflammatory disease of the tonsils, pharynx, and floor of the mouth; trench mouth.

**viosterol,** a preparation of vitamin D made from irradiated ergosterol in vegetable oil used as a substitute for cod-liver oil.

**viral,** relating to a virus, or caused by a virus.

**viremia,** viruses found in the blood.

**virile,** characteristic of a man; masculine or manly; having copulative power.

**virilism,** relating to male secondary characteristics in a female.

**virility,** the state of possessing normal sex characteristics in a male.

**virologist,** one who specializes in virology.

**virology,** the branch of science concerned with viruses and virus diseases.

**virucide,** an agent that destroys viruses.

**virulence,** the degree of pathogenicity possessed by microorganisms to produce disease.

**virulent,** infectious or highly poisonous; having a rapid and malignant course.

**viruliferous,** conveying or producing a virus.

**virus,** a minute infectious organism that causes disease in all life forms and which depends upon a living host for its metabolism and replication.

**viscera,** the interior organs within the cavities of the body, especially the abdomen and thorax.

**visceral,** pertaining to the viscera.

**visceralgia,** neuralgia of any of the viscera.

**viscerogenic,** originating in the viscera.

**viscid,** adhering and thick; having a glutinous or sticky quality.

**viscosimeter,** a device for measuring the viscosity of fluids.

**viscosity,** state of being sticky and resistant to flow.

**viscous,** thick, sticky, or gummy; having a glutinous quality.

**viscus,** any interior organ of the three large body cavities, especially the abdomen.

**vision,** sight; seeing; faculty of sensing light and color; an imaginary sight.

**visual,** pertaining to vision.

**visual acuity,** clarity of vision; sharpness.

**visual field,** the total area in which objects may be seen by the fixed eye.

**visual purple,** purple pigment in the rods of the retina; rhodopsin.

**vital,** pertaining to vital functions or processes; necessary to life.

**vital signs,** referring to temperature, pulse, respiration (TPR).

**vital statistics,** pertaining to a record of births, marriages, disease, and deaths in a population.

**vitamin,** an organic substance which occurs in natural foods and is necessary in trace amounts for normal metabolic functioning of the body.

**vitamin A,** fat-soluble vitamin occurring in two forms: retinol and dehydroretinol, found in egg yolk, fish-liver oils, liver, butter, cheese and many vegetables, necessary for night vision and for protecting epithelial tissue.

**vitamin $B_c$,** folic acid.

**vitamin B complex,** an important group of water-soluble vitamins isolated from liver, yeast, and other sources which include thiamine, riboflavin, niacin, niacinamide, the vitamin $B_6$ group, biotin, pantothenic acid, folic acid and others. The vitamin B complex group affects growth, appetite, lactation, and the gastrointestinal, nervous, and endocrine systems.

**vitamin $B_1$,** thiamine.

**vitamin $B_2$,** riboflavin.

**vitamin $B_6$,** pyridoxine.

**vitamin $B_{12}$,** cyanocobalmin, extracted from liver which is essential for red blood cell formation.

**vitamin C,** ascorbic acid which aids in growth, weight gain, appetite, blood-building, and prevents disease, such as scurvy.

**vitamin D,** fat-soluble vitamins found in fish-liver oils, milk products, eggs, and ultraviolet irradiation of ergosterol, necessary for absorption of calcium and phosphorus, valuable in normal bone formation of the skeleton and teeth.

**vitamin E,** a fat-soluble vitamin necessary in the body for reproduction, muscular development, and resistance of red blood cells to hemolysis, found in wheat germ, cereals, egg yolk, and beef liver.

**vitamin G,** riboflavin.

**vitamin H,** biotin.

**vitamin K,** found in green vegetables, important for normal clotting of the blood.

**vitellin,** a protein found in egg yolk.

**vitiligo,** destruction of melanocytes which form white patches on various sites of the body.

**vitreous,** pertaining to the vitreous humor of the eye; vitreous body; vitreous chamber.

**vitreous body,** a transparent jelly-like mass that fills the vitreous chamber; vitreous humor.

**vitreous chamber,** the cavity of the eyeball behind the lens.

**vitreous humor,** the transparent gelatinous substance that fills the chamber or cavity behind the lens of the eye; vitreous body.

**vivisect,** to dissect the body of an animal.

**vivisection,** the dissection of a living animal for purposes of demonstrating or studying physiological facts or for pathological investigation of diseases.

**vocal cords,** either of two tissue bands projecting into the cavity of the larynx which vibrate and produce vocal sounds of speech.

**voice,** the sounds uttered by living beings produced by vocal cord vibrations.

**void,** to urinate.

**vola,** a hollow surface, such as the sole of a foot or palm of a hand.

**volar,** the palm or foot surfaces.

**volaris,** palmar; concerning the palm of the hand.

**volition,** the act of choosing, or power of willing.

**volume,** a space occupied by a substance; the capacity of a container.

**voluntary,** pertaining to or under the control of the will.

**voluntary muscles,** voluntary musles are attached to the skeleton and are innervated by nerves coming from the brain or spinal cord; muscles subject to being controlled by the will.

**volvulus,** twisting of the bowel causing intestinal obstruction.

**vomer,** a bone of the skull which forms a large part of the nasal septum.

**vomitory,** an emetic; inducing vomiting.

**vomitus,** the ejected matter in vomiting.

**vox,** the voice.

**vulnerability,** susceptibility to injury, or disease.

**vulnerable,** easily injured.

**vulnus,** an injury or a wound.

**vulsella,** vulsellum, a special forceps with clawlike hooks.

**vulva,** external female genitalia, including the mons pubis, labia majora and minora, clitoris, and vestibule of the vagina.

**vulvectomy,** surgical excision of the vulva.

**vulvitis,** inflammation of the vulva.

**vulvovaginal,** pertaining to the vulva and vagina.

**vulvovaginitis,** inflammation of the vulva and vagina.

# W

**wad,** a mass of fibrous material such as cotton, used for a surgical dressing or for packing.

**waist,** the section between the ribs and the hips in the human body.

**Waldeyer's ring,** the ring of tonsillar lymphatic tissue that surrounds the nasopharynx and oropharynx.

**walleye,** leukoma of the cornea; strabismus; exotropia.

**ward,** a large hospital room containing several or many patients.

**wart,** epidermal tumor originating from a virus; verruca.

**Wassermann test,** a test which detects syphilis.

**wash,** a solution for cleansing or for bathing a part; eyewash, or mouthwash.

**waste,** gradual decay, or reduction of bodily susbtance, health, or strength; to emaciate; excrement.

**wasting,** enfeebling, or causing loss of bodily strength.

**water,** a colorless, odorless, tasteless liquid, necessary to life of humans and animals; used in preparation of medicinal substances, as an aqueous solution.

**water brash,** gastric burning pain; heartburn.

**waters,** amniotic fluid; bag of water surrounding the fetus.

**water-soluble,** capable of dissolving in water, as many organic compounds.

**wave,** any wavelike pattern.

**wax,** a plastic substance obtained from plants or insects; cerumen, or ear wax.

**waxy,** pertaining to wax, or to the degeneration of body tissue resulting from accumulations of waxlike insoluble protein; characteristic of amyloid.

**weak,** lacking strength.

**wean,** the process of discontinuing breast feeding and substituting other nourishment.

**wen,** a sebaceous cyst; pillar cyst.

**wet-nurse,** a woman who suckles other infants.

**wheal,** a round, localized area of edema on the skin attended by severe itching which vanishes quickly; a lesion of urticaria.

**wheeze,** difficult breathing with a whistling sound resulting from narrowing of the lumen of a respiratory passageway.

**whelk,** a wheal; a pustule, nodule, tubercle, or pimple.

**whiplash,** an acute cervical sprain or injury caused by a sudden jerking of the head, as in an automobile accident.

**whipworm,** a parasitic nematode of the genus Trichuris.

**white blood cell,** leukocyte; white blood corpuscle.

**white matter,** nerve tissue of the brain and spinal cord.

**whitlow,** a felon; infected finger.

**W.H.O.,** World Health Organization.

**whooping cough,** an infectious disease marked by catarrh of the respiratory tract with a peculiar cough, caused by Bordetella pertussis, especially in children.

**will,** having the power to control one's actions or emotions.

**windpipe,** the trachea.

**wisdom tooth,** the last molar tooth on each side of the jaw which usually erupts around the 25th year.

**witch hazel,** used as an astringent.

**withdrawal,** a pathological retreat from people and the world of reality; symptoms that occur when one abstains from drugs to which one is addicted; abstention from drugs.

**withdrawal symptoms,** a term used to describe effects of drug withdrawal in patients who have become addicted, which include nausea, vomiting, abdominal pain, tremors, and convulsions.

**wolffian body,** an embryonic body on each side of the spinal column; mesonephros.

**womb,** uterus.

**woolsorter's disease,** a pulmonary form of anthrax which develops in handlers of contaminated wool.

**word blindness,** inability to comprehend printed or written words, a form of aphasia; alexia.

**word salad,** the use of a mixture of words and phrases that lack meaning or logic, commonly seen in schizophrenia.

**worm,** a soft-bodied elongated invertebrate without limbs.

**wound,** an injury to the body caused by a physical means with rupture of normal skin and flesh.

**wrinkle,** a small crease or fold in the skin.

**wrist,** the joint between the forearm and hand; carpus.

**wrist drop,** a paralysis of the extensor muscles of the hand and fingers.

**writer's cramp,** an occupational disability caused by excessive writing.

**wryneck,** a contracted state of one or more neck muscles, resulting in an abnormal position of the head; torticollis.

**Wunderlich's curve,** a typical fever curve significant in typhoid fever.

# X

**xanthemia,** yellowish pigment in the blood.

**xanthine,** a nitrogenous compound, related to uric acid, present in the blood and certain tissues of the body.

**xanthinuria,** an excretion of xanthine in large amounts with the urine.

**xanthochromia,** yellowish discoloration of patches of the skin or of the spinal fluid.

**xanthocyanopia,** a condition in which a person cannot distinguish between red and green, but can distinguish between yellow and blue; a form of color blindness.

**xanthocyte,** a cell that contains yellow pigment.

**xanthoderma,** yellow skin.

**xanthodont,** yellow teeth.

**xanthoma,** a condition marked by small, yellow nodules of the skin, especially of the eyelids.

**xanthopsia,** yellow vision.

**xanthosis,** jaundice.

**X chromosome,** one of the two sex chromosomes carrying female characteristics, which occur in pairs in the female cell and zygote, and with one Y chromosome in a male cell and zygote.

**xenodiagnosis,** a diagnosis or means of determining parasitic disease in humans by feeding an uninfected host on material believed to be infected and observing the results.

**xenogenesis,** reproduction of offspring unlike either parent.

**xenogenous,** a condition caused by a foreign body or toxin.

**xenomenia,** bleeding from other sites during menstruation.

**xenophobia,** abnormal fear of strangers.

**xenophonia,** an alteration in voice production, as in lack of bodily strength.

**xenopthalmia,** inflammation of the eye caused by a foreign body.

**xeransis,** a loss of moisture of the skin causing dryness.

**xerocheilia,** dryness of the lips.

**xeroderma,** excessive dryness of the skin; a form of ichthyosis.

**xerophthalmia,** an abnormal condition of the eye marked by dryness and thickening of the lining membrane of the lid and eyeball due to a deficiency of vitamin A.

**xerostomia,** dryness of the mouth.

**xiphisternum,** the lower portion of the sternum or xiphoid process.

**xiphoid,** relating to the sword-shaped xiphisternum.

**xiphoiditis,** inflammation of the cartilage xiphoid process.

**X-linked,** sex-linked, or transmitted by genes on the X-chromosome.

**X-ray,** to examine by roentgen rays.

**X-ray therapy,** used to treat certain diseases, as cancer.

**Xylocaine,** trademark for lidocaine, used in medicinal preparations.

**xylometazoline,** used as a topical nasal decongestant.

**xylose,** a pentose used in diagnostic tests of intestinal absorption.

**xysma,** membranous material in stools of diarrhea.

**xyster,** a surgical instrument used in surgery to scrape bone.

# Y

**yaw,** a primary lesion of the skin due to yaws.

**yawn,** an involuntary opening of the mouth with a long inhalation, due to fatigue or drowsiness.

**yawning,** deep inspiration with the mouth wide open, resulting from fatigue or boredom.

**yaws,** an infectious tropical disease, marked by eruptions of tubercles on the skin, and rheumatism, caused by the spirochete Treponema pertenue.

**Y bacillus,** a bacillus that causes dysentery.

**Y chromosome,** one of a pair of sex chromosomes, an X and Y, that carry male characteristics.

**yeast,** a viscid substance composed of aggregated cells of small unicellular sac fungi, used to supplement B-complex vitamins.

**yellow body,** the corpus luteum formed in the cavity of the graafian follicle after the expulsion of the ovum, and which persists dùring pregnancy.

**yellow fever,** an acute infectious disease marked by jaundice, vomiting, epigastric tenderness, hemorrhages, and fever, transmitted by the bite of a female mosquito.

**yoke,** a connecting structure.

**yolk,** stored in the form of protein and fat granules in the ovum, as a nutrient.

**Young's rule,** a children's dose of medication is determined by adding 12 to the age and dividing the result by the age, making the quotient the denominator of a fraction, the numerator of which is 1. The proportion of adult medication to be given to a child is represented by the fraction.

**youth,** the period of adolescence.

# Z

**zein,** protein derived from maize or corn.

**Zeiss' gland,** a sebaceous gland at the free edge of the eyelid.

**zelotypia,** a morbid interest in any project or cause.

**zero,** the point on a thermometer or other scale at which the graduation begins.

**zestocausis,** cauterization with steam.

**zinc chloride,** used as an astringent, antiseptic, and escharotic.

**zinc oxide,** used mostly in the form of ointment and as an antiseptic and astringent.

**zoanthropy,** a mental condition in which one has the delusion that he is an animal.

**zoetic,** pertaining to life; vital.

**zona,** a band or girdle; herpes zoster; zone.

**zonesthesia,** having the sensation of constriction, as by a girdle.

**zoonosis,** a disease transmissible to man by animals.

**zoophagous,** living on animal food.

**zoophobia,** pathological aversion toward animals.

**zooplasty,** transplantation of tissue from lower animals to the human body.

**zootherapeutics,** veterinary medicine.

**zoster,** herpes zoster; shingles.

**zosteriform,** resembling herpes zoster.

**zygapophysis,** one of the articular processes of the neural arch of a vertebra, usually occurring in pairs.

**zygoma,** the prominence of the cheekbone.

**zygomatic,** pertaining to the zygoma.

**zygomatic arch,** the formation on each side of the cheeks composed of each malar bone articulating with the zygomatic process.

**zygomatic process,** a thin projection that extends from the temporal bone; that part of the malar bone which forms the zygoma.

**zygote,** the union of male and female gametes to produce a new single-celled individual or zygote.

**zymase,** an enzyme found in yeast.

**zyme,** a fermenting substance.

**zymogen,** a substance that develops into an enzyme.

**zymology,** the science concerned with fermentation.

**zymolysis,** the change produced or the fermentative action of enzymes.

**zymolytic,** pertaining to zymolysis.

**zymose,** an enzyme responsible for the changes of a disaccharide into a monosaccharide.

**zymosis,** fermentation; an infectious disease.

**zymosthenic,** increasing the functional activity of an enzyme.

**zymotic,** pertaining to fermentation; relating to an infectious disease.

# INDEX

# INDEX

**A**bdomen
  adhesions and, 410, 411
  aortic aneurysm in, 64-65
  anesthesia for surgery for, 32
  celiac disease and, 260-261
  Cesarean section and, *see*
    Childbirth cramps
      acute gastritis and, 515-516
      appendicitis and, 33
      gastroenteritis and, 489-490
      indigestion and, 514
      intrauterine devices and, 45-46
      laxative and, 33
      regional ileitis and, 489-490
      ulcerative colitis and, 495
  distention
    intestinal obstruction and, 496
    megacolon and, 497
  heartburn and, 514
  indigestion and, 514
  laparoscope and, 155
  ovarian cysts and, 206
  pain in
    chronic gastritis and, 516
    colic, 276
    doctor called for, 514
    duodenal disorders and, 513
    dysentery and, 403
    follicle cysts and, 203-204
    food allergy and, 26
    gall bladder disease and, 222, 224
    infectious hepatitis and, 326
    intestinal obstruction and, 496
    laxatives and, 349, 455
    Meckel's diverticulum and, 491
    pancreatic cancer and, 401
    pancreatitis and, 397
    peritonitis and, 410-411
    pregnancy complications and,
      441-442
    rheumatic fever and, 466-467
    salpingitis and, 200
    "spastic colitis" and, 494
    stomach disorders and, 513, 514
    volvulus and, 492
  plastic surgery and, 422
  purplish streaks on skin of, 12,
    419-420
  pyloric stenosis and, 520
  taps, 315
  tumors within
    hernia and, 247
    paracentesis and, 315
    sonography and, 500
  *see also* Appendix; Fallopian tubes;
    Gall bladder; Hernia; Kidneys;
    Large intestine; Liver; Ovaries;
    Pancreas; Peritonitis; Pregnancy;
    Small intestine; Spleen; Stomach;
    Urinary bladder; Uterus
Abdominal lipectomy, 422

Abdominoperineal resection, 461-462
Abortion, 197-199
  complete, 198
  curettage for, 190
  dangers of, 198
  description, 197
  endometritis and, 191
  fibroids and, 192-195
  habitual, 198
  incomplete, 198
  induced, 197
  inevitable, 198
  legal aspects of, 199
  missed, 198
  operative procedures for, 199
  self-treatment, 199
  sexual intercourse and, 199
  spontaneous, 197, 199
  syphilis and, 559
  threatened, 198, 199
  travel and, 428
  tubal pregnancy and, 201-202
Abrasions, first aid for, 218
Abruptio placentae, 438-439, 445-446
Abscess, 5-7
  antibiotics for, 5
  Bartholin, 177-178
  blood poisoning and, 50-51
  brain, 147, 376
  breast, 94-95, 441
  carbuncle distinguished from, 5
  cause, 5, 7
  cysts and, 337
  diverticulitis and, 493
  draining, 7
  ear canal, 145, 146
  epididymitis and, 343
  felon, 229
  laryngeal obstruction and, 530
  lung, 333, 336, 545, 570
  lymph gland, 52
  ointments for, 7
  osteomyelitis and, 79
  ovarian, 200
  paronychia, 229
  parotid gland, 468
  pilonidal cyst, 416, 417
  rectum and anus and, 460
  regional ileitis and, 489-490
  salpingitis and, 200
  squeezing, 5, 6, 7
  susceptibility to, 5
  teeth, 331
    middle ear pain due to, 146, 147
  tonsil and, 424-425
  *see also* Infections
Absorption, *see* Large intestine; Small
  intestine
Abstinence, 42
Accidents
  alcoholism and, 19

  amputation and, 70
  liability case and, 4
Acetone, acidosis and, 132
Achalasia, 158, 159
Achlorhydria, 615
Acid
  first aid for swallowed, 218, 219
  stomach and
    aging and, 515
    alcohol and, 515
Acid-base status, 310
Acidosis, 133, 308
  metabolic, 310-311
  respiratory, 310
  Acne, 476-477
  radiation therapy for, 569
Acoustic nerve tumors, 151
Acromegaly, 419, 420
ACTH, *see* Adrenocorticotropic
  hormone
Activated charcoal, swallowed poisons
  and, 219
Active immunity, 252
  *see also* Immunizations and
    vaccinations
Acute appendicitis, 33
Acute cholecystitis, 222
  *See also* Gall bladder
Acute gastritis, 515-516
Acute urinary retention, 451
Acute yellow atrophy of the liver, 324
"Adaptation diseases," 360
Addiction, *see* Alcohol abuse; Drug
  addiction
Addison's disease, 12
Adenoids
  acute inflammation, 523-524
  description, 523
  infection of the, 524
    common cold and, 543
    glandular enlargement in neck
      and, 523-524
    middle ear infection and, 147
    removal (adenoidectomy), 524, 525, 526
      middle ear infection and, 148
    *see also* Tonsils
Adenoma
  of breast, 95
  growth hormone, 418-420
  of lung, 337, 338
  of pancreas, 399-400
  pituitary, 418-421
Adenomatous disease, 95
Adhesions, abdomen and, 410, 411
Adolescence, 8
  age of puberty, 8
  allergy and, 20, 21
  breast development in, 8, 9
    boys and, 9, 95
  delayed, 10, 14
  homosexual tendency and, 473

hormones for inducing, 10
intellectual development during, 10
late, 10
marriage during, 10
masturbation during, 10
organs responsible for, 9
ovaries and, 203
parents and, 9
peer relationships and, 9
perspiration and, 478
precocious, 10, 14
psychological changes in, 9, 10
sex education and, 10
sexual urges in, 10
scoliosis, 74-75
significance of, 8
skin and, 9, 476-477
tuberculosis and, 538, 540-541
voice changes and, 8, 10
see also Menstruation
Adrenal glands, 11-13
  cancer and, 13
  Conn's syndrome, 12
  cortex, 11
    Addison's disease, 12
    Cushing's disease, 12
    function, 12
  description, 11, 12
  malfunctioning, 11, 12
  medulla
    function, 11
    pheochromocytoma and, 11
  noradrenalin, 11
  prostate cancer and, 453
  stress and, 360
  surgical removal (adrenalectomy), 13
  transplants, 13, 535-536
  tumors, 12-13
  x-ray study of, 12
  see also Adrenalin
Adrenalin, 11
  for asthma, 25
  effects of, 11
  for hives, 27
  local anesthesia and, 30
Adrenocorticotropic hormone (ACTH),
350-351
  allergy and, 22
  arthritis and, 38, 350-351
African sleeping sickness, 403
Afterbirth (placenta), see Childbirth
Aging, 14-17
  alcohol consumption and, 15
  Alzheimer's Disease and, 16-17
  arteriosclerosis and, 16
  childbirth and, 15
  childhood and, 14
  choking and, 211
  constipation and, 455
  emotional disturbances and, 15
  exercise and, 14, 15, 16
  forestalling, 15
  gray hair and, 16
  heart trouble and, 16
  high blood pressure and, 16
  impotence and, 510, 511
  intellectual facilities and, 16
  laboratory tests indicating, 14
  longevity, 14, 15-16
  marriage and, 15
  menopause
    artificially stimulated menstrual
      cycle and, 16

  early, 16
  nutrition, 15
    caloric needs, 135
    vitamin needs, 562
  obesity and, 16
  organs and, 14, 15, 16
  physical labor and, 15
  physical therapy for, 415
  premature, 16
  prior illness, 14
  prolapse of the rectum and, 461
  prostate enlargement and, 451
  rehabilitation for, 414-415
  senility and, 14
  sexual activity and, 14
    potency, 15
    sperm count, 511
  skin and, 16
  sleep adequacy and, 15
  slowing process, 16
  smoking and, 15
  start of, 14
  stomach disorders and, 514, 515
  stress and, 361
  surgery and, 15
  warm climate and, 15
Agoraphobia, 355
AHF (antihemophilic factor), 51
AIDS, 285-286
Air pollution, lungs and, 330
Alarm system, Intensive Care Unit and,
292
Albumin, see Urination
Alcohol abuse, 18-19
  Alcoholics Anonymous, 19
  Antabuse (disulfiram), 19
  blackout (alcoholic amnesia), 18
  causes of, 18
  coma and, 368
  controlled drinking and, 19
  definition, 18
  delirium tremens and, 18-19
  gastroenteritis and, 489
  heredity and, 18
  larynx cancer and, 529
  lithium carbonate and, 19
  longevity and, 18
  nervous system damage from, 18
  neuropathy and, 362-363
  organs affected by, 18
  pancreatitis and, 397, 399
  predisposition to, 18
  pregnancy and, 19
  prevention, 18
  psychiatric therapy and, 19
  stages of, 18
  tests for, 18
  tranquilizers and, 19
  treatment, 19
Alcohol consumption
  aging and, 15
  arteriosclerosis and, 56
  chronic gastritis and, 516
  as depressant, 351
  epilepsy and, 368
  gouty arthritis and, 39
  heart and, 232
  indigestion and, 514
  kidney disease and, 295
  liver
    cirrhosis, 324-325
    fatty, 325

  infectious hepatitis relapse and,
    326
  obesity and, 136
  pregnancy and, 287, 427
  preoperative routines and, 447-448
  sexual relations and, 474-475
  stomach acidity and, 515
  tongue and, 322
  ulcer and, 517, 519
  urethral infection and, 555
Alcoholics Anonymous, 19
Alcoholism, see Alcohol abuse
Aldomet, Raynaud's disease and, 57
Alkali, first aid for swallowed, 218
Alkalosis, 308
  metabolic, 311
  respiratory, 310
Allergens, 20
Allergy, 20-28
  adenoidectomy and, 524
  to animal hairs, 22, 25
  atopic dermatitis and, 26
  blood transfusions and, 309
  bronchitis and, 545
  byssinosis and, 335
  causes, 20, 21, 22
  common cold and, 543
  conjunctivitis and, 165
  contact dermatitis and, 20, 26
  to cosmetics, 162, 476
  croup and, 260
  curing, 20
  dangers of, 20, 21
  definition, 20
  diagnosing, 20, 21, 22
  to dust, 21, 22, 23, 24
  to dyes, 21
  eczema and, 20, 26
  eyes and, 162
  to feathers, 21
  gastroenteritis and, 489
  to grasses, 21
  hay fever, 20, 21, 22-23, 24-25
  heredity and, 20
  hives, 20, 26-27, 28
  hoarseness and, 544
  immunizations and, 253
    antitoxins, 21
    measles vaccine and, 255
    mumps vaccine and, 256
  incidence, 21
  to insect stings, 21, 27
  to mold spores, 21, 22
  nasal polyps, 391
    sinusitis and, 392
  to perfumes, 21
  physical, 28
  to plastics, 21
  poison ivy as, 26, 482-483
  to pollens, 21, 22-23, 25
  prevention, 20
  pruritus ani and, 460
  as psychosomatic illness, 356
  recurrence, 21, 24
  rhinitis, 20, 23
  seasonality, 21, 22-23
  sinus infections and, 23
  to smoke, 162
  to soap, 162
  stress and, 360
  sudden, 21
  tendency toward, 21
  tonsillectomy and, 524

treatment, 22
  antihistamines, 22, 24
  injections, 22, 24, 25
  length of, 20
  specialist for, 22
  steroids, 22, 24, 350-351
  *see also* Asthma; Drug allergy; Food
    allergy
Allopurinol, for gouty arthritis, 39
Alopecia areata, 480
Alzheimer's disease, 16-17
Amaurotic familial idiocy (Tay-Sachs
  disease), 264-265
  testing for, 288
Ambulation, as postoperative measure,
  448
Amebiasis, 402-403
American Medical Association
  Information Service, 474
Amnesia, alcoholic, 18
Amniocentesis, *see* Pregnancy
Amoebic dysentery, *see* Dysentery
Amphetamines, obesity and, 134
Ampicillin, typhoid fever and, 280
Amputation
  bone tumor and, 91
  gangrene and, 7
  limbs and, 72
  of penis, 340
  rehabilitation and, 414-415
  replantation surgery and, 463-464
Amylase
  blood chemistry for, 308
  pancreatitis and, 397
Analgesics, 347-348
  anesthesia and, 31
  resistance to, 346
  *see also* Aspirin
Anemia, 48-50
  atrophic gastritis and, 516
  bleeding and, 49
  blood count for, 48, 305
  blood transfusions and, 306
  bone marrow and, 49-50, 306
  cancer and, 50, 104
  cirrhosis and, 325
  danger of, 48
  fatty liver and, 325
  heart muscle impairment and, 233
  hemorrhoids and, 456
  Hodgkin's disease and, 53
  hookworm disease and, 404
  infection susceptibility and, 5
  kinds of:
    Cooley's (Mediterranean), 49, 502,
     503
    deficiency, 49, 563
    folic acid deficiency, 562
    hemolytic, 49, 502
    iron deficiency, 49
    pernicious, 49, 561
    sickle-cell, 48-49, 502
    toxic, 50
    vitamin $B_{12}$ deficiency, 49
  leukemia and, 53
  malnutrition and, 49
  menstruation and, 48, 183
  ovarian tumor and, 206
  premature babies and, 387, 388
  preoperative measures and, 447-448
  rheumatoid arthritis and, 38
  schistosomiasis and, 403
  spleen overactivity and, 502

stomach removal and, 520
stool analysis and, 315
treatment of, 50
ulcerative colitis and, 495
vitamins and, 49
Anesthesia, 29-32
  anesthesiologist, 29-31, 32
  childbirth and, 29
  children and, 32
  endotracheal, 31, 32
  "induction of, " 29
  "preanesthetic evaluation and
    premedication," 29
  for specific operations, 32
  types, 29-30
    balanced, 29
    caudal, 30, 32
    epidural, 30
    general inhalation, 29, 32
    intravenous, 30
    local, 30, 32
    spinal, 30, 32
    topical, 30-31, 32
Anesthesiologist, 29, 30, 31, 32
Anesthetic ointments
  hemorrhoids and, 441
  leukoplakia of vulva and, 178
Aneurysm, *see* Blood vessels
Angina, Ludwig's, 530
Angina pectoris, 232, 237-239, 243-244
  arteriosclerosis and, 55
Angiocardiography, 235, 566
Angioedema, *see* Hives
Angiogram
  of brain, 371
  brain tumor and, 377
  kidney disease and, 300
Angioma, 378
Animal bites, *see* Bites
Ankle
  fracture, 84, 90
  replacement of joint, 84
  swelling
    preeclampsia and, 443-444
    pregnancy and, 430, 442
Anoscope, polyps and, 458
Antacid drugs
  effectiveness of, 515
  gastritis and, 516
  gastroenteritis and, 516
  morning sickness and, 429
  ulcer and, 517-518
Anterior resection, 461-462
Anthracosis, 334
Anthrax, 284-285
Antibiotics, 346-347
  allergy to, 5, 346
  prescriptions, 7
  self-medication, 5, 346
  vaginitis caused by, 182
  *see also specific antibiotics, e.g.,*
    *penicillin*
Antibodies, 306
Anticoagulant drugs, 238
  coronary thrombosis and, 238
  phlebitis and, 334
  thrombophlebitis and, 60
Antidiuretic hormone, diabetes
  insipidus and, 420
Antigens, 306
Antihemophilic factor (AHF), 51
Antihistaminic drugs, 392

allergy and, 22
  drug, 27
  food, 26
  hay fever and, 23-24
  insect, 27
  physical, 28
for common cold, 543
conjunctivitis and, 165
for contact dermatitis, 26
Antilymphocytic globulin (ALG), organ
  transplants and, 536
Antirabies injection, 209
Antiseptics
  animal or human bites and, 209
  styes and, 166
Antispasmodic drugs
  acute gastritis and, 516
  gastroenteritis and, 516
  indigestion and, 514
  morning sickness and, 429
  mucous colitis and, 494
  pyloric stenosis and, 520
Antithyroid drugs, 532
Antitoxin
  allergy to, 21
  diphtheria, 117, 128
Antivenin, 209
Anus, *see* Hemorrhoids; Rectum and
  anus
Anxiety
  alcoholism and, 18
  headache and, 369
  tranquilizers and, 348
Anxiety neurosis, 354-355, 358
Aorta
  aneurysm in, 58-59
    replacement and, 65
  coarctation, 241, 242
  sonography for abnormalities of, 500
Apathy, hypopituitarism and, 421
Aphasia, 366
Apoplexy, *see* Stroke
Appendicitis, 33-36
  acute, 33
  antibiotics for, 34
  cause, 33
  complications, 34
  diagnosis, 33
  enema and, 33
  incidence, 33
  indigestion and, 33
  laxatives and, 33, 411, 455
  peritonitis and, 33-36, 410
  pinworms and, 405
  recurrent, 33
  surgery (appendectomy) for, 33-36
  symptoms, 33
  whipworms and, 404
Appendix, 33-34
  ruptured, 33-36
  *see also* Appendicitis
Appetite
  appendicitis and, 33
  cirrhosis and, 325
  depression and, 357
  drugs for reducing, 349-350
  esophageal tumor and, 160
  gastritis and, 516
  indigestion and, 514
  infectious hepatitis and, 326
  neurasthenia and, 354
  pancreatic cancer and, 401
  peritonitis and, 410

radiation sickness and, 569
regional ileitis and, 489-490
stomach disorders and, 513, 521
tuberculosis and, 538-539, 540
*see also* Fasting
Arm
brachial neuropathy, 363
fracture, 88-89, 215
plastic surgery and, 422
replantation surgery and, 464
Arrhythmia
cardiac, 239-240, 245
paroxysmal, 240
Arsenic, syphilis and, 559
Arteries
aneurysm, 58-59
arteriogram for, 566
grafts, 62-63, 64-65
hardening of, *see* Arteriosclerosis
*see also* Coronary artery disease;
Renal artery
Arteriogram, 566
arteriosclerosis and, 55
kidney tumor and, 300
renal artery obstruction and, 63-64
Arteriosclerosis, 55-56
alcohol consumption and, 18, 56
aneurysm and, 58
causes of, 55, 56
cerebral
fainting and, 368
Parkinsonism and, 370
cerebral hemorrhage and, 378
cerebral thrombosis, 366
cholesterol and, 15, 55, 56, 310
coronary artery disease and, 237
diabetes mellitus and, 132
diagnosis of, 55
impotence and, 473
long life and, 15, 16
physical activity and, 56
preventing, 55
renal blood vessel and, 63-64, 295
retinal thrombosis and, 176
smoking and, 56
stress and, 360
stroke and, 379
surgery for, 62-64
amputation and, 70-72
blood vessel transplant and,
536-537
bypass, 62-63
endarterectomy, 62, 536-537
grafts, 62-63
internal mammary artery implant,
63
sympathectomy, 62
symptoms, 55
tendency toward, 55
treatments, 55-56
Arteriovenous aneurysm (A-V), 59
Arteriovenous fistulas, 68
Arteriovenous malformations, 367
Arthritis, 37-40
gonorrhea and, 557
psychosomatic illness and, 356
of spine, 72
Still's disease and, 38
stress and, 361
treatment
antibiotics, 37
arthroplasty, 83-84
climate, 37

drugs, 37, 38, 347, 351
heat therapy, 37, 412
rehabilitation and, 414
spas, 37
surgery, 38, 39, 83
teeth removal, 37
tonsillectomy, 37
types, 37
bacterial, 40
gouty, 37, 39
osteoarthritis, 38-39
rheumatoid, 38
traumatic, 39-40
Arthrography, 568
torn knee cartilage and, 78
Arthroplasty, 83-85
elbow, 85
hip, 86
shoulder, 85
Arthroscopy, torn knee cartilage and,
78
Artificial insemination, 509-510
Artificial respiration
drowning and, 212-214
electric shock and, 214
fainting, dizziness, or vertigo and,
214
gas poisoning and, 216
swallowed poison and, 218-219
*see also* Cardiopulmonary
resuscitation
Asbestos, 334
Asbestosis, 334
Ascaris (roundworm), 405
Ascorbic acid (Vitamin C), *see*
Vitamins
Asiatic flu, 547-548
Aspiration, bursitis and, 76
Aspiration pneumonia, 333
Aspirin
allergy to, 27, 347
arthritis and, 37, 38
mumps and, 121
postspinal headache and, 32
rheumatic fever and, 467
sinusitis, 392
Asthma, 20, 22, 23, 25-26, 27, 28
bronchiectasis and, 546
bronchitis and, 545
emphysema and, 332
hay fever and, 23
psychosomatic illness and, 356
sputum analysis and, 314-315
Astigmatism, *see* Eyes
Ataxia, multiple sclerosis and, 370
Atelectasis, 331-332
of the newborn, 266-267
Athlete's foot, 477-478
"Athlete's heart," 240
Atomic fallout, effect of, 569
Atopic dermatitis, *see* Eczema
Atresia, congenital, 157
Atrophic gastritis, 516
Audiogram, 147
Audiometer, 145
Autoimmune reactions, thyroiditis as,
532
Autointoxication, 488
Automatic respiratory devices,
Intensive Care Unit and, 292
Autonomic (sympathetic) nervous
system, 362, 363
*see also* Nervous diseases

Autotransplant, 535

Baby, *see* Child Behavior; Childbirth;
Infancy; Infant feeding; Newborn;
Pregnancy
Bacillary dysentery, 495
Back
fracture of, 216
pain in lower, 72-73
*see also* Spine
Backache
fibroids and, 194
pregnancy and, 430
pyelonephritis and, 297
Bacteremia, 50
Bacteria, 279
abscesses caused by, 5
altering genes in, 291
septicemia and, 5, 50-51
*see also* Infections
Bacterial arthritis, 40
Bacterial endocarditis, 241, 245
Bacterial infections, *see* Infections
Bad breath, 319-320
*see also* Breath
Bagassosis, 335
Baking lamp, heat treatment and, 412
Balance, equilibrium and, 151
Balanced anesthesia, 29
Baldness, 479-480
Barbiturates, 348
need for, 356
overdose, 219
Bartholin glands, 177-178
Basal metabolic rate, 531
Basal temperatures, ovulation and, 507
"Baseball" finger, 227
Bathing, skin and, 478
BCG (bacillus Calmette-Guérin), 541
*see also* Tuberculosis
Beard, precocious development of, 10
Bedwetting (enuresis), 112-113, 295
Bees, allergy to sting, 21, 27
Behavior, *see* Child behavior;
Emotional disturbances; Infancy
Belching
duodenal disorders and, 513
food allergy and, 26
stomach disorders and, 513
ulcer and, 517
Bell's palsy (facial paralysis), 364
Benemid, gouty arthritis and, 39
Benzedrine, 351
Benzene, bone marrow injury and, 50
Beriberi, 49, 362-363, 561
Bile, 221
peritonitis and, 410
*see also* Gall bladder; Liver
Bile ducts
cholangiogram of, 567
pancreatic cancer and, 401
*see also* Gall bladder
Biliary cirrhosis, 324
Biliary dyskinesia, 226
Bilirubin, blood chemistry for, 308
Biopsy, 314
cancer and, 104
breast, 96
cervical, 188
cone, 188
penis, 340
colonoscopy and, 154-155
endometrial, 191, 507-508

endoscopy and, 154
excisional, 314
frozen section, 314
Hirschsprung's disease and, 262
needle, 314
sarcoidosis and, 335
testicular, 510
see also Laboratory tests
Birth control, 41-47
decision to use, 41
educating about, 42
methods, 42
abstinence, 42
coitus interruptus (withdrawal), 42, 43
condoms, 42, 43-44
contraceptive jellies, 42, 45
diaphragm, 42, 44-45
douches, 42, 44
intrauterine devices (IUD), 42, 45-46, 200
oral contraceptives (pills), 42, 46, 185, 509
rhythm, 42-43
sterilization, 42, 47
need for, 41
see also Pregnancy; Sexual intercourse
Birth defects, see Congenital deformities
Birthmark, 484
Bismuth, syphilis and, 559
Bites
animal
allergy to, 21, 27
first-aid treatment, 209
rabies, 256-257, 283-284
human
first-aid treatment for, 209
hand and, 229
insect, 209, see also specific insects
snakes, 210
"Black eye," 162
Blackheads
acne and, 477
adolescence and, 9
"Black lung," 334
Blackout, 18
Bladder, see Gall bladder; Urinary bladder
Bleeding
anemia and, 49
blood vessel tumor and, 485
diverticulum of esophagus and, 159
hemophilia and, 51-52
leukemia and, 53
polycythemia rubra vera and, 50
scurvy and, 561
tendencies, 51-52
tourniquet for, 60
see also Hemorrhage
Blepharoplasty, 422
Blindness, see Eyes
Blood
bone marrow and, 48
injury to, 50
test, 306
cancer spread through, 103
cholesterol in, 135
circulation
amputation and, 70, 72
chilblain and, 481
massage and, 413

clotting, see also Thrombosis
hemophilia and, 51-52
lacerations and, 60-62
platelets and, 48
polycythemia rubra vera and, 50
coagulation
adrenalin and noradrenalin and, 11
Vitamin K and, 561-562
coughing up, 151, 330
lung cancer and, 337
definition, 48
hemoglobin, 48
malaria and, 404
plasma, 48
platelets, 48
red blood cells, 48
sepsis of the newborn and, 267
in the sputum, 545
lung embolus and, 58
in stool, 456
hemorrhoidectomy and, 457
rectal cancer and, 461
sugar in, see Diabetes mellitus
urine and, 296
white blood cells (leukocytes), 48
see also Anemia; Blood diseases; Blood vessels; Laboratory tests; Liver; Spleen
Blood bank, 309
Blood chemistry tests, 309-310
eclampsia and, 444
hyperparathyroidism and, 407
hypoparathyroidism and, 408
preeclampsia and, 443
Blood count
anemia and, 49
appendicitis and, 33
hematological blood tests and, see Laboratory tests
polycythemia rubra vera and, 50
Blood culture, 310
septicemia and, 50-51
Blood diseases, 50-53
see also specific blood diseases
Blood gases, 310
analyzer, 310
Blood poisoning (septicemia), 5, 50
blood culture and, 310
lymph gland infection and, 52
sepsis of the newborn, 267
spleen removal and, 504-505
Blood pressure
definition, 235
high (hypertension), 235, 236
arteriosclerosis and, 55
birth control pills and, 46
blood vessel transplant and, 536-537
cerebral hemorrhage and, 378
Conn's syndrome and, 12
coronary artery disease and, 239
Cushing's syndrome and, 12, 418-419
danger of, 235
diet for, 138
eclampsia and, 444
emotional disturbances and, 235
heart muscle and, 232-233
induced labor and, 432
kidney disease and, 294-295, 296
long life and, 16
nosebleeds and, 394

obesity and, 135-136, 235
psychosomatic illness and, 356, 360
stress and, 360
stroke and, 366, see also Nervous diseases
symptoms, 235-236
temporary, 236
toxemia and, see Pregnancy
treatment for, 235
low, 236
measurement of, 235
normal level, 236
pheochromocytoma and, 11
pregnancy and, 426-427, 428
Blood test
alcohol intoxication and, 18
dysentery and, 403
erythroblastosis and, 263
infectious mononucleosis and, 283
kidney function and, 294
phenylketonuria and, 290
spleen diseases and, 502
syphilis, 557, 558
tetany of the newborn and, 267
tonsillectomy and, 525
typhoid fever and, 279
whooping cough, 126
Blood transfusions, 306-309
abortion and, 198
anemia, 50, 305, 306
bladder operations and, 552
brain surgery and, 377
chemical imbalance and, 292
exchange, see Erythroblastosis
gall bladder operations and, 225
intrauterine, 309
lung injuries and, 337
malaria and, 404
mastectomy and, 97
operations and, 454
postoperative measure, 449
preoperative measure, 448
postpartum hemorrhage and, 440
premature babies and, 388, 448
serum hepatitis and, 327
spleen removal and, 504
stomach operations and, 522
tubal pregnancy and, 202
Blood vessels
aneurysm, 58-59, 367, 378
aortic, 61
graft for, 537
of heart, 243
surgery for, 62, 64-65, 378
arteriovenous fistulas, 68
Buerger's disease, 57, 62
bypass procedures, see Bypass operations
embolism, 58
birth control pills and, 46
cerebral, 378
coronary thrombosis and, 238
pulmonary, 334
surgery for, 64
hemangioma (blood vessel tumor), 67-68, 393, 483, 484-485
lip, 316
liver and, 327
tongue, 322
heredity and, 66
lacerations, 60, 62
malformation of, 378

preeclampsia and, 444
Raynaud's disease, 56-57, 62
thrombosis, 58, see also Stroke
    coronary, see Coronary artery
        disease
    retinal, 176
    surgery for, 64
    thrombophlebitis and, 60
transplants for, 536-537
    endarterectomy, 379, 536
see also Arteries; Cirrhosis of the
    liver; Grafts; Neurosurgery;
    Varicose veins
"Blue baby," 236, 312
Blue Cross insurance, 1
Body lice, 481
Body odors, 478
Boil
    carbuncle and, 5
    ear canal pain and, 145
    see also Abscess
Bone marrow
    blood produced by, 48
    frozen section biopsy of, 314
    Hodgkin's disease and, 54
    injury to, 50
    leukemia and, 53
    spleen removal and, 504, 505
    study, 306
Bones
    bursitis and, 75-76
        bunions, 76-77
    cysts, 407, 408
    exercise for conditions of, 413-414
    frozen section biopsy of, 314
    graft, 86, 92
    infection (x ray of), 568
    leprosy and, 282
    nodules and rheumatic fever, 466
    osteitis fibrosa cystica, 81, 407, 408
    osteomalacia, 81
    osteomyelitis, 79
    osteoporosis, 81
    osteotomy, 83
    Paget's disease (osteitis deformans),
        80-81
    reconstructive surgery on, 81, 83
    rehabilitation and, 414-415
    segmental bone resection, 92
    skeleton, 71
    torn knee cartilage, 78-79
    tumors, 91-92
        amputation and, 70, 72
    x ray of, 567-568
    see also Fractures
Bone scan, 570
    cancer spread and, 103
Booster shots, 252
Bottle feeding, see Infant feeding
Botulism, gastroenteritis and, 489
Boutonniere finger, 227
Bowel movements
    after childbirth, 440
    change in, 455, 461, 497
    daily, 455, 486
    endometriosis and, 197
    failure of, 496
    fissure in anus and, 459
    fistula operation and, 460
    hemorrhoid operation and, 457
    irregular, 456
    radium treatment of the cervix and,
        189

rectocele and, 180
regular, 455
spinal cord injury and, 382
spinal cord tumors and, 380
see also Constipation; Diarrhea;
    Large intestine; Rectum and Anus
Bowels, see Large intestine; Small
    intestine
Boxer's fracture, 228
Boys, puberty in, 8
    breast enlargement and, 9, 95
    see also Adolescence
Brachial neuropathy, 363
Brain
    abscess, 376
        middle ear infection and, 147-148
    alcoholism and, 18
    aneurysm in, 58
    angiography of, 371, 377
    appearance of, 372
    atelectasis of the newborn and, 267
    CAT scan of, 365, 371, 377, 565-566,
        570
    cerebral arteriosclerosis and, see
        Arteriosclerosis
    cerebral edema, 376
    cysts, 371
    electroencephalography (EEG), 371
    embolus to, 58, see also, Stroke
    frozen section biopsy of, 314
    gas poisoning and, 216
    hallucinatory drugs and, 351
    hemorrhage (cerebral), 366, 378
    hydrocephalus, 380
    hyperactivity and, 115
    inflammation, see also Encephalitis;
        Meningitis; Meningoencephalitis;
        Poliomyelitis
        chickenpox and, 116
    injury to, 374, see also Cerebral palsy
    neurosurgery (craniotomy), 372, 373
        access to, 372
        aneurysms, 379
        blood vessel malformation, 378
        cerebral hemorrhage, 378
        embolus, 379
        infections, 376
        injury to brain and, 374, 375
        small stroke, 379
        tumors, 376-378
    spinal taps and, 315
    thrombus in, 64
    tranquilizers and, 348
    tumors, 365, 376-378
        angiography and, 371
        CAT scan and, 377, 565-566
        coma and, 368-369
        convulsions and, 378
        electroencephalography and, 371
        hearing and, 378
        location of, 377
        operation for, 377
        pituitary gland malfunction and,
            421
        radiation therapy for, 378
        speech and, 378
        symptoms, 377
        vision and, 378
    see also Mental deficiency
Branchial cysts, 530
Brassiere, see Breasts
Break bone fever (dengue fever), 281
"Breakthrough bleeding," 46

Breast cancer, 95, 96
    adrenalectomy and, 13
    avoiding, 96
    breast injury and, 94
    breast reconstruction and, 422
    curing, 97
    diagnosis, 95-96
        biopsy, 96
        frozen section examinations, 96
        mammogram, 96, 567
    family tendency toward, 97
    follow-up examination and, 97
    incidence of, 100
    males and, 95
    nursing and, 93
    pregnancy and, 97
    treatment of, 97
        chemotherapy, 97, 106
        hormones, 105
        lump removal, 96, 97
        mastectomy, 95-97
        pituitary gland removal, 420
        radiation therapy, 97
    see also Breasts
Breast milk, see Nursing
Breasts, 93-99
    adolescence and, 8, 93
        boys and, 9, 95
        menstruation and, 8
    benign tumor, 95, 96, 97
    birth control pills and, 46
    brassiere for, 93
        breast-feeding and, 270
        breast reconstruction, 99
        mastectomy, 97
        pregnancy and, 427
    cancer, see Breast cancer
    cysts, 95
    enlarging, 93, 97
    examination, 94
    hair removal from, 94
    heredity and, 93
    infections, 94-95
        postpartum period and, 440-441
    male, 95
    menstruation and, 8, 94, 185
    nipples
        inverted, 93-94, 428
        milk secretion cessation and, 418
        nursing and, 270
        pregnancy and, 426, 427
        reconstructing, 99
    nursing and, see Infant feeding
    plastic surgery of, 97-99
    postpartum period
        breast-feeding, see Infant feeding
        engorgement, 440
        infections and, 440-441
    pregnancy, 426, 427
        breast shape and, 93
        nipples and, 426
    reconstruction, 422
        brassieres for, 99
        flaps and, 424
        nipples, 99
    self-examination, 94
    shape of, 93, 94
    swelling in newborn, 385
    symmetry of, 93
Breath
    bad breath, 319-320
    shortness of
        anemia and, 50
        heart failure and, 233

Breath-holding behavior, 108-109
Breathing
  cardiopulmonary resuscitation and, 620
  larynx and, 527
    obstruction, 529
  newborn difficulties with, 384
Breathing airways, as postoperative measure, 448
Breech delivery, 431, 436, 439
Bright's disease (glomerulonephritis), 296
Brill's disease, 281
Bronchial asthma, see Asthma
Bronchial tube, 544-545
  foreign body and, 566
  frozen section biopsy of, 314
  see also Bronchitis
Bronchiectasis, 336, 545-546
  asthma and, 26
  bronchitis and, 544-545
  cystic fibrosis and, 335
  sputum and, 546
Bronchitis, 544-545, 547
  common cold and, 544
  emphysema and, 332
  hoarseness and, 544
  respiratory acidosis, 310
  smoking and, 15
  sputum and, 545
  tracheitis and, 529
Bronchography, 545, 566
Bronchopneumonia, 333
Bronchoscopy, 155, 545, 546
  atelectasis of the newborn and, 267
  massive atelectasis and, 331-332
Brucellosis, 282
Bubonic plague, see Plague
Buerger's disease, 57-58
  sympathectomy for, 62
Bunions, 76-77
Burns, 422
  electric shock and, 214
  first-aid treatment for, 210-211
  larynx and, 530
  reconstruction and, 422, 423-424
  see also Plastic surgery
Bursitis, 75, 76
  bunions and, 76, 77
  heat therapy and, 412
  x-ray therapy for, 569
Butazolidin, for arthritis, 37, 39
Bypass operations, 379
  axillofemoral, 63
  carotid artery plaques and, 379
  coronary artery, 62-64, 243-244, 245
    arteriosclerosis and, 62-63
    coronary artery disease and, 238
  femoropopliteal, 63
  iliofemoral, 62
  renal artery obstruction and, 63-64
  see also Grafts
Byssinosis, 335

Caffeine, 351
Calamine lotion, chickenpox and, 116
Calcium
  blood chemistry for, 308
  deposits of and bursitis, 76
  newborn and, 388
  nursing mother and, 269
  pregnancy and, 427, 429

tetany of the newborn and, 267
  see also Parathyroid glands
Callus, 91
Calories, values of, 143-144
  see also Diet; Obesity; Underweight
Cancer, 100-106
  age groups and, 100
  anemia and, 50
  birth control pill and, 46
  blood chemistry test and, 310
  causes of, 100-101
  cure of, 104
  definition of, 100
  detection, 2
  diagnosis
    biopsy, 104
    CAT scan and, 103-104
    frozen section examination, 104
    microscopic report, 102-104
  endoscopy and, 154
  environment and, 100
  family tendency toward, 100
  heredity and, 287
  immunotherapy and, 105
  incidence, 100, 101
  informing patient of, 104
  Intensive Care Unit and, 292
  interferon and, 291
  lymph glands and, 52
  noninvasive (in situ), 188
  nonsurgical treatment of, 105, 106
    chemotherapy, 105
    hormone therapy, 106, 350
    radiation therapy, 105
  nuclear scan for, 570
  obesity and, 100, 136
  pain relief surgery for, 382
  preventing, 103
  recovery from, 105
    chances for, 104
    follow-up examinations and, 105
    metastasis and, 104
    pregnancy and, 105
  size, 104
  smoking and, 15
  spread, 101, 104, 105
  surgical treatment, 104
    recuperation, 104
    recurrence, 105
    removal of cancer and, 104-105
  untreated, 104
  virulence of, 101
  as virus, 105-106
  weight loss and, 104
  see also Biopsy; Radiation therapy;
    specific organs and sites
Canker sores, food allergy and, 26
Carbohydrates, diet for low, 142-143
Carbon dioxide snow hemangioma and, 67-68
Carbuncle, 5
  abscess distinguished from, 5
  cause, 5
Cardiac arrest, cardiopulmonary resuscitation and, 219-220
Cardiac arrhythmia, 239-240, 245
Cardiac Care Unit (CCU), 245-246
Cardiac catheterization, 234-235
Cardiac decompensation, see Heart failure
Cardiac massage, cardiopulmonary resuscitation and, 220
Cardiac monitoring equipment, Intensive Care Unit and, 292

Cardiopulmonary resuscitation (CPR), 220
  swallowed poisons and, 218
Carpal tunnel syndrome, 228
Cartilage, torn knee, 78-79
Caruncle of the urethra, 553-554
Cast, for fractures, 86
"Cast in the eye" (strabismus), see Eyes
Castor oil, foreign body in ear and, 214
Castration complex, 355
Cataracts, see Eyes
Catarrhal jaundice, see Infectious hepatitis
Catarrhal laryngitis (croup), 260, 528, 530, 544
Catheterization
  cardiac, 234-235
  postpartum period and, 440
  ureteral stones and, 299
  vaginal plastic operations, 181
  see also Urination
CAT scan (Computerized Axial Tomography), 565-566
  advantage of, 565
  sonography and, 566
  use of, 2
    brain, 565
    pancreas, 399
  x-ray exposure and, 565
  see also specific sites
Caudal anesthesia, 30, 32
Cauterization
  cervical, 187
  nosebleeds and, 394
Cavities, teeth, 331
Celiac disease, 260-261, 278
  stool analysis and, 315
Cellulose, obesity and, 134
Centipede, first aid for bite from, 209
Central nervous system, 362, 363, 372
  see also Nervous system;
    Neurosurgery; specific nervous
    diseases; Spine
Cerebral arteriosclerosis, see Arteriosclerosis
Cerebral edema, 376
Cerebral embolism, 366
Cerebral hemorrhage, 366-367, 378
Cerebral palsy, 79, 364-365
  exercises for, 413-414
  mental deficiency and, 359
Cerebral thrombosis, 366
Cerebrospinal fluid
  hydrocephalus and, 380
  leak through nose, 374
  spinal tap and, 370
Cerebrovascular accidents (strokes), see Stroke
Certified Registered Nurse Anesthetists (C.R.N.A.'s), 29
Cerumen (ear wax), 145, 149
Cervicitis, 186
Cervix, 186-189
  after childbirth, 441
  blocking sperm, 509
  cancer of, 187-189, 192, 196, 207, 339, 479
  cauterization of, 186-187
  cervicitis, 186
  description, 186
  erosion and, 187, 188, 430
  hysterogram, 194

measles and, 129
Papanicolaou smear, 187, 188, 189, 313-314
polyp, 187-188
pregnancy and, 426
Cesarean section, see Childbirth
Cesium isotope, 570
Chagas' disease, 403
Chancre, syphilis and, 557-558
see also Venereal diseases
Charcoal (activated), swallowed poisons and, 219
Checkup, see Physical examination
Chemicals
blood chemistry and, 309-310
burns (first-aid treatment for), 210
contact dermatitis and, 26
fumes (emphysema), 332
imbalance, see also Kidneys
hormones and, 350
Intensive Care Unit and, 292
poisoning
fatty liver and, 325
toxic hepatitis and, 327
Chemotherapy, 105
Chest
pain
heart attack and, 239
laxatives and, 349
lung cancer and, 337
x rays of, 566
Chewing
myasthenia gravis and, 80
nerve connected with, 362
Chickenpox (varicella), 116-117, 128, 252
genital herpes and, 560
shingles and, 479
Chilblain, 481
Child behavior
bedwetting, 112-113
breath-holding, 108-109
fears, 110-111
head-banging, 108
hyperactivity, 114-115
learning disability, 114
masturbation, 109-110
nailbiting, 108
nightmares, 110
night terrors, 110
parenting and, 115
sleep, 114
sleepwalking, 110
speech defects, 111
teeth-grinding, 108
temper tantrums, 109
thumbsucking, 107-108
tics, 109
see also Infancy
Childbirth
abnormal presentation, 431
age of, 15
cervical cancer and, 188
anesthesia for, 29, 434
breech delivery, 431, 436, 439
cerebral palsy and, 364-365
Cesarean section, 29, 438-440
abruptio placentae and, 446
anesthesia for, 29, 439
birth control, 41
breech presentation and, 436
cardiac patient and, 442
fetal distress and, 438

hyaline membrane disease and, 266
indications for, 438-439
myomectomy and, 195
pelvimetry x ray for, 567
placenta previa, 445
preeclampsia and, 444
pregnancy after, 440
prolapsed cord and, 437
vaginal plastic operations and, 180-181
dysmenorrhea and, 185
endometritis and, 191
episiotomy, 434-435, 441
fetal distress, 434, 438
forceps delivery, 435-436
hemorrhoids after, 441
hysterectomy after, 196
infection susceptibility and, 5
labor, 430-435
induced, 432-433, 446
inertia labor, 437-438
multiple births and, 437
postpartum hemorrhage, 440
prolapsed cord, 439
mental retardation and, 289
multiple births, see Pregnancy
natural (prepared), 433-435
nature of, 428-429
normal mechanisms (head presentation), 430-431
pelvimetry x ray for, 567
placenta (afterbirth), 435
abruptio placentae, 439
placenta previa, 431, 438, 445
postpartum hemorrhage, 440
postpartum period, 440-441
prematurity, see Newborn
prolapsed cord, 437, 439
stillbirth (erythroblastosis) and, 263
uterine prolapse and, 179-180
vagina and, 179
see also Birth Control; Congenital deformities; Infant feeding; Newborn; Pregnancy
Children
analgesics and, 348
anesthesia and, 32
bowel habits in, 455
constipation, 455
brain tumors in, 378
choking and, 211
diseases, see specific diseases
drug safety and, 345
growth retardation in
growth hormone and, 421
growth hormone tumor and, 418-419
heart trouble and, 231
immunization schedule, 252, see also Immunizations and vaccinations
informed consent and, 447
nose fracture in, 390
nutrition
diets, 274-275
eating habits, 10
reducing diet for, 136
vitamin needs, 562
plastic surgery on, 395, 422-423
radiation therapy and, 568
spleen removal and, 502, 504
tuberculosis and, 538, 540-541

vulvovaginitis and, 182
weight gain in, 136
see also Adolescence; Child behavior
Chin, plastic surgery for receding or protruding, 422, 535
Chlamydia infections, urethral infections and, 555
Chloral hydrate, 348
Chlorides, blood chemistry for, 308
Chloromycetin
tularemia and, 281
typhoid fever and, 280
Chloroquine, malaria and, 280, 404
Choking
first-aid treatment for, 211-212
from foreign body in the larynx or trachea, 156, 529
Cholangiogram, 567
Cholecystitis, 222
see also Gall bladder
Cholecystogram, 222, 567
Cholecystomy, 224
see also Gall bladder
Cholera, 285
diarrhea and, 488
gastroenteritis and, 489
vaccination, 257, 258, 285
Cholesterol
arteriosclerosis and, 15, 55-56, 310
blood chemistry for, 308, 309-310
heart disease and, 239
low-cholesterol diet, 138
Chondromas, 91
Chorea (St. Vitus' dance), rheumatic fever and, 466
Chromophobe adenoma, 418
Chromosomes, hallucinatory drugs and, 351-352
Chronic gastritis, 516
Chronic lung tuberculosis, see Tuberculosis
Chronic pharyngitis, 527
Chronic ulcerative colitis, 486, 488, 495
Cigarette cough, 545
Cimetidine, 515, 518
Cinefluorograms, 564
Cineradiograms, 564
Circulation, see Arteries; Blood; Blood vessels; Heart
Circumcision, 339-340, 385-386
cervical cancer and, 188
hemophilia and, 51
Cirrhosis of the liver, 52, 324-325, 327-328
alcoholism and, 18
blood vessel surgery for, 66
esophageal varicosities and, 159
mesocaval shunt and, 65, 537
spleen enlargement and, 502, 503
see also Liver
Claudication, 55
Claustrophobia, 355
Cleft palate, 317, 318
nursing and, 269
plastic surgery and, 422
Climate
arthritis and, 37
asthma and, 26
Climax, sexual, 474
Clinoril, 37, 38
Clitoris, 177, 178
Clomid, 437, 507

Closed cardiac massage, 220
Clot, *see* Thrombus
Clothing
  contact dermatitis and, 26
  scarlet fever spread by, 125, 130
  typhoid fever and, 279
Clubfoot, 69-70
Coarctation of the aorta, 241, 242
Cobalt treatments, 13, 568-570
  bladder tumor, 552
  breast removal, 97
  cancer, 104
  *see also* Radiation therapy
Cocaine, topical anesthesia and, 30-31
Cocoa, caffeine in, 351
Codeine, sinusitis and, 392
Cod liver oil, infant feedings and, 273
Coffee, caffeine in, 351
Cognitive psychotherapy, 356-357
Coitus interruptus, 42, 43
Colchicine, for gouty arthritis, 39
Cold
  allergy to, 28
  burns from, 210
  chilblain and, 481
  frostbite from, 211
  Raynaud's disease and, 56-57
  *see also* Common cold
Cold sores (herpes simplex), 478-479, 560
Colic, crying and, 107, 276
Colitis, 494-496
  amoebic, *see* Dysentery
  blood in stool, 456
  chronic ulcerative, 486, 488, 495
  colonoscopy and, 155
  description, 494
  dysentery, 495-496
  functional, 494
  intestinal obstruction and, 496, 497
  laxatives and, 349
  mucous, 494-495
  organic, 424
  as psychosomatic illness, 536
  spastic, 494
  stool analysis for, 315
  stress and, 361
Collarbone, 215
Colloid goiter, 532
Colon
  sigmoidoscopy for, 154
  *see also* Large intestine
Colonic irrigations, 488
Colonoscopy, 154
  bowel polyps and, 458, 498
  description, 498
  hemorrhoids and, 457
  mucous colitis and, 494
  prolonged diarrhea and, 488
  ulcerative colitis and, 495
Colostomy, *see* Large intestine
Colostrum, 269
Coma, 368-369
  brain injury and, 374
  diabetes mellitus and, 131
  eclampsia and, 444
  encephalitis and, 365
  meningitis and, 365
Common bile duct, *see* Gall bladder
Common cold, 543-544, 547
  bronchitis and, 544
  hoarseness and, 544
  influenza and, 547

middle ear infection and, 147
  nosebleeds and, 394
  sinusitis and, 392
  sore throat and, 526
Compensation cases, 3-4
Complete blood count, 305
Compulsion neurosis, 355
Computerized axial tomography, *see* CAT scan
Conception, *see* Pregnancy; Sexual intercourse
Concussion, 374
Condoms, 42, 43-44
Conduction deafness, 149-150
Conductive heat, heat treatments and, 412
Cone biopsy, 188
Confinement, *see* Childbirth
Confusion, hyperinsulinism and, 399
Congenital anemias, 49
Congenital atresia, 157
Congenital deafness, 149
Congenital deformities
  birth control and, 41
  branchial cysts, 530
  causes of
    drugs, 69, 288
    German measles, 119, 256
    radiation, 288
    x rays, 569
  cerebral palsy, 364
  cervical rib, 363
  cervicitis, 186
  cleft palate, 317-318
  clubfoot, 69-70
  congenital bronchiectasis, 546
  deafness (congenital), 149
  definition, 287
  of ear, 152, 153
  epilepsy, 367
  epispadias, 554, 555
  of esophagus, 156-157, 159
  of Fallopian tubes, 201
  hammer toe, 78
  of hand, 229
  harelip, 317
  of heart, 568
    congenital heart disease, 236, 241, 243
    valves, 332-333
  hemolytic anemia, 502
  hip dislocation, 69, 70
  Hirschsprung's disease, 262, 497
  hypospadias, 554, 555
  kidneys and, 300-301
  limb deformities, 70
  lung cysts, 337
  male sterility and, 510
  Meckel's diverticulum, 491
  phocomelia, 70
  pilonidal cysts, 416
  polydactylism, 70
  spinal cord, 380
  spondylolisthesis, 75
  treating
    plastic surgery, 422, 424
    rehabilitation, 414
  urethral stricture, 553
  varicocele, 343-344
  wry neck (torticollis), 76
  *see also* Pregnancy
Congenital fistula, 68
Congenital heart disease, 241

Congenital hemolytic anemia (hemolytic jaundice), 502, 503
Congenital laryngeal stridor, 268
Conjunctivitis, 165
  allergic, 165
  gonorrhea and, 165
  infectious ("pink eye"), 165
  measles and, 129
  red eyelid margins and, 162
  traumatic, 165
Conn's syndrome, 12
Consanguinity, 288
Constipation
  aging and, 455
  appendicitis and, 33
  blood in stool and, 456
  celiac disease and, 260-261
  children and, 455
  chronic, 455, 486, 488
  description, 486
  fissure in ano and, 459
  food allergy and, 26
  hernia and, 247
  infants and, 276
  lubricants for, 455, 488, *see also* Mineral oil
  pregnancy and, 429
  prolapse of the rectum and, 461
  recurrent, 455
  reducing diet and, 135-136
  "spastic colitis" and, 494
  ureteral stones and, 299
  *see also* Bowel movements; Enema; Large intestine; Laxatives; Rectum and anus; Stool
Contact dermatitis, 20, 26
Contact lenses, 163
  cataracts and, 170, 171
  nearsightedness and, 163
  soft, 163
Contact reactions, as physical allergy, 28
Contraception, *see* Birth control
Contraceptive jellies, foams, and suppositories, 42, 45
Contrast media, 565
Contusions, first aid for, 218
Convalescent serum, 252
Convergent strabismus ("lazy" eye), 172
Convulsions
  amaurotic familial idiocy and, 264
  barbiturates and, 348
  brain tumor and, 365, 377, 378
  eclampsia and, 362
  encephalitis and, 365
  first-aid treatment for, 368
  hyperinsulinism and, 399
  idiocy and, 359
  pneumonia and, 127
  rabies and, 283
  roseola and, 130
  tetanus and, 284
  tetany of the newborn and, 267
  *see also* Epilepsy
Cooley's anemia, 49
  spleen and, 502
Copper, Wilson's disease and, 290
Cordotomy, 382
Cornea, *see* Eyes
Corns, 77
Coronary artery disease, 233, 236-239
  angina pectoris, 232, 236-239, 243

arteriosclerosis and, 237
conditions predisposing toward, 239
coronary artery thrombosis, 62, 64,
  232, 233, 234, 237-239, 243-244,
  245
  arteriosclerosis and, 55-56
  endarterectomy for, 62
coronary insufficiency, 237
coronary occlusion, see Heart attack
definition of, 237
diet and, 239
men and, 239
physical exertion and, 239
smoking and, 239
surgery and, 238, 241, 242, 243-245
  see also Bypass operations
  see also Heart disease
Coronary insufficiency, 237
Coronary occlusion, see Heart attack
Coronary thrombosis, see Coronary
  artery disease
Corpus luteum cyst, 204
Corrosives, esophagus and, 157
Cortex, see Adrenal glands
Corticotropin secreting adenomas, 418
Cortisone, 267, 350-351
  see also Steroids
Cosmetics, 476
  allergy to, 162, 476
    contact dermatitis, 26
  infections from, 5
Cosmetic surgery, 422
  see also Plastic surgery
Cough
  asthma and, 25
  blood, 330
  bronchiectasis and, 546
  bronchitis and, 545
  celiac disease and, 261
  choking and, 211
  chronic pharyngitis and, 527
  cigarette, 545
  common cold and, 543
  croup and, 260
  emphysema and, 332
  hernia and, 247
  influenza and, 547
  laryngitis and, 544
  lung cancer and, 337
  massive atelectasis and, 331
  measles and, 129
  mucus and, 330
  nosebleeds and, 394
  silicosis and, 334
  tracheitis and, 529
  tuberculosis and, 538-539, 540
  whooping, 126-127
  see also Lungs
CPR, see Cardiopulmonary
  resuscitation
Crabs, 482
Cradle cap, 384
Cramps, abdominal, see Abdomen
Cranial nerves, 362
  organs supplied by, 362
Craniopharyngioma, 420
Craniotomy, pituitary tumor and, 420
  see also Neurosurgery
Creatinine, blood chemistry for, 308
Cretinism, 531
Crossed eyes (strabismus), see Eyes
Croup (catarrhal laryngitis), 260, 528,
  530, 544

Crying, in infants, 107
Cryosurgery
  cataract removal and, 170
  detached retina and, 174
  hemangioma and, 67-68
Cryptorchidism, 341-342
Culdoscope, 155
Curettage, see Dilatation and curettage
Cushing's disease, 12
Cutaneous ureterostomy, 552
Cyanosis, emphysema and, 332
Cyclic therapy, 192
  endometrial hyperplasia and,
    191-192
  ovarian dysfunction and, 203
Cyclopropane, childbirth and, 29-30,
  434
Cystadenomas, of breast, 95
Cystectomy, 552
Cystic fibrosis (mucoviscidosis), 262,
  335
Cystic mastitis, chronic, 95
Cystitis, 549
  bladder stones and, 551
Cystocele, 180, 181
  cystitis and, 549
Cystogram, 567
Cystoscopy, 155, 450, 549-550
  bladder tumor and, 552
  ureteral stones and, 299
  ureteroceles and, 303
Cystotomy, 452-453, 551
  ureteral strictures and, 553
Cysts
  Bartholin, 177
  bone, 408
  brain, 371
  branchial, 530
  breast, 95
  follicle, 203-204
  ganglion, 485
  jaw, 319
  kidney, 300
  liver, 327
  lung, 337-338
  osteitis fibrosa cystica, 81
  ovarian, 204-206
  pancreatic, 400
  pilonidal, 416-417
  sebaceous, 483-484

Dandruff, 480-481
Dark-field examination, 306
Deafness, see Ears
Defecation, see Bowel movements
Deficiency anemia, 49
Dehydration
  cholera and, 285
  impaired kidney function and, 294
  tongue and, 321
  ulcerative colitis and, 495
Delirium tremens (D.T.'s), 18-19
Delivery, see Childbirth
Dementia praecox, see Schizophrenia
Demerol, 30
Demyelination, multiple sclerosis and,
  370
Dengue fever, 281
Dental care, see Teeth
Deodorants
  contact dermatitis and, 26
  effectiveness, 478
  infections from, 5

Deoxyribonucleic acid (DNA), 287
Depilatories, 480
Depression, 354, 355, 356, 357, 358
  alcoholism and, 18
  menopause and, 207
  neurasthenia and, 354
  postpartum period and, 441
  psychotherapy for, 19, 415
  sexual desire and, 475
  stimulating drugs and, 351
de Quervain's disease, 228
Deranged knee, 78-79
Dermabrasion, 477
Dermal cysts, 483
Dermatitis
  atopic, 26
  contact, 26
Dermoid cyst, of ovary, 205
Developmental disability, see Mental
  deficiency
Deviated septum, 390-391
Dexedrine, 351
Diabetes insipidus, 420-421
Diabetes mellitus, 131-133
  amputation and, 70
  antidiabetic oral medication for, 132
  arteriosclerosis and, 55, 132
  avoiding, 131-132
  cause, 131
  coma and, 369
  Conn's syndrome and, 12
  coronary artery disease and, 239
  definition, 131
  diagnosis, 131
    blood chemistry for, 308
    glucose tolerance blood test, 131,
      308, 310
    urine analysis and, 131, 132, 311
  diet, 133
  eyes and, 175
    cataracts and, 170
  impotence and, 511
  incidence, 131
  infection and, 5, 132
    gangrene and, 7, 133
    kidneys and, 297
  insulin for, 131-132, see also
    Pancreas
    acidosis and, 132-133, 310-311
    bacteria-producing, 291
    function of, 397
    overdose, 368
  insulin shock (hypoglycemia), 132,
    212, 310, 397, 399-400
    blood chemistry for, 308
    fainting and, 368
  life span and, 133
  neuropathy from, 362-363
  pancreas removal and, 401
  pancreatitis and, 399
  physical activity and, 133
  predisposing factors in, 131
  pregnancy and, 133, 427, 442-443
    induced labor and, 432
  surgery and, 133
  symptoms, 131
  tuberculosis and, 539
  uncontrollable, 133
  urination frequency and, 295
Dialysis equipment
  arteriovenous fistula and, 68
  Intensive Care Unit and, 292
  see also Kidneys

Diaphragm
  as contraceptive, 42, 45
  hernia of, 247-248, 250, 251
Diarrhea
  acute gastritis and, 516
  antibiotics and, 489
  anxiety neurosis and, 354-355
  bloody
    Meckel's diverticulum and, 491
    ulcerative colitis and, 495
  celiac disease and, 261
  cholera and, 285
  description, 488
  dysentery and, 402
  food allergy and, 20, 26
  gastroenteritis and, 489, 516
  hookworm disease and, 404
  infants and, 277
  metabolic acidosis and, 310-311
  prolapse of the rectum and, 461
  recurrent, 455
  regional ileitis and, 489-490
  "spastic colitis" and, 494
  stool analysis and, 315
  toxic shock syndrome and, 185
  ulcerative colitis and, 495
  whipworm and, 404
  see also Bowel movements; Large
    intestine; Rectum and anus; Stool
Diathermy, 412
  for arthritis, 37
Dicumarol, 239
Diet
  acne and, 9
  aging and, 135
  bowel movement regularity and, 455
  breast-feeding and, 269
  celiac disease and, 261
  charts
    ambulatory ulcer, 141
    caloric values, 143-144
    elimination for allergies, 142
    gout (low purine), 140
    high-calorie (gaining), 141
    high-residue (high-roughage), 139
    liquid, 140
    low-calorie (reducing), 137
    low-carbohydrate, 142-143
    low-cholesterol, 138
    low-residue (low-roughage), 139
    low-salt (high blood pressure), 138
  chronic gastritis and, 516
  complexion and, 476
  constipation and, 455, 488
  coronary artery disease and, 239
  cystitis and, 549
  diabetes mellitus and, 131-133
  diverticulosis and, 493
  duodenal disorders and, 513
  gall bladder disease and, 221-226
  gastrectomy and, 513-514
  gouty arthritis and, 37, 39
  hay fever and, 25
  hemorrhoidectomy and, 457
  indigestion, 514
  infants and young children, 273-275,
    see also Infant feeding
    constipation and, 276
    cow milk allergy and, 278
    diarrhea and, 277
    mucous colitis and, 494
  kidney disease and, 295-296
    stones, 299

pancreatitis and, 397
peptic ulcer and, 517-518
pregnancy and, 427, 429
regional ileitis and, 490
rheumatoid arthritis and, 38
stomach acidity and, 515
stomach disorders and, 513
ulcer and, 518
ulcerative colitis and, 495
urethral infection and, 555
weight reduction, see Obesity
see also Fluids; Obesity;
  Underweight; Vitamins
Differential blood count, 305-307
Digitalis, heart failure and, 234
Dilantin, 363
Dilatation and curettage (D and C), 190,
  191, 198
  endometrial hyperplasia and,
    190-192
Diodoquin, amoebic dysentery and,
  403
Diphtheria, 117, 118, 128
  croup and, 260
  Schick test, 253
  vaccination, 252, 257, 258
Disability, 3-4
  see also Physical therapy;
    Rehabilitation; specific diseases
Diseases
  periodic health examination and, 2
  stress and, 360-361
  see also Immunizations and
    vaccinations; specific diseases
Disseminated sclerosis, see Multiple
  sclerosis
Diverticulosis, 493
  colonoscopy for, 155
Diverticulitis, 488, 493-494
  bladder fistula and, 551
  colonoscopy for, 155
Diverticulum
  bladder stones and, 551
  of the esophagus, 158-159
  of the urethra, 554
Dizziness
  anxiety neurosis and, 354-355
  brain tumor and, 365
  first-aid treatment for, 214
  head injury and, 376
  neurasthenia and, 354
  pregnancy and, 430
  see also Vertigo
Doctor
  child's fear of, 111
  compensation cases and, 3-4
  confiding in, 3
  fees, 1
  health examination tests decided
    by, 2
  hospital choice and, 1
  medical records and, 2-3
  nursing service advice from, 2
  selecting, 1
Dog bite, rabies and, 256-257, 258,
  283-284
  see also Bites
Dominant characteristic, 287, 289
Douches, 42, 44, 45
  abortion and, 199
  acidic vagina and, 509
  after childbirth, 441
  birth control and, 42, 44, 45

bleeding after, 188
cauterization of cervix and, 187
cervicitis and, 186
dilatation and curettage and, 191
intercourse and, 179, 509
pessary and, 180
pregnancy and, 430
Down's syndrome, 289, 290, 359
Dreams
  erotic, 472
  nightmares and, 110
Drinking, see Alcohol abuse; Alcohol
  consumption
Dropsy, cirrhosis and, 325
Drowning
  first-aid treatment for, 212-213, 214
  reflex reactions and, 28
Drug addiction, 346
  hallucinatory drugs, 351-352
  infectious hepatitis and, 326
  tranquilizers, 348-349
Drug allergy, 21, 25, 27
  to analgesics (aspirin), 347-348
  to antibiotics, 346
  to hormones, 350
  to steroids, 22, 24
Drugs
  advertisements about, 345
  alcoholism and, 19
  breast-feeding and, 269
  chemotherapy, 106
  children and, 345
  expiration, 345
  government control of, 345
  immunity to, 346
  in home medicine cabinet, 345
  over-the-counter, 345
  overdose, 218, 346, 348
    antibiotics, 346-347
    barbiturates, 348
    laxatives, 349
    narcotics, 349
    sleeping pills, 368
    stimulating drugs, 351
    tranquilizers, 348, 356
  pregnancy and, 69, 236, 287, 346,
    430
  prescription renewal, 346
  professional advice on taking, 345
  reading label on, 345
  reuse, 345
  self-medication, 345
    analgesics, 347
    stimulating drugs, 351
    sulfa drugs, 347
    tranquilizers, 348
  weight-gain and, 134, 136
  weight-reduction and, 349-350
  see also specific drugs; specific drug
    groups, e.g., Antibiotics
Duodenitis, 515, 516-517
Duodenum
  alcohol and, 18
  disease
    diagnosis of, 513
    diet and, 513-514
    emotional symptoms and, 514
    proclivity toward, 513
    symptoms of, 513
  duodenal (peptic) ulcer, see Ulcer
  function, 513
  gallstone retrieval from, 226

gastroduodenoscopy and, 154
inflammation of the (duodenitis), 515, 516-517
Dupuytren's contracture, 228
Dust
    allergy to, 21, 22, 23, 25
    pneumonoconiosis and, 418
Dwarfism, 421
Dyes
    allergy to, 21
    contact dermatitis and, 26
Dysentery
    amoebic, 403, 495
        gastroenteritis and, 489
        liver and, 324
        sexual contact and, 402
    bacillary, 495
Dysmenorrhea, 185
Dyspareunia (painful intercourse), see Sexual intercourse
Dyspepsia, see Indigestion

Ears, 145-153
    acoustic nerve for, 362
        tumors, 151
    anatomy, 146
    brain tumor and, 378
    congenital deformities of, 152-153
    deafness, 148-151
        cause for, 148
        central, 149
        conductive (middle ear), 149-151
        congenital, 149
        fenestration operation, 150
        German measles and, 288
        hearing aid for, 149-150
        otosclerosis and, 150-151
        perceptive (inner ear), 149
        stapedectomy, 150-151
        surgery for, 150
        talking and, 111-112, 149
        tympanoplasty, 151
    ear canal pain, 145
    eardrum
        middle ear infection and, 147, 148
        myringotomy, 147
        perforated, 149
        tympanoplasty, 151
    equilibrium and, 151
    Eustachian tube
        middle ear infections and, 147
        obstruction, 569
    foreign body in, 214
    hearing, 145
        adenoids and, 524
        heredity and, 15
        mastoidectomy and, 148
        mastoiditis and, 148
        Ménière's syndrome, 151-152
        middle ear infection and, 147-148
        noise damage, 145
        tests, 145, 147
    infection
        chickenpox and, 116
        lymph glands and, 52
        measles and, 121, 129
        rheumatic fever and, 465
    mastoid
        mastoidectomy, 148
        middle ear infection and, 147
    Ménière's syndrome, 151-152, 369
    middle ear, 145-146
        adenoids inflammation and, 523-524

deafness and, 149-150
infection (otitis media), 116, 147-148, 544
myringotomy and, 147
pain in, 146
tonsil inflammation and, 523-524
of newborn, 384
plastic surgery of, 152-153, 422, 425
replantation surgery, 464
vertigo and, 151, 369
wax (cerumen), 145
    impacted, 149
Eating habits, 514-515
    adolescence and, 10
    indigestion and, 514
    see also Diet; Obesity; Underweight
Echinococcus cyst, 324, 327, 406
Echocardiogram, 234
ECHO virus disease, 285
Eclampsia, 444-445
Ectopic pregnancy, see Pregnancy
Ectropion, 167-168
Eczema, 20, 26, 478
    atopic dermatitis as, 26
    psychosomatic illness and, 356
    smallpox vaccination and, 254
    varicose veins and, 67
Edema, cerebral, 376
Eggs, see Food allergy
Ejaculation, 43
Elbow
    arthroplasty for, 84, 85
    bursitis and, 76
    psoriasis and, 482
Elderly, see Aging
Electric shock, first-aid treatment for, 214
Electrocardiogram, 231, 234, 239, 240
Electrocauterization, cervicitis and, 186-187
Electroencephalography (EEG), 371
Electrolysis, 480
    breast hair and, 94
Electroshock therapy, 357-358
Elephantiasis, 405
Embolism, see Blood vessels
Emergencies, see First-aid treatments
Emotional disturbance, 405
    adolescence and, 9-10
    aging and, 15
    allergy and, 21, 24
    bedwetting and, 112, 295
    colitis and, 494-495
    epilepsy and, 368
    fainting and, 368
    gouty arthritis and, 39
    heart and, 232
    high blood pressure and, 235
    hyperactivity and, 115
    impotence and, 511
    indigestion and, 514
    infertility and, 509
    lower back pain and, 73
    menopause and, 207
    menstruation and, 184
    migraine and, 369
    peptic ulcer and, 518
    pregnancy and, 430
    Raynaud's disease and, 56-57
    sexual intercourse and, 177, 472
    stomach acidity, 515
    tics as, 109

underweight and, 136
    see also Mental illness; Stress
Emphysema, 332
    asthma causing, 26
    bronchiectasis and, 546
    cystic fibrosis and, 335
    respiratory acidosis and, 310
    smoking and, 15
Empyema, 336
Encephalitis, 365
    Asiatic flu and, 548
    chickenpox and, 116, 128
    coma and, 368-369
    German measles and, 128
    gonorrhea and, 557
    infectious mononucleosis and, 283
    measles and, 121, 129
    mumps and, 129
    Parkinsonism and, 370
    smallpox vaccination and, 254
    whooping cough and, 130
Encephalography, 370-371
Endarterectomy, 379, 536-537
    arteriosclerosis and, 62
    stroke and, 62, 536-537
Endocarditis, 245
    bacterial, 241
Endocrine glands, 418
    obesity, 134
    underweight, 136
    see also Hormones; specific disorders; specific glands; specific hormones
Endometrial biopsy, 191, 507-508
Endometrial hyperplasia, 190, 192, 195, 196, 203
Endometrial polyps, 195
Endometriosis, 197
    blocked Fallopian tubes and, 508
    dysmehorrhea and, 185
    of ovary, 205
Endometritis, 191
Endometrium, see Uterus
Endoscope, 154-155
    duodenal disease and, 513, 516
    gallstone removal and, 226
    stomach disease and, 513
        cancer and, 521
    see also specific kinds of endoscopy, e.g., Colonoscopy
Endotracheal anesthesia, 31, 32
Endotracheal tube, elective tracheotomy and, 530
Enema
    abdominal pain and, 33
    before x ray, 566
    constipation and, 455
    frequency of, 488
    heat stroke and, 216
    megacolon and, 497
    mucous colitis, 494
    as postoperative routine, 449
    as preoperative routine, 499
Entamoeba histolytica, liver and, 324
Entropion, 167-168
Enuresis, 112-113, 295
Ephedrine, 351
Epidemic hepatitis, see Infectious hepatitis
Epidemic (infectious) jaundice, 281-282
Epidemic parotitis, see Mumps
Epidemic typhus fever, 281

Epididymis
    epididymitis, 343
    prostatectomy and, 454
Epididymitis, 343
Epidural anesthesia, 30
Epigastric hernia, 247
Epiglottis
    choking and, 211
    congenital laryngeal stridor, 268
    larynx and, 527
Epilepsy, 367-368
    barbiturates and, 347
    causes of, 367
    control of, 367-368
    convulsions in, 212
    cure, 368
    electroencephalography and, 371
    grand mal seizure, 367
    having children and, 368
    heredity and, 368
    incidence, 368
    Jacksonian seizures, 367
    petit mal seizures, 367
    precautions and, 368
    psychomotor seizures, 367
    symptoms of, 367
Epinephrine, 25, 27
Episiotomy, 434-435
Epispadias, 554, 555-556
Equilibrium, 151
Ergot, abortion and, 199
Erythroblastosis (Rh-factor disease),
    263-264, 311-312
    exchange transfusions for, 263-264,
        309, 312
    intrauterine transfusion, 309
    mental retardation and, 289
Esophagitis, 157
Esophagoscopy, 154, 155, 156
Esophagus, 156-160
    achalasia (spasm of esophagus),
        158, 159
    birth deformities and, 156-157
        congenital atresia, 157
        congenital web of esophagus, 157
        tracheoesophageal fistula, 156
    corrosives swallowed and, 157
    description, 156
    diverticulum of, 158, 159
    esophagoscopy and, 154, 155, 156
    food stuck in, 156
    hiatus hernia of, 157
    hot foods and, 156
    peptic ulcer, see Ulcers
    regurgitation, 156
    ruptured, 157-158
    swallowing inability, 156
    throat tightness and, 156
    tumor of, 160
    varicose veins of, 159
        cirrhosis and, 325
    vomiting alkalis or acids and, 218
    see also Duodenum; Stomach
Espundia, 403
Estrogen, 203
    birth control pills and, 46
    hyperplasia and, 191
    osteoporosis and, 81
    senile vaginitis and, 182
Ethambutol, 542
Ether, 29
Ethmoid sinuses (ethmoidectomy), 392
Ethrane (enflurane), 30, 31

Eustachian tube, see Ear
Examination, see Physical examination
Exanthem subitum (roseola), 124, 130
Excisional biopsy, 314
Exenteration operation, cervical cancer
    and, 189
Exercise
    aging and, 14, 16
    heart disease and, 14
    longevity and, 14
    middle age and, 15
    obesity and, 134
    osteoarthritis and, 39
    thrombophlebitis and, 59-60
    see also Physical therapy
Extradural hemorrhage, 375
Extrasystole, 239
Extremities
    amputation, 72
    diabetes mellitus and, 132
    heart failure and, 233
    see also Ankle; Feet; Finger;
        Fracture; Hands; Legs; Toes
Eye banks, cornea transplants and,
    166, 175
Eyedrops
    abrasion of cornea and, 166
    atropine, 168
    chalazion and, 166
    conjunctivitis and, 165
    cortisone, 166, 168
    detached retina and, 175
    eyestrain and, 161
    glaucoma and, 169
    iritis and, 168
    to newborn, 385
    strabismus surgery and, 173
Eyeglasses
    astigmatism and, 165
    cataract removal and, 171
    eyestrain and, 161
    facial paralysis and, 364
    farsightedness and, 164
    nearsightedness and, 163
    strabismus and, 172
    see also Contact lenses
Eyelids
    cysts (chalazion), 166-167
    ectropion, 167-168
    entropion, 167-168
    itching, 162
    plastic surgery for burns of, 422, 423
    styes, 166-167
    swelling, 162
    trachoma, 176
Eyes, 161-176
    arteriosclerosis and, 55
    astigmatism, 164-165
        contact lenses and, 163
        eyestrain and, 165
    "black eye," 162
    blindness
        amaurotic familial idiocy and,
            264-265
        corneal transplantation and, 166
        detached retina and, 174
        diabetes mellitus and, 175
        German measles and, 289
        glaucoma and, 168
        heredity and, 15
        iritis and, 168
        Niemann-Pick disease and, 265
        retinal thrombosis and, 176

    retrolental fibroplasia and, 266
    trachoma and, 176
    brain condition and, 369
        tumor and, 365, 377
    bulging of the, 162
        hyperthyroidism and, 521-532, 534
    burns, 211
    cataracts, 169-171
        cause, 170
        contact lenses and, 170, 171
        diabetes mellitus and, 175
        diagnosis, 170
        eyeglasses and, 171
        intraocular lenses and, 170
        surgery, 170-171
    color, 161
    cornea
        conjunctivitis and, 165
        foreign body in, 165
        keratomileusis and, 163
        laceration of, 165-166
        scratch in, 166
        trachoma, 176
        transplants, 166, 535
        ulcer of, 166
    dacryocystitis, 168
    diabetes mellitus and, 132, 175
    examination, 161
    eyeball
        foreign body in, 165
        glaucoma and, 168-169
        spots floating in front of eyes and,
            162
    farsightedness (hyperopia), 164
        convergent strabismus and, 172
        detecting, 164
    foreign bodies in, 214
    glaucoma, 168-169
    hay fever and, 23
    iris
        eye color and, 161
        iritis, 168
    itching, 162
    lens, 169-170
    nearsightedness (myopia), 162-164
        contact lenses for, 163
        detached retina and, 164
        detecting, 163
        divergent strabismus and, 172
        exam and, 163
        eyeglasses and, 163
        surgery for, 163
    nerves connected with, 362
    normal, 161, 162
    pupils
        in children, 161
        shock and, 219
    retina
        amaurotic familial idiocy and, 264
        description, 173
        detached, 163-164, 173-175
        glioma of, 175-176
        retinal thrombosis, 176
        tear, 173-175
    spots before the, 162
        hyperinsulinism and, 399
        preeclampsia and, 443
        pregnancy complications and,
            441-442
    strabismus (crossed eyes), 171-173
        cause, 171-172
        convergent ("lazy" eye), 172
        danger of, 172

divergent, 171-172
medical treatment, 172
patch for, 172, 173
prevention, 172
surgery for, 172, 173
styes, 166-167
sympathetic ophthalmia, 176
tearing, 161
trachoma, 176
tumors, 175-176
detached retina and, 174-175
gliomas, 175-176
melanoma, 175
Vitamin A deficiency and, 561
see also Conjunctivitis; Newborn
Eyestrain, 161, 162
astigmatism and, 164-165

Face
acromegaly and, 419-420
adenoid enlargement and, 523-524
aging and
brown spots and, 476
plastic surgery and 422, 425
animal or human bites and, 209
burns of and reconstruction, 422,
423, 424
fractured bone on, 215
infections of, 5, 52
nerve connected with, 362
parotid gland tumor removal and,
469-470
pimples on, 6
plastic surgery, wrinkles and, 476
trigeminal neuralgia (tic douloureux)
and, 363-364
see also Skin
Facial paralysis (Bell's palsy), 364
Fainting, 368
first-aid treatment for, 214
hyperinsulinism and, 399
pregnancy complications and, 430, 442
Fallopian tubes (uterine tubes), 199-202
blocked, 508-509
description, 199-200
hysterogram of, 567
peritonitis and, 410
salpingitis, 200-201
surgical sterilization and, 47
tubal (ectopic) pregnancy, 201-202
Family planning, see Birth control
Farmers' lung, 335
Farsightedness, see Eyes
Fasting
gastroenteritis and, 516
indigestion and, 514
preoperative routines and, 447
stomach x rays and, 566
Fatigue, 354
allergy and, 21, 24
bronchitis, 544-545
headache and, 369
heart failure and, 233
infection susceptibility and, 5
menopause and, 207
muscular, 11
muscular dystrophy and, 80
myasthenia gravis and, 79-80
pregnancy and, 428, 441
sexual desire and, 475
tuberculosis and, 538, 539
Fat necrosis, breast and, 95
Fatty Liver, 325

Fatty tumors (lipomas), 483, 485
Fears, children and, 110-111
Feces, see Stool
Feet
athlete's foot, 477-478
clubfoot, 69-70
flat (pes planus), 77
fracture of, 90
ganglion and, 485
infection, 52
plantar warts, 77, 484
pregnancy complications and, 430,
441-442
see also Legs; Metatarsal; Toes
Felon, 229
Female organs, 190, 193
after childbirth, 441
aging and, 16
culdoscope and, 155
deformities of and plastic surgery,
422
removal and sexual activity, 472
see also Childbirth; Douches;
Hysterectomy; Menstruation;
Pregnancy; Sexual intercourse;
specific organs; Sterility; Venereal
disease
Femoral hernia, 247
Femoropopliteal graft, 63
Fenestration operation, deafness and,
150-151
Fertility, see Birth control; Fertilization;
Pregnancy; Sterility
Fertility pills, 437
multiple births and, see Pregnancy
Fertilization, 42-43, 506-507
see also Pregnancy
Fetal distress, see Childbirth
Fetal heartbeat, 426
fetal distress and, 437
monitoring, 434
see also Pregnancy
Fetology, 430
Fever
blankets for, 121
convulsion associated with, 368
Fibrillation, of heart, 240-241
Fibroadenomas, of breast, 95
Fibroids, of uterus, 192-194, 196, 431,
439, 508, 509
Fibromas, 483, 485
of lip, 316
of ovary, 205
of tongue, 322
of vaginal wall, 179
Fibula, fracture of, 89
Filariasis, 405
Finger
dislocated, 216
ganglion and, 485
osteoarthritic nodes on joint, 39
polydactylism, 70
Raynaud's disease and, 57
replacement of joint, 84
replantation surgery and, 463, 464
see also Hands
Fingernails, blueness of and heart
failure, 233
Fingertip injury, 227
First-aid treatments
abrasions, 218
bites
animal or human, 209

insect, 209
snake, 210
burns, 210-211, 214
cardiopulmonary resuscitation
(CPR), 219-220
choking, 211-212, 529
Heimlich maneuver, 211-212, 219
colic, 276
concussion, 374
contusions, 218
convulsion, 212, 368
dislocation, 216
dizziness, 214
drowning, 212, 213, 214
eyes
foreign body in, 165
scratch in, 165-166
fainting, 214
foreign bodies, 214
in eyes, 165
strangulation and, 219
fracture, 87, 215-216
arm, 215
back, 216
collarbone, 215
compound, 215
jaw, 215, 318-319
leg, 215-216
shock and, 219
shoulder, 215
skull, 215
frostbite, 211
gas poisoning, 216
heat exhaustion, 216-217
heat stroke, 216
hemorrhage, 217-218
lacerations, 218
neck injury, 216
nosebleed, 394
poisoning, 213, 218-219
radiation exposure, 219
shock, 219
electric, 214
splinters, 214
sprain, 216
stab wounds, 214-215
strangulation, 219-220
suffocation, 213, 219
tracheotomy (emergency), 530
vertigo, 214
Fissure in ano, 459
Fistula
arteriovenous, 68
bladder, 550-551
tracheoesophageal, 156-157
Fistula in ano, 459, 460
Fits, see Convulsions
5—FU, 522
Flagyl, trichomonas infections and, 182
Flaps, 423-424
free, 423, 424
Flashes (hot), menopause and, 207
Flatfeet (pes planus), 77
Fleas
plague and, 282
rickettsial disease and, 281
Flies
polio spread by, 123
typhoid fever spread by, 279
Flu, see Influenza
Fluids
accumulation (heart failure) and, 233
acute gastritis and, 516

cholera and, 285
common cold and, 543
cystitis and, 549
diet, 140
epilepsy and, 368
gastroenteritis and, 515-516
kidney function and, 294
at mealtime, 514
Ménière's disease and, 369
postoperative measure and, 449
prostatic infections and, 450
pyelonephritis and, 442
retention (dysmenorrhea) and, 185
urethral infection and, 555
Fluke worms, 405
Fluoroscopy, 564
duodenal disease and, 513
stomach disease and, 513
Fluothane (halothane), 434
Foams, as contraceptives, 42, 45
Follicle cysts, 203-204
Fontanelle, of newborn, 384, 385
Food
contamination
amebiasis and, 402-403
gastroenteritis and, 489
infectious hepatitis and, 326
typhoid fever and, 279
poisoning, 489
Food allergy, 21, 25, 26
atopic eczema and, 26
to cow's milk, 277, 278
diarrhea in infants and, 277
eggs
German measles vaccination and, 119
measles vaccination and, 255
mumps vaccination and, 256
elimination diet for, 142
hives and, 27
rhinitis and, 23
to spices, 27
Foodpipe, see Esophagus
Foot, see Feet
Forceps delivery, 435-436
Foreign bodies, first aid for
in larynx, 530
in lung (bronchitis), and, 545
in trachea, 529
treatments for, 214-215
X-ray examination and, 565, 567
Formula, bottle-feeding and, see Infant feeding
Fractures, 84-91
ankle, 84, 90
arm, 88
comminuted, 85, 90
compound, 85, 90
delayed union, 87
foot, 90
hand, 228
healing of, 91
incomplete (greenstick), 85
jaw, 318-319
leg, 89, 91
nose, 389-390
pathologic, 90
pelvic region, 89
shock and, 219
shoulder, 88
simple, 85
skull
deafness and, 149

depressed, 374-375
spinal column, 381-382
treatment
cast, 85, 88-90
results, 87, 90
setting, 85-86, 87, 90
traction, 86, 88, 89
whirlpool bath, 413
x ray of, 91, 567-568
see also First-aid treatments
Free flaps, 423-424
Frigidity, 472-473
Frontal sinus, surgery on the, 392
Frostbite, first-aid treatment for, 211
Frozen section biopsy, 314
cancer and, 104
of breast, 96
of ovary, 206
Full-thickness grafts, 423, 425
Fundal plication, 249
Fungus infections, 477-478
see also specific infections

Galactocele, 95
Galactosemia, 289
Gall bladder, 221-226
attack, 514
chemical disturbance, 221
cholecystography of, 567
common bile duct, 221
functional disorder of, 222
gallstone in, 222-225, 226
gastroduodenoscopy and, 154
spasms (biliary dyskinesia), 226
surgery and, 224-225
description, 221, 223
disease, 221-224
cancer, 224
causes, 221
diagnosis, 222
diet for, 221, 222, 224, 225
as food allergy, 26
incidence, 221
peritonitis and, 410-411
preventing, 222
symptoms, 222
functional disorder, 222
gallstones, 221-224
cancer and, 224
in common bile duct, 222, 224-226
diagnosing, 222
inflammation and, 222
jaundice and, 224, 225
liver damage and, 324
pancreatitis and, 397
pregnancy and, 221
sonography and, 500-501
treatment, 224-226
visualization, 567
inflammation, 221
surgery
liver and, 329
removal (cholecystectomy), 221, 224
Gallstones, see Gall bladder
Gamma globulin, 252, 255-256
chickenpox and, 116
infectious hepatitis and, 326
measles and, 120, 129
Ganglion, 229, 483, 485
Gangrene
amputation and, 7, 70
Buerger's disease and, 57-58

diabetes mellitus and, 133
gall bladder disease and, 222, 224
hemorrhoids and, 456
intussusception and, 492
Raynaud's disease and, 57
strangulated hernia and, 249
thrombosis and, 58
torsion of the testicle, 343
volvulus and, 492
Gas gangrene antitoxin, compound fracture and, 90
Gas poisoning, first-aid treatments for, 216
Gastrectomy, 513-514
duodenal ulcer, 520
stomach cancer and, 521-522
subtotal, 518-519
Gastric analysis, 312-313
Gastric (peptic) ulcer, see Ulcer
Gastritis
acute, 515-516
atrophic, 516
chronic, 516
stomach acidity and, 517-518
Gastroduodenoscopy, 154
Gastroenteritis, 489, 515-516
Gastrointestinal (food) allergy, see Food allergy
Gastroscopy, 154, 155
chronic gastritis and, 516
peptic ulcer and, 517
Gaucher's disease, spleen and, 502, 503
General inhalation anesthesia, 29, 31-32
Genetic counseling, 288, 291
mental deficiency and, 360
sickle-cell anemia and, 49
Genetic engineering, 291
Genetic medicine, 290-291
Genital herpes, see Venereal diseases
Genital lice, 481, 482
Genitals, see specific male and female organs; Venereal diseases
German measles (rubella), 118-119, 128
cleft palate and, 317
congenital deafness and, 149
congenital heart disease and, 236
mental retardation and, 288
pregnancy and, 288
vaccination, 252, 256, 258
Giant, growth hormone tumor and, 418-419
Giant cell tumors, 91
Gibraltar fever, 282
Gill slits (branchial cysts), 530
Glands, see Endocrine glands; Lymph glands
Glandular fever, see Infectious mononucleosis
Glaucoma, 168-169
Gliadin, celiac disease and, 261
Glioma, 377
of eye, 175-176
Globulin, blood chemistry for, 308
Glomerulonephritis, 296
Glossitis, 321
Glucose tolerance test, 131, 308, 310
Gluteal hernia, 248
Gluten products, celiac disease and, 260
Goiter, see Thyroid gland
Gold isotope, 569

Gold salts, for rheumatoid arthritis, 38
Gonorrhea, *see* Venereal diseases
Gout, 298
    blood chemistry for, 308
    diet for, 140
Gouty arthritis, 37, 39
Graft
    aortic aneurysm and, 65
    arterial, 62-63, 64-65
    blood vessel transplants and,
      535-536, 537
    bone, 86, 92
    patch, 62
    skin, *see* Reconstructive surgery
    tendons and, 227
    *see also* Bypass operations; Shunt
Grand mal seizures, epilepsy and, 367
Grass, allergy to, 21
Grippe, *see* Influenza
"Ground itch," hookworms and, 404
Group therapy, 357
Growth
    chart, 9
    menstruation and, 8
    pituitary gland and, 418
Growth hormone tumors, 418-419
Guinea pig inoculations, 315
Guthrie's test, 290
Gynecomastia, 95

Hair
    adolescence and facial, 8
    allergy to animal, 21
    baldness, 479-480
    dandruff, 480-481
    dyeing and, 480
    electrolysis, 480
    excessive growth of, on women, 480
    graying, 16
      premature, 480
    hirsutism, 203
    loss of (alopecia), 480
      leprosy and, 282
    of newborn, 384
    radiation therapy and, 569
    seborrheic dermatitis, 480-481
    shampoo frequency, 480
    split-thickness graft and, 425
Hallucinations, delirium tremens and,
    18-19
Hallucinatory drugs, 351-352
Halothane, 29-30, 31
Hammer toe, 78
Handedness, changing, 111
Handicapped, *see* Physical therapy;
  Rehabilitation; *specific diseases*
Hands, 227-229
    anatomical snuffbox of, 218
    arthritis of, 83
    artificial, 72
    birth deformities of, 229
    burns, 422, 425
    carpal tunnel syndrome, 228
    chapped, 476
    de Quervain's disease, 228
    Dupuytren's contracture, 228
    ganglion, 229
    human bites and, 229
    infection, 52, 229
    injuries
      dislocated finger, 227-228
      fingertip, 227
      fracture, 228

      incidence, 227
      "jammed" finger, 227-228
      nerve, 227
      skier's thumb, 228
      tendon, 227
    pinched nerve, 228
    skin cancer and, 485
    surgery
      reconstructive, 422, 423, 424
      replantation, 464
      trigger fingers, 228
      tumors, 228-229
Harelip, 317
    breast-feeding and, 269
Harrington rods, 75
Hay fever, *see* Allergy
Head
    injuries to, 374-376, *see also*
      Neurosurgery
      concussion, 374, 376
    of newborn, 384
    pituitary gland malfunction and,
      420-421
    *see also* Brain
Headache
    allergy and, 20, 369
    analgesics and, 347-343
    laxatives and, 349
    migraine, 369
    significance of, 369
Head-banging, 109
Head lice, 481
Health examination, *see* Physical
  examination
Health insurance, 1-2
Hearing, *see* Ears
Hearing aids, 149-150
Heart, 231-246
    adrenalin and, 11
    alcohol consumption and, 18-19, 232
    aneurysm and, 243
    angiocardiography, 235
    arrhythmias of, 233, 239-240, 245
      extrasystole, 239-240
      paroxysmal, 240
    arteriosclerosis and, 55-56
    bacterial endocarditis and, 241, 245
    "blue baby" and, 236, 243
    Cardiac Care Unit (CCU), 245-246
    cardiac catheterization, 234-235
    cardiopulmonary resuscitation and,
      219-220
    cholesterol and, 135
    coarctation of aorta, 242, 243
    congenital heart disease, 236, 241
      angiocardiography of, 568
    echocardiogram of, 234
    electrocardiogram of, 231, 234, 239,
      240
    embolism and, 58, 466
    endocarditis and, 466
    fibrillation of, 240-241, 466
    fluoroscope and, 231, 234
    hyperthyroidism and, 531-532
    impaired function, 231, 232-233
      asthma and, 26
      diabetes mellitus and, 132
      exercise and, 14
      longevity and, 16
      pregnancy and, 442
      sexual intercourse and, 472
    medications and, 232
    mitral commissurotomy, 242

    murmurs, 241
    myocarditis, 465
    obesity and, 15, 135, 232
    pain in, 232
    palpitations, 240
      anemia and, 50
      anxiety neurosis and, 354-355
    patent ductus arteriosus, 242, 243
    pericarditis, 241-243
    physical exertion and, 231
    pulmonic stenosis, 241
    radionucleotide studies of, 234
    rheumatic fever and, 465-467
    septal defects, 241, 242
    smoking and, 15, 232
    sonography and, 500-501
    stress test of, 234
    "strong," 231
    structure, 230, 231, 233
    surgery, 241-245
      benefits from, 241-243
      coronary bypass operation for,
        62-63, 243-245
      Intensive Care Unit and, 292-293
      internal mammary artery implant
        operation and, 63
      transplant, 245, 534, 535-536
    valves and, 232-233
      care, 245
      infection (bacterial endocarditis),
        241
      rheumatic fever and, 232-233,
        465-466
      rheumatic heart disease and, 241,
        242, 243, 465
      surgery and, 245
    x ray of (angiocardiography), 231,
      234, 565-567, 568
    *see also under* Coronary
Heart attack (coronary occlusion), 237,
  239
    birth control pill and, 46
    indigestion and, 514
    smoking and, 232
Heart block, 240, 243
Heartburn, 514
    chronic gastritis and, 516
    duodenal disorders and, 513
    gall bladder disorder and, 222
    indigestion and, 514
    pregnancy and, 430
    stomach disorders and, 513, 514
    ulcer and, 517
Heart failure (cardiac decompensation),
  233-234, 245
    emphysema and, 332
Heart muscle, myocarditis and, 245, 465
Heat
    allergy to, 28
    cystic fibrosis and, 261-263
Heat exhaustion, first-aid treatment for,
  216-217
Heat stroke, first-aid treatment for, 216
Heat therapy, *see* Physical therapy
Heimlich maneuver, 211-212, 219, 530
Hemangioma, *see* Blood vessels
Hematological blood tests, *see*
  Laboratory tests
Hematology, 105
Hematoma, breast and, 95
Hemiplegia, 366
Hemodialysis, arteriovenous aneurysm
  and, 59

Hemoglobin, 48, 306
  sickle-cell anemia and, 48-49
  *see also* Blood
Hemolytic anemia, 49
Hemolytic disease of newborn,
  *see* Erythroblastosis
Hemolytic jaundice, 502, 503
Hemophilia, 41, 51-52
Hemoptysis, tuberculosis and, 541
Hemorrhage
  anemia and, 306
  aneurysm and, 59
  cerebral, 378
  chronic gastritis and, 516
  cirrhosis of the liver and, 325
  compound fracture and, 215
  convulsions and, 212
  diverticulitis and, 493
  esophagus and, 159
  extradural, 375
  eyes and, 176, 385
  first-aid treatment for, 217-218
  hemophilia and, 51-52
  intestinal tract and, 217
  intracranial, 376, 378
  liver and, 325, 327
  lung injury and, 337
  Meckel's diverticulum and, 491
  peptic ulcer and, 517
  polycythemia and, 50
  pregnancy and
    abruptio placentae, 445-446
    ectopic, 201-202
    placenta previa, 438-439, 445
    postpartum period and, 441
    preeclampsia and, 444
  scalp wound, 374
  shock, 219
  spleen disease and, 502
  stab wounds, 214-215
  subdural, 374-375
  thrombocytopenic purpura and, 502
  tonsillectomy, 306, 526
  tuberculosis and, 538-539
  varicose veins and, 67
  Vitamin K deficiency and, 561-562
  *see also* Bleeding
Hemorrhagic disease of the newborn,
  267
Hemorrhoidectomy, 457
Hemorrhoids, 66, 456-457, 458
  anemia and, 49
  causes, 456
  colonoscopy and, 457
  during pregnancy, 429
  incidence, 456
  prevention, 456
  recurrence, 457-458
  symptoms, 456
  treatment, 456
Heparin, 62, 239, 334, 464
Hepatitis
  infectious (A or B), 326
    vaccination, 252, 258
  infectious mononucleosis and, 283
  jaundice and, 224
  serum (hemologous serum jaundice),
    327
  toxic, 327
  viral, 7
Heredity, 287-289
  aging and, 14
  alcoholism and, 18

allergies and, 24, 26
  hay fever, 23
amniocentesis and, 290-291
breasts and, 93
cancer and, 287
congenital anemias, 49, 502
  Cooley's, 49
  hemolytic, 49
  Mediterranean, 49
  sickle-cell, 48
coronary artery disease, 239
cystic fibrosis, 335
deformities, 287
  avoiding, 288
  gene and chromosome
    examination, 290-291
  likelihood of, 291
  marriage and, 287, 288
deoxyribonucleic acid (DNA), 287
dominant characteristics, 287-289
Down's syndrome, 359
epilepsy, 368
eye disorders and, 162, 164, 168, 170,
  172
genetic counseling, 288, 291
genetic engineering, 290-291
genetic medicine, 290-291
gouty arthritis and, 39
height and, 288
hemophilia, 51
high blood pressure, 235
intelligence, 288
longevity and, 288
Mendelian law and, 287, 289
mental disorders, 355
multiple births, 437
multiple polyposis, 458
muscular dystrophy, 369
personality and, 288
recessive characteristics, 287, 288
syphilis, 557, 558
traits, 288
varicose veins, 59, 66
*see also* Congenital deformities
Hermaphrodite, 471
Hernia, 247-251
  birth and, 247
  causes, 247
  cystocele, 180, 181
  of diaphragm, 247, 250
  hiatus, 157
  hydrocele, 342-343
  inguinal, 247, 248, 249, 250-251
  medical treatment of, 248, 251
  rectocele, 180, 181
  scrotum swelling in newborn, 386
  strangulated, 249
    intestinal obstruction and, 496
  surgery for, 249-251
    Canadian method, 251
    recurrence and, 251
  umbilical, 247, 249
  undescended testicle and, 341-342
Herniated slipped disk, 363, 381
Heroin, overdose, 219
Herpes
  genital, *see* Venereal diseases
  simplex (cold sore), 478-479, 560
  zoster (shingles), 479, 560
  *see also* Chickenpox
Heterophile agglutination test, 283
Hiatus hernia, 157
Hiccups, infant and, 275

Hip
  arthroplasty, 84, 86
  bursitis, 76
  congenital dislocation, 69, 70
  *See also* Fractures
Hirschsprung's disease (megacolon),
  497
Hirsutism, ovarian dysfunction and, 203
Hives, 20, 22, 27, 28
Hoarseness, 528, 544
Hodgkin's disease, 53-54
  chemotherapy for, 106
  non-Hodgkin's lymphoma, 54
  spleen removal and, 503
Homosexuality, 473
  syphilis and, 557
Homotransplant, 534, 535, 537
  *see also* Transplantation of organs
Hong Kong flu, 547-548
Hookworms, 405
Hormone-producing tumors, 205
Hormones, 350-351, 418, 476
  *see also* Sex hormones; *specific*
    *endocrine glands; specific*
    *hormones*
Hospital insurance, 1-2
Hospitals, 1-2, 449
Huhner test, 509
Hyaline membrane disease (respiratory
  distress syndrome), 266, 388
Hydrocele, 342-343, 386
Hydrocephalus, 380
  pituitary gland malfunction and, 421
Hydrocortisone, bursitis and, 76
Hydrophobia, *see* Rabies
Hydrotherapy, *see* Physical therapy
Hymen, 177
  hymenotomy, 177
  menstruation and, 177, 184
Hymenotomy, 177
Hypercholesterolemia, 310
Hyperimmune serum
  mumps, 129
  whooping cough and, 127, 130
Hyperinsulinism (insulin shock),
  *see* Diabetes mellitus
Hyperopia (farsightedness), *see* Eyes
Hyperparathyroidism, 407, 408
  osteitis fibrosa cystica and, 81
Hypersensitivity, *see* Allergy
Hypersplenism, 502, 503
Hypertension (high blood pressure), *see*
  Blood pressure
Hyperthyroidism, *see* Thyroid gland
Hypertrophic gastritis, 516
Hypnotism, 355-356
Hypodermic needles
  infectious hepatitis and, 326
  serum hepatitis and, 327
Hypoglycemia (insulin shock), *see*
  Diabetes mellitus
Hypoparathyroidism, 408-409
  blood chemistry for, 308
Hypopituitarism, 421
Hypospadias, 554, 555-556
Hypothermia, heart surgery and, 244
Hypothyroidism, *see* Thyroid gland
Hysterectomy, 195-197
  abruptio placentae and, 446
  cervical cancer and, 189, 196
  endometrial polyps and, 191
  endometriosis and, 196, 197
  fibroids and, 195

hyperplasia and, 191-192, 196
indications for, 196
menopause and, 196
ovaries and, 196
prolapse of the uterus and, 180
types, 195
uterine cancer and, 192, 196
vaginal, 179-180, 195
Hysteria, 356
Hysterogram, 191, 194, 508, 567

Icterus index, 308
Idiocy, 359
Idiot savant, 359
Ileal bladder operation, 552, 553
Ileostomy, 486
ulcerative colitis and, 495
Ileotransverse colostomy, 490
Iliofemoral bypass operation, 63
Image intensifier, 564
Imbeciles, 359
Immunity
active, 252
colostrum and, 269
diphtheria and, 118
to drugs, 346
passive, 252
transplantation, 535
Immunizations and vaccinations
allergy to, 253
booster shots, 252, 256
cholera, 257, 258, 285
convalescent serum and, 252
diphtheria, 118, 128, 252-253, 258
Schick test, 253
gamma globulin, 252, 255-256
German measles, 119, 128, 252, 256, 258
infectious hepatitis, 252, 258
influenza, 258, 547
measles, 120, 129, 252, 255-256, 258
mumps, 122, 129, 252, 256, 257, 258
plague, 257, 258
poliomyelitis, 123-124, 129, 252, 255, 257, 258
Sabin oral vaccine, 255
Salk vaccine, 255
rabies, 256-257, 258, 284
reactions to, 253, 255, 256
Rocky Mountain spotted fever, 258, 281
schedule, 252, 257
smallpox, 252, 253-254, 257, 258
tetanus, 252, 257, 258
travel and, 257, 280
tuberculosis, 256, 541
tests for, 253
typhoid fever, 252, 256, 258, 279-280
typhus fever, 257, 258, 281
whooping cough, 127, 130, 252, 258
yellow fever, 257, 258, 280
Immunotherapy, 105
Impetigo, 477
of the newborn, 385
Impotence, see Sexual intercourse
Imuran, 536
Incisional biopsy, 314
Incisional hernia, 247
Incontinence, see Urination
Increased intracranial pressure, 374-375
Indocin, 37, 38
Induced labor, 432-433
Inertia labor, 437-438

Infancy
allergies, 20-21
atopic dermatitis, 26
cow milk, 278
anemia and, 48
behavior
breath-holding, 108-109
crying, 107
pacifier use, 108
sleep, 113-114
thumbsucking, 107-108
bowel movements, 276
constipation, 276
diarrhea, 277-278
"blue baby," 236, 312
celiac disease, 278
circumcision, 339-340
colic, 276
dacryocystis in, 168
hernias in, 247, 249
see also Congenital deformities;
Immunizations and vaccinations;
Newborn; specific diseases
Infant feeding
bottle-feeding, 270-272
diarrhea and, 277-278
eliminating, 275
position of baby, 275
premature babies and, 387-388
sterilization, 271, 275
thrush, 268
weight loss in, 385
breast-feeding, 269-270
bowel movements, 275
breast infections, 94
breast pump, 270
"caked" breasts, 270
colostrum, 269
contraindications, 269
drugs and, 269
infections, 440, 441
medications for, 93
nipple care, 270, 440; for "cracked," 270; for inverted, 93
passive immunity and, 252
start of milk flow, 269, 440
tetany of the newborn and, 267
weaning, 93, 270, 418, 440
weight loss in, 385
hiccups, 275
orange juice, 273
premature baby and, 387-388
regurgitation, 275
solid foods, 273
adding new, 275
canned, 275
cereal, 273
chopped (junior foods), 275
fresh, 275
fruits, 273-274
liquids and, 275
schedule, 273-274
self-feeding, 275
vitamins and, 272
Infantile paralysis, see Poliomyelitis
Infarct, 366, 378
Infections, 5-7
anemia and, 49
antibiotics for, 5, 7
avoiding serious, 5
blood count and, 48, 305
blood poisoning and, 50-51
cause, 5, 7

curing, 5, 7
dangerous areas of, 5
diabetes and, 131
draining, 7
limb amputation and, 7, 70, 72
ointments and, 7
pus formation and, 5
recurrence prevention, 7
susceptibility to, 5
vaccines and, 7
Vitamin A and, 561
see also Abscess; Antibiotics;
Gangrene; Lymph glands; specific infections; Spleen
Infectious (epidemic) jaundice, 281-282
Infectious hepatitis, see Hepatitis
Infectious mononucleosis, 283
infectious hepatitis and, 326
liver and, 324
spleen enlargement and, 502
Infectious and virus diseases, 279
see also specific diseases
Infertility, see Sterility
Influenza, 547
Asiatic and Hong Kong and, 547-548
bronchitis and, 545, 547
common colds and, 543, 547
sore throat and, 526
"swine," 548
vaccination, 258, 547, 548
Informed consent, 447
Infrared machines, heat treatments and, 412
Inguinal hernia, 247, 248, 251
INH (isonicotinic acid hydrazide), 542
Inhalation anesthesia, see General inhalation anesthesia
Inheritance, see Heredity
Inherited immunity, 252
see also Immunizations and vaccinations
Injury
compensation for, 3-4
as liability case, 4
see also specific injuries
Inner ear deafness, 149
Innovar, 30
Insanity, 355
marriage and, 287, 288
Insect bites, see Bites; specific insects
Insomnia, 356
barbiturates and, 348
caffeine and, 351
neurasthenia and, 354
Insulin, see Diabetes mellitus
Insurance
compensation, 3-4
health, 1
liability, 4
medical record information and, 2-3
Intellectual development
adolescence and, 9-10
aging and, 16
alcoholism and, 18
during pregnancy, 19
epilepsy, 367
heredity and, 288
Intelligence quotient (IQ), 358-359
Intensive Care Unit (ICU), 292-293
Cardiac Care Unit (CCU), 245-246
Intercourse, see Sexual intercourse
Interferon, 291
Internal hernia, 248

Interstitial cystitis, 549
Intestinal obstruction, 496-497
Intestines, see Large intestine; Small
   intestine
Intoxication, see Alcohol abuse
Intracranial hemorrhage, 374-376, 378
Intracranial pressure, increased, 374-375
Intraductal papillomas, 95
Intraocular lens, 170
Intrauterine devices (IUD's), 42, 45-46,
   200
Intrauterine transfusion, 309
Intravenous anesthesia, 30
Intravenous cholangiography, 222
Intravenous urography, 567
Intussusception, 491-492
Invasive procedure, 447
Involutional melancholia, 357
Iodine
   colloid goiter and, 532
   hyperthyroidism and, 531-532
   toxic goiter and, 532
   see also Radiation therapy
Ipecac (syrup of), 218
Iridectomy, 169
Iris, see Eyes
Iritis, 168
Iron
   menstruation and, 48
   newborn and, 388
   pregnancy and, 427
Iron deficiency anemia, 49
   see also Anemia
Irritable colon, 494
Irritability
   barbiturates and, 348
   hyperthyroidism and, 531-532
Ischemia, 366
Isoniazid, 302
Isonicotinic acid hydrazide (IAH), 542
Isotopes, radiation therapy and, 569-570
Itching
   in anus, 460-461
   chickenpox and, 116
   hives and, 27
   pityriasis rosea and, 482
   poison ivy and, 483
   psychosomatic illness and, 356
   scabies and, 481

Jacksonian seizures, epilepsy and, 367
"Jammed" finger, 227
Jaundice, 324
   blood chemistry for, 308, 309-310
   blood transfusions, 306, 308, 309
   cirrhosis and, 325
   diagnosis, 222, 224
   erythroblastosis and, 263
   gallstones and, 224, 225, 226
   hemolytic, 502, 503
   hepatitis and, 221, 224
   homologous serum, 327
   infectious (epidemic), 281-282
   infectious mononucleosis and, 283
   liver cancer and, 325
   in newborns, 384
   nosebleeds and, 394
   pancreatic cancer and, 401
   phototherapy and, 263
   Vitamin K deficiency, 561-562
Jaws, 318-319
   cysts of, 319
   fractures of, 318-319

infection of, 318
Joints
   arthrography of, 568
   arthroplasty for, 83-84
   exercises for conditions of, 413-414
   fusion of, 83
   ganglion and, 485
   heat therapy and, 412
   hydrotherapy and, 413
   massage, 413
   reconstructive surgery on, 81, 83
   rehabilitation and, 414-415
   rheumatic fever and, 465, 466
   tapping, 40
   torn knee cartilage, 78-79

Kala azar, 403
Karotype, 290, 291
Keloid, 481
   radiation therapy for, 569
Keratomileusis, 163
Kidneys
   blood chemistry for, 308
   congenital defects, 300-301
   cysts, 300
   dialysis, 304
      uremia and, 297
   disease
      albumin in the urine and, 295
      alcohol consumption and, 295
      arteriovenous aneurysm and, 59
      causes, 294
      diabetes mellitus and, 132
      diagnosis, 300, 311, 500, 567
      diet for, 295
      gouty arthritis and, 39
      high blood pressure and, 294-295
      intravenous urography of, 567
      oteomalacia and, 81
      salt restriction and, 295
      smoking and, 295
      sonography, 500
      urination frequency and, 295
      urine analysis, 311
   "dropped" ("floating"), 302
   glomerulonephritis and, 296
      cystitis and, 549
   injuries, 301
   location and structure, 294, 295
   metabolic acidosis and, 310
   nephrosis, 296-297, 350
   normal functioning, 294
   prostate enlargement and, 451
   pyelonephritis (kidney infections),
      297-298, 442
   removal (nephrectomy), 300
   renal artery obstruction and, 63-64
   scanning, 570
   stones, 298-299
      bladder stones and, 551
      composition of, 298
      diet, 299
      formation of, 298
      gouty arthritis and, 39
      hyperparathyroidism and, 407
      recurrence, 299
      surgical removal, 298
      symptoms, 298
      ureteral stones, 299
   transplantation, 303-304, 535
   tuberculosis of the, 301-302
   tumors, 299-300
      Wilm's, 106, 299-300

uremia, 297
   coma and, 369
   water secretion and
      diabetes insipidus and, 420
      pituitary gland and, 418
   see also Nephritis
Kidney stones, see Kidneys
Kilovolt, 568
Klinefelter's syndrome, 289
Knees
   arthroplasty for, 84
   bursitis in, 76
   psoriasis and, 482
   tapping, 40
   torn cartilage of, 78-79
   water on the, 39
   see also Joints
Koplik's spots, measles and, 120, 129
Korsakoff's psychosis, alcoholism and,
   18
Kveim test, 335

Labor, see Childbirth; Pregnancy
Laboratory tests, 305-315
   abdominal taps (paracentesis), 315
   as aging indicator, 14
   allergy and, 21
   appendicitis and, 33
   blood chemistry, 309-310
   blood cultures, 51, 310
   blood gas analyzer, 310-311
   bone marrow analysis, 306
   cirrhosis of the liver, 325
   gastric analysis, 312, 313
   glucose tolerance test, 131, 310
   guinea pig inoculations, 315
   hematological blood tests, 305-306
      complete blood count, 305
      differential blood count, 305
      lead poisoning and, 306
      sedimentation rate, 306
   infectious hepatitis, 326
   Intensive Care Units and, 292
   liver function and, 329
   lung taps (thoracentesis), 315
   Papanicolaou smear, 187-188, 189,
      313-314
   parasitic diseases, 402, 403
   pregnancy tests, 311, 427
   pus cultures, 315
   Rh test, 311-312
   serologic tests, 306
   spinal taps, 315
   sputum analysis, 314-315
   stool analysis, 315
   streptococcus sore throat, 526
   syphilis and, 183
   typhoid fever, 279
   urine analysis and, 131, 311
   vaginitis, 182
   whooping cough, 126
   see also Biopsy
Labyrinthitis, middle ear infection and,
   147
Laceration
   of blood vessels, 60, 62
   first aid for, 218
Laparoscope, 47, 155
   ovarian cyst and, 205
Large bowel, see Large intestine
Large intestine
   bowel strangulation, 249
   colostomy, 461-462, 499

diverticulitis and, 493
 ileotransverse, 490
 preliminary, 496
description, 486, 487
diverticulitis, 488, 493-494
diverticulosis, 493-494
Hirschsprung's disease (megacolon),
 497
intussusception, 491-492
tumors, 496, 497-498, 499
 bladder fistula and, 550-551
 cancer, 102, 103
 colostomy, 499
 location, 497
 polyps, 498
 recurrence, 499
ureters transplanted into, 552
volvulus, 492, 496
water absorption and, 486
 see also Bowel movements; Colitis;
 Colon
Laryngectomy, 529
Laryngoscopy, 527
Larynx, 527-529
 acute laryngitis and, 527, 544
 congenital laryngeal stridor, 268
 croup, 544
 description, 527
 diphtheria and, 117
 drowning and spasms of, 213
 frozen section biopsy of tissue of, 314
 hoarseness, 528, 544
 inspection of, 527
 obstruction of the, 530
 tracheotomy and, see Trachea
 tumors of the, 528-529
 diagnosis, 528
 incidence, 528
 symptoms, 528
 treatment for, 528-529
Laser beam coagulation, see Photocoagulation
Laxatives, 349, 455
 abdominal pain and, 33, 411
 before x ray, 566
 danger of, 345
 diarrhea and, 488
 habit, 349
 indigestion and, 514
 mucous colitis and, 494
 overdose, 349
 pregnancy and, 429
"Lazy" eye (convergent strabismus), 172
Lead
 bone marrow injury and, 50
 neuropathy and, 362-363
 poisoning, 306
Learning disability, 114
Legs
 amputating, 72
 bowed in newborn, 386
 fracture, 89, 91, 215, 216
 replantation surgery and, 464
 thrombophlebitis and, 60
 see also Feet; Varicose veins
Leiomyoma (fibroids), of uterus, 194-195,
 196, 431, 439, 508, 509
Leishmaniasis, 403
Leprosy, 282-283
Leukemia, 52-53
 blood count and, 305
 chemotherapy and, 105-106
 nosebleeds and, 394

phosphorus and, 570
 spleen enlargement and, 502
 virulence of, 101
Leukocytes, see White blood cells
Leukoplakia, 320-321, 322
 of vulva, 178
Liability cases, 4
Libido (sexual desire), see Sexual
 intercourse
Lice, 481-482
 relapsing fever, 281
 rickettsial diseases and, 281
Lienorenal shunt, 65, 66
Life expectancy, see Longevity
Ligaments, bursitis and, 75
Ligation
 tubal, 47
 of varicose vein, 60, 66, 67
Light
 allergy to, 28
 measles and, 120
"Lightening," 428
Limb
 absent (phocomelia), 69, 70
 amputation of, 7, 70-72, 91, see also
 Replantation surgery
 artificial, 72
 brain tumor and, 365, 378
 embolus to, 58
 extra, 69, 70
 joint fusion to stabilize, 83
 multiple sclerosis and, 370
 phantom, 72
 spinal cord tumors and, 380
 weakness, 364
Limp, congenital hip dislocation and, 70
Linear accelerator, prostate cancer and,
 453
Lipase, pancreatitis and, 397
Lipomas, 483, 485
Lips, 316-318
 blueness
 heart failure and, 233
 laryngeal obstruction and, 529-530
 cancer of, 316-317
 cleft palate, 317-318
 cold sores on, 478-479, 560
 harelip, 317
 infections on, 5, 6, 7, 316
 syphilitic, 316
 swollen, 316
 tumors of, 316
 upper
 hair on, 8
 infections of, 5, 6, 7
 pimples on, 6
 see also Cleft palate
Liquids, see Fluids
Lisping, in children, 111
Lithium, 358
Lithium carbonate, alcoholics and, 19
Litholapaxy, 551
Liver
 abscess, 324, 327, 570
 acute yellow atrophy of, 324
 amoebic dysentery and, 324
 blood circulation through esophageal
 varicosities and, 159
 cancer of, 325, 327
 alcohol consumption and, 101
 cysts, 327
 description, 323

disorders
 alcoholism and, 15, 18
 birth control pills and, 46
 blood chemistry for, 308
 causes, 323
 diagnosis, 324
 halothane damage, 30
 scanning, 570
 sonography, 500
 urine analysis, 311
 erythroblastosis and, 263
 extracts (chronic gastritis) and, 516
 fatty, 325
 frozen section biopsy of tissue of, 314
 gallstones and, 324
 heart disease and, 324
 hemangioma in, 67-68
 Hodgkin's disease and, 54
 infection, 324
 infectious mononucleosis, 283, 324
 injuries, 327
 jaundice, 324
 leukemia and, 53
 lymphoma and, 53
 Niemann-Pick disease, 265
 parasites and, 324
 surgery, 327-329
 transplant, 535, 536, 537
 tumors, 327-328
 see also Cirrhosis of the liver;
 Hepatitis
Lobar pneumonia, 333
Lobectomy, 336-338, 546
Lobotomy, 357
Local anesthesia, 30, 32
Lochia, 441
Lockjaw, see Tetanus
Locomotor ataxia (tabes), 366, 558
Longevity, 14-16
 alcoholism and, 18
 coronary bypass operation and, 243
 determination of, 14
 diabetes mellitus, 133
 exercise and, 14
 heredity and, 288
 marriage and, 15
 nutrition and, 15
 obesity and, 16, 135
 organ transplants and, 537
 smoking and, 15
 see also Aging
Lower back pain, 72-73
 slipped disk, 73
LSD, 351
Ludwig's angina, 530
Lumbago
 exercises for, 413-414
 whirlpool baths and, 413
Lumbar hernia, 248
Lumbar puncture, see Spinal tap
Lumbar sympathectomy, Buerger's
 disease and, 57
Lungs, 330-338
 abscess, 333, 545, 570
 air pollution and, 330
 atelectasis of the newborn, 266-267
 blood clots (embolus) to, 58, 334, 570
 bronchiectasis, 330, 336
 bronchoscopy, 545-546
 cancer, 337-338
 asbestos fibers and, 334-335
 chest x ray and, 566
 coughing up blood and, 330
 incidence, 100

lung taps and, 315
  smoking and, 15, 100-101, 330, 338
  sputum analysis, 314-315
cold air and, 330
cystic fibrosis (mucoviscidosis), 335
cysts of, 336, 337, 338
dust diseases (pneumonoconioses),
  334-335
emphysema, 330, 332, 336
frozen section biopsy of, 314
hot air and, 330
infections, 336
  cystic fibrosis and, 262
injuries to, 336-337
operations, 336, 337, 338
  bronchiectasis and, 546
  pulmonary resection, 552
  removal of one, 330
  transplants, 535-536
pulmonary infarction, 333-334
sarcoidosis, 335
scanning, 570
scoliosis and, 75
sonography, 500
spontaneous pneumothorax
  (collapse of lung), 332
structure, 330, 331
tap, 315
thrombus in, 64
tumors, 336, 337-338
see also Bronchitis; Pneumonia;
  Tuberculosis
Lupus, 482
Lye, swallowing, 157
Lymphadenitis, 52
Lymphangiography, 566
Lymphangiomas, liver and, 327
Lymphangitis, 52
Lymphatic channel, infection and, 52
Lymph glands, 52
  cancer and, 52, 101
  frozen section biopsy of, 314
  functions, 52
  infections of, 52
  infectious mononucleosis and, 283
  leukemia and, 53
  lymphangiography and, 566
  roseola and, 130
  sonography and, 500-501
  spleen enlargement and, 502
  tuberculosis and, 52
Lymphoma, 53
  Hodgkin's disease, 53-54
  non-Hodgkin's lymphoma, 54

Malaria, 280, 403-404
  spleen enlargement and, 502
Male organs
  adolescence and, 8
    precocious, 10
  deformities and plastic surgery of,
    422
  impotency and, 15, see also Sexual
    intercourse
  vasectomy, 454
  see also Sexual intercourse; specific
    organs; Sterility; Venereal diseases
Malignancy, see Cancer; specific
  organs and sites
Malnutrition
  achalasia and, 159
  anemia and, 49
  cystic fibrosis and, 262

fatty liver and, 325
hookworm disease and, 404
infection susceptibility and, 5
infectious hepatitis and, 326
menstruation and, 183
osteomalacia and, 81
pneumonia and, 333
pregnancy and, 289
Malta fever, 282
Mammography, see Breast cancer
Mammoplasty, 422
Manic-depressive disorder, 358
Mantoux test, for tuberculosis, 253
Maple syrup urine disease, mental
  retardation and, 289
Marital relations, see Sexual
  intercourse
Marriage
  during adolescence, 10
  epilepsy and, 368
  longevity and, 15
  mental illness in family and, 355
  sex advice before, 473
Massage, see Physical therapy
Massive atelectasis, 331-332
Mastectomy, 95-97
"Master gland," see Pituitary gland
Mastoid, see Ear
Mastoidectomy, 148
Masturbation, see Sexuality
Maxillary sinus, surgery of the, 392
Measles (rubeola), 119-121
  encephalitis and, 365
  vaccination, 252-253, 255-256, 257,
    258
Meckel's diverticulum, 491
Meconium, 434
  fetal distress and, see Childbirth
Medicaid, 1
Medical record, 2-3
Medicare, 1
Medications and drugs, see Drugs
Mediterranean anemia, 49
  spleen and, 502, 503
Mediterranean fever, 282
Medulla, see Adrenal glands
Megacolon (Hirschsprung's disease),
  262, 497
Melanoma
  of eye, 175
  skin grafts and, 424
Mellitus, fatty liver and, 325
Meloplasty, 422
Memory
  alcoholic amnesia and, 18
  epilepsy, 367
Mendelian law, 287, 289
Meniere's syndrome, 151-152, 369
Meningiomas, 377
Meningitis, 365-366
  coma and, 368-369
  gonorrhea and, 557
  middle ear infection and, 148
  syphilitic, 365
Meningocele, 380
Meningoencephalitis, mumps and, 122
Meningomyelocele, 380
Menopause, 206-208
  age, 207
  aging and, 16
  artificial, 207
  bleeding after, 192, 207
  description, 206

fibroids and, 192, 194
hysterectomy and, 196
male, 512
onset, 183
ovaries removal and, 206
pregnancy and, 207
symptoms, 207
throat tightness in, 156
treatment, 207
weight gain and, 135
Menstruation, 183-185
  adolescence and, 8-9
    informing child about, 185
  after childbirth, 441
  analgesics and, 347
  anemia and, 48
  artificially stimulated at menopause,
    16
  barren period of month, 506
  birth control pills and, 185
  blood appearance, 184
  breasts and, 94
  bringing on, 183-184
  cervical cancer and, 189
  cervical polyps and, 187
  cervicitis and, 186
  description, 183
  douching and, 179
  duration, 184
  dysmenorrhea, 184-185
  endometrial hyperplasia and, 191
  endometrial polyp and, 191
  endometriosis and, 197
  excessive bleeding, 184
  fertile period of month, 506
  fibroids and, 194
  growth and, 8
  hymen and, 177, 184
  hysterectomy and, 196
  intrauterine devices and, 45
  irregular, 184, 191
  late, 10
  missing, 183
  onset, 8, 183
  ovarian dysfunction and, 203
  ovulation, 43
    failure, 507
  precocious, 10
  premenstrual tension, 185
  prolactin-secreting adenomas and,
    418
  radiation and, 565
  regularity of, 8
  rhythm method of birth control and,
    42-43
  salpingitis and, 200
  scant bleeding, 184
  sex hormones and, 203
  sexual intercourse during, 474
  tampons and, 185
    toxic shock syndrome, 185
  vagina and, 179, 183-184
    vaginitis and, 182
  see also Menopause; Pregnancy
Mental illness
  anxiety neurosis, 354-355
  birth control and, 41, 47
  castration complex, 355
  dependency and, 355
  depression, 354, 355, 356, 357, 358
    psychotherapy and, 415
  electroshock therapy, 357-358
  group therapy, 357

heredity and, 355
hypnotism and, 355-356
hysteria, 356
incidence, 354
insanity, 355
insomnia and, 356
involutional melancholia, 357
manic-depressive disorders, 358
marriage and, 355
"nervous breakdown," 354
neurasthenia 354
neuroses, 354
    compulsion, 355
    constipation and, 486
    diarrhea, 488
    frigidity, 472-473
    nymphomania, 472
    obsessions, 355
    phobias, 355
    plastic surgery of nose and, 395
Oedipus complex, 355
paranoia, 358
postpartum psychosis, 358
pregnancy and, 358
pruritus ani, 460
psychiatric hospitalization, 356
psychoanalysis, 357
psychoses, 354, 357
psychosomatic illnesses, 356
schizophrenia, 354, 358
sexual problems and, 355
sleep and, 356
suicide and, 355
surgery for, 357, 380
tranquilizers and, 356
see also Emotional disturbances;
    Psychiatry; Psychotherapy
Mental retardation, 359-360
    cretinism, 531
    Down's syndrome, 359
    German measles and, 288
    idiocy, 359
    idiot savant, 359
    imbeciles, 359
    inherited or congenital conditions,
        289-290
    metabolic disorders, 290, 359
    mild retardation, 359
    moron, 359
    pregnancy and, 359
    see also Mental illness
Mesh graft, 424-425
Mesocaval shunt, see Shunt
Metabolic acidosis, 308, 310
Metabolic alkalosis, 308, 310-311
Metabolic diseases
    blood chemistry for, 308
    impaired kidney function, 294
    mental retardation and, 289-290
Metabolism, 531
    blood chemistry and, 310
    imbalance (delirium tremens) and,
        18-19
    malnutrition, 15
    obesity and, 134
    overactive (pheochromocytoma) and,
        11
    parathyroid glands and, 407
    see also Thyroid gland
Metatarsal
    bunions and, 77
    corns, 77
    fracture of, 90

Metronidazole, 403, 404
Mev, 568
Microsurgery, replantation surgery
    and, 463-464
Middle ear, see Ear
Migraine, 369
    as allergy, 20
    see also Headache
Milk
    allergy to, 277, 278
    brucellosis and, 282
    diphtheria and, 117
    galactosemia and, 290
    poliomyelitis and, 123
    typhoid fever and, 279
    see also Infant feeding
"Milk alkali syndrome," 311
Milk cysts (galactocele), 95
Mineral oil
    bowel functions and, 455
    constipation and, 276, 488
    fissure in ano and, 459
    foreign body in ear and, 214
    foreign body in eye and, 214
    pregnancy and, 429
    vitamin absorption and, 563
Minerals
    adrenal cortex and, 12
    blood chemistry and, 309
    impaired kidney function and, 294
"Miner's lung," 334
Miscarriage, see Abortion
Mite
    rickettsial diseases and, 281
    scabies, 481
Mitral commissurotomy, 242
Mitral stenosis, 241, 242
Mold spores, allergy to, 21, 22, 23, 25
Moles, 483, 484
    electrolysis on, 480
    of lip, 316
    malignant, see Melanoma
Mongolism, see Down's syndrome
Mononucleosis, see Infectious
    mononucleosis
Morning sickness, 429
Moron, 359
Morphine, overdose, 219
Mosquito
    dengue fever and, 281
    malaria and, 280
    yellow fever and, 280
Motion sickness
    barbiturates and, 348
    tablets for morning sickness, 429
Motrin, 37
Mouth
    bad breath, 319-320
    canker sores in, 26
    care of newborn, 384
    cleft palate plastic surgery, 422
    leukoplakia and cancer and,
        320-321, 322
    peritonsillar abscess, 524-525
    pyorrhea, 320
    thrush, 268
    trench mouth, 320
    Vitamin B$_2$ deficiency and, 561
    see also Jaws; Lips; Salivary glands;
        Teeth; Tongue
Mouth-to-mouth artificial respiration,
    see Artificial respiration;
    Cardiopulmonary resuscitation

Mucous colitis, 494
Mucous membranes
    Addison's disease and, 12
    parasites entering through, 402
Mucoviscidosis, see Cystic fibrosis
Multiple births, see Pregnancy
Multiple polyposis, 458
Multiple sclerosis, 370
Mumps (epidemic parotitis), 121-122,
    129
    deafness and, 149
    encephalitis and, 365
    orchitis, 510
    parotid gland and, 468
    reduced sperm count and, 510
    vaccination, 252, 256, 257, 258
Murmurs, heart, 241
Muscle relaxants, 29
    lower back pain and, 73
Muscles
    adolescence and, 8
    analgesics and, 347
    bursitis and, 75
    fractures and, 413
    frozen section biopsy of, 314
    hypoparathyroidism and, 408
    neuromuscular disorders, 79-81
        see also specific disorders
    reconstructive surgery on, 81
    neuropathy of, 363
    physical therapy for, 413
    rehabilitation, 414-415
    rheumatic fever and, 466-467
    spasms, 412
    sprains, 412
    system, 82
    wry neck (torticollis), 76
Muscular dystrophy, 79-80, 369-370
    exercises for, 413-414
Myambutol, 302
Myasthenia gravis, 80
Myelography, 381, 568
Myocarditis, 128, 232-233, 245, 548
Myomas, 497
Myomectomy, 195
Myopia (nearsightedness), see Eyes
Myringotomy, 147

Nailbiting, 108
Naprosyn, 37, 38
Narcosis, 30
    see also Sleep
Narcotics, 349
    anesthesia and, 29
    labor pain and, 434
    lung injuries and, 336-337
    as postoperative measure, 449
    as preoperative routine, 447
    resistance to, 346
    sex and, 475
Nasal polyps, 391, 393-394
Nasal sinuses, see Nose
Natural childbirth, see Childbirth
Navel
    omphalitis, 268
    umbilical hernia and, 247, 249
Nearsightedness, see Eyes
Neck
    bleeding from, 217-218
    Cushing's syndrome and, 419-420
    first aid for injury to, 216
    glandular swelling in, 524
    meningitis and, 365-366

nerve connected with, 362
stiffness
ECHO virus disease and, 285
poliomyelitis and, 129
thyroiditis and, 532
vein distention and, 233
wry (torticollis), 76
exercises for, 413-414
Needle biopsy, 314
Negligence, liability cases and, 4
Neonatologist, 29
Nephrectomy, 300
Nephritis, 125, 130, 296
see also Kidneys
Nephrosis, 296-297, 350
Nerve blocks, Buerger's disease and,
57
Nerves
diabetes mellitus and, 132
leprosy and, 282
paralysis and electrical stimulation,
413
rehabilitation, 414-415
Vitamin B₁ and, 561
Nervous diseases
brain scan and, 371
CAT scan and, 371
electroencephalography (EEG), 371
spinal tap and, 370
stimulating drugs and, 351
see also Neurosurgery; specific
diseases
Nervous system, 362, 363
alcohol abuse and, 18
function, 362, 372
stimulating drugs and, 351
structure, 362, 363
central nervous system, 372
Peripheral nerves, 372, 382-383
syphilis and, 558-559
see also Neurosurgery
Nervous tension, see Stress
Neuralgias, analgesics and, 347-348
Neurasthenia, 354
Neuritis (neuropathy), 362-363, 548,
561
Neurofibromas, 377
Neuropathy, see Neuritis
Neurosis, see Mental illness
Neurosurgery, 372
see also specific organs and sites of
Nevi, see Moles
Newborn
bathing, 386
bluish spot at base of spine of, 385
bowed legs in, 386
breasts swollen in, 385
breathing difficulty in, 384
ear care, 384
eyes, 384
blood spots in, 385
color of, 385
crossed appearance of, 385
discharge from, 385
eye drops, 385, 557
flash pictures, 387
focusing, 385
marks over, 385
puffiness, 385
fontanelle, 384, 385
head, 384, 385
impetigo, 385
jaundice (physiologic), 384

mouth care, 384
normalcy determination, 384
nose care, 384, 385
pacifier for, 387
premature babies, 387-388
anemia in, 388
antibiotics to, 388
bathing, 388
care required, 387
cribs heated for, 387
defects in, 387
definition, 387
dietary supplements for, 388
feeding, 387-388
hospital facilities for, 387
hyaline membrane disease, 266,
388
leaving hospital, 387
mental development, 388
nursing and, 269
oxygen supply to, 387
retrolental fibroplasia, 266
survival chances, 387
time in incubator, 387
transporting, 387
pyloric stenosis, 520-521
rectal area care, 386
room temperature for, 386
scalp care, 384
scrotum swelling (hydrocele),
342-343, 386
skin of, 384-385
syphilis and, 558
taken out-of-doors, 387
"tongue-tie" in, 384
umbilical cord area, 386
vaginal area care, 386
visitors to, 386
vitamins and, 562
weight loss in, 385
see also Childbirth; Circumcision;
Congenital deformities; Infancy;
Infant feeding; Pregnancy
Nicotinic acid, 151, 561
Niemann-Pick disease, 265
Nightmares, 110
Night terrors, 110
Nipples, see Breasts
Nitrous oxide, 29, 34, 434
Nodular goiter, 531
Noise, hearing loss and, 145, 149
Non-Hodgkin's lymphoma, 54
Nose
cancer and, 393-394
basal cell cancer, 485
common cold and, 543
deviated septum, 390-391
foreign body in, 214
fractured, 389-390
hay fever and, 23
infection, 7
lymph glands and, 52
middle ear pain and, 146
rhinitis and, 23
influenza and, 547
nasal polyps, 391, 391-392, 393
nasal sinuses, 391-393
cancer of, 393-394
description, 391, 393
ethmoid sinuses surgery, 392
frontal sinus surgery, 392
sinusitis, 391-392
sphenoid sinus surgery, 392

surgery of, 392-393
tumor of, 393-394
of newborn, 385-386
plastic surgery (rhinoplasty),
394-396, 422
building up a nose for, 395-396
burns and, 422
deformities corrected by, 394-395,
422
dressings and packings removal
from, 396
nasal swelling, 396
normal breathing and, 396
repeating, 396
scars visible after, 395
selecting desired type for, 395, 396
submucous resection and, 391
replantation surgery and, 464
saddlenose, 535
structure, 388, 389
tumors of, 393-394
see also Sinusitis
Nosebleeds, 389, 394
Nose drops, sinusitis and, 392
Novocain, 30, 57, 76, 315, 376, 434
Nuclear radiation, first aid for exposure
to, 219
Nuclear scanning, 570
Nurses
floor, 2
home, 2
Intensive Care Unit and, 292-293
practical, 2
special-duty, 2
Nursing, see Breast feeding
Nutrition, see Diet; Vitamins
Nymphomania, 472
Nystatin, 268

Obesity, 134-136
aging and, 16
arteriosclerosis and, 55, 56
birth control pills and, 46
breast shape and, 93
cancer and, 100, 136
coronary heart disease and, 135, 239
diabetes mellitus and, 131
emotions and, 135
heart strain and, 15
hernia and, 248
high blood pressure and, 136
life span and, 135
lower back pain and, 73
osteoarthritis and, 39
ovarian dysfunction and, 203
weight loss and, 134-136
children and, 136
constipation and, 135-136
diet for, 137, 143-144
drugs and, 134, 349-350
exercise and, 134
failure of, 135
method of, 134
"miracle diets," 135
salt intake and, 136
spot reducing, 136
treatments for, 135-136
vitamins for, 562
Oedipus complex, 355
Ointments
burns and, 210
infections and abscesses and, 7
Old age, see Aging

Omphalitis, 268
Oncology, 105
   see also Cancer
Operations, see Surgery
Ophthalmologist, 161
   see also Eyes
Ophthalmoscope, 170
Optical instruments, see Endoscopy
Optometrist, 161
   see also Eyes
Oral contraceptives, 42, 46, 46-47, 185,
   509
Orchidopexy, 342
Orchitis
   male infertility and, 510
   mumps and, 129
Orgasm
   intercourse without, 43
   withdrawal and, 43
   see also Sexual intercourse
Oriental sore, 403
Orthoptics, 172, 173
Osteitis deformans, 80-81
Osteitis fibrosa cystica, 81
   hyperparathyroidism and, 407-408
Osteoarthritis, 38-39
Osteogenic sarcomas, 91
Osteomalacia, 81
Osteomas, 91
Osteomyelitis, 79, 376
Osteoporosis, 81
Osteotomy, 83
Otitis media (middle ear infection), 116,
   147-148
Otoplasty, 422
Otosclerosis, 149, 150
Ovaries, 202-206
   aging and, 14
   cancer of, 106, 196, 204-206
   corpus luteum cyst, 204
   description, 202
   dysfunction, 203
   hormone-producing tumors, 205
   hysterectomy and, 196
   mumps and, 122, 129
   salpingitis and, 200, 203
   sonography, 500
   see also Ovulation
Overdose, see Drugs
Overweight, see Obesity
Ovulation, 42-43, 203
   birth control pills and, 46
   failure of, 507
   see also Menstruation; Ovaries;
   Pregnancy
Oxygen
   anesthesia and, 29, 31
   hyaline membrane disease and, 266
   lung injuries and, 337
   massive atelectasis and, 331-332
   poisoning (retrolental fibroplasia),
   266
   premature babies and, 387
   tent, 528
Oxytocin, 418

Pacemakers, heart block and, 240
Pacifier, 108, 387
Paget's disease (osteitis deformans),
   80-81
Pain
   abdominal, see Abdomen
   analgesics and, 347-348

childbirth and, 434
   fainting and, 368
   narcotics and, 349
   shock and, 219
   surgery to relieve, 382
Pain-relieving drugs, see Analgesics
Palate
   diphtheria and, 128
   hay fever and, 23
Palpitations, see Heart
Pancreas, 397-401
   abscess, 399
   cancer of, 401
   cysts, 397, 400
   description, 397, 398
   frozen section biopsy of, 314
   hyperinsulinism (hypoglycemia), 397,
   399-400
   pancreatitis, 397-399, 400, 410
     mumps and, 129
   sonography of, 500-501
   tumors, 401
     benign, 400
   Zollinger-Ellison syndrome, 400
   see also Diabetes mellitus
Pancreatitis, 308, 397-399, 400, 410
   mumps and, 129
Pansinusitis, 391
Papanicolaou smear, 187, 188, 313-314
Papillomas
   intraductal, 95
   of lip, 316
   of tongue, 322
   urinary bladder and, 551
   of vocal cord, 528
Para-aminosalicylic acid (PAS), 302,
   542
Paracentesis (abdominal taps), 315
Paralysis
   brain tumor and, 377
   Conn's syndrome and, 12
   encephalitis and, 365
   facial, 470
   hydrotherapy and, 413
   mental deficiency and, 359
   rehabilitation, 414-415
   spinal cord and, 380, 381, 382
   of vocal cords, 530
   see also Stroke
Paralysis agitans, see Parkinsonism
Paranoia, 358
Parasites, 402-403
   diseases, 402-403, see also specific
   diseases
Parathormone, see Parathyroid glands
Parathyroid glands, 308, 407-409
   description, 407
   frozen section biopsy of, 314
   operating upon, 407-408
   overactivity (hyperparathyroidism),
   407-408
   removal, 408-409
   thyroid surgery and, 408-409
   tumor, 81, 407-408
   underactivity (hypoparathyroidism),
   408-409
Paresis, 366
   syphilis and, 558
Parkinsonism, 372, 379-380
   rehabilitation, 415
Paronychia, 229
Parotid glands, 468
   see also Salivary glands

PAS (para-aminosalicylic acid), 302,
   542
Patent ductus arteriosus, 241, 242
Paternity, determination, 287
Pathologist, 305
   see also Laboratory tests
Pathology tests, see Laboratory tests
Pediatrician, 29
Pedicle graft, 424
Pellagra, 561
Pelvimetry, 567
Penicillin
   diphtheria and, 117, 128
   eyedrops and, 385
   resistance to, 346
Penis
   cancer, 340
   circumcision, 339-340, 386
   infection and, 555
   structure, 339, 340
Pentothal, 29, 30
Peptic ulcer, see Ulcer
Pericarditis, 233, 241-243, 245
Perineal prostatectomy, 451
Period, see Menstruation
Peripheral nervous system, 362, 363,
   372
Perirectal abscess, 460
Peritoneal cavity, 410
Peritonitis
   abdominal taps and, 315
   adhesions and, 410-411
   appendectomy and, 34-35
   blocked Fallopian tubes and, 508
   cause, 410
   description, 410
   diverticulitis and, 423
   gonorrheal, 182, 560
   hernia strangulation and, 249
   intestinal obstruction and, 496
   intussusception and, 491
   large intestine surgery and, 499
   peptic ulcer and, 517
   prevention, 411
   recovery, 411
   salpingitis and, 200
   symptoms, 410
   treatment, 411
   tubal pregnancy and, 201
   volvulus and, 492
Peritonsillar abscess, 524
Pernicious anemia, 49
   gastric analysis and, 312
   tongue and, 321
   Vitamin $B_{12}$ deficiency and, 561
Perspiration
   anxiety neurosis and, 354-355
   brucellosis and, 282
   cystic fibrosis and, 262, 335
   delirium tremens and, 18-19
   excessive, 478
   heat exhaustion and, 216
   hyperthyroidism and, 531-532
   pulmonary tuberculosis and, 540
   shock and, 219
Pertussis, see Whooping cough
Pes planus (flat feet), 77
Pessary, 180
   tipped womb and, 189-190
Petit mal seizures, epilepsy and, 367
Petroleum
   first aid for swallowed, 218, 219
   skin cancer and, 485

"Phantom limb," 72
Pharyngitis (sore throat), see Throat
Pharynx, see Throat
Phenylketonuria (PKU), 289-290, 359
Pheochromocytoma, 11
Phlebitis
  birth control pills and, 46
  pulmonary infarction and, 334
Phlebothrombosis, 59-60
Phlebotomy, polycythemia vera and, 50
Phobias, 355
Phocomelia, 70
Phosphatase, blood chemistry for, 308
Phosphorus
  blood chemistry for, 308
  isotope, 570, see also Radiation
    therapy
  skin cancer and, 485
Photocoagulation, 174
  diabetes mellitus and, 175
  retinal thrombosis and, 176
Phototherapy, erythroblastosis and,
  263
Phrenic nerve crush, 336
Physiatrists, 415
  see also Rehabilitation
Physical examination
  cancer prevention and, 103
  infection avoidance and, 5
  pregnancy and, 426-427
Physical therapy, 412-414, 415
  aging and, 415
  description, 412
  electrical stimulation, 412, 413
  exercise, 412, 413-414
  heat treatments, 412, 413
    elderly, and 415
  hydrotherapy, 413
  manipulation, 412
  massage, 413
    skin tone and, 476
  ultraviolet (UV) light therapy, 413, 415
    acne and, 477
    skin and, 477
  see also Rehabilitation
Physiologic jaundice, 384
Physiotherapy
  lower back pain and, 73
  osteoarthritis and, 39
  rheumatoid arthritis and, 38
  wry neck (torticollis), 76
Piles, see Hemorrhoids
Pilocarpine, muscular dystrophy and,
  80
Pilonidal cysts, 416-417
Pinch grafts, 423-424
Pineal gland, tumor of, 10
"Pink eye," 165
Pinworms, 405
Pituitary gland, 418-426
  adolescence and, 9, 10
  description, 418, 419
  diabetes insipidus and, 420
  dwarfism, 421
  hormones secreted by, 418
  ovarian dysfunction and, 203
  removal and breast cancer, 420
  thyroid cancer and, 531
  tumors and, 418, 419, 420
    acromegaly, 419-420
    adenomas, 418-419
    chromophobe type, 418

corticotropic-secreting tumors of,
    418, 419
  Cushing's syndrome, 419-420
  growth hormone tumors, 418-420
  medications for, 420
  prolactin-secreting adenomas, 418
  radiation therapy and, 420
  recurrence, 420
  surgical treatment, 420
  underactivity (hypopituitarism),
    420-421
  underweight and, 136
  x ray of, 12
Pityriasis rosea, 482
PKU (phenylketonurial), 289-290, 359
Placenta previa, 431, 438-439, 445
Plague, 282
  vaccination, 257, 258, 259
Planned Parenthood, 42
Plantar warts, 77, 484
Plasma, 48
  see also Blood
Plasmochin, malaria and, 404
Plastic operations, see Plastic surgery;
  Vagina
Plastic surgery
  children and, 422-423
  conditions involving, 422-423
  cosmetic surgery results, 422
  description, 422
  outcome of operation and, 422-423
  plastic surgeon for, 422
  trans-sex operations and, 471
  see also Reconstructive surgery;
    specific organs or sites, e.g.,
    Breasts
Platelets, 48
  see also Blood
Pleoptics, 172
Pneumoencephalography, 370-371
Pneumonectomy, 338, 546
Pneumonia, 333
  Asiatic flu and, 548
  bronchiectasis and, 546
  bronchitis and, 545
  chickenpox and, 116
  common cold and, 544
  encephalitis, 365
  influenza and, 547
  liver infection and, 324
  measles and, 121
  tracheitis and, 529
  tracheoesophageal fistula and,
    156-157
  viral, 7, 333
  vomiting petroleum and, 218
  whooping cough and, 127, 130
Pneumonic plague, 282
Pneumoconioses (dust diseases),
  334-335
Poison Control Center, 218
Poisoning
  first-aid treatment for, 218-219
  food, 488
  lead, 306
  oxygen (retrolental fibroplasia) and,
    261
  see also Blood poisoning
Poison ivy, 26, 483
Poliomyelitis (infantile paralysis), 79-80,
  122-124, 129
  tonsillectomy and, 524
  vaccination, 252, 255, 257, 258
    Sabin, 255
    Salk, 255

Pollen, allergy to, 21, 22, 23, 25
  see also Allergy
Polycystic kidney disease, 300
Polycythemia vera, 50
  phosphorus and, 570
Polydactyly, 229
Polyneuritis, 363
Polyp
  cervical, 187-188
  colonoscopy and, 155
  endometrial, 191, 195
  of large intestine, 498
  nasal, 391
  of rectum and anus, 456, 458, 459
  of vagina, 179
Polypectomy, 391
Portacaval shunt, see Shunt
Postoperative measures, 448-449
  appendectomy, 35-36
  cataract removal, 171
  detached retina, 175
  gall bladder operation, 225
  hemorrhoidectomy, 457-458
  large intestine surgery, 499
  peptic ulcer, 519
  pilonidal cyst removal, 417
  polyp removal, 459
  radium treatment of cervix, 188, 189
  spleen removal, 504
  strabismus, 173
  tracheotomy, 530
  vaginal plastic surgery, 181
  varicose vein surgery, 67
  see also Preoperative measures
Postpartum hemorrhage, 440
Postpartum period, see Childbirth
Postpartum psychosis, 358
Postspinal headache, 32
Potassium, blood chemistry for, 308
Potency, see Sexual intercourse
Practical nurses, 2
"Preanesthetic evaluation and
  premedication," 29
Preeciampsia, 443-444
Pregnancy
  abdomen enlargement, 428
  abruptio placentae, 445-446
  adolescence and, 10
  alcohol consumption and, 19, 287, 427
  allergy and, 21, 25
  amniocentesis, 290-291, 471
    Down's syndrome and, 265
    sex determination and, 471, 500
  anemia and, 427
  backaches and, 430
  bathing, 428
  breast care, 428
    breast lumps, 97
    breast reconstruction, 97-98
    inverted nipples, 93-94
  calcium and, 427
  cancer recurrence and, 105
  cerebral palsy, 364
  cervical cancer and, 189
  cervicitis and, 186
  classes of instruction for parents,
    426
  clothing to wear during, 427-428
  conception, 506, 507, 508
  constipation and, 429
  dental care and, 429
  diabetes mellitus and, 426, 442-443
  diagnosis, 426

diet, 427, 429
dizzy spells during, 430
douching and, 430
drugs and, 69, 236, 288, 289, 292, 346, 430
due date determination, 427
ectopic (tubal), 184, 200, 201-202
    abortion and, 202
    sonogram for, 500
    test for, 311
endometriosis and, 197
fertilization, 42
fetal movements, 426, 428
fibroids and, 195
frigidity and, 473
gall bladder problems and, 221, 225
German measles and, 119, 288
heartburn and, 430
heart disease in, 442
hemorrhoids and, 429, 456
hernia and, 247, 251
    umbilical, 247
hysterectomy and, 196
internal examination and, 427
iron and, 427
kidney infection and, 297
leg cramps and, 430
"lightening," 428
medical history and, 426
menopause and, 207
mental deficiency and, 359
mental disease and, 358
"morning sickness" (nausea and vomiting), 426
multiple births, 437
    causing, 437
    diagnosis, 437
    fertility pills, 437
    fraternal twins, 437
    identical twins, 437
    labor management, 437
    obstetrical management of, 437
    quadruplets, 437
    triplets, 437
    twins, 437
myomectomy and, 195
ovarian cysts and, 203, 206
paternity determination, 287
pelvic measurements and, 429
pelvimetry, 567
physical activity and, 427
physical examination and, 426-427, 428
physical signs, 426
placenta previa, 431, 438, 445
poliomyelitis and, 122, 123-124
preeclampsia and, 443-444
prolapse of the uterus and, 181
radiation and, 288
rest periods, 428
Rh factor and, 311-312
saliva production, 429
salt intake and, 427
sex hormones and, 203
sexual intercourse and, 428
smoking and, 427
sonography and, 500
spleen removal, 504
swimming during, 428
symptoms of, 426
syphilis and, 559
tests, 183, 311, 427
thrombophlebitis and, 59

thyroid condition and, 534
toxemia, 430, 443
travel during, 428
tuberculosis and, 540
urination during, 429
vaginal bleeding, 426, 428
vaginal discharge during, 430
vaginitis and, 182, 268
varicose veins, 429-430
visits to obstetrician, 426-427, 428
vitamins taken during, 427, 561
weight
    gain, 427
    without intercourse, 474
    see also Abortion; Birth control; Childbirth; Congenital deformities; Heredity; Menstruation; Newborn
Premature ejaculation, 473, 511
Prematurity, see Newborn
Preoperative measures
    appendectomy, 35
    before entering hospital, 447-448
    cataract operation, 171
    gall bladder surgery, 225
    in hospital, 447-448
    informed consent and, 447
    peptic ulcers, 447
    spleen removal, 503
    strabismus, 173
    thyroid operation, 533
    see also Postoperative measures
Prepared (natural) childbirth, see Childbirth
Primaquine, malaria and, 280
Procaine, local anesthesia and, 30
    see also Novocain
Proctoscopy, 154
Progesterone, 203
    birth control pills and, 46
    cyclic therapy and, 203
    hyperplasia and, 191-192
Progressive muscular atrophy, 80
Prolactin adenomas, 418
Prolapsed cord, 437, 439
Prolapse of the rectum, 461
Prolapse of the uterus, 179-180
Prostaglandins, abortion and, 199
Prostatectomy, 451, 452, 453-454
Prostate gland, 450-454
    cancer of the, 105, 453-454
    description, 450
    enlarged
        benign (prostatism), 451-453
        cystitis and, 549
        urination frequency and, 295
    epididymitis and, 343
    examination of, 450
    infection of (prostatitis), 450
    operation (prostatectomy), 451, 452, 453-455
        impotence and, 453
        incontinence, 453-454
    stones in, 454
Prostatism, 451-453
Prostatitis, 450
Prostigmin, myasthenia gravis and, 80
Protein, blood chemistry for, 308
Pruritus ani, 460-461
Pseudohermaphrodite, 471
Pseudomembranous enterocolitis, 489
Psittacosis pneumonia, 333
Psoriasis, 482
Psychedelic drugs, 351-352

Psychiatric hospitalization, 356
Psychiatry, 354
    alcohol abuse and, 18-19
    homosexuality and, 473
    need for, 355
Psychoanalysis, 357
Psychologist, 354
Psychomotor seizures, epilepsy and, 367
Psychoses, 354, 357
    delirium tremens, 18-19
    Korsakoff's, 18-19
Psychosomatic illnesses, 356, 361
Psychotherapy, 356-358
    dyspareunia and, 474
    frigidity and, 473
    impotence and, 512
    mucous colitis and, 494
    Parkinsonism and, 370
    pruritus ani and, 461
    sexual incompatibility, 474
    sexual malfunction and, 474-475
        premature ejaculation and, 511
    ulcerative colitis and, 495
    see also Psychiatry
"Ptomaine" poisoning, 516
Puberty, 8
    see also Adolescence
Pubic hair, adolescence and, 8
Pulmonary edema, respiratory acidosis and, 310
Pulmonary embolism, 333-334
Pulmonary emphysema, see Emphysema
Pulmonary fibrosis, respiratory acidosis and, 310
Pulmonary infarction, 333-334
Pulmonary resection, 542
Pulmonary tuberculosis, see Tuberculosis
Pupils, see Eyes
Purgatives, see Laxatives
Purine, diet for low, 140
Purpura, nosebleeds and, 394
Pus
    cultures, 315
    draining, 7
    see also Abscess; Infections
Pyelograms, kidney tumor and, 300
Pyelonephritis, 297-298, 442
Pyloric stenosis, 520-521
Pyorrhea, 320

"Q" fever, 281
Quadruplets, as multiple births, see Pregnancy
Quarantine
    diphtheria and, 118
    scarlet fever and, 125
    whooping cough and, 127
Quarterway houses, 19
"Quickening" (fetal movements), 426, 428
Quinidine, paroxysmal arrhythmia and, 240
Quinine, 149, 404
Quinsy sore throat, 524

Rabbit fever (tularemia), 281
Rabies (hydrophobia), 283-284
    vaccination, 284
Rad, 568
Radiation
    atomic fall out effect, 569

first aid for exposure to, 219
pregnancy and, 288
Radiation therapy, 420, 568-570
  acne and, 477, 569
  atomic energy and, 568
  bladder tumors and, 552
  bone tumor and, 92
  brain tumors and, 378
  breast cancer and, 97
  bursitis and, 569
  cataracts and, 170
  cervical cancer and, 188-189
  description, 568
  effect of, 568
  esophageal tumor and, 160
  Eustachian tube obstruction and, 569
  glioma and, 176
  hazards from, 568
  hemangioma and, 68
  Hodgkin's disease and, 54
  hypopituitarism and, 421
  isotopes, 569-570
    cobalt, 54, 529, 570
    iodine, 570
    phosphorus, 570
  of keloid, 481, 569
  kilovolt, 568
  laryngeal cancer and, 529
  "mev," 568
  non-Hodgkin's lymphoma and, 54
  normal cells and, 569
  organ transplants and, 536
  ovarian tumor and, 205-206
  pituitary gland and, 12, 420
  prostate cancer and, 453
  "r," 568
  "rad," 568
  radium applicator, 569
  radon, 569
  reproductive system and, 569
  skin cancer and, 104, 485
  skin grafts and, 485
  spinal cord tumors, 381
  thyroid gland and, 532, 569
  tongue cancer and, 322
  toxic anemia and, 50
  treatment number, 568
  use of, 568
  uterine cancer and, 192
  warts and, 569
  see also Cobalt treatments
Radio-frequency current, 363-364
Radiologist, 564
  see also X-ray examinations
Radionucleotide studies, of heart, 234
Ragweed, 23
  hay fever and, 21, 22-23
  low counts, 25
Rats
  infectious (epidemic) jaundice and,
    281-282
  plague and, 282
Raynaud's disease, 56-57
  sympathectomy for, 62
Reactive depressions, 357
Reattachment of an amputated part,
  replantation surgery and, 464
Reconstructive surgery, 81, 83, 422-425
  composite grafts, 423
  flaps, 423, 424
    free, 423, 424
  pedicle graft, 424

skin grafts
  color of, 424, 425
  conditions needing, 424
  donor site reuse, 425
  full-thickness grafts, 423, 425
  mesh graft, 425
  moles and, 484
  as normal skin, 425
  pinch grafts, 423-424
  principles followed in obtaining,
    425
  quality of, 425
  split-thickness grafts, 423, 425
  success of, 425
  sunburn of, 425
  tissues from other individuals, 423
  see also Plastic surgery
Rectocele, 180, 181
Rectum and anus, 455-462
  abscesses, 460
  bleeding from, 498
  cancer of the, 461-462
    colostomy, 461
    diagnosis of, 461
    diarrhea and, 455
    incidence, 461
    polyps, 458-459, 461
    sigmoidoscopy and, 457
    surgical treatment, 461
    symptoms, 461
  fissure in ano, 459
  fistula in ano, 459, 460
  polyps, 456, 458-459, 461
  proctoscopy and, 154
  prolapse of the rectum, 461
  pruritus ani, 460-461
  rectocele, 180, 181
  see also Bowel movements;
    Constipation; Diarrhea;
    Hemorrhoids; Large intestine; Stool
Recurrent fever, 281
Recurrent hernia, 247
Red blood cells, 48
  see also Blood
Reducing diet, see Diet; Obesity
Regional anesthesia, 30
Regional enteritis, see Regional ileitis
Regional ileitis, 489-491
Regurgitation
  acid indigestion and, 514
  heartburn and, 514
  infants and, 275
  see also Vomiting
Rehabilitation, 412-415
  aging and, 414-415
  best use of, 414-415
  description, 412
  goals of, 414
  improvement and, 414
  psychological factors used, 415
  see also Physical therapy
Rejection reaction, 535-536
  kidney transplant and, 304
Rejuvenation operations, 15
Renal cell carcinoma, 300
Renal failure, see Kidney
Replantation surgery, 463-464
  plastic surgery and, 422
Reproductive organs, radiation therapy
  and, 565, 569
  see also specific male and female
    organs
Residue diet, 493

high, 139
low, 139
Respiration, see Breathing
Respiratory acidosis, 310
Respiratory alkalosis, 310
Respiratory Distress Syndrome, 266
Retardation, see Mental retardation
Reticuloendothelial cells, spleen
  removal and, 504
Retina, see Eyes
Retinoscopy, 163, 164
Retrolental fibroplasia, 266
Retropubic prostatectomy, 451, 454
Rheumatic fever, 465-467
  cause, 465
  dental care and, 467
  description, 465
  heart and, 465-466
    valves, 466
  joints and, 465
  recurrence and, 466-467
  scarlet fever and, 125, 130
  symptoms, 466
  treatment, 466-467
    ACTH and, 350-351
    cortisone and, 350-351
Rheumatic heart disease, 241, 243,
  465
  pregnancy and, 442
Rheumatism, 37
  see also Arthritis
Rheumatoid arthritis, 38
Rh-factor disease, see Erythroblastosis
Rhinitis (allergic), 20, 23, 27
Rhinoplasty (plastic surgery of nose),
  see Nose
RhoGAM, 264, 312
  see also Erythroblastosis
Rh test, 311-312
  pregnancy and, 427
  see also Erythroblastosis
Rhythm method, birth control and, 42-43
Rhytidoplasty, 422
Riboflavin, see Vitamins
Ribs
  fracture, 332
  removal of, 338
Rickets, 561
Rickettsial diseases, 281
Rickettsialpox, 281
Rocky Mountain spotted fever, 281
  vaccination, 281
Rose fever, 23
Roseola (Exanthem subitum), 124, 130
Roughage, see Residue
Roundworm (Ascaris), 404, 405
Rubella, see German measles
Rubeola, see Measles
Rubin Test, 508
Rupture, see Hernia
Ruptured invertebral disks, 381
Sabin oral vaccine, 123, 255
  see also Poliomyelitis
Sacroiliac sprain, 72
"Saddle nose," plastic surgery and, 394
Salicylates, 37
  see also Aspirin
Saliva, pregnancy and, 429
Salivary glands, 468-470
  description, 468
  parotid gland
    abscess within, 468
    tumor removal, 469

sublingual glands tumor, 470
submaxillary glands
    abscess, 469
    infections, 468
    stones and, 468-469
    tumors, 470
tumors, 469-470
    see also Mouth
Salk vaccination, 123, 255
    see also Poliomyelitis
Salpingitis, 200-201
Salt
    blood chemistry for, 308
    cholera and, 285
    heart failure and, 234
    heat exhaustion, 216-217
    low-salt diet, 138
        Ménière's syndrome and, 151
    menstruation and, 185
    nephrosis and, 297
    preeclampsia and, 444
    pregnancy and, 427
    weight reduction and, 136
Sarcoidosis, 335
Sarcoma, of uterus, 192, 195
Scabies, 481
Scalp
    dandruff and, 162
    infection and lymph glands, 52
    laceration of, 374
    of newborn, 384
    psoriasis, 482
    replantation surgery and, 464
    seborrhea, 162
    tinea capitis, 479
    see also Hair
Scanning, nuclear, 570
Scaphoid bone, fracture of, 228
Scarlatina, see Scarlet fever
Scarlet fever (scarlatina), 124-125, 130,
    258
    deafness and, 149
Scars, plastic surgery and, 422
    children and, 422-423
Schick test, 118, 128, 253
Schistosomiasis, 403
Schizophrenia, 354, 358
Sciatica, 72, 363
Scintillation counter apparatus, 570
Scoliosis, 74-75
Scorpion, first aid for bite from, 209
Scrotum, 340
    swelling of newborn, 386
    variocele, 343-344
Scrub typhus, 281
Scurvy, 49, 52, 561
    nosebleeds and, 394
Seatworm, see Pinworm
Sebaceous cysts, 483-484
Seborrheic dermatitis, 480-481
Sedatives
    anesthesia and, 29
    preoperative routines and, 447
    see also Barbiturates; Tranquilizers
Sedimentation rate, 306
Self-examination, of breasts, 94
Senile vaginitis, 182
Senility, physical aging and, 14
Sensitivity, see Allergy
Sepsis of the newborn, 267-268
Septal defects, 241, 242
Septicemia, see Blood poisoning
Serologic test, 306

Serum hepatitis, see Hepatitis
Serums, allergy to, 21, 22
Sex
    changing, 471
    determination, 471
    hermaphrodite, 471
    pseudohermaphrodite, 471
Sex education, 10
Sex hormones
    adolescence and, 9, 10
        acne, 476-477
    adrenal cortex and, 12
    female
        breasts and menstruation and, 94
        menopause and, 16, 207, 208
        menstrual irregularities, 184
        menstruation and, 183
        multiple births, 437
        premenstrual tension and, 185
        prostate cancer and, 453
        sex change and, 471
    homosexuality and, 473
    hormone-producing tumors and, 205
    male
        impotence, 511
        sex change and, 471
        sterility and, 511
        undescended testicle and, 342
    sexual desire and, 472
    see also Cyclic therapy; specific sex
        hormones, e.g., Estrogen
Sex organs, see specific male and
    female organs
Sexual intercourse
    abortion and, 198-199
    after childbirth, 441
    aging and, 14, 15
    artificial insemination, 509
    bleeding after, 186, 188
    cauterization of cervix and, 186
    cervical cancer and, 188
    climax, 474
    clitoris and, 177
    desire (libido)
        adolescence and, 10
        alcohol and, 475
        decreased, 475
        drugs and, 475
        female organ removal and, 472
        fulfillment and, 474
        hormones and, 472
        men and, 472
        variability of, 472
    douching, 179
        alkaline before, 509
    endometriosis and, 197
    excessive, 474
    first act for a woman, 474
    frigidity, 472-473
    heart condition and, 472
    hymen and, 177
        hymenotomy and, 177
    hysterectomy and, 196
    impotence, 15, 473, 511
        age of, 511
        causes of, 511
        description, 511
        hormones and, 511
        incidence, 511
        male menopause, 512
        prostate removal and, 453
        sterility and, 511

    treating, 512
    incompatibility, 474
    incomplete, 474
    inhibitions and misinformation and,
        473-474
    low sperm count and, 509
    menopause and, 207
    menstruation and, 474
    middle age and, 475
    necessity of, 472
    nymphomania, 472
    orgasm
        conception and, 506
        without, 43
    painful (dyspareunia), 177, 474
        Bartholin cyst and, 177
        dyspareunia and, 177
        salpingitis and, 200
        senile vaginitis and, 182
        urethral diverticulum and, 554
        vaginal spasm and, 177
    pregnancy and, 428
    premature ejaculation, 473, 511
    prolapse of the uterus and, 179
    prostatic infections and, 450
    sexual attitudes and, 472
    sexual malfunction and, 472, 474-475
    urethral infection and, 555
    vagina and, 179
        plastic operations and, 181
        Trichomonas infections and, 182
    widows and widowers and, 475
    see also Birth control; Pregnancy;
        Venereal diseases
Sexuality
    before marriage and, 473-474
    children and
        masturbation and, 109-110, 472
        puberty and, 8
        sex information to, 471
    duration of, 475
    erotic dream, 472
    homosexuality, 473
    information and, 474
    masturbation
        adolescence and, 10
        attitude toward, 472
        children and, 109-110, 472
    maximum sexual activity age and,
        472
    medical advice and, 473
    mental illness and, 355
    sex education, 473
Shaking palsy, see Parkinsonism
"Shingles" (herpes zoster), 364, 479,
    560
Shock
    abruptio placentae and, 445-446
    blood transfusion for, 309
    burns and, 210
    chemical imbalance and, 292
    definition of, 360
    embolus and, 58
    first-aid treatment for, 219
        electric, 214
    hemorrhage and, 218
    insulin, see Diabetes mellitus
    lung injuries and, 337
    pancreatitis and, 397
    paroxysmal arrhythmia and, 240
    pulmonary infarction and, 334
    spontaneous pneumothorax and, 332
    tubal pregnancy and, 201-202

Shoulder
  arthroplasty, 84, 85
  bursitis and, 76
  dislocated, 216
  fracture of, 215
Shunt
  arteriovenous fistulas and, 68
  lienorenal, 66
  mesocaval, 65
    cirrhosis of the liver and, 325,
      328-329, 537
    esophageal varicosities and, 159
  portacaval, 66
    cirrhosis of the liver and, 325, 328
Sickle-cell anemia, 48-49
  spleen and, 502
  testing for trait, 288
Sight, see Eyes
Sigmoid colon, volvulus and, 492
Sigmoidoscope, 154, 457
  bowel tumors and, 498
  mucous colitis and, 494
  polyps and, 458, 498
  prolonged diarrhea and, 488
  rectal cancer and, 461
  ulcerative colitis and, 495
Silicosis, 334
Silo-filler's disease, 335
Sinusitis, 20, 391-392
  allergy and, 22
  bronchitis and, 545
  chronic pharyngitis and, 527
  common cold and, 544
  glandular enlargement in neck and,
    524
  middle ear pain and, 146
  nosebleeds and, 394
  tonsillitis and, 523-524
Sinusotomy, 392
Skeleton, 71
  see also Bones
Skier's thumb, 228
Skin
  acne, 9, 476-477
  adolescence and, 9
  aging and, 16
  allergy and, 20
  athlete's foot, 477
  bathing and the, 478
  blood vessel tumors of the
    (hemangioma), 483, 484-485
  body odors, 478
  cancer, 104, 485
    cause, 485
    moles and, 48
    plastic surgery and, 422-423
    signs of, 485
    skin grafts and, 423
    sun overexposure and, 476
  chapped hands and, 476
  chilblain, 481
  clay packs and, 476
  cold sores (herpes simplex), 478-479
  cosmetics and, 476
  diet and, 476
  dry, 476
  eczema, 478
  fibrous tumors (fibromas), 483, 485
  frozen section biopsy of, 314
  "hormone" creams and, 476
  hypopituitarism and, 421
  impetigo, 477
  keloid, 481
  large pores, 476

leprosy and, 282
lice, 481-482
lupus and, 482
massage, 476
moles, 484
mud baths and, 476
newborn, 384-385
parasites entering through, 402
pellagra and, 561
perspiration and, 478
pityriasis rosea and, 482
planing, 477
poison ivy and, 482-483
psoriasis and, 482
radiation treatments and, 568-569
ringworm and, 479
scabies and, 481
sebaceous cysts of, 483-484
"shingles" (herpes zoster) and, 479
shock and, 219
skin creams and, 476
subcutaneous tissues and the, 483
surgical conditions of the, 483
tularemia and, 281
ultraviolet rays and, 413, 476
vaseline and, 476
vitamin deficiency and, 476
vitiligo, 482
warts, 483, 484
wrinkle prevention and, 476
  see also Grafts; Hair; Plastic
    surgery; Reconstructive surgery
Skin grafts, see Reconstructive surgery
Skin planing (dermabrasion), 477
Skull
  fracture, 215, 318
    depressed, 374, 375
  neurosurgery
    increased intracranial pressure
      and, 374-376
    infections and, 376
    intracranial hemorrhage and, 376
  osteomyelitis of, 376
Sleep, 354-355
  aging and, 15
  children and, 113-114
    bedwetting, 112-113
    hours for, 113
    nightmares, 110
    night terrors, 110
    sleepwalking, 110
  depression and, 357
  drugs producing, 30
    barbiturates and, 348
    coma, 368
    resistance to, 346
  hyperthyroidism and, 531
  insufficient, 162
  manic-depressive disorders and, 358
  need for, 356
  preoperative routines and, 447
  teeth-grinding in, 108
"Sleeping sickness," see Encephalitis
Sleepwalking, in children, 110
Slipped disk, 72, 73, 413-414
  herniated, 363, 381
Small bowel, see Small intestine
Small intestine
  chronic ulcerative colitis, 486, 488,
    495
  description, 486, 487
  gastroenteritis, 489, 515-516
  intussusception, 491-492

length, 486
Meckel's diverticulum, 491
necessity of, 486
regional ileitis, 489-490
tumors of, 497, 498, 499
ureters transplanted into, 552
volvulus, 492, 496
water absorbed through, 486
Smallpox, vaccination, 252, 253-254,
  257, 258
Smoking
  arteriosclerosis and, 56
  breast feeding and, 269
  Buerger's disease and, 57
  cardiac irregularity and, 240
  chronic gastritis and, 516
  chronic pharyngitis and, 527
  "cigarette cough," 545
  coronary artery disease and, 239
  heart and, 232
  kidneys and, 295
  larynx cancer and, 529
  leukoplakia and, 320
  lip cancer and, 316
  longevity and, 15
  lung cancer and, 101, 330, 337
  pregnancy and, 287, 427
  preoperative routines and, 447
  Raynaud's disease and, 57
  tongue cancer and, 321
  thyroid surgery and, 534
  tuberculosis and, 541
  ulcer and, 518
  underweight and, 136
  upper respiratory illnesses and, 545
Snake, first aid for bite from, 210
Sodium salicylate, for rheumatoid
  arthritis, 38
Sodium, see Salt
Sonography, 500-501
  CAT scan and, 566
  description, 500
  fibroids and, 194
  gall bladder disease and, 222
  image creation, 500
  interpreting, 500
  kidney disease and, 300
  method, 500
  ovarian cyst and, 204
  pancreas and, 399, 400
  pregnancy and, 426, 431, 500-501
    breech presentation, 436
    multiple births, 437
    placenta previa, 445
    tubal, 202
  x rays and, 500
South American spotted fever, 281
"Spastic colitis," 494
Spasticity
  amaurotic familial idiocy and, 264
  multiple sclerosis and, 370
Speech
  brain tumor and, 378
  cleft palate and, 318
  creating, 527
  defects, 111
  diphtheria and, 118
  therapy, 414
  see also Larynx
Spenoid sinus, surgery on the, 392
Sperm
  artificial insemination and, 509-510
  cervix blocking, 509   (continued)

see also Penis; Pregnancy; Sexual intercourse; Testicles
Spinal anesthesia, 30, 31, 32
Spinal canal, myelography of, 568
Spinal cord
  function, 372
  infection, see Poliomyelitis
  injury, 381-382, 415
  neurosurgery, 372
    birth deformities, 380
    pain relief and, 382
    ruptured disk, 381
    tumors, 381
  spinal nerve roots, 362
  tumors of, 380-381
Spinal-fusion, see Spine
Spinal tap, 315, 365, 370
Spine
  arthritis of, 72
  curvature of the (scoliosis), 74-75
  lower back pain and, 72-74
  osteoporosis and, 81
  scoliosis, 74-75
  slipped disk, 72, 73
  spinal fusion operation, 73
    scoliosis and, 75
    spondylolisthesis and, 75
  spondylolisthesis, 75
  sprain, 72
  wry neck, 76
  x ray of, 74
  see also Back
Spirochetal jaundice, 281-282
Spleen, 502-505
  accessory spleens, 504
  cirrhosis of the liver and, 325
  conditions enlarging, 502
  description, 502-503
  diseases and disorders of, 502-503
    distinguishing between, 502
    spleen removal and, 503, 504
    symptoms of, 502
    treatment, 502-503
  erythroblastosis and, 263
  frozen section biopsy of, 314
  Hodgkin's disease and, 53
  infectious mononucleosis and, 283
  leukemia and, 53
  lymphoma and, 53
  Niemann-Pick disease, 265
  overactive, 502
  polycythemia vera and, 50
  removal of the (splenectomy), 503, 504
    pregnancy and, 504
  rupture of the, 502
  splenic puncture, 505
  tumors of the, 502
Splenectomy, 503, 504
Splenorenal shunt, cirrhosis of the liver and, 328
Splinters, first-aid treatment for, 214
Splints, first aid and, 215
Split-thickness graft, 423, 425
Spondylolisthesis, 75
Spontaneous pneumothorax, 332
Sprain
  first-aid treatments for, 216
  whirlpool baths and, 413
Sprue, stool analysis and, 315
Sputum, 545
  analysis, 314-315
  bronchitis and, 545

tracheitis and, 529
tuberculosis and, 539, 540
Stab wound
  first aid for, 214-215
  heart and, 243
  spontaneous pneumothorax and, 332
Stapedectomy, 150
Steam inhalations
  laryngitis and, 528, 544
  sinusitis and, 392
Sterility, female, 506-510
  acidic vagina and, 509
  artificial insemination, 509-510
  "barren period" of the month, 506, 507
  blocked Fallopian tubes, 508-509
  causes, 506
  cervix blocking sperm and, 509
  contraceptive pills and, 509
  definition, 506
  emotional disturbances and, 509
  endometrial hyperplasia and, 191
  "fertile period" of the month, 506, 507
  fibroids of the uterus and, 194, 509
  gonorrhea and, 183, 560
  hormonal imbalance and, 508
  Huhner test, 509
  hysterogram, 508
  incidence, 506
  ovarian cysts and, 509
  ovarian dysfunction and, 203
    ovulation failure, 507
  radiation and, 565
  Rubin test, 508
  salpingitis and, 200
Sterility, male, 473, 510-511
  age of, 511
  description, 506, 510
  epididymitis and, 343
  gonorrhea and, 560
  incidence, 506
  potency and, 511
  remarriage and, 511
  significance of, 510
  sperm count (ejaculate) and, 510, 511
  testicular inability, 510
  treatment of, 511
  varicocele and, 344, 511
Sterilization, 42, 47
  women, 155
Steroids
  allergy to, 22, 24
  for asthma, 25
  for contact dermatitis, 26
  for drug allergy, 27
  for facial paralysis, 364
  for nephrosis, 297
  See also specific steroids, e.g., Cortisone
Still's disease, 38
Stimulating drugs, 351
Stomach, 513-521
  acidity, 515, 516
    digestion, 520
  alcohol and, 18
  acute gastritis and, 515-516
  cancer, 312, 521-522
    atrophic gastritis and, 516
    stomach ulcer and, 517, 518
  chronic gastritis and, 516
  description, 513
  disease
    aging and, 514

diagnosis of, 513
emotional conditions and, 514
food combinations and, 513
minimizing, 513
symptoms of, 513
dyspepsia, see Indigestion
gastric analysis, 312-313
gastroduodenoscopy, 154
gastroenteritis, 489, 515-516
gastroscopy, 154
peptic ulcer, see Ulcer
pyloric stenosis, 520-521
removal of part of (gastrectomy), 513-514
x ray of, 566
see also Duodenum
Stomach tubes
  peptic ulcer and, 519
  as postoperative measure, 449
  as preoperative measure, 448
Stones
  gallstones, see Gall bladder
  kidney, see Kidney
  prostate gland and, 454
  salivary glands and, 468-469
  ureteral, 299
  uric acid, 298, see also Gout
Stool
  analysis, 315
  appendicitis and, 33
  black, 455
    chronic gastritis and, 516
    laxatives and, 349
  blood in, 455, 457, 461, 488
  celiac disease and, 261
  change in, 455
  cystic fibrosis and, 335
  laxatives and, 349
  mucus and, 455
    spastic colitis and, 494
    ulcerative colitis and, 495
  parasitic diseases and, 402, 404, 405, 406, see also specific diseases
  straining at, 456, 461
  see also Constipation; Diarrhea; Large intestine; Rectum and anus
STP, 351
Strabismus, see Eyes
Strains, whirlpool baths and, 413
Strangulated hernia, intestinal obstruction and, 496
Strangulation, first-aid treatment for, 219
Streptococcus
  scarlet fever and, 124, 130
  sore throat and, 526
  throat culture for, 124
Streptomycin, 542
Stress, 360-361
  "adaptation diseases," 360
  adrenal glands and, 11
  aging process and, 361
  allergy and, 360
  barbiturates and, 348
  concept of, 360
  emotional reactions to, 360
  frequency of urination and, 295
  headache and, 369
  high blood pressure and, 360
  menopause and, 207
  menstruation and, 184-185
  peptic ulcer and, 517
  physical disease, 360

psychosomatic disorders and, 360
rheumatoid arthritis and, 38
role of health in, 361
sexual desire and, 475
spastic colitis and, 494
susceptibility to, 14
tranquilizers and, 348
work conditions and, 354
see also Emotional disturbances
Stress test, 234
Stretching, see Traction
Stricture of the urethra, 553
Stroke (cerebrovascular accident),
   366-467, 378
aneurysm and, 367
arteriovenous malformation and, 367
cerebral hemorrhage, and, 366
cerebral thrombosis and, 366
coma and, 368-369
definition, 368
electroencephalography and, 371
embolism and, 58
   cerebral, 366-367
endarterectomy and, 62, 536
ischemia and, 366
pituitary gland malfunction and, 420-421
rehabilitation and, 414, 415
"small" (infarct), 366, 378
transient ischemic attacks, 366
Strontium isotope, 570
Stuttering, children and, 111
St. Vitus' dance (chorea), rheumatic
   fever and, 466
Styes, of eyelids, 166
Subarachnoid space, 367
Subacromial bursitis, 76
Subcutaneous tissues, surgical
   conditions of, see Skin
Subdeltoid bursitis, 76
Subdural hemorrhage, 374-375
Sublingual glands, 468
   see also Salivary glands
Submaxillary glands, 468
   see also Salivary glands
Submucous resection, of the nasal
   septum, 391
Subtotal gastrectomy, 518-519
Suffocation
first-aid treatment for, 212-213, 219
quinsy sore throat and, 524
heart failure and, 233
hyaline membrane disease and, 266
tracheotomy and, 529, 530
Suicide, 19, 355, 357
Sulfa drugs, 347
Sulfone drugs, 283
Sun
acne and, 477
brown facial spots and, 476
overexposure to, 476
   cold sores and, 479
   lip cancer, 316
   skin cancer and, 485
   skin grafts and, 425
   vitiligo and, 482
see also Skin
Sunburns, first aid for, 210
Sunscreens, 476
Sunstroke, first-aid treatment for, 216
Suprapubic prostatectomy, 451, 452
Surgery
aging and, 15
children's fears of, 111

Intensive Care Unit prior to, 293
see also Anesthesia; Postoperative
   procedures; Preoperative
   procedures; specific organs, sites,
   disorders, and types of surgery,
   e.g., Plastic surgery
Suture removal, as postoperative
   measure, 449
Swallowing
achalasia and, 159
choking and, 211-212
corrosives and, 157
esophageal tumors and, 160
esophagitis and, 157
inability, 156
myasthenia gravis and, 80
nerve connected with, 362
pharyngitis and, 526
rabies and, 283
sharp object, 157-158
thyroiditis and, 532
"Swine" flu, 548
Sympathectomy
arteriosclerosis and, 62
Buerger's disease and, 57, 62
Raynaud's disease and, 57, 62
Sympathetic nervous system, 362, 363
see also Nervous diseases
Sympathetic ophthalmia, 176
Syndactyly, 229
Syphilis, see Venereal diseases

Tabes (locomotor ataxia), 366
syphilis and, 558
Tagamet, 516, 518
"Tagging" with an isotope, 570
Tampons, toxic shock syndrome and,
   185
Tapeworms, 405-406
TAT, see Tetanus antitoxin
Tay-Sachs disease, see Amaurotic
   familial idiocy
Tear duct, blocked, 162
Tearing, see Eyes
Teeth, 321
abscess, 321
bad breath and, 319-320
cavities, 321
extraction, 241
lip cancer and jagged, 316
nursing mother and, 269
pregnancy and, 429
premature loss of, 16
preoperative routines and, 448
rheumatic fever and, 467
Teeth-grinding, in sleep, 108
Temperature, see Fever
Temper tantrums, in children, 109
Tension, see Stress
Terminal ileitis, see Regional ileitis
Testicles
adolescence and, 9
biopsy, 510
   frozen section, 314
cancer, 106
hydrocele, 342-343, 386
injuries to, 341
mumps and, 122
orchitis, 510
prostate cancer and, 453
sperm production and, 510, 511
torsion (twist) of, 343
tumors, 341

undescended, 341-342, 510
Tetanus (lockjaw), 284
vaccination, 252, 253, 257, 258, 284
Tetanus antitoxin (TAT)
animal bite and, 209
compound fracture and, 90
Tetany, hypoparathyroidism and, 408, 409
see also Convulsions
Tetany of the newborn, 267
Tetracycline, 282, 285, 403
T4, 531
Thalidomide, congenital heart disease
   and, 236
Thiamine, see Vitamins
"Third-party action," 4
Thoracentesis (lung taps), 315
Thoracoplasty, 338
Throat
branchial cysts (gill slits), 530
common cold and, 543, 544
culture
   diphtheria, 128
   scarlet fever, 124
   streptococcus, 124
   whooping cough, 126
hay fever and, 23
nerve connected with, 362
pain
   adenoid inflammation and,
      523-524
   tonsil inflammation and, 523-524
sore (pharyngitis), 524, 526-527
   chronic, 527
   diphtheria and, 117, 128
   infectious mononucleosis and, 283
   influenza and, 546-547
   middle ear pain and, 146
   poliomyelitis and, 129
   quinsy, 524
   rheumatic fever and, 465
   scarlet fever and, 124, 130
   streptococcus and, 526
   syphilis and, 558
spasms in and rabies, 283
tightness in women, 156
trench mouth and, 320
see also Adenoids; Larynx; Mouth;
   Salivary glands; Tonsils; Thyroid
   gland; Trachea
Thromboangitis obliterans, see
   Buerger's disease
Thrombocytopenic purpura, 52, 502,
   503
Thrombophlebitis, 59-60
surgery for, 64
varicose veins and, 67
Thrombosis, see Blood vessels;
   Coronary artery disease
Thrush, 268
Thumbsucking, 107-108
Thymus gland, organ transplants and,
   536
Thyroid gland, 531-534
activity determination, 531
adolescence and, 10
blood chemistry for, 308
bulging eyes and, 162
cancer and, 532-534
description, 531
enlargement and radiation therapy
   and, 569
frozen section biopsy of, 374
function, 531

goiter, 531, 532
 colloid, 531-532
 hoarseness and, 528
 hyperthyroidism and, 531, 532,
 533-534
 nodular, 531
 recurrence of, 533
 surgery for, 532-534
 thyroiditis and, 532
 iodine isotope and, 570
 malfunction cause, 531
 obesity and, 134
 ovarian dysfunction and, 203
 overactivity (hyperthyroidism), 531
 psychosomatic illness and, 356,
 361
 thyroid extract and, 134
 thyroidectomy, 532-533, 534
 need for, 532-533
 parathyroid function and, 408-409
 thyroid scan, 531, 570
 underactivity (hypothyroidism), 531
 underweight and, 136
Thyroiditis, 532
Thyroxin, see Thyroid gland
Tibia, fracture of, 89
Tic douloureux, 363-364, 379
Tick fever, 281
Ticks
 relapsing fever and, 281
 rickettsial diseases and, 281
 Rocky Mountain spotted fever and,
 258, 281
 tularemia and, 281
Tics, as child behavior, 109
Tinea capitis, 479
Tinea cruris, 479
Tine test, 253
Tipped womb, 189-190
Toes
 bunions on, 76, 77
 corns on, 77
 fractures of, 90
 hammer toe, 78
 infection and lymph glands and, 52
 polydactylism and, 70
 see also Feet
Tongue, 321-322
 cancer, 321, 322
 changes in, 321
 frozen section biopsy of, 314
 glossitis, 321
 leukoplakia and, 320-321, 322
 nerve connected with, 362
 thrush and, 268
 "tongue-tie" of newborn, 384
 tumors, 322
Tonometer, 169
Tonsils
 abscesses, 524
 acute inflammation, 523-524
 description, 523
 tonsillectomy, 524, 525-526
 anesthesia for, 32
 arthritis and, 37
 bronchitis and, 545
 hay fever and, 25
 hoarseness and, 544
 middle ear pain and, 147
 rheumatic fever and, 465
 tonsillitis and, 524
 tonsillitis, 524
 common cold and, 543

glandular enlargement in neck
 and, 523-524
 trench mouth and, 320
 see also Adenoids
Topical anesthesia, 30-31, 32
Torsion of the testicle, 343
Torticollis, see Wry neck
Total Body Scanner, see CAT scan
Total disability, 3
Tourniquet
 bleeding and, 60, 62
 compound fractures and, 215
 hemorrhage and, 217-218
 insect bites and, 209
 snake bites and, 210
Toxemia of pregnancy, see Pregnancy
Toxic anemias, 50
Toxic goiters, 531
Toxic hepatitis, 327
Toxic shock syndrome, 185
Trachea (windpipe), 529
 choking and, 156, 211-212
 endotracheal anesthesia and, 32
 tracheitis, 529
 tracheotomy (tracheostomy), 260,
 292, 529-530
 choking and, 212
 croup and, 260
 diphtheria and, 117
 elective, 530
 emergency, 530
 laryngeal spasm and, 213
 laryngectomy, 529
 laryngitis and, 528
Tracheitis, 529
 common cold and, 544
Tracheobronchitis, Asiatic flu and, 548
Tracheoesophageal fistula, 156-157
Tracheostomy (tracheotomy), see Trachea
Tracheotomy, see Trachea
Trachoma, 176
Tranquilizers, 207, 348-349, 356
 alcohol consumption and, 19
 mucous colitis and, 494-495
Transplantation immunity, 535, 536
Transplantation of organs, 535-537
 adrenal glands and, 13
 from an animal to a human, 535
 cornea and, 166
 heart and, 245, 534, 535
 kidneys and, 303-304
 life span extension and, 537
 new organ reaction and, 536
 from one part of a patient's body to
 another (autotransplant), 535
 rejection reaction, 535-536
 transplantation immunity, 535, 536
 see also Grafts
Transurethral prostatectomy, 453
Transurethral resection, 454
Traumatic arthritis, 39
Traumatic fistula, 68
Trench fever, 281
Trench mouth, 320
 tongue and, 321
Trichinosis, 404
Trichomonas infection
 of the urethra, 555
 of the vagina, 182, 403
Trigeminal neuralgia, 363-364, 379
Trigger fingers, 228
Triplets, as multiple births, see
 Pregnancy

Truss, hernia and, 248-249
T3, 531
Tubal ligation, 47
Tubal (ectopic) pregnancy, see
 Pregnancy
Tuberculosis, 336, 338, 538-542
 age and, 538
 breast infection and, 95
 blocked Fallopian tubes and, 508
 bronchitis and, 545
 chronic lung (pulmonary), 539, 540
 "active" case, 540
 diagnosis and, 540
 inactive, 540
 pregnancy and, 540
 prognosis, 540-541
 spread of, 541
 control of, 538
 coughing up blood and, 330
 description, 538
 diagnosis, 539
 epididymitis and, 343
 fistulas and, 460
 gastric analysis and, 312-313
 guinea pig inoculation with, 315
 infants and, 539, 540
 iritis and, 168
 kidneys and, 301-302
 lymph glands and, 52
 meningitis and, 365
 osteomyelitis and, 79
 prevention, 538
 primary infection, 539
 salpingitis and, 200
 silicosis and, 334
 skin and, 482
 spread, 538
 sputum and, 314-315, 330, 545
 susceptibility to, 538, 539
 symptoms of, 538-539
 tests for, 539
 treatment, 502-503, 541-542
 vaccination against (BCG), 256, 541
 x ray and, 566
Tuboplasty, 508
Tularemia (rabbit fever), 281, 333
Tumor, see Radiation therapy; specific
 organs and sites; specific tumors
Turner's syndrome, 289
Twins, as multiple birth, see Pregnancy
Tympanoplasty, 151
Typhoid fever, 279-280
 carrier, 279
 diarrhea and, 488
 encephalitis and, 365
 gastroenteritis and, 489
 liver infection and, 324
 vaccination, 252, 256, 258, 279
Typhus, 281
 epidemic, 281
 scrub, 281
 vaccination, 257, 258

Ulcer
 of cornea, 166
 peptic, 157, 347, 348, 517-520
 alcohol consumption and, 18
 aspirin and, 347, 348
 avoiding, 517
 cancer and, 518, 521
 causes, 517
 description, 517
 diagnosis, 517

diet for ambulatory, 141
endoscopy and, 154
esophagitis and, 157
gastric analysis, 312-313
harmful effects of, 517
healing and, 517-518
hyperinsulinism and, 399
incidence, 517
operations for, 518-520
peritonitis and rupture of, 410
proclivity, 517
psychosomatic illness and, 356, 361
recurrence, 518
symptoms, 517
types of, 517
Zollinger-Ellison syndrome and, 400
Ulcerative colitis, chronic, 488, 495
Ultrasound, see Sonogram
Ultraviolet (UV) light therapy, see Physical therapy
Umbilical cord
care of in newborn, 386
prolapsed, 437
separation of baby from, 435
Umbilical hernia, 247, 249
Umbilicus, see Navel
Unconsciousness, see Coma
Underweight, 136
causes, 136
children and, 136
diet for, 141
drugs and, 136
emotions and, 135, 136
smoking and, 136
vitamins and, 136
Undescended testicle, 341-342
Undulant fever, 282
Upper respiratory diseases, 543-548
see also Larynx; specific diseases; Throat
Urates, gouty arthritis and, 37, 39
Urea nitrogen, blood chemistry for, 308
Uremia, 297
coma and, 369
Ureter
stones in, 299
transplanted, 552
ureterocele, 303
see also Kidneys
Ureterocele, 303
Ureterosigmoidostomy, 552, 553
Urethra, 339, 553-556
caruncles of the, 553-554
cystitis and, 549
description, 553
diverticulum of the, 554
epispadias, 554, 555-556
female and, 553
gonorrhea and, 559
hypospadias, 554, 555-556
infections of, 555
male and, 553
strictures and, 553
see also Urinary bladder
Uric acid
blood chemistry for, 308
stones, 298, 299
Urinary bladder
bladder fistula, 551
cordotomy and, 382
cystitis, 429, 549

cystocele and, 180, 181
cystoscopy, 155, 549, 550, 567
bladder stones and, 551
description, 549
incomplete emptying of, 451
infection and urethral diverticulum, 555
paralysis and spinal cord deformities and, 380, 382
prostate enlargement and, 451
spinal cord tumors and, 380
stones (calculi), 551
cystitis and, 550
tumors of the, 551-552
cystitis and, 550
papillomas, 551-552
treatment, 551-552, 553
see also Catheterization; Urethra; Urination
Urination
albumin and, 443
bedwetting, 112-113
bladder fistula and, 550-551
bloody, 554
bladder stones and, 551
bladder tumors and, 551-552
cystitis and, 549
gonorrhea and, 559
kidney injury and, 301
kidney tumors and, 300
ureter tumors and, 302
catheterization
as postoperative measure, 440, 449
as preoperative routine, 448
cloudiness, 296
cystocele and, 180
decreased, 443
diabetes mellitus and, 131
frequent, 451
urethra infection and, 555
gonorrhea and, 182, 559
hysterectomy and, 196
inability
bladder stones and, 551
urethral stricture and, 553
obstruction to the passage of
urethral diverticulum and, 554
painful, 296
cystitis and, 549
urethral stricture and, 553
pregnancy and, 426, 429, 442, 443-444
prolapse of the uterus and, 179
prostate enlargement and, 451
prostate operations and, 453
pyelonephritis and, 297, 442
radium treatment of cervix and, 189
salpingitis and, 200
sugar in, see Diabetes mellitus
ureteral stone and, 299
vaginal plastic operations and, 181
see also Catheterization; Urethra; Urinary bladder
Urticaria, see Hives
Uterine tubes, see Fallopian tubes
Uterus (womb), 189-197
abruptio placentae and, 445-446
cancer, 192, 196, 207, 339
curettage of, 190, 191, 192, 195, 198
description, 189, 190, 193
endometrial biopsy and, 507-508

endometrial hyperplasia and, 191-192, 195, 196, 203
endometrial polyp and, 191, 195
endometriosis and, 197
endometritis and, 191
fibroids (leiomyomas) of, 194-195, 196, 431, 439, 508
hysterogram of, 191, 567
infantile, 190
intrauterine device and, 42, 45-46
myomectomy of, 195
oxytocin from, 418
pregnancy and, 189, 426
prolapse, 179, 180
sarcoma of, 192, 195
sonography and, 500
tipped, 189-190

Vaccination, see Immunizations and vaccinations
Vagina, 178
acidic, 509
cancer of, 179
care of newborn, 386
cystocele and, 180, 181
cysts of, 179
description, 179
discharge
during pregnancy, 430
postpartum (lochia), 441
douching, 44, 45, 430
fibromas of, 179
fungus infection of, 430
hysterectomy and, 179-180, 196-197
plastic operations of, 181, 196, 439
trans-sex operations and, 471
polyps of, 179
pregnancy complications and, 442
rectocele and, 180, 181
spasms of, 177
trichomonas vaginitis, 182, 403
vaginitis, 182
vulvitis, 178
yeast infection, 268
Vaginitis, 182
Vagotomy, 518
Valium, intravenous anesthesia and, 30
Varicella, see Chicken pox
Varicocele, 66, 343-344, 511
reduced sperm count and, 511
Varicose veins, 66-67
birth control pills and, 46
inherited, 59
injections for, 66
ligation or stripping of, 60
pregnancy and, 428, 429-430
surgery and, 61, 66, 67
thrombophlebitis and, 59-60
untreated, 67
varicocele and, 343-344
see also Esophagus; Hemorrhoids
Vascular disorders, see Arteries; Blood vessels; specific disorder
Vascular surgery, see Blood vessels
Vas deferens
prostatectomy and, 454
surgical sterilization and, 47
vasectomy, 47, 454
Vasectomy, 47, 454
Venereal diseases, 557-560
description, 557
gonorrhea, 182-183, 559-560
blocked Fallopian tubes and, 508
complications, 560

conjunctivitis and, 165
contracting, 559
diagnosis, 559
endometritis and, 191
epididymitis and, 343
eyedrops to newborn and, 385
female and, 182, 183
hysterectomy and, 196
male infertility and, 510
organs affected by, 557
peritonitis and, 411
prostate gland and, 450
recurrence, 560
reduced sperm count and, 510
salpingitis and, 200
symptoms, 559
syphilis and, 557
treatment for, 559
urethral infections and, 555
urethral strictures and, 553
heart valve dysfunction and, 232-233
herpes, 560
cervical cancer and, 188
meningitis and, 365
mental retardation and, 289
sex education and, 10
syphilis, 183, 557-559
aneurysm and, 58
blood test for, 306, 558
breast infection and, 95
chancre, 557-558
female and, 183
gonorrhea and, 557
heredity and, 558
incidence of, 557
iritis and, 168
marriage and, 559
of the nervous system, 366, 558
organs affected by late, 558
pregnancy and, 427, 559
preventing, 558
recovery, 559
symptoms, 557
treatment, 558
transmitting, 557, 558
Ventral hernia, 247
Ventriculoperitoneal shunt, 380
Verrucae, see Warts
Vertigo, 151, 369
brain tumor and, 365
first-aid treatment for, 214
Ménière's syndrome, 151-152, 369
Viruses, 279
cancer and, 100-101, 105-106
gastroenteritis and, 489
see also specific virus diseases
Virus pneumonia, 7, 333
Vision, see Eyes
Vital signs, Intensive Care Unit
monitoring of, 292-293
Vitamins, 561-563
A
deficiency, 561
eyesight and, 563
foods rich in, 562
to newborns, 562
overdose, 562
weight gain and, 563
addition of, 561
administration of, 562
anemia and, 49, 563
B₁ (thiamine)
anemia and, 49

breasts and menstruation, 94
deficiency, 561
foods rich in, 562
to newborns, 562
B₂ (riboflavin)
deficiency, 561
foods rich in, 562
B₆ (pyridine)
foods rich in, 562
B₁₂
anemia and, 49
deficiency, 561
foods rich in, 562
C (ascorbic acid)
anemia and, 49
common cold and, 543
deficiency, 561
foods rich in, 562
to newborns, 562
children's needs, 562
chronic gastritis and, 516
common cold and, 543, 563
D
deficiency, 561
foods rich in, 562
hypoparathyroidism and, 408
to newborns, 562
overdose, 562
pregnancy and, 562
deficiency, 561, 562
causes, 561
curing, 561
diseases caused by, 561-562, see
also specific diseases
menstruation and, 183
pills for, 562
skin condition and, 476
definition, 561
E
deficiency, 561
foods rich in, 562
pregnancy and, 562
elderly's needs, 562
folic acid
deficiency, 561
foods rich in, 562
infants and, 272, 562
injection of, 562
K
adenoidectomy and, 525
deficiency, 561-562
foods rich in, 562
gall bladder surgery and, 225
hemorrhagic disease of the
newborn and, 267
pregnancy and, 562
tonsillectomy and, 525
mineral oil and, 455, 563
minimum daily requirements, 562
necessity of, 561
niacin (foods rich in), 562
nicotinic acid deficiency, 561
nursing mother and, 269
overdose, 562
pregnancy and, 562
morning sickness and, 429
premature baby and, 388
reducing diet and, 562
sickle-cell anemia and, 49
spleen removal and, 504
"therapeutic formula," 562
tongue and, 321
weight gain and, 136

Vitiligo, 482
Vitrectomy, 175
Vocal cords, 527, 528
see also Larynx
Voice box, see Larynx
Volvulus, 492, 496
Vomiting
appendicitis and, 33
diverticulum of esophagus and, 156,
159
food allergy and, 20
infants and, 278
morning sickness and, 429
pyloric stenosis and, 520
stomach contents, 156
for swallowed poison, 218
undigested food, 156
see also Esophagus
Vulva, 177
cancer of, 178-179
leukoplakia, 178
vulvitis, 178
vulvovaginitis, 182
Vulvectomy, 178-179
Vulvitis, 178
Vulvovaginitis, 182

Warts, 393, 483, 484
plantar, 77
Wassermann test, 557
Water
adrenal cortex and, 12
cholera spread and, 285
colloid goiter and iodine content of,
531
hydrotherapy, see Physical therapy
infant feeding and, 270, 272
infectious hepatitis spread by, 326
kidneys and, 418
on the knee, 40
poliomyelitis spread by, 123, 129
small intestine and, 486
typhoid fever spread by, 279
see also Fluids
Wax (cerumen), in ears, 145, 150
Weight, see Obesity
Weil's disease, 281-282
Wens, see Sebaceous cysts
Wheals, hives with, 27
Whiplash, exercises for, 413-414
Whipworm, 404
White blood cells, see Laboratory tests
Whooping cough (pertussis), 126-127,
130
common cold and, 543
encephalitis and, 365
hoarseness and, 544
vaccination, 252, 258
cystic fibrosis and, 335-336
Widal test, 279
Wilm's tumors, 106, 299-300
Wilson's disease, 290
Windpipe, see Trachea
Withdrawal (coitus interruptus), 42, 43
Womb, see Uterus
Wood's light, 479
World Health Organization, malaria
and, 403-404
Worm diseases, 404-406
see also specific diseases
Wrinkles, plastic surgery and, 476
Wrist, replacement of joint, 84

Wry neck (torticollis), 76
  exercises for, 413-414

Xeroradiogram, 564
X ray examination, 564-570
  of adrenal glands, 12
  of arteries (arteriograms), 566
  arteriosclerosis and, 55
  atelectasis of the newborn and,
    266-267
  back pain (lower) and, 74
  barium for gastrointestinal tract, 566
  of the bile ducts (cholangiogram),
    567
  bladder stones and, 551
  body parts visualized by, 564
  of bone infection, 568
  of bone marrow injury, 50
  of bone tumor, 91, 568
  bowel cancer and, 498, 499
  brain tumor and, 365, 377
  of breasts (mammography), 567
  bronchitis and, 545
  of cartilage injury, 568
  celiac disease and, 261
  of the chest, 565-566
  childbirth (pelvimetry x ray) and, 567
  of chromophobe tumor, 418
  chronic gastritis and, 516
  colitis and, 494
  of colon, 497
  contrast media for, 565
  Cooley's anemia and, 502
  of craniopharyngioma, 501
  cystic fibrosis and, 335
  definition, 564

diarrhea (prolonged) and, 488-489
duodenal disease and, 516
enema before, 566
of Fallopian tubes (hysterogram), 567
fluoroscopy, 564
foreign bodies visualized by, 564-567
of fracture, 85, 87, 91, 567-568
of gall bladder (cholecystography),
  222, 567
  gallstones, 226, 567
gases visualized by, 565
of hand, 227
of heart (angiocardiography), 231,
  566
hernia of diaphragm and, 566
Hirschsprung's disease and, 262,
  497
hyperparathyroidism and, 407
image intensifier, 564
Intensive Care Unit and, 292
intestinal obstruction and, 496
of joints (arthography), 568
of kidneys (intravenous urography),
  294, 567
laxative before, 566
of lungs, 333, 337, 566
of lymphatic vessels
  (lymphangiography), 566
maxillary sinus surgery and, 392
moving picture, 564
nasal fracture and, 389
overdose, 565
peptic ulcer and, 517
peritonitis and, 410
possession of, 564
pregnancy and, 288

pulmonary infarction and, 334
pyloric stenosis and, 520
radiologist, 564
regional ileitis and, 489
sarcoidosis and, 335
sinusitis and, 392
skull fracture and, 374
sonogram and, 500-501
of the spinal canal (myelography),
  568
spondylolisthesis and, 75
spontaneous pneumothorax and,
  332
stomach disease and, 513, 521
technician, 564
treatments, see Radiation therapy
tuberculosis and, 253, 538, 540, 541,
  566
of urinary bladder (cystogram), 567
  bladder stones, 551
of uterus (hysterogram), 567
of veins, 566
volvulus and, 492
xeroradiogram, 564
see also CAT scan; Endoscopy;
  Radiation therapy; Sonography;
  specific kinds of x rays
Xylocaine, 31

Yeast infection, thrush and, 268
Yellow fever, 280
  vaccination, 257, 258, 280

Zollinger-Ellison syndrome, 400
Zyloprim, for gouty arthritis, 39

# ACKNOWLEDGEMENTS TO SOURCES OF ILLUSTRATIONS

The editor wishes to express his appreciation to Georg Thieme Verlag of Stuttgart; Sylvia and Lester Bergman; and Shirley Baty for the many fine illustrations that have been used in this encyclopedia. Thanks are also expressed to the following individuals and organizations for illustrative material reproduced in this work: Dr. Otto Kestler; The American Cancer Society, Inc., New York; The Maico Co.; The New York University Medical Center; and The March of Dimes, New York.